D1769387

Thyroid Disease

Endocrinology, Surgery, Nuclear Medicine, and Radiotherapy

Second Edition

Thyroid Disease
Endocrinology, Surgery, Nuclear Medicine, and Radiotherapy

Second Edition

Editor

Stephen A. Falk, M.D., F.A.C.S.
Clinical Associate Professor of Surgery
University of Rochester School of Medicine and Dentistry
Rochester, New York

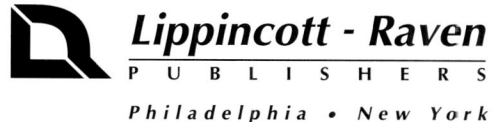

Lippincott - Raven
PUBLISHERS
Philadelphia • New York

Acquisitions Editor: Kathey Alexander
Developmental Editor: Anne M. Sydor
Manufacturing Manager: Dennis Teston
Production Manager: Lawrence Bernstein
Production Editor: Colophon
Cover Designer: Jeane Norton
Indexer: Beta Computer Indexing
Compositor: Lippincott–Raven Electronic Production
Printer: Kingsport

© 1997 by Lippincott-Raven Publishers. All rights reserved. This book is protected by copyright. No part of it may be reproduced, stored in a retrieval system, or transmitted, in any form or by any means—electronic, mechanical, photocopy, recording, or otherwise—without the prior written consent of the publisher, except for brief quotations embodied in critical articles and reviews. For information write **Lippincott-Raven Publishers, 227 East Washington Square, Philadelphia, PA 19106-3780.**

Chapter 10 compiled by Donald L. St. Germain, M.D. Copyright 1993, Dartmouth-Hitchcock Medical Center, with modifications.

Materials appearing in this book prepared by individuals as part of their official duties as U.S. Government employees are not covered by the above-mentioned copyright.

Printed in the United States of America

9 8 7 6 5 4 3 2 1

Library of Congress Cataloging-in-Publication Data

Thyroid disease: endocrinology, surgery, nuclear medicine, and radiotherapy/editor, Stephen A. Falk. — 2nd ed.
    p.   cm.
    Includes bibliographical references and index.
    ISBN 0-397-51705-X
    1. Thyroid gland—Diseases.   I. Falk, Stephen A., 1945–   .
[DNLM: 1. Thyroid Diseases.   WK 200 T5464 1997]
RC655. T4827   1997
616.4′4—dc21
DNLM/DLC
for Library of Congress

Care has been taken to confirm the accuracy of the information presented and to describe generally accepted practices. However, the authors, editors, and publisher are not responsible for errors or omissions or for any consequences from application of the information in this book and make no warranty, express or implied, with respect to the contents of the publication.

The authors, editors, and publisher have exerted every effort to ensure that drug selection and dosage set forth in this text are in accordance with current recommendations and practice at the time of publication. However, in view of ongoing research, changes in government regulations, and the constant flow of information relating to drug therapy and drug reactions, the reader is urged to check the package insert for each drug for any change in indications and dosage and for added warnings and precautions. This is particularly important when the recommended agent is a new or infrequently employed drug.

Some drugs and medical devices presented in this publication have Food and Drug Administration (FDA) clearance for limited use in restricted research settings. It is the responsibility of the health care provider to ascertain the FDA status of each drug or device planned for use in their clinical practice.

To my Teachers and Family—Marcia, Ben, and Elizabeth

Contents

Foreword to the First Edition Jerome M. Hershman .... *xi*
Preface .... *xiii*
Acknowledgments .... *xv*
Contributors .... *xvii*

Part I. Historical Introduction

1. Thyroidology—Reflections on Twentieth-Century History 1
   Alvin L. Ureles and Zachary R. Freedman

Part II. Basic Clinical Sciences

2. Embryology and Surgical Anatomy of the Lower Neck and Superior Mediastinum . 15
   John T. Hansen

3. Physiology of Thyroid Hormone Synthesis, Secretion, and Transport 29
   Jonathan S. LoPresti and Peter A. Singer

4. Clinical Approach to Thyroid Function Testing 41
   Peter A. Singer

5. Parathyroid Function and Calcium Homeostasis 53
   Jessica C. Rockwell and Daniel T. Baran

6. Pathology of Thyroid Disease 65
   Virginia A. LiVolsi

7. Fine-Needle Biopsy of the Thyroid 105
   Michael M. Kaplan and Joel I. Hamburger

8. Uptake Tests, Thyroid and Whole Body Imaging with Isotopes 113
   George A. Wilson and Robert E. O'Mara

9. Diagnostic Imaging of the Thyroid Gland 135
   Arnold M. Noyek, David M. Finkelstein, Ian J. Witterick, and Joel C. Kirsh

Part III. Molecular Biology of the Thyroid Gland

10. Molecular Basis of Thyroid Disease 183
    Donald L. St. Germain

    Glossary for Chapter 10 203

11. Molecular Biology of the Thyroid Stimulating Hormone Receptor 209
    Shigenobu Nagataki and Yuji Nagayama

12.	Thyroid Hormone Resistance Syndromes	223
	Stephen J. Usala	
13.	Oncogenes and Thyroid Cancer	231
	Michael T. McDermott	

Part IV. Hyperthyroidism

14.	Hyperthyroidism: Systemic Effects and Differential Diagnosis	241
	Amy L. O'Donnell and Stephen W. Spaulding	
15.	Medical Management of Hyperthyroidism: Theoretical and Practical Aspects	253
	Jeffrey I. Mechanick and Terry F. Davies	
16.	Iodine-131 Treatment of Hyperthyroidism	297
	Sidney H. Sobel and Roland Bramlet	
17.	Surgical Treatment of Hyperthyroidism	319
	Stephen A. Falk	
18.	Thyroid-Associated Ophthalmopathy: Etiology and Pathogenesis	341
	Tomasz Bednarczuk, John S. Kennerdell, and Jack R. Wall	
19.	Thyroid-Associated Ophthalmopathy: Treatment	359
	Ronald R. Reed	

Part V. Hypothyroidism

20.	Clinical Manifestations and Differential Diagnosis of Hypothyroidism	379
	Alice C. Chiu and Steven I. Sherman	

Part VI. Thyroiditis: Nodular and Congenital Thyroid Disease

21.	Thyroiditis	393
	Paul D. Woolf	
22.	Solitary Thyroid Nodule: Concepts in Diagnosis and Treatment	411
	George L. A. From and Victor G. Lawson	
23.	Multinodular Goiter	431
	George L. A. From and Victor G. Lawson	
24.	Management of Substernal Thyroid Disease	447
	William Lawson, Anthony J. Reino, and Hugh F. Biller	
25.	Management of Thyroid Disorders Involving the Airway	457
	Victor G. Lawson	
26.	Congenital Thyroid Cysts and Ectopic Thyroid	467
	Charles M. Myer III and Robin T. Cotton	

Part VII. Treatment with Thyroid Hormone

27.	Replacement and Suppressive Treatment with Thyroid Hormone	475
	Sheldon S. Waldstein	

Part VIII. Thyroid Cancer

28. Thyroid Cancer: Controversies and Etiopathogenesis 495
Sharon L. Collins

29. Evaluation and Surgical Treatment of Papillary and Follicular Carcinoma 565
Elliot W. Strong

30. Thyroglobulin in Benign and Malignant Thyroid Disease 587
Andre J. Van Herle and Katja Anna Van Herle

31. Iodine-131 and External Radiation in the Treatment of Local and Metastatic Thyroid Cancer 601
Martin Schlumberger, Claude Parmentier, Florent de Vathaire, and Maurice Tubiana.

32. Medullary Thyroid Carcinoma and the Multiple Endocrine Neoplasia Syndromes . 619
Donald T. Donovan and Robert F. Gagel

33. Anaplastic Carcinoma, Lymphoma, Unusual Malignancies, and Chemotherapy for Thyroid Cancer 645
M. William Audeh, Leslie Memsic, and Allan Silberman

34. Management of Thyroid Carcinoma Invading the Upper Aerodigestive System 657
Judith M. Czaja and Thomas V. McCaffrey

Part IX. Surgery of the Thyroid Gland

35. General and Regional Anesthesia for Thyroid Surgery 667
Wen-hsien Wu, Jay Jong-il Choi, and Steven S. C. Cheng

36. The Technique of Thyroidectomy by Cervical and Thoracic Approaches 681
Eric A. Birken, Stephen A. Falk, and Richard H. Feins

37. Complications of Thyroid Surgery: An Overview 697
Stephen A. Falk

38. Nonmetabolic Complications of Thyroid Surgery 705
David D. Caldarelli and Andrew J. Lerrick

39. Metabolic Complications of Thyroid Surgery: Hypocalcemia and Hypoparathyroidism; Hypocalcitonemia; and Hypothyroidism and Hyperthyroidism 717
Stephen A. Falk

40. Complications of Thyroid Surgery: Thyrotoxic Storm 739
Leonard Wartofsky and Mark E. Peele

Subject Index 747

Foreword to the First Edition

Thyroid Disease: Endocrinology, Surgery, Nuclear Medicine, and Radiotherapy is a comprehensive volume dealing with all aspects of thyroid disease. Stephen Falk, the editor, has accomplished the difficult task of integrating into a single volume contributions from workers with different points of view to consider all facets of thyroid disease management. The authors are seasoned clinicians with extensive practical experience. There are chapters dealing with relevant basic science, thyroid function tests, disorders of thyroid function, and thyroid tumors, and there is an extensive review of the etiology and pathogenesis of each condition.

The chapters present the details of management of each thyroid disorder. Although there is an emphasis on surgical management, medical treatment is also discussed in detail. Surgical therapy of all aspects of goiter and thyroid cancer are thoroughly covered. Complications of therapy are reviewed in many contexts. Each chapter includes an up-to-date review of the literature, and in most chapters there are extensive citations. The book is abundantly illustrated.

In this authoritative and comprehensive volume, the reader will find all of the answers to questions and problems encountered in dealing with patients with thyroid disease.

Jerome M. Hershman, M.D.
Chief, Endocrinology Division
West Los Angeles Veterans
Administration Medical Center
Professor of Medicine
U.C.L.A. School of Medicine
Los Angeles, California

Preface

The clinical manifestations of thyroid disease are so protean that afflicted patients present to every kind of generalist and specialist. Consequently, many disciplines contribute to the diagnosis and treatment of the patient with thyroid disease. What we have endeavored to produce in *Thyroid Disease: Endocrinology, Surgery, Nuclear Medicine, and Radiotherapy, Second Edition,* is a scholarly and clinically oriented state-of-the-art reference volume, integrating the special perspectives of the many disciplines that are commonly confronted with the clinical manifestations of thyroid disease—physiology and endocrinology, surgery, nuclear medicine, radiation and medical oncology, diagnostic radiology, embryology and anatomy, anatomic and clinical pathology, immunology, ophthalmology, pediatrics, anesthesiology, and others. This was the goal of both editions. I hope that this integrated work will foster a multidisciplinary approach that can offer the best care for the patient with thyroid disease.

I chose the contributing authors for this project based on their expertise, writing ability, and enthusiasm. The charge to the contributors was to formulate their chapters as thorough, well-referenced compilations of established knowledge and up-to-date treatments of new concepts and material. By adhering to specific guidelines, I could assure that *Thyroid Disease: Endocrinology, Surgery, Nuclear Medicine, and Radiotherapy, Second Edition,* would read as an integrated work and have the authority of a multiauthored text. However, the guidelines were meant to indicate the core or essential material to be covered. The contributors were encouraged to include related aspects of their topics, either novel or established, theoretical or practical, controversial or dogmatic.

There are significant changes in the second edition. Since the first edition was published in 1990, all chapters were brought completely up to date. To reflect the great strides in understanding thyroid disease which molecular biology offers, a new section titled, "Molecular Biology of the Thyroid Gland," has been added; this section is edited and partly authored by Donald L. St. Germain, M.D. and consists of four chapters. The first chapter, "Molecular Basis of Thyroid Disease," contains a glossary of molecular biology terms and serves as a foundation and overview for the next three chapters—"Molecular Biology of the Thyroid-Stimulating Hormone Receptor," "Thyroid Hormone Resistance Syndromes," and "Oncogenes and Thyroid Cancer." This section covers basic and advanced material, as do all other chapters of the book; it also covers its topic in a didactic and understandable manner, especially for the reader without expertise in molecular biology.

Other changes for this edition are the organization of the table of contents into sections. The contributors and I have expended much care and effort to make every chapter well-organized, readable, thorough, and clinically applicable. Many of the chapters are superbly written works of exceptional scholarship that highlight the contributors broad mastery of their topics. We hope we have met the high expectations of our readers.

This book integrates the medical and surgical aspects of thyroid disease. One goal is to offer the reader a complete source of information on thyroid disease—a one-stop reference for the novice and sophisticate alike, containing information that previously could be found only in scattered reports in the literature and chapters in various books.

This volume can be used as a practical, clinically-oriented text and as a reference. It will be of interest and use to a wide variety of physicians and residents-in-training: endocrinologists, internists, surgeons, nuclear medicine specialists, radiation and medical oncologists, pathologists, ophthalmologists, pediatricians, family physicians, and anesthesiologists—in short, to any physician who sees and treats patients with thyroid disease.

Stephen A. Falk, M.D., F.A.C.S.

Acknowledgments

I wish to thank the following people:

My staff, Char Yarger, Val Frere, Sandra Dayton, L.P.N., and Linda Burns, R.N., who showed great dedication and effort in the organization and realization of this book; Lana Rudy, M.A., M.L.S., the librarian at Werner Health Sciences Library, Rochester General Hospital, Rochester, New York, who offered great assistance in providing thousands of articles and abstracts needed for the writing and editing of this book; Anne M. Sydor, Ph.D., of Lippincott–Raven Publishers, who served as a superb Developmental Editor; and my patients.

I am also grateful to the contributing authors with whom I have worked for their enthusiasm, knowledge, and scholarship. It was an honor for me to associate with such an illustrious group of authorities in the field of thyroid medicine and surgery. To the contributing authors I give my gratitude and, I anticipate, the gratitude of the readers of this book.

Contributors

M. William Audeh, M.D Cedars-Sinai Cancer Center, 8700 Beverly Boulevard, Los Angeles, California 90033

Daniel T. Baran, M.D. Professor of Orthopedics, Medicine, and Cell Biology, Department of Medicine and Orthopedics, University of Massachusetts Medical Center, 55 Lake Avenue North, Worcester, Massachusetts 01655

Tomasz Bednarczuk, M.D. Department of Endocrinology, Medical Research Center, Polish Academy of Science, 02-097 Warsaw, Poland

Hugh F. Biller, M.D. Chairman, Department of Otolaryngology, Mt. Sinai Medical Center, 1 Gustave Levy Place, Box 1189, New York, New York 10023

Eric A. Birken, M.D., F.A.C.S. Clinical Assistant Professor of Surgery, University of Rochester School of Medicine and Dentistry, 4 Coulter Road, Clifton Springs, New York 14432

Roland Bramlet, Ph.D. Rochester, New York 14610-3363

David D. Caldarelli, M.D. Professor and Chairman, Department of Otolaryngology/Bronchoesophagology, Rush-Presbyterian-St. Luke's Medical Center, 1653 West Congress Parkway, Room 201 Senn, Chicago, Illinois 60612

Steven S.C. Cheng, M.D. Department of Anesthesiology, University of Medicine and Dentistry of New Jersey Medical School, 185 South Orange Avenue, Newark, New Jersey 07103

Alice C. Chiu, M.D. Section of Endocrinology, Baylor College of Medicine, One Baylor Plaza, Room 537E, Houston, Texas 77030

Jay Jong-il Choi, M.D. Department of Anesthesiology, University of Medicine and Dentistry of New Jersey Medical School, 185 South Orange Avenue, Newark, New Jersey 07103

Sharon L. Collins, M.S., M.D., F.A.C.S. Department of Otolaryngology—Head and Neck Surgery, Loyola University of Chicago Medical Center, 2160 S. First Avenue, Maywood Illinois 60153; and Chief, Section of Otolaryngology—Head and Neck Surgery, Hines VA Hospital, Hines, Illinois

Robin T. Cotton, M.D. Professor, Department of Otolaryngology, University of Cincinnati, College of Medicine; and Director, Department of Otolaryngology, Children's Hospital Medical Center, 3333 Burnet Avenue, Cincinnati, Ohio 45229

Judith M. Czaja, M.D. Clinical Fellow, Department of Otolaryngology—Head and Neck Surgery, University of Cincinnati, 231 Bethesda Avenue, Cincinnati, Ohio 45267-0528

Terry F. Davies, M.D., F.R.C.P. Department of Medicine, Division of Endocrinology, Mt. Sinai School of Medicine, 1 Gustave Levy Place, New York, New York 10029

Donald T. Donovan, M.D. Professor of Medicine, Bobby R. Alford Department of Otorhinolaryngology and Communicative Sciences, Baylor College of Medicine, 6550 Fannin Street, Suite 1727, Houston, Texas 77030

Stephen A. Falk, M.D., F.A.C.S. Clinical Associate Professor of Surgery, University of Rochester School of Medicine and Dentistry, 350 Sandringham Road, Rochester, New York 14610

Richard H. Feins, M.D. University of Rochester School of Medicine and Dentistry, 601 Elmwood Avenue, Rochester, New York 14642

David M. Finkelstein, M.D., F.R.C.S.(C) Department of Surgery, Division of Otolaryngology, York County Hospital, 679 Davis Drive, Suite 105 Newmarket, Ontario, Canada L3Y 5G8

Zachary Freedman, M.D. The Genesee Hospital, 222 Alexander Street, Suite 5500, Rochester, New York 14607

George L.A. From, M.D., F.R.C.P.(C) Associate Professor of Medicine, University of Toronto, The Toronto Hospital, MC8-441, 339 Bathurst Street, Toronto, Ontario, Canada M5G 2C4

Robert F. Gagel, M.D. Professor of Medicine and Chief, Department of Endocrine Neoplasia and Hormonal Disorders, The University of Texas M.D. Anderson Cancer Center, 1515 Holcombe Boulevard, Box 15, Houston, Texas 77030

Joel I. Hamburger, M.D. 6114 Pickwood Drive, West Bloomfield, Michigan 48034

John T. Hansen, Ph.D. Department of Neurobiology and Anatomy, University of Rochester School of Medicine and Dentistry, 601 Elmwood Avenue, Rochester, New York 14642

Michael M. Kaplan, M.D. Departments of Medicine and Nuclear Medicine, William Beaumont Hospital, 6900 Orchard Lake Road, #203, West Bloomfield, Michigan 48622-3425

John S. Kennerdell, M.D. Department of Ophthalmology, Allegheny General Hospital and Medical College of Pennsylvania, and Hahnemann University, Pittsburgh, Pennsylvania 15212

Joel C. Kirsh, M.D., F.R.C.P.(C) Department of Diagnostic Imaging, The Credit Valley Hospital, Mississauga, Ontario, Canada L5M 2N1

Victor G. Lawson, M.D., F.R.C.S.(C), F.A.C.S. Central Kentucky Otolaryngology—Head and Neck Surgical Associates, Bluegrass Medical Center, 24 Clinic Drive, Suite B, Paris, Kentucky 40361

William Lawson, M.D., D.D.S. Professor, Department of Otolaryngology—Head and Neck Surgery, Mt. Sinai Medical Center, Box 1189, 1 Gustave Levy Place, New York, New York 10023 and Staff Physician and Chief, Section of Otolaryngology, Veteran's Administration Medical Center, Bronx, New York

Andrew J. Lerrick, M.D. Assistant Professor, Department of Otolaryngology/Bronchoesophagology, Rush-Presbyterian-St. Luke's Medical Center, Rush Medical College, 1653 West Congress Parkway, Chicago, Illinois 60612

Virginia A. LiVolsi, M.D. Vice Chair for Anatomic Pathology, Professor of Pathology and Laboratory Medicine, University of Pennsylvania Medical Center, 3400 Spruce Street/6 Founders Pavilion, Philadelphia, Pennsylvania 19104-4328

Jonathan S. LoPresti, M.D., Ph.D. Associate Professor of Medicine, Division of Endocrinology, Diabetes, and Hypertension, University of Southern California School of Medicine, 2025 Zonal Avenue, GNH-6602, Los Angeles, California 90033

Thomas V. McCaffrey, M.D., Ph.D. Professor, Department of Otolaryngology, Mayo Clinic, 200 First Street, S.W., Rochester, Minnesota 55905

Michael T. McDermott, M.D. Clinical Professor of Medicine, Department of Endocrinology, University of Colorado Health Sciences Center, 4200 East 9th Avenue, Denver Colorado, 80262

Jeffrey I. Mechanick, M.D. Department of Medicine, Division of Endocrinology, Mount Sinai School of Medicine, 1 Gustave Levy Place, New York, New York 10029

Leslie Memsic, M.D. Cedars-Sinai Cancer Center, 8700 Beverly Boulevard, Los Angeles, California 90033

Charles M. Myer, III, M.D. Professor, Department of Otolaryngology, University of Cincinnati, College of Medicine; and Department of Pediatric Otolaryngology, Children's Hospital Medical Center, 3333 Burnet Avenue, Cincinnati, Ohio 45229

Shigenobu Nagataki, M.D.   The First Department of Internal Medicine, Nagasaki University School of Medicine, 1-7-1 Sakamoto, Nagasaki, 852 Japan

Yuji Nagayama, M.D.   Department of Pharmacology 1, Nagasaki University School of Medicine, 1-12-4 Sakamoto, Nagasaki, 852 Japan

Arnold M. Noyek, M.D., F.R.C.S.(C), F.A.C.S.   Otolaryngologist-in-Chief, University of Toronto, Mount Sinai Hospital, 600 University Avenue, Toronto, Ontario, Canada M5G 1X5

Amy L. O'Donnell, M.D.   Department of Veterans Affairs Western New York Healthcare System, Research Service (151), 3495 Bailey Avenue; and Department of Medicine, State University of New York at Buffalo, Buffalo, New York, Buffalo, New York 14215

Robert E. O'Mara, M.D.   University of Rochester School of Medicine and Dentistry; and Chief, Division of Nuclear Medicine, Strong Memorial Hospital, 601 Elmwood Avenue, Box 620, Rochester, New York 14642

Claude Parmentier, M.D.   Department of Nuclear Medicine, Institut Gustave-Roussy, Rue Camille DesMoulins, 94805 Villejuif Cedex, France

Mark Peele, M.D.   Division of Cardiology, Brooke Medical Center, Fort Sam Houston, San Antonio, Texas 78234-5012

Ronald R. Reed, M.D.   500 Kreag Road, Pittsford, New York 14534

Anthony J. Reino, M.D., F.A.C.S.   Assistant Clinical Professor, Department of Otolaryngology—Head and Neck Surgery, The Mt. Sinai Medical Center Box 1189, 1 Gustave Levy Place, New York, New York 10023; and Staff Physician and Associate Director, Veteran's Administration Medical Center, Bronx, New York

Jessica C. Rockwell, M.D.   Assistant Clinical Professor of Medicine, Columbia University at Cooperstown, Mary Imogene Bassett Hospital, 1 Atwell Road, Cooperstown, New York 13326

Martin Schlumberger, M.D.   Department of Nuclear Medicine, Institut Gustave-Roussy, Rue Camille DesMoulins, 94805 Villejuif Cedex, France

Steven I. Sherman, M.D.   University of Texas, M.D. Anderson Cancer Center, Baylor College of Medicine, 1515 Holcombe Boulevard, Box 15, Houston, Texas 77030

Allan Silberman, M.D.   Cedars-Sinai Cancer Center, 8700 Beverly Boulevard, Los Angeles, California 90033

Peter A. Singer, M.D.   Department of Medicine, Division of Endocrinology, Diabetes, and Hypertension, University of Southern California School of Medicine, 1355 San Pablo Street, Los Angeles, California 90033

Sidney H. Sobel, M.D., F.A.C.R.   Clinical Associate Professor of Radiation Oncology, University of Rochester School of Medicine and Dentistry, 601 Elmwood Avenue, Rochester, New York 14642; and Director, Finger Lakes Community Cancer Center, Clifton Springs Hospital and Clinic, 2 Coulter Road, Clifton Springs, New York 14432

Stephen W. Spaulding, M.D., C.M.   Department of Veterans Affairs Western New York Healthcare System, Research Service (151), 3495 Bailey Avenue; and Department of Medicine, State University of New York at Buffalo, Buffalo, New York 14215

Donald L. St. Germain, M.D.   Departments of Medicine and Physiology, Dartmouth Medical School, One Medical Center Drive, Lebanon, New Hampshire, 03756

Elliot W. Strong, M.D., F.A.C.S   Attending Surgeon, Head and Neck Service, Memorial Sloan Kettering Cancer Center 1275 York Avenue; and Professor of Surgery, Cornell University Medical College, New York, New York 10021-6007

Maurice Tubiana, M.D.   Department of Nuclear Medicine, Institut Gustave-Roussy, Rue Camille DesMoulins, 94805 Villejuif Cedex, France

Alvin L. Ureles, M.D. *University of Rochester School of Medicine and Dentistry; Chief, Thyroid Laboratory, The Genesee Hospital, 222 Alexander Street, Rochester, New York 14607*

Stephen J. Usala, M.D., Ph.D. *Clinical Associate Professor, Texas Technical University Health Sciences Center School of Medicine, Suite A, 1900 S. Coulter Drive, Amarillo, Texas 79106*

Andre J. Van Herle, M.D. *Professor of Medicine, Division of Endocrinology, Department of Medicine, UCLA School of Medicine, 10833 Le Conte Avenue, Los Angeles, California 90095-1682*

Katja Anna Van Herle, M.D., M.S.P.H. *Chief Resident, Department of Medicine, UCLA School of Medicine, 10833 Le Conte Avenue, Los Angeles, California, 90095-1682*

Florent de Vathaire, M.D. *Department of Epidemiology, Institut Gustave-Roussy, Rue Camille DesMoulins, 94805 Villejuif Cedex, France*

Sheldon S. Waldstein, M.D. *Professor of Medicine, Northwestern University Medical School; and Chairman, Division of Medicine, The National Center for Advanced Medical Education, 541 N. Fairbanks Court, 6th Floor, Chicago, Illinois 60611-3319*

Jack R. Wall, M.D., Ph.D. *Department of Ophthalmology, Allegheny General Hospital and Medical College of Pennsylvania, and Hahnemann University, Pittsburgh, Pennsylvania 15212*

Leonard Wartofsky, M.D., M.A.C.P. *Chairman, Department of Medicine, The Washington Hospital Center, 110 Irving Street, N.W., Washington, D.C. 20010-2975; Professor of Medicine and Physiology, Uniformed Services University of the Health Sciences; and Clinical Professor of Medicine, Georgetown, George Washington, and Howard University Schools of Medicine*

George A. Wilson, M.D. (Deceased) *Associate Professor of Radiology, University of Rochester School of Medicine and Dentistry, Rochester, New York 14642*

Ian J. Witterick, M.D., F.R.C.S.(C) *Department of Otolaryngology, University of Toronto, Mount Sinai Hospital, 600 University Avenue, Toronto, Ontario, Canada M5G 1X5*

Paul D. Woolf, M.D. *Professor of Medicine, Pathology, and Laboratory Medicine, University of Rochester School of Medicine, 601 Elmwood Avenue, Box 693, Rochester, New York 14642*

Wen-hsien Wu, M.D. *Chairman, Department of Anesthesiology, University of Medicine and Dentistry of New Jersey Medical School, 185 South Orange Avenue, Newark, New Jersey 07103*

CHAPTER 1

Thyroidology— Reflections on Twentieth-Century History

Alvin L. Ureles and Zachary R. Freedman

"In Darkness Dwells the People Which Knows Its Annals Not" Prof. Ulrich B. Phillips
(Inscription on the William Clements Library, University of Michigan)

We have been invited to set the scene and highlight some thoughts as to where we've been, where we are now, and where we may be going in thyroidology, an invocation to the important proceedings that are to follow.

THE PRELUDE

Let it not be said that we came into this century empty-handed. By the mid nineteenth century, most of the fanciful theories about the nature of the thyroid and its struma had been discarded. In 1836, the English morphologist T. W. King (1) presented detailed descriptions of the thyroid follicle, delineating its lymphatics and blood supply, and included some intelligent guesses about the nature of colloid. Cruveilhier (2) established the thyroid as a ductless gland, and he and Virchow made note of its vesicles. There was no more talk of "bronchocoele" among the savants of medicine.

Serious attention began to be paid to environmental factors as a cause for goiter, particularly certain foods, drinking water, and stress. By 1812, Gay-Lussac (3) had discovered the element iodine, a product of his restless curiosity over the seaweed-bred mother liquor that was corroding the copper vats of Napoleon's troubled gunpowder industry. It was a momentous discovery.

There soon followed a series of epiphanies that often characterize our profession. Seaweed, kelp, and marsh seawater ameliorated goiter. This was known for centuries, but the mechanism was obscure. Perhaps the secret was in the iodine content.

Prout (4), in England, tested iodine's toxicity on himself in 1816, then tried it successfully in the treatment of goiter. It then became standard therapy in London's St. Thomas Hospital. Coindet (5), in France, in 1820, similarly made systematic studies with tincture of iodine and proved its therapeutic efficacy. By 1833, Boussingault (6) was prescribing iodized salt for the prevention and treatment of goiter. And so it was that decades before we had any substantive understanding of the pathophysiology of the hyperplastic thyroid, we had an efficacious treatment for it. Little wonder that iodine became a "miracle drug" and in this context was much abused. Toxicity became rampant through its indiscriminate use. There were reports of serious morbidity and deaths. It rapidly fell into disrepute. But, as the century drew to a close, it was rescued by Bauman (7), who carefully documented the relationship of iodine to various states of thyroid dysfunction, out of which was to develop a firmer rationale for its use.

By the 1870s, valuable insights into the nature of thyroid failure began to emerge from London. Fagge (8) demonstrated the absence of thyroid function as a cause of sporadic and congenital cretinism. William Gull (9), the curmudgeon of Guy's Hospital, and his gentle counterpart, William Ord (10), clarified the clinical and pathological role of the thyroid in myxedema.

The ultimate confirmation of these clinical conclusions came in 1891, when G. R. Murray (11) showed that a hypodermic extract of sheep's thyroid in a glycerin emulsion reversed and cured human myxedema. This was followed shortly by the discovery by Fox (12) and Mackenzie (13) that crude animal thyroid taken by mouth was dramatically therapeutic. The news spread fast throughout Europe, but not in time for Osler, now at

A. L. Ureles: University of Rochester School of Medicine and Dentistry; The Genesee Hospital, Rochester, New York 14607.

Z. R. Freedman: The Genesee Hospital, Rochester, New York 14607.

Johns Hopkins, to include it in his 1892 publication of *The Principles and Practice of Medicine*.

No less a contribution was made by the vivid sequential descriptions of exophthalmic hyperthyroidism by Flajani (14) (1802) and Caleb Parry's (15) posthumous report (1825), neither clinician fully appreciating the role of the "bronchocoele" in cardiac failure and in the other debilitating symptoms of the disease. This enlightenment remained for the keen eye of the Irishman Robert J. Graves (16) (1835), and the subsequent insights of the German Karl A. von Basedow (17) (1840), who promulgated the "Merseburg triad" of goiter, exophthalmos, and palpitations, and went so far as to prescribe the iodide-rich mineral waters of the region to cure the disease. No clinician, even today, should examine a patient with endocrine exophthalmos without paying passing homage to such names as Moebius (1886, disordered convergence), Stellwag (1880, widened palpebral fissure and stare), and von Graefe (1850, lid lag and retraction) (18). All the great names of Europe added to the clinical picture—Marie, Charcot, Trousseau, and Stokes, to name but a few. It was some 50 years after Graves' description, however, before such thoughtful observers as Horsley (19) (1886) were to suggest that an overactive "hypersecreting" thyroid gland, elaborating its own humor, was the basis for the disease.

With this breakthrough, the stage was set for studies revealing the "metabolic effects" of thyroid extract. By 1893, Muller (20) had introduced evidence that the thyroid played a role in the oxidation of food and the rate of protein metabolism. Metabolic rates of hyper- and hypothyroid states were clearly differentiated. The disorders began to take on new meaning. Two years later, another famous German, Magnus-Levy (21), showed, by measuring the exchange of oxygen and carbon dioxide, that these metabolic insights were correct. Thereupon was laid the groundwork for the quintessential function of thyroid hormone. It was a substance that "regulated" the chemical activities of the body.

But where was thyroid surgery during the nineteenth century? The answer is best recounted in the meticulous review on the subject by William Stewart Halsted, who in the autumn of his career wrote "The Operative Story of Goiter: The Author's Operation" (22). For over a thousand years, any operative attack on the thyroid gland was considered breathtaking heroics, fraught with danger to the patient and almost certain bereavement for the family. Thyroidectomy placed a cloud of professional butchery over the head of the surgeon who might be tempted to indulge himself. As late as 1850, the French Academy of Medicine proscribed any attempt to remove the thyroid surgically. The procedures previously performed successfully were for the most part simple enucleations of nodules, partial resections, or artery ligations. All totaled, only 106 bona fide thyroidectomies had been documented by mid century, with mortality rates as high as 40% (22), mostly resulting from exsanguination and sepsis.

This grim picture was turned around by the pivotal discovery of a quiet, modest country doctor from Georgia, Crawford W. Long, who was the first to use sulfuric ether as an anesthetic in his surgery (1842). What brought this to world attention (and brought high visibility to Boston's reputation), was W. T. G. Morton's flamboyant demonstration of ether's efficacy at the Massachusetts General Hospital in 1846. Although the question of priority may never be resolved, the fact of "anesthesia," as Oliver Wendell Holmes came to name it, changed the course of surgery and human suffering forever (23).

Twenty years later, in 1867, a second giant leap occurred when the beloved teacher and investigator Joseph Lister published his five papers in *Lancet*, characterizing "The Antiseptic System" (24). Within months, the dreaded complications of sepsis in thyroid surgery were in retreat and all of Europe's major surgical theaters became enveloped in a miasma of carbolic acid. This improved state of affairs continued for two decades until, in 1883, Gustav Neuber of Kiel (25) put on cap and gown and introduced "asepsis" as an important alternative to "antisepsis."

Finally came the simple but important victory of hemostasis. Jules Pean of France not only invented the vaginal extirpation of fibroids, but, in 1874, invented the operative hemostat.

Thus, by the last quarter of the nineteenth century, the circle was completed. Pain was conquered. Sepsis slid into the shadows. The bloodbath was over. The scene was set for the giants of twentieth-century surgery to begin cultivating their fame. It began in Europe and remained there for a long time, principally because the major surgical centers in the New World were unaccountably slow to accept the revelations of antisepsis and asepsis.

In Vienna, Billroth, who prior to 1877 had proceeded with thyroidectomy reluctantly and with great discouragement, emerged as the world leader in this operation (26). His mortality rate dropped to 8%. Patients and students flocked to Austria. The clinical experience grew exponentially. Early lessons were sharply enunciated: the recurrent laryngeal nerve must be identified and isolated; it must not be wounded. Total extirpation of the gland leads to prompt tetany, a lesson taken up by his assistant von Eiselberg, who went on to clarify the relationship of the phenomenon to the parathyroid.

The greatest contribution, however, came in Bern, where Theodor Kocher (27), a careful, skillful academician, guided the "new surgery" into a high level of respect. His students went to the laboratory to solve problems. The conservation of tissue and avoidance of trauma became the linchpins of operative technique. Billroth's speed was no longer the goal. Kocher's meticulous attention to detail became the norm. He published widely. By 1889, his mortality rate was reduced to 2.4%. At the end of the century it was 0.18%. By his death in 1917, over 5000 cases had passed through his world-renowned clinic.

Halsted's salute to him was that he taught us the lessons of induced operative myxedema, and how to recognize, manage, and treat various forms of hyperthyroidism and thyroid cancer. He gave us the detailed blueprints for incision, ligature, and extirpation.

It remained for von Mikulicz (28), a student of Billroth, to add the finishing touches to our modern operation. By the end of the century, his technique for bilateral partial resection had clearly asserted itself as a method for avoiding hypothyroidism, nerve paralysis, and tetany.

By this time, the impressive young American student referred to previously, William Stewart Halsted, had made intensive rounds of the European theaters, absorbing the teachings of Billroth and Kocher, and perfecting his laboratory skills under Wolfler, whose extensive monograph on the thyroid remains a classic to this day. Halsted returned to the United States in 1880. He began his career problematically as a bon vivant New York practicing surgeon caught in the grips of a debilitating cocaine addiction. Under the watchful eyes of close friends (including William Welch), he transferred to Baltimore, where he slowly evolved into the legendary, and first, Johns Hopkins Professor of Surgery. Students, such as Cushing and Bartlett, and colleagues, such as Welch and Osler, held his surgical, laboratory, and teaching skills in the highest regard.

When he died in 1922, he had personally launched American surgery on its way, pioneered the course for the acceptance of Listerism, polished surgical thyroidectomy to its present art, given the surgical world its rubber gloves, and primed the pathway for such great American thyroid specialists of our century as Mayo, Lahey, and Crile (25).

THE TWENTIETH CENTURY

The flywheel of progress was now in full gear and we shall be able to only lightly graze its rapid spin. In doing this we shall have to omit the names and contributions of many worthy investigators.

Basics

The concept of a follicular cell secretion being incorporated into colloid, and its subsequent resorption and elimination into the bloodstream, was fathered by Carlson and Woelfel (29) in 1910. Colloidal storage and release was further developed by Uhlenhuth, who tracked thyroid metamorphosis and growth from the salamander to man (30). Thus, the thyroid parenchymal cell was found to have a unique behavior unlike other glandular cells that store their products within their own confined cytoplasm. Severinghaus (31) pointed out the unusual phasic character of the thyroid with different follicles in different stages of activity at any one time.

In 1932, Nonidez (32) discovered the parafollicular cells, recognized their extrathyroidal origin, and suspected they might secrete another type of hormone. (He was right!) In addition, he described the complex neuroanatomy of the thyroid. Previously, the Hopkins anatomist Major (33) in 1909 had worked out the vascular maze of the gland, and Wilson (34) in 1929 had clarified the lymphatic network.

Chemistry

Although a frantic search for the thyroid hormone began in the latter part of the nineteenth century with various extractions and manipulations of thyroglobulin, serious biochemistry began with Oswald's isolation of diiodotyrosine in 1911 (35). Four years later, on Christmas day, Kendall (36) crystallized the pure hormone and named it "thyroxin." A decade later (1926), Harrington improved the yield and in a brilliant flurry of biochemical insight characterized the material as a hydroxyphenyl ether of tyrosine, containing four atoms of iodine. The following year, with Barger (37), he synthesized the hormone and predicted that its *in vivo* synthesis would involve similar steps, that is, the oxidative coupling of diiodotyrosine. Thus, the long search for the "central substance" was resolved, except for the unsettling observation that crude thyroid was more calorigenic than could be accounted for by its thyroxine content. The unraveling of this conundrum was to await the second half of our century.

Hormonal Function

As early as 1921, Plummer (38) recognized that the fundamental action of thyroxine (T_4) was its acceleration of metabolic activity in all body cells. Numerous *in vivo* and *in vitro* experiments confirmed this. The effect of T_4 on the metamorphosis of amphibia had been noted by Gudernatsch as early as 1912 (39).

There followed in the 1920s a broader understanding of myxedema protein, its water-retaining properties, and the effects of T_4 on protein turnover and water mobilization by Byron (40). Joe Aub, in Boston, began investigating calcium metabolism and was first to note bone loss in hyperthyroidism, a subject of increasing concern to us today (41). In collaboration with Meyer and McTiernan, he further showed that T_4 acted directly on body cells and not indirectly through other systems, such as the adrenal or nervous system (42).

As early as 1934, Herman Blumgart noted the inverse ratio of cholesterol to metabolic rate. He also showed a positive therapeutic effect of thyroidectomy on a subset of patients with end-stage angina pectoris (43), confirming the reduced oxygen demands on the heart in patients with hypothyroidism. Within the next decade, almost every conceivable tissue and organ had been subjected to an evaluation of thyroid hormone effects. The results were confirmatory. The actions of the hormone were pervasive and ubiquitous.

Thyrotropin

As we might suspect, in retrospect, both light and confusion was generated over the early observations on thyrotropin (TSH). By 1927, the Smiths (44), in a series of fine studies in hypophysectomized animals, demonstrated thyroid atrophy along with other peripheral endocrine gland failure. Aron (45) and Loeb and Bassett (46) in 1929 followed up with the identification of a substance that qualified (by bioassay) as thyrotropin, although by the 1950s a pure substance had not been clearly identified. Still, it was evident that the pituitary made, among others, a specific glycoprotein that had the ability to stimulate hyperplasia and hyperfunction in the thyroid. But it was not sustained, and it was peculiarly absent in the hyperplasia and hyperfunction of Graves' disease. The precise identification of TSH and the solution to this paradox had to await the rewarding techniques of protein and receptor purification, polypeptide analysis, and immunological science.

Metabolism

The early decades of this century were dominated by a determined search for diagnostic tools to take advantage of our newfound clinical acumen and therapeutic success. The observation that thyroid hormone played a major role in influencing basal metabolism, body heat, and gas exchange, together with the development by Benedict (47) of a practical instrument, with standardized nomograms and surface area formulas by DuBois (48), channeled our profession into one of those mindless misapplications of basic science that we are wont to succumb to recurrently. Thousands of "modern" doctors engaged in primary care set out to unmask thyroid disorders by meeting patients at the crack of dawn in their respective private offices to check their basal metabolic rates. Breathing oxygen was harmless, and the descending track of the pen on the motorized drum made a convincing graph of consumption. It sounded like science. It looked like science. And it was, in the careful hands of researchers such as Boothby and Rynearson. But as a general tool, it was, at best, a very loose test of thyroid function, particularly where it counted—in early onset disease. It was frequently carried out under less than ideal conditions, with many modifying and exacerbating factors at work, all difficult to measure and control. Thus, the data were most often flawed.

To this very day we still see patients in clinic who had been placed on a lifetime of animal thyroid at an early age, all on the basis of dubious numbers obtained from an instrument long relegated to medical oblivion. What was needed was a quantitative test in which we could trust and believe. For this we had to wait until the 1940s, a time great strides were taking place in the arena of iodine physiology and chemistry.

Iodine

When, in 1910, David Marine showed that "cancer" in brook trout was merely fish goiter secondary to iodine deficiency, it once again reawakened the flagging interest in iodine for goiter prevention and treatment (49). There soon followed his famous "Akron experiment" with O. P. Kimball (50), in which dietary enrichment with iodide brought about a precipitous drop in goiter in schoolchildren (1916 to 1920). McClendon's (51) correlation of goiter with iodine content of drinking water in World War I draftees made headlines. Health officer G. W. Goler also made headlines (1923) when he added 7.5 kilograms of iodide to the Rush Reservoir in Rochester, New York (52). The incidence of goiter decreased accordingly, in spite of the public furor about "invasions of privacy" (53). Out of all this, at long last, came an assured place for iodine in the prophylaxis of goiter.

Although iodine in the treatment of toxic goiter had its advocates in the nineteenth century, not until the 1920s did serious clinical studies support its role in therapy [Neisser (54), Loewy and Zondek (55)]. Means' group, in Boston, showed that iodine worked directly on the thyroid gland and not against the thyroid hormone (56). Boothby and Rynearson (57) showed that the metabolic rate of patients with exophthalmic goiter was modulated by iodine treatment. It was H. S. Plummer (58), however, who demonstrated conclusively in 1923 the importance of iodine in the treatment of toxic goiter and its value in the preoperative preparation of the toxic patient for surgery. Not only did iodine control the devastating symptoms of the disease, but the incidence of thyroid storm dropped dramatically. The hyperplasia and vascularity of the gland regressed. Thyroidectomy was safer and surer in most good surgeons' hands.

The other avenue of iodine research, diagnosis, was slower in starting and was troubled by the difficulties in developing accurate methods for the quantitative analysis of the minuscule amount of protein-bound hormonal iodine found in human serum. Numerous studies in the late 1930s confirmed that this protein-bound component gave the most precise description of the secretory activity of the thyroid gland. Precipitation and butanol extraction was even more precise. The arguments raged over the optimal methodologies, with numerous strategies concocted to avoid the many pitfalls of the assay. In the end, by the

1940s, we had a valuable addition to our diagnostic armamentarium, thanks to the early labors of such talents as Perkin and Hurxthal (59), Grauer and Saier (60), and Riggs and Man (61), to name but a few. We could now finally sort out thyrotoxicosis in young children, psychotics, patients with heart failure and pulmonary disease, or other concomitant catabolic illnesses, all of whom could not be evaluated by the most scrupulously conducted metabolism test. In addition, this new tool opened up a fledgling understanding of factors that influenced thyroxine binding. The truly great strides in iodine research, however, had to await what became one of the most important and exciting chapters in the history of basic medical and clinical research—the provision of radioactive isotopes for the study of the pathophysiology of disease and for its diagnosis and therapy.

Radioactive Iodine

No brief review, such as this, can do justice to the cascade of investigations that followed the introduction of cyclotron-produced radioisotopes of iodine by Fermi in 1934 (62). Two groups—Saul Hertz from Harvard, working with Roberts and Evans (63) from the Massachusetts Institute of Technology, ran head-to-head with Hamilton, Soley, and Lawrence (64) in Berkeley, California—provided our profession with the basic data and applications for the new isotopes. These were all short-lived nuclides, requiring handy access to a physics laboratory, temporarily delaying the budding science of nuclear medicine several years until post–World War II, when radioactive iodine-131, with its duet of gamma and beta emissions and an 8-day half-life, became available, from the atomic pile, to all investigators.

Within the decades of the 1940s and 1950s, significant clinical experience was accumulated in the diagnosis and treatment of thyrotoxicosis [Hertz (65), Hamilton (66), Soley (67), and Chapman (68)]. Treatment for primary and metastatic thyroid cancer proved feasible [Seidlin and Marinelli (69), Rawson (70), and Beierwaltes (71)].

Improved methodologies, such as autoradiography, chromatography, and electrophoresis, helped to produce important advances in mapping the pathways of iodine and thyroid hormone physiology [Taurog, Chaikoff (72)], culminating in the discovery and synthesis of triiodothyronine by Gross and Pitt-Rivers (73) (1952).

The invention of the scintillation crystal and the Anger gamma camera (74) (1958) allowed us to dispatch our inefficient Geiger-Müller tubes and rectilinear scanning equipment to the medical museums. Metastable technetium-99m proved to be a valuable addition to the diagnostic laboratory. In time, after a struggle for purification was overcome, iodine-123, with its 13-hour half-life, soft x-ray, and absent destructive beta ray emission, became commercially available, fulfilling our hopes for the ideal isotope. The thyroidal uptake and distribution of radioiodine-123 and technetium-99m became standard fare all over the world for evaluating hyperthyroidism and the thyroid nodule.

The laboratory kept pace with the clinic. As the 1960s began, iodine-125, which was first described in 1951, came into production and was added to the list [Myers and Vanderleeden (75)]. It filled important requisites for *in vitro* studies with its 60-day half-life and soft radiation. It proved to be a fine labeling agent.

By 1964, Murphy and Pattee (76) developed a displacement method to measure more specifically thyroid hormone in the blood. It was the forerunner of one of the most significant laboratory breakthroughs of the century, the development by Rosalind Yallow and Sol Berson of the radioimmunoassay technique (77), which, though centered on the measurement of insulin (1962), was quickly translated to the measurement of thyroxine and its chemical family. It is interesting that these two Nobel prize winners, who had spent the better part of their investigative lives in the thyroid arena, developed a major contribution to thyroidology while busying themselves in another field.

With every improvement, the chase to pin down free thyroxine and free triiodothyronine became more inspired. Recant and Riggs (1952) had hypothesized, on the basis of inconsistent thyroxine levels with various clinical disorders, that protein binding in the blood could mitigate and obscure the true active free thyroid hormone component (78). The proof came in the tedious, demanding technique of equilibrium dialysis or ultrafiltration, in which the free component was separated from its protein linkage, captured, and measured [Ingbar and Braverman (79), Sterling and Brenner (80) (1965 to 1966)]. This test, though never applicable to the general laboratory, remains, for many, the gold standard in measuring the free T_4 or T_3 (triiodothyronine) components. A more practical method of looking at both the free and the bound fractions was developed by Milton Hamolsky in 1959 (81) in what became known confusingly (but through no fault of his own) as the T_3 uptake (i.e., a procedure that displaced labeled T_3 to the red cell and later to resin). The product of this uptake and the measured total T_4 formed a useful mathematical correlate of thyroid function. Ultimately, radioimmunoassay [Chopra (82), in 1972] and enzyme-linked immunoadsorbent assay [Schall (83), in 1978] were added to our bag of tricks for solving these clinical questions.

Antithyroid Agents

The use of pharmacologic doses of iodide had left in its wake the confusing observation that at least a subset of people did not benefit from its administration. They developed iodide goiter and myxedema, or, paradoxically, they developed iodide-induced thyrotoxicosis. In addition, there were the unpredictable hypersensitivity reactions of iodism and the dangerous "iodine escape" phenomenon in those patients with Graves' disease who had initially responded. This led to the systematic search for other agents to modulate thyroid secretion.

The clues came in the late 1920s with the experimental observations in rabbits, by Chesney (84), of hyperplastic goiters induced by cabbage diets. Sodium thiocyanate used in the early treatment of hypertension was noted to cause a similar type of hyperplasia. These observations were linked in the next decade by Hercus and Perves (85) who characterized the cabbage (Brassicae) principle as a thionamide. In the early 1940s, Richter and Clisby (86), using taste-testing experiments with phenylthiourea in rats, noted the induction of goiters and hypothyroidism and recognized that a promising agent had appeared on the scene. When, in turn, hypophysectomy or oral thyroid prevented this hyperplasia, the mechanisms of its antithyroid action began to be elucidated [Astwood (87), in 1944]. By the end of the 1940s, the various thionamide compounds had been sorted out for activity and toxicity. Methimazole and propylthiouracil emerged as the drugs of choice for treatment in primary thyrotoxicosis [Stanley and Astwood (88)] in the United States, and carbimazole in Europe. There followed a proliferation of literature establishing optimal doses, safety, and precautions. No novel agents have yet displaced these pioneering drugs.

Thyroid Cancer

The story of thyroid malignancy has had a curious history, with diagnosis and treatment beset with disputatious dogma. Pathologic classification in the 1800s is difficult to interpret in light of our present knowledge. The term *sarcomatous degeneration* was applied liberally to anaplastic lesions, and often simply *thyroid tumor* was applied to the rest. In Halsted's extensive compilation of documented thyroidectomies, the first notation on the presence of "thyroid cancer cells" was in 1862 (Gosselin, Paris). Chiari in Prague reported 55 "sarcomas" (our quotes) and 11 carcinomas in 7700 postmortems (22).

Problems of interpretation in the past, though for the most part resolved, remain to this day and relate to the unique features and behavior of thyroid malignancies. Follicular cancers appear to dominate in endemic goiter areas, papillary cancers in nonendemic regions [Ward (89), in 1935]. Unlike in other cancers, 5- and 10-year "cures" are less meaningful in what are essentially indolent growths. Yet these sleeping crabs may suddenly and inexplicably become more aggressive, encroach and/or metastasize, recur, and, more ominously, transform into highly lethal, undifferentiated cancers. Metastases sometimes do not mirror the mother lesion. Arguments still abound over when blood vessel invasion is an artifact versus a real fact. Some benign-looking follicular goiters may spread their benign-looking histopathology to local nodes, or find their way to the lungs or bones. They may even be functional, and a large-enough tumor burden may cause an added debilitating thyrotoxicosis. Local nodal metastases are often less ominous than local invasion. Finally, along with the confusion over the multifocal origin of papillary follicular cancer, we have the problem of "occult" disease, which, though very common, is "harmless" (except when it is not) (90).

At the 1948 Brookhaven Conference on Radioactive Iodine, Ben Duffy suggested to the senior author of this chapter (Ureles) that he check the records of a young thyroid cancer patient from the Massachusetts Institute of Technology, whom he was treating at that time for lung metastases. He suggested that the patient might have had thymic irradiation as an infant. It turned out that Ben was quite correct. In 1950, with P. J. Fitzgerald, he reported 28 cases in *Cancer* to illustrate this fascinating correlation he had noted (91). It was one of those landmark observations that often receive little attention except in retrospect. In 1951, Lou Hempelman was told about these findings. He was looking for a radiation biology project to work on and this excited his interest. The result was a series of four excellent intensive surveys from 1955 to 1975, all confirming this concept and, with numerous other subsequent investigators, Hempelman interdicted radiation exposure to the normal developing infant and adolescent thyroid for all time (92).

Advances in Recent Decades

A torrent of major discoveries has followed in recent decades. The 1950s began with numerous studies clarifying the action and role of T_3 after its discovery by Gross and Pitt-Rivers. The *in vitro* conversion of thyroxine to T_3 began to shape our view of the latter as the active hormone (93). The remarkably rapid and increased activity of T_3 over thyroxine was clearly established (94).

The advantage of the antithyroid drugs in preparing thyrotoxic patients for surgery was confirmed (95), and their long-term use without surgery was established as another option for treatment (96). Radioactive iodine treatment for Graves' disease began to replace surgical intervention in many centers (97).

The assays for studying thyrotropin, although still bioassays in nature, were considerably improved. The use of thyrotropin as a diagnostic tool was firmly established (98). TSH was shown not to be the exophthalmos-producing substance of Graves' disease, which some had claimed (99). Corticosteroids proved useful in treating infiltrative exophthalmos (100) and myxedema (100a). The inability to suppress the toxic thyroid with thyroxine was discovered [Greer and Smith (101)] and formed the basis of an important test of the toxic thyroid's autonomy from pituitary control.

Congenital defects in hormonal synthesis were beginning to unfold, as cretins and hypothyroid children were studied all over the world (102). V. K. Summers (103), in England, defined myxedema coma once and for all as a truly recognizable medical emergency.

Nodular goiter as a potential source of thyroid malignancy was highlighted, triggering a groundswell of surgical excisions (104). Radical neck dissection for thyroid cancer came under increasing attack and more conservative procedures were explored (105). More metastatic thyroid cancer was reported to be successfully treated with radioiodine [Dobyns (106)] and suppressed with thyroxine [Balme (107)].

Quantitative mathematical concepts of iodine metabolism, storage, and turnover were developed [Berson (108)].

There then appeared a paper by Freedberg, Kurland, and Hamolsky (1955) documenting, within the technology of the time, that there may be a rare subset of hypometabolic patients, with normal thyroid function, who responded selectively to oral T_3, possibly because of a failure to deiodinate T_4 (109). Tittle, coining the phrase *metabolic insufficiency*, published a similar paper the following year (110). These reports unwittingly created a brief but intense flurry of uncritical clinical "hyperpharmacy," in which numerous tired, achy, sluggish patients were placed by their physicians on large-dose trials of oral T_3 to "cure" their metabolic insufficiency. Fortunately the fad was short-lived.

By 1957, the augmenting and depressant effects of estrogen (111) and androgen (112), respectively, on thyroxine binding had been identified. It was the year, however, that Deborah Doniach, together with I. M. Roitt (113), in England, recognized Hashimoto's thyroiditis as a disturbance of autoimmunity, with humoral and cell-mediated changes, involving thyroglobulin and the thyroid follicle. It was the beginning [along with the important immune-animal model of Rose and Witebsky (114)] of a new road toward solving the pathophysiologic mechanisms of some of the major thyroid diseases. Crile (115) and others presented a classification of the different forms of thyroiditis and their treatment, especially with adrenocortical steroids in subacute thyroiditis.

The following year, another stellar observation came out of the Commonwealth. D. D. Adams, in New Zealand, had discovered an abnormal "late acting" thyroid stimulator (LATS), distinctly different from TSH (116). LATS was identified in the serum of numerous thyrotoxic patients and could stimulate guinea pig thyroid. The findings were soon confirmed by others. There were, however, some confounding problems. What was LATS? Where did it come from? Why didn't we find it in all Graves' disease patients? The answers were to be found in the decades ahead, as immunological research began to merge with endocrinology.

The modulating effects of reserpine and guanethidine in hyperthyroidism were established, and the useful role of this group of pharmacologic agents in the treatment of thyroid crisis was beginning to be recognized (117).

The decade ended with the description of familial increased and decreased thyroxine-binding disorders [Beierwaltes (118), Tanaka (119)]. The first hopes were raised that myxedema coma might be treatable with intravenous triiodothyronine (120).

The 1960s began with numerous studies that reinforced and expanded on previous observations. New syndromes of congenital hypothyroidism were described in which isolated defects in the metabolic pathway were identified (121).

Since its inception, the treatment of the thyrotoxic patient with radioiodine was frustrated by the high frequency of resultant hypothyroidism. There was a plethora of such reports (122). Numerous formulas, innovations, and strategies had been developed to select the precise dose to accomplish the task without recurrence of disease or thyroid failure. It was all to no avail. In the 1960s we examined the results of all these mathematical excursions, which proved only to delay a large group of patients from ultimately developing signs of thyroid ablation. The bottom line was that many centers accepted the fact that Graves' disease was a disorder involving the entire gland and that to treat the disease effectively with radioiodine they accepted the trade-off, treating patients promptly with ablating doses, replacing them with oral thyroxine, and obviating the future problem of patients "drifting" into hypothyroidism.

Nagging concerns that radioactive iodine treatment of thyrotoxicosis might lead to the induction of leukemia, thyroid cancer, or some other malignancy were put to rest by a large cooperative study conducted by the United States Public Health Service [follow-up on 36,000 cases, Saenger (123)].

Winship (124) analyzed 562 cases of thyroid cancer in children between the ages of 4 months and 14 years of age from all over the world. The results proved to us what we already suspected, which was that in children, as in patients over 40, this malignancy can be a devastating mortal disease.

In 1962, D. D. Adams (125) was heard from again, this time recognizing another "unique" thyroid stimulator that was neither TSH nor LATS. The trail was getting hotter! In 1963, Roger Guillemin (126), in Paris, opened up a new chapter in our understanding of the hypothalamic–pituitary–thyroid axis with his discovery of a peptide thyroid-releasing factor of hypothalamic origin. Numerous analogies were to be found in other endocrine pathways. Neuroendocrinology became a clinical as well as a research science.

In 1961, Sipple (127) noted a possible relationship between familial pheochromocytoma and thyroid cancer. Hazzard (128), 3 years previously, had provided the grist by recognizing medullary carcinoma as a distinct entity. A series of papers quickly followed that identified the familial nature of the nonsporadic form, associated multiple endocrine neoplasias (types IIA and IIB), the relationship to calcitonin, provocative testing, and paraneoplastic syndromes. It was the beginning of a vast literature (129).

Conflicting reports continued on the relative merits of the effect of oral T_4 in suppressing thyroid nodules (130).

Methodologies improved steadily. The radioimmunoassay of thyrotropin [Utiger (131)] and free thyroxine [Ingbar and Braverman (132)] gave a new precision to diagnosis.

Beta-blockers (particularly propranolol) became the standard method of controlling thyrotoxic patients while awaiting definitive therapy, even though this drug indication was not recognized by the Food and Drug Administration (133). It became a vital part of the regimen in treating patients with thyroid crisis (134). Guanethidine and reserpine faded into the background.

McKenzie and others, working on the etiology of Graves' disease, began to close in on the concept that thyroid stimulators, which had attracted so much attention, were antibodies representing another autoimmune process (135).

The syndrome of primary hypothyroidism, amenorrhea, and galactorrhea was differentiated from Chiari-Frommel syndrome by Ross and Nusynowitz (136), opening the door to an understanding of prolactin–thyroid relationships.

The 1970s brought an accurate radioimmunoassay for the elusive T_3 [Chopra (137)], and clear documentation of T_3 toxicosis [Hollander (138)]. Cellular chemical mechanisms that turned on via protein kinase activation were further elucidated (139). There was clarification of choriocarcinoma (molar)-TSH versus chorionic-TSH, LATS, and pituitary-TSH [Hershman (140)].

A new imaging procedure burst onto the scene in the form of thyroid echography, using high-frequency probes that could define thyroid nodules with a resolution of 0.5 centimeter or more [Blum (141)]. These scans were particularly valuable in delineating cystic from solid lesions, although attempts to characterize tissue signatures in the latter group proved unavailing.

There was a rapid evolution of the technology through the decade (i.e., static A mode to B mode to real time). In addition, echography of the orbital muscles proved useful in evaluating Graves' ophthalmopathy, with the surprising finding that 90% of Graves' disease patients, with or without clinically evident eye changes, had distinct bilateral changes on scanning [Werner (142)].

Just as the biochemistry of the 1960s focused on the pathways and enzymatic links of the thyronines in their cellular and extracellular milieu, the molecular biology of the 1970s began to concentrate on the phenomena of hormonal nuclear receptor sites and binding affinities [De Groot (143)]. The idea that TSH elicits its specific action on cyclic AMP (cAMP) via nonspecific kinase and prostaglandin suggested that a specific landing field must exist on the cell surface membrane. A world of veteran and rookie investigators entered the field. Another hunt was on.

The role of T_3, reverse T_3, and the interrelationships of nonthyroidal illness was further clarified by Chopra's group in California (144).

In 1972, Dussault and Leberge developed a sensitive method for the detection and screening of hypothyroidism in newborns (145). By 1974, Alan Klein's team at the University of Pittsburgh, had demonstrated that cord blood TSH could successfully screen for congenital hypothyroidism (146). Both groups correctly predicted the merits of screening for the prevention and reduction of mental retardation caused by this disease. With some variation in methodologies, the screening concept spread quickly over North America and thence to all parts of the globe, happily saving millions of dollars in future institutional costs and, most importantly, stopping the prospective development of congenital cretinism.

A variety of important studies on thyroid-stimulating antibodies (TSab) emerged in mid decade using an array of receptor assay techniques, closing the circle on the mechanism of Graves' disease [Onaya, Orgiazzi, Holmes, Bech, McKenzie, Zakarija (147)]. Retro-orbital radiation for early endocrine exophthalmos resurfaced as a therapeutic option [Ravin (148)]. Thyrotoxicosis with lymphocytic thyroiditis and a low radioiodine uptake was firmly documented by Gluck's group (149) in Texas. This was the progenitor paper of what was later to be called "painless thyroiditis" (150) and then extended to encompass "transient postpartum thyroiditis" by Amino's team (151) in Tokyo.

Gershengorn and Weintraub (152), at the National Institutes of Health (NIH), described a new syndrome of hyperthyroidism: inappropriate secretion of TSH by a resistant pituitary (1975). Refetoff (153), in 1969, had previously described familial generalized T_4 resistance. Many other reports followed in the 1970s. These were new recognitions of puzzling forms of hyperthyroxinism. In 1970, Hamilton et al. (154) described a patient with pituitary hyperthyroidism resulting from a thyrotropin-producing pituitary chromophobe adenoma. Confirmations of this clinical entity soon followed. Additional families with elevated thyroxine-binding globulins and hormone values were also documented. All of this meant that an elevated T_4 required more and more critical evaluation and clinical reasoning.

The first successful attempt to treat a hypothyroid fetus by intrauterine injections of thyroxine was detailed by Van Herle's group (155) at the University of California (1975). That group, in another pivotal paper that same year, used a sensitive radioimmunoassay to show that significantly elevated thyroglobulin values could serve as a marker in differentiated thyroid carcinoma. It would prove useful in metastatic disease (156) and recurrence (157).

In the latter half of the 1970s, a simple direct diagnostic procedure arose upon the scene like a morning sunrise. It changed the life of the thyroidologist for all time. Fine-needle-aspiration (FNA) cytology had been gaining advocates in Europe for many years. Indeed, we had explored this idea with large-bore biopsy needles in the 1950s. The acceptance of FNA in our country had to await the development of capable cytology technicians under the supervision of knowledgeable pathologists. In addition, there was a tradition in our literature, although poorly documented, propagated by such surgical-pathology luminaries as Lawrence Sloan and Virginia Frantz, that needle biopsy was inadvisable because of tumor "seeding" (158). Subsequent events proved this to be furthest from the truth. The extensive series of Galvan (159) in Germany, Miller and Hamburger (160) in Michigan, Walfish (161) in Toronto, and Gershengorn's team (162) at NIH, dispelled, once and for all, any doubts. We had an "old" new way of looking at the thyroid that was going to put fresh meaning into the terms *thyroid nodule* and *goiter*. It was no passing fancy.

The 1980s were characterized by the unrelenting probing of cell behavior in thyroid disease, with a concatenation of spellbinding research. Youngblood's Chapel Hill team (163) found a distinctly different thyrotropin-releasing hormone (TRH)-like substance in placental tissue that may regulate the fetal pituitary–thyroid axis. Spitz (164) found an abnormal megaTSH resulting from a biosynthetic error in the pituitary. In this disorder, patients are euthyroid in spite of elevations in the TSH radioimmunoassay.

New understanding of the pathophysiology of certain primary myxedemas came out of the discovery of growth-blocking antibodies by Drexhage et al. (165), who had already noted certain characteristic (but somewhat controversial) growth-stimulating antibodies as a cause of goiter (165a). These latter antibodies, unlike the thyroid stimulating antibodies of Graves' disease, appear to act via a pathway that does not involve cAMP.

Okita et al. (166), in Toronto, demonstrated deficiencies in specific suppressor T lymphocytes in lymphocytic thyroiditis. This allows thyroid-directed forbidden clones of organ specific helper T lymphocytes to destroy tissue directly and indirectly, reinforcing our evolving concepts of the mechanisms of autoimmune disease.

More syndromes of hyperthyroxinemia that could be mistaken for thyrotoxicosis were elaborated upon, including those associated with familial dysalbuminemia [Docter (167) and Rajatanavin (168)] and familial dysprealbuminemia [Moses (169)]. Jansen et al. (170) described a new syndrome of hyperthyroxinemia resulting from decreased peripheral triiodothyronine production.

In the 1980s, amiodarone, a new efficient antiarrhythmic with an extraordinarily high iodine content, arrived on the scene from Europe. Clinical observations soon followed, closely recapitulating all the other insults noted over the decades from stable iodine, such as induced thyrotoxicosis, induced hypothyroidism, and iodide goiter [Dickstein (171)]. Some cynic has said that the only thing we learn from history is that we learn nothing from history. This is a case in point.

Not surprisingly, as the autoimmune mechanisms of Graves' disease have centered on target-specific immunoglobulins, the long-suspected immunological abnormality of Graves' ophthalmopathy appears to be confirmed. Ophthalmopathic immunoglobulins have been identified and assays developed to measure them [Atkinson (172)]. Cyclosporine, however, appears to be more promising than older, more toxic immunosuppressants [Weetman (173)].

After desiccated thyroid preparations had all but been driven off the market, we were left with synthetic thyroxines as our replacement drug. After a minor flurry over changes in purification and bioavailability, most preparations appear to be comparable. However, all can produce the phenomenon of "chemical hyperthyroidism," in which patients are euthyroid with elevated T_4s and normal T_3s (174).

An additional bonus to the immunoglobulin story was the further identification of IgGs with selective growth-stimulating properties [van der Gaag (175)]. These IgGs are found in all types of functioning, nonfunctioning, and euthyroid goiters, suggesting that an entire gamut of thyroid disease is associated with an autoimmune background. In addition, it is clear that membrane-directed antibodies in such disorders as Graves' disease are heterogeneous and multifunctional [i.e., some are clearly thyroid stimulating (TSAb), some are inhibitors of TSab and TSH (TSHIAb), and some are enhancers of TSH-binding (TSHEAb)]. The net effect of the various concentrations of these at any one time may well determine whether or not a given patient is better, worse, or in remission [Zakarija (176)].

The 1980s focused our attention on osteoporosis, particularly in women, and legitimate questions were raised about the effects of thyroid replacement as a potentiator of bone loss [Ettinger (177), Krolner (178), Coindre (179)]. The increased turnover of bone in hyperthyroidism had been well established for decades. Although the histomorphometric findings are disturbing indeed in thyroxine-replaced hypothyroid patients, there are no controlled clinical data in our thyroid cancer patients, to date (e.g., patients highly suppressed with thyroxine) that demonstrate a "clinically significant" increased incidence of central or distal bone fracture.

The 1980s came to a close with new data emanating from an improved, highly sensitive, two-site TSH immunoradiometric assay that allows us to diagnose accurately all phases of thyroid activity in one laboratory package [Spencer (180)]. In a world in which the cost of medical care looms as an ever-present concern, this would be most welcome (181).

The final decade of the twentieth century is the decade of molecular thyroidology. Using the myriad techniques of molecular biology, through analysis of gene expression and the structure–function relationships of various peptides and molecules, we have witnessed advances in our fundamental knowledge of normal and abnormal thyroid physiology. These advances occurred in the areas of thyroid stimulatory hormone (TSH), the thyrotropin receptor (TSH-R), defective thyroid hormone synthesis, defects in serum binding proteins, and resistance to thyroid hormone. We march awestruck to the twenty-first century.

Thyroid Stimulating Hormone

Advances have included greater knowledge of basal and regulated TSH gene expression, including TSH beta subunit and alpha gene transcription (182). Although rare, autonomous production of TSH-producing pituitary tumors has been described (183,184). Tumor cell lines have been deficient in TR-beta. Also, defective biosynthesis of TSH has been linked with Pit-1 mutations, both autosomal recessive and dominant forms (185–187). Congenital hypothyroidism, with low TSH and low T_4, an autosomal recessive trait, has been characterized to TSH beta mutations. Deletion of TSH beta is found more commonly in Japanese populations, a mutation preventing the dimerization between mutant TSH beta and the common alpha subunit (188,189).

The Thyrotropin Receptor

The 1990s have yielded significant advances in our understanding of the genetic regulation of the TSH-R. The gene promoter of the TSH-R has been characterized.

Investigations have linked the relationship of TSH-R to possible autoimmunity, especially Graves' ophthalmopathy, as well as to mutations activating the TSH receptor to produce hyperfunctioning thyroid adenomas and hereditary toxic thyroid hyperplasia (190).

Congenital hyperthyroidism, without evidence for autoimmunity, has been linked to TSH-R mutations. Both autosomal dominant and sporadic mutations occur in patients with goiter and elevated T_4 and suppressed TSH. These mutations, occurring in the transmembrane and intracellular loops of the TSH receptor, result in constitutional activation of the receptor, with increased cAMP production (191,192). In addition, somatic mutations in the TSH-R have been found in patients with "hot nodules." The net result is clonal cell proliferation and increased T_4 secretion (190,193–195).

Inactivation of the TSH-R has also been characterized. This results in resistance to TSH, with congenital hypothyroidism but elevated TSH levels. Two families with autosomal recessive inheritance have been described with mutations in the extracellular TSH-binding domain (190,196).

Defective Thyroid Hormone Synthesis

Molecular thyroidology has allowed the identification of defective thyroglobulin synthesis and secretion that result in congenital goiter and low T_4 levels. These have been found to be autosomal recessive in families with a high prevalence of consanguinity. However, no identifiable mutations have been reported (197).

Mutations in the thyroperoxidase (TPO) gene have been identified in patients with hypothyroidism, goiter, and elevated TSH levels. Appropriately, these individuals have an increased perchlorate discharge (198).

Serum Binding-Protein Deficits

In most individuals, the condition of elevated thyroid-binding globulins (TBGs) is acquired, secondary to estrogen or advanced AIDS. There have been no known genetic defects defined. However, deficient synthesis of TBGs has been associated with inheritance, affecting 1 in 15,000 males, who present with low T_4 and normal free T_4 and TSH levels. Female carriers have a reduced level of TBG (to 50%). Mutations have included frame-shift mutations and amino acid substitutions that alter TBG stability. A variety of mutations can cause partial TBG stability (199,200).

Other abnormalities have included mutations in TBPA (transthyretin) as well as in albumin in the syndrome referred to as familial dysalbuminemic hyperthyroxinemia (FDH). Most defects are autosomal dominant and recently shown to be caused by an ARG 218 HIS mutation in several different families.

Resistance to Thyroid Hormone

Mutations in the thyroid receptor beta have been characterized as autosomal dominant and have been localized to three regions within the carboxyterminus. The mutations reduce thyroid hormone binding and/or transactivation. Inactive mutant receptors bind to DNA and block the function of normal receptors. Affected individuals have relatively few signs of hyperthyroidism, despite increased thyroid hormone levels and inappropriately normal TSH levels (201).

CONCLUSION

And the advances continue. We have an increased understanding of the role of thyroid hormone in prenatal and neonatal neurologic development, as well as of thyroid function in patients with systemic illness, the so-called euthyroid sick syndrome. We can only marvel at what technological innovations will occur in the years ahead that will increase our knowledge of the genetics of normal and abnormal thyroid physiology.

We have, in summary, come a long way in this wonderful century, blessed with tools and insights never dreamed of by our worthy predecessors. Where will we be at the turn of the century, as we close these bountiful and productive years? Is it reasonable to hope that the bloom of immunology and genetic engineering still lies ahead, enabling us to manipulate the defects of thyroid disease in our favor, both post hoc and preventively? Is it too much to predict that, in the decades before us, we will have discovered precisely what turns on the loaded gun of autoimmunity and pulls the trigger so unexpectedly? Will the surgical blade and the therapeutic isotope be retired to the sidelines? Will the mystery of thyroid cancer, so different in evolution and biologic behavior from other cancers, resolve before our eyes and yield to some unique pharmacologic strategy? Will *cretinism* be a term buried in history? Will we find a way to graft a thyroid gland so that it will not be rejected? The questions go on and on. The answers are locked in the future. But, as we hope this chapter has helped to demonstrate, it is a future supported by a very distinguished past and a very energetic present.

REFERENCES

1. King TW. Observations on the thyroid gland. *Guy's Hosp Rep* 1836;1:429.
2. Cruveilhier J. *Antomic pathologigue du corps humain.* Paris: JB Bailliere, 1836; T II Liv XXXV Pl IV.
3. Crosland MP. *Dictionary of scientific biography,* vol 5. 1972;317–327.
4. Prout WM. *Chemistry, meteorology and the functions of digestion. Bridgewater treatise 18.* London: WM Pinckney, 1834;100.
5. Coindet JR. Decouverte d'un nouveau remede contra le goitre. *Ann Chim Phys* 1820;15.
6. Boussingault JB. Memoire sur les saline iodiferes des Andes. *Ann Chim Phys* 1833;54:163.
7. Bauman E. Ueber das normale Vorkommen des Jods im Thierkorper. III mitt. Der Iodgehalt der Schilddrusen von Menschen und Thiereen. *Hoppe-Seyler's Ztschr Physiol Chem* 1896;22:1.
8. Fagge CH. On sporadic cretinism occurring in England. *Medico-Chir Tr* 1871;54:155.
9. Gull W. A cretinoid state supervening in adult life in women. *Tr Clin Soc* London, 1875;7:180.
10. Ord WM. On myxoedema, a term proposed to be applied to an essential condition in the "cretinoid" affection occasionally observed in middle-aged women. *Medico-Chir Tr* 1878;61:57.
11. Murray GR. Note on the treatment of hypodermic injections of an extract of the thyroid gland of a sheep. *Br Med J* 1891;2:796.
12. Fox EL. A case of myxedema treated by taking extract of thyroid by mouth. *Br Med J* 1892;2:941.
13. Mackenzie HWG. A case of myxedema treated with great benefit by feeding with fresh thyroid glands. *Br Med J* 1892;2:940.
14. Flajani GF. *Collezione d'osservazioni e reflessioni di chirurgia.* Rome 1802;3:270.
15. Parry CH. *Collections from the unpublished papers of the late Caleb Hilliel Parry.* London. 1825;2:111.
16. Graves RJ. Clinical lectures (part II). *London Med Surg J* 1835;7:516.
17. Von Basedow CA. Exophtalmos durch Hypertrohie des Zellgewebes in der Augenhohle. *Wchnschr ges Heilk* 1840;6:197.
18. Von Graefe HA. Vorlag uber die Basedow'sche Krankeit. *Klin Monatsbl Augenh* 1864;2:183.
19. Horsley V. Remarks on the function of the thyroid gland. A critical and historical review. *Br Med J* 1892;1:215,265.
20. Muller F. Beitrage zur Kenntniss der Besedow'schen Krankheit. *Deutsches Arch Klin Med* 1893;51:335.
21. Magnus-Levy A. Ueber den respiratorischen gewechselunter dem einfluss der thyreoiden sowie unter verschiedenen pathologischen zustanden. *Berl Klin Wchnschr* 1895;32:650.
22. Halsted WS. The operative story of goiter: the author's operation. *Johns Hopkins Rep* 1720;XIX:71.
23. Graham H. *The story of surgery.* New York: Doubleday Doran, 1939;322–325.
24. Lister J. *The collected papers of Joseph Baron Lister.* (2 vols) London: Clarendon, 1909.
25. Nuland SB. *Doctors: the biography of medicine.* New York: Alfred A. Knopf, 1988;382.
26. Wolfer A. Die Kropfextirpationen an Hofr. Billroth's Klinik von 1877 bis 1881. *Wein med Wochenschr* 1882;xxxii:5.
27. Kocher T. Ueber ein drittes Tausend Kropfextirpationen. *Arch klin Chir* 1906;lxxix:786.
28. Mikulicz J. Beitrag zur Operation des Kropfes. *Wein med Wochenschr* 1886;xxxvi:1,40,70,97,100.
29. Carlson AJ, Woelfel A. On the internal secretion of the thyroid gland. *Am J Physiol* 1910;26:32.
30. Uhlenhuth E. The secretion process in the living thyroid gland. *Anat Rec* 1926;32:224.
31. Severinghaus AE. Cytological observations on secretion in normal and activated thyroids. *Ztschur Zellforsch mikr Anat* 1933;19:653.
32. Nonidez JF. Further observations on parafollicular cells of mammalian thyroid. *Anat Rec* 1932;53:339.
33. Major RH. Studies on the vascular system of the thyroid gland. *Am J Anat* 1909;9 475.
34. Wilson GE. The nature of the so-called microcapillaries of the thyroid gland and other secreting epithelia. *Anat Rec* 1929;42:243.
35. Oswald A. Gewinning von 3-5 Dijodotyrosin aus Jodeiweiss. *Ztschr Physiol Chem* 1911;70:310.
36. Kendall EC. The isolation in crystalline form of the compound containing iodin which occurs in the thyroid. *Trans Assoc Am Physicians* 1915;30:420.
37. Harrington CR, Barger G. Chemistry of thyroxine no 111 constitution and synthesis of thyroxine. *Biochem J* 1927;21:169.
38. Plummer HS. Interrelationship of the function of the thyroid gland and of its active agent thyroxin in the tissues of the body. *JAMA* 1921;77:243.
39. Gudernatsch JF. Fullerungs Versuche an Amphibienlarven. *Zentralbl Physiol* 1912;26:323.
40. Byron FB. The nature of myxoedema. *Clin Sci* 1934;1:273.
41. Aub JC, Bauer W, Ropes M, et al. The relation of the thyroid gland to calcium metabolism. *Trans Assoc Am Physicians* 1927;42:344.
42. Meyer OO, McTiernan C, Aub JC. The effect of thyroxin upon the metabolism of isolated normal and malignant tissue. *J Clin Invest* 1933;12:723.
43. Blumgart HL, Levine SA, Berlin DD. Congestive heart failure and angina pectoris: the therapeutic effect of thyroidectomy on patients without clinical or pathologic evidence of thyroid toxicity. *Arch Intern Med* 1933;51:866.
44. Smith PE. Hypophysectomy and a replacement therapy in the rat. *Am J Anat* 1930;45:205.
45. Aron M. Action de la prehypophyse sur la thyroide chez le Cobaye. *Conpt Rend Soc Biol* 1929;102:682.
46. Loeb L, Bassett RB. Effect of hormones of anterior pituitary on thyroid gland in the Guinea pig. *Proc Soc Exp Biol Med* 1932;29:1128.
47. Benedict FG. A Portable respiration apparatus for clinical use. *Med Surg J* (Boston) 1918;28:667.
48. DuBois EF. *Basal metabolism in health and disease.* 1st ed. Philadelphia: Lea & Febiger, 1924.
49. Marine D. Further observation and experiment on the so-called thyroid cancer of brook trout. *J Exp Med* 1910;12:310.
50. Marine D, Kimball OP. The prevention of simple goiter in man. *Arch Intern Med* 1920;20:661.
51. McClendon JF, Hathaway RS. Inverse ratio between iodine in food and drink and goiter, simple and exophthalmic. *JAMA* 1924;82:1668.
52. Health Bureau, Rochester, New York. *Monthly bulletin.* 1923;May:2.
53. Kohn L. Goiter, iodine and George W Goler: the Rochester experiment. *Bull Hist Med* 1975;49:389.

54. Neisser E. Ueber Jodbehandlung bei Thyreotoxikose. *Berl Klin Wchnschr* 1920;57:461.
55. Loewy A, Zondek H. Morbus Basedowii und Jodtherapie. Klinischhe und Gasanalytische Beobachtungen. *Deutche med Wchnschr* 1921; 47:1387.
56. Means JH, Thompson WO, Thompson PK. On the nature of the iodine reaction in exophthalmic goiter. *Trans Assoc Am Physicians* 1928; 43:146.
57. Boothby WM, Rynearson EH. Increase in circulation rate produced by exophthalmic goiter. *Arch Intern Med* 1935;55:547.
58. Plummer HS. Results of administering iodin to patients having exophthalmic goiter. *JAMA* 1923;80:1953.
59. Perkin HJ, Hurxthal LM. The fraction of iodine in the blood in thyroid disease. *J Clin Invest* 1939;18:733.
60. Grauer RC, Saier E. A comparison of the distilling and dry ashing methods for the determination of blood iodine. *Endocrinology* 1939; 24:553.
61. Riggs DS, Man EB. A permanganate acid ashing method for iodine determinations. *J Biol Chem* 1940;134:193.
62. Fermi E. Radioactivity induced by neutron bombardment. *Nature* 1934;133:757.
63. Hertz S, Roberts A, Evans RD. Radioiodine as an indicator in the study of thyroid physiology. *Proc Soc Exp Biol Med* 1938;38:510.
64. Hamilton JG, Soley MH. Studies in iodine metabolism by use of a new radioactive isotope of iodine. *Am J Physiol* 1939;127:557.
65. Hertz S, Roberts A. Application of radioactive iodine in the therapy of Graves' disease. *J Clin Invest* 1942;21:624.
66. Hamilton HB, Werner SC. The effects of sodium iodide, 6-propyl thiouracil and 1-methyl-2-mercaptoimidazole during radioiodine therapy of hyperthyroidism. *J Clin Endocrinol* 1952;12:1083.
67. Soley MH, Miller ER. Treatment of Graves' disease with radioactive iodine. *Med Clin North Am* 1948;January:1–15.
68. Chapman EM, Evans RD. Radioactive iodine in hyperthyroidism. *JAMA* 1946;131:86.
69. Seidlin SM, Marinelli LD, Oshry E. Radioactive iodine therapy: effect on functioning metastases of adenocarcinoma of the thyroid. *JAMA* 1948;132:838.
70. Rawson RW, et al. The effect of total thyroidectomy on the function of metastatic thyroid cancer. *J Clin Endocrinol* 1948;8:826.
71. Beierwaltes WH. Indications and contraindications to the treatment of thyroid cancer with radioactive iodine. *Ann Intern Med* 1952;37:23.
72. Taurog A, Chaikoff IL, Fuller DD. The mechanism of iodine concentration by the thyroid gland. *J Biol Chem* 1947;171:189.
73. Gross J, Pitt-Rivers R. The identification of 3,5,3′-L-triiodothyronine in human plasma. *Lancet* 1952;1:439.
74. Anger HO. Scintillation camera. *Rev Sci Instrum* 1958;29:27.
75. Meyers WG, Vanderleeden JC. Radioiodine-125. *J Nucl Med* 1960; 1:149.
76. Murphy BEP, Pattee CJ. Determination of thyroxine utilizing the property of protein binding. *J Clin Endocrinol* 1964;24:187.
77. Berson SA, Yallow RS. General principles of radioimmunoassay. *Clin Chem Acta* 1968;22:51.
78. Recant L, Riggs DS. Thyroid function in nephrosis. *J Clin Invest* 1952;31:789.
79. Ingbar SH, Braverman LE, Dawber NA, et al. A new method for measuring the free thyroid hormone in human serum and an analysis of the factors that influence its concentration. *J Clin Invest* 1965;44:1679.
80. Sterling K, Brenner MA. Free thyroxine in human serum: simplified measurement with the aid of magnesium precipitation. *J Clin Invest* 1966;45:153.
81. Hamolsky MW, Stein M, Freedberg AS. The thyroid hormone–plasma protein complex in man. 11: A new method for study of "uptake" of labelled hormonal components by human erythrocytes. *J Clin Endocrinol* 1957;17:33.
82. Chopra IJ. A radioimmunoassay for measurement of thyroxine in unextracted serum. *J Clin Endocrinol Metab* 1972;34:938.
83. Schall RF Jr, Fraser AS, Hansen HW, et al. A sensitive manual enzyme immunoassay for thyroxine. *Clin Chem* 1978;24:1801.
84. Chesney AM, Clauson TA, Webster B. Endemic goiter in rabbits. 1. Incidence and characteristics. *Bull Johns Hopkins Hosp* 1928;43:261.
85. Hercus CE, Pervis HD. Studies on endemic and experimental goiter. *J Hyg* 1936;36:182.
86. Richter CP, Clisby KH. Toxic effects of bitter-tasting phenylthiocarbamide. *Arch Path* 1942;33:46.
87. Astwood EB. The chemical nature of compounds which inhibit the function of the thyroid gland. *J Pharmacol Exp Ther* 1943;78:79.
88. Stanley MM, Astwood EB. Determination of the relative activities of antithyroid compounds in man using radioactive iodine. *Endocrinology* 1947;41:66.
89. Ward R. Malignant goiter: a survey of geographical types. *West J Surg* 1935;43:494.
90. Ureles AL. Cancer of the endocrine glands: thyroid cancer. In: *Clinical oncology—a multidisciplinary approach.* 6th ed. *Am Cancer Society,* 1983;326–336.
91. Duffy BJ Jr, Fitzgerald PJ. Cancer of the thyroid in children: a report of 28 cases. *J Clin Endocrinol Metab* 1950;10:1296.
92. Hempelman LH, Hall WJ, Phillips M, et al. Neoplasms in person treated with x-rays in infancy: fourth survey in 20 years. *J Natl Cancer Inst* 1975;55:519.
93. Pitt-Rivers R, Stanbury JB, Rapp B. Conversion of thyroxin to 3,5,3′-triiodothyronine in vivo. *J Clin Endocrinol* 1955;15:616–620.
94. Asper SP, Selenkow HA, Planondon CA. The metabolic activity of 3,5,3′-L-triiodothyronine in myxedema. *Proc Am Soc Clin Invest* 1953;May:7.
95. Bartels EC. Hyperthyroidism—evaluation of treatment with antithyroid drugs followed by subtotal thyroidectomy. *Ann Intern Med* 1952; 37:1123–1134.
96. Solomon DH, Beck JC, Vanderlan WP, et al. Prognosis of hyperthyroidism treated by antithyroid drugs. *JAMA* 1953;152:201–205.
97. McCullagh P. Radioactive iodine in the treatment of hyperthyroidism. *Ann Intern Med* 1952;37:739–744.
98. Skansee B. Use of thyrotropin in differential diagnosis of primary and secondary hypothyroidism. *Acta Endocrinol* 1953;13:358–370.
99. Simkin B, Starr P. Failure of short-term administration of thyrotropic hormone to produce exophthalmos in man. *Proc Soc Exp Biol Med* 1953;84:90.
100. Kinsell LW, Partridge J, Fireman N. The use of ACTH and cortisone in the treatment and differential diagnosis of malignant exophthalmos: a preliminary report. *Ann Intern Med* 1949;38:913.
100a. Inch RS, Rolland CF. Localized pretibial myxedema treated with cortisone. *Lancet* 1953;2:1039.
101. Greer MA, Smith GE. Method for increasing accuracy of radioiodine as a test of thyroid function by use of desiccated thyroid. *J Clin Endocrinol* 1954;14:1374–1384.
102. McGirr EM, Hutchinson JH. Radioactive iodine studies in nonendemic cretinism. *Lancet* 1953;1:1117–1120.
103. Summers VK. Myxedema coma. *Br Med J* 1953;2:366–368.
104. Cattell RB, Colcock BP. Present day problems of cancer of the thyroid. *J Clin Endocrinol* 1953;13:1408–1415.
105. Crile G Jr. Adenoma and carcinoma of the thyroid gland. *N Engl J Med* 1953;249:585–590.
106. Dobyns BM, Maloof F. Study and treatment of 119 cases of carcinoma of thyroid with radioactive iodine. *J Clin Endocrinol* 1951;11: 1323–1360.
107. Balme HW. Metastatic cancer of the thyroid successfully treated with thyroxin. *Lancet* 1954;1:812–813.
108. Berson SA, Yallow RS. Quantitative aspects of iodine metabolism. *J Clin Invest* 1954;33:1533–1552.
109. Freedberg AS, Kurland GS, Hamolsky MW. Effect of L-triiodthyronine alone and combined with L-thyroxine in nonmyxedematous hypometabolism. *N Engl J Med* 1955;253:57–60.
110. Tittle CR. Effects of 3,5,3′ L-triiodothyronine in patients with metabolic insufficiency: preliminary report. *JAMA* 1956;162:271–274.
111. Engstrom W, Markardt B. Influence of estrogen on thyroid function. *J Clin Endocrinol* 1954;14:215–222.
112. Keitel HG, Sherer MG. Marked depression of plasma protein-bound iodine concentration in absence of clinical hypothyroidism during testosterone medication. *J Clin Endocrinol* 1957;17:854–861.
113. Doniach D, Roitt IM. Autoimmunity in Hashimoto's disease and its implications. *J Clin Endocrinol* 1957;17:1293–1304.
114. Rose NR, Witebsky E. Studies on organ specificity: changes in thyroid glands of rabbits following active immunization with rabbit thyroid extracts. *J Immunol* 1958;76:417.
115. Crile G Jr, Schneider RW. Diagnosis and treatment of thyroiditis with special reference to use of cortisone and ACTH. *Cleve Clin Q* 1952; 19:219–224.
116. Adams DD. Presence of abnormal thyroid stimulating hormone in serum of some thyrotoxic patients. *J Clin Endocrinol* 1958; 18:699–712.

117. Darnaud C, Denard Y, Moreau G, et al. Effect of reserpine on hyperthyroidism: attempt at interpretation and therapeutic implications. *Presse Med* 1959;67:457–460.
118. Beierwaltes W, Robbins J. Familial increase in thyroxine-binding sites in serum alpha globulin. *J Clin Invest* 1959;38:1683–1688.
119. Tanaka S, Starr P. A euthyroid man without thyroxine-binding-globulin. *J Endocrinol* 1959;19:485–487.
120. Nordqvist P, Dhuner KG, Stenberg K, et al. Myxedema coma and CO_2 retention. *Acta Med Scand* 1960;166:189–194.
121. Choufoer JC, Kassenaar AA, Querido A. Syndrome of congenital hypothyroidism with defective dehalogenation of iodotyrosines: further observation and discussion of pathophysiology. *J Clin Endocrinol* 1960;20:983–1002.
122. Segal R, Silver S, Yohalem SB, et al. Myxedema following radioactive iodine therapy of hyperthyroidism. *Am J Med* 1961;354–364.
123. Saenger EL, Thoma GE, Tompkins EA. Incidence of leukemia following treatment of hyperthyroidism: preliminary report of the cooperative thyrotoxicosis follow-up study. *JAMA* 1968;205:855.
124. Winship T, Rosvoll RV. Childhood thyroid carcinoma. *Cancer* 1961;14:734–743.
125. Adams DD, Perves HD, Sirett NE, et al. Presence of short acting abnormal thyroid stimulator in blood of a thyrotoxic patient. *J Clin Endocrinol* 1962;22:623–626.
126. Guillemin R, Yamozaki E, Gard DA, et al. In vitro secretion of thyrotropin (TSH) stimulation by a hypothalamic peptide (TRF). *Endocrinology* 1963;73:564–572.
127. Sipple JH. The association of pheochromocytoma with carcinoma of the thyroid gland. *Am J Med* 1961;31:163–166.
128. Hazzard JB, Harok WA, Crile G Jr. Medullary (solid) carcinoma of the thyroid: a clinicopathologic entity. *J Clin Endocrinol* 1959;19:152–161.
129. Keiser HR, Beaven MA, Doppeman J, et al. Sipple's syndrome: medullary thyroid carcinoma, pheochromocytoma and parathyroid disease. *Ann Intern Med* 1973;75:561–579.
130. Glassford GH, Fowler EF, Cole WH. Treatment of nontoxic goiter with desiccated thyroid: results and evaluation. *Surgery* 1965;58:621–625.
131. Utiger R. Radioimmunoassay of human plasma thyrotropin. *J Clin Invest* 1965;44:1277–1286.
132. Ingbar SH, Braverman LE, Dawber NA, et al. New method for measuring free thyroid hormone in human serum and analysis of factors that influence its concentration. *J Clin Invest* 1965;44:1679–1689.
133. Hadden DR, Montgomery DAD, Shanks RG, et al. Propranolol and iodine-131 in management of thyrotoxicosis. *Lancet* 1968;2:852–854.
134. Buckle RM. Treatment of thyroid crisis by beta-adrenergic blockade. *Acta Endocrinol* 1968;57:168–176.
135. McKenzie JM. Experimental production of thyroid stimulating antithyroid antibody. *Endocrinology* 1968;83:877–884.
136. Ross F, Nusynowitz ML. Syndrome of primary hypothyroidism, ammenorrhea and galactorrhea. *J Clin Endocrinol* 1968;28:591–595.
137. Chopra J, Solomon D, Beall GN. Radioimmunoassay for measurement of triiodothyronine in human serum. *Acta Endocrinol* 1971;67:793–800.
138. Hollander CS, Shenkman L, Mitsuma T, et al. Hypertriiodothyroninemia as a premonitory sign of thyrotoxicosis. *Lancet* 1971;2:731–732.
139. Spaulding S, Burrow GW. Several adenosine 3′,5′-monophosphate dependent protein kinases in the thyroid. *Endocrinology* 1972;91:1343–1349.
140. Hershman JM. Hyperthyroidism induced by trophoblastic thyrotrophin. *Mayo Clin Proc* 1972;47:913–918.
141. Blum M, Goldman AB, Herskovic A, et al. Clinical applications of thyroid echography. *N Engl J Med* 1972;287:1164–1169.
142. Werner SC, Coleman DJ, Franzen LA. Ultrasonic evidence of consistent orbital involvement in Graves' disease. *N Engl J Med* 1974;290:1447–1450.
143. De Groot LJ, Torresani J. Triiodothyronine binding to isolated liver cell nuclei. *Endocrinology* 1975;96:357–369.
144. Chopra IJ, Chopra V, Smith S, et al. Reciprocal changes in serum concentration of 3,3′,5′-triiodothyronine (reverse T-3) and 3,3′,5-triiodothyronine (T-3) in systemic illness. *J Clin Endocrinol Metab* 1975;41:1043–1049.
145. Dussault JH, Leberge C. A new method for detection of hypothyroidism in the newborn. *Clin Res* 1972;20:918.
146. Klein AH, Agustin AV, Foley TP. Successful laboratory screening for congenital hypothyroidism. *Lancet* 1974;2:77–79.
147. McKenzie JM. Thyroid stimulating antibody in Graves' disease. *Thyroid Today* 1980;3(5).
148. Ravin JG, Sisson JC, Knapp WT. Orbital radiation for ocular changes of Graves' disease. *Am J Ophthalmol* 1975;79:285–288.
149. Gluck FB, Nusynowitz ML, Plymate S. Chronic lymphocytic thyroiditis, thyrotoxicosis, and low radioactive iodine uptake. *N Engl J Med* 1975;293:624–628.
150. Papapetrou P, Jackson I. Thyrotoxicosis due to silent thyroiditis. *Lancet* 1975;1:361–363.
151. Amino N, Miya K, Takuma T, et al. Transient hypothyroidism after delivery in autoimmune thyroiditis. *J Clin Endocrinol* 1976;42:296.
152. Gershengorn MG, Weintraub BD. Thyrotropin-induced hyperthyroidism caused by selective pituitary resistance to thyroid hormone: new syndrome of "inappropriate" secretion of TSH. *J Clin Invest* 1975;56:633–642.
153. Refetoff S, DeWind LT, DeGroot LJ. Familial syndrome combining deaf mutism, stippled epiphysis, goiter, and abnormally high PBI: possible target organ refractoriness to thyroid hormone. *J Clin Endocrinol Metab* 1967;27:279.
154. Hamilton CR, Adams LC, Maloof F. Hyperthyroidism due to thyrotropin producing pituitary chromophobe adenoma. *N Engl J Med* 1970;283:1077.
155. Van Herle AJ, Young RT, Fisher D, et al. Intrauterine treatment of hypothyroid fetus. *J Clin Endocrinol Metab* 1975;40:474–477.
156. Van Herle AJ, Uller RP. Elevated serum thyroglobulin: marker of metastases in differentiated thyroid carcinomas. *J Clin Invest* 1975;56:272–277.
157. LoGerfo P, Stillman T, Colaccio D, et al. Serum thyroglobulin and recurrent thyroid cancer. *Lancet* 1977;1:881–882.
158. Werner SC. *The thyroid—a fundamental and clinical text*. New York: Paul Hoeber, 1955;378.
159. Galvan G, Pohl GB, Skerbisch I. Die Feinnaelpunktion Kalter Strumaknoten bei 4555 Patienten eines Strumaendemiegebiets. *Schweiz Med Wochenschr* 1976;106:1247–1251.
160. Miller JM, Hamburger JI, Kini S. Diagnosis of thyroid nodules. *JAMA* 1979;241:481–484.
161. Walfish PG, Hazani E, Strawbridge HTG. Combined ultrasound and needle aspiration cytology in the assessment and management of hypofunctioning thyroid nodule. *Ann Intern Med* 1977;87:270–274.
162. Gershengorn MC, McClung MR, Chu EW, et al. Fine needle aspiration cytology in the preoperative diagnosis of thyroid nodules. *Ann Intern Med* 1977;8:265–269.
163. Youngblood WW, Humm J, Lipton MA, et al. Thyrotropin-releasing hormone like bioactivity in placenta. *Endocrinology* 1980;106:541–546.
164. Spitz IM, LeRoith D, Herschit, et al. Increased high-molecular weight thyrotropin with impaired biologic activity in a euthyroid man. *N Engl J Med* 1981;304:278–282.
165. Drexhage HA, Bottazzo GF, Bitensky L, et al. Thyroid growth-blocking antibodies in primary myxedema. *Nature* 1981;289:594–596.
165a. Zakarija M, McKenzie JM: Editorial—do thyroid growth promoting immunoglobulins exist? *J Clin Endocrinol Metab* 1990;70:308–310.
166. Okita N, Row VV, Volpe R. Suppressor T lymphocyte deficiency in Graves' disease and Hashimoto's thyroiditis. *J Clin Endocrinol Metab* 1981;52:528–533.
167. Docter R, Bos G, Krenning EP. Inherited thyroxine excess: a serum abnormality due to an increased affinity for modified albumin. *Clin Endocrinol* 1981;15:363–371.
168. Rajatanavin RR, Young RA, Taylor C, et al. Familial dysalbuminemic hyperthyroxinemia: a syndrome that can be confused with thyrotoxicosis. *N Engl J Med* 1982;306:635–639.
169. Moses AC, Lawlor J, Haddow J, et al. Familial euthyroid hyperthyroxinemia resulting from increased thyroxine binding to thyroxine binding prealbumin. *N Engl J Med* 1982;306:966–969.
170. Jansen M, Krenning EP, Oostdyk W, et al. Hyperthyroxinemia due to decreased peripheral triiodothyronine production. *Lancet* 1982;2:849–851.
171. Dickstein G, Amikam S, Riss E, et al. Thyrotoxicosis induced by amiodarone, a new efficient antiarrhythmic drug with high iodine content. *Am J Med Sci* 1984;288:14–17.
172. Atkinson S, Holcombe M, Kendall-Taylor P. Ophthalmopathic immunoglobulin in patients with Graves' ophthalmopathy. *Lancet* 1984;2:374–376.
173. Weetman AP, Ludgate M, Mills PV, et al. Cyclosporin improves Graves' exophthalmopathy. *Lancet* 1983;2:486.

174. Rendell M, Salmon D. "Chemical hyperthyroidism": the significance of elevated serum thyroxine levels in L-thyroxine treated individuals. *Clin Endocrinol* 1985;22:693–700.
175. van der Gaag RD, Drexhage HA, Wiersenga WM, et al. Further studies on thyroid growth-stimulating immunoglobulins in euthyroid nonendemic goiter. *J Clin Endocrinol Metab* 1985;60:972.
176. Zakarija M, McKenzie JM. The spectrum and significance of autoantibodies reacting with the thyrotropin receptor. *Endocrinol Metab Clin North Am* 1987;16:343–363.
177. Etttinger B, Wingerd J. Thyroid supplements: effect on bone mass. *West J Med* 1982;136:473–476.
178. Krolner B, Vesterdal-Jorgenson J, Pors NS. Spinal bone mineral content in myxedema and thyrotoxicosis: effect of thyroid hormones and antithyroid treatment. *Clin Endocrinol* 1983;18:439–446.
179. Coindre JM, David JP, Revere L, et al. Bone loss in hyperthyroidism with hormone replacement: a histometric study. *Arch Intern Med* 1986;146:48–53.
180. Spencer CA. Clinical utility of sensitive TSH assays. *Thyroid Today* 1986;ix(2).
181. Bayer MF, Kriss JP, McDougall IR. Clinical experience with sensitive thyrotropin measurements: diagnostic and therapeutic implications. *J Nucl Med* 1985;26:1248–1256.
182. Endocrine Society. Thyrotropin molecular biology: update 1994. In: Shupnik MA, Ridgway EC, Chin WW. Braverman LE, Refetoff S, eds. *Endocrine reviews monographs. 3. Clinical and molecular aspects of diseases of the thyroid.* 1994;1:18–22.
183. Gesundheit N, Petrick PA, Nissim M, Dahlberg PA, Doppman JL, Emerson CH, Braverman LE, Oldfield EH, Weintraub BD. Thyrotopin-secreting pituitary adenomas: clinical and biochemical heterogeneity. Case reports and follow-up of nine patients. *Ann Intern Med* 1989;111:827–835.
184. Glycoprotein hormone pituitary tumors. In: Jameson JL, Kay TWH, Mazzaferri E, eds. *Advances in endocrinology and metabolism.* 1991; 125–147.
185. Pfaffle RW, DiMattia GE, Parks JS, Brown MR, Wit JM, Jansen M, Van der Nat H, Van den Brande JL, Rosenfeld MG, Ingraham HA. Mutations of the POU-specific domain of Pit-1 and hypopituitarism without pituitary hypoplasia. *Science* 1992;257:1118–1121.
186. Radovick S, Nations M, Du Y, Berg LA, Weintraub BD, Wondisford FE. A mutation in the POU-homeodomain of Pit-1 responsible for combined pituitary hormone deficiency. *Science* 1992;257:1115–1118.
187. Tatsumi K, Miyai K, Notomi T, Kaibe K, Amino N, Mizuno Y. Cretinism with combined hormone deficiency caused by a mutation in the PIT1 gene. *Nat Genet* 1992;1:56–58.
188. Dacou-Voutetakis C, Feltquate DM, Drakopoulou M, Kourides IA, Dracopoli NC. Familial hypothyroidism caused by a nonsense mutation in the thyroid-stimulating hormone beta-subunit gene. *Am J Hum Genet* 1990;46:988–993.
189. Hayashizaki Y, Hiraoka Y, Endo Y, Miyai K, Matsubara K. Thyroid-stimulating hormone (TSH) deficiency caused by a single base substitution in the CAGYC region of the beta-subunit. *EMBO J* 1989; 8:2291–2296.
190. Vassart G, Parma J, van Sande J, et al. The thyrotropin receptor and the regulation of thyrocyte function and growth: update 1994. In: Braverman LE, Refetoff S, eds. *Endocrine reviews monographs. 3. Clinical and molecular aspects of diseases of the thyroid.* The Endocrine Society. 1994;3:77–80.
191. Kopp P, van Sande J, Parma J, Duprez L, Gerber H, Joss E, Jameson Jl, Dumont JE, Vassart G. Brief report: congenital hyperthyroidism caused by a mutation in the thyrotropin-receptor gene. *N Engl J Med* 1995;332:150–154.
192. Parma J, Duprez L, van Sande J, Paschke R, Tonacchera M, Dumont J, Vassart G. Constitutively active receptors as a disease-causing mechanism. *Mol Cell Endocrinol* 1994;100:159–162.
193. Parma J, Duprez L, van Sande J, Cochaux P, Gervy C, Mockel J, Dumont J, Vassart G. Somatic mutations in the thyrotropin receptor gene cause hyperfunctioning thyroid adenomas. *Nature* 1993;365: 649–651.
194. Porcellini A, Ciullo I, Laviola L, Amabile G, Fenzi G, Avvedimento VE. Novel mutations of thyrotropin receptor gene in thyroid hyperfunctioning adenomas. Rapid identification by fine needle aspiration biopsy. *J Clin Endocrinol Metab* 1994;79:657–661.
195. Russo D, Arturi F, Wicker R, Chazenbalk GD, Schlumberger M, DuVillard JA, Caillou B, Monier R, Rapoport B, Filetti S, et al. Genetic alterations in thyroid hyperfunctioning adenomas. *J Clin Endocrinol Metab* 1995;80:1347–1351.
196. Sunthornthepvarakui T, Gottschalk ME, Hayashi Y, Refetoff S. Brief report: resistance to thyrotropin caused by mutations in the thyrotropin-receptor gene. *N Engl J Med* 1995;332:155–160.
197. Medeiros-Neto G, Targovnik HM, Vassart G. Defective thyroglobulin synthesis and secretion causing goiter and hypothyroidism. *Endocr Rev* 1993;14:165–183.
198. Abramowicz MJ, Targovnik HM, Varela V, Cochaux P, Krawiec L, Pisarev MA, Propato FV, Juvenal G, Chester HA, Vassart G. Identification of a mutation in the coding sequence of the human thyroid peroxidase gene causing congenital goiter. *J Clin Invest* 1992;90: 1200–1204.
199. Refetoff S, Nicoloff JT. Thyroid hormone transport and metabolism. In: DeGroot LJ, ed. *Endocrinology.* Philadelphia: WB Saunders, 1995.
200. Bartalen L. Thyroid hormone-binding proteins: update 1994. Braverman LE, Refetoff S, eds. *Endocrine reviews monographs. 3. Clinical and molecular aspects of diseases of the thyroid.* The Endocrine Society. 1994;6:140–142.
201. Refetoff S, Weiss RE, Usala SJ. The syndromes of resistance to thyroid hormone. *Endocr Rev* 1993;14:348–399.

CHAPTER 2

Embryology and Surgical Anatomy of the Lower Neck and Superior Mediastinum

John T. Hansen

EMBRYOLOGY OF THE NECK AND RELATED VISCERA

A thorough understanding of the embryology of the neck and its visceral structures requires an appreciation of the development of the branchial arches and pharyngeal pouches. Development of the branchial arch complex in the human begins around the fourth week of embryonic development. Human embryos have five branchial arches, which correspond to arch numbers 1, 2, 3, 4, and 6 of the primitive vertebrate branchial arches, although many anatomists consider the fusion of arches 4 and 6 as comprising a single fourth arch. The branchial arch apparatus consists of (a) branchial arches, (b) pharyngeal pouches, (c) branchial grooves, and (d) branchial membranes. Each branchial arch consists of mesoderm derived from the paraxial mesoderm of somitomeres or occipital somites and is covered externally by ectoderm and internally by endoderm. Migration of ectodermally derived neural crest cells into the branchial arches results in discrete swellings, which demarcate each arch.

Therefore, externally the branchial region is characterized by the appearance of a distinctive branchial groove separating intervening branchial arches on the ventrolateral aspect of the neck. Internally, each arch contains an outpocketing of the primitive foregut endoderm, referred to as a pharyngeal pouch (Fig. 1). The neural crest cells, which initiate branchial arch formation, are unique in that, despite their ectodermal origin, they are a major contributor to the mesenchyme in the embryonic head.

Mesenchymal condensations consisting of neural crest–derived ectomesenchyme form the cartilaginous precursors to some of the bony derivatives of the first and second branchial arches, whereas the bony and cartilaginous derivatives of the third and fourth arches arise from lateral plate mesoderm. The mesoderm of each branchial arch contributes to the muscles of mastication and facial expression, several other muscles innervated by the trigeminal nerve, one muscle innervated by the glossopharyngeal nerve, and all of the muscles of the pharynx and larynx innervated by the vagus nerve. Moreover, each arch is associated sometime during its development with one of the aortic arches and with the development of the visceral derivatives of the pharyngeal pouches.

Infrahyoid Muscles

As embryonic development in the neck continues, the derivatives of the branchial arch system become covered anteriorly by several pairs of "strap" muscles, or infrahyoid muscles, derived from the somites of the cervical region. These somites are segmentally innervated by the ansa cervicalis of the cervical plexus (ventral primary rami of spinal nerves C1 to C4). The infrahyoid muscles are not direct derivatives of the branchial arch musculature but originate from the cervical somites and migrate around the neck, forming attachments to the hyoid bone and thyroid cartilage, or sternum.

Thyroid Gland

The thyroid gland begins its development during the fourth embryonic week, and is the first endocrine gland to appear in the human embryo. The thyroid anlage be-

---

J. T. Hansen: Department of Neurobiology and Anatomy, University of Rochester School of Medicine and Dentistry, Rochester, New York 14642.

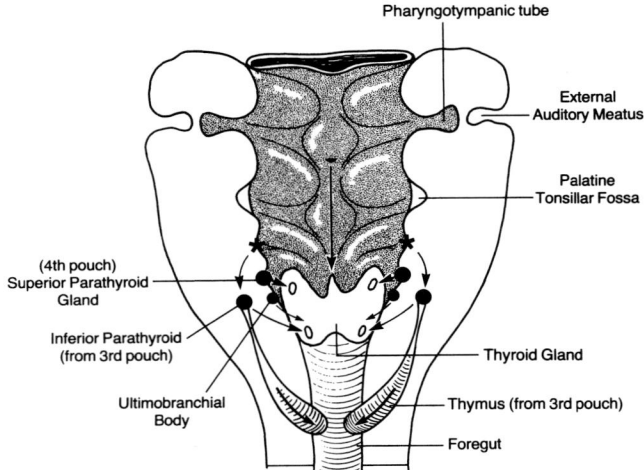

FIG. 1. Schematic representation of the pharyngeal pouch derivatives, showing the migration of the thyroid, parathyroid, and thymus glands. As the thyroid gland descends from the foramen cecum, the parathyroid glands attach themselves to the passing thyroid. (Redrawn, with permission, from ref. 19.)

gins as a thickened median endodermal derivative just caudal to the future site of the median tongue bud (see Fig. 1). As the embryo elongates and undergoes differential growth, the thyroid diverticulum migrates anteriorly and inferiorly to the hyoid bone and laryngeal cartilages, tethered by a slender thyroglossal duct (Fig. 2).

The thyroglossal duct normally breaks down by the end of the fifth week and the thyroid gland continues its downward migration. By the seventh week of embryonic development, the thyroid diverticulum has assumed its adult position anterior to the trachea. This diverticulum forms a bilobed gland, with the two lobes connected by a small isthmus. Often a small amount of thyroid tissue extends superiorly from the isthmus and is known as the pyramidal lobe. This pyramidal lobe is present in about 50% of all humans and more commonly is associated with the left side of the isthmus. Aberrant thyroid tissue may be found anywhere along its migratory pathway, but most often it is found just posterior to the foramen cecum of the tongue (lingual thyroids).

Parathyroid Glands

The parathyroid glands develop directly from the pharyngeal pouch system (see Fig. 1). Paired inferior parathyroid glands develop from the third pair of pharyngeal pouches in concert with the thymus anlage. Thymic development begins near the end of the fourth week, and the inferior parathyroids form early in the fifth week. Together, the inferior parathyroid glands and thymus migrate inferiorly during elongation and differential growth of the neck region. Normally, the inferior parathyroid glands separate from the thymus tissue and migrate medially to assume their adult position posteriorly and inferiorly on the lateral lobes of the thyroid gland. The superior parathyroid glands actually develop somewhat inferior to the inferior parathyroids, as derivatives of the fourth pair of pharyngeal pouches. However, the superior parathyroid glands migrate only a short distance inferiorly and then become attached to the thyroid diverticulum as it migrates inferiorly anterior to the trachea. The superior parathyroid glands come to rest posteriorly and superiorly behind the lateral lobes of the thyroid gland. Because the migratory route of the inferior parathyroid glands is longer and its migration is associated with that of the thymus gland, the inferior parathyroid glands often are found anywhere along the normal migratory route of the thymus gland, and they may even follow the thymus into the superior mediastinum (see later).

Ultimobranchial Body Formation

Just caudal to the development of the superior parathyroids from the fourth pharyngeal pouch, small invaginations appear that become the rudiments of the ultimobranchial bodies. Late during the fifth week of development, these rudiments detach from the pharyngeal wall and become embedded in the posterior aspect of the thyroid gland as it migrates inferiorly to its definitive location. Once in the thyroid gland, the ultimobranchial cells differentiate into the C cells (parafollicular cells), which produce calcitonin.

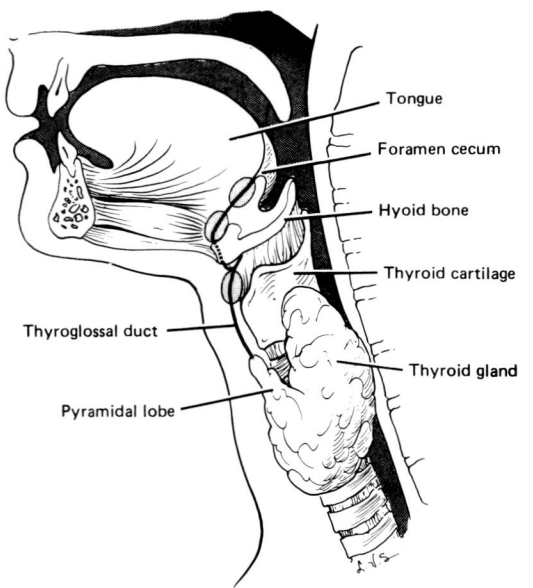

FIG. 2. Sagittal view showing descent of the thyroid gland from the foramen cecum. The course of the thyroglossal duct is also indicated. (Reproduced, with permission, from ref. 20.)

FASCIAL COMPARTMENTS IN THE NECK

The fascial layers of the neck below the level of the hyoid bone consist of a layer of superficial fascia and three distinct layers of deep fascia (Fig. 3). The superficial fascia includes the subcutaneous tissue and its associated fat and, in the case of the head and neck, the muscles of facial expression.

In the neck, this superficial fascia envelops the platysma muscle. Deep to the superficial fascia is the deep cervical fascia, which is thicker and is divided anatomically into three layers: the superficial or investing layer, the pretracheal layer, and the prevertebral layers. A fourth fascial compartment also exists in the neck and includes the carotid sheaths, which are formed by condensations of the adjacent fascial layers.

Superficial Fascia

In the neck, the superficial fascia includes the subcutaneous tissue, associated fat, and the platysma muscle. This fascial layer is continuous with the superficial fascia over the clavicle, and it extends to the deltoid and pectoral regions. The superficial fascia also extends posteriorly to the midline. The superficial fascia is thin anteriorly on the neck but becomes much thicker and fibrous on the back of the neck.

Deep Fascia: Superficial (Anterior or Investing) Layer

The superficial layer of the deep fascia completely invests the neck like a nylon stocking. This fascial layer attaches posteriorly to the ligamentum nuchae and spinous processes of the cervical vertebrae, and extends anteriorly around the neck to invest both the trapezius and sternocleidomastoid muscles (see Fig. 3). This fascial sleeve meets the fascial layer from the other side in the anterior midline by passing in front of the strap (infrahyoid) muscles. Superiorly, the superficial layer of deep cervical fascia attaches to the hyoid bone and inferior border of the mandible, and inferiorly it attaches to the sternum, clavicle, acromion, and spine of the scapula. Just above its attachment to the sternum, the superficial layer of fascia splits into an anterior and a posterior lamina, which attach to the anterior and posterior aspects of the sternum. The space between these two lamina is the suprasternal space (of Burns). Although the external and anterior jugular veins may appear to lie in the subcutaneous superficial fascia, in reality they lie in the superficial sheet of this investing layer of the deep cervical fascia. If possible, the anterior jugular veins should be avoided when incising this fascial layer, although this may be difficult when the veins lie in the midline.

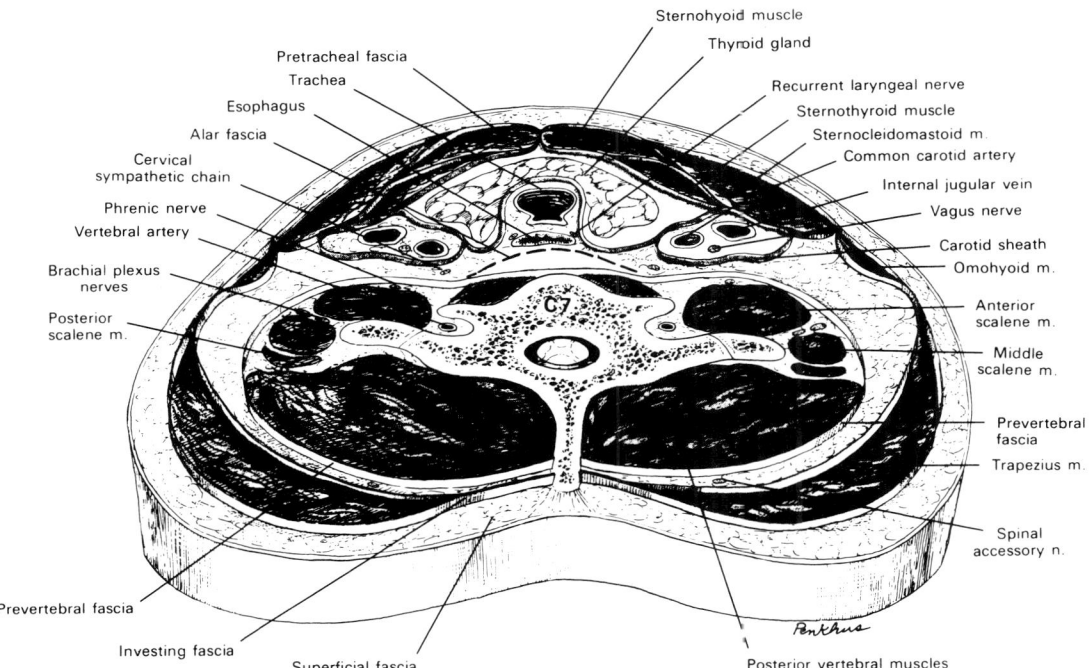

FIG. 3. Cross section of the neck at the level of the seventh cervical vertebra. Note the superficial fascia and the layers of the deep cervical fascia, which include the investing, pretracheal and prevertebral layers. m, muscle; n, nerve. (Reproduced, with permission, from ref. 3.)

Deep Fascia: Pretracheal (Middle) Layer

This thin, delicate fascial layer passes anterior to the thyroid gland and trachea (hence its name pretracheal), but posterior to the strap muscles (see Fig. 3). It extends superiorly along with the infrahyoid muscles to its attachment to the thyroid cartilage and hyoid bone. Inferiorly, the pretracheal fascia passes behind the manubrium of the sternum and becomes continuous with the fibrous pericardium over the great vessels emanating from the heart. Laterally, the pretracheal fascia is continuous with the anterior portion of the carotid sheaths. At the level of the thyroid gland, the pretracheal fascia splits to envelop the gland, thus contributing to its capsule. The vessels supplying the thyroid gland lie deep to the pretracheal fascial layer.

Deep Fascia: Prevertebral (Posterior) Layer

The prevertebral layer of the deep cervical fascia begins at the spinous processes of the cervical vertebrae and ligamentum nuchae, invests the posterior vertebral muscles (e.g., splenius capitis, cervicis), the lateral vertebral muscles (scalene muscles and levator scapulae), and the anterior vertebral muscles (e.g., longus colli, capitis). This fascial layer passes posterior to the esophagus and trachea, and just anterior to the vertebral column (see Fig. 3). Laterally, the prevertebral layer of fascia extends to form the posterior aspect of the carotid sheath. Where the prevertebral fascia lies behind the esophagus and trachea it is often referred to as the retrovisceral fascia. However, the retrovisceral fascia is really two layers, a posterior lamina (the true prevertebral fascia) and the alar fascia.

Superiorly, the prevertebral fascia extends to the base of the skull and inferiorly courses to the superior mediastinum. In the superior mediastinum, the prevertebral fascia divides into a posterior layer, which becomes continuous with the anterior longitudinal ligament on the vertebral bodies, and an anterior layer, which blends with the posterior surface of the esophagus at about the level of the sternal angle. Further laterally, the prevertebral fascia forms the axillary sheath, which encloses the axillary vessels and brachial plexus.

Carotid Sheaths

The carotid sheaths envelop the internal jugular vein, common carotid artery, and vagus nerve. These fascial sheaths lie between the pretracheal and prevertebral fascial layers. Anteriorly, the carotid sheath is fused with the superficial or investing layer of the deep cervical fascia. Anteriomedially, the carotid sheath is fused with the pretracheal fascia, and posteriorly with the prevertebral fascia.

MUSCLES OF THE ANTERIOR NECK

Infrahyoid Muscles

The infrahyoid or strap muscles of the neck include four pairs of muscles that attach to the hyoid bone and thyroid cartilage. Together, these muscles form the floor of the muscular triangle and include the sternohyoid, sternothyroid, thyrohyoid, and omohyoid muscles (Fig. 4). These muscles are invested by the superficial (investing) fascia of the deep cervical fascia and covered more anteriorly by the superficial cervical fascia, or subcutaneous tissue, which also contains the platysma. Retraction of the sternohyoid and sternothyroid muscles reveals the underlying thyroid gland and trachea. Lateral and superficial to the sternothyroid muscle, one sees the superior belly of the omohyoid (Gr. *omos,* shoulder) muscle. Deep to the omohyoid's attachment to the hyoid bone lies the thyrohyoid muscle. All four pairs of infrahyoid muscles are innervated by muscular branches from the ansa cervicalis (ventral rami of C1, C2, C3), with the thyrohyoid nerve innervating the muscle of the same name descending directly off of the hypoglossal nerve.

Occasionally, the sternohyoid and sternothyroid muscles are divided for better surgical exposure to the thyroid gland, especially if the muscles are fused to the underlying gland. Unfortunately, the level at which the muscular nerve branches enter these muscles is not uniform. Hollinshead (1) describes an upper nerve branch that enters the sternohyoid and sternothyroid muscles at the level of the thyroid cartilage, and a second set of muscular branches that enter the same muscles slightly above the level of the jugular (suprasternal) notch. Therefore, bisecting these muscles approximately halfway between the lower border of the thyroid cartilage and the jugular notch should spare the innervation to these muscles. Together, the infrahyoid muscles depress the larynx and hyoid bone after their elevation during swallowing (deglutition).

One final pair of muscles, and more importantly their innervation, deserves attention. These muscles are the paired cricothyroid muscles, which are innervated by the external branch of the superior laryngeal nerve. Functionally, the cricothyroids produce elongation of the vocal folds, thereby creating tension on the folds. This function is accomplished by anteriorly tilting the thyroid cartilage on the cricoid cartilage. These small muscles are innervated by the external laryngeal branch of the superior laryngeal nerve, which usually is found lying medial to the superior thyroid artery coursing in the sternothyroid-laryngeal triangle. However, in about 21% of 400 specimens examined, the external laryngeal nerve was aberrant and found either lying upon the superior thyroid artery or looping through and about its small arterial branches, just superior to the lateral pole of the thyroid gland (2). Injury to this nerve may be associated with voice fatigue (especially in public speakers), inability to reach high-pitched sounds

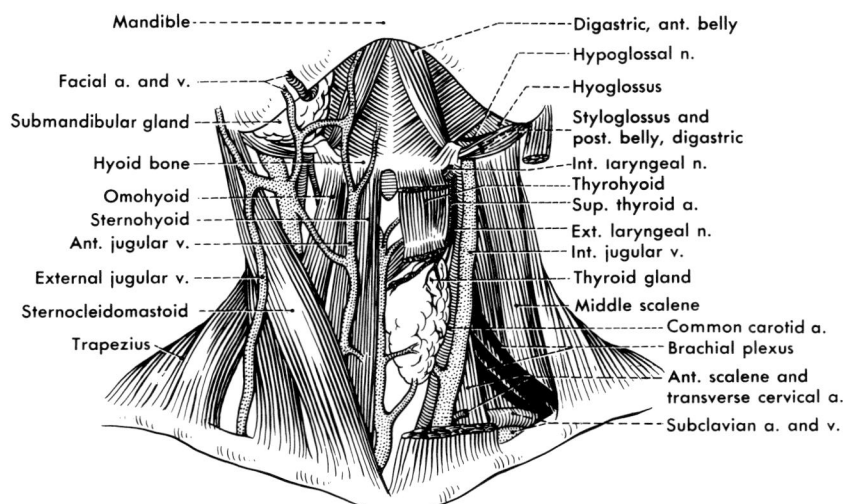

FIG. 4. Anterior view of the neck. On the left side of the neck the sternocleidomastoid and most of the infrahyoid muscles, submandibular gland, and other superficially located structures have been removed. a, artery; n, nerve; v, vein. (Reproduced, with permission, from ref. 1.)

(especially in professional singers), postdeglutition cough, choking, or aspiration pneumonitis (2). This small "spider web–like" nerve may be especially vulnerable if the lateral lobes of the thyroid gland are enlarged and extend superiorly toward the superior thyroid vessels.

Blood Supply

The blood supply to the infrahyoid muscles is principally by muscular branches of the inferior thyroid artery. This artery also supplies blood to some of the deeper prevertebral muscles. The ascending cervical branch of the inferior thyroid artery also supplies blood to the muscles in the neck. Muscular branches from the superior thyroid artery supply the superior aspects of the strap muscles, especially the sternohyoid, sternothyroid, and superior belly of the omohyoid muscle.

The venous drainage of the strap muscles is via tributaries of the external jugular and internal jugular veins (see Fig. 4). Variations in this venous system are common (axiom: veins are variable). The anterior surface of the infrahyoid muscles usually is drained largely by the anterior jugular vein and its tributaries. These veins ultimately converge superior to the sternal notch and drain into the jugular venous arch, which then flows into the terminal portion of the external jugular vein or subclavian veins. Small venous tributaries of the superior, middle, and inferior thyroid veins also may drain blood from the infrahyoid muscles.

THYROID GLAND

The thyroid gland consists of right and left (lateral) lobes, connected in the middle by a narrow isthmus (Fig. 5). Often, the isthmus exhibits a conical lobe, the pyramidal lobe, that may ascend as high as the hyoid bone (Figs. 5,6). When present (about 50% of the time), the pyramidal lobe demarcates the midline migratory route of the thyroid gland (see Fig. 2), and it is associated more often with the left side of the isthmus. Occasionally, a fibrous or muscular band is attached to the pyramidal lobe and, when present, is termed the levator glandulae thyroideae. Small accessory thyroid glands may be present either above the lateral lobes or the isthmus. The human thyroid gland is variable in size. It normally weighs 20 to 30 g, is somewhat larger in women, and may become enlarged during pregnancy (3).

Normally, the lateral lobes of the thyroid gland are conical in shape, with the apex of the cone extending rostrally. Each lobe is approximately 5 cm in length and may extend inferiorly as far as the fifth or sixth tracheal rings. The most posterior extension of the lateral lobes of the gland, which lie at the level of Berry's ligament, are termed the tubercles of Zuckerkandl and are important for their relationship to the recurrent laryngeal nerves (see later) (4). The isthmus of the gland connects the caudal two thirds of the lateral lobes and usually measures about 1.25 cm in breadth, lying just anterior to the second and third tracheal rings. The lateral lobes lie along the lateral aspect of the larynx, reaching the level of the middle of the thyroid cartilage (see Fig. 5). The thyroid gland is encased within a fibrous capsule derived from the pretracheal (middle) layer of the deep cervical fascia. The origin of the thyroid gland's capsule is controversial and has been variously referred to as the pretracheal fascia, perithyroid sheath, thyroid fascia, and false thyroid capsule (1). Apparently, there is no clear agreement in the literature as to what actually constitutes the thyroid fascia. However, the fascia surrounding the thyroid gland should not be confused with the true connective tissue capsule of the gland, which is the term appropriately reserved for the connective tissue surrounding the surface of the gland and sending septa between the various lobes of the gland. Using this ter-

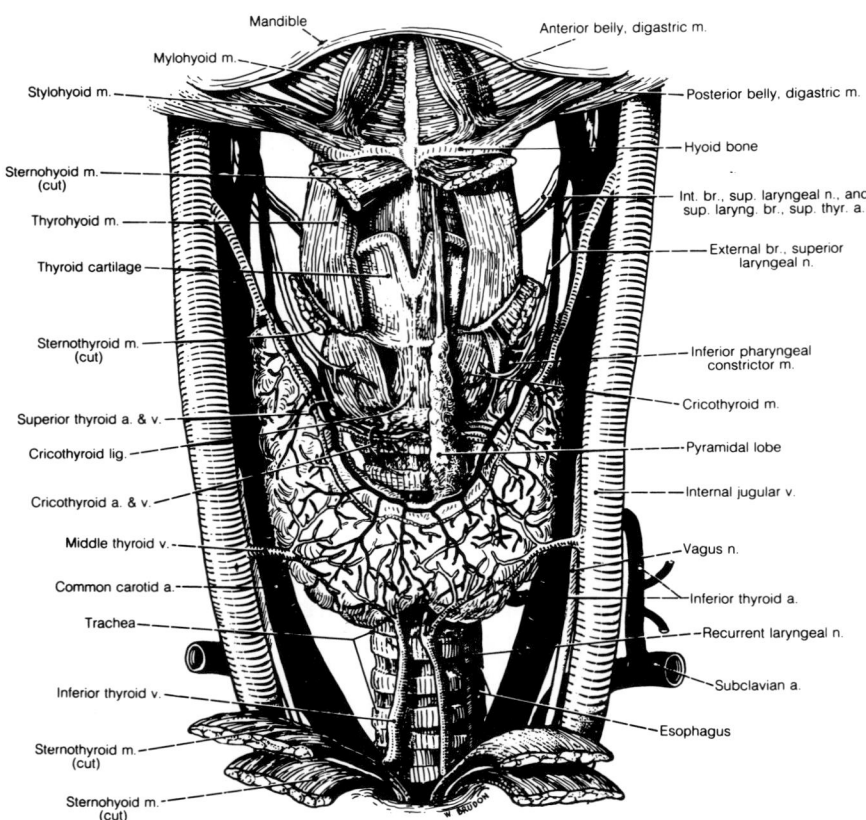

FIG. 5. Arterial supply, venous drainage, and innervation of the thyroid gland and adjacent structures. Muscles have been reflected. a, artery; m, muscle; n, nerve; v, vein. (Reproduced, with permission, from ref. 21.)

minology, Hollinshead (1) refers to the capsule as an "integral" part of the gland, inseparable from the parenchyma except by sharp dissection. The pretracheal fascia anteriorly extends above the isthmus and invests the pyramidal lobe if present (anterior suspensory ligament) (4). This anterior fascial extension also envelops a group of lymph nodes termed the Delphian lymph nodes (part of the anterior cervical lymph nodes).

Variations

Variations commonly associated with the thyroid gland are related to its development. These variations include small "ectopic" accessory glands associated with the migratory route of the gland from the foramen cecum at the base of the tongue, or they consist of cysts or fistulae that result from remnants of the thyroglossal duct (see Fig. 2). A lingual thyroid may persist near the origin of the gland anlage from the foramen cecum, but the number of reports is infrequent (1 case in 3000) (5).

Suprahyoid, infrahyoid, and prethyroid accessory glands may lie all along the normal migratory route of the thyroid anlage. Rarely, thyroid tissue may migrate inferiorly to a retrosternal position in the superior mediastinum adjacent to the great vessels. When present, the muscular slip of the levator glandulae thyroideae is observed descending from the pharynx or hyoid bone. This anomalous slip of tissue frequently occurs on the left side, and its embryonic derivation is problematic. Eisler (6) categorizes the levator of the thyroid gland into one of three groups: (a) anterior levators derived from the cricothyroid muscle and innervated by the external branch of the superior laryngeal nerve; (b) lateral levators derived from the thyrohyoid muscle (or the infrahyoid group of muscles together) and innervated by a branch from the ansa cervicalis; or (c) posterior levators derived from the inferior constrictor of the pharynx and innervated, like the anterior ones, by the superior laryngeal nerve.

Blood Supply

The thyroid gland has an extremely rich blood supply, in fact, one of the richest in the body considering its size. It is supplied by four main arteries, the paired superior and the paired inferior thyroid arteries (see Figs. 5,8). The superior thyroid arteries may originate from the uppermost portion of the common carotid artery or, more commonly, as the first or second branch of the external carotid artery. The superior thyroid artery lies close to the external branch of the superior laryngeal nerve as they both descend into the neck. Because of the artery's close association with this nerve, clamping of the superior thyroid artery may damage

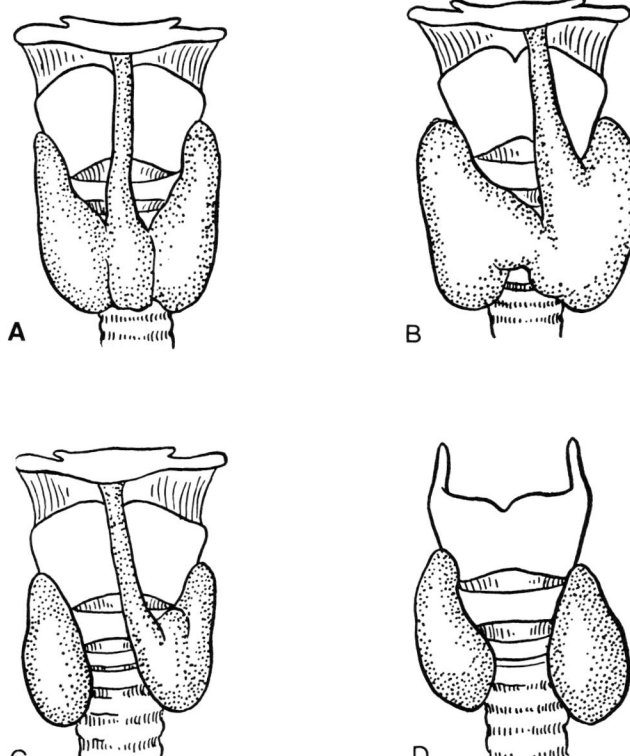

FIG. 6. Several unusual forms of the thyroid gland. A, B, and C all have large pyramidal lobes that extend to the hyoid bone. In B and C the lobe is asymmetrically attached to the thyroid gland. In C and D, the isthmus is lacking. (Reproduced, with permission, from ref. 1.)

the nerve if the latter is not first recognized. Consistent branches of the superior thyroid artery include a small infrahyoid branch, a branch to the sternocleidomastoid muscle, a superior laryngeal artery that accompanies the internal branch of the superior laryngeal into the thyrohyoid membrane, and a cricothyroid branch. As the superior thyroid arteries approach the thyroid gland, the arteries divide into anterior and posterior branches, which then distribute numerous small branches to the gland and anastomose with their counterparts from the opposite side.

The inferior thyroid arteries are more variable and may even be absent on one side in about 0.2% to 6% of cases (7,8). An absence occurs more frequently on the left side. Normally, the inferior thyroid artery arises from the thyrocervical trunk (quite variable) and ascends into the neck on the medial aspect of the anterior scalene muscle, deep to the prevertebral fascia. The artery then loops medially and downward to the anterior surface of the longus colli muscle, penetrates the prevertebral fascia, and crosses the vertically ascending recurrent laryngeal nerve (Fig. 7, and see Fig. 11). Typically, the inferior thyroid artery divides into two branches: an upper branch to the posterior aspect of the gland and a lower branch to the lower pole of the gland. Anastomoses across the midline as well as between the inferior and superior thyroid arteries are common. Additional blood supply to the thyroid gland may occur from smaller arteries including the ascending cervical artery, tracheal, pharyngeal, and esophageal branches, and the inferior laryngeal artery that accompanies the recurrent laryngeal nerve (1).

In 1.5% to 12.2% of the cases, a thyroid ima artery may be present (7). When present, this artery arises most commonly on the right side and ascends in front of the trachea (hence its importance in tracheostomy). It may be thought of as an "aberrant" inferior thyroid artery. The origin of the thyroid ima artery is variable; most commonly it arises either from the brachiocephalic, right common carotid, or directly from the aortic arch. Rarely, the artery may arise from the internal thoracic (mammary) artery. The thyroid ima artery may be only a small twig, or it may be large enough to replace the inferior thyroid artery (1).

Two or three large pairs of veins drain the thyroid gland (Fig. 8, and see Fig. 5). These veins anastomose freely within the gland parenchyma. The superior thyroid vein emerges from the upper pole of the gland, accompanies the superior thyroid artery, and typically empties into the internal jugular vein or common facial vein at about the level of carotid bifurcation. The middle thyroid vein is variable in both size and occurrence. Middle thyroid veins are found in slightly more than 50% of the bodies examined and arise from the lateral side of the gland, cross the common carotid artery anteriorly, and usually drain into the internal jugular vein (9). The inferior thyroid veins form two trunks that emerge from the lower portion of the gland. The right trunk passes anterior to the brachiocephalic artery and drains into the right brachiocephalic vein. The left trunk drains in front of the trachea into the left brachiocephalic vein (see Fig. 8). Frequently, the right and left inferior thyroid veins may join and drain by a common stem (thyroid ima vein) into the left brachiocephalic vein. Anastomoses between the inferior thyroid veins are common and often form a plexus of veins in front of the trachea (plexus thyroideus impar) (1). When present, this plexus may be a source of bleeding in a tracheostomy.

PARATHYROID GLANDS

Typically, humans possess two pairs of parathyroid glands, a superior pair and an inferior pair (see Fig. 7). But a recent surgical study of 503 autopsy cases demonstrated that four parathyroid glands were found in only 84% of the cases (Fig. 9) (10). More than four glands were found in 13% of the cases, and only three parathyroids were identified in 3%. In the 13% in which more than four glands were found, most were either rudimentary or divided (two split glands lying close to one another). Of the 64 cases with more than four glands, 18 cases had five glands, 3 had six, 1 had seven, 1 had eight, and 1 had eleven parathyroid glands.

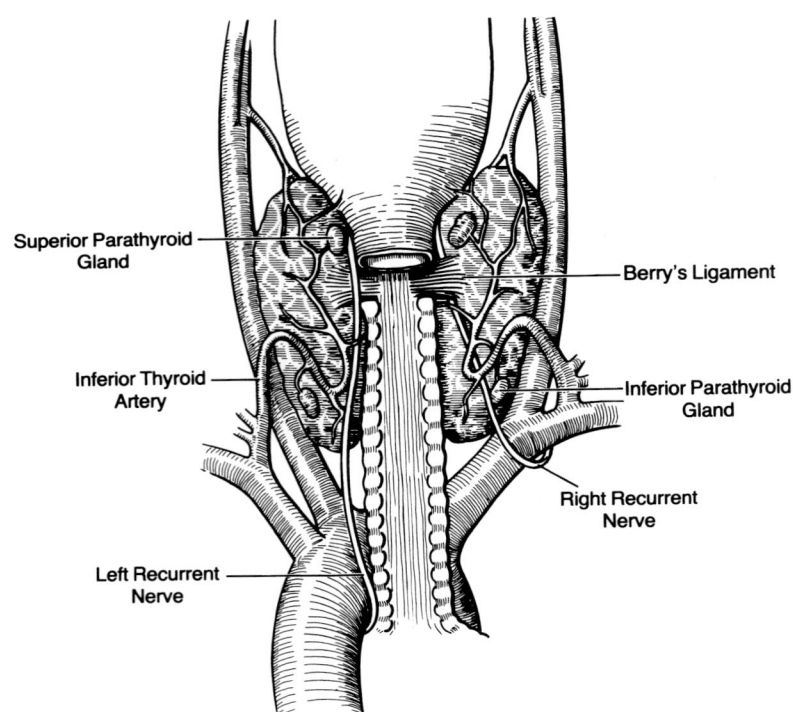

FIG. 7. Common positions of the parathyroid glands on the posterior aspect of the thyroid gland. Note the blood supply to the thyroid and parathyroid glands. On the right side, the recurrent laryngeal nerve is shown passing anterior to the inferior thyroid artery and Berry's ligament. On the left side, the recurrent nerve passes posterior to both structures. This pattern is variable (see text). (Redrawn, with permission, from ref. 13.)

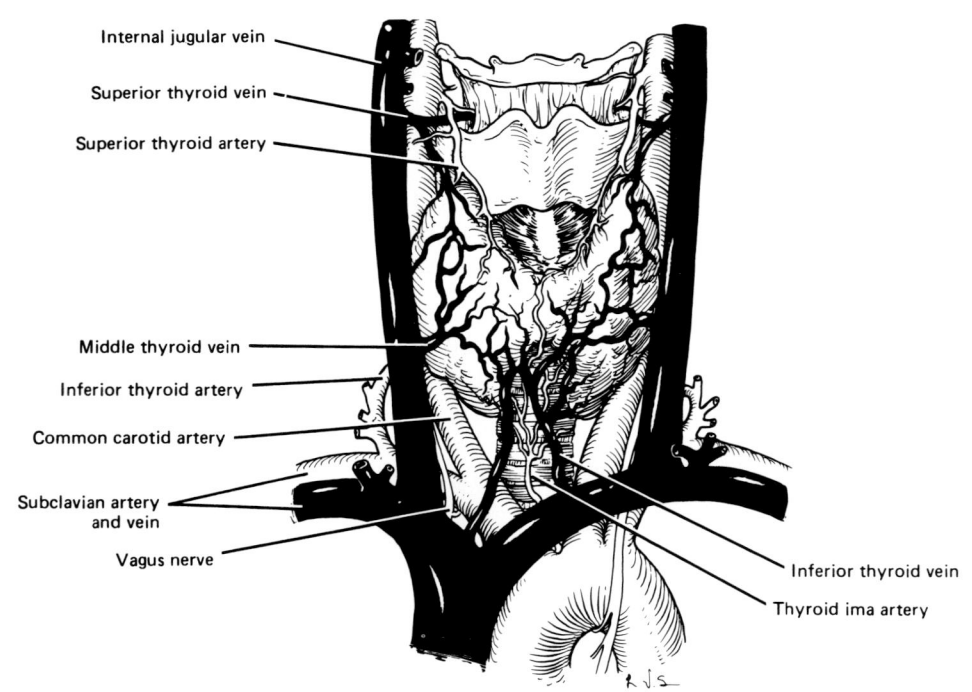

FIG. 8. Arterial supply and venous drainage of the thyroid gland. (Reproduced, with permission, from ref. 20.)

Anatomically, the superior parathyroid glands are the most consistent. About 80% lie within a circumscribed circle approximately 2 cm in diameter, 1 cm superior to the intersection of the recurrent laryngeal nerve and the inferior thyroid artery (10). The superior parathyroid glands often lie within the fascial covering of the thyroid gland and are freely movable upon the thyroid capsule (note the distinction between the fascia covering the thyroid gland and the thyroid capsule). Occasionally, the parathyroids lie within the thyroid capsule itself. On the other hand, the inferior parathyroid glands, because of their embryologic migration with the thymus anlage (see Fig. 1), are significantly more variable in their anatomic location (see Fig. 9). About 61% of the inferior parathyroid glands are located either inferior, lateral, or posterior to the lower pole of the thyroid gland (10). Commonly, inferior parathyroids are found in the thyrothymic ligament, a fibrous band of connective tissue that connects the lower thyroid pole and the upper thymic horn (10a). In approximately 26% of cases, parathyroids also may be found in the cervical portion of the thymus gland. Anywhere from 2% to 4% of the inferior parathyroids are located further inferior, associated with the thymus gland in the superior mediastinum (Figs. 9,10). A number of studies describe varying numbers and anatomic locations for parathyroid tissue, but the reports obtained from cadaveric material should be suspect because of the difficulty in finding parathyroids in previously fixed material (1).

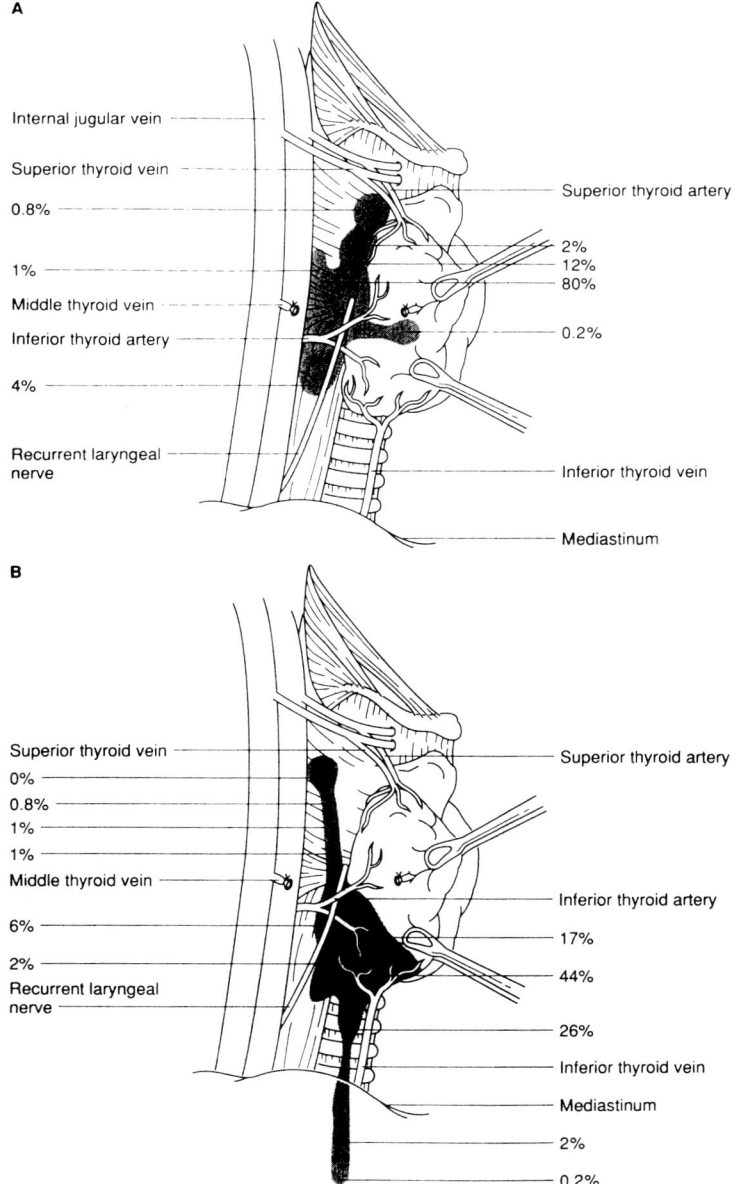

FIG. 9. Sites of normal and aberrant parathyroids. Location of superior parathyroid **(A)** and inferior parathyroid **(B)** glands from 503 autopsy cases. The shaded areas show the most common distribution sites and the numbers are the percentage of the glands found at each site. (Reproduced, with permission, from ref. 10.)

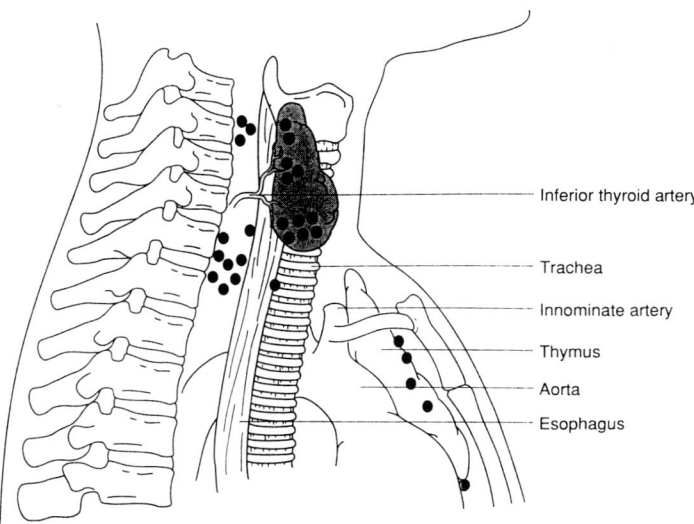

FIG. 10. Sites of parathyroid glands that were missed on initial exploration but identified on subsequent operation. (Reproduced, with permission, from ref. 22.)

In light of the variable positions of the parathyroid glands, especially the inferior pair, their location with respect to the thyroid capsule deserves some attention. Generally speaking, the superior parathyroids lie either within the prevertebral fascia covering the posterior aspect of the thyroid gland or in the true capsule of the gland itself. The inferior parathyroid glands, on the other hand, either lie below the inferior thyroid artery as it lies on the posterior surface of the thyroid gland (i.e., the parathyroids lie anterior to the thyroid fascia), or they lie above the inferior thyroid artery and hence outside the thyroid fascia. Only rarely are inferior parathyroids embedded within the gland itself (11).

Blood Supply

It is generally accepted that the parathyroid glands receive their blood supply from the thyroid arteries, and most frequently the inferior thyroid artery (see Fig. 7). Nevertheless, ligation of the inferior thyroid artery does not always compromise the blood supply to the parathyroid tissue (1). This may be because of the abundant anastomoses that exist between the parathyroids. Anastomoses occur not only with the thyroid arteries but also with the arteries of the larynx, pharynx, esophagus, and trachea. Some surgeons contend that once the parathyroid gland is identified, the blood supply has probably already been compromised. Therefore, many surgeons suggest dissecting the parathyroids with an attached vascular pedicle in an effort to maintain a blood supply (5).

Preservation of the inferior thyroid artery, the major source of blood to the parathyroids, also should be left intact. Attention should be paid to dissecting and ligating the smaller branches of the inferior thyroid artery while leaving the vascular supply to the inferior parathyroids intact. Similarly, the superior parathyroids should be left intact with their vascular pedicle. Dissection around the parathyroids should always proceed with great caution because the parathyroid glands are notoriously fragile and easily injured. Should the blood supply to the parathyroids become compromised, the glands may be resected, minced into several small cubes, and autografted into the sternocleidomastoid muscle or the forearm musculature (5). The venous drainage of the parathyroid glands is unremarkable and occurs via the superior, middle, and inferior thyroid veins.

LARYNGEAL NERVES

The vagus nerves course inferiorly from their exit at the jugular foramen toward the mediastinum and pass inferiorly through the neck in the carotid sheath along with the common carotid artery and the internal jugular vein (see Fig. 5). In addition to several small pharyngeal branches, the cervical vagus nerve gives rise to the superior laryngeal nerve. This nerve passes posterior, or deep, to the internal and external carotid arteries (see Fig. 5). The superior laryngeal nerve often divides high in the neck, usually near the internal carotid artery. The larger internal branch of the superior laryngeal nerve passes inferomedially to enter the larynx by passing through the thyrohyoid membrane. This nerve branch is sensory to the upper portion of the larynx above the level of the vocal folds. The smaller external branch of the superior laryngeal nerve passes deep to the external carotid artery, where it joins the superior thyroid artery as this latter structure descends toward the thyroid gland. This external branch innervates the small cricothyroid muscle (see Fig. 5) and may also send a small branch of its own to the inferior pharyngeal constrictor muscle. The cricothyroid muscles are important in that they help to maintain tone of the true vocal folds. Damage to the external branch of the superior laryngeal nerve may compromise this function. As noted, because the external branch courses with the superior thyroid artery, care must be exercised to preserve this nerve before the superior thyroid artery is ligated. Damage to the external branch and the consequent denervation of the cricothyroid muscle may be especially traumatic for patients who rely heavily on their voice, such as public speakers or singers (2,12). When damaged, the timbre of the voice is lost, the voice tires easily, and it is less resonant. High-pitched sounds are especially difficult to make.

Recurrent Laryngeal Nerves

The recurrent, or inferior, laryngeal nerves are of primary importance in the anatomy of the neck and superior mediastinum. The right recurrent laryngeal nerve arises in the lower neck by leaving the vagus nerve as the vagus passes anterior to the right subclavian artery (see Fig. 7). The recurrent nerve loops below and around the right subclavian artery and then ascends upward to the larynx. On the left side, the recurrent laryngeal nerve arises from the vagus as the vagus crosses the anterior surface of the aortic arch in the mediastinum. This recurrent branch loops around the aortic arch and likewise passes upward toward the larynx (see Fig. 7). Near their origins from the vagus nerve, the recurrent branches give rise to several small cardiac branches and then continue their course superomedially, in or lateral to the groove between the trachea and the esophagus (the tracheoesophageal groove) (1). As the recurrent branches ascend in the tracheoesophageal groove, they give off small nerve branches to the trachea and the esophagus.

As the recurrent laryngeal nerves course superiorly in the neck, they come into direct relationship with the inferior thyroid arteries. These arteries arise lateral to the nerves and then course medially to the thyroid gland (Fig. 11, and see Fig. 7). Unfortunately, the relationship of the recurrent laryngeal nerves and the inferior thyroid arteries is variable. On either side, the recurrent nerve may pass anterior to the artery, posterior to the artery, or between the first major subdivisions of the inferior thyroid artery (13) (see Figs. 7,11). A number of studies have documented this variable anatomic relationship, often with no clear consensus of opinion. However, Hollinshead (1) summarized the major configuration of these two structures by concluding that on the right side the recurrent nerve frequently (about 50% of the time) passes between either the main or minor branches of the inferior thyroid artery. The nerve passes posterior to the artery on the right side in only about 25% of the cases. On the left side, the recurrent branch more commonly passes behind, or posterior to, the inferior thyroid artery (50% of the cases), and it rarely passes anterior to the artery or its minor branches (10% to 12% of cases).

Moreover, the anatomic relationship of the recurrent laryngeal nerves to the trachea also may be variable. Berlin (14) observed that the right recurrent branch may lie as much as 1 cm lateral to the trachea, and he found that the right recurrent nerve is in the tracheoesophageal groove or sulcus only 59% of the time. On the left side, the recurrent branch is in the tracheoesophageal groove 70% of the time.

As the recurrent laryngeal nerves approach the larynx, they come into direct relationship with the thyroid gland. At this point, the lateral lobes of the thyroid gland are attached to the upper two or three tracheal rings by a condensation of pretracheal fascia called Berry's ligament (suspensory or lateral ligament, sometimes incorrectly called the posterior suspensory ligament) (15) (see Figs. 7,11). Berry's ligament is important in that the recurrent laryngeal nerve on each side passes either deep to this ligament (75% of cases) or through the ligament (25%). Berlin's study (14) even suggests that, in about 7% to 10% of the cases, the recurrent nerves may actually pass through the substance of the thyroid gland for a short distance (see Fig. 11). Nevertheless, identification of the recurrent laryngeal nerves usually can be made at the level of this important landmark. Once the recurrent nerves enter the larynx (below the level of the vocal folds), or just outside the larynx, they divide into anterior and posterior branches. Once again, some of the early anatomic studies are confusing and inconsistent, but King and Gregg (16) describe the nerve as dividing externally in as many as 25% of the cases and mention that the two branches may be as far apart as 0.6 cm. In contrast, Armstrong and Hinton (17) report an incidence of external division of the recurrent nerves in 73% of the cases. Apparently, there is no significant difference in the incidence of extralaryngeal division between the right and left nerves.

On rare occasions, the recurrent laryngeal nerve may arise from the cervical vagus approximately at the level of the thyroid gland itself. When this occurs, the nerve does not loop around the subclavian artery but passes directly to the larynx by coursing posterior to the common carotid artery. This anomaly occurs far more frequently on the right side, where it is always associated with an anomalous retroesophageal subclavian artery (1).

The recurrent laryngeal nerves innervate all of the muscles of the larynx except the cricothyroid, which is innervated by the external branch of the superior laryngeal nerve. The recurrent laryngeal nerves also are sensory to the mucosa of the larynx below the level of the vocal folds. Importantly, the only abductors of the vocal folds are the posterior cricoarytenoid muscles, and denervation of these muscles or trauma to the recurrent laryngeal nerves that innervate these muscles may compromise the function of these abductors. If denervated, the vocal folds

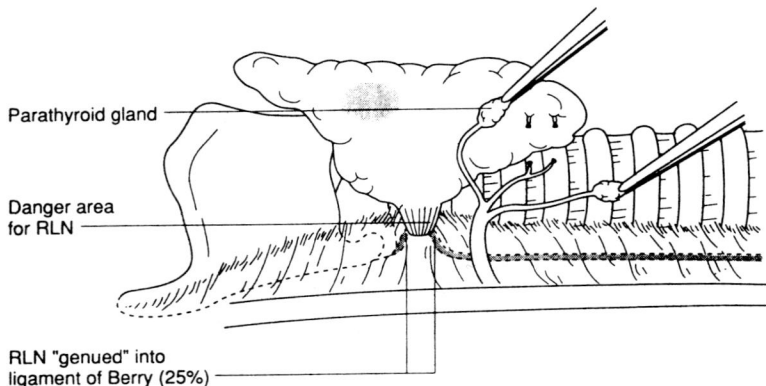

Parathyroid gland

Danger area for RLN

RLN "genued" into ligament of Berry (25%)

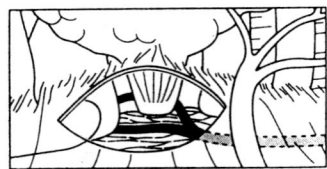

Anterior branch of bifed RLN within ligament of Berry

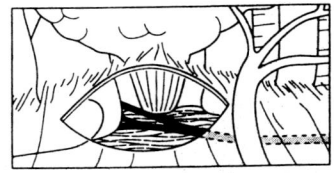

RLN normal course lateral to ligament of Berry

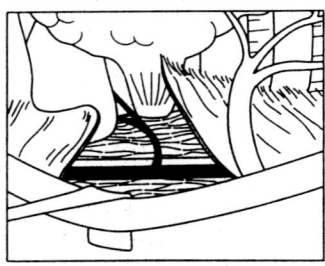

Non-RLN arising from vagus (1%) on right side

FIG. 11. Variations in the distal course of the recurrent laryngeal nerve (RLN) and its relationship to Berry's (suspensory or lateral) ligament and the thyroid gland. (Reproduced, with permission, from ref. 4.)

tend to approximate one another in an adducted position. Under normal conditions (i.e., without significant laryngeal edema), the airway remains open but inspiratory stridor may occur. The ability to speak, however, will be compromised, producing hoarseness of the voice (5). Dyspnea also may occur.

THYMUS GLAND

The normal extent of the thymus gland in the neck is limited. The thymus consists of two lobes connected in the midline by a variable amount of connective tissue. The thymus gland extends partly into the neck and partly into the thorax. In the neck, the thymus gland lies anterior to the trachea and esophagus, but deep to the origins of the sternohyoid and sternothyroid muscles. In the thorax, the thymus lies anterior to the great vessels emanating from the heart and just beneath the sternum in a compartment known as the superior mediastinum. The full anatomic extent of the thymus gland is normally from about the fourth costal cartilage in the thorax to the lower border of the thyroid gland in the neck.

Because of the embryologic origin of the thymus gland from the third pharyngeal pouch and its migratory route through the neck into the superior mediastinum, small accessory pieces of thymic tissue often are found in the lower neck region along the gland's embryonic migratory route. Harman (18) has described one case in which the thymus extended superiorly into the neck to the level of the thyroid cartilage. One of these apical extensions of the lateral lobe of the thymus actually reached the angle of the mandible. Under normal conditions, however, extensions of thymic tissue this high into the neck are rare. When present, they are usually referred to as a cervical thymus (1). With respect to the anatomy associated with thyroid surgery, it is most important to remember that parathyroid tissue may be associated with the thymus gland either in the lower neck or in the superior mediastinum (see Figs. 9,10).

TRACHEA AND ESOPHAGUS

The trachea begins just below the level of the cricoid cartilage anterior to the sixth cervical vertebra, and it extends inferiorly in the midline into the thorax. Some important anterior relationships to the trachea include the thyroid gland and its isthmus (crossing the anterior surface of the trachea at the level of the second, third, and fourth tracheal cartilages), inferior thyroid veins (if present), the thyroid ima artery, tracheal lymph nodes, and the infrahyoid muscles (see Figs. 3,5,7,8). Laterally, the trachea is related to the lobes of the thyroid gland, the great vessels in the neck, and posterolaterally the recurrent laryngeal nerves. Posteriorly in the neck lies the esophagus.

The esophagus begins at the inferior border of the cricoid cartilage, being continuous superiorly with the pharynx. The superior-most portion is its narrowest point. Unlike the midline trachea, the esophagus deviates somewhat to the left in the cervical region. On its anterior surface, the esophagus is near the trachea. Anterolateral are the lobes of the thyroid gland, the inferior thyroid arteries, and the carotid sheath. Because of the lateral curvature of the esophagus to the left, the left recurrent laryngeal nerve often lies on the anterior surface of the esophagus, whereas the right recurrent laryngeal nerve lies along the right margin of the esophagus (1). In this normal position, the recurrent laryngeal nerves are often said to lie in the tracheoesophageal groove. Posteriorly, the esophagus lies upon the vertebral column and is separated from this latter structure by several layers of fascia.

Blood Supply and Innervation

The blood supply to the cervical portions of the trachea and esophagus is principally via the inferior thyroid arteries. Additional arteries supplying blood to the esophagus may include the subclavian, ascending pharyngeal, transverse cervical, vertebral, costocervical trunk, and common carotid arteries. Rich anastomoses exist between the arteries of the trachea and the esophagus.

The innervation of the trachea and esophagus in the neck is via the recurrent laryngeal nerves. These nerves give off small branches to both structures as the main nerve trunk ascends toward the larynx.

ACKNOWLEDGMENTS

The author thanks Anita Matthews for redrawing several of the figures, and Michael Vilardo, M.D., for helping to research this chapter.

REFERENCES

1. Hollinshead WH. *Anatomy for surgeons, vol 1. The head and neck*, 2nd ed. New York: Harper & Row, 1968.
2. Moosman DA, DeWeese MS. The external laryngeal nerve as related to thyroidectomy. *Surg Gynecol Obstet* 1968;127:1011–1016.
3. Clemente CD. *Gray's anatomy*, 30th ed. Philadelphia: Lea & Febiger, 1985.
4. Thompson NW. Thyroid gland. In: Greenfield LJ, Mulholland MW, Oldham KT, Zelenock GB, eds. *Surgery. Scientific principles and practice*. Philadelphia: JB Lippincott, 1993;1163–1187.
5. Kaplan EL. Thyroid and parathyroid. In: Schwartz SI, ed. *Principles of surgery, vol 2.* New York: McGraw-Hill, 1989;1613–1685.
6. Eisler P. Der M. Levator glandulae thyreoideae und verwandte praelaryngeale muskelbildungen. *Anat Anz* 1900;17:183–196.
7. Faller A, Scharer O. Uber die variabilitat der arteriaw thyreoideae. *Acta Anat* (Basel) 1947;4:119–122.
8. Hunt PS. A reappraisal of the surgical anatomy of the thyroid and parathyroid glands. *Br J Surg* 1968;55:63–66.
9. Bachhuber CA. Complications of thyroid surgery: anatomy of recurrent laryngeal nerve, middle thyroid vein, and inferior thyroid artery. *Am J Surg* 1943;50:96–100.
10. Akerstrom G, Malmaeus J, Bergstrom R. Surgical anatomy of human parathyroid glands. *Surgery* 1984;95:14–21.
10a. Ashley SW, Wells SA. Parathyroid glands. In: Greenfield LJ, Mulholland MW, Oldham KT, Zelenock GB, eds. *Surgery. Scientific principles and practice*. Philadelphia: JB Lippincott, 1993;1187–1209.
11. Walton AJ. The surgical treatment of parathyroid tumors. *Br J Surg* 1931;19:285–291.
12. Harrison TS. The thyroid gland. In: Sabiston DC, ed. *Textbook of surgery, vol 1*. Philadelphia: WB Saunders, 1986;579–610.
13. Hollinshead WH. Anatomy of the endocrine glands. *Surg Clin North Am* 1952;32:1115–1140.
14. Berlin DD. The recurrent laryngeal nerves in total ablation of the normal thyroid gland. *Surg Gynecol Obstet* 1935;60:19–26.
15. Lore JM. Surgery of the thyroid gland. In: Tenta LT, Keyes GR, eds. *Symposium on surgery of the thyroid and parathyroid glands, vol. 13*. Philadelphia: WB Saunders, 1980;69–83.
16. King BT, Gregg RL. An anatomical reason for the various behaviors of paralyzed vocal cords. *Ann Otol Rhinol Laryngol* 1948;57:925–944.
17. Armstrong WG, Hinton JW. Multiple divisions of the recurrent laryngeal nerve. *Arch Surg* 1951;62:532–539.
18. Harman NB. "Socia thymi cervicalis," and thymus accessorius. *J Anat Physiol* 1901;36:47–53.
19. Sadler TW. *Langman's medical embryology*, 7th ed. Baltimore: Williams & Wilkins, 1995.
20. Lindner HH. *Clinical anatomy*. Norwalk, CT: Appleton & Lange, 1989.
21. Woodburne RT, Burkel WE. Essentials of human anatomy, 8th ed. New York: Oxford University Press, 1988.
22. Brennan MF, Doppman JL, Marx SJ, Spiegel AM, Brown EM, Aurbach GD. Reoperative parathyroid surgery for persistent hyperparathyroidism. *Surgery* 1978;83:669–676.

CHAPTER 3

Physiology of Thyroid Hormone Synthesis, Secretion, and Transport

Jonathan S. LoPresti and Peter A. Singer

The thyroid axis determines the thyroid status of any given individual by regulating the availability of thyroid hormone to all tissues. The system is organized into two components: the thyroid gland, which is primarily responsible for the synthesis, storage, and secretion of thyroxine (T_4) and triiodothyronine (T_3), and the peripheral arm, which controls the metabolism of T_4 and T_3 after their release into the circulation. Integration of the thyroid gland and the periphery to maintain euthyroidism is coordinated at the anterior pituitary gland, with thyrotropin (TSH) mediating thyroid hormone output from the thyroid gland. TSH regulates a series of enzymatic reactions within the thyroid gland that are responsible for the generation of T_4 and T_3, including the synthesis of thyroglobulin (Tg), the uptake and organification of iodide, the iodination of Tg to form T_4 and T_3, its storage in the gland as colloid, and the hydrolysis of the stored Tg to release T_4 and T_3 into the circulation. Thyroxine is a prohormone, with little intrinsic hormonal activity, and it must be converted to the potent 3,5,3'-triiodothyronine (T_3) to render biologic action.

Peripheral thyroid hormone metabolism, through an enzymatic cascade of deiodination and conjugation of T_4 and its metabolites, is responsible for the production and regulation of circulating T_3 levels, its delivery to the tissues, and the availability of T_3 at the nucleus, the site of thyroid hormone action. This chapter describes this thyroid axis in healthy euthyroid adults.

Included is a description of the enzymatic steps required for the synthesis and release of thyroid hormone from the thyroid gland and the role that TSH plays in its

---

J. S. LoPresti and P. A. Singer: Department of Medicine, Division of Endocrinology, Diabetes, and Hypertension, University of Southern California School of Medicine, Los Angeles, California 90033.

regulation. In addition, prereceptor thyroid hormone metabolism, including the role of serum binding proteins and the various deiodinating and conjugating enzyme systems responsible for regulating T_3 concentrations, is discussed. The well-orchestrated alterations in the thyroid axis that occur in fasting and illness are summarized. Finally, the integration of the central and peripheral thyroid axis at the level of the anterior pituitary gland is described.

THYROID HORMONE BIOSYNTHESIS

The primary function of the thyroid gland is the synthesis and secretion of T_4, although it does secrete small amounts of the active form of the thyroid hormone T_3, as well. All steps required for the formation of thyroid hormone are localized within the thyroid follicular cells. A polarity in the production of thyroid hormone exists: Tg synthesis and iodination occur at the apical end, and thyroid hormone is released in the basal portion of the cell. An intact hypothalamic–pituitary–thyroid axis and a ready source of iodide are required for the normal production of T_4 and T_3 by the thyroid gland. Any interruption in this axis, or deficiency in the availability of iodide, compromises the synthetic ability of the thyroid gland. This section discusses the synthesis and secretion of thyroid hormone and the factors that regulate these events.

Iodide Metabolism

Approximately 100 to 150 μg of inorganic iodide is needed per day for normal thyroid hormone biosynthesis (1). The main source of iodide is the diet, with daily intake averaging 300 to 700 μg in the United States because of the iodination of salt, bread, milk, and other foodstuffs.

In addition, iodide concentrations are high in many commonly used medications which, when administered, can dramatically increase iodide exposure. Iodide deficiency, however, is still a significant health problem in many parts of the world where no dietary iodide supplementation has been implemented. A higher incidence of goiter and hypothyroidism is present in these areas. It should be noted that excessive intake of iodide can promote thyroid dysfunction, including Hashimoto's thyroiditis, hypothyroidism in patients with a prior history of thyroid surgery or thyroid disease, and thyrotoxicosis in individuals with a preexisting goiter (2).

The total body iodide pool of about 9000 µg is quite large because of the substantial stores present in the thyroid gland. Eight thousand micrograms is located in the colloid and serves as a source of iodide when iodide intake is low. The remainder is divided between that contained in the circulation as thyroid hormone (600 µg) and the free iodide present in the extracellular fluid (150 µg). Dietary iodide is almost completely absorbed by the gastrointestinal tract and enters the extracellular iodide pool where it is available for uptake by the thyroid gland. Other sources include the iodide generated during the metabolism of thyroid hormone and the small amount that leaks from the thyroid gland during the normal release of T_4 and T_3. The iodide not utilized in the synthesis of new thyroid hormone is rapidly cleared by the kidneys, with only a small amount lost in the feces. In the euthyroid subject ingesting a normal diet in the United States, an equilibrium exists between the iodide ingested and that excreted.

Iodide Transport

Inorganic iodide is transported into the follicular cell by an iodide pump located in the basolateral membrane (3). This appears to be an active transport system in that the pump has the ability to concentrate serum iodide against a large chemical gradient and involves a Na+/K+-ATPase-mediated sodium transport requiring ATP for energy (4). The iodide pump is under the control of TSH: increases in TSH secretion augment the uptake of iodide into the follicular cell. In addition to that located in the thyroid, this active transport system for iodide is also located in the salivary glands, mammary glands, and gastric mucosa (4). Iodide transport into the thyroid gland can also be influenced by the serum iodide level: iodide deficiency increases pump activity and iodide excess inhibits iodide uptake. These various mechanisms ensure that there are adequate iodide levels in the thyroid gland to maintain normal thyroid hormone synthesis.

Thyroglobulin Biosynthesis

Thyroglobulin is a large glycoprotein composed of two smaller subunits, with a molecular weight of 660,000 daltons. Ten percent of the mass of the Tg molecule consists of carbohydrate moieties (5). The gene that controls the formation of Tg is located on chromosome 8 (6). Synthesis of Tg begins on polysomes located in the rough endoplasmic reticulum, the major organelle present in the follicular cell, and is completed in the Golgi apparatus (7,8). Once Tg synthesis is finished, exocytotic vesicles are formed from the Golgi membrane to transport the Tg to the apical surface of the follicular cell, where iodination and transfer to the colloid for storage occur. Thus, there is a basal-to-apical movement of Tg within the follicular cell (8). All of these steps of Tg synthesis appear to be under the control of TSH.

Iodination of Thyroglobulin

The formation of thyroid hormone takes place within the Tg molecule at the apical surface of the follicular cell. It requires two separate oxidative reactions that are catalyzed by one enzyme, thyroid peroxidase (TPO), located in the apical plasma membrane of the cell. The steps include binding of iodide to tyrosyl residues to form iodotyrosyls, and their subsequent coupling to produce iodothyronines. As in the synthesis of Tg, the process of thyroid hormone generation is controlled by TSH.

Autoradiographic studies have shown that iodide, once taken up in the basal portion of the follicular cell, rapidly moves to the apical surface and into the follicular lumen (9). Once in the lumen of the cell, the iodide is converted to its more reactive form, I_2. This peroxidation of iodide is catalyzed by TPO and appears to be a requisite for the iodination of tyrosines within the Tg molecule (10). Only a small percentage of the tyrosyl residues are available for iodination, with those tyrosines located in the amino-terminus of the molecule being preferentially iodinated.

Coupling of iodotyrosines within the Tg molecule, an oxidative reaction, produces the thyroid hormones. T_4 is the combination of two diiodotyrosines (DITs), and T_3 results from the union of one monoiodotyrosine (MIT) and one DIT (Fig. 1). As in the iodination of tyrosyl residues, the coupling of the iodotyrosines is catalyzed by the thyroid peroxidase enzyme (11). A peroxide-generating system found on the apical plasma membrane of the follicular cell is necessary for the TPO-mediated iodotyrosyl coupling to occur (12). Iodide availability can also regulate thyroid hormone formation. When iodide is in abundant supply, T_4 is the major thyroid hormone found in the Tg, whereas in states of relative iodide deficiency, more T_3 is detected in the Tg molecule. This appears to be an attempt by the thyroid gland to maintain homeostasis as well as to conserve iodide. TSH likely regulates these TPO-mediated reactions.

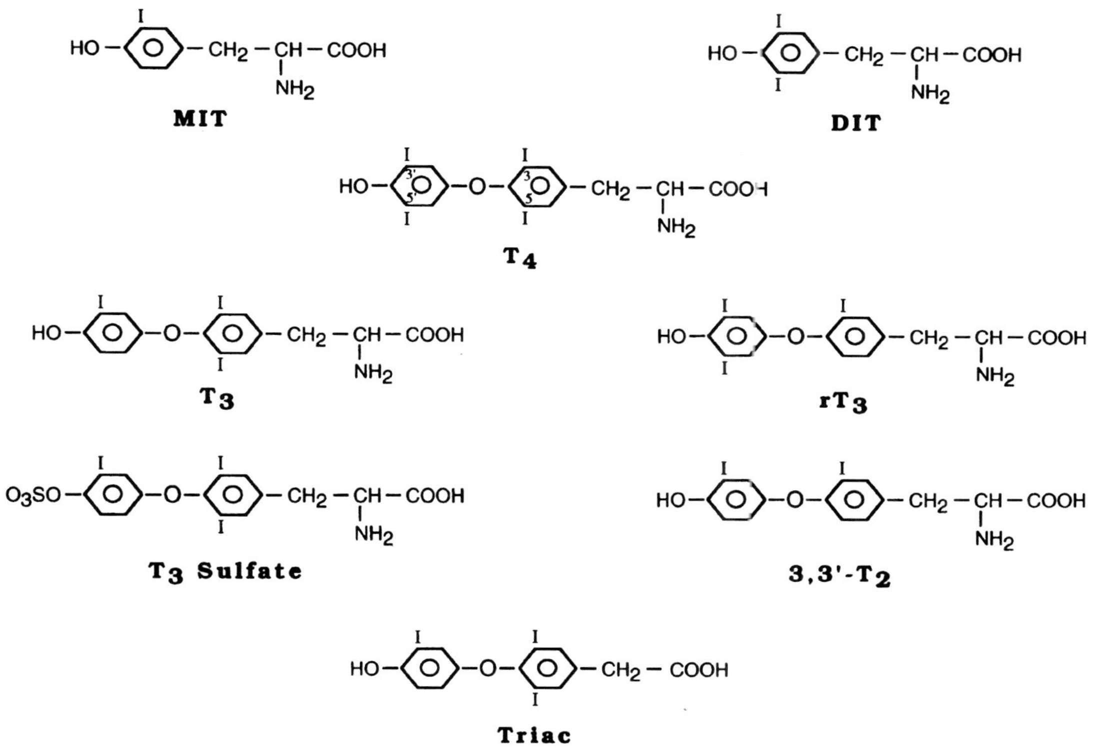

FIG. 1. Structures of the major thyronine metabolites and of the iodotyrosyls, MIT and DIT (present in iodinated thyroglobulin). The terminology of the location of the iodides is shown on the structure of T_4.

Thyroid Hormone Release

The sequence of events that determines the proportion of T_4 and T_3 released from the thyroid gland is also TSH dependent. It involves the resorption of the stored Tg from the colloid in the follicular lumen of the cell, and its transport from the apical to the basolateral surface of the follicular cell where the secretion of thyroid hormone into the circulation occurs. Enzymatic degradation of the Tg by intracellular lysosomes frees the T_4 and T_3 molecules contained within the Tg, with T_4 being the preferred secretory product. A 5'-deiodinase enzyme within the cell can influence the amounts of T_4 and T_3 released: activation of this enzyme converts T_4 to T_3, leading to preferential T_3 secretion by the thyroid gland.

The initial step in this process is the resorption of the stored Tg into the follicular cell by a specialized type of endocytosis called micropinocytosis (13). There is an invagination of the apical plasma membrane into small vesicles, which fuse to form colloid droplets, which are then transported to the basal surface of the cell for thyroid hormone secretion. The resorbed Tg must undergo hydrolysis within lysosomes in order for the thyroid hormones to be released from the colloid droplets.

The vesicles formed during Tg resorption by micropinocytosis reach the basolateral surface of the cell via endosomal transport (14). Lysosomes fuse with the colloid droplets, and the peptidases within them catalyze the degradation of Tg to release T_4, T_3, MIT, and DIT. The majority of the iodide released during Tg breakdown is recycled and acts as an intrathyroidal source of iodide for future synthesis of thyroid hormone (15). The T_4 and T_3 liberated from the Tg remain free within the follicular cell and are available for release into the circulation. This likely occurs by an active transport mechanism as TSH stimulates the release of thyroid hormone from the thyroid gland (16).

The major secretory product of the human thyroid gland is T_4, with only small amounts of T_3 being released. The intake of iodide influences the DIT-to-MIT ratio in the Tg. DIT is the preferential iodotyrosine formed when iodide is readily available, leading to the secretion of T_4. However, as iodide sources diminish, MIT is characteristically produced, which leads to more T_3 formation and T_3 release. In addition, the thyroid gland contains a 5'-deiodinase that can locally convert T_4 to T_3 and increase the proportion of T_3 released into the circulation (17). This intrathyroidal 5'-deiodinase is controlled by TSH, which enhances T_3 secretion during periods of TSH stimulation (i.e., primary hypothyroidism, or the TSH-stimulating immunoglobulin present in Graves' disease) (Fig. 2).

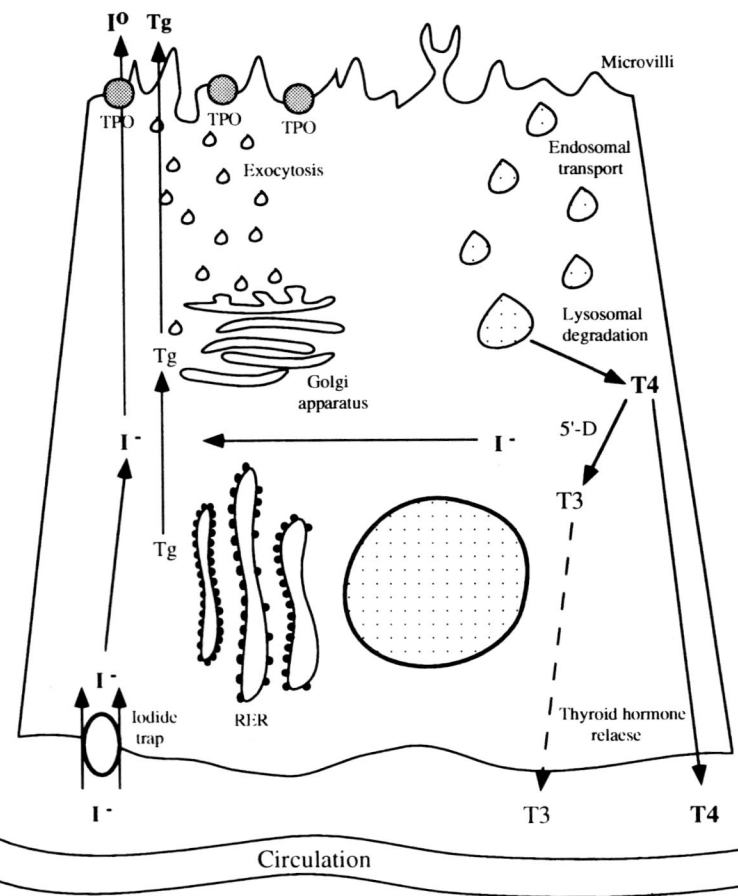

FIG. 2. Steps in the synthesis and secretion of the thyroid hormones. Note the basal-apical-basal nature of this process. Iodide is trapped at the basal surface of the cell and moves quickly to the apical surface. Thyroglobulin (Tg) is initially synthesized in the endoplasmic reticulum (RER), and synthesis is completed in the Golgi apparatus. Tg is transported to the apical surface by exocytosis. Iodination of the Tg is catalyzed by the thyroid peroxidase (TPO) at the apical portion of the cell. After reuptake into the cell as colloid droplets, the Tg moves to the basal surface by endosomal transport. T_4 and T_3 are released from the Tg via lysosomal degradation. The T_4 and T_3 are then secreted into the circulation at the basal membrane. TSH regulates all these steps of thyroid hormone synthesis and release.

In summary, the synthesis and secretion of thyroid hormone from the thyroid gland is a highly regulated process primarily controlled by TSH. It is designed to produce T_4, which, after its release, serves as a precursor to the active form of thyroid hormone, T_3. In essence, the thyroid gland functions as a supply of thyroid hormone. However, under conditions of iodide deficiency or hyperstimulation by TSH, the gland can become the major source of circulating T_3 in order to conserve iodide as well as to maintain euthyroidism. This autoregulation of the thyroid gland, acting in conjunction with the peripheral metabolism to be discussed later, maintains metabolic homeostasis in humans.

PERIPHERAL THYROID HORMONE METABOLISM

Peripheral thyroid hormone metabolism is a complex process designed to regulate the level of circulating T_3 and its availability to the tissues. Compared to other mammals, which rely more heavily on the thyroid gland for their T_3 needs, humans have this extrathyroidal source of T_3 developed that allows greater local (i.e., individual tissue) regulation of thyroid hormone requirements in health and illness. The serum binding proteins are one facet in this peripheral strategy of thyroid hormone activation. Thyroxine-binding globulin (TBG), transthyretin (TTR) or thyroxine-binding pre-albumin (TBPA), and albumin retain the thyroid hormones in the circulation and help deliver them to their sites of metabolism and action (18). A second component is the generation of T_3 by its conversion from T_4 by a 5'-deiodinase located outside the thyroid gland (19). However, recent studies have demonstrated that the production of T_3 is more complicated than previously suspected, and the regulation of the serum T_3 concentration involves both its formation from T_4 and its subsequent disposal, in a push–pull phenomenon. These other metabolic pathways of T_3 disposal include the inactivation routes of deiodination and sulfate conjugate formation, as well as the path of acetic acid analog generation (19). The production of 3,3',5'-triiodothyronine [reverse T_3 (rT_3)] and T_4-sulfate from T_4, the non-T_3 routes of T_4 disposal, also helps regulate circulating T_3 levels in humans. This section describes the major binding proteins and their role in the transport of the thyroid hormones in the circulation and their delivery to tissues, as well as the enzymatic pathways involved in thyroid hormone metabolism and their interactions in determining serum and tissue T_3 concentrations. Also, the influence of nonthyroidal illness on peripheral thyroid hormone metabolism will be discussed.

Serum Binding Proteins

Most thyroid hormone circulates bound to binding proteins, so that only 0.03% of T_4 and 0.3% of T_3 is unbound, or free, and available to the tissues for either thyroid hormone action or degradation (18). The serum proteins that function as thyroid hormone binding proteins are TBG, TTR, and albumin. Eighty percent of T_4 is bound to TBG, 15% is bound to TTR, and the remaining 5% is bound to albumin. Binding to these proteins is noncovalent and reversible, and it is consistent with the law of mass action (Fig. 3). Any change in binding protein levels will acutely alter the free T_4 level, but eventually a new equilibrium will be reached and a normal free T_4 concentration will be achieved if the hypothalamic–pituitary axis is intact. In addition, apolipoproteins can also bind thyroid hormone, but their role in the transport of thyroid hormone is unclear (20). It is apparent, however, that TBG serves as the primary thyroid hormone binding protein in the euthyroid range of serum T_4 values.

Thyroxine binding globulin (TBG) is a 54-kDa glycoprotein synthesized and secreted by the liver (21). The gene responsible for the regulation of TBG resides on the long arm of the human X chromosome (22). The TBG molecule consists of a 359-amino-acid polypeptide chain and four polysaccharide units consisting of five to nine sialic acid residues. Normally, TBG has a single binding site for thyroid hormone that has a tenfold greater affinity for T_4 than for T_3 (23). Only about one-third of the TBG molecules carry thyroid hormone in a euthyroid individual. TBG serves as the major thyroid binding protein because of its 100-fold greater affinity for T_4 than that of TTR, even though TBG circulates at a concentration that is about 20-fold less than that of TTR. Because of these properties of TBG, the total serum T_4 value measured is dependent on the level of TBG, although if equilibrium is maintained, the free T_4 levels are normal.

Various factors can change the concentration of TBG and alter the total serum T_4 levels (Table 1). The most common cause of an elevated TBG value is the high estrogen state seen with pregnancy and with the use of oral contraceptive pills (24). The rise in TBG appears to result both from enhanced synthesis of TBG by the liver and from a slowing of the clearance of TBG from the circulation. Other drugs that increase TBG concentrations include heroin, methadone, clofibrate, 5-fluorouracil, and nicotinic acid (25–28).

Certain diseases also can elevate TBG levels. Diverse forms of liver disease are the most commonly encountered causes of increased TBG levels; these include acute and chronic viral hepatitis, primary biliary cirrhosis, and hepatocellular carcinoma (29,30). Presumably, enhanced hepatic synthesis of TBG is responsible for the observed rise in TBG. Recently, infection with the human immunodeficiency virus (HIV) has been reported to increase TBG concentrations, but the mechanism responsible is unknown (31). An inherited excess of TBG has also been described (32).

Reductions in circulating TBG levels are also commonly observed, with acute and chronic nonthyroidal illnesses being the most frequent etiologies of this acquired decrease in TBG values (33). Other causes of low TBG are nephrotic syndrome due to a tubular leak of the protein, chronic pharmacologic glucocorticoid administration, the use/abuse of androgens and anabolic steroids, and a congenital deficiency of TBG (32,34–36). Despite these alterations in TBG concentrations, free T_4 and TSH levels are normal and the patients remain euthyroid if the hypothalamic–pituitary axis is intact.

Transthyretin (TTR) is a 55-kDa protein composed of a tetramer of four identical 127-amino-acid subunits, but it contains no carbohydrate moieties. TTR is synthesized and secreted by the liver and contains two iodothyronine binding sites. However, only one of these sites carries T_4 (TTR does not bind T_3). The function of TTR in the transport of thyroid hormone in euthyroid humans appears to be limited in the presence of TBG, because its removal from serum has no influence on free T_4 values (37).

Albumin is a 66.5-kDa, 585-amino-acid protein synthesized by the liver. It has the ability to bind many hor-

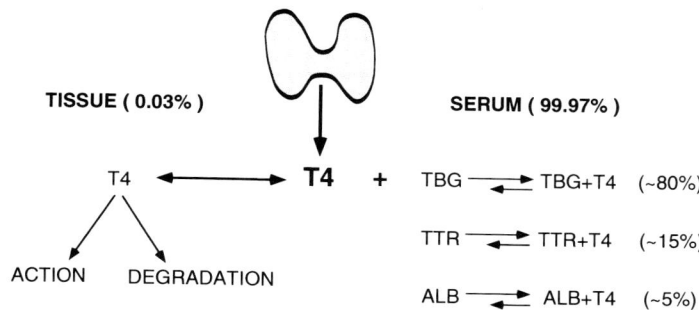

FIG. 3. T_4-binding protein interaction. TBG is the major protein involved in thyroid hormone transport in the circulation. Note that only 0.03% of the T_4 circulates in the free state and is available to the tissues for thyroid hormone action or degradation. The law of mass action governs this relationship.

TABLE 1. *Factors that alter serum TBG concentrations*

Elevation	Reduction
Sex steroids	Sex steroids
Hyperestrogenic states	Androgens
Oral contraceptive pills	Anabolic steroids
Pregnancy	
Other drugs	Drugs
5-Fluorouracil	Glucocorticoids
Heroin/methadone	
Clofibrate	
Nicotinic acid	
Disease	Disease
Acute and chronic viral hepatitis	Nonthyroidal illness (acute, chronic)
Primary biliary cirrhosis	Nephrotic syndrome
Hepatocellular carcinoma	
HIV infection	
Congenital excess	Congenital deficiency

mones and drugs, although all of these interactions appear to be nonspecific and weak in nature. Its removal from serum (similar to that of TTR) does not change free T_4 concentrations. However, because of its high serum concentrations, albumin does play a minor role in the transport of thyroid hormone (38).

In summary, the evolution of serum thyroid hormone binding proteins and their affinity for T_4 and T_3 has facilitated the conversion of the thyroid-gland-dominant source of T_3 present in lower mammals to that of the peripheral source of T_3 established in humans. For this transfer to have occurred, there must have developed at least four roles for the proteins in thyroid hormone metabolism. The first was to maintain an adequate store of circulating thyroid hormone, minimizing the reliance on the thyroid gland for the body's source of thyroid hormone. The second was to minimize exposure of the thyroid hormone to their disposal sites. The third was a distribution system of the thyroid hormones to the location(s) of their activation, and the fourth, the delivery by the binding proteins of thyroid hormones to the tissues in which they would perform the thyroid hormone activity. The absolute necessity of binding proteins in sustaining peripheral thyroid hormone metabolism is unsure, as individuals with a congenital absence of these proteins are euthyroid. However, this euthyroidism occurs at the expense of increased hormone turnover and iodide requirements, making the serum binding proteins a key development in nature's attempt to conserve iodide in an iodide-deficient environment.

Thyroid Hormone Metabolism

Thyroxine, the relatively weak hormone secreted by the thyroid gland, must be converted to the potent T_3 for full thyroid hormone expression. This conversion increases the binding affinity of the hormone to the nuclear thyroid receptor protein by a factor of at least tenfold. The prereceptor metabolism of T_4 after its release from the thyroid gland is responsible for this activation step. In addition to the generation of T_3 from T_4, the regulation of circulating levels of T_3 and the delivery to the tissues also rely on other metabolic pathways of hormonal disposal (conjugation, acetic acid formation). The major players in this complex process are the serum binding proteins discussed previously, and the thyroid hormones T_4, T_3, and rT_3, and their alternate metabolic products, including the sulfate conjugates and the acetic acid analogs (see Fig. 1). The interaction among these metabolic pathways is responsible for maintaining thyroid homeostasis. This system also allows for local control of thyroid hormone needs as well as moment-to-moment variations in thyroid hormone requirements at the tissue level.

Thyroxine

Thyroxine (T_4) is synthesized and secreted solely by the thyroid gland. Normally, a euthyroid human will produce and metabolize approximately 90 to 100 µg of T_4 per day. This daily production of T_4 remains steady for most of adult life, which accounts for the relatively constant L-T_4 replacement doses required by hypothyroid patients. T_4 primarily circulates bound to TBG, with only 0.03% existing in the free state and available for conversion to T_3 or to those sites where T_4 undergoes metabolic inactivation. Because of this intense binding of T_4 to TBG, the extrathyroidal turnover of T_4 is slow, with the serum half-life for T_4 being 7 days. Also, this means that T_4 primarily resides in the circulation and not in the intracellular compartment, a prerequisite for the human's reliance on the peripheral metabolism of thyroid hormone for the body's active thyroid hormone needs (39) (Table 2).

Triiodothyronine

Whereas the source of T_4 is the thyroid gland, the origin of triiodothyronine (T_3) is more complicated. The euthyroid adult produces 30 to 35 µg of T_3 per day, with 20% arising from direct thyroidal secretion and the remaining 80% being derived by a monodeiodination of T_4 in the peripheral tissues. This conversion of T_4 to T_3 is catalyzed by a spe-

TABLE 2. *Thyroid hormone kinetics*

	T_4	T_3	rT_3
Concentration (mean)	7.5 µg/dL	120 ng/dL	15 ng/dL
Volume of distribution (L)	10	35	90
Metabolic clearance rate (L/day)	1.2	25	150
Serum half-life	7 days	1 day	4 hr
Production rate (µg/day)	100	30	20

cific 5′-deiodinase enzyme, but the tissue(s) responsible is unknown. Like T_4, the vast majority of T_3 circulates bound to TBG, but with a much lower affinity than that seen for T_4. This explains the kinetic differences observed between T_3 and T_4. T_3 has a 50-fold lower serum concentration than T_4, with a free fraction of 0.3% (in contrast to 0.03% for T_4), and a serum half-life of 1 day. Because of this less avid binding to TBG, most of the body's store of T_3 resides in the intracellular compartment, where it is able to render thyroid hormone action (see Table 2) (39).

Reverse Triiodothyronine

Reverse T_3 (rT_3) is the third major circulating thyroid hormone. Like T_3, rT_3 is produced in the peripheral tissues, but it is generated by an inner rather than outer ring deiodination of T_4. This reaction is catalyzed by a specific 5-deiodinase enzyme system. In contrast to T_3, rT_3 has no inherent biologic activity, and its generation from T_4 is considered an inactivation step in thyroid hormone metabolism. The adult produces about 20 μg of rT_3 per day, which also circulates bound to TBG but has a rapid serum half-life of 4 hours. It seems that the formation of rT_3 is primarily a disposal pathway in the peripheral metabolism of T_4 (see Table 2) (40).

Alternate Routes of Metabolism

The sum of the blood production rates of T_3 and rT_3 (the monodeiodinative products of T_4 disposal) account for 70% of the peripheral metabolism of T_4 (40). The remainder occurs by conjugation of T_4 to sulfate, by deamination and decarboxylation to form the acetic acid analog tetrac, and by ether-link cleavage (19). In addition, after their formation from T_4, T_3 and rT_3 can both undergo further metabolism: they can be deiodinated to form 3,3′-diiodothyronine (T_2).

Triiodothyronine, but not rT_3, can also be conjugated with sulfate to form T_3-sulfate (T_3S), and it can be converted to its acetic acid analog, triac (19). The enzymes responsible for these reactions are the phenolsulfotransferases found in many tissues throughout the body and the L-aminotransferase located in the liver, respectively (19). The subsequent metabolic products of T_3 and rT_3 must be taken into account when assessing overall thyroid hormone metabolism, because it is likely that not all of the T_3 and rT_3 formed within the tissues reaches the circulation and, as a result, the blood production rates reported for T_3 and rT_3 underestimate the total body formation of these thyroid hormones (41). These represent the alternate routes of disposal and they function in regulating circulating T_3 levels (Fig. 4).

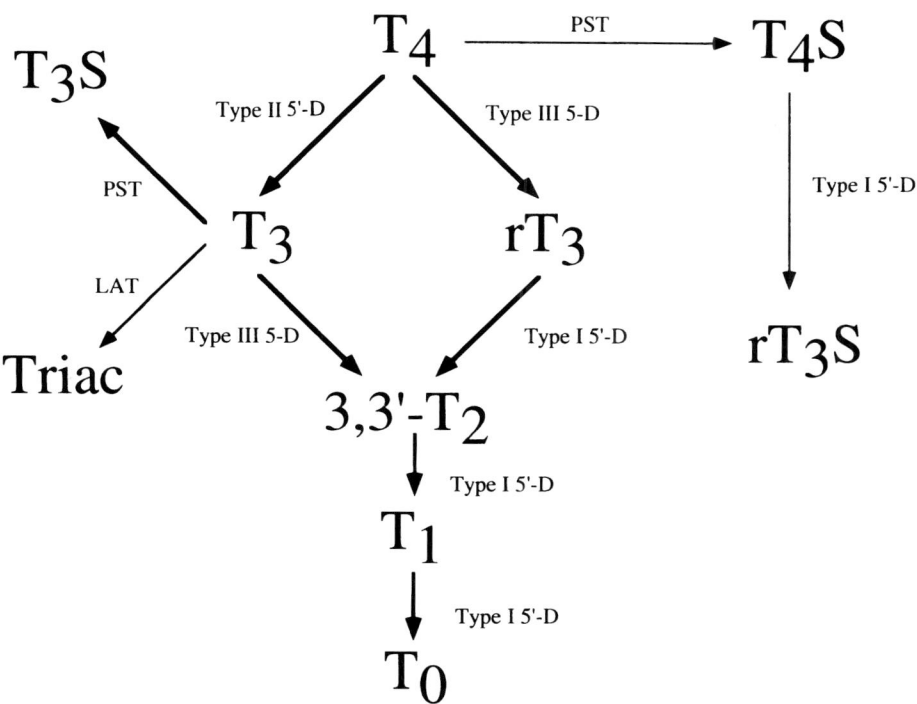

FIG. 4. Peripheral thyroid hormone metabolism in humans. Phenolsulfotransferase (PST) catalyzes thyronine sulfate formation, and L-aminotransferase (LAT) is responsible for producing triac from T_3.

TABLE 3. *Iodothyronine deiodinases*

	Type I 5'-D	Type II 5'-D	Type III 5-D
Location	Liver, kidney, thyroid	CNS, pituitary, placenta, brown adipose tissue	Placenta, CNS, skin
Substrate preference	rT_3>sulfated thyronines >T_4>T_3	T_4>rT_3>T_3	$T_4 \geq rT_3$
PTU	Inhibits	No effect	No effect
Selenium	Present	Absent	Present
Km for T_4	High	Low	Low

Abbreviations: PTU, propylthiouracil; Km, dissociation constant.

Iodothyronine Deiodinases

There are currently two classes of thyronine deiodinases, which are characterized by their enzyme kinetics (Table 3) (42). They have been divided into types I and II outer ring, or 5'-deiodinases, and the inner ring, or 5-deiodinase, termed type III. A detailed description of the molecular characteristics of these enzymes can be found in Chapter 10, Molecular Basis of Thyroid Disease.

Type I 5'-deiodinase (type I 5'-D) is located in the liver, kidney, and thyroid gland. Primarily viewed as an outer ring deiodinase, the type I 5'-D also has the ability to remove an inner ring iodide (42). A defining characteristic of this enzyme is its ability to be inhibited by the antithyroid drug, propylthiouracil (PTU). It has recently been shown that selenium is a necessary component and must be present for the enzyme to function normally (43). rT_3 and the sulfated thyronine conjugates are the preferred substrates for this enzyme, although it is also capable of converting T_4 to T_3 (42). This suggests that the type I 5'-D functions more as a disposal rather than as an activating enzyme in thyroid hormone metabolism. Indeed, the Km for T_4 is quite high and, as a result, T_4 would likely function as a source of T_3 only when T_4 values are in the thyrotoxic range. Despite these obvious kinetic limitations, it has not been disproven that the type I 5'-D can serve as a source of circulating T_3 in euthyroid humans.

Type II 5'-deiodinase (type II 5'-D) is distinct from the type I 5'-D in both its tissue location and its enzymatic characteristics. It is found in the CNS, placenta, and the pituitary gland. In contrast to type I 5'-D, this enzyme is not inhibited by PTU, nor does it contain selenium (42). The enzyme displays a low Km for T_4, suggesting that T_4 is the preferred substrate for the type II 5'-D. In contrast to type I 5'-D, rT_3, T_3, and the sulfated thyronines serve as poor substrates for the enzyme. Because of these kinetic characteristics, some authors have speculated that type II 5'-D is primarily responsible for regulating the conversion of T_4 to T_3, and hence it is responsible for serum T_3 levels (40). Because of its limited tissue distribution, however, it is difficult to accept that it is the sole enzymatic source of circulating T_3 in humans.

Type III 5-deiodinase (type III 5-D) is located in the CNS, skin, and placenta, and it serves as an inner ring deiodinase. This enzyme is not inhibited by PTU, but, like type I 5'-D, type III 5-D is a selenium-containing enzyme. T_4 and T_3 are the preferred substrates for the type III deiodinase (42). As a result, it appears that this enzyme is responsible for the generation of rT_3 from T_4, as well as for inactivating T_3 by catalyzing it to T_2 in local tissues. Type III 5-D seems to be an enzyme devoted to controlling thyroid hormone action by determining the final availability of T_3 to the tissues, either by diverting T_4 to rT_3 or producing T_2 from T_3.

Addendum

Recent evidence has shown that the type II 5'-deiodinase also is a selenium-containing enzyme and is distributed in many tissues (57).

Regulation of Iodothyronine Metabolism

The goal of peripheral thyroid hormone metabolism is to maintain circulating and tissue T_3 levels appropriate for the thyroid hormone requirements in health and illness. It involves both activating (production of T_3) and inactivating (generation of rT_3, T_2, and sulfated thyronine conjugates) pathways of metabolism. The interactions among these metabolic routes ultimately determine the T_3 concentration and availability to the tissues.

Seventy percent of the prohormone T_4 produced daily by the thyroid gland undergoes either inner ring or outer ring monodeiodination to form the inactive rT_3 or the biologically active T_3, catalyzed by the type III 5-D and type II 5'-D (and possibly type I 5'-D) enzymes, respectively. The formation of rT_3 appears to be a terminal route of disposal, as the rT_3 is rapidly cleared from the serum via outer ring deiodination to T_2 by type I 5'-D located in the liver and kidney (40). The T_2 that is formed is completely deiodinated, presumably by the same type I 5'-D, to produce a thyronine nucleus devoid of iodide. This stripping of the iodide from the rT_3 molecule is important in the conservation of iodide.

On the other hand, T_3 has a more diverse route of disposal after its formation from T_4 than does rT_3. Nature has likely evolved these multiple pathways of T_3 metabolism to finely regulate T_3 availability at the tissue level. Like rT_3, T_3 can undergo deiodination to form T_2. In contrast to rT_3, the conversion of T_3 to T_2 is likely catalyzed by type III 5-D located in the tissues where T_3 renders its hormonal action. This functions as a local regulator of thyroid hormone availability. The T_2 that is formed from T_3 is then handled in a manner similar to that of the T_2 that is produced from rT_3. This T_2 production accounts for only 50% of the total T_3 disposal, whereas more than 50% of rT_3 is routed to T_2. The remaining T_3 is primarily conjugated with a sulfate to produce T_3S, with a small proportion being converted to its acetic acid analog, triac (44). These two pathways are, in the main, inactivating routes of T_3 metabolism. In addition, these metabolites are preferred substrates for type I 5'-D and are efficiently deiodinated and rapidly cleared from the circulation. As a consequence, T_3S and triac function both in iodide conservation and in regulating T_3 availability to the tissues. The regulation of circulating T_3 concentrations, and the thyroid status of any given individual, is a push (T_4 to T_3)–pull (T_3 to T_2, T_3S, and triac) phenomenon, with conversion of T_4 to T_3 dominant in determining the T_3 levels in healthy individuals (see Fig. 4).

Mechanism of Action

It is currently believed that the unbound or free T_3 crosses the cell membrane to enter the cell by passive diffusion to render thyroid hormone action in the nucleus (45). In addition, recent evidence suggests that specific T_3 receptors are present on the cell membrane and can function as an active mechanism for transporting T_3 intracellularly (46). It is likely that passive transport serves as the main route for T_3's entry into the cell, because it appears that the free T_3 levels in the cytosol and nucleus are nearly the same as seen in the serum. Because of this equilibrium between the serum and the cell, the circulating free T_3 concentrations reflect the thyroid state of any individual.

The physiologic actions of thyroid hormone are growth, differentiation, calorigenesis, and TSH suppression. These effects are mediated by T_3 receptors located in the nucleus of the cell. Four T_3 nuclear receptors have been well described to date and are designated the $\alpha 1$, $\alpha 2$, $\beta 1$, and $\beta 2$ isoforms (47). The $\alpha 1$ and $\beta 1$ receptors are present in most tissues throughout the body, and binding of T_3 to them promotes thyroid hormone action, presumably by increasing mRNA and protein synthesis. The $\beta 2$ receptor is unique to the pituitary and is central in the negative feedback regulation of TSH by thyroid hormone. In contrast, the $\alpha 2$ isoform is inhibitory by nature and likely acts as a negative regulator of thyroid hormone action. The distribution of the various T_3 receptors and the nuclear T_3 content determine the thyroid status of an individual. Mutations in the β receptors, which diminish the ability of T_3 to bind to the nucleus, have been described in the syndrome of resistance to thyroid hormone. Affected individuals display varying degrees of growth and mental retardation as well as hypothyroidism (48). This experiment of nature underscores the central role that the nuclear T_3 receptors play in the action of thyroid hormone in humans.

Nonthyroidal Illness

The alterations in thyroid hormone metabolism in the presence of either illness or caloric deprivation are a well-orchestrated and predictable adaptive response to reduce metabolic demands and conserve protein stores (49). The initial change observed in all patients is a fall in serum T_3 levels, producing the so-called low T_3 state of nonthyroidal illness. This is accompanied by a rise in circulating rT_3 values. Currently, it is believed that the decrease in T_3 values results from a reduction in the conversion of T_4 to T_3 via an inhibition of the 5'-D enzyme responsible for generating T_3. The reciprocal increase in the rT_3 concentration results from a slowing in its clearance secondary to a reduction in type I 5'-D activity. As the illness becomes more severe, a decline in serum T_4 concentrations is observed, producing the low T_3–low T_4 state (49). The fall in T_4 level appears to result from a change in the affinity of TBG for T_4 such that T_4 does not bind as avidly to TBG. The mechanisms responsible for this loss of binding affinity include a structural change in the TBG molecule and the production of an inhibitor that interferes with the normal T_4-TBG interaction (49) (see Chapters 10 and 12).

Recent evidence suggests that shunting of T_3 to its alternate disposal pathways also lowers the serum T_3 concentration in fasting and illness. Studies have demonstrated an increase in the generation of both T_3S and triac during a short-term fast. In addition, elevated serum levels of T_3S have been observed in severely ill patients. What eventual role the hypertrophy of these alternate routes of T_3 disposal will play in the genesis of the low T_3 state needs to be elucidated (49).

Summary

The prereceptor metabolism of thyroid hormone is a poorly understood process that is designed to regulate circulating T_3 levels, the availability of T_3 to the nucleus, and ultimately the thyroid hormone needs of the individual. It is composed of serum binding proteins that maintain a large circulating store of the prohormone T_4, as well as aid in the delivery of the thyroid hormones to their sites of action and disposal. Also, a series of enzymes that catalyze the production of the active hormone (T_3) and the inactive metabolites (rT_3, T_2, and the thyronine conjugates) are involved. All of these components work in concert to maintain the thyroid status appropriate to the availability of foodstuffs and the health of the patient.

HYPOTHALAMIC–PITUITARY–THYROID AXIS

Communication between the thyroid gland and the peripheral tissues where thyroid hormone undergoes its metabolism is essential to achieve and sustain euthyroidism. It is primarily accomplished at the level of the hypothalamus and anterior pituitary gland in healthy humans. The physiologic regulators responsible for integrating the normal function of the thyroid gland and the periphery include the hypothalamic hormone thyrotropin-releasing hormone (TRH), TSH, a glycoprotein hormone secreted from the anterior pituitary gland, and the serum free-T_4 concentration. These factors interact in a classical negative feedback mechanism to ensure that an adequate supply of T_4 is available in the circulation for its conversion to the active hormone, T_3.

TRH, a three-amino-acid peptide, was first isolated and synthesized in the late 1960s. Primarily concentrated in the median eminence and paraventricular nuclei of the hypothalamus, it is released into the hypothalamic portal circulation and serves as the dominant positive regulator of TSH synthesis in, and release from, the thyrotroph cells in the anterior pituitary gland (50). After the intravenous administration of TRH to humans, a prompt rise in circulating TSH is noted, with peak levels of TSH being attained 30 minutes after injection (51). *In vitro* studies have shown that TRH enhances TSH synthesis at both the transcriptional and the translational levels, and that it stimulates the secretion of any pre-formed TSH from the thyrotrophs (52). TRH also modulates the bioactivity of the TSH by altering the final glycosylation of the TSH molecule released, with TRH being necessary for the secretion of bioactive TSH (53). The chronic administration of TRH to patients with hypothalamic-hypothyroidism improves the ability of circulating TSH to stimulate the thyroid gland to secrete T_4. TRH itself is under the negative feedback influence of circulating thyroid hormones, where TRH mRNA levels are inversely proportional to circulating T_3 values (54).

Thyrotropin is a glycoprotein hormone synthesized and secreted by the thyrotroph cell population located in the anterior pituitary, and it influences all enzymatic steps required for the synthesis and secretion of T_4 (and T_3) from the thyroid gland (see previous discussion). Structurally, TSH consists of two distinct subunits, designated the α and β chains, which are linked by a covalent bond. The α-subunit is common to all glycoprotein hormones, including LH, FSH, and hCG, whereas the β-subunit confers specific bioactivity to the molecule. In addition, post-translational alteration of the glycosylation of the TSH molecule occurs, which influences TSH bioactivity (53).

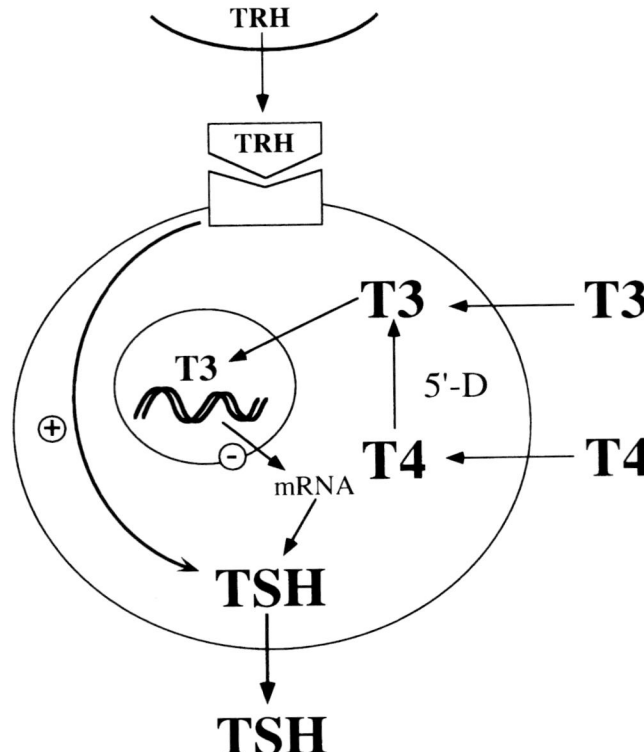

FIG. 5. Regulation of TSH release from the thyrotroph. Note that the nuclear T_3 arises from local T_4 to T_3 conversion in the cell.

The circulating TSH level reflects the net of the negative influence of thyroid hormone and the positive stimulation of TRH on TSH synthesis and release from the thyrotroph (50). Whereas peripheral tissues rely on circulating T_3, the thyrotroph depends on the local generation of T_3 from T_4 for its thyroid hormone needs. Larsen and colleagues (55) have estimated that 50% of nuclear T_3 arises from local conversion of T_4 catalyzed by a unique type II 5′-D within the thyrotroph, and 50% comes directly from the circulation (Fig. 5). This contrasts with peripheral tissues, where at least 80% of the nuclear T_3 is derived from serum. In the thyrotroph, binding of T_3 to the β2 thyroid hormone receptor initially decreases the synthesis of the β-subunit of TSH and eventually reduces the production of the α-subunit (56). Countering this negative influence of T_3 on the thyrotroph is the stimulatory effect of TRH on TSH biosynthesis. The TRH tone at the thyrotroph is also influenced by thyroid hormone as T_3 decreases TRH generation in the hypothalamus (54). A reduction in the nuclear content of T_3 diminishes this negative influence and promotes TSH synthesis and release by the thyrotroph. Other neurotransmitters and hormones (i.e., dopamine, somatostatin, and glucocorticoids), all of which have inhibitory actions on TSH

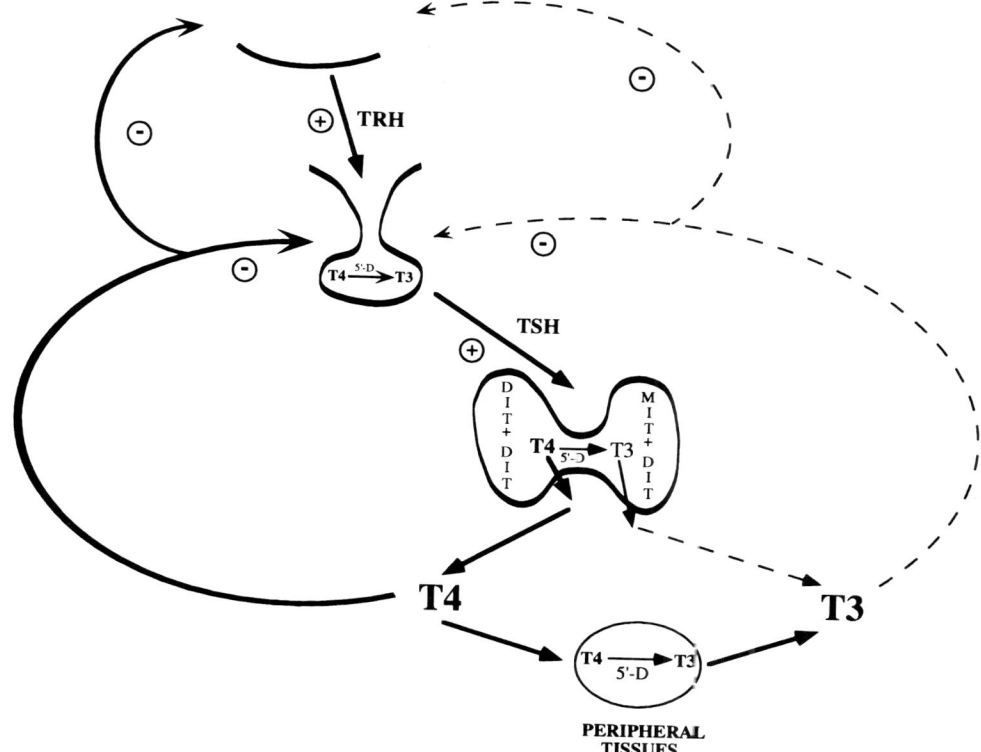

FIG. 6. Integrated thyroid axis in humans.

synthesis and release, can also influence the production of TSH and likely play a role in the fine-tuning of serum TSH levels (50).

Coordinating the function of the thyroid gland (synthesis and secretion of T_4) and the peripheral metabolism of thyroid hormone (generation and regulation of circulating T_3) occurs at the level of the pituitary gland. The dependence of the anterior pituitary on the circulating T_4 concentration for its primary source of T_3 is key to integrating the thyroid axis in humans. Having the thyrotroph sense changes in the free T_4 level, and altering TSH synthesis and release accordingly (drop in T_4 and increase in TSH or rise in T_4 and decrease in TSH), ensures that the proper amount of T_4 is produced by the thyroid gland to sustain a normal free circulating T_4 concentration. This, in turn, assures that there is an adequate supply of T_4 to the peripheral tissues to generate the active thyroid hormone, T_3, and maintain the thyroid status appropriate for the health of the individual (Fig. 6).

ACKNOWLEDGMENTS

This study was supported by grant DK-11721 and General Clinical Research Centers Program grant M01-RR-43 from the National Institutes of Health.

REFERENCES

1. Dunn JT, VanderHaar F. *A practical guide to the correction of iodine deficiency.* International Council for Control of Iodine Deficiency Disorders, 1990.
2. Roti E, Vagenakis AG. Effect of excess iodide: clinical aspects. In: Braverman LE, Utiger RD, eds. *The thyroid: a fundamental and clinical text*, 6th ed. Philadelphia: JB Lippincott, 1991;390–402.
3. Chambard M, Verrier B, Gabrian J, Mauchamp J. Polarization of thyroid cells in culture: evidence for the basalateral localization of the iodide "pump" and the thyroid-stimulating hormone receptor-adenylcyclase complex. *J Cell Biol* 1983;96:1172–1177.
4. Wolff J. Congenital goiter with defective iodide transport. *Endocr Rev* 1983;4:240–254.
5. Arima T, Spiro MJ, Spiro RG. Studies of the carbohydrate units of thyroglobulin. Evaluation of their microheterogeneity in the human and calf proteins. *J Biol Chem* 1972;247:1825–1835.
6. Avvedimento VE, DiLauro R, Monticelli A, et al. Mapping of human thyroglobulin gene on the long arm of chromosome 8 by in situ hybridization. *Hum Genet* 1985;71:163–166.
7. Vassart G, Dumont J. Identification of polysomes synthesizing thyroglobulin. *Eur J Biochem* 1973;32:332–330.
8. Roth J, Taatjes D, Lucocq J, et al. Demonstration of an extensive transtubular network continuous with the Golgi apparatus stack that may function in glycosylation. *Cell* 1985;43:287–295.
9. Ekholm R, Wollman SH. Site of iodination in the rat thyroid gland deduced from electron microscopic autoradiographs. *Endocrinology* 1975;97:1432–1443.
10. Taurog A. Thyroid peroxidase-catalyzed iodination of thyroglobulin: inhibition by excess iodide. *Arch Biochem Biophys* 1970;139:212–220.
11. Deme D, Pommier J, Nunez J. Kinetics of thyroglobulin iodination and of hormone synthesis catalyzed by thyroid peroxidase. Role of iodide in the coupling reaction. *Eur J Biochem* 1976;70:435–440.
12. Bjorkman U, Ekholm R, Denef J-F. Cytochemical localization of hy-

drogen peroxide in isolated thyroid follicles. *J Ultrastruct Res* 1981; 71:105–115.
13. Bernier-Valentin F, Kostrouch Z, Rabilloud R, et al. Coated vesicles from thyroid cells carry iodinated thyroglobulin molecules. First indication for an internalization of the thyroid prohormone via a mechanism of receptor-mediated endocytosis. *J Biol Chem* 1990;265:17373–17380.
14. Kostrouch Z, Munari-Silem Y, Rajas F, et al. Thyroglobulin internalized by thyrocytes passes through early and late endosomes. *Endocrinology* 1991;129:2202–2211.
15. Dunn AD, Crutchfield HE, Dunn JT. Proteolytic processing of thyroglobulin by extracts of thyroid lysosomes. *Endocrinology* 1991;128: 3073–3080.
16. Tietze F, Kohn LD, Kohn AD, et al. Carrier-mediated transport of monoiodotyrosine out of thyroid cell lysosomes. *J Biol Chem* 1989; 264:4762–4765.
17. Ishii H, Inada M, Tanaka K, et al. Induction of outer and inner ring monodeiodinases in human thyroid gland by thyrotropin. *J Clin Endocrinol Metab* 1983;57:500–505.
18. Schussler GC. Thyroxine-binding proteins. *Thyroid* 1990;1:25–34.
19. Engler D, Burger AG. The deiodination of the iodothyronines and their derivatives in man. *Endocr Rev* 1984;5:151–184.
20. Benvenga S, Gregg RE, Robbins J. Binding of thyroid hormone to human plasma lipoproteins. *J Clin Endocrinol Metab* 1988;67:6–16.
21. Marshall JS, Pensky J. Studies on thyroxine-binding globulin (TBG) III. Some physical characteristics of TBG and its interaction with thyroxine. *Arch Biochem Biophys* 1971;146:76–83.
22. Trent JM, Flink IL, Morkin E, et al. Localization of the human thyroxine-binding globulin gene to the long arm of the X chromosome (Nq21-22). *Am J Hum Genet* 1987;41:428–435.
23. Hocman G. Human thyroxine binding globulin. *Rev Physiol Biochem Pharmacol* 1981;81:428–435.
24. Ain KB, Refetoff S. Relationship of oligosaccharide modification to the cause of serum thyroxine binding globulin excess. *J Clin Endocrinol Metab* 1988;66:1037–1043.
25. Webster JB, Coupal JJ, Cushman P Jr. Increased serum thyroxine levels in euthyroid narcotic addicts. *J Clin Endocrinol Metab* 1973;37: 928–934.
26. McKerron CG, Scott RL, Asper SP, Levy RI. Effects of clofibrate (Atromid S) on the thyroxine-binding capacity of thyroxine-binding globulin and free thyroxine. *J Clin Endocrinol Metab* 1969;29:957–961.
27. Beex L, Ross A, Smals P Kloppenborg P. 5-Fluorouracil-induced increase of total thyroxine and triiodothyronine. *Cancer Treat Rep* 1977; 61:1291–1295.
28. Cashin-Hemphill L, Spencer CA, Nicoloff JT, et al. Alterations in serum thyroid hormonal indices with colestipol-niacin therapy. *Ann Intern Med* 1987;107:324–329.
29. Schussler GC, Schaffner F, Karn F. Increased serum thyroid hormone binding and decreased free hormone in chronic active liver disease. *N Engl J Med* 1978;299:510–515.
30. Kalk WJ, Kew MC, Danilewitz MD, et al. Thyroxine binding globulin and thyroid function tests in patients with hepatocellular carcinoma. *Hepatology* 1982;2:72–76.
31. LoPresti JS, Fried JC, Spencer CA, Nicoloff JT. Unique alterations of thyroid hormone indices in AIDS. *Ann Intern Med* 1989;110:970–975.
32. Burr WA, Ramsden DB, Hofenberg R. Hereditary abnormalities of thyroxine-binding globulin concentration. *Q J Med* 1980;49:295–313.
33. Bellabarba D, Inada M, Varsano-Aharon N, Sterling K. Thyroxine transport and turnover in major nonthyroidal illness. *J Clin Endocrinol Metab* 1968;28:1023–1030.
34. Robbins J, Rall JE, Petermann ML. Thyroxine-binding by serum and urine proteins in nephrosis. Qualitative aspects. *J Clin Invest* 1957;36: 1333–1342.
35. Oppenheimer JH, Werner SC. Effect of prednisone on thyroxine-binding proteins. *J Clin Endocrinol Metab* 1966;26:714–721.
36. Federman DD, Robbins J, Rall JE. Effects of methyltestosterone on thyroid function, thyroxine metabolism and thyroxine-binding protein. *J Clin Invest* 1958;37:1024–1030.
37. Pages RA, Robbins J, Edelhoch H. Binding of thyroxine and thyroxine analogs to human serum prealbumin. *Biochemistry* 1973;12:2773–2779.
38. Tabachnick M, Giorgio NA Jr. Thyroxine–protein interactions. II. The binding of thyroxine and its analogues to human serum albumin. *Arch Biochem Biophys* 1964;104:563–569.
39. Nicoloff JT, Low JC, Dussault JH, Fisher DA. Simultaneous measurement of thyroxine and triiodothyronine peripheral turnover kinetics in man. *J Clin Invest* 1972;51:473–483.
40. LoPresti JS, Eigen A, Kaptein E, et al. Alterations in 3,3′,5′-triiodothyronine metabolism in response to propylthiouracil, dexamethasone, and thyroxine administration in man. *J Clin Invest* 1989;84:1650–1656.
41. LoPresti JS, Anderson KP, Nicoloff JT. Does a hidden pool of reverse triiodothyronine (rT3) production contribute to total thyroxine (T4) disposal in high T3 states in man. *J Clin Endocrinol Metab* 1990;70: 1479.
42. Kohrle J, Hesch D. Leonard JL. Intracellular pathways of iodothyronine metabolism. In: Braverman LE, Utiger RD, eds. The thyroid. A fundamental and clinical text. Philadelphia: JB Lippincott, 1991;144–189.
43. Berry MJ, Larsen PR. The role of selenium in thyroid hormone action. *Endocr Rev* 1992;13:207–219.
44. LoPresti JS, Nicoloff JT. Triiodothyronine sulfate (T3S): a major regulator of T3 metabolism in man. *J Clin Endocrinol Metab* 1994;78: 688–692.
45. Mendel CM. The free hormone hypothesis: a physiologically based mathematical model. *Endocr Rev* 1989;10:232.
46. Docter R, Krenning EP, Bernard HF, Hennemann G. Active transport of iodothyronines into human cultured fibroblasts. *J Clin Endocrinol Metab* 1987;65:624.
47. Brent GA, Moore DA, Larsen PR. Thyroid hormone regulation of gene expression. *Ann Rev Physiol* 1991;53:17–35.
48. Refetoff S. Thyroid hormone resistance syndromes. In: *The thyroid*, 6th ed. Philadelphia: JB Lippincott, 1991;1280–1294.
49. LoPresti JS, Nicoloff JT. Nonthyroidal illnesses. In: Endocrinology, 3rd ed. Philadelphia: WB Saunders, 1995;665–675.
50. Marley TE. Neuroendocrine control of thyrotropin secretion. *Endocr Rev* 1989;2:396–436.
51. Haigler E, Putman J, Hershman J, Baugh C. Direct evaluation of pituitary thyrotropin reserve utilizing synthetic thyrotropin releasing hormone. *J Clin Endocrinol Metab* 1991;33:573–581.
52. Shupnik MA, Greenspan SL, Ridgeway EC. Transcriptional regulation of thyrotropin subunit genes by thyrotropin-releasing hormone and dopamine in pituitary cell cultures. *J Biol Chem* 1986;261: 12675–12679.
53. Beck-Peccoz P, Amr S, Menezes-Ferreira M, Faglia G, Weintraub B. Decreased receptor binding of biologically inactive thyrotropin in central hypothyroidism: effect of treatment with thyrotropin-releasing hormone. *N Engl J Med* 1985;312:1085–1089.
54. Kakucska I, Rand W, Lechan RM. Thyrotropin-releasing hormone gene expression in hypothalamic paraventricular nucleus is dependent upon feedback regulation by both triiodothyronine and thyroxine. *Endocrinology* 1992;130:2845–2850.
55. Larsen PR, Silva JE, Kaplan MM. Relationship between circulating and intracellular thyroid hormones: physiological and clinical implication. *Endocr Rev* 1981;2:87–107.
56. Shupnik MA, Ridgway EC. Thyroid hormone controls thyrotropin gene expression in rat anterior pituitary cells. *Endocrinology* 1987; 121:619–628.
57. Croteau W, Davey JC, Galton VA, St. Germain DL. Cloning of the mammalian type II deiodinase. A selenoprotein differentially expressed and regulated in human and rat brain and other tissues. *J Clin Invest* 1996;98:405–417.

CHAPTER 4

Clinical Approach to Thyroid Function Testing

Peter A. Singer

Thyroid disorders are among the most common conditions encountered in clinical practice. Because of subtle clinical features associated with some forms of thyroid dysfunction, the clinician must decide which test (or tests) is best suited to diagnose or exclude a disorder. Nowadays, in the era of cost containment and evolving diagnostic and treatment guidelines, the physician may actually be limited in his or her ability to choose among available tests. The purpose of this chapter is to describe currently available thyroid tests (Table 1) and to discuss their utility in diagnosing and managing individuals with thyroid abnormalities.

IN VITRO TESTS OF THYROID FUNCTION

Serum Total Thyroxine

Since the development of highly specific and sensitive radioimmunoassays for circulating thyroxine (T_4) in the early 1970s by Chopra and associates (1), radioimmunoassay has remained the standard method for measuring serum total T_4, although nonisotopic methods are also employed. Previous methods, none of which are used today, included the protein-bound iodine (PBI) test, the butanol extractable iodine (BEI) test, and T_4 measurement by column or by competitive protein binding. The serum total T_4 is the most commonly requested thyroid function test, and it is often used as a "screen" for thyrometabolic status (2). Although the serum total T_4 measurement generally reflects the functional status of the thyroid gland, a number of factors may alter total T_4 levels without changing the individual's thyrometabolic status. The most common of these, in the ambulatory individual, is a change in concentration of thyroxine-binding globulin (TBG). High or low TBG states with their respective increases and decreases in total T_4 concentrations do not affect metabolic status.

Elevated serum total T_4 levels with euthyroidism are also seen in familial dysalbuminemic hyperthyroxinemia, an autosomal dominant disorder characterized by preferential binding of T_4 to an abnormal serum albumin (3). Serum total triiodothyronine (T_3) levels remain normal, and individuals with this disorder are euthyroid, as reflected by normal serum free T_4 and thyroid-stimulating hormone (TSH) levels.

Elevated total T_4 levels may also occur when there is production of endogenous antibodies to T_4, especially in patients with Hashimoto's thyroiditis or other autoimmune disorders, and also occasionally in patients with Waldenstrom's macroglobulinemia associated with a benign monoclonal gammopathy (4).

Another condition of elevated total T_4 levels is peripheral resistance to thyroid hormone, first described by Refetoff and associates (5). Individuals with this condition may have goiter, and they may also be hyperactive in behavior. Also, in contrast to other conditions of hyperthyroxinemia with a normal thyrometabolic state, serum free T_4 levels are also elevated. Nevertheless, patients with this disorder are euthyroid. This genetic disorder, although rare, has led to inappropriately treating for hyperthyroidism.

Nonthyroidal illnesses (NTI) also may be associated with elevated serum total T_4 levels. As many as 20% of patients admitted to psychiatric hospitals have been noted to have mildly elevated serum T_4 levels (6). Hyperemesis gravidarum is also frequently associated with elevated serum total T_4 levels (7). In states of NTI associated with high total T_4 concentrations, the levels usually return to normal within days to a few weeks.

Nonthyroidal illness may also be associated with low serum total T_4, especially in patients with significant ill-

P. A. Singer: Department of Medicine, Division of Endocrinology, Diabetes, and Hypertension, University of Southern California School of Medicine, Los Angeles, California 90033.

TABLE 1. Commercially available thyroid function tests

In vitro tests	In vivo tests
Tests of thyroid function	Radioactive iodine uptake test (RAIU)
Total thyroxine (T$_4$, TT$_4$)	Thyrotropin-releasing hormone test (TRH)
Total triiodothyronine (T$_3$, TT$_3$)	Perchlorate discharge test[b]
Free thyroxine (FT$_4$)	Triiodothyronine (T$_3$) suppression test[b]
Free triiodothyronine (FT$_3$)[a]	
Triiodothyronine resin uptake test (T$_3$RU)	
Free thyroxine (or free triiodothyronine) index (FT$_4$I, FT$_3$I)	
Reverse triiodothyronine (rT$_3$)[a]	
Thyrotropin (TSH)	
Serologic tests for specific disorders	
Antimicrosomal antibodies (AMA)	
Antithyroglobulin antibodies (ATA)	
Thyroid-stimulating antibodies (TsAb)	
Endogenous antibodies to T$_4$ and T$_3$[a]	
Thyroglobulin (Tg)	
Calcitonin (CT)	

[a]Infrequently used.
[b]Outmoded, but available.

nesses (8). Following recovery, serum total T$_4$ levels return to normal (9).

Table 2 lists the causes of euthyroid hyperthyroxinemia. It is important to recognize these disorders to avoid unnecessary and inappropriate treatment.

Thus it should be emphasized that there are pitfalls in relying on the serum total T$_4$ as a completely reliable index of thyroid status.

Free T$_4$ Measurements and Estimates

The gold standard of thyrometabolic status is measurement of serum free T$_4$ (FT$_4$) by equilibrium dialysis (10). When measured by the dialysis method, the free T$_4$ is not affected by changes in binding protein concentrations, or by nonthyroidal illness. Unfortunately, the equilibrium dialysis method is cumbersome and expensive, and it is therefore not routinely performed. Commercial FT$_4$ levels are most commonly measured by immunoassay techniques, but their reliability is less than optimal, because they may be affected by illness or significant changes in binding proteins (11,12). Thus, the clinical usefulness of free T$_4$ measurements by any method may be limited (13).

Although thyrometabolic status is best reflected by the free T$_4$ level, from a clinical point of view, an estimate (or index) of free T$_4$ is generally adequate. The free T$_4$ index is obtained by multiplying the serum total T$_4$ and an indirect assessment of TBG. Serum TBG is generally estimated by either of two methods, one termed the thyroid uptake test (TU) and the other, the T$_3$ uptake test (T$_3$U) (14). The free T$_4$ index (FT$_4$I) is calculated by taking the quotient of the total T$_4$ and TU, or by the product of the T$_4$ and T$_3$U. The TU is directly proportional to TBG levels in serum, whereas the T$_3$U is inversely proportional to TBG levels (15). The result, using either method, is that variances in serum TBG levels are largely eliminated and the calculated FT$_4$I accurately reflects actual free T$_4$ status. For example, if the T$_3$U is employed, the FT$_4$I may be calculated as follows: FT$_4$I = T$_4$ · (T$_3$U$_{measured}$/T$_3$U$_{mean\ normal}$).

The normal range of T$_3$U may be 25% to 35%; therefore, the mean normal would be 30%. It should be noted that extreme changes in TBG levels, or the presence of severe nonthyroidal illness, may result in poor correlation between calculated and measured FT$_4$ levels.

Serum Total Triiodothyronine

Triiodothyronine (T$_3$) is measured in serum by radioimmunoassay. Like T$_4$, T$_3$ is bound to TBG, although less avidly. Nevertheless, alterations in TBG levels result

TABLE 2. Hyperthyroxinemia without hyperthyroidism

	Serum hormone levels					
Condition	T$_4$	FT$_4$I	FT$_4$	T$_3$	FT$_3$I	TSH
TBG excess	↑	n	n	↑	n	n
Acute nonthyroidal illness[a]	↑	↑	↑,n	↓,n	↓,n	n
Abnormal binding to albumin	↑	↑	n	n	n	n
Increased TBPA	↑	↑	n	n	n	n
Medications[b]	↑	↑	n,↑	n,↓	n,↓	n
Peripheral resistance to thyroid hormone	↑	↑	↑	↑	↑	n,↑
Endogenous antibodies to T$_4$[c]	↑	↑	n	n	n	n

[a]Usually mild and transient.
[b]See Table 3.
[c]Usually associated with Hashimoto's thyroiditis.
Abbreviations: T$_4$, thyroxine; FT$_4$I, free thyroxine index; FT$_4$, free thyroxine; T$_3$, triiodothyronine; FT$_3$I, free triiodothyronine index; TSH, thyrotropin; TBG, thyroxine-binding globulin; TBPA, thyroxine-binding prealbumin; ↑, elevated; ↓, decreased; n, normal or unchanged.

in changes in total T_3 (but not free T_3) concentrations. Therefore, as with serum T_4, an estimate (or index) of free T_3 may be obtained by employing the same formula used in calculating the FT_4I.

Because the majority of T_3 is derived from peripheral metabolism of T_4, clinical states or pharmacologic agents that impair normal T_4 metabolism result in lower total T_3 levels (Table 3).

The principal uses for obtaining the serum T_3 are to determine the severity of hyperthyroidism, and to confirm the diagnosis of suspected thyrotoxicosis in which serum T_4 levels are normal or equivocal. In addition, the serum T_3 may be indicated in evaluating patients with autonomously functioning thyroid adenomas, where so-called T_3 toxicosis may be present. Such patients may have normal or borderline elevated serum T_4 levels, along with suppressed serum TSH levels (16).

There is no role for measuring serum T_3 levels as a screen of thyroid function, or as an index of the degree of severity of hypothyroidism (17).

Serum Thyrotropin

The development of the first serum thyroid-stimulating hormone (TSH), or thyrotropin, assay by Odell and colleagues (18) in 1965 was a major advance in the assessment of thyroid function, because it demonstrated that individuals with primary hypothyroidism had elevated serum levels of TSH. The ability to measure TSH resulted in the virtual elimination of the cumbersome and often painful TSH-stimulation test for the diagnosis of hypothyroidism. Although early assays for TSH by radioimmunoassay were capable of detecting elevated serum TSH levels in patients with primary hypothyroidism, they were often unsuitable for accurately measuring TSH in euthyroid or hyperthyroid individuals. Within several years, more sensitive assays for TSH were developed, and, with these, the majority of euthyroid individuals had detectable TSH, so that by the early 1970s the serum TSH became the standard for distinguishing hypothyroid patients from euthyroid individuals. The functional sensitiv-

TABLE 3. *Effects of drugs on thyroid function*

Drug and site of action	Serum hormone level				Comment
	T_4	FT_4	T_3	TSH	
Hypothalamic-pituitary axis					
Dopamine	↓	↓	↓	∨	
L-dopa	n	n	n	n	TSH changes seen only in hypothyroidism
Metoclopramide	n	n	n	n	Transient TSH changes
Amphetamines	↑	↑	↑,n	↑	Transient effects
Glucocorticoids	n	n	n	↓	Central effects on TSH mild
Synthesis and/or release of thyroid hormone					
Methimazole, propylthiouracil	↓	↓	↓	↑	Antithyroid drugs
Sulfonamides, sulfonylureas, ketoconazole, phenylbutazine	↓	↓	↓	↑	
Lithium carbonate	↓	↓	↓	↑	Usually with Hashimoto's thyroiditis
Iodides	↓	↓	↓	↑	Usually with Hashimoto's thyroiditis
Iodides	↑	↑	↑	↓	Usually with underlying nodular goiter
Binding protein changes					
Estrogens, clofibrate, perphenazine, heroin, methadone	↑	n	↑	n	Increased TBG
Androgens, danazole, glucocorticoids, L-asparaginase	↓	n	↓	n	Decreased TBG
Phenytoin, fenclofenac, phenylbutazone, salicylates	↓	n	↓	n	Salicylates may ↑ FT_4 slightly
Thyroid hormone metabolism					
Propylthiouracil, glucocorticoids, propranolol	n	n	↓	n	Peripheral inhibition of T_4 to T_3; propranolol may decrease cell uptake of T_4 resulting in ↑ T_4
Amiodarone, iopanoic acid, ipodate	↑	↑	↓	↑	Peripheral and pituitary inhibition of T_4 to T_3; ipodate (and possibly amiodarone) decreases cell uptake of T_4
Heparin	n,↑	n,↑	n	n	Displace T_4 from TBG, and decrease cell uptake of T_4 effects minor, and after IV bolus of heparin
Phenytoin, rifampin, phenobarbital	↓	↓	n	n,↑	Accelerate T_4 disposal; ↑ TBG in L-T_4-treated hypothyroidism
Gastrointestinal absorption					
Cholestyramine, cholestipol, soybean flour	↓	↓	↓	↑	Inhibition of L-T_4 absorption; effects only in L-T_4-treated patients

Abbreviations: ↑, elevated; ↓, decreased; n, unchanged; T_4, thyroxine; FT_4, free thyroxine; T_3, triiodothyronine; TSH, thyroid-stimulating hormone (thyrotropin).

ity of such early assays, however, did not allow for differentiation between hyperthyroidism and euthyroidism. Subsequent assays of the 1970s, however, were more sensitive, in that euthyroid individuals rarely had TSH levels below normal, and virtually all hyperthyroid patients had suppressed TSH concentrations (19,20). Despite these improvements in TSH assays, their clinical usefulness was limited because they were complex to perform, and they had a relatively lengthy "turnaround" time. While relatively sensitive, they were not generally available to clinicians.

Recent Developments in TSH Assays

Until 10 years ago, nearly all clinical TSH assays were performed by radioimmunoassay. By the mid 1980s, many commercial laboratories began using more sensitive immunometric TSH methods, with either monoclonal or polyclonal antibodies. The functional sensitivity of such assays was 0.1 mU/L, tenfold more sensitive than radioimmunoassay methodology. For the first time, measurement of serum TSH allowed the differentiation between hyperthyroid and euthyroid individuals (21,22). Because of the greater sensitivity provided by immunometric methods, TSH terminology has changed, and the term *sensitive* TSH emerged (23).

In recent years, nonisotopic immunometric TSH assays have been developed, using a chemiluminescent label. These newer assays have a functional sensitivity of 0.01 mu/L, which is 10 times greater than the previously most "sensitive" TSH, and 100 times more sensitive than radioimmunoassay methods. TSH assays with a sensitivity of 0.01 mu/L are currently termed *third generation,* and an increasing number of commercial and hospital laboratories are using this assay (24).

Clinical Applications of TSH Assays

1. *To diagnose primary hypothyroidism.* The presence of an elevated TSH is confirmation of primary hypothyroidism. The degree of hypothyroidism should be assessed by obtaining a serum T_4. TSH levels are also elevated in patients with subclinical hypothyroidism, in which serum total T_4 is normal or borderline low.

2. *To assess thyroid hormone replacement therapy.* The goal of treatment of primary hypothyroidism with levothyroxine is normalization of both serum T_4 and TSH levels. Current TSH assays can detect over-replacement with levothyroxine, because TSH concentrations will be low. This has clinical relevance, inasmuch as current evidence suggests that patients with suppressed TSH levels, even in the presence of normal serum T_4 levels, may experience disproportionate loss of bone mineral content. This appears to be especially so in postmenopausal women (25–27). In addition, chronic over-replacement with levothyroxine may be associated with cardiac abnormalities, including supraventricular arrhythmias and ventricular septal hypertrophy (28,29).

3. *To assess TSH suppression in thyroid cancer.* Thyroid-suppressive therapy is part of the routine management of certain patients with well-differentiated (papillary and follicular) thyroid carcinoma, because growth of these tumors may be TSH responsive (30). Treatment with levothyroxine is titrated to suppress TSH while attempting to avoid clinical hyperthyroidism. The availability of third-generation TSH measurements has rendered this task much simpler than before, because previous TSH suppression could be confirmed only by demonstrating the absence of serum TSH response to exogenous thyrotropin-releasing hormone (TRH) administration. With few exceptions, suppressed TSH levels, when measured in third-generation assays, correlate with absent TSH responses (31).

4. *To assess suppressive therapy of nodular goiter.* TSH measurements are useful for following patients with either solitary or multinodular goiter, in whom suppressive thyroid hormone therapy is sometimes employed. Although the efficacy of levothyroxine suppression for benign goiter is not universally accepted, it still is frequently employed (32). Hence, it is important to have accurate TSH measurements to avoid excess dosing.

5. *For diagnosis of subclinical hyperthyroidism.* Patients with few or equivocal symptoms and signs of hyperthyroidism, with normal or borderline elevated total T_4 and total T_3 levels, and with suppressed serum TSH levels have subclinical hyperthyroidism (33). Before the advent of sensitive TSH assays, such individuals usually went undiagnosed. Current evidence suggests that such individuals, especially those past 60 years of age, have a fourfold greater risk of developing cardiac arrhythmias, especially atrial fibrillation (29).

Pitfalls of TSH Measurements

There are a number of conditions in which the serum TSH does not accurately reflect thyrometabolic status. The clinician needs to be aware of these states to avoid making incorrect conclusions, to initiate therapy where necessary, and to avoid treatment if unnecessary.

1. *Nonthyroidal illness ("sick euthyroid" syndrome).* Although the serum total T_4 and free T_4 index may be abnormal in patients with nonthyroidal illness, the serum TSH unfortunately may fail to clarify the thyroid status in a significant proportion of patients. Spencer and colleagues (34) have shown that approximately 10% of euthyroid patients admitted to the hospital have abnormal TSH levels (two thirds low, one third elevated). Of individuals with markedly suppressed TSH levels, the majority were being treated with either pharmacologic doses of glucocorticoids or dopamine, both of which are inhibitors

of TSH (see later). In the group with elevated TSH levels, those with nonthyroidal illness had normal serum total T_4 levels. Once clinical recovery occurs, TSH levels return to normal (35). The clinical importance is that abnormal serum TSH levels must be interpreted with caution in hospitalized patients, and the serum TSH should not be employed as the only thyroid function test in such circumstances.

2. *Changing thyroid status.* Thyroid status must be stable for the serum TSH to be considered reliable. Although a suppressed TSH level is indicative of hyperthyroidism in the untreated individual, patients who are being treated with antithyroid drugs, or those who have undergone thyroid ablation with radioactive iodine for hyperthyroidism, may exhibit suppressed TSH levels for several months after serum T_4 and T_3 have reached normal or subnormal levels; this reflects prolonged suppression of the hypothalamic–pituitary–thyroid axis (36,37). A similar phenomenon may occur in patients who had previously been taking supraphysiologic doses of thyroid hormone (38).

Hypothyroid patients recently begun on levothyroxine therapy also may have discordant serum TSH and T_4 levels because of the delay in fall of TSH after initiation of therapy. Thus, normal serum T_4 and elevated TSH levels, after a month or so of therapy, would not necessarily reflect underreplacement with levothyroxine (39). This underscores the recommendation that dose changes should be made no more frequently than every 6 to 8 weeks unless the clinical situation dictates otherwise (40).

In addition to the discrepancies in TSH and T_4 levels observed with recent initiation of treatment of hypothyroidism, variable compliance with taking levothyroxine may also give misleading results. Patients who take medication intermittently, or who take it consistently for only a few weeks prior to an office visit, may have a relatively normal serum T_4, and elevated serum TSH levels.

3. *Central hypothyroidism.* Hypothyroidism due to either hypothalamic or pituitary disease (central, or secondary hypothyroidism) is characterized by low serum T_4 and normal TSH levels (41). Therefore, relying on the serum TSH to screen for possible hypothyroidism in such patients would result in a failure to make the correct diagnosis. Fortunately, most individuals with central hypothyroidism exhibit additional hormonal manifestations of pituitary insufficiency, or have symptoms of a mass effect (such as visual acuity or visual field abnormalities), decreasing the likelihood that the diagnosis would be overlooked.

4. *Hyperthyroidism associated with inappropriate TSH secretion.*
   a. TSH-secreting pituitary tumor. Serum TSH levels are elevated or inappropriately normal in patients with hyperthyroidism due to TSH-producing tumors (42). Although such lesions are rare, comprising only approximately 0.5% of all pituitary tumors, it is important to be aware of this disorder. TSH-producing tumors are typically macroadenomas, resulting in mass-effect symptoms, and therefore they are usually diagnosed. Nevertheless, inappropriate treatment for Graves' disease or other forms of hyperthyroidism does occur in patients in whom TSH levels are not initially obtained.
   b. Central resistance to thyroid hormone. This rare genetic disorder is characterized by elevated serum T_4 and T_3 and inappropriately normal, or mildly elevated, TSH concentrations (43). As with patients with TSH-producing pituitary tumors, awareness of this disorder will avoid inappropriate therapy. Patients with this disorder can be differentiated from patients with TSH-producing tumors, because the latter have elevated serum levels of the alpha subunit (44).

Can the Serum TSH be used as a "Screening" Thyroid Function Test?

The fact that the serum TSH is abnormal in both hypothyroidism and hyperthyroidism would seem to make it ideally suited as a screen of thyroid status, because, with rare exceptions, a normal TSH level would suggest normal thyroid hormone homeostasis. Indeed, experience in ambulatory individuals suggests that a normal TSH virtually excludes the possibility of thyroid dysfunction (45). Also, the serum TSH is more sensitive than the serum T_4 as a test for thyroid dysfunction, because the TSH can detect subclinical thyroid disorders, in which serum total T_4 (and T_3) are usually normal. Thus, as a result of advances in TSH methodology, serum measurements of thyroid hormones may become relegated to the "second line" in the assessment of suspected thyroid dysfunction. Although some experts have suggested that measurement of serum total T_4 and/or the FT_4I may be as useful as the serum TSH as a screen of thyroid status (2), others feel that the serum TSH is preferable (40,46). Figure 1 shows a suggested algorithm for using the TSH in the evaluation of thyroid function. In addition, Figure 2 depicts how changes in free T_4 levels affect TSH concentrations.

When Should T_4 and T_3 Determinations Be Performed?

The above discussion is not intended to imply that measurements of total T_4 and T_3 are unnecessary in the evaluation of thyroid dysfunction. Indeed, the serum TSH does not correlate with degree of thyroid dysfunction. In clinical hyperthyroidism, the serum T_4 and T_3 provide complementary information as to the severity of the disorder, as does the serum T_4 in hypothyroidism. When hyperthyroidism is suspected, an estimate of the free T_4 is a reasonable first step in the evaluation (Fig. 3).

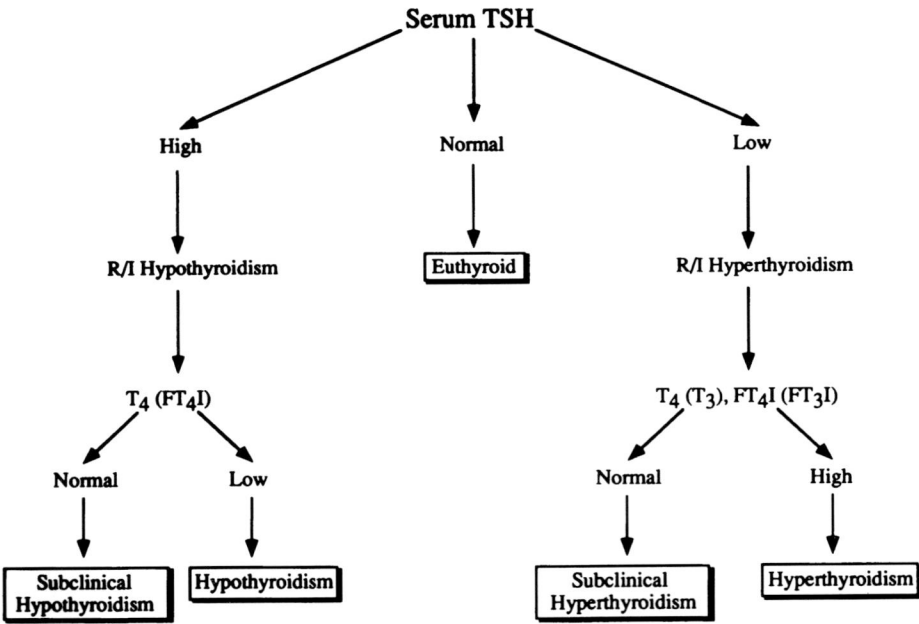

FIG. 1. Suggested algorithm for the use of the serum TSH as an outpatient screen for thyroid dysfunction. The serum TSH is also useful as an initial test when hypothyroidism is suspect. R/I, rule in.

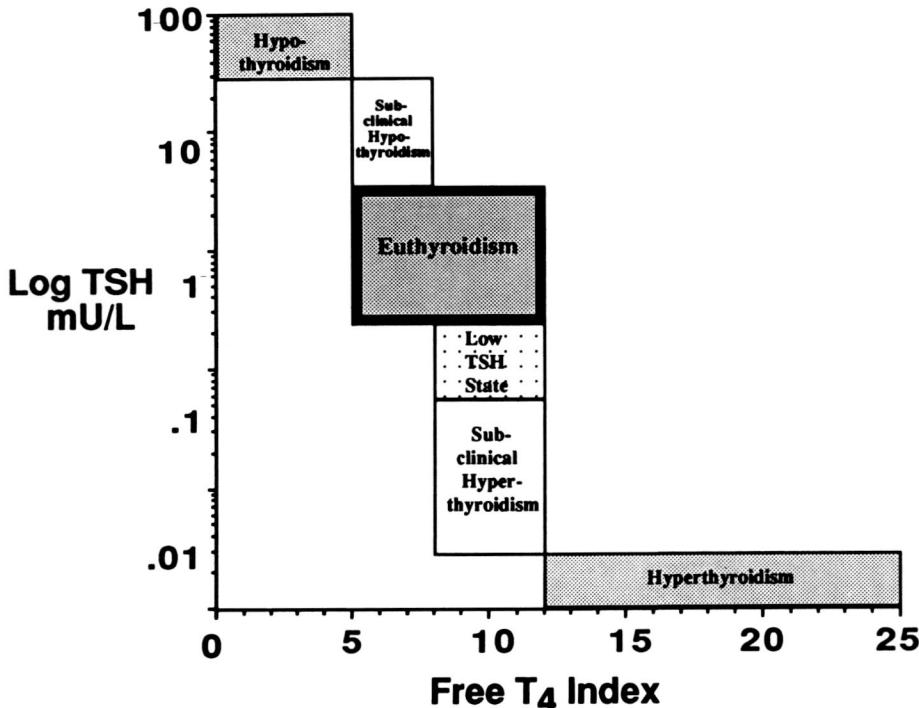

FIG. 2. The relationship between free T_4 and serum TSH is shown. Note that there is a clear separation of TSH values between euthyroidism and hyperthyroidism, or hypothyroidism. The low TSH state is more ill defined, and it may not represent a clinical disorder.

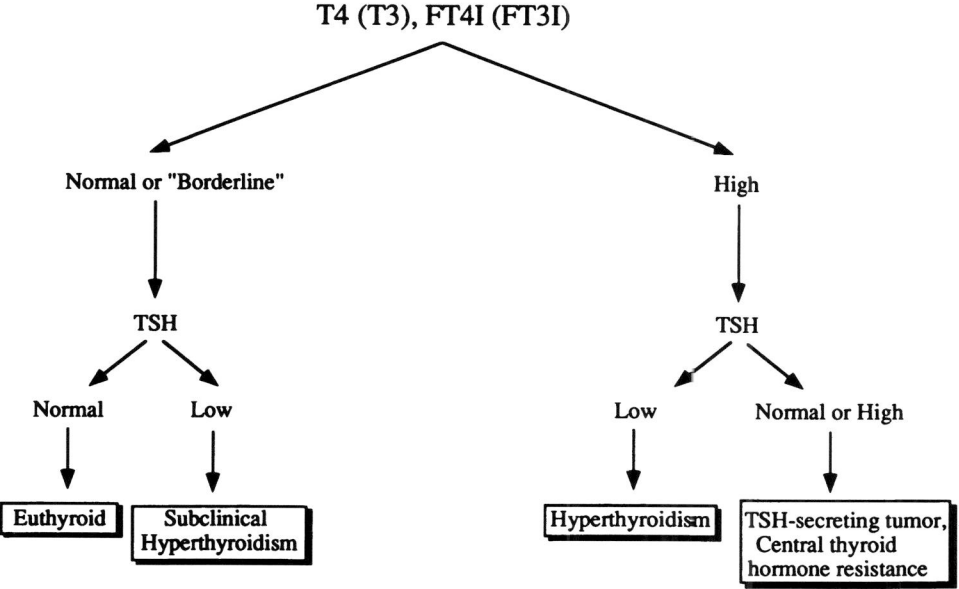

FIG. 3. Evaluation of suspected hyperthyroidism. When there is clinical suspicion for hyperthyroidism, an estimate of free T_4 (T_3) status may be the best initial test. The serum T_3 and FT_3I are optional, as indicated by parentheses. A low TSH implies TSH suppression. This schema does not differentiate between the various types of hyperthyroidism.

In addition, TSH values may not accurately reflect changing thyroid status during treatment of hyper- or hypothyroidism. Thus, measurement of serum thyroid hormone levels become necessary to evaluate thyroid status.

OTHER SEROLOGIC TESTS OF THYROID FUNCTION

Thyroid Antibodies

Circulating antithyroid antibodies, specifically antimicrosomal (AMA) and antithyroglobulin (ATA) antibodies, are usually present in patients with autoimmune thyroid disease (47). Until recently, hemagglutination techniques were employed for measuring antibodies, but much more sensitive immunoassay methods are currently being used. Since the introduction of immunoassay techniques, the term *antithyroperoxidase* (anti-TPO) has become interchangeable with AMA. Antimicrosomal antibodies are detectable in more than 90% of patients with chronic autoimmune thyroid disease, and nearly 100% of individuals with Hashimoto's thyroiditis and more than 80% of patients with Graves' disease have positive titers (48). Although antithyroglobulin antibodies are more specific than AMA, they are less sensitive, and therefore they are not as useful in the detection of autoimmune thyroid disease (49). Elevated levels of AMA are also frequently positive in a variety of other organ-specific autoimmune diseases, such as lupus erythematosus, rheumatoid arthritis, autoimmune pernicious anemia, Sjögren's syndrome, type I diabetes mellitus, and Addison's disease (50). In addition, elevated AMA levels are more prevalent in first-degree relatives of individuals with autoimmune thyroid disease (51).

Approximately 15% of adults (especially women) in the United States have elevated AMA titers (52). The prevalence of positive AMA titers increases with age, as does the incidence of primary hypothyroidism. The presence of a positive AMA titer should alert the clinician to the possibility of hypothyroidism. Individuals with positive AMA and elevated TSH levels, even with normal serum total T_4 levels (i.e., subclinical hypothyroidism), have a 3% to 5% per year likelihood of developing clinical hypothyroidism (52–55). Not only may measurements of AMA levels be useful in the diagnosis of individuals with suspected autoimmune thyroid disease, but they also may have prognostic value when used in conjunction with the serum TSH.

Thyroid-Stimulating Antibodies

The immune pathogenesis of Graves' disease was first suspected in the mid-1950s, when it was observed that injecting sera of Graves' patients into rats produced a prolonged uptake of radioactive iodine in the rat thyroid glands. Hence the term *LATS*, or long-acting thyroid stimulator, was coined (56). Later, LATS was characterized as a 7S immunoglobulin, and, in recent years, several assays have been developed for the detection of LATS, or thyroid-stimulating antibodies (TSAb). Two types of assays are commonly used—one dependent on generation of cyclic adenosine monophosphate (cAMP), and the other a radioreceptor method that relies on the TSH-binding inhibitory properties of the immunoglobulin. The cAMP-generating assay is termed thyroid-stimulating immunoglobulin (TSI), and it is detectable in 90% to 95% of hyperthyroid patients with Graves' disease. The other assay (dependent on TSH-binding inhibition) detects both stimulating and blocking antibodies. Termed TBII, it is detected in up to 85% of patients with hyperthyroid Graves' disease (44).

Thyroid-stimulating-antibody measurements are not indicated for the routine diagnostic evaluation of suspected Graves' disease, but they may be useful when the diagnosis of Graves' is not evident. Also, TSAb measurements may be helpful if the diagnosis of hyperthyroidism associated with pregnancy (in which radioactive iodine uptake tests are contraindicated) is not clear-cut. TSAb levels, especially with the TBII test, should also be obtained in patients with Graves' disease during pregnancy to help predict the possibility of neonatal thyrotoxicosis or hypothyroidism. Significantly elevated titers of TBII (i.e., greater than 70%) are associated with a greater likelihood of hyperthyroidism in the neonate (57).

Serum Thyroglobulin

Thyroglobulin (Tg) is elevated in the sera of patients with nearly all types of thyroid disorders, thus limiting its use as a diagnostic test (58). Its greatest clinical utility is in the management of patients with well-differentiated (papillary and follicular) thyroid carcinoma. An elevated or rising Tg level (after initial surgical and ablation therapy) suggests persistence or recurrence of tumor (59). Thyroglobulin is measured by radioimmunoassay or by immunometric techniques. Although antithyroid antibodies may cause interference with accurate Tg measurements in up to 10% of individuals, in such patients measurements of both Tg and anti-Tg antibodies can be used concurrently to provide information regarding the tumor status (59). The use of Tg measurements is discussed more fully in Chapter 30.

Serum Calcitonin

Calcitonin is a polypeptide secreted by the parafollicular (C) cells of the thyroid gland, and it is elevated in patients with medullary carcinoma of the thyroid (MTC). Calcitonin levels are used to follow patients with diagnosed MTC, and as an adjunct to screen family members of affected individuals with MTC (60). The clinical use of serum calcitonin measurement is discussed in greater detail in Chapter 32.

IN VIVO THYROID FUNCTION TESTS

Radioactive Iodine Uptake Test

The thyroidal radioactive iodine uptake (RAIU) test is performed by administering an isotope of iodine (usually ^{123}I) orally and then measuring the percentage of the ^{123}I trapped by the thyroid gland. The test is usually performed 24 hours after administration of the isotope, although it can be done earlier. Before the development of sensitive and specific assays for thyroid hormones, the RAIU was used as an adjunct to differentiate hyper- from hypothyroid states, with elevated and low RAIU values implying hyper- and hypothyroidism, respectively. Today, though, its principal utility is in differentiating hyperthyroidism into high or low uptake states. A more complete discussion of the RAIU is included in Chapter 8.

Thyrotropin-Releasing Hormone Test

Administration of synthetic TRH intravenously results in an increase in TSH concentrations in normal individuals. In states of thyroid hormone excess, exogenous TRH fails to elicit an increase in TSH. The principal uses of the TRH test had been to assess the degree of suppression of TSH, and to differentiate secondary (pituitary) from tertiary (hypothalamic) hypothyroidism (61). The availability of third-generation TSH assays has largely eliminated the need for TRH testing, because individuals with suppressed TSH levels do not respond to exogenous TRH (31). In those individuals in whom the TRH test is felt to be indicated, however, the test is done by obtaining a basal TSH level, and then TSH levels at 30 and 60 minutes after the IV injection of 200 to 500 mcg of synthetic TRH (Protirelin). The TSH response to TRH may be absent or blunted in patients with severe illness, advanced age (especially men), administration of corticosteroids or IV dopamine, or depression (62).

Triiodothyronine Suppression Test

The T_3 suppression test was traditionally used to test disorders associated with autonomous thyroid function, such as Graves' disease or hyperfunctioning thyroid adenomas. It is infrequently used nowadays, although it may still have some utility in individuals with suspected autonomous thyroid function.

The T_3 suppression test is performed by obtaining a baseline RAIU, and after 1 week of 75 to 100 mcg of oral T_3, the RAIU is repeated. Euthyroid individuals suppress the RAIU to less than 50% of baseline values, whereas autonomous function is characterized by a lack of suppression. The T_3 suppression test should probably be avoided in elderly individuals or those with suspected underlying heart disease, to avoid the possibility of precipitating angina pectoris or cardiac arrhythmia.

EFFECTS OF PHARMACOLOGIC AGENTS ON THYROID FUNCTION

Many drugs used in the treatment of nonthyroidal disease have either *in vitro* or *in vivo* effects on thyroid function. Pharmacologic agents may alter thyroid function at any of the following sites:

1. The hypothalamic–pituitary axis.
2. The thyroid gland.
3. Binding proteins.
4. Deiodinative sites.
5. The gastrointestinal tract.

This section will discuss commonly used agents that may have clinical effects. A more comprehensive list is included in Table 3.

Agents Affecting the Hypothalamic–Pituitary Axis

As mentioned earlier in this chapter, dopamine may play a minor role in the physiologic regulation of TSH secretion, and, when administered pharmacologically, it decreases TSH secretion (63). Although dopamine administration has little, if any, effect on T_4 and T_3 concentrations, its administration in patients with undiagnosed primary hypothyroidism might result in an incorrect diagnosis by virtue of its suppressive effect on TSH. Withdrawal of dopamine in hypothyroidism results in a return of TSH to previously elevated levels. Dopamine may also suppress TSH to undetectable levels in patients with severe NTI (64). Similarly, levodopa administration can cause a decrease in TSH levels in patients with primary hypothyroidism, but it does not alter T_4, FT_4, or T_3 levels (65). Metoclopramide hydrochloride, a dopamine antagonist commonly used in the treatment of patients with gastrointestinal disorders, may result in transient, albeit minor, increases in TSH levels (66).

Octreotide, a synthetic analog of somatostatin used for treatment of patients with acromegaly, decreases TSH concentrations but does not result in hypothyroidism. In general, the effects on TSH inhibition are not sustained over the duration of octreotide therapy (67).

Pharmacologic doses of glucocorticoids also lower serum TSH levels, but without resulting in hypothyroidism (68).

Amphetamine abuse may result in increased thyroid hormone levels, possibly related to an increase in TSH secretion (69). Patients abusing such stimulants often appear hypermetabolic, and their serum T_4 levels may be mildly increased, thus causing hyperthyroidism to be diagnosed erroneously. The effects of amphetamines on thyroid function are transient and relatively minor.

Agents Affecting the Thyroid Gland

Among the agents that directly affect the thyroid gland, iodides have the most important clinical effects (70). Iodides may produce either hypothyroidism (by inhibiting thyroid hormone release), or hyperthyroidism (by serving as a substrate for thyroid hormone biosynthesis) (71).

Patients with chronic autoimmune (Hashimoto's) thyroiditis are particularly sensitive to the inhibitory effects of iodides, whereas individuals with multinodular goiter, especially those coming to the United States from iodine-deficient areas, are more likely to become hyperthyroid when exposed to iodides (72).

Amiodarone, a potent antiarrhythmic agent that is 37% iodide (by weight), has been of particular interest to endocrinologists because of its diverse effects on clinical thyroid function In North America, hypothyroidism has been reported to occur in approximately 10% of patients taking amiodarone, especially in patients with underlying Hashimoto's thyroiditis, whereas iodide-induced hyperthyroidism appears to occur in only 1% to 2% of North American patients taking amiodarone (73,74). By contrast, in geographic areas of iodide deficiency, individuals taking amiodarone develop hypo- and hyperthyroidism at rates of approximately 2% to 3%, and 10%, respectively (75–77).

Even in the absence of underlying thyroid disease, amiodarone consistently alters serum thyroid hormone levels. Observed changes include elevations in serum T_4, FT_4, and the FT_4I, and lower total T_3 levels. Serum T_4 and FT_4 levels increase within 1 to 3 weeks after initiation of amiodarone treatment, reach a peak within 1 to 3 months, and remain increased throughout the duration of treatment (78). Approximately 40% of patients taking amiodarone have greater than normal serum T_4, FT_4, and FT_4I, all the while remaining in a euthyroid state, as evidenced by normal TSH concentrations (79). These changes probably occur because of the inhibitory effects of amiodarone on peripheral thyroid hormone metabolism (see later)

Lithium carbonate, which is used in the treatment of depression, inhibits thyroid hormone synthesis and release, and it may produce hypothyroidism in 15% to 50% of patients, especially in those with Hashimoto's thyroiditis (80,81). The mechanism of lithium's action is similar to that which occurs with iodides. Patients receiving lithium should be periodically monitored to detect hypothyroidism. Ketoconazole, a commonly employed agent known to affect adrenal steroid biosynthesis, has recently been reported to cause clinical hypothyroidism, probably by virtue of its inhibitory effects on thyroid hormone biosynthesis (82).

Hypothyroidism, as well as transient painless thyroiditis, has been reported to occur in patients receiving interleukin-2 for the treatment of neoplasms (83). Alpha interferon used for the treatment of hepatitis C is associated with the development of positive titers of AMA, as well as both transient hyper- or hypothyroidism (84–86). Thyroid autoantibodies were present in the majority of those who developed hypothyroidism, suggesting susceptibility in patients with underlying Hashimoto's thyroiditis.

Recently, adverse effects of cigarette smoking on thyroid function have been observed. Smoking may increase the severity of hypothyroidism in patients who already have the disease, by directly affecting both thyroid hormone synthesis and secretion, and perhaps also by inhibiting the peripheral action of thyroid hormone (87).

Agents Altering Metabolism and/or Cell Uptake of Thyroid Hormone

Propranolol (88), glucocorticoids (89), and the iodide-containing agents iopanoic acid and amiodarone (78) inhibit peripheral deiodination of T_4 to T_3, resulting in a reduction of serum T_3 levels. Iopanoic acid, ipodate, and amiodarone also inhibit intrapituitary T_4-to-T_3 conversion, resulting in a decrease of negative feedback on TSH secretion, and a small increase in serum TSH, T_4, and free T_4 levels. These agents have also been shown to cause an increase in serum total T_4 and free T_4 levels by interfering with cell uptake of T_4, an effect that has also been noted with large doses of propranolol (90).

Aminoglutethimide, a drug currently used as an adjunct in the treatment of breast, prostate, and adrenal carcinomas, may be associated with the development of primary hypothyroidism, possibly by inhibiting thyroxine synthesis. A recent study documented that 9 of 29 patients with prostate cancer treated with aminoglutethimide developed clinical and biochemical features of hypothyroidism (91).

Phenytoin, an agent that may affect thyroid function by several mechanisms, appears to enhance T_4 metabolism. Hypothyroid patients who take phenytoin therefore require a larger replacement dose of levothyroxine (92). This may also occur in patients taking other medications that increase the hepatic metabolism of thyroxine, including phenobarbital, carbamazepine, and the antituberculosis medication rifampin (93,94).

Agents Affecting Thyroid Binding Proteins

Pharmacologic agents may affect serum thyroid hormone levels either by altering the concentration of the binding proteins, or by inhibiting thyroid hormone binding to the proteins (Table 3) (see also Table 1 in Chapter 3). Clinically, estrogens are the most important, and increases in serum T_4 and T_3 levels are dose dependent (95). Low-dose oral contraceptives, for example, produce a relatively minor effect on TBG levels. Other agents known to increase TBG, such as clofibrate or perphenazine, result in only minor increases in TBG levels and therefore serum T_4 and T_3 levels.

Androgenic steroids are the agents most commonly implicated in the low TBG state (96). Pharmacologic doses of glucocorticoids may decrease TBG levels by accelerating its disposal. As mentioned in Chapter 3, both free thyroid hormone levels and TSH levels are unaffected by changes in TBG concentrations. It recently has been observed, however, that hypothyroid women with breast cancer who are on androgen therapy have a decrease in levothyroxine requirement (97). Whether or not this reflects androgen effects on thyroid hormone metabolism is not known. Chronic nicotinic acid administration may result in lower serum TBG and total T_4 levels, while maintaining euthyroidism (98).

Of the agents that inhibit binding of thyroid hormones to TBG, phenytoin may be the most relevant clinically. Chronic treatment with phenytoin results in lower serum total T_4 and FT_4 levels, while serum T_3 and TSH concentrations remain normal. Phenytoin lowers serum T_4 (but not T_3) by displacing it from TBG.

Salicylates, including the nonsteroidal anti-inflammatory agent salsalate, may lower serum T_4 levels by inhibiting binding to TBG (99). Salsalate has been reported to lower T_4 levels as much as 40%, and conventional salicylates administered in therapeutic range may result in a 20% to 30% decrease in serum total T_4 levels (99). Salicylate administration may cause a slight and brief increase in free T_4 levels. Furosemide, in IV doses of larger than 80 mg, also results in a transient slight increase of serum free T_4, and a decrease in total T_4 levels (100).

Agents That Affect Gastrointestinal Absorption of Thyroid Hormone

Several drugs, including the hypolipidemic agents cholestyramine and cholestipol, inhibit gastrointestinal absorption of exogenous thyroid hormone (101). Aluminum-hydroxide-containing antacids also interfere with levothyroxine absorption (102), as does the anti-inflammatory agent sucralfate (103). Ferrous sulfate also appears to interfere with levothyroxine absorption, especially when the agents are administered together (104). Because iron supplements are routinely given in pregnancy, it is important to remind pregnant women to take levothyroxine and iron at least 4 hours apart.

ACKNOWLEDGMENT

The author gratefully acknowledges the expert secretarial assistance of Elsa C. Ahumada.

REFERENCES

1. Chopra IJ. A radioimmunoassay for measurement of thyroxine in unextracted serum. *J Clin Endocrinol Metab* 1972;34:938–947.
2. Helfand M, Crapo LM. Screening for thyroid disease. *Ann Intern Med* 1990;112:840–849.
3. Moses AC, Lawler J, Haddow J, Jackson IMD. Familial euthyroid hyperthyroxinemia resulting from increased thyroxine-binding to thyroxine-binding prealbumin. *N Engl J Med* 1982;306:966–969.
4. Sakata S, Nakamura S, Miura K. Auto-antibodies against thyroid hormone or iodothyronines: implications in diagnosis, thyroid function, treatment and pathogenesis. *Ann Intern Med* 1985;103::579–589.
5. Refetoff S, DeWind T, DeGroot LJ. Familial syndrome combining deaf-mutism stippled epiphyses, goiter, and abnormally high PBI: possible target organ refractoriness to thyroid hormone. *J Clin Endocrinol Metab* 1967;27:2779–2794.
6. Morley JE, Shafer RB. Thyroid function screening in new psychiatric admissions. *Arch Intern Med* 1982;143:591–593.
7. Goodwin TM, Montoro M, Mestman JH. Transient hyperthyroidism and hyperemesis gravidarum: clinical aspects. *Am J Obstet Gynecol* 1992;167:648–652.
8. Lum SMC, Kaptein EM, Nicoloff JT. Influence of nonthyroidal illnesses on serum thyroid hormone indices in hyperthyroidism. *West J Med* 1983;138:670–675.
9. Hamblin PS, Dyer SA, Mohr VS, Legrand BA, Lim, CF, Tuxen DV, et al. Relationship between thyrotropin and thyroxine changes during recovery from severe hypothyroinemia or critical illness. *J Clin Endocrinol Metab* 1986;62:717–722.
10. Nelson JC, Tomel RT. Direct determination of free thyroxine in undiluted serum by equilibrium dialysis. *Clin Chem* 1988;34:1737.
11. Spencer CA. Clinical evaluation of free T$_4$ techniques. *J Endocrinol Invest* 1986;9:57–66.
12. Hay ID, Bayer MF, Kaplan MM, Klee GG, Larsen PR, Spencer CAl. American Thyroid Association assessment of current free thyroid hormone and thyrotropin measurements and guidelines for future clinical assays. *Clin Chem* 1991;37:2002.
13. Kaptein EM. Clinical applications of free thyroxine determinations. *Clin Lab Med* 1993;13:653–672.
14. Larsen PR, Alexander NM, Chopra IJ, Hay ID, Hershman JM, Kaplan MM, et al. Revised nomenclature for tests of thyroid hormones and thyroid related proteins in serum. *J Clin Endocrinol Metab* 1987;64:1089.
15. Larsen PR, Alexander NM, Chopra IJ, et al. Revised nomenclature for tests of thyroid hormones and thyroid related proteins in serum. *J Clin Endocrinol Metab* 1987;64:1089.
16. Bitton RN, Wexler C. Free triiodothyronine toxicosis: a distinct entity. *Am J Med* 1990;88:531–533.
17. Surks MI, Chopra IJ, Mariash CN, Nicoloff JT, Solomon SH. American Thyroid Association Guidelines for use of laboratory tests in thyroid disorders. *JAMA* 1990;263:1529–1532.
18. Odell WD, Wilber JF, Paul WE. Radioimmunoassay of thyrotropin in human serum. *J Clin Endocrinol Metab* 1965;25:1179–1188.
19. Ridgway EC, Weintraub BD, Cevallos JL, Rack MC, Mallof F. Suppression of pituitary TSH secretion in the patient with a hyperfunctioing thyroid nodule. *J Clin Invest* 1973;52:2783–2792.
20. Wehmann RE, Rubenstein HA, Nisula BC. A sensitive convenient radioimmunoassay procedure which demonstrates that serum TSH is suppressed below the normal range in thyrotoxic patients. *Endocr Res* 1979;6:249–255.
21. Spencer CA. Clinical utility and cost effectiveness of sensitive thyrotropin assays in ambulatory and hospitalized patients. *Mayo Clin Proc* 1988;63:1214–1222.
22. Klee GG, Hay ID. Assessment of sensitive thyrotropin assays for an expanded role in thyroid function testing: proposed criteria for analytic performance and clinical utility. *J Clin Endocrinol Metab* 1987;64:461–471.
23. Gorman CA. Letter to the Editor: Revised nomenclature for tests of thyroid hormone and thyroid-related proteins in serum. *J Clin Endocrinol Metab* 1987;64:1089–1092.
24. Spencer CA, Nicoloff JT. Serum TSH measurement: a 1990 status report. *Thyroid Today* 1990;13:1–12.
25. Ross DS. Subclinical hyperthyroidism: possible danger of overzealous thyroxine replacement therapy. *Mayo Clin Proc* 1988;63:1223–1229.
26. Wartofsky L. Does replacement thyroxine therapy cause osteoporosis? *Adv Endocrinol Metab* 1993;4:157–175.
27. Ross DS. Hyperthyroidism, thyroid hormone therapy and bone. *Thyroid* 1994;4:319–326.
28. Biondi B, Fazo S, Carella C, et al. Cardiac effects of long term thyrotropin-suppressive therapy with levothyroxine. *J Clin Endocrinol Metab* 1993;77:334–338.
29. Sawin CT, Geller A. Wolf PA, et al. Low serum thyrotropin concentrations as a risk factor for atrial fibrillation in older persons. *N Engl J Med* 1994;331:1249–1252.
30. Dulgeroff AJ, Hershman JM. Medical therapy for differentiaed thyroid carcinoma *Endocr Rev* 1994;15:500–515.
31. Spencer CA, LoPresti JS, Patel A, Guttler RB, Eigen A, Shen D, et al. Applications of a new chemiluminometric thyrotropin assay to subnormal measurements. *J Clin Endocrinol Metab* 1990;70:453–460.
32. Cooper DS. Thyroxine suppression therapy for benign nodular disease. *J Clin Endocrinol Metab* 1995;80:331–334.
33. Ross DS. Subclinical hyperthyroidism. In: Braverman LE, Utiger RD, eds. *Werner and Ingbar's the thyroid: a fundamental and clinical text*, 6th ed. Philadelphia: JB Lippincott, 1991:1249–1255.
34. Spencer CA, Eigen A, Shen D, Duda M, Qualis S, Weiss S, Nicoloff JT. Specificity of sensitive assays of thyrotropin (TSH) used to screen for thyroid disease in hospitalized patients. *Clin Chem* 1987;33:1391–1396.
35. Faber J, Kirkegaard C, Rasmussen B, Westin H, Busen-Sorensen M, Jensen IW. Pituitary-thyroid axis in critical illness. *J Clin Endocrinol Metab* 1987;65:315–320.
36. Toft AD, Irvine WJ, Hunter WM, Ratcliffe JG, Seth J. Anomalous plasma TSH levels in patients developing hypothyroidism in the early months after 131I therapy for thyrotoxicosis. *J Clin Endocrinol Metab* 1974;39:607.
37. Uy HL, Reasner CA, Samuels MH. Pattern of recovery of the hypothalamic-pituitary-thyroid axis following radioactive iodine therapy in patients with Graves' disease. *Am J Med* 1995;99:173.
38. Singer PA, Nicoloff JT, Stein RB, Jaramillo J. Transient TRH deficiency after prolonged thyroid hormone therapy. *J Clin Endocrinol Metab* 1978;47:512–518.
39. Nicoloff JT, Spencer CA. The use and misuse of the sensitive thyrotropin assay. *J Clin Endocrinol Metab* 1990;71:553–558.
40. Singer PA, Cooper DS, Levy EG, Ladenson PW, Braverman LE, Daniels G, et al. Treatment guidelines for patients with hyperthyroidism and hypothyroidism. *JAMA* 1995;273:808–812.
41. Pinchera A, Martino E, Faglia G. Central hypothyroidism. In: Braverman LE, Utiger RD, eds. *Werner and Ingbar's the thyroid: a fundamental and clinical text*, 6th ed. Philadelphia: JB Lippincott, 968–984.
42. Smallridge RC. Thyrotropin secreting pituitary tumors. *Endocrinol Metab Clin North Am* 1987;16:765–792.
43. Refetoff S, Weiss RE, Usala SJ. The syndromes of resistance to thyroid hormone. *Endocr Rev* 1993;14:348–399.
44. Oppenheim DS. TSH and other glycoprotein producing pituitary adenomas: alpha-subunit as a tumor marker. *Thyroid Today* 1991;14:1–11.
45. Chopra IJ, Hershman JM, Pardridge WM, Nicoloff JT. Thyroid function in nonthyroidal illnesses. *Ann Intern Med* 1983;98:946–957.
46. Klee GG, Hay ID. Biochemical thyroid function testing. *Mayo Clin Proc* 1994;69 469–470.
47. Brown J, Solomon DH, Beall GN, Teraski PI, Chopra IJ, Van Herle AJ, et al. Autoimmune thyroid disease—Graves' and Hashimoto's. *Ann Intern Med* 1978;88:379–391.
48. Kaufman KD, Filetti S, Seto P, Rapport B. Recombinant human thyroid peroxidase generated in eukaryotic cells: a source of specific antigen for the immunological assay of antimicrosomal antibodies in the sera of patients with autoimmune thyroid disease. *J Clin Endocrinol Metab* 1990;70:724.
49. Beever K, Bradbury J, Phillips D, McLachlan SM, Pegg C, Goral A, et al. Highly sensitive assays of autoantibodies to thyroglobulin and to thyroid peroxidase. *Clin Chem* 1989;35:1949–1954.
50. Ruf J, Feldt-Rasmussen U, Hegedus L, Ferrand M, Carayon P. Bispecific thyroglobulin and thyroperoxidase autoantibodies in patients with various thyroid and autoimmune diseases. *J Clin Endocrinol Metab* 1994;79:1404.
51. Sheonfeld Y, Schwartz RS. Immunologic and genetic factors in autoimmune diseases. *N Engl J Med* 1984;311:1019–1029.
52. Sawin CT, Chopra D, Azizi F, Mannix JE, Bacharach P. The aging thy-

roid: increased prevalence of elevated serum thyrotropin in the elderly. *JAMA* 1979;242;247–250.
53. Gordin A, Lamberg BA. Spontaneous hypothyroidism in symptomless autoimmune thyroiditis: a long term follow up study. *Clin Endocrinol* 1981;15:537–543.
54. Tunbridge WM, Brewis M, French JM, Appleton D, Bird T, Clark F, et al. Natural history of autoimmune thyroiditis. *Br Med J* 1981;282:258–262.
55. Rosenthal MJ, Hunt WC, Garry PJ, Goodwin JS. Thyroid failure in the elderly: microsomal antibodies as discriminant for therapy. *JAMA* 1987;258:209–213.
56. Adams DD, Purves HD. Abnormal responses in the assay of thyrotropin. *Proc Univ Otago Med Sch* 1956;34:11–12.
57. Zakarija M, McKenzie JM. Pregnancy associated changes in the thyroid stimulating antibody of Graves' disease and the relationship to neonatal hyperthyroidism. *J Clin Endocrinol Metab* 1983;57:1036–1040.
58. Van Herle A. Serum thyroglobulin measurement in the diagnosis and management of thyroid disease. *Thyroid Today* 1981;4:1–5.
59. Spencer CA, Wang CC. Thyroglobulin measurement: techniques, clinical benefits, and pitfalls. *Endocrinol Metab Clin North Am* 1995;24:841–863.
60. Pommier RF, Brennan MF. Medullary thyroid carcinoma. *The Endocrinologist* 1992;2:393–405.
61. Snyder PJ, Jacobs LS, Rabello MM, et al. Diagnostic values of thyrotropin releasing hormone in pituitary and hypothalamic diseases. *Ann Intern Med* 1974;81:751–757.
62. Ivor MD, Jackson MRCP. Thyrotropin-releasing hormone. *N Engl J Med* 1982;306:145–155.
63. Morley JE. Neuroendocrine control of thyrotropin secretion *Endocr Rev* 1981;2:396–436.
64. Kaptein EM, Spencer CA, Kamiel MB, Nicoloff JT. Prolonged dopamine administration and thyroid hormone economy in normal and critically ill subjects. *J Clin Endocrinol Metab* 1980;51:387–393.
65. Rapoport B, Refetoff S, Fang VS, Friesen HG. Suppression of serum thyrotropin (TSH) by L-dopa in chronic hypothyroidism: interrelationships in the regulation of TSH and prolactin secretion. *J Clin Endocrinol Metab* 1973;36:256–262.
66. Healey DL, Burger HG. Increased prolactin and thyrotrophin secretions following oral metoclopramide: dose-response relationships. *Clin Endocrinol (Oxf)* 1977;7:195–201.
67. Itoh S, Tanaka K, Kimagae M, Takeda F, Morio K, Kogure M, et al. Effect of subcutaneous injection of a long acting analogue of somatostatin (SMS 201-995) on plasma thyroid stimulating hormone in normal human subjects. *Life Sci* 1988;42:2691–2699.
68. Brabant A, Brabant G, Schuemeyer T, et al. The role of glucocorticoids in the regulation of thyrotropin. *Acta Endocrinol* 1989;121:95–100.
69. Morley JE, Shafer RB, Elson MK, Slag MF, Raleigh MJ, Brammer GL, et al. Amphetamine-induced hyperthyroxinemia. *Ann Intern Med* 1980;3:707–709.
70. Braverman LE. Iodine and the thyroid: 33 years of study. *Thyroid* 1994;4:351–356.
71. Vagenakis AG, Braverman LE. Adverse effects of iodides on thyroid function. *Med Clin North Am* 1975;59:1075–1088.
72. Braverman LE. Iodine induced thyroid disease. *Acta Med Austriaca* 1990;17(suppl 1):29–33.
73. Figge HL, Figge J. The effects of amiodarone on thyroid hormone function: a review of the physiology and clinical manifestations. *J Clin Pharmacol* 1990;30:588–595.
74. Lombardi A, Martino E, Braverman LE. Amiodarone and the thyroid. *Thyroid Today* 1990;13:1–7.
75. Martino E, Safran M, Aghini-Lombardi F, et al. Environmental iodine intake and thyroid dysfunction during chronic amiodarone therapy. *Ann Intern Med* 1984;101:28–34.
76. Borowski GD, Garofano CD, Rose LI. Effect of long term amiodarone therapy on thyroid hormone levels and thyroid function. *Am J Med* 1985;78:443–450.
77. Hawthorne GC, Campbell NPS, Geddes JS, et al. Amiodarone induced hypothyroidism: a common complication of prolonged therapy: a report of eight cases. *Arch Intern Med* 1985;145:1016–1019.
78. Melmed S, Nademanee K, Reed AW, Henrickson J, Singh BN, Hershman JM. Hyperthyroxinemia with bradycardia and normal thyrotropin secretion after chronic amiodarone administration. *J Clin Endocrinol Metab* 1981;53:997–1001.
79. Amico JA, Richardson V, Alperts B, Klein I. Clinical and chemical assessment of thyroid function during therapy with amiodarone. *Arch Intern Med* 1984;144:487–490.
80. Spaulding SW, Burrow GN, Bermudez F, Himmerlhock JM. The inhibitory effect of lithium on thyroid hormone release in both euthyroid and thyroid toxic patients. *J Clin Endocrinol Metab* 1972;35:905–911.
81. Bocchetta A. Bernardi F, Pedditzi M, et al. Thyroid abnormalities during lithium treatment. *Acta Psychiatr Scand* 1991;83:193–198.
82. Kitching NH. Hypothyroidism after treatment with ketoconazole. *Br Med J* 1986;293:993–994.
83. Kung AWC, Jones MB, Lai CL. Effects of interferon-gamma therapy on thyroid function, T-lymphocyte subpopulations and induction of autoantibodies. *J Clin Endocrinol Metab* 1990;71:1230–1234.
84. Schultz M, Muller R, von zur Muhlen A, Brabant G. Induction of hyperthyroidism by interferon-α-2b. *Lancet* 1989;1:1452.
85. Primo J, Hinojosu J, Moles JR, et al. Development of thyroid dysfunction after α-interferon treatment of chronic hepatitis C. *Am J Gastroenterol* 1993;88:1976–1977.
86. Baudin E, Marcellin P, Pouteau M, et al. Reversibility of thyroid dysfunction induced by recombinant alpha interferon in chronic hepatitis C. *Clin Endocrinol (Oxf)* 1993;39:657–661.
87. Muller B, Zulweski H, Huber P, et al. Impaired action of thyroid hormone associated with smoking in women with hypothyroidism. *N Engl J Med* 1995;333:964–969.
88. Reeves RA, From GLA, Paul W, Leenen FHH. Nadolol, propranolol and thyroid hormones: evidence for a membrane-stabilizing action of propranolol. *Clin Pharmacol Ther* 1985;37:157–161.
89. LoPresti JS, Eigen A, Kaptein E, Anderson DP, Spencer CA, Nicoloff JT. Alterations in 3,3′5′-triiodothyronine metabolism in response to propylthiouracil, dexamethasone, and thyroxine administration in man. *J Clin Invest* 1989;84:1650–1656.
90. Cooper DS, Daniels GH, Ladenson PW, Ridgway EC. Hyperthyroxinemia in patients treated with high dose propranolol. *Am J Med* 1982;73:867–871.
91. Figg WD, Thilbault A, Sartor AO, et al. Hypothyroidism associated with aminoglutethimide in patients with prostate cancer. *Arch Intern Med* 1994;154:1023–1025.
92. Blackshear JL, Shultz AL, Napier JS, Stuart DD. Thyroxine replacement requirements in hypothyroid patients receiving phenytoin. *Ann Intern Med* 1983;99:341–342.
93. Cavalieri RR, Pitt-Rivers R. The effects of drugs on the distribution and metabolism of thyroid hormone. *Pharmacol Rev* 1987;33(2):55–80.
94. Isely WL. Effect of rifampin therapy on thyroid function tests in a hypothyroid patient on replacement with L-thyroxine. *Ann Intern Med* 1987;107:5117–518.
95. Heath H, Lee RB, Diamond RC, Wartofsky L. Conjugated estrogen therapy and tests of thyroid function. *Ann Intern Med* 1974;81:351–354.
96. Deyssig R, Weissel M. Ingestion of androgenic anabolic steroids induces mild thyroidal impairment in male body builders. *J Clin Endocrinol Metab* 1993;76:1069–1071.
97. Arafah BM. Decreased levothyroxine requirements in women with hypothyroidism during androgen therapy for breast cancer. *Ann Intern Med* 1994;121:247–251.
98. Shakir KMM, Kroll S, April BS, Drake AJ, Eisold JF. Nicotinic acid decreases serum thyroid hormone levels while maintaining a euthyroid state. *Mayo Clin Proc* 1995;70:556–558.
99. Bishnoi A, Carlson HE, Gruber BL, Kauffman LD, Bock JL, Lidonnici K. Effects of commonly prescribed nonsteroidal anti-inflammatory drugs on thyroid hormone measurements. *Am J Med* 1994;96:235–238.
100. Stockigt JR, Lim CF, Barlow JW, Mohr VS, Toplis DJ, Hamblin PS, et al. Interaction of furosemide with serum thyroxine binding sites: in vivo and in vitro studies and comparision with other inhibitors. *J Clin Endocrinol Metab* 1985;60:1025–1031.
101. Kaplan MM. Interactions between drugs and thyroid hormones. *Thyroid Today* 1981;4:1–6.
102. Liel Y, Sperber AD, Shany S. Nonspecific intestinal adsorption of levothyroxine by aluminum hydroxide. *Am J Med* 1994;97:363–365.
103. Havrankova J, Lanaie R. Levothyroxine binding by sucralfate. *Ann Intern Med* 1992;117:445–446.
104. Campbell NRC, Hasinoff BB, Stalts H, Rao B, Wong NC. Ferrous sulfate reduces thyroxine efficacy in patients with hypothyroidism. *Ann Intern Med* 1992;117:1010–1013.

CHAPTER 5

Parathyroid Function and Calcium Homeostasis

Jessica C. Rockwell and Daniel T. Baran

CALCIUM PHYSIOLOGY: OVERVIEW

Calcium homeostasis is an important requirement of living organisms. Calcium ions participate in intracellular activities, intercellular communication through channels and ion exchange pumps, neurotransmitter release, and hormone-receptor interactions, as well as neuromuscular excitation, membrane potentials, and the coagulation cascade. Calcium is essential for normal bone development and mineralization, and the skeleton serves as the major reservoir of calcium and phosphate ions. The clinical consequences of abnormal calcium balance can range from mild to life threatening. Acute hypocalcemia can result in laryngospasm and death; chronic hypocalcemia can cause increased neuromuscular irritability and seizures. Acute hypercalcemia can result in death from asystole; chronic hypercalcemia can result in a variety of disorders, such as nephrolithiasis, psychiatric disturbances, pancreatitis, peptic ulcer disease, and an array of somatic complaints (1–3). Calcium and phosphate balance is tightly controlled through the interactions of parathyroid hormone (PTH) and 1,25-dihydroxyvitamin D_3 [$1,25(OH)_2D_3$] (calcitriol).

Less than 1% of total body calcium is associated with extracellular fluids; 99% is stored in bone. More than 50% of plasma calcium is bound to protein, primarily albumin, and a small fraction is bound to anions such as citrate and lactate. It is the free, ionized fraction of total calcium that is biologically active. Alterations in pH affect the binding of calcium to albumin, and changes in serum proteins affect total serum calcium.

The average diet contains 500 to 1500 mg calcium per day. Calcium is absorbed in the small intestine by active transport and facilitated diffusion. Efficiency of absorption varies inversely with the amount of calcium ingested. The absorbed calcium is in equilibrium with body stores and filtered through the kidney. Reabsorption of calcium in the kidney is highly efficient, with 150 to 300 mg excreted in the urine per day; 250 to 500 mg calcium is exchanged between plasma and bone daily (Fig. 1).

PHOSPHATE

Phosphate metabolism is closely related to calcium balance. Phosphate is predominantly an intracellular anion. Of total body phosphorus, 80% is stored in bone and less than 0.1% in the extracellular fluid. Phosphate is critical to many intracellular functions and is an integral component of nucleic acids, phospholipids, and proteins. Phosphate is absorbed with calcium in the intestine and is released from bone during active resorption. The primary route of phosphate excretion is renal, and its rate of excretion is dependent on glomerular filtration and PTH levels. Hypophosphatemia stimulates the enzyme 1α-hydroxylase to increase $1,25(OH)_2D_3$ production and gastrointestinal absorption of phosphate. Chronic hypophosphatemia resulting from excess antacid ingestion or conditions of renal phosphate wasting can impair bone mineralization and result in osteomalacia. Hyperphosphatemia from renal insufficiency can lead to hypocalcemia by the formation of calcium-phosphate complexes. This leads to a fall in serum calcium and secondary hyperparathyroidism (4). Unlike calcium, the serum phosphorus concentration is variable and is affected by age, sex, nutritional status, and changes in pH.

J. C. Rockwell: Columbia University at Cooperstown, Mary Imogene Bassett Hospital, Cooperstown, New York 13326.

D. T. Baran: Department of Medicine and Orthopedics, University of Massachusetts Medical Center, Worcester, Massachusetts 01605.

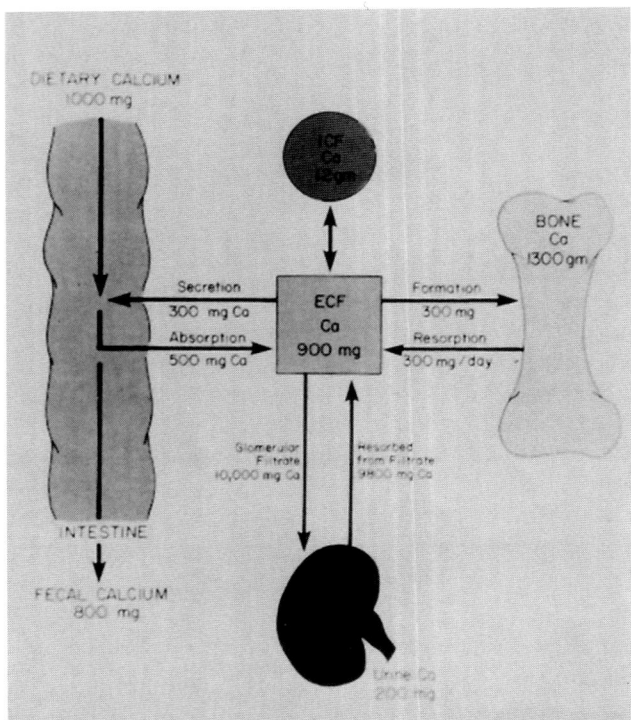

FIG. 1. Average daily intake, absorption, distribution, and excretion of calcium. ECF, extracellular fluid; ICF, intracellular fluid.

MAGNESIUM

Calcium homeostasis is also affected by magnesium, which is the most abundant intracellular divalent cation. Magnesium is important as a cofactor for numerous enzymatic reactions and the regulation of neuromuscular activity. An adult contains approximately 25 g of magnesium, and two thirds resides in the skeleton. In bone, magnesium is located on the crystal surface, and only a fraction is exchangeable with extracellular magnesium. Only 1% of the body's magnesium is in the extracellular compartment. This explains the fact that serum magnesium levels are a poor reflection of total body magnesium. Magnesium homeostasis is not hormonally mediated, as is that of calcium and phosphate. Magnesium balance is a reflection of intestinal absorption and fractional excretion by the kidney.

Magnesium is important for normal PTH secretion from the parathyroid glands. When magnesium levels are very low, PTH secretion is inhibited. Hypomagnesemia is an important consideration in some patients with hypocalcemia.

Magnesium deficiency has become more widely recognized in association with certain drugs, malnutrition, alcoholism, and diabetes mellitus, as well as electrolyte and calcium disorders. Magnesium therapy is being used for a larger number of medical conditions, including preeclampsia, hypocalcemia, ischemic heart disease, and cardiac arrhythmias (5).

HORMONAL REGULATION OF CALCIUM BALANCE

Secretion of PTH is stimulated by low calcium levels in the plasma and in the cytoplasm of the parathyroid cell (6,7). Target organs of PTH are the kidneys and skeleton, and PTH exerts indirect effects on the intestine through the action of $1,25(OH)_2D_3$. Renal effects of PTH are decreased proximal tubular reabsorption of phosphate, increased calcium reabsorption in the distal tubules, and increased activity of mitochondrial 1α-hydroxylase, which hydroxylates 25-hydroxyvitamin D_3 (25-OHD$_3$) to form $1,25(OH)_2D_3$, the most potent metabolite of vitamin D (8). It stimulates absorption of calcium and phosphate in the small intestine and may feed back on the parathyroid glands to alter PTH secretion. Increased plasma calcium levels suppress PTH secretion. PTH and $1,25(OH)_2D_3$ also act on bone to increase resorption, releasing stored calcium and phosphate from bone matrix. PTH and $1,25(OH)_2D_3$ exert their effects on bone by stimulating osteoblasts, via interaction with receptors, to secrete factors that activate osteoclasts. The interactions of calcium, PTH, and vitamin D are tightly regulated through feedback inhibition (Fig. 2). Alterations in calcium or vitamin D intake, parathyroid gland or renal function, or gas-

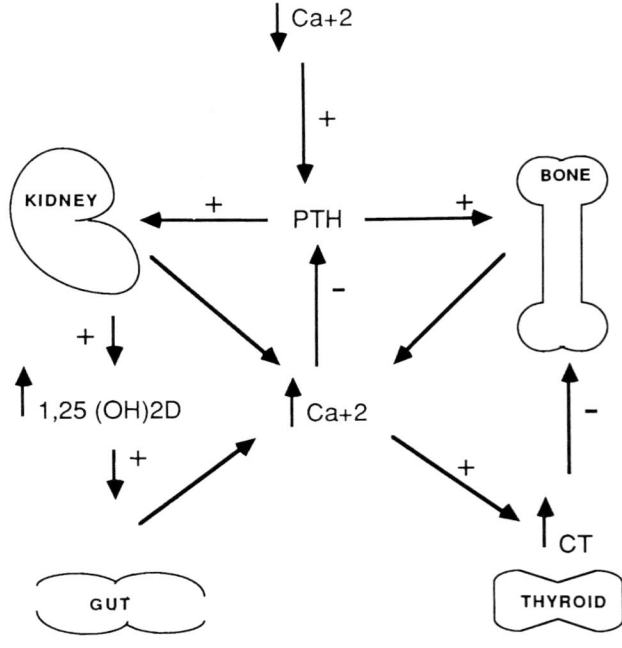

FIG. 2. Hormonal interactions and multiorgan response to changes in serum calcium. CT, calcitonin; ↑, increase; ↓, decrease; +, stimulate; –, suppress.

trointestinal absorption have an impact on calcium homeostasis and bone metabolism.

PARATHYROID HORMONE

Parathyroid hormone is produced and secreted by the chief cells of the parathyroid glands. PTH is produced as a large preprohormone of 115 amino acids. Proteolysis during intracellular secretion of the hormone yields a pre-PTH molecule and the intact hormone (90 and 84 amino acids, respectively) (6,7). Peripheral metabolism of the intact molecule is rapid and occurs in the liver and parathyroid cell to yield multiple PTH fragments. The biologically active PTH fragment consists of the N-terminal region (amino acids 1 to 34), which has a very short half-life. The mid-molecule and C-terminal fragments (amino acids 44 to 69 and 34 to 84, respectively) are not bioactive and their clearance is dependent on glomerular filtration, resulting in longer half-lives than the bioactive fragment. C-terminal fragments make up 70% to 95% of circulating PTH, whereas intact PTH makes up 5% to 30% of circulating PTH, and N-terminal fragments are minimal in the circulation.

Radioimmunoassays for PTH have been developed to measure the C-terminal, mid-molecule, N-terminal, and intact hormone (9–11). The C-terminal assay, although quite sensitive in patients with normal renal function, measures only bioinactive hormone and is not useful to differentiate low from normal levels. The mid-molecule assay is extremely sensitive but is also affected by abnormal renal function. The N-terminal assay, although quite specific for hyperparathyroidism if elevated, is very insensitive because of the very short half-life of this PTH fragment in serum. The intact PTH assay, which is a two-site immunoradiometric assay (IRMA), is currently the most sensitive and specific assay available for evaluating patients with altered calcium balance. When evaluating patients and clinical data, it is important to know what type of PTH assay is being used. The intact PTH assay is able to distinguish low from normal PTH levels. This is important in evaluating the etiology of hypocalcemia and differentiating hypoparathyroidism from other causes of hypocalcemia in which PTH is normal or elevated, as occurs in states of PTH resistance or secondary hyperparathyroidism. In addition, the intact PTH assay is helpful in differentiating patients with hypercalcemia of malignancy or other nonparathyroid causes of hypercalcemia from parathyroid-mediated hypercalcemia. The rapid rate of intact PTH clearance allows for direct assessment of the secretory activity of the parathyroid glands in response to changes in serum calcium and other secretagogues (12). For example, an intact-PTH level can be obtained intraoperatively on patients undergoing parathyroidectomy for hyperparathyroidism, to document removal of the adenoma.

Parathyroid hormone interacts with cell membrane receptors to activate adenylate cyclase, causing increased production of adenosine 3′,5′-cyclic monophosphate (cAMP) (6). PTH-induced cAMP production precedes hormone-induced phosphaturia. Measurement of urinary (nephrogenous) cAMP, therefore, is a method of evaluating the bioactivity of PTH.

The most potent secretagogue for PTH is decreased serum or parathyroid cell calcium. Falling or low serum calcium stimulates PTH secretion, and release of preformed PTH occurs seconds after an acute fall in ionized calcium. Catecholamines can modulate PTH secretion. Beta-agonists augment and beta-antagonists inhibit PTH secretion. The effect of beta-agonists in augmenting PTH secretion is additive to the stimulatory effect of hypocalcemia.

Magnesium is essential for adequate PTH secretion and end-organ response (13,14), and it is important in 1α-hydroxylase activity. When serum magnesium levels fall to less than 0.4 mmol/L, the parathyroid glands do not secrete hormone adequately in response to hypocalcemic stimuli, cAMP production in response to exogenous PTH is low, and 1α-hydroxylase activity is reduced. Sustained correction of serum calcium will not occur until magnesium is adequately replaced.

Parathyroid hormone has both anabolic and catabolic effects on bone. Anabolic effects presumably occur at physiologic levels. The use of intermittent injections of PTH to increase bone mass in osteoporotic patients is currently being evaluated. The catabolic effects are well characterized. Increased levels of PTH increase bone resorption by enhancing the activity of osteoclasts, which results in release of calcium and phosphate from bone matrix. The prompt release of PTH in response to hypocalcemia and the readily available source of calcium in bone are essential to normal calcium homeostasis.

VITAMIN D

1,25-Dihydroxyvitamin D_3 acts as a steroid hormone (15,16). It is essential to the maintenance of calcium balance. Vitamin D is biologically inactive. Activation requires 25-hydroxylation in the liver and 1α-hydroxylation in the kidney. The kidney is the only site (in the healthy non-pregnant state) in which clinically important 1α-hydroxylation takes place. Normally, 1,25(OH)$_2$D$_3$, the most potent form of vitamin D, exerts negative feedback on its own production through a suppressive effect on the enzyme 1α-hydroxylase. Elevated 1,25(OH)$_2$D$_3$ levels also activate an alternate pathway of vitamin D metabolism in the kidney by stimulating the enzyme 24-hydroxylase to produce 24,25-dihydroxyvitamin D_3, which is essentially inactive.

It is known that 1,25(OH)$_2$D$_3$ exerts its physiologic effect through interaction with its steroid receptors. It has been shown to affect expression of the PTH gene: low levels of $1,25(OH)_2D_3$ stimulate, and elevated levels suppress, gene expression. If patients with renal failure are given pharmacologic doses of calcitriol, excess PTH production can be suppressed and thus secondary hyperparathyroidism averted (4). The vitamin D receptor has been localized in a variety of cells, including enterocytes of the small intestine, osteoblasts, and renal tubular cells. Additionally, $1,25(OH)_2D_3$ receptors have been isolated in cells not associated with calcium balance, such as keratinocytes of the skin, hematopoietic lymphoid cells in the bone marrow, and islet cells of the pancreas (15).

Nonclassical effects of vitamin D are also apparent (17). Vitamin D has been found to stimulate cell differentiation and suppress cell proliferation. It is proving to be clinically useful in patients with psoriasis, a disorder involving excess proliferation of keratinocytes. When given topically or enterally to patients with psoriasis, there is marked improvement. Vitamin D stimulates differentiation of HL-60 cells (a human leukemic cell line), rendering them benign. The hormone also acts on cell membranes to cause immediate intracellular effects through interactions with the sodium–hydrogen antiport system and membrane phospholipids. The physiologic and clinical consequences of these nonclassical effects have yet to be fully elucidated.

Clinical syndromes of abnormal vitamin D metabolism are well recognized. High $1,25(OH)_2D_3$ levels result in hypercalcemia. Excessive vitamin D intake or increased 1α-hydroxylase activity, as occurs in sarcoidosis or other granulomatous disorders, can cause hypercalcemia (18). The macrophages present in the granulomas have the capacity to 1α-hydroxylate 25-OHD, resulting in elevated levels of $1,25(OH)_2D_3$ and increased gastrointestinal absorption of calcium and phosphate.

Syndromes of low $1,25(OH)_2D_3$ levels occur as a result of vitamin D deficient diets, lack of exposure to sunlight (a common occurrence in the elderly), and malabsorption syndromes. Disorders of vitamin D metabolism may result from deficient substrate, impaired hydroxylation, or resistance to the active metabolite. Rickets is caused by deficient vitamin D levels during childhood, resulting in impaired growth and bowing of the long bones. Osteomalacia is the adult form of bone disease caused by vitamin D deficiency.

CALCITONIN

Calcitonin (CT) is a 32-amino-acid peptide produced in the parafollicular (C) cells of the thyroid (19). It is secreted in response to elevated plasma calcium levels, and it acts on bone to inhibit the activity and proliferation of osteoclasts. CT also acts on the kidneys to decrease reabsorption of electrolytes, resulting in enhanced excretion of calcium, phosphate, magnesium, and sodium. CT acts through adenylate cyclase and the production of cAMP as a second messenger. Gastrointestinal hormones (e.g., gastrin and pentagastrin) also stimulate secretion of CT. Studies on normal and thyroidectomized dogs given an oral load of calcium show that hypercalcemia occurs in thyroidectomized dogs but not controls, suggesting a relationship between dietary calcium, gastrointestinal activity, and CT secretion. CT may act to buffer the hypercalcemic effects of an oral calcium load.

Extrathyroidal C cells and CT production have been identified in multiple organs, including the thymus, lungs, urinary bladder, gastrointestinal tract, and central nervous system. The physiologic role of the extrathyroidal C cells and CT production is unclear, but it may be related to a common neuroectodermal origin. The CT production at extrathyroidal sites contributes to circulating CT levels. Patients who have undergone total thyroidectomy have measurable but reduced levels of circulating CT (20).

Calcitonin is of primary importance in the setting of rapid bone resorption and calcium release, in which the magnitude of CT secretion is the greatest. CT inhibits osteoclastic bone resorption. The effect on bone resorption by CT is lost over time owing to an "escape phenomenon," likely secondary to down-regulation of the CT receptor. This is an important issue clinically when using CT for the treatment of hypercalcemia, in which it is beneficial acutely but has a short-lived effect. CT also exerts analgesic effects in some patients with osteoporotic crush fractures, presumably because of enhanced production of endorphins. Medullary carcinoma of the thyroid (MCT) is derived from the C cells and is characterized by elevated CT levels. Studies on patients with MCT, however, show normal calcium, phosphate, and PTH concentrations.

The primary function of CT in humans is unclear. CT appears to preserve the skeleton at times of increased need, as in pregnancy, lactation, and growth, and it may buffer a hypercalcemic response to an oral calcium load, although this is not well established in humans. Because there are no known syndromes of abnormal calcium balance in humans caused by excess or deficient CT, there is no evidence that deficient CT levels, such as occur after thyroidectomy, are detrimental. The role of CT in the development of osteoporosis is controversial. CT levels have been reported to be low, normal, and elevated in osteoporotic patients. Basal and stimulated CT levels are lower in women and decline with age, and after thyroidectomy or ^{131}I treatment. However, CT deficiency, as occurs after thyroidectomy, does not appear to increase the incidence of osteoporosis when more sensitive CT assays are used and thyroid hormone replacement is maintained in the euthyroid range (21–24).

Calcitonin is currently approved for the treatment of Paget's disease, osteoporosis, and hypercalcemia. Newer pharmacologic preparations may have improved and broader clinical applications.

HYPERCALCEMIA

Hypercalcemia occurs as a result of increased bone resorption (which releases calcium into the circulation), impaired renal clearance of calcium, and increased gastrointestinal absorption of calcium. Malignancy and primary hyperparathyroidism account for 85% of all causes of hypercalcemia. Measurement of PTH is crucial to evaluate a patient with hypercalcemia.

Primary hyperparathyroidism (PHPT) is a relatively common disorder causing hypercalcemia at a frequency of 1 case per 1000 (25,26). In an outpatient study, it was reported to occur in 1% of women over age 60 (27). It is seen in middle-aged individuals, with a predominance in women. Symptoms may be indolent, and they range from nonspecific to severe. Younger patients are more likely to be asymptomatic. With the advent of routine blood calcium screening, hyperparathyroidism is now identified before severe secondary disorders develop. In the past, a significant percentage of patients with hyperparathyroidism presented with bone disease (47% to 79%) and nephrolithiasis (3% to 21%). In more recent reviews, the majority of patients (57%) are diagnosed incidentally with no symptoms, whereas 7% present with nephrolithiasis. None present with bone disease as their primary symptom (25).

Primary hyperparathyroidism results from excess secretion of PTH despite elevated calcium levels. Patients develop hypercalcemia from increased renal tubular reabsorption of calcium, increased intestinal absorption of calcium due to increased $1,25(OH)_2D_3$ production, and increased bone resorption. Patients are commonly hypophosphatemic as a result of the phosphaturic effect of PTH. PTH also causes proximal tubular bicarbonate wasting and can result in a renal tubular acidosis. A single parathyroid adenoma is present in 80% to 85% of cases, parathyroid hyperplasia in 10% to 15%, and parathyroid carcinoma in less than 5%. The last tends to occur in a younger age group, and it presents with greater elevation of serum calcium and PTH (28).

Secondary hyperparathyroidism occurs in renal insufficiency (most commonly) and vitamin D–deficient states. The parathyroid glands are hyperplastic. Renal insufficiency induces excess PTH production to compensate for hypocalcemia. The latter results from hyperphosphatemia resulting from reduced renal clearance of phosphate and impaired 1α-hydroxylation of 25-hydroxyvitamin D in the kidney. Vitamin D–deficient states can be caused by abnormalities at multiple levels, as discussed previously. Excess PTH production is a compensatory mechanism to correct the hypocalcemia of vitamin D deficiency.

Malignancy-associated hypercalcemia can occur as a result of bone metastasis or from humoral factors. Lytic bone metastases are associated with hypercalcemia and are commonly seen in breast and lung cancer. Multiple myeloma is classically associated with bone changes, although only 40% of patients develop hypercalcemia. Mediators of the bone destruction in myeloma include lymphotoxin, interleukin-1, and interleukin-6 (29–32).

The predominant mediator of humoral hypercalcemia is parathyroid hormone related peptide (PTHrp) (33). This PTH-like substance was first recognized because of the presence of increased nephrogenous cAMP without elevated PTH levels. PTHrp has since been identified. It is homologous to PTH at the amino terminus. Eight of the first 13 amino acids are identical to those of PTH. This is the critical region needed for activation of the PTH receptor. PTHrp is longer than PTH and exists in three forms (139,141, and 173 amino acids each). PTHrp, like PTH, increases serum calcium, causes phosphaturia, and stimulates production of $1,25(OH)_2D_3$. It is typically found in squamous cell tumors, renal cell cancer, and breast cancer. It has also been identified in islet cell tumors, T-cell leukemia and lymphoma, and pheochromocytomas. PTHrp does play a role in normal physiology. It is normally present in epidermal keratinocytes, and it is secreted into milk in high concentrations. PTHrp is present in fetal tissue and is likely vital to normal bone and cartilage formation.

Familial hypocalciuric hypercalcemia (FHH) is an autosomal dominant disorder causing hypercalcemia (34). Patients are hypercalcemic, with inappropriately normal or elevated PTH levels; in contrast to PHPT, however, they are hypocalciuric and do not exhibit the adverse sequelae of hypercalcemia. They are not cured by neck exploration. FHH is due to a heterozygous gene mutation likely affecting an extracellular calcium-sensing receptor, which results in an altered set-point for the parathyroid response to changes in serum calcium. Neonatal severe hyperparathyroidism is a rare disorder, which is fatal without parathyroidectomy. It is presumed to be the homozygous form of the gene defect for FHH (35).

Lithium carbonate, used commonly to treat bipolar disorders, affects calcium homeostasis and may cause hypercalcemia (36). Patients on lithium, similar to patients with FHH, have elevated PTH levels and are hypocalciuric. Lithium may also affect bone metabolism (37). Thiazide diuretics are occasionally associated with hypercalcemia. Most patients with persistent hypercalcemia who are taking thiazides, however, have latent PHPT. Thiazides act by reducing tubular secretion of calcium in the distal tubules, resulting in reduced clearance of calcium. Thiazides can precipitate hypercalcemia in patients on lithium therapy as well as those with undiagnosed hyperparathyroidism (38).

Calcium balance can be altered by other nonparathyroid endocrine diseases (Table 1). Hyperthyroidism in particular is associated with hypercalcemia attributed to increased bone turnover (39–41). Hypercalcemia occurs in up to 20% of patients with hyperthyroidism. Serum calcium and phosphate levels are elevated, and urinary

TABLE 1. *Classification of hypercalcemia*

Elevated PTH
  PHPT (%)
    Adenoma, 80–85
    Hyperplasia, 10–15
    Carcinoma, <5
  Lithium-induced
  Familial hypocalciuric hypercalcemia
Malignant hypercalcemia
  Humoral (PTH-related peptide)
  Lytic/bone metastasis
Vitamin D–related
  Intoxication
  Granulomatous disorders
Endocrine-associated
  Hyperthyroidism
  Addison's disease
  Pheochromocytoma (MEN II)
Increased bone turnover
  Immobilization in the face of high bone turnover
    (e.g., Paget's disease)
  Vitamin A intoxication
Reduced renal clearance of calcium
  Thiazides
Miscellaneous
  Milk alkali syndrome

Abbreviations: MEN, multiple endocrine neoplasia; PHPT, primary hyperparathyroidism; PTH, parathyroid hormone.

excretion of calcium and phosphate is increased, whereas serum PTH and $1,25(OH)_2D_3$ levels are suppressed. Adrenal insufficiency is occasionally associated with hypercalcemia; however, the mechanism is unclear (3). Parathyroid function is normal in adrenal insufficiency. Hemoconcentration and volume depletion are the presumed causes of hypercalcemia in this disease. Reduced glomerular filtration resulting in increased tubular reabsorption of calcium may also play a role. Pheochromocytoma has been associated with hypercalcemia. In addition to the known association of pheochromocytoma with hyperparathyroidism in the multiple endocrine neoplasia (MEN) II syndromes, hypercalcemia has occurred in isolated pheochromocytoma. The etiology has previously been attributed to hemoconcentration and volume contraction, although more recently, PTHrp has been implicated as the cause of hypercalcemia in patients with pheochromocytoma.

Therapy

Treatment of hypercalcemia (Table 2) depends in part on the etiology. In general, it is important to increase renal clearance of calcium, decrease bone turnover, and reduce intestinal absorption of calcium (42). Saline hydration causes increased calcium loss in the urine at the proximal tubule, and loop diuretics block calcium reabsorption in the distal tubules. Bisphosphonates (pamidronate and etidronate), CT, and mithramycin act through different mechanisms to reduce bone resorption, and they may be required in a patient who has not responded to hydration and diuresis alone. Pamidronate and etidronate bind to hydroxyapatite and impair osteoclast function to prevent bone resorption. They are associated with few side effects. CT is quite effective in reducing serum calcium acutely, primarily by inhibition of bone resorption and also by enhanced calcium excretion in the kidney (43). However, tachyphylaxis to the effect develops rapidly. Mithramycin has been used to treat hypercalcemia, but its use is limited by bone marrow, hepatic, and renal toxicity (44). Glucocorticoids are useful in some cases of hypercalcemia. Patients with hypercalcemia due to PHPT do not respond to glucocorticoids. Oral phosphates can serve as adjunctive therapy in patients with normal renal function. They work by binding calcium in the gut. Intravenous phosphorus is contraindicated in the setting of hypercalcemia. The non-

TABLE 2. *Therapy for hypercalcemia*

Agent		Dosage	Side effects
Primary			
Hydration	Isotonic saline	2.5–6 L/day	Volume overload
Diuretics	Loop diuretics (furosemide)	10–20 mg IV every 4–8 hr	Electrolyte deficiencies
Secondary			
Bisphosphonates	Pamidronate	15–45 mg/day for 6 days or 45–90 mg IV over 24 hours	Fever, pain, GI upset
	Etidronate	7.5 mg/kg for 3–7 days	
Mithramycin		25 µg/kg over 4–6 hours every 24–48 hours	Renal, hepatic, bone marrow Local with extravasation
Calcitonin		4–8 IU/kg every 4–6 hours	Nausea, flushing
Gallium nitrate		200 mg/m² for 5 days	Nephrotoxic Contraindicated in patient receiving aminoglycosides
Occasionally useful			
Glucocorticoids		200–300 mg IV for 3–5 days	
Oral phosphate		1–2 gm PO per day	Diarrhea

steroidal agent indomethacin is theoretically effective in treating humoral hypercalcemia of malignancy when the etiology is a result of osteoclast-activating factor or prostaglandin production, although its usefulness in clinical situations is often less than optimal (42). Gallium nitrate has recently been approved for the treatment of malignancy-associated hypercalcemia (45). It is associated with renal toxicity, especially in patients concomitantly treated with aminoglycosides.

HYPOCALCEMIA

Hypocalcemia can occur for multiple reasons (46) (Table 3). Nonendocrine causes are most often seen in critically ill, hospitalized patients (47). The most common cause is low serum albumin, although the ionized fraction of calcium is normal. Metabolic or respiratory alkalosis will reduce ionized calcium levels due to increased protein binding, and patients may develop symptomatic hypocalcemia. Risk factors for hypocalcemia in hospitalized patients include renal failure, multiple transfusions, gastrointestinal bleeding, and abdominal surgery. Pancreatitis is associated with hypocalcemia, although the etiology remains obscure. Tumor lysis and rhabdomyolysis are associated with hypocalcemia, secondary to the hyperphosphatemia that is characteristic of these disorders.

Postsurgical Hypocalcemia

Hypocalcemia after parathyroid or thyroid surgery is common. It is most often transient and asymptomatic. The frequency of symptomatic hypocalcemia and the likelihood of developing permanent hypocalcemia are affected by the underlying diagnosis and by the extent of thyroid or parathyroid resection.

In patients undergoing total thyroidectomy, hypocalcemia has been found to occur in up to 83% of patients (48–50). Of these, only 13% require treatment, two thirds transiently and one third permanently. The most common cause of transient, asymptomatic hypocalcemia after thyroid surgery is a fall in serum albumin from stress and hemodilution. Thyroid cancer, Hashimoto's disease, and Graves' disease are associated with a tenfold increase in risk of hypocalcemia. The cause of postoperative hypocalcemia has been attributed to inadvertent parathyroid resection and vascular compromise. Graves' disease–related autoimmune fibrosis affecting parathyroid tissue and increased bone resorption are additional precipitants (51).

Hypocalcemia after parathyroid surgery has been attributed to effects of anesthesia, hormone changes induced by the stress of surgery, hemodilution from intravenous fluids, excess parathyroid gland removal, vascular insufficiency to the normal glands, bone hunger following successful surgery, and hypercalcemic suppression of nonadenomatous parathyroid tissue (52). The "hungry bone syndrome" (HBS) is frequently implicated as the etiology of postoperative hypocalcemia in patients with PHPT. After parathyroid surgery, the sudden fall in PTH abolishes the excess stimulation of osteoclasts. However, the compensatory increase in osteoblast activity to remineralize the skeleton persists. The net effect is increased skeletal calcium deposition. The HBS has been found to occur in 12.6% of patients with PHPT (53). Patients at risk for developing HBS are older, and they have a longer history of PHPT, higher serum calcium, alkaline phosphatase, PTH, and blood urea nitrogen levels preoperatively, and larger adenomas. Symptomatic hypocalcemia, consisting of paresthesias, tetany, and a positive Chvostek's sign lasting several weeks, has been reported despite attempts to maintain normocalcemia and normomagnesemia. This has been attributed to longstanding PHPT with neuromuscular adaptation to hypercalcemia. The rapid fall in serum calcium levels to the normocalcemic range induces neuromuscular irritability (54).

Hypoparathyroidism

Primary hypoparathyroidism is a disorder of inadequate PTH secretion in response to hypocalcemia. Decreased

TABLE 3. Differential diagnosis of hypocalcemia

Inadequate parathyroid hormone
    Congenital hypoparathyroidism
    Acquired hypoparathyroidism
        Autoimmune
        Postsurgery
        Metastasis
    Hypomagnesemia
Impaired response to PTH
    Magnesium deficiency
    Renal failure
    Pseudohypoparathyroidism
Vitamin D–related
    Deficient sun exposure
    Fat malabsorption or deficient fat intake
    Defective metabolism
        Vitamin D–dependent rickets type I (deficient 1α-hydroxylase)
    Defective end-organ response to 1,25(OH)$_2$D$_3$
        Vitamin D–resistant rickets (previously termed vitamin D–dependent rickets type II)
Other
    Hyperphosphatemia (renal failure, tumor lysis, rhabdomyolysis)
    Pancreatitis (formation of calcium and phosphate soaps—questionable)
    "Hungry bones" following surgical care of PHPT
    Alkalosis (normal total calcium with reduced ionized calcium)
    Posttransfusion (chelation effect)
Spurious
    Hypoalbuminemia (normal ionized calcium)

Abbreviation: PTH, parathyrohormone.

$1,25(OH)_2D_3$ levels, as a result of hyperphosphatemia and the low PTH levels, exacerbate the hypocalcemia because of inadequate intestinal absorption of calcium and reduced bone resorption. Hypoparathyroidism may occur from autoimmune destruction of the parathyroid glands, as a consequence of previous surgery, from iron deposition, or (rarely) from metastatic disease involving the parathyroid glands (55).

Pseudohypoparathyroidism is a form of hypoparathyroidism in which there is resistance to PTH (56). Hypocalcemia is present despite PTH levels that are high normal or clearly elevated. Patients usually display a characteristic somatic phenotype of short stature, low intelligence, and short fourth metacarpals or metatarsals. Pseudohypoparathyroidism occurs in two forms. Type I is a disorder of the PTH receptor in which there is a deficiency of a guanine nucleotide regulatory protein. Patients are unable to respond to exogenous PTH with a rise in nephrogenous cAMP. Type II pseudohypoparathyroidism is not a result of a receptor abnormality, but of an inadequate response to the intracellular messenger cAMP. The abnormal phenotype is more common in type I patients, and they may also be resistant to other hormones, such as thyroid-stimulating hormone (TSH) and prolactin secretion in response to exogenous thyrotropin-releasing hormone (TRH).

Hypomagnesemia causes hypocalcemia by affecting PTH secretion and inducing end-organ resistance to the hormone. Magnesium deficiency occurs in states of malabsorption or malnutrition. Aminoglycosides and certain chemotherapeutic agents (e.g., cisplatin) cause magnesium deficiency by affecting renal tubular function and increasing magnesium clearance (57).

Diagnosis

The evaluation of a patient with hypocalcemia involves consideration of the conditions listed in Table 3. A thorough history and physical examination and an appreciation of the clinical setting will guide the workup. The initial laboratory evaluation should include calcium, albumin, phosphate, and magnesium levels. An ionized calcium level is helpful, as it measures the active form of calcium and eliminates the impact of serum proteins on total calcium. Subsequent evaluation of the hypocalcemic patient by measurement of PTH levels and vitamin D metabolites will be dictated by the these results, the history, and the clinical setting (for example, renal failure, previous neck exploration, or a history of malabsorption).

Therapy

Treatment of hypocalcemia (Table 4) depends on the severity and rate of onset. Patients with a serum calcium of less than 3 mg/dL, seizures, or tetany must be treated emergently with intravenous calcium. Calcium gluconate (10%) is supplied in 10-mL vials containing 93 mg elemental calcium. Calcium chloride is supplied in 10-mL vials and contains 272 mg elemental calcium. One or two ampules of calcium gluconate (93 to 186 mg) can be diluted in 50 to 100 mL dextrose and infused over 10 to 15 minutes (to avoid venous irritation). After the initial bolus for severe hypocalcemia or in the stable patient requiring IV replacement, an infusion of 1 to 2 mg/kg per hour (10 ampules calcium gluconate in 1 liter = 930 mg) should be initiated, with improvement of hypocalcemia expected in 6 to 12 hours (resolution of symptoms and serum calcium greater than 7 mg/dL). If the patient is unable to take oral calcium supplements, a maintenance infusion of 0.3 to 0.5 mg/kg per hour can be given. Dietary or oral supplements should provide 1.5 to 2.5 g of calcium per day. Calcium preparations vary in the content of elemental calcium per tablet. Calcium carbonate contains more elemental calcium per dose than calcium gluconate or lactate, thus requiring the ingestion of fewer tablets. Vitamin D replacement may be required to treat hypocalcemia. Vitamin D preparations vary in price, potency, rate of onset of action, and half-life. All of these factors are important in monitoring therapy, which may be lifelong. With all preparations, the therapeutic-to-toxic ratio is small, and thus the risk of inducing hypercalcemia is significant. Serum calcium should be monitored regularly and maintained in the low-normal range.

Ergocalciferol is the most frequently administered preparation because of its availability and low cost. The dose is 50,000 to 100,000 U/day. This preparation has a slow onset of action because it must be 25- and 1α-hydroxylated, and it has a long half-life because it is stored in fat. Calcitriol [$1,25(OH)_2D_3$] and dihydrotachysterol (DHT), a synthetic analog of $1,25(OH)_2D_3$, have more rapid onset of action and shorter half-lives, but they are more potent and more expensive for long-term management of hypocalcemia. The dose of calcitriol is 0.25 to 1.0 µg/day, and the dose of DHT is 0.25 to 1.0 mg/day. If magnesium deficiency is present, this must be corrected as well. Parenteral replacement of magnesium can be given intravenously or intramuscularly. Magnesium sulfate is provided in 10% or 50% solutions, which contain 0.5 g/5 ml or 0.5 gm/ml of magnesium, respectively (0.5 g = 4 mEq). The total replacement dose of magnesium is 2 to 4 mEq/kg, which is administered over 3 to 5 days by giving 1 mEq/kg in the first 24 hours, followed by 0.5 mEq/kg over the next 3 to 4 days. For intramuscular replacement, a schedule of 16 mEq every 4 to 6 hours for the first 24 hours, followed by 8 mEq every 6 hours for 3 to 4 days, is recommended. For intravenous replacement, 40 mEq per liter (5 ampules of 10% or 1 ampule of 50% $MgSO_4$ per liter saline) giving 2 liters over the first 24 hours followed by 1 liter over 24 hours for 3 to 4 days.

TABLE 4. Drugs for acute and chronic management of hypocalcemia

Drug	Treatment of choice	Alternate treatment	Assessment	Comments
		Acute (patient with tetany, seizures)		
Calcium, parenteral	Calcium gluconate 10%,[a] two ampules in 100 ml, D5W over 10–15 min	Calcium chloride 10%,[b] 1/2 ampule (5 ml) over 10–15 min	Monitor SCa, SPi, SMg, ECG; S albumin, ionized calcium PTH if appropriate	If SMg low, replace (see below)
		Stable patient		
Calcium, parenteral	Calcium gluconate 10%, 1–2 mg/kg per hr over 6–12 hr		Monitor SCa every 4 hr; stop infusion or reduce to maintenance when SCa >8.0 mg/dl; check for Chvostek and Trousseau signs	
		Maintenance		
Calcium, parenteral	Calcium gluconate 10%, 0.3–0.5 mg/kg per hr			
		Chronic		
Calcium, oral	Calcium carbonate: Os-Cal 500 (500 mg),[c] Tums (200 mg), Extra Strength Tums (400 mg)	Calcium lactate 625 mg (80 mg),[c] calcium gluconate 1 g (90 mg)[c]		Dosage: 1.0–2.5 g elemental calcium/day; calcium carbonate preferred because concentration of elemental calcium per tablet is greatest requiring ingestion of fewer tablets
Vitamin D	Ergocalciferol (Drisdol) 50–100,000 U/d	Dihydrotachysterol (DHT) 250–1000 µg/d; 1,25 (OH)$_2$D (Rolcaltrol) 0.25–1.00µg/d	With all vitamin D preparations, monitor for hypercalcemia	Ergocalciferol: inexpensive; must be 25-and 1α-hydroxylated; slow onset of action; long half-life DHT: less potent than 1,25(OH)$_2$D; does not require 1α-hydroxylation. 1,25 (OH)$_2$D; does not require 25- or 1α-hydroxylation; very potent; short half-life; expensive
Magnesium, parenteral	Magnesium sulfate 10%;[d] day 1: 1 mEq/kg per 24 hr, 16 mEq IM q 4–6 hr or 3–4 mEq/hr IV; days 2–5: 0.5 mEq/kg per 24 hr, 8 mEq IM q 6 hr or 1–2 mEq/hr IV		With all magnesium preparations, rule out renal insufficiency; if present, monitor levels closely	
Magnesium, oral	Magnesium gluconate 500 mg (2.2 mEq);[c] magnesium, oxide 400 mg (20 mEq)[c] 1–2 tabs qd			May cause diarrhea

Abbreviations: D5W, 5% dextrose in water; S, serum; Ca, calcium; Pi, inorganic phosphate; Mg, magnesium; ECG, electrocardiogram; PTH, parathyroid hormone; 1,25(OH)$_2$D, 1α,25-dihydroxyvitamin D; IM, intramuscular; IV, intravenous; q, every.
[a]1 g in 10-ml ampule provides 90 mg elemental calcium.
[b]1 g in 10-ml ampule provides 272 mg elemental calcium.
[c]Numbers in parentheses are amount of the element per tablet.
[d]1 g in 10-ml ampule provides 98 mg or 8.13 mEq elemental magnesium. (Magnesium sulfate 50% = 49.3 mg/ml.)

Oral magnesium supplementation is limited by diarrhea, but it may be provided by magnesium oxide (400 mg) at one or two tablets per day (20 to 40 mEq) (58,59).

When replacing calcium and magnesium in the acute setting, it is important to monitor blood levels frequently; to monitor the electrocardiogram, particularly in patients on digoxin (because calcium potentiates the toxic effects of digoxin); and to be certain of the patient's renal status to assure adequate clearance of magnesium and phosphate. The long-term management of the patient with hypocalcemia requires regular monitoring of therapy. The goal should be to maintain calcium levels in the low-normal range, and the patient should wear a medical alert bracelet.

REFERENCES

1. Stevenson JC. Fluid and electrolyte disorders: calcium. *Br J Hosp Med* 1984;32:71–72,75–76.
2. Martin TJ. Drug and hormone effects on calcium release from bone. *Pharmacol Ther* 1983;21:209–228.
3. Wilson JD, Foster DW. *Williams' textbook of endocrinology,* 7th ed. Philadelphia: WB Saunders, 1981.
4. Pitts TO, Piraino BH, Mitro R, et al. Hyperparathyroidism and 1,25-dihydroxyvitamin D deficiency in mild, moderate and severe renal failure. *J Clin Endocrinol Metab* 1988;67:876–881.
5. McLean RM. Magnesium and its therapeutic uses: a review. *Am J Med* 1994;96:63–76.
6. Habener JF, Rosenblatt M, Patts JT Jr. Parathyroid hormone: biochemical aspects of biosynthesis, secretion, action, and metabolism. *Physiol Rev* 1984;64:985–1053.
7. Pocotte SL, Ehrenstein G, Fitzpatrick LA. Regulation of parathyroid hormone secretion. *Endocr Rev* 1991;12:291–301.
8. Kurokawak K. The kidney and calcium homeostasis. *Kidney Int* 1994;45:597–605.
9. Blind E, Schmidt-Gayk H, Scharla S, et al. Two-site assay of intact parathyroid hormone in the investigation of primary hyperparathyroidism and other disorders of calcium metabolism compared with a midregion assay. *J Clin Endocrinol Metab* 1988;67:353–360.
10. Hackeng WHL, Aps P, Netelenbos JC, Aps CJM. Clinical implications of estimation of intact parathyroid hormone (PTH) versus total immunoreactive PTH in normal subjects and hyperparathyroid patients. *J Clin Endocrinol Metab* 1986;63:447–453.
11. Armitage EK. Parathyrin (parathyroid hormone): metabolism and methods for assay. *Clin Chem* 1986;32:418–424.
12. Brent GA, LeBoff MS, Seely EW, Conlin PR, Brown EM. Relationship between the concentration and rate of change of calcium and serum intact parathyroid hormone levels in normal humans. *J Clin Endocrinol Metab* 1988,67:944–950.
13. Cronin RE, Knochel JP. Magnesium deficiency. *Adv Intern Med* 1983;28:509–533.
14. Fuss M, Cogan E, Gillet C, et al. Magnesium administration reverses the hypocalcemia secondary to hypomagnesemia despite low circulating levels of 25-hydroxyvitamin D and 1,25-dihydroxyvitamin D. *Clin Endocrinol (Oxf)* 1985;22:807–815.
15. DeLuca H. The vitamin D story: a collaborative effort of basic science and clinical medicine. *FASEB J* 1988;2:224–236.
16. Reichel H, Koeffler HP, Norman AW. The role of the vitamin D endocrine system in health and disease. *N Engl J Med* 1989;320:980–991.
17. Cancela L, Nemere I, Norman AW. 1a,25(OH)$_2$ vitamin D$_I$: a steroid hormone capable of producing pleiotropic receptor mediated biological responses by both genomic and nongenomic mechanisms. *J Steroid Biochem* 1988;30:33–39.
18. Insogna KL, Dreyer BE, Mitnick M, Ellison AF, Broadus AE. Enhanced production rate of 1,25-dihydroxyvitamin D in sarcoidosis. *J Clin Endocrinol Metab* 1988;66:72–75.
19. Emmertsen K. Medullary thyroid carcinoma and calcitonin. *Dan Med Bull* 1985;32:1–28.
20. Becker KL, Snider RH, Moore CF, Monaghan KG, Silva OL. Calcitonin in extrathyroidal tissues of man. *Acta Endocrinol (Copenh)* 1979;92:746–751.
21. McDermott MT, Kidd GS. The role of calcitonin in the development and treatment of osteoporosis. *Endocr Rev* 1987;8:377–390.
22. Lowery WD, Thomas CG Jr, Awbrey BJ, Rosentstein BD, Talmage RV. The late effect of subtotal thyroidectomy and radioactive iodine therapy on calcitonin secretion and bone mineral density in women treated for Graves' disease. *Surgery* 1986;100:1142–1148.
23. Hurley DL, Tiegs RD, Wahner HW, Heath H III. Axial and appendicular bone mineral density in patients with long-term deficiency or excess calcitonin. *N Engl J Med* 1987;317:537–541.
24. McDermott MT, Kidd GS, Blue P, Ghaed V, Hofeldt FD. Reduced bone mineral content in totally thyroidectomized patients: possible effect of calcitonin deficiency. *J Clin Endocrinol Metab* 1983;56:936–939.
25. Mundy GR, Cove DH, Fisken R. Primary hyperparathyroidism: changes in the pattern of clinical presentation. *Lancet* 1980;1:1317–1320.
26. Mallette LE. Review: primary hyperparathyroidism an update: incidence, etiology, diagnosis and treatment. *Am J Med Sci* 1987;293:239–249.
27. Heath H, Hodgson SF, Kennedy MA. Primary hyperparathyroidism. *N Engl J Med* 1980;302:189–193.
28. Shane E, Bilezikian JP. Parathyroid carcinoma: a review of 62 patients. *Endocr Rev* 1982;3:218–226.
29. Mundy GR, Bertolini DR. Bone destruction and hypercalcemia in plasma cell myeloma. *Semin Oncol* 1986;13:291–299.
30. Garrett IR, Durle BGM, Nedwin GE, et al. Production of lymphotoxin, a bone-resorbing cytokine, by cultured human myeloma cells. *N Engl J Med* 1987;317:526–532.
31. Thomson BM, Saklatvala J, Chambers TJ. Osteoblasts mediate interleukin-1 stimulation of bone resorption by rat osteoclasts. *J Exp Med* 1986;164:104–112.
32. Bataille R, Jourdan M, Zhang XG, Klein B. Serum levels of interleukin-6, a potent myeloma cell growth factor, as a reflection of disease severity in plasma cell dyscrasias. *J Clin Invest* 1989;84:2008–2011.
33. Burtis WJ, Brady TG, Orloff JJ, et al. Immunochemical characterization of circulating parathyroid hormone-related protein in patients with humoral hypercalcemia of cancer. *N Engl J Med* 1990;322:1106–1112.
34. Marx SJ, Spiegel AM, Levine MA, et al. Familial hypocalciuric hypercalcemia: the relation to primary parathyroid hyperplasia. *N Engl J Med* 1982;307:416–426.
35. Aida K, Koishi S, Inoue M, et al. Familial hypocalciuric hypercalcemia associated with mutation in the human Ca^{2+}-sensing receptor gene. *J Clin Endocrinol Metab* 1995;80:2594–2598.
36. Mallette LE, Eichhorn E. Effects of lithium carbonate on human calcium metabolism. *Arch Intern Med* 1986;146:770–776.
37. Baran DT, Schwartz MP, Bergfeld MA, Teitelbaum SL, Slatopolsky E, Avioli LV. Lithium inhibition of bone mineralization and osteoid formation. *J Clin Invest* 1978;61:1691–1696.
38. Gammon GD, Docherty JP. Thiazide-induced hypercalcemia in a manic-depressive patient. *Am J Psychiatry* 1980;137:1453–1454.
39. Mosekilde L, Christensen MS. Decreased parathyroid function in hyperthyroidism: interrelationships between serum parathyroid hormone, calcium-phosphorus metabolism and thyroid function. *Acta Endocrinol (Copenh)* 1977;84:566–575.
40. Jastrup B, Mosekilde L, Melsen F, Lund BJ, Sorensen OH. Serum levels of vitamin D metabolites and bone remodeling in hyperthyroidism. *Metabolism* 1982;31:126–132.
41. Mundy G, Shapiro JL, Brandelin JG, Canalis EM, Raisz LG. Direct stimulation of bone resorption by thyroid hormones. *J Clin Invest* 1976;58:529–534.
42. Mundy GR, Wilkinson R, Heath DA. Comparative study on available medical therapy for hypercalcemia of malignancy. *Am J Med* 1983;74:421–432 .
43. Binstock ML, Mundy GR. Effect of calcitonin and glucocorticoids in combination on the hypercalcemia of malignancy. *Ann Intern Med* 1980;93:269–272.
44. Henley JW, Ibbertson HK. Current concepts in the medical management of metabolic bone disease. *Drugs* 1974;8:246–249.
45. Hall TJ, Chambers TJ. Gallium inhibits bone resorption by a direct effect on osteoclasts. *Bone Miner* 1990;8:211–216.
46. Juan D. Hypocalcemia: differential diagnosis and mechanisms. *Arch Intern Med* 1979;139:1166–1171.

47. Chernow B, Zaloga G, McFadden E, et al. Hypocalcemia in critically ill patients. *Crit Care Med* 1982;10:848–851.
48. Scanlon EF, Kellogg JE, Winchester DP, Larsen RH. The morbidity of total thyroidectomy. *Arch Surg* 1981;116:568–571.
49. Wingert DJ, Friesen SR, Iliopoulos Jl, Pierce GE, Thomas JH, Hermreck AS. Post-thyroidectomy hypocalcemia. *Am J Surg* 1986;152:606–611.
50. Falk SA, Birken EA, Baran DT. Temporary postthyroidectomy hypocalcemia. *Arch Otolaryngol Head Neck Surg* 1988;114:168–174.
51. Michie W, Duncan T, Hamer-Hodges DW, et al. Mechanism of hypocalcemia after thyroidectomy for thyrotoxicosis. *Lancet* 1971;1:508–514.
52. Zamboni WA, Folse R. Adenoma weight: a predictor of transient hypocalcemia after parathyroidectomy. *Am J Surg* 1986;152:611–615.
53. Brasier AR, Nassbaum SR. Hungry bone syndrome: clinical and biochemical predictors of its occurrence after parathyroid surgery. *Am J Med* 1988;84:654–660.
54. Fonseca VA, Bloom RD, Dick R, Dandona P. Tetany despite normocalcemia and normomagnesemia following parathyroidectomy. *Postgrad Med J* 1987;63:885–886.
55. Horwitz CA, Laird Meyers WP, Foote FW. Secondary malignant tumors of the parathyroid glands. *Am J Med* 1972;52:797–808.
56. Levine MA, Downs RW Jr, Moses AM, et al. Resistance to multiple hormones in patients with pseudohypoparathyroidism. *Am J Med* 1983;74:545–556.
57. Keating MJ, Sethi MR, Bodey GP, Samaan NA. Hypocalcemia with hypoparathyroidism and renal tubular dysfunction association with aminoglycoside therapy. *Cancer* 1977;39:1410–1411.
58. Orland MT, Saltman RJ, eds. *Manual of medical therapeutics,* 25th ed. Boston: Little, Brown, 1986.
59. Flink EB. Nutritional aspects of magnesium metabolism. *West J Med* 1980;133:304–312.

CHAPTER 6

Pathology of Thyroid Disease

Virginia A. LiVolsi

The thyroid gland is affected by pathological lesions of varied morphologies, which can be divided into two types: those that show a diffuse pattern and those that produce nodules.

Diffuse thyroid lesions are those that are associated with nonneoplastic conditions affecting the gland: hyperplasia and thyroiditis. Nodular lesions comprise those disorders that consist of nonneoplastic hyperplasias as well as benign and malignant tumors. This chapter will review the pathology of the thyroid and will describe its normal appearance and changes in diseased states. The emphasis will be on those disorders that present as clinical nodules and in which the clinical and pathological differential diagnoses include malignancies.

Embryologically, the thyroid consists of two portions: (a) the median anlage from the foramen cecum of the tongue, which descends to its anterior neck position in association with the thyroglossal duct (the latter atrophies, although remnants of thyroid tissue may persist along this pathway of descent); and (b) the lateral anlage of the thyroid derived from the fourth–fifth branchial pouch complex, which includes the ultimobranchial body, the source of the parafollicular (or C) cells. Fusion of the median with the lateral anlage occurs in the upper and midlateral thyroid, where the C cells are found in the adult human gland (1).

In 14% to 28% of adult thyroids, and more frequently in those of neonates and infants, solid cell nests (clusters of epithelial cells sometimes with associated lymphocytes) are found; these represent the residuum of the ultimobranchial body (2–6).

Mal-descent during fetal life can result in several abnormalities. Lingual thyroid results when the thyroid retains its primitive location at the base of the tongue (7–9).

Thyroid tissue can be found along the pathway of the thyroglossal duct (10–14). Studies indicate that 63% of thyroglossal duct cysts contain normal thyroid tissue in their walls (14). Ectopic thyroid may also be found in the larynx or trachea (15–17). When descent of the median anlage is accentuated, normal thyroid can be found substernally, in the pericardium, or even in the heart itself (18–21).

Because of the intimate developmental relationships, derivatives of the branchial or pharyngeal pouches (parathyroid tissue, salivary gland remnants, and thymus) can sometimes be found in the thyroid (22). Developmental considerations also explain the finding of normal thyroid tissue in the cervical fat or muscle (22,23). Fat, cartilage, and muscle may occasionally be found within the thyroid capsule (23–25). These minor abnormalities of development must be remembered lest they be confused with infiltrative neoplastic growth.

Lateral aberrant thyroid (26–28), or thyroid located lateral to the jugular veins, *if unassociated with lymph node,* may be seen as part of anomalous development. Thyroid tissue, even if normal in appearance, anywhere within lymph nodes lateral to the jugular vein represents metastatic papillary thyroid carcinoma and is not a developmental anomaly. Many pathologists, but not all (29–33), accept normal thyroid follicles as an embryologic rest within capsules of medially located nodes (14,31,33). This thyroid tissue consists of normal follicles; no papillae of psammoma bodies are found and the tissue is in the nodal capsule (14).

ANATOMY OF THE THYROID

The normal adult thyroid consists of two lobes connected by an isthmus. The normal gland weight ranges from 14 to 18 g and depends on the sex and size of the individual, as well as on appropriate iodine intake (34,35). Thyroid tissue is light brown in color and firm in consistency. Nodules are not uncommon in the adult gland and can be found grossly in about 10% of the endocrinologi-

---

V. A. LiVolsi: Department of Pathology and Laboratory Medicine, University of Pennsylvania Medical Center, Philadelphia, Pennsylvania 19104-4328.

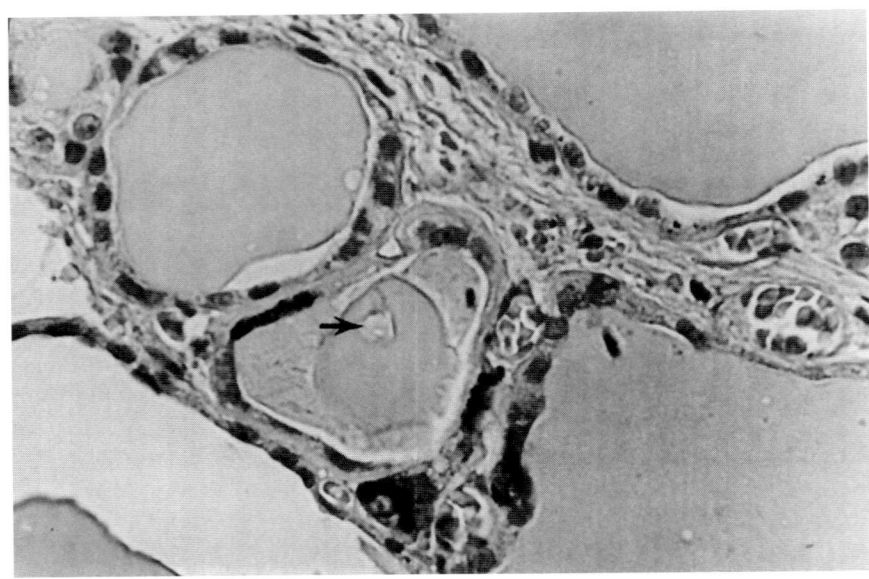

FIG. 1. Normal thyroid. Note calcium oxalate crystal *(arrow)* in colloid. (H & E, ×150.)

cally normal population (36–38). Microscopically, the thyroid is composed of follicles lined by epithelial cells that surround the central colloid; 20 to 40 follicles make up a lobule. Birefringent crystalline material (shown by chemical analysis and x-ray diffraction analysis to be calcium oxalate) can be found commonly in the colloid of normal or diseased thyroids (Fig. 1) (39). Between the follicular epithelial cells are calcitonin-containing parafollicular, or C, cells. Difficult to identify by usual stains, the normal C cells can be identified by immunostaining for calcitonin (Fig. 2) (40–43).

Ultrastructural studies (44,45) of normal thyroid show follicular cells arranged in a single layer around the central colloid. The cells contain liposomes and a complement of endoplasmic reticulum and small mitochondria. The nuclei are round with homogeneous chromatin (44). In the interstitium, numerous fenestrated capillaries are noted.

The C cells are always separated from the follicular epithelium by a basement membrane. In the cytoplasm, numerous double-membrane-bound neurosecretory granules containing calcitonin are found (40,41).

DIFFUSE THYROID ENLARGEMENTS

Thyroiditides

Although occasionally presenting as nodules or asymmetric enlargement of the gland, thyroiditis commonly involves the thyroid diffusely.

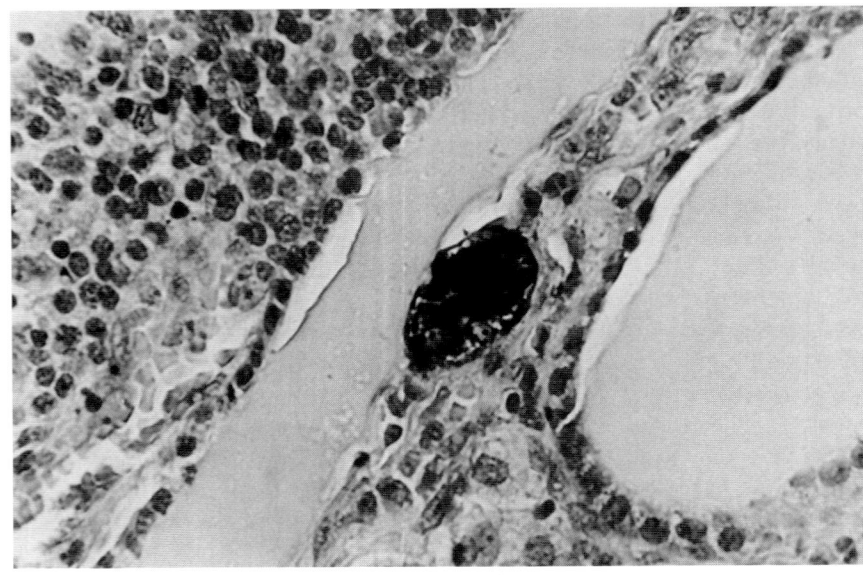

FIG. 2. Darkly stained C cell in normal gland. (Calcitonin immunoperoxidase, ×150.)

Acute thyroiditis (i.e., infection of the gland) occurs in young malnourished children, elderly debilitated adults, or immunocompromised individuals (46,47). Grossly, the thyroid may be focally or diffusely softened. Purulent foci will be noted. Microscopically, acute inflammation with microabscess formation, necrosis, and microorganisms is seen. In immunocompromised patients, fungal organisms are often identified.

Microorganisms that may cause acute thyroiditis include bacteria (46,47), fungi [*Candida, Aspergillus, Cryptococcus, Actinomyces,* and *Coccidioides* (48–51)] and, rarely, mycobacteria, spirochetes, and parasites (52–55). Cytomegalovirus and pneumocystis infections of the thyroid have been described in patients with acquired immunodeficiency syndromes (AIDS) (56,57).

In man, the routes of infection to the thyroid are (a) direct extension from a focus in the head or neck, and (b) hematogenous spread (46,47). Takai et al. (58) described a syndrome of acute supportive thyroiditis associated with left pyriform sinus fistula.

Granulomatous subacute thyroiditis probably represents the response of the thyroid to systemic viral infection (46,59–65); some authors suggest that it represents actual viral infection of the gland. The disease is not thought to be autoimmune in nature, and the mild increases in antithyroid antibody titers that may be found in affected patients usually disappear with resolution of the clinical symptoms and may represent epiphenomena secondary to thyroid damage (60,66,67). A viral causation for this disorder can be supported by both clinical and epidemiologic studies. Epidemics of subacute thyroiditis have been reported. Greene (60) documented cases of subacute thyroiditis–associated infection with mumps, measles, influenza, Coxsackievirus, mononucleosis, and adenovirus (68–71).

Pathologically, subacute thyroiditis is characterized by asymmetrical or diffuse involvement of the gland. Irregular white-tan lesions or several small poorly demarcated nodules may simulate carcinoma (46,61,65). Microscopically, early in the disease, there is loss of the follicular epithelium and colloid depletion. Leakage of stored hormone occurs, and clinical hyperthyroidism may result. The inflammatory response, composed initially of polymorphonuclear leukocytes and even microabcesses, progresses until lymphocytes, plasma cells, and histiocytes make up the major portion of inflammatory cells. The follicular epithelium is replaced by a rim of histiocytes and giant cells. Recovery is associated with regeneration of follicles from the viable edges of the involved areas (46, 61,65,72).

Palpation thyroiditis (multifocal granulomatous folliculitis) is found in most surgically resected thyroids (85% to 95%), and it probably represents the thyroid response to minor trauma. The histologic features of this lesion include multiple isolated follicles or small groups of follicles that show partial or circumferential loss of epithelium and replacement of the lost epithelium by inflammatory cells, predominantly macrophages (73).

AUTOIMMUNE THYROID DISEASE

The spectrum of autoimmune thyroid disease includes diffuse toxic goiter frequently with associated exophthalmos (Graves' disease) on the one hand and hypothyroidism-associated lymphocytic thyroiditis (Hashimoto's disease) on the other. However, in between, various lesions associated with hyper-, hypo-, or euthyroidism can be found.

The work of Volpe, Davies, and others (74–85) suggests that autoimmune thyroid disease involves an *inherited defect* in immune surveillance. Antigen-specific suppressor T-cell function is disturbed; a specific randomly mutating clone of helper T cells induces antibody-producing B cells. The interferon in turn causes human leukocyte antigen (HLA)-DR expression on thyroid epithelial cells (74,78,80), so that the epithelium can act *directly* as antigen-presenting cells and perpetuate the immune response (74,78,80–82). The role of autoantibodies may aggravate thyroid destruction (79,83–85).

Pathology of Autoimmune Disease

The presence of lymphoid cells in the substance of the thyroid parenchyma probably reflects an abnormal immunologic state. However, the interrelationships among classic chronic thyroiditis, its variants, and nonspecific thyroiditis are problematic.

The morphologic and immunopathological overlap between nonspecific lymphocytic thyroiditis and Hashimoto's disease suggests that they represent a spectrum of autoimmune injury.

In *chronic lymphocytic (Hashimoto's) thyroiditis* (86–90), the gland is firm and symmetrically enlarged, weighing from 25 to 250 g. Normal thyroid lobulation is accentuated by interlobular fibrosis. The thyroid has a tan-yellow appearance attributed to its abundant lymphoid tissue. The thyroid follicles are small and atrophic. Colloid appears dense or may be absent (Fig. 3). Follicular cells are metaplastic and include oncocytic (Hürthle cell), clear cell, and squamous types (86–90). In the stroma and in atrophic follicles, lymphoplasmacytic infiltrates with well-developed germinal centers are found.

The proportion of B and T cells within the thyroid differs from that in the peripheral blood, which is normal. The T-to-B-cell ratio in blood is between 70% and 80%, to 20%, and in the thyroid it is between 40% and 45%, to 50% (91). T lymphocytes within the thyroid are predominantly the suppressor type, whereas the peripheral blood of these patients contains mostly helper T cells.

The fibrous or *fibrosing variant of Hashimoto's thyroiditis* makes up 10% to 12% of cases and affects elderly

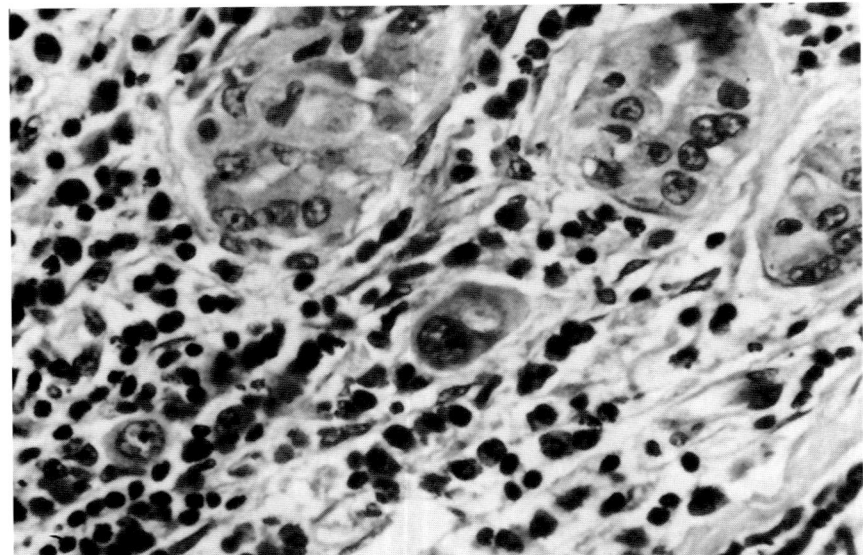

FIG. 3. Classic Hashimoto's thyroiditis. Note atrophic follicles, absence of colloid, and infiltrate of lymphocytes, plasma cells, and immunoblasts *(lower left)*. (H & E stain, ×200.)

patients who present with goiters and hypothyroidism (89,90). Pathologically, the thyroid architecture is destroyed with severe follicular atrophy, dense keloid-like fibrosis, and prominent squamous or epidermoid metaplasia of the follicular epithelium.

The gland of *fibrous atrophy* (idiopathic myxedema) is tiny, often weighing only 2 to 5 g. Destruction of the thyroid parenchyma with fibrous replacement and follicular atrophy occurs (90); lymphocytic infiltrates are prominent. Squamous metaplasia of follicles is seen as well, although this change may reflect not a true metaplasia but hyperplasia of ultimobranchial body rests.

Painless Thyroiditis with Hyperthyroidism

Recent clinical, immunologic, and pathological studies have confirmed that painless thyroiditis is an autoimmune disease (92–102). Mizukami et al. (97) analyzed 26 biopsies from patients with painless thyroiditis. All showed follicular disruption and lymphocytic infiltration, but stromal fibrous and oxyphilic changes were rare. Subset analysis of the intrathyroidal lymphocytes showed similarities to Hashimoto's thyroiditis (97).

Focal Nonspecific Thyroiditis

Lymphocytic infiltration of the thyroid is found more frequently at autopsy and in surgical specimens since the addition of iodide to the water supplies of the United States about 60 years ago (103–108). Iodide (iodine) may combine with a protein, act as an antigen, and evoke an immune response localized to the thyroid gland. Whether these lymphocytic infiltrates imply the meaning of autoimmune thyroiditis is unclear. Postmortem studies indicate an incidence of focal lymphocytic thyroiditis of about 15% to 20% in women and rarely in men (104–106). Kurashima and Hirokawa (105) believe that focal lymphocytic infiltration of the thyroid represents an immunological disorder associated with aging.

Focal aggregates of lymphocytes are noted, and occasionally germinal-center formation, but oncocytes are rarely present. Follicular atrophy is also rare (105,107).

Other Entities with Lymphocytes in the Thyroid

Diffuse Toxic Goiter

Lymphoid infiltration, sometimes associated with follicular-center formation, are often seen in patients with classic hyperthyroid Graves' disease (109). Usually, the lymphoid cells are found only in the interfollicular stroma and do not encroach upon the follicles themselves. The follicles show marked epithelial hyperplasia unless presurgical iodide treatment has been administered. Fibrosis is unusual.

Toxic Nodular Goiter

In glands with hyperfunctioning follicular nodules, lymphocytic collections can be seen, in unusual cases, outside the capsule of the nodule (110,111).

Drug-Associated Thyroiditis

Some drugs may affect thyroid morphology. Often, it is not possible to determine if the drug has induced the thyroiditis or has uncovered preexisting subclinical thyroid disease. Certain drugs have been associated with morphologic changes. Goiter commonly develops in patients treated for prolonged periods with lithium (112,113); hypothyroidism occurs in 3% to 12% of such cases (113).

Thyroid functional abnormalities have been recognized in patients taking amiodarone (114–121). Alves et al. (114) reported that in 104 patients on chronic amiodarone treatment, 32% developed hyperthyroidism and 23% hypothyroidism. The histologic changes described by Smyrk et al. (121) included follicular damage and disruption, epithelial cell vacuolization, and macrophagic and lymphocytic reaction to degeneration follicles. By electron microscopy, a lamellar configuration was seen in a few lysosomes (121).

Atkins et al. (122) described hypothyroidism occurring in several patients receiving interleukin-2 (IL-2) and lymphokine-activated killer (LAK) cell therapy for advanced cancers. They postulated that the therapy unmasked a subclinical autoimmune thyroiditis; the hypothyroidism appeared associated with a favorable tumor response in these patients.

FIBROSING THYROID LESIONS

Included in this category are the fibrosing (fibrous) variant of Hashimoto's thyroiditis and fibrous atrophy, which were discussed above.

Riedel's disease (invasive fibrous thyroiditis) has been included among the thyroiditides, but incorrectly, because this really is not a disorder of the thyroid but one that involves the thyroid (89,90,123–135). Invasive fibrous thyroiditis is an extremely rare entity, with an incidence of 0.05% of surgical thyroid diseases (125). Schwaegerle et al. (126) reviewed the literature on Riedel's disease and added seven cases from their own material. They found a female preponderance (83%). Thyroid function was noted to be normal in 64%, depressed in 32%, and overactive in 4% (126). The major symptom is a painless goiter and dyspnea.

Descriptions of the thyroid range from stony hard to woody ("ligneous thyroiditis") (123–135). When the lesion is confined to the neck, no systemic abnormalities are found; however, in some patients, the neck lesion represents part of a systemic disease; retroperitoneal, mediastinal, or retro-orbital fibrosis as well as sclerosing cholangitis may occur. In the Schwaegerle et al. (126) review, 34% of patients with Riedel's disease reported after 1960 had other fibrosing lesions (127–130,134). Familial cases with multifocal involvement have been described (127). No etiologic relationship to drugs has been suggested for isolated Riedel's disease (135).

Grossly, the fibrosis involves all or part of the thyroid and is described as woody and very hard (89,90,126). Extension of the fibrosis beyond the thyroid is characteristic. Histologically, the involved portions of the gland are destroyed and replaced by keloid-like fibrous tissue, associated with lymphocytes and plasma cells (89,90,126). The fibrous tissue extends into muscle, nerves, and fat, entraps vessels, and in about 25% of cases also encases the parathyroid glands (126). There is an associated vasculitis (predominantly a phlebitis) with frequent thrombosis (126,131,135). In 25% of cases of Riedel's disease, an adenoma is identified centrally in the fibrotic mass (125). Although the relationship between the adenoma and the fibrous reaction is unknown, the fibrous tissue proliferation may be a reaction to the adenoma or its products.

Quantitative studies (89) of the immunoglobulin-containing cells in fibrous Hashimoto's thyroiditis show that cells containing kappa light chains outnumbered lambda-containing cells (64% versus 36%), whereas in Riedel's disease lambda-containing cells were 71% of the population. In Hashimoto's thyroiditis, IgA cells made up 15% of the immunocytes, whereas IgA-containing plasma cells comprised 47% of the immunocyte population in Riedel's disease. The immunologic evaluation supports the separation of the distinctive Riedel's disease lesion from other thyroiditides.

Radiation Fibrosis

Reaction of the thyroid to radiation can result in a variety of complications that are related to dose in cases of external radiation to the gland. When radioiodine is administered, hypothyroidism is common and the incidence increases with time (136–145).

Pathological changes occur in the thyroid after external radiation in about 75% of cases and include foci of follicular hyperplasia (88%), lymphocytic infiltration (67%), oncocytic metaplasia (42%), fibrosis (25%), and adenomatous nodule formation (51%) (142–145).

Months or years after radioiodine, a grossly shrunken and fibrotic gland results that histologically shows fibrosis, follicular atrophy, oncocytic and squamous metaplasia, lymphocytic infiltration, and nuclear abnormalities (141–144). Vascular change (intimal thickening and sclerosis of arterial walls, often with inflammatory cell cuffing) is characteristic of radiation damage (141,144).

Amyloid

Amyloid is found in thyroid in three different settings. The most common of these is the amyloid in the stroma of medullary thyroid carcinoma. Amyloid goiter (146–149) is a tumefactive mass of amyloid associated with a foreign body giant cell response and with adipose tissue. It is associated with systemic amyloidosis (148). Another complication of systemic amyloidosis is amyloid deposition in the thyroid stroma and in glandular and periglandular blood vessels. Hypothyroidism may result (148,149).

Some patients (14% to 24%) with scleroderma will experience thyroid dysfunction as a result of interfollicular fibrosis, and 5% show evidence of chronic lymphocytic thyroiditis (150–152). The fibrosis may be caused by vascular sclerosis, common in scleroderma (153).

PIGMENTS IN THE THYROID

Pigmentation of the thyroid may be caused by iron (hemosiderin) deposition in sites of bleeding, and it may be found in disorders of iron metabolism such as hemosiderosis (154). In the former, the pigment is found in macrophages, whereas in the latter it is present in the follicular epithelium (155–164).

Minocycline-Associated Pigment (Black Thyroid)

In patients on chronic minocycline therapy, deposition of minocycline-associated pigment produces coal-black coloration to the thyroid. Histologically, a granular dust-like precipitate of black-brown pigment is noted in the apical portions of the follicular epithelial cells (155–164). Only rarely are abnormalities of thyroid function noted in these cases (156).

NODULAR THYROID ENLARGEMENTS

This category includes the common lesions of the thyroid that present as solitary or multiple nodules, benign nodular goiter, toxic nodules, and benign and malignant neoplasms. The nodular thyroid lesions are of most interest to surgeons and patients, because the major differential diagnostic possibility is cancer. This section describes the gross and microscopic morphology of the various thyroid nodular lesions; ancillary diagnostic techniques that aid the pathologist in precise classification of specific tumors are described. In many of the malignant tumors, specific morphologic features have been proven to be or are suggestive of prognostic importance.

Lesions Characterized by a Papillary Pattern

Papillary lesions include papillary carcinoma, papillary hyperplasia (often associated with hyperfunction), and papillary change in an adenoma or adenomatous follicular nodule.

Papillary Carcinoma of the Thyroid

In the United States, thyroid carcinoma accounts for about 1% of all cancers and 0.2% of cancer deaths (165,166). Most of these cancers are of the papillary type. This is the most common malignant tumor of the gland in countries having iodine-sufficient or iodine-excess diets (167–172), and it comprises about 80% of thyroid malignancies in the United States. Included in this figure are all papillary cancers, mixed papillary and follicular cancer, and the follicular variant. Despite differences in appearance, all of these tumors share biologic and clinical features that necessitate their being grouped together (173–186) and distinguished from pure follicular cancer.

These common tumors tend to be biologically indolent, and they have an excellent prognosis (>90% survival at 20 years) (173–186). The tumors invade lymphatics leading to multifocal lesions and to regional node metastases. Venous invasion rarely occurs; metastases outside the neck are unusual (5% to 7% of cases) (176,180–183).

Papillary carcinoma can occur at any age, although most tumors are diagnosed in patients in the third and fifth decades (173,176,180,182,183,187,188). It has rarely been diagnosed as a congenital tumor (184). Women are reported to be affected more than men in ratios from 2:1 to 4:1 (182,183,187,188).

Etiologic Factors

Etiologic factors for papillary carcinoma are not well established. The addition of iodine to the diet in endemic goiter areas in Europe has been associated with a decreased incidence of follicular cancer and an increase in papillary carcinoma (167–172). External radiation probably plays a role in the development of papillary cancer (189–194). The recent epidemic of pediatric thyroid cancer after the nuclear accident at Chernobyl in the Ukraine adds further evidence to this relationship (190). A history of external radiation in a patient who develops thyroid papillary cancer is not associated with a less favorable prognosis; Samaan et al. (194) compared nonradiated and radiated groups and found that although the latter had more extensive disease at diagnosis, the prognoses in both groups were similar.

Some authors believe that patients with Graves' disease have a higher than expected incidence of papillary cancer (195–197); other studies disagree (198).

Many studies indicate that up to one third of papillary cancers arise in the setting of chronic thyroiditis (199). However, these studies tend to lack serologic proof of preexisting thyroiditis. Follow-up studies of patients with documented thyroiditis indicate that the tumor that arises much more frequently in these glands is malignant lymphoma, not papillary cancer (see later). Because papillary cancer and thyroiditis are both common conditions, the possibility of coincidental coexistence is more likely than an etiologic relationship.

Occasionally, papillary cancers arise in benign nodules or adenomas (173,175,198). This may result merely from

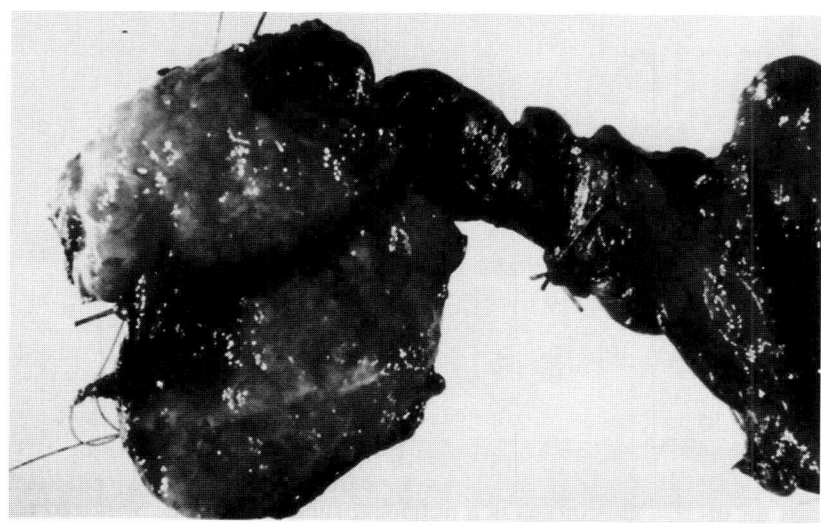

FIG. 4. Gross confined papillary carcinoma is partly replacing one lobe of this thyroid.

a malignant tumor arising in a nodular area of the gland instead of in a nonnodular zone (i.e., it is likely to be a random event of location, rather than indicating a causal relationship).

The association of papillary carcinoma and parathyroid adenoma and/or hyperplasia has been described by several authors. Both types of lesions are associated with a history of low-dose external radiation to the neck (200–202).

Pathology

The gross appearance of papillary thyroid cancer is quite variable (173,175,176,180,198). This has led to classification of the tumor based on gross type: small (occult), intrathyroidal (encapsulated and diffuse), and extrathyroidal (massive) (173,175,178,181,198).

The tumors in occult papillary cancer [for pathology, the preferred terms are *small papillary cancer* or *papillary microcarcinoma* (173,175,178,181,198,203–211)] measure 0.1 to 1.5 cm (198,210,211). Vickery et al. (175) indicated that most of these small tumors measure 4 to 7 mm. Harach et al. (209) noted that 35.6% of autopsied patients in Finland had occult papillary carcinoma. These authors suggested that tumors measuring under 5 mm be considered a normal finding and be left untreated. However, lymph node metastases from lesions less than 0.5 cm are known (207,208,211). Distant metastases, although very rare, are also documented (211). It is therefore appropriate to diagnose these small lesions as carcinomas. The small papillary carcinoma is a nonencapsulated, sclerotic, white-to-tan nodule often located subcapsularly. Histologically, the tumors may be totally follicular or they may show papillary areas as well. Sclerosis may be prominent; the lesions often infiltrate the surrounding thyroid.

Clinical papillary cancers may be located anywhere in the gland (173,175,181,198). The intrathyroidal lesions (comprising about 70% of papillary cancers) that usually measure over 1.5 cm appear as firm nonencapsulated or partly encapsulated lesions (Fig. 4). Calcification may be present. Gross cystic changes may be noted (173,175, 198,212,213). Occasionally gross papillations will be seen. Areas of hemorrhage and cholesterol clefts may be found (175,176,178,181,198). Necrosis is uncommon in the usual papillary cancer in the absence of prior needle biopsy.

Some papillary carcinomas are very large (5 cm or greater) and extend grossly beyond the thyroid capsule into cervical soft tissues (173,175,178,198).

Encapsulated papillary carcinomas resembling adenoma grossly make up about 8% to 13% of the group (175,178,181,198,210,214,215).

Microscopically, papillary carcinomas share certain features. The neoplastic papilla contains a central core of fibrovascular (occasionally just fibrous) tissue, lined by one or occasionally several layers of cells with crowded oval nuclei. In contrast, hyperplasia of thyroid follicles may sometimes exaggerate into papillary change; there is infolding of the lining epithelium composed of columnar cells with basal round and uniform nuclei. There is either no central core or a core of edematous or myxomatous paucicellular stroma, often including small follicles (subfollicle formation) (175).

Psammoma bodies that represent the ghosts of dead papillae (216,217) are differentiated from dystrophic calcifications by lamellations. True psammoma bodies are formed by focal areas of infarction of the tips of papillae attracting calcium that is deposited upon the dying cells. Progressive infarction of the papilla and ensuing calcium deposition lead to lamellation (216–219). Psammoma bodies are usually present within the cores of papillae or

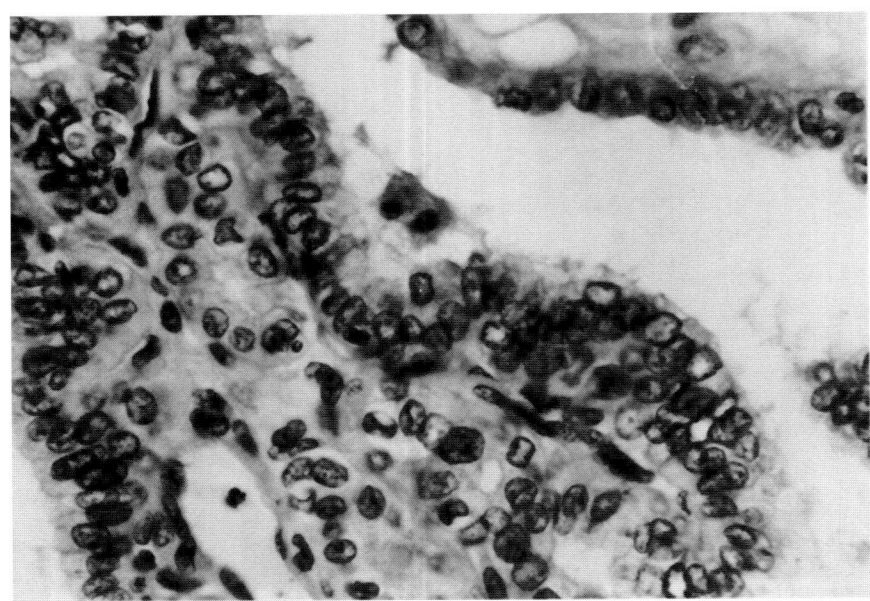

FIG. 5. Papillary carcinoma. The characteristics of the nuclei are evident. Note clearing of chromatin and overlapping of nuclei. In lower left is small vessel in fibrovascular core of papilla. (H & E stain, ×200.)

in the tumor stroma, but not within the neoplastic follicles. Only rarely are psammoma bodies found in benign conditions in the thyroid (216–223).

The nuclei of papillary cancer cells have been described as clear, ground-glass, and empty or Orphan Annie–eyed (Fig. 5). These nuclei are larger and more oval than normal follicular nuclei, and they contain hypodense chromatin (173,175,198,223–227). In papillary cancer, these nuclei often overlap one another. Intranuclear inclusions of cytoplasm are often found. Another characteristic of the papillary cancer nucleus is the nuclear groove (225–227). Although grooves can be seen in nuclei of other thyroid lesions, the grooved nucleus is present consistently and in many cells in papillary cancer (224–228).

Most of these tumors are composed predominantly or focally of papillary areas (173,175,198,222,223). A large number contain follicular areas as well (Fig. 6) (173, 178,181,198,222,223,229). Clear nuclei are found in over 80% to 85%, and nuclear grooves are seen in almost all the cases. Mitoses are exceptional in the usual papillary carcinoma cells (175,223). Psammoma bodies are found in about 40% to 50% of cases (173,175,181,198,222, 223,229), but their presence in thyroid tissue indicates that a papillary carcinoma is present somewhere in the

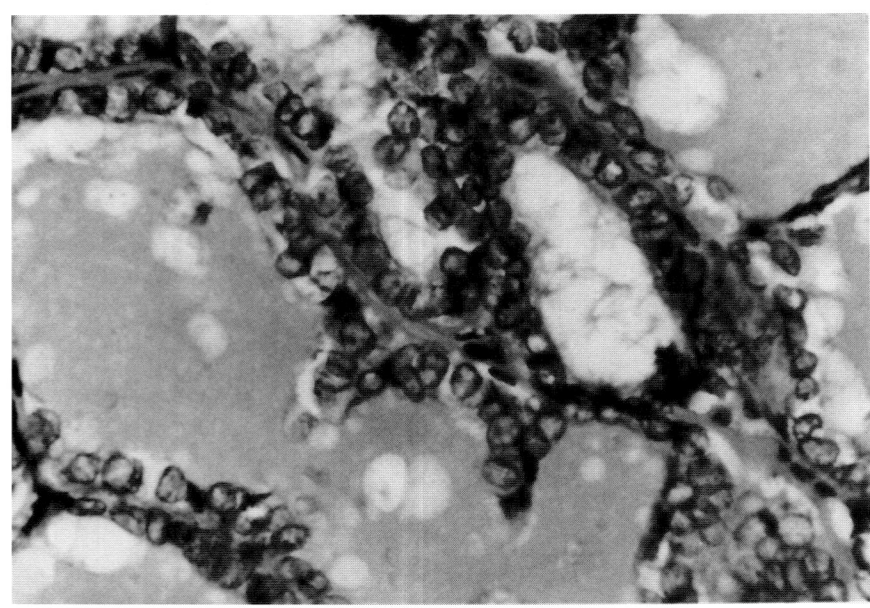

FIG. 6. Follicular variant of papillary carcinoma. Totally follicular pattern is present, but note nuclei similar to those present in Figure 5. (H & E stain, ×200.)

gland. The finding of psammoma bodies in a cervical lymph node is strong evidence of a papillary cancer in the thyroid.

Many papillary carcinomas (about 15% to 45%) contain foci of squamous differentiation (173,198,223,229). Almost all papillary carcinomas show areas of desmoplasia, either in the central portions of the tumor or at the peripheral zones of the lesions (173,175,181,198,223,229). Even in encapsulated lesions, sclerosis is seen in areas of capsular penetration.

Scattered lymphocytes are common at the invasive edges of the tumor (173,178,198,223,229). Rarely, an intense lymphocytic infiltrate is seen, but it is localized to the invasive tumor foci and does not indicate a preexisting underlying chronic thyroiditis. Volpe (75) suggests that these immunocytes are reacting to altered cell-surface antigens on the tumor cells or to abnormal tumor-cell products. Increased numbers of antigen-presenting dendritic cells are found near these lesions (230). A recent study indicates that patients whose thyroid tumors contain large numbers of lymphocytes enjoy a better prognosis than those without lymphoid infiltrates (231).

Papillary carcinoma invades the glandular lymphatics (173,175,181,198,223,229,232,233). This probably accounts for two commonly noted features of this tumor: the so-called multifocality of the tumor and a high incidence of regional node metastases. The monoclonal nature of papillary carcinoma has been confirmed by Hicks et al. (234) and Namba et al. (235) using molecular biology techniques. It is likely that the multifocality of papillary carcinoma is a result of intrathyroidal lymphatic spread. (The uncommon pathological finding of multiple microcarcinomas in a gland surgically excised for benign nodules may, however, be explained by multiclonality of the malignant foci; no studies attempting to explain this finding are yet available).

What does *multifocality* mean for therapy and prognosis? Some argue that because of multifocal microscopic lesions in the gland, the entire gland should be excised (236–242); others indicate that more conservative surgery (lobectomy or lobectomy and isthmusectomy) followed by thyroid suppression is adequate, because the tumors are often hormonally controllable (236–242). The low frequency of local recurrence in the opposite thyroid lobe (241) and the long-term follow-up studies of conservatively treated patients showing excellent results suggest that the second viewpoint is the wiser (236–242). Of course, treatment of extrathyroidal or massive papillary cancer requires more radical procedures (243,244).

Venous invasion can be identified in up to 7% of papillary cancers (175,178,244,245). Whether this finding alone is predictive of a more aggressive behavior is unclear.

Regional lymph node metastases are extremely common (50% or more) at initial presentation of usual papillary cancer. Most studies (175,180,194,246–248), but not all (188), indicate that this feature does not adversely affect long-term prognosis.

Some patients present with cervical node enlargement and have no clinically or grossly obvious thyroid tumor. Not infrequently, the nodal metastasis involves one node that may be cystic (203,212,248). The histology of the nodal metastases in papillary cancer may appear papillary, mixed, or follicular. The thyroid primary in these cases may be microscopic, and it is usually found on the ipsilateral side of the nodal metastasis. Because such tiny tumors can give rise to, and indeed present as, node metastases, it is the opinion of this author that all papillary microcarcinomas be diagnosed as carcinomas. When the microcarcinoma is an incidental finding in a lobe removed for a benign nodule, the clinical risk to that patient of metastases or other complications of a malignancy is very low (203,205).

Tumor grading is of no use in papillary thyroid cancer, because over 95% of these lesions are grade 1 (176,187). In some tumors, either in the primary site or in recurrences, areas of poorly differentiated cancer characterized by solid growth of tumor, mitotic activity, and cytologic atypia can be found. Such lesions have a much more guarded prognosis (229). Anaplastic change in a papillary cancer can occur, although it is uncommon (173,198,249).

Distant metastases of papillary carcinoma to lungs and bones (175,181,198,250–253) occur in 5% to 7% of cases. Despite the presence of multiple metastases, however, survival may still be prolonged, especially if the metastases can be treated with radioiodine (251–253). In ordinary papillary carcinoma, death is uncommon (180,187,253).

The electron microscopic appearance of papillary carcinoma includes a nucleus with dispersed chromatin and highly infolded nuclear membrane (corresponding to the nuclear groove seen at the light microscopic level), intranuclear inclusions, and many mitochondria and numerous cytoplasmic filaments (254–256).

Immunostaining shows that most papillary cancers (92% to 100%) contain thyroglobulin, thyroxine, and triiodothyronine (257). Low-molecular-weight keratin is found in virtually all papillary carcinomas (258–262). Utilizing microwave antigen retrieval techniques, some authors have found that high-molecular-weight keratins are also found in papillary carcinoma (262). This is a potentially useful way of distinguishing follicular variants of papillary cancer from true follicular neoplasms.

Some authors have shown that flow cytometry may be useful to assess prognosis in papillary cancer, because aneuploid tumors often are associated with a more aggressive clinical course (263–266). However, because most papillary thyroid cancers are diploid, this test is of limited value.

Poor prognostic factors in papillary carcinoma include older age at diagnosis, male sex, large tumor size, and extrathyroidal growth (181,187,188,267–274). Pathological variables associated with a more guarded prognosis include less differentiated or solid areas, vascular invasion, and aneuploid cell population (175,180,198,223,273).

Subtypes of Papillary Carcinoma

Follicular Variant. Grossly and histologically, the tumor in the follicular variant may appear encapsulated (173,175,178,181,198,223,275). Despite the almost total follicular pattern in the primary site, features that suggest a tumor is a follicular variant of papillary cancer include characteristic nuclei, psammoma bodies, and desmoplastic response at invasive areas. The prognosis of the follicular variant is apparently similar to usual papillary cancer, but there may be a greater risk for this variant to metastasize outside the neck (176,223,273,276).

Tall Cell Variant. Hawk and Hazard (178) found the tall cell variant made up about 10% of the papillary cancers they studied. The tumor is large (>6 cm), extends extrathyroidally, and shows mitotic activity, necrosis, and vascular invasion more often than usual papillary cancer (178,277). The tumor tends to occur in elderly patients.

The tall cell is twice as tall as it is wide, and its cytoplasm is often quite eosinophilic (277). The tumors show an extensive papillary pattern (Fig. 7). The prognosis for this variant is less favorable than for usual papillary cancer. Local recurrences with invasion of the trachea are seen; this complication may prove fatal (178,187,277).

Columnar Cell Variant. Only eight published cases of columnar cell variant are known. Most of the patients have been men; the mortality rate is 90% at 5 years (278–280). Histologic features of this lesion include extreme papillarity, tall columnar cells, and nuclear stratification.

Diffuse Sclerosis Variant. Diffuse sclerosis variant, which often affects children and young adults, may present as bilateral goiter. The tumor permeates the gland, outlining the intraglandular lymphatics. Tumor papillae have associated areas of squamous metaplasia. Numerous psammoma bodies are found. Lymphocytic infiltrates are found around the tumor foci (198,223,273,281–284). The lesions tend to recur in the neck and have a somewhat more serious prognosis than usual childhood papillary cancer. Carcangiu et al. (282) compared eight cases of this variant to their entire series of 241 cases of papillary cancer, and they found a higher frequency of nodal metastases (100% versus 37.5%) and of distant metastases (54% versus 14%), and less likelihood of disease-free survival (25% versus 77%) at the 8-year follow-up.

Encapsulated Variant. Encapsulated variant presents grossly as an adenoma and comprises from 8% to 13% of papillary cancers (175,198,210,214,215,223,273). Microscopically, such lesions can also show total encapsulation; however, there are cytologic features of papillary cancer, including nuclear changes and psammoma bodies. Some of these lesions show focal invasion into the capsule (215,285).

Rare variants of papillary cancer in which prognostic data are not well established include the solid type (286), the clear cell type (286,287), and the oxyphilic variant (288,289). The last of these appears to have a prognosis similar to usual papillary cancer, but the number of cases with sufficient follow-up data is scant.

The molecular biology of papillary cancer is discussed elsewhere in this text. However, interesting results have been reported about translocations of *ret* oncogene in some papillary carcinomas (290). The percentage of cases with translocation varies with different populations

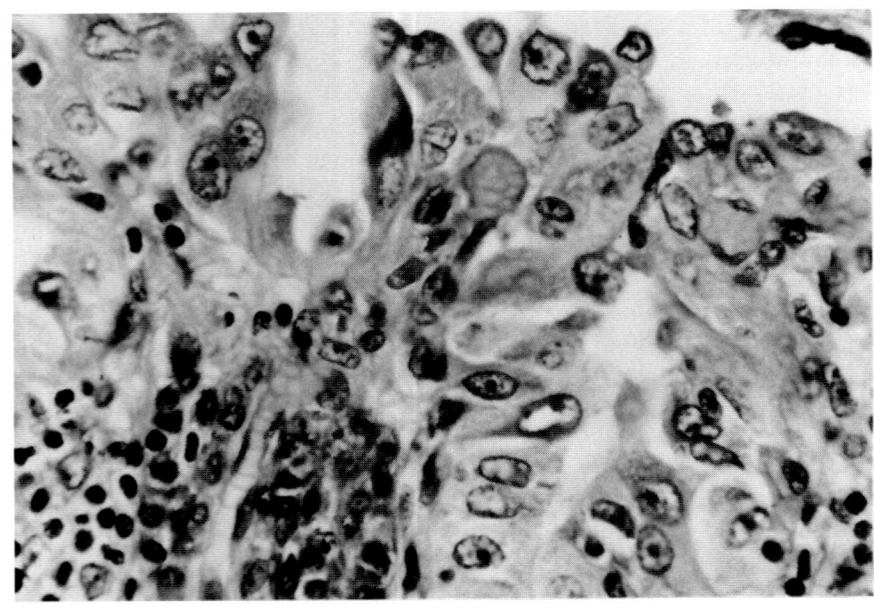

FIG. 7. Tall cell variant papillary cancer. Note large cells that appear elongated. Also note *(lower left)* lymphoplasmacytic infiltrate in core of papilla. (H & E stain, ×200.)

studied. The clinical significance of translocation is not fully known, although some reports indicate that tumors with translocated *ret* have a poor prognosis.

Papillary Hyperplasia

Papillary hyperplasia, seen in untreated autoimmune hyperthyroidism (Graves' disease), congenital errors of thyroid metabolism, and hyperfunctioning foci in goitrous glands, shows overgrowth of the follicular epithelium. The cell growth involves both hypertrophy and hyperplasia; infoldings (i.e., papillations) form. Diffuse papillary hyperplasia is distinguished from papillary carcinoma by the preservation of the gland architecture, the diffuse character of the lesion, and the normal nuclei. In toxic nodular goiter, the changes are similar but the lesion tends to be more focal. Nuclear characteristics differentiate the lesion from cancer.

Papillary Hyperplasia in Follicular Nodule

Well-circumscribed solitary thyroid nodules may show a microscopic appearance of papillary growth. However, the papillae contain extremely edematous stalks with follicles in them. The nuclei are round and not clear; there are no psammoma bodies. Some of these nodules produce a warm or hot appearance on scan (175,198,291). At times, areas in nodular goiters show a focally similar papillary appearance; these areas are often associated with hemorrhage and edema.

Although *papillary adenoma* has been used as a diagnostic term for these lesions, it should not be used, because it has been applied to a number of lesions, from hyperplastic ones to encapsulated papillary carcinomas, leading to confusion.

Lesions with Follicular Architecture

The majority of thyroid lesions (physiologic hyperplasia, benign nodular lesions, and neoplasms) display a macro- or microfollicular pattern. The thyroid lesions in this histologic category include those found in patients with congenital disorders of thyroid metabolism (dyshormonogenetic goiter) and disorders of the thyroid in diffuse toxic goiter [autoimmune hyperthyroidism (Graves' disease)]. In some of these conditions, hypothyroidism is found, in others, hyperfunction, and in still others, euthyroidism is present.

When the thyroid cannot produce normal amounts of thyroid hormone, the pituitary secretes increased amounts of thyrotropin (TSH), which, in turn, directs the thyroid follicular cells to produce more thyroid hormones—thyroxine and triiodothyronine (T_4 and T_3). The cells undergo hyperplasia and hypertrophy. The thyroid gland enlarges; in some cases, nodules form.

The morphology of the thyroid in patients with dyshormonogenesis is similar despite the different biochemical abnormalities (292–296). The glands are usually enlarged and nodular; secondary changes including hemorrhage and fibrosis can be found. Microscopically, the changes consist of extreme follicular hyperplasia. Most nodules show microfollicular or trabecular patterns. Clear cell change may be seen. Cytologic atypia is very common and may be so severe as to suggest a malignancy. However, true invasive growth is extremely rare (297,298).

Hyperthyroidism

Autoimmune hyperthyroidism occurs predominantly in women (with a ratio of about 9:1) (75,299–303). Patients with Graves' disease show a genetic predisposition to the disease, and their relatives have an unusually high incidence of other autoimmune disorders (303). The gland is infiltrated by lymphocytes (304). Similarities to Hashimoto's thyroiditis include an apparently genetically determined defect in suppressor T cells with consequent proliferation of thyroid-directed B cells, which produce antithyroid autoantibodies. These antibodies [thyroid receptor immunoglobulins (TRAbs)] are directed against the thyrotropin receptor complex of the follicular epithelial cell, which they stimulate to grow and function (305). Hence, the gland enlarges and secretes increased amounts of thyroid hormones, resulting in clinical hyperthyroidism.

Grossly, the thyroid in Graves' disease is diffusely and usually symmetrically enlarged, with weights of 50 to 150 g. Vascularity is markedly increased. Low-power histologic examination shows *retention* of lobular architecture, prominent vascular congestion, and follicular hyperplasia. The follicular cells are columnar with enlarged nuclei. Colloid is virtually absent. When colloid is present, it is scanty and scalloping of the colloid (a fixation artifact) is seen where it abuts the epithelium. Papillary infoldings of the follicular epithelium are also seen (304). In the stroma, lymphocytes, often arranged in follicular or germinal centers, are found. Within the follicular centers, B cells predominate; T lymphocytes, especially helper subsets, are seen in a perifollicular location.

Therapy-induced changes in histology include decreased vascularity and involution of the follicular epithelium with repletion of colloid after iodide therapy; beta-blocking drugs and thiouracil do not alter the morphology (304,306).

Nodular Thyroid Disease and Hyperthyroidism

Descriptions of clinical hyperthyroidism in patients with nodular glands have been attributed to Plummer and

Goetsch (307). The gland may be multinodular, or only a solitary mass may be present.

Toxic Nodular Goiter

In toxic nodular goiter, the clinical symptom complex of hyperthyroidism is associated with a nodular gland (308). This cause of hyperthyroidism is more commonly seen in older individuals. The histology is similar to diffuse toxic goiter, with the changes occurring within nodules.

Toxic Nodule (Adenoma, Carcinoma)

Rarely, a solitary nodule functions autonomously and produces clinical hyperfunction (291). Most of these are benign nodules; only rare examples of documented follicular carcinomas producing hyperthyroidism are known (291,308–312).

Follicular Thyroid Nodules

Nodular Goiter

The incidence of nodular goiter depends on the criteria used to define it. About 2% to 6% of the population has a clinical mass (36,37). About 10% of thyroids removed at autopsy contain nodules, usually multiple, but up to 40% to 50% of thyroids harbor microscopic nodules (36,37.313–316). Although multinodular goiter can be associated with hyperfunction (317), usually the patient is euthyroid.

Grossly nodular goiters range from slightly to massively enlarged glands (weights of 50 to over 800 g can be found) with intact capsules and a bumpy external surface (Fig. 8). Sectioning reveals multiple nodules of varying consistency, separated by variable amounts of normal-appearing thyroid. The nodules are composed chiefly of brown thyroid tissue; fibrous bands and calcification are noted. Microscopically, colloid lakes alternating with normal to hyperplastic-appearing foci of thyroid, hemorrhage, siderosis, fibrosis, calcification, and even bone are found. Variable amounts of lymphocytic infiltrate will also be found, possibly reflecting an immunological abnormality (318). The initiating events in the development and progression of nodular goiter have been studied by Studer et al. (319–326), who suggest that certain follicular cells or groups of cells are intrinsically more rapidly growing than their neighbors. The initial proliferation is polyclonal, involving one follicle, or more likely a group of follicles. Adjacent follicles remain quiescent. In the process, vascular compression in the stroma leads to focal ischemia, necrosis, and inflammatory changes. At later times, the same process may affect another group of follicles until large zones of the thyroid are affected. As the process continues, the secondary phenomena (hemorrhage, fibrosis, and calcification) take place. While these changes occur, the hormonal stimuli to the gland continue. Distortion of the vascular supply and the presence of dilated follicles filled with colloid interfere with the distribution of iodide and thyrotropin. Some parts of the gland will be exposed to excess thyrotropin, and focal hyperplasia may occur; other areas will have relative iodide and/or thyrotropin deficiency, leading to zones of atrophy.

What can be said about solitary follicular nodules that histologically, at least, appear identical to the multiple nodules seen in nodular goiter? Are these, then, regenerative, proliferative nodules, but not neoplasm? Or, alternatively, do they represent true benign follicular adeno-

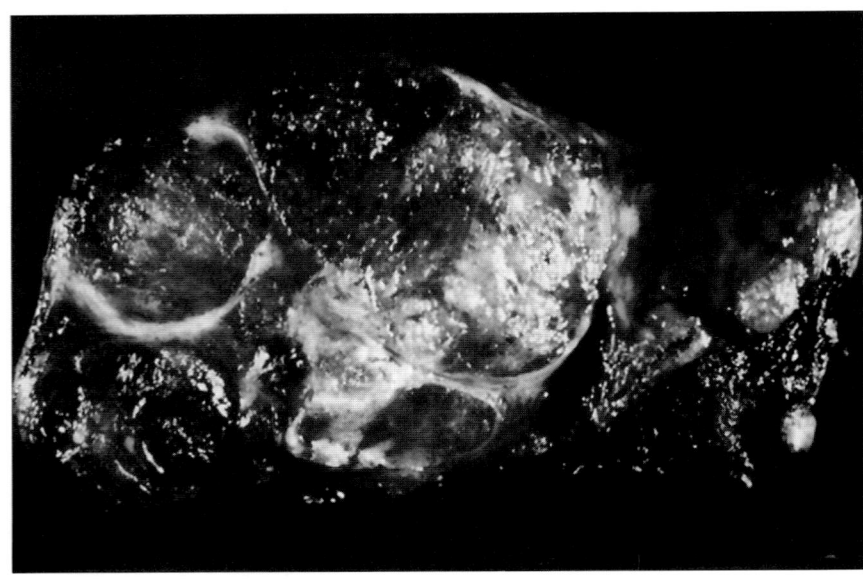

FIG. 8. Multinodular goiter: classic gross appearance.

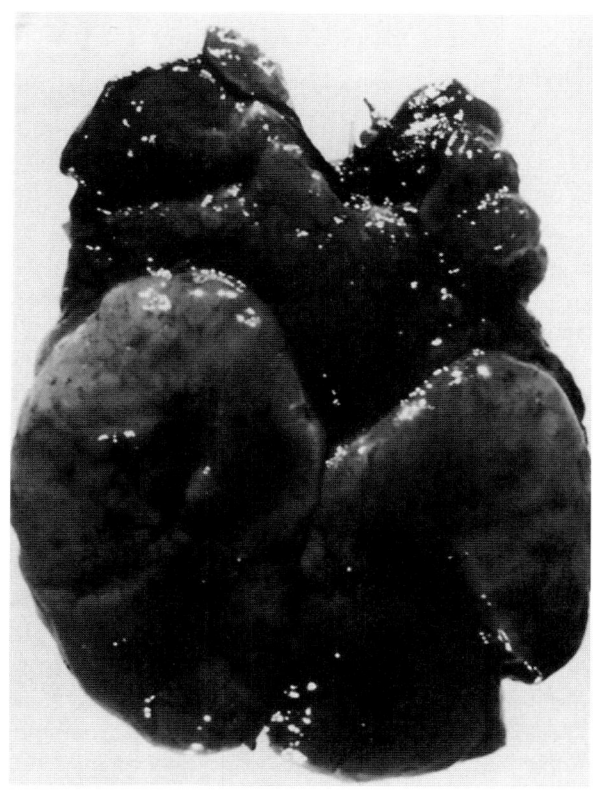

FIG. 9. Follicular adenoma (gross photograph).

mas? Many pathologists prefer the less definitive term *adenomatous* or *adenomatoid follicular nodule* for such lesions, avoiding the issue of histogenesis.

Hicks et al. (234) and Namba et al. (235), using restriction fragment length polymorphism techniques, found that solitary thyroid follicular nodules were clonal; hence, they are follicular adenomas. Recent studies of multinodular goiters have shown that 70% of these apparently hyperplastic nodules are clonal (327); furthermore, several different nodules in one multinodular goiter seem to represent the same clone. The biologic meaning of these data remains to be defined; whether these findings will have clinical relevance is unclear.

Follicular Adenoma

A follicular adenoma or solitary adenomatous or adenomatoid nodule is defined as a benign encapsulated mass of follicles, usually showing a uniform pattern throughout the confined nodule (Fig. 9) (222,229,328). Adenomas are solitary; indeed, if there are multiple nodules in a lobe or a thyroid gland, it is probably more appropriate to diagnose multinodular goiter with adenomatous change (adenomatous hyperplasia). The features that Meissner (328) used to distinguish histologically between adenoma and adenomatous nodules included encapsulation, uniformity of pattern within the adenoma, and compression of the surrounding gland by the adenoma and its capsule.

Descriptive terms that have been used to delineate the patterns seen in follicular adenomas include *macrofollicular, simple, microfollicular, fetal, embryonal,* and *trabecular* (Fig. 10). However, because these patterns have no clinical import, it is not necessary to subdivide thyroid adenomas. Relatively common changes found in adenomas include hemorrhage, edema, and fibrosis, especially in the central portions of the tumor.

Whether or not some solitary follicular nodules have the biologic potential to become carcinoma is unknown;

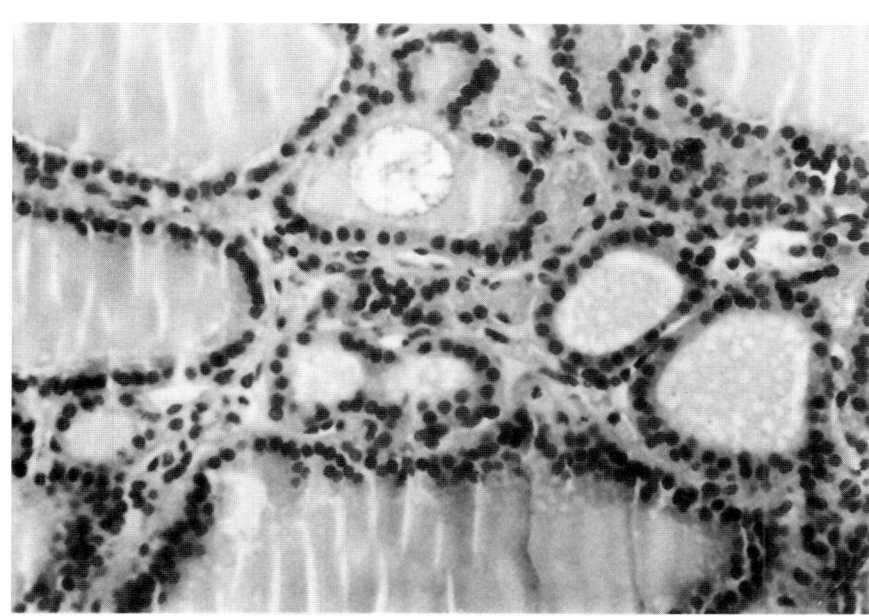

FIG. 10. Relatively uniform appearance in center of follicular adenoma. (H & E stain, ×150.)

the finding of an aneuploid cell population in 27% of such lesions has suggested to some authors that some of these may represent carcinoma *in situ* (329). The solitary follicular lesion that is removed by lobectomy and that, when adequately studied, shows no evidence of invasion, will neither recur nor metastasize.

Occasionally, a follicular adenoma contains bizarre cells; that is, it shows random, often marked, cytologically atypical cells with huge hyperchromatic nuclei; sometimes multinucleated cells may be seen. These lesions are benign (229).

Atypical Follicular Adenoma

Atypical follicular adenoma, a term proposed by Hazard and Kenyon (330), includes those follicular tumors that show pathologically disturbing features (spontaneous necrosis, infarction, numerous mitoses, or unusual cellularity), but do not show invasive characteristics. The overwhelming majority of the atypical adenomas behave in a benign fashion clinically (229,330–333).

Follicular Carcinoma of the Thyroid

Follicular carcinoma comprises about 2% to 5% of thyroid cancer (167,168,335,336); however, in iodide-deficient areas, this tumor is more prevalent, making up 25% to 30% of thyroid cancers (167,168,335). When iodide is added to the diet, papillary cancer increases and follicular carcinoma becomes less common (167).

Clinically and pathologically, follicular carcinoma is a solitary mass in the thyroid. Follicular carcinoma has a marked propensity of vascular invasion (not lymphatics). It is possible that follicular cancers produce certain factors that alter the venous endothelium, allowing the tumor easy access (337). In any event, follicular carcinoma avoids lymphatics; hence, true embolic lymph node metastases are exceedingly rare.

Follicular carcinoma disseminates hematogenously and metastasizes to bone, lungs, brain, and liver (271, 338–342). Follicular cancer metastases will usually be treatable by radioiodine if there is no normal thyroid tissue present in the neck. For this reason, many surgeons consider total thyroidectomy appropriate therapy for encapsulated follicular cancers.

Because it is very difficult if not impossible to render a definitive cancer diagnosis with a fine-needle aspiration (FNA) sample or a frozen section of such a tumor, delayed-completion thyroidectomy may be necessary.

Alternatively, because the disease-free interval after lobectomy and/or cure of these encapsulated lesions is so great, completion thyroidectomy may represent overtreatment in a large percentage of these patients (331,339,340,343). Some therapists prefer radioablation of the residual thyroid, either when the definite diagnosis of cancer is made or if and when metastases first appear (331).

Total thyroidectomy appears warranted in those individuals who present with metastatic disease and in whom the primary is still untreated.

Lymph node dissection is not recommended, because these tumors do not spread to nodes; abnormal-appearing or enlarged nodes should be sampled, however.

Patients who have follicular carcinoma that is widely invasive fare poorly (186,331,338–341). However, those individuals with encapsulated follicular tumors confined to the thyroid enjoy a prolonged survival (greater than 80% at 10 years) (186,331,338,341,344,345). Several studies have addressed those factors (clinical and pathological) that are associated with a worse outcome (176,181,186,252,331, 332,334,341–346). These factors include old age at diagnosis, male sex, extrathyroidal growth or metastasis at time of diagnosis, extensive vascular invasion, solid or trabecular growth pattern, and aneuploid cell population. An extremely significant complication that may occur in patients with follicular cancer is transformation into anaplastic cancer (341–347); this may occur *de novo* in an untreated follicular lesion, or in metastatic foci.

Pathology. The widely invasive follicular carcinoma is a tumor that is clinically and surgically recognized as a cancer; the role of the pathologist in its diagnosis is to confirm that it is of thyroid origin and is a follicular neoplasm. Lang et al. (334,341) noted that 80% of the patients with widely invasive cancers developed metastases and about 20% died of tumor. Woolner et al. (181) found a 50% fatality rate for widely invasive tumors, compared with only 3% for those with minimal invasion (181,257).

The minimally invasive follicular carcinoma can be diagnosed by the pathologist only upon examining well-fixed histologic sections (348). These lesions are not diagnosable by FNA cytology, because the diagnosis requires the demonstration of invasion at the edges of lesion; therefore, sampling of the center of the lesion, as with FNA, cannot be diagnostic.

Similar problems exist in evaluating such lesions by frozen section. Some authors (349) have recommended that intraoperative assessment of such lesions involve the examination of frozen sections from three or four separate areas of the nodule. This wastes resources and rarely gives useful diagnostic information. The surgeon should have removed the lobe involved by the nodule, and, if it is a follicular carcinoma that is only minimally invasive, the appropriate therapy has probably already been accomplished. Because only a small number of these lesions shows evidence of invasion at the time of permanent section (i.e., the majority of them are benign), and because overdiagnosis is more dangerous for the patient than is the delay in making a definitive diagnosis, we discourage frozen section evaluation for these nodules (350,351).

The distinction between minimally invasive follicular carcinoma and angioinvasive encapsulated follicular car-

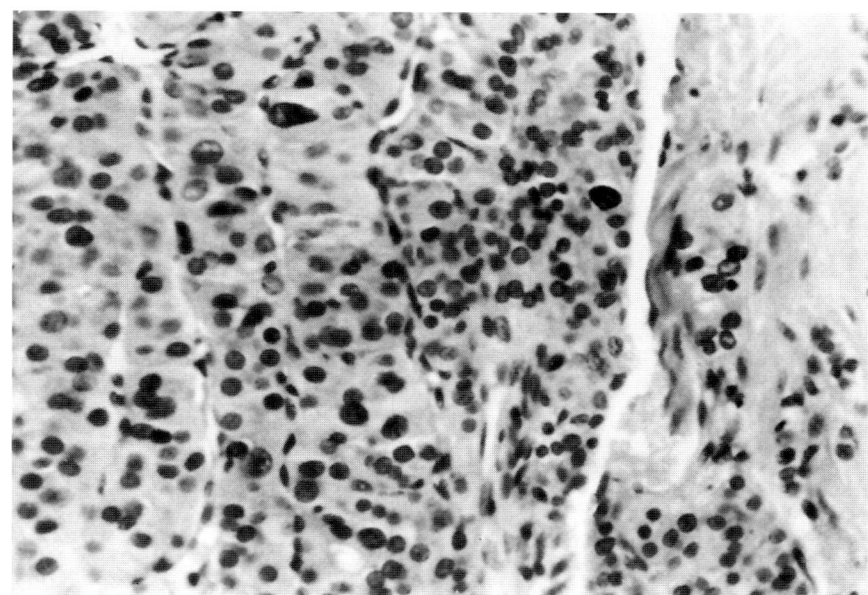

FIG. 11. Follicular carcinoma. Note solid trabecular pattern. (H & E stain, ×150.)

cinoma is important. It is the author's practice to diagnose as minimally invasive follicular carcinoma those tumors that are encapsulated and in which invasion of the capsule or penetration of the capsule is found, but in which no vascular invasion is identified. Those tumors in which vessel invasion is seen, at or beyond the level of the tumor capsule, are diagnosed as angioinvasive follicular carcinoma. (Most follicular cancers that show vascular invasion will demonstrate capsular invasion also; occasional examples do not.) The latter group of tumors can be biologically aggressive; anywhere from 33% to 50% of them will recur and/or metastasize at 10 years of follow-up (352).

Grossly, the minimally invasive follicular carcinoma resembles a follicular adenoma. The lesion is well encapsulated, and the thickness of the capsule is prominent (331,338,341,353,354). Microscopically, the tumor demonstrates a microfollicular or trabecular pattern with regular, small round follicles (Fig. 11) (331,341). Hemorrhage, necrosis, or even tumor infarction may be noted, and significant mitotic activity is often found.

What are the minimum criteria for making this diagnosis? Invasion of the capsule, through the capsule, and invasions into veins in or beyond the capsule represent the diagnostic criteria for carcinoma in a follicular thyroid neoplasm (Fig. 12). The criterion for vascular inva-

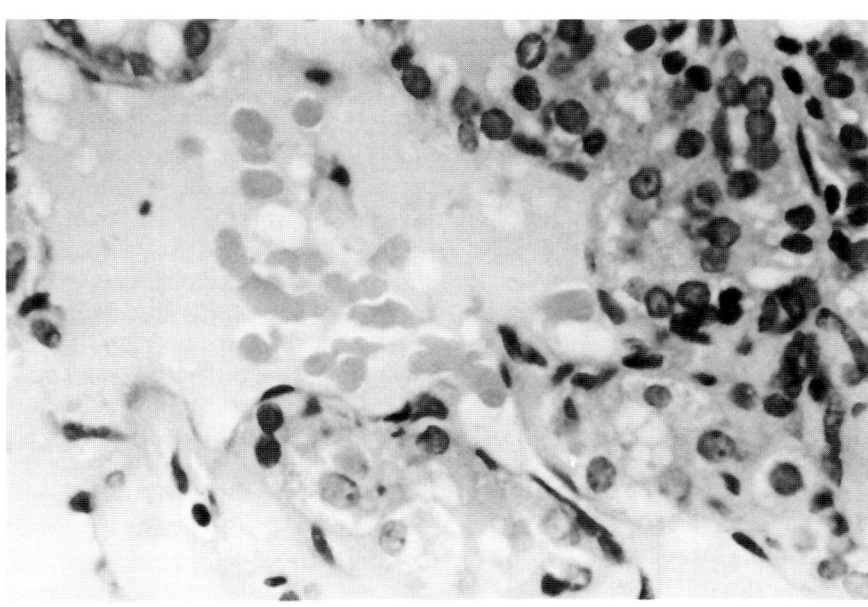

FIG. 12. Capsular vein shows red blood cells and tumor (right) admixed. (H & E stain, ×200.)

sion applies solely and strictly to veins in or beyond the capsule, because tumor plugs within capillaries in the substance of the tumor have no apparent diagnostic and prognostic importance (341).

The definition of capsular invasion has evoked great debate among pathologists. Some require vascular invasion to render a diagnosis of follicular carcinoma; others need penetration through the capsule of the tumor, and still others need invasion into the capsule (331,334,338,341,353).

Kahn and Perzin (332) found in their series that only capsular invasion was associated with metastatic disease. Evans (338) and Schroder et al. (353) agreed that capsular invasion was an important diagnostic criterion. Lang et al. (334,341) and Franssila et al. (331) require penetration of the capsule to diagnose a follicular tumor as carcinoma. Iida (354) noted that distinguishing capsular invasion from trapping may prove difficult; he required that the invasive tongues of tumor sever and deflect the collagen fibers in the capsule.

Is capsular invasion insufficient for the diagnosis of follicular cancer? Kahn and Perzin (332) found that 1 in 7 patients (14%) with only capsular invasion demonstrated metastases. Evans (331) noted that only capsular invasion was present in 3 of 7 patients (43%) with metastases. However, in these three cases, metastases were already present at the initial diagnosis (Fig. 13) (331,337).

On the other hand, those authors who diagnose tumors with capsular invasion only as atypical adenoma indicate a benign clinical course after thyroid lobectomy. Periods of follow-up differ among various series.

Recurrences or metastases can appear within 5 years after thyroidectomy (331–334,341), but some encapsulated follicular carcinomas notoriously can present as metastases many years after initial resection.

None of the modern ancillary techniques assists in defining benign from malignant follicular tumors. Ultrastructural, morphometric, and flow cytometric analyses have not helped in distinguishing these lesions (329,355).

Hürthle Cell Lesions

Hürthle cells are derived from follicular epithelium and are characterized morphologically by large size, distinct cell borders, voluminous granular cytoplasm, large nucleus, and prominent nucleolus (356). Ultrastructural studies have shown that the cytoplasmic granularity is produced by huge mitochondria filling the cell (357,358). Studies by Tremblay (359,360) have shown that these cells contain high levels of oxidative enzymes.

These cells can be found in a number of conditions in the thyroid and they cannot be considered specific for any disease entity: nodular goiter, nonspecific chronic thyroiditis, longstanding hyperthyroidism, chronic lymphocytic thyroiditis (Hashimoto's disease), and nodules and neoplasms (86,90,141,143,356,361,362).

Nodules of Hürthle cells are not all neoplastic. In fact, the majority represent Hürthle cell change of preexisting follicular adenomatous nodules in goiters or thyroiditis (362).

The clinical behavior of Hürthle cell neoplasms has elicited debate in the literature. Some authors cite 80% or more of these lesions as benign, whereas others consider all such lesions malignant (363–367). Because most Hürthle cell neoplasms are follicular in pattern, the criterion for distinguishing benign from malignant is the same as for follicular neoplasms (i.e., the identification of invasion) (367–370). However, the pathological

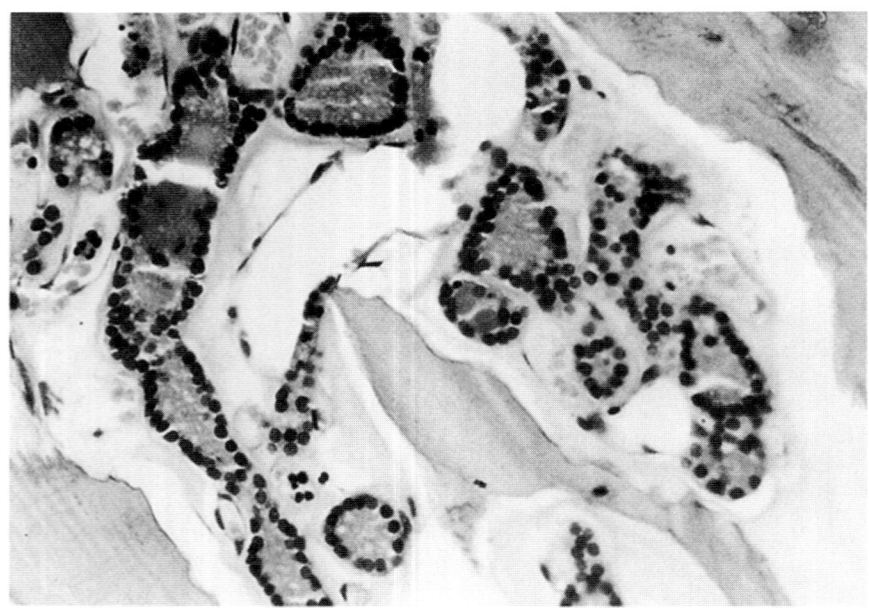

FIG. 13. Bone metastasis of follicular thyroid cancer in vertebra. Note follicular differentiation—thyroglobulin stain was positive. Primary tumor had been removed 24 years before. (H & E stain, ×150.)

criterion for malignancy is met more frequently for tumors composed of Hürthle cells than for their non-Hürthle counterparts. Thus, whereas 2% to 3% of solitary encapsulated follicular tumors of the thyroid show invasive characteristics, 30% to 40% of such lesions showing Hürthle cell cytology will show such features. In addition, whereas true follicular carcinomas of the thyroid rarely, if ever, metastasize embolically to lymph nodes, about 30% of Hürthle cell carcinomas do (367,369).

Most Hürthle cell neoplasms of the thyroid are solitary mass lesions that show complete or partial encapsulation. They are distinguished from the surrounding thyroid by their distinctive brown to mahogany color (370). Rarely, a Hürthle cell neoplasm may undergo spontaneous infarction, especially after FNA (371,372).

The claim that all Hürthle cell neoplasms should be considered malignant or potentially malignant, especially if 2 cm or greater in size (363–365), is no longer considered valid. Many studies from the United States and Europe (362,365–367,371–374) indicate that benign Hürthle cell neoplasms exist (Fig. 14). Nuclear atypia, multinucleation, cellular pleomorphism, mitoses, and histologic pattern of the lesion are not predictive of behavior (365,366,373–384). Large size should be of concern, because 80% of those Hürthle cell tumors that are 4 cm or greater will show histologic evidence of malignancy. Pathologic criteria for malignancy—vascular invasion, transcapsular penetration, destructive capsular invasion—can predict the clinical behavior of these tumors (364,367,383,384). The distinction between benign and malignant Hürthle cell tumors is made by the pathologic evaluation of the mass, applying strict criteria as noted above for non-Hürthle follicular tumors. In the absence of invasion, a Hürthle cell thyroid tumor should be considered benign. Total thyroidectomy is not needed for all Hürthle cell neoplasms (364,367,383,384).

In the histologically defined carcinomas, flow cytometric data may provide prognostic aid. Histologic carcinomas that show an aneuploid pattern may behave more aggressively than those that are diploid (380–381).

Rare tumors with Hürthle cell cytology are papillary carcinomas both by morphologic appearance and by clinical behavior (288,289). The finding of oncocytic cytology in an otherwise classical papillary carcinoma does not indicate an aggressive lesion when compared for size and stage with non-oncocytic papillary cancers. Caution must be used, however, not to confuse Hürthle cell papillary carcinoma with the tall cell variant of papillary carcinoma, which, as discussed previously, is an aggressive thyroid tumor.

C-Cell Lesions

The hormone calcitonin was discovered and characterized in the early 1960s; the thyroid C cell was described in many animal species at the end of the nineteenth and in the early twentieth century. In the early 1960s, pathologists were defining the morphology of the tumor now known as medullary carcinoma (385–387). In 1966, Williams (387) proposed that medullary carcinoma might be derived from the C cell and predicted that if the C cell was the source of calcitonin, the tumors might also produce this hormone.

The C cells are derived embryologically from the remnants of the ultimobranchial body and ultimately from the neural crest (1,42,388–390). In humans, C cells are found along the lateral aspects of the thyroid lobes in the upper two thirds of the gland (1). The C cells comprise less than

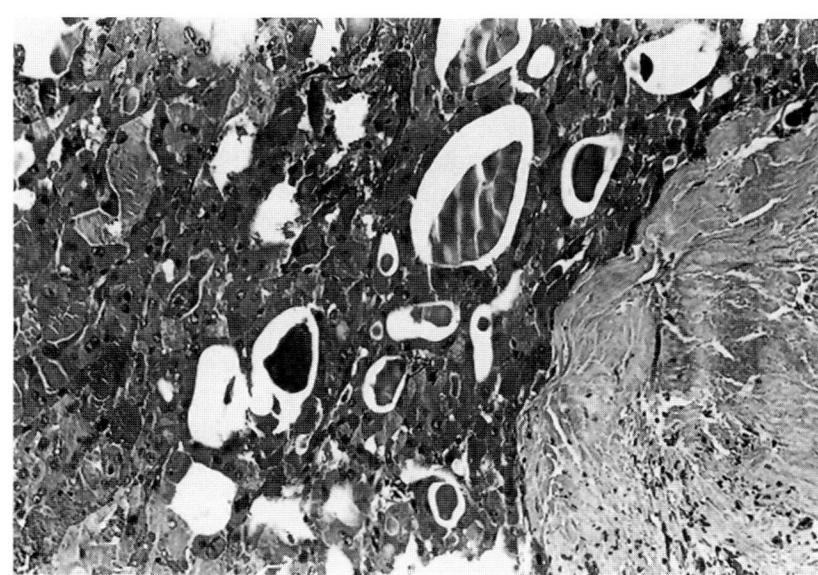

FIG. 14. Circumscribed Hürthle cell nodule. No invasion seen. (H & E stain, ×100.)

0.1% of the thyroid mass in humans (41,391–393). Wolfe et al. (391,392) showed excellent correlation between immunohistochemical localization of these cells and calcitonin content of the area of the thyroid in which they were found. The number of C cells in the thyroid differs according to age (391,392,394), with infants and young children having larger numbers of these cells than adults. The definition of the normal number of C cells in an adult thyroid remains controversial (391,392,395–397). Clusters of C cells in adults have been described in endocrinologically normal adults (395). O'Toole et al. (397) examined thyroid glands from forensic autopsies and recognized a trend toward increased numbers of these cells in older individuals (over age 60); however, they noted large standard deviations. This remains a problem area for pathologists; fortunately for them, the identification of excess numbers of C cells (i.e., C-cell hyperplasia) in the thyroid glands of patients with medullary carcinoma is now a moot point. With the availability of an excellent genetic test for *ret* oncogene mutations to detect familial medullary cancer and the precursor, C-cell hyperplasia, histopathologists do not have to guess which patients have the familial forms of this thyroid tumor (398–403).

Medullary Thyroid Carcinomas

Medullary thyroid carcinoma is unusual and comprises from 3% to 10% of all thyroid malignancies; in the general population, the lower figure is probably more accurate (229,404–409). There is no known or suspected etiology for medullary carcinoma. However, in a small but significant minority of cases, a genetic basis for the tumor can be identified. About 10% to 20% of patients with medullary carcinoma have a positive family history of thyroid tumors, or evidence of hypercalcemia or pheochromocytoma. The clinical features are similar in both sporadic and familial cases that are symptomatic (181,229,404–417). Medullary carcinoma can affect patients of any age; most affected individuals are adults with an average age of about 50 years. However, in familial cases, children can be affected; also, in these instances, the age of diagnosis tends to be younger (mean age, about 20 years).

Although in the sporadic variety there is a slight male predominance, in familial cases the sex ratio is 1, because an autosomal dominant mode of inheritance is present.

Most patients will present with a thyroid nodule that is painless but firm. In up to 50% of cases, obvious nodal metastases will be present at the time of diagnosis. Distant metastases, such as to lung, bone, or liver, may also be noted initially in about 15% to 25% of cases (404–418). When the tumor produces excess hormone other than calcitonin, the presenting symptoms may be related to that hormone hypersecretion [e.g., adrenocorticotropic hormone (ACTH), prostaglandin] (419–423).

In the familial forms, there are associated endocrine and/or neuroendocrine lesions. Sipple's syndrome [multiple endocrine neoplasia (MEN) type II or IIA] (400–403, 424–436) is familial (transmitted as autosomal dominant with an almost complete penetrance), and consists of medullary thyroid cancer and C-cell hyperplasia, adrenal pheochromocytoma and adrenal medullary hyperplasia, and parathyroid hyperplasia (425–436). Although most affected patients have the complete syndrome, not every patient need manifest all of these lesions. Recent studies have shown that the gene responsible for familial medullary carcinoma, as well as for multiple endocrine neoplasia type II and IIB, is located on chromosome 10 (400–403,437–439).

Multiple endocrine neoplasia type IIB consists of medullary thyroid carcinoma and C-cell hyperplasia, pheochromocytoma, and adrenal medullary hyperplasia, and mucosal neuromas, gastrointestinal ganglioneuromas, and musculoskeletal abnormalities (435,440–457). These patients may have familial disease (over 50% do) (440–457); some cases arise apparently as spontaneous mutations. These patients have biologically aggressive medullary carcinoma and may succumb to metastases at an early age. MEN IIB shows similarity to von Recklinghausen's disease, because in neurofibromatosis similar lesions are found in the gastrointestinal tract, and pheochromocytomas are common (457). Nerve growth factor has been identified in some medullary carcinoma of these patients; it has been postulated that this product of the tumor may be responsible for the neural lesions seen in the MEN IIB patients (458,459). However, the neural lesions often precede by many years the development of medullary cancer (446).

The pathologist may contribute to the determination of familial rather than sporadic disease if, upon examining a medullary carcinoma of the thyroid, he notes multifocal and/or bilateral tumors and the presence of C-cell hyperplasia (430,460–462). Specific point mutations in the *ret* oncogene define the phenotype of the familial medullary cancer syndrome (398–403). When the mutations are identified, early total thyroidectomy can be offered to avoid the development of the carcinoma in these individuals (400).

In some sporadic medullary cancers, *ret* oncogene mutations in regions similar to those in familial disease have been identified (463,464).

Pathology

The tumor is usually located in the area of highest C-cell concentration (i.e., the lateral upper two thirds of the gland). In familial cases, multiple small nodules may be detected grossly, and lesions in the isthmus may be found rarely (404–412). The tumors range in size from barely visible to several centimeters. Many medullary carcinomas are grossly circumscribed; some

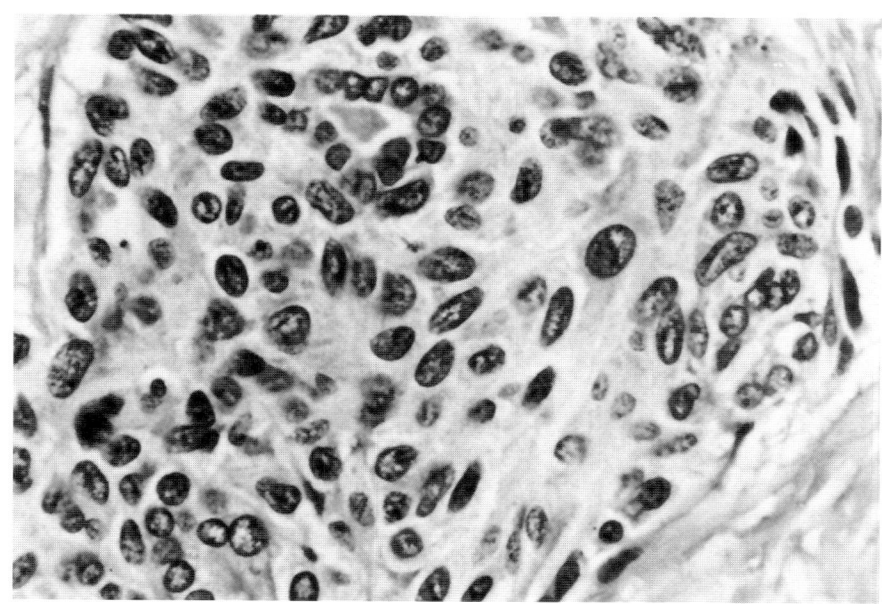

FIG. 15. Classic appearance of medullary carcinoma with small round and spindle-shaped cells admixed. (H & E stain, ×150.)

show infiltrative borders. Some tumors show necrosis and hemorrhage.

The typical medullary carcinoma may be microscopically circumscribed or more likely will be freely infiltrating into the surrounding thyroid. The pattern of growth is of tumor cells arranged in nests separated by varying amounts of stroma. The tumor nests are composed of round, oval, or spindle-shaped cells; there often is isolated cellular pleomorphism or there may even be multinucleated cells (Fig. 15). The nuclei are uniform; the nuclear/cytoplasmic ratio is low. Intranuclear cytoplasmic inclusions are commonly noted (465); mitoses can be seen. The tumor stroma characteristically contains amyloid, although this is not necessary for the diagnosis (Fig. 16). The tumors commonly invade lymphatics and veins. Some medullary carcinomas are grossly and microscopically encapsulated (181, 229,466). Mendelsohn and Oertel (467) reported a series of encapsulated thyroid lesions classified as atypical adenomas and showed that many of these were medullary cancers containing immunoreactive calcitonin. The follow-ups of encapsulated medullary carcinomas indicate that they have a more benign prognosis than usual medullary tumors.

Saad et al. (466) defined several histologic subtypes of medullary carcinoma: insular, trabecular, carcinoma-like,

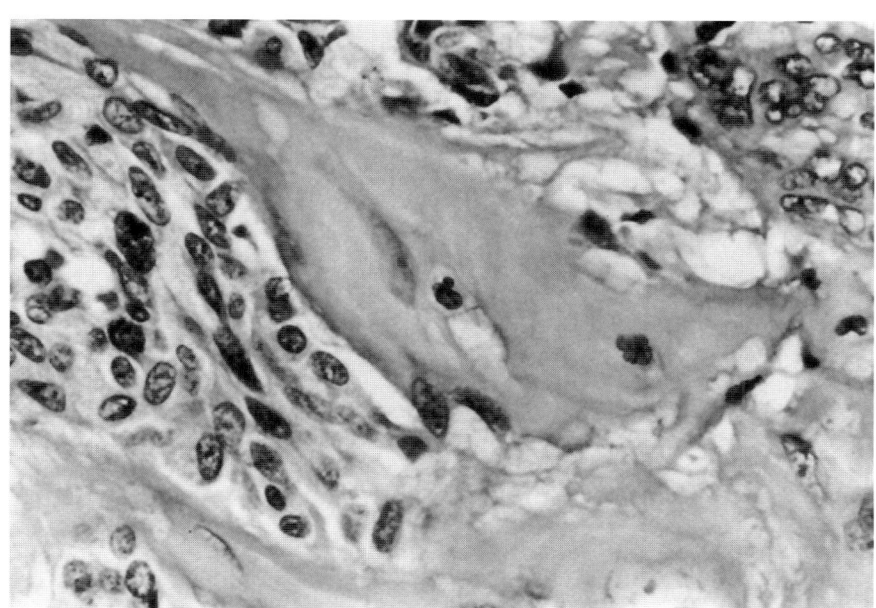

FIG. 16. Same case as Figure 15. In the center, note amorphous material that is amyloid. (H & E stain, ×150.)

and amyloid-rich. However, other variations have been described. Additional subtypes include papillary (468,469), glandular or follicular (470), small cell (469), giant cell (471), clear cell (472), oncocytic (473,474), and squamous (474). Of all these (and some have only been described as case reports of individual tumors), the small cell type shows a more aggressive biologic behavior (469).

Other variations in medullary carcinoma include the production of various hormones (419,420,474–484), vasoactive substances (385,479,480,485–487), mucin (488, 489), and melanin (490–492).

Occasional lesions (and often these are small cell type) do not contain immunoreactive calcitonin. In order to accept a calcitonin-free tumor as a medullary carcinoma, it should arise in a familial setting or occur in a thyroid with unequivocal C-cell hyperplasia. Immunoreactivity for calcitonin gene-related peptide would add proof of the histogenic nature of such a lesion (469,493,494).

Prognostic Factors

From the clinical standpoint, stage is the most important variable for prognosis (181,229,404,405,414,419,460,466, 486,487,495–502). A tumor confined to the thyroid without nodal or distant metastases is associated with prolonged survival. Several workers have found that younger patients (under age 40), especially women, fare somewhat better than the whole group of medullary cancer patients (466,499,500). Patients who are discovered by screening because they are members of affected families often have very small tumors and can be cured by thyroidectomy (503–519). Patients with Sipple's syndrome tend to have less aggressive tumors than the sporadic group (430), whereas the patients with MEN type IIB have aggressive lesions and a survival rate of less than 5% at 5 years (520,521). With the advent of genetic testing of family members in affected kindreds, early diagnosis before the development of medullary cancer is possible. Thyroidectomy at an early age can therefore result in cures (400).

Pathological features that have been related to prognosis include tumor pattern, amyloid content, pleomorphism, necrosis, and mitotic activity (522–526). Small cell medullary carcinomas and those tumors with extensive areas of necrosis and marked cellular pleomorphism are associated with poor prognosis. Encapsulated tumors and tumors with uniform cytology and abundant amyloid tend to be indolent tumors (466,469,522).

Immunostaining results have significant predictive value in medullary carcinoma. Tumors that show diffuse and intense calcitonin staining tend to be indolent, and those with little staining behave as rapidly metastasizing lesions (466,486,487,495,499–501,511,524,525).

In both primary and metastatic sites, there is an inverse relationship between calcitonin and carcinoembryonic antigen (CEA), with the latter being retained and calcitonin immunoreactivity decreasing as tumor becomes more widely metastatic (495,499,500,524,526).

Schroder et al. (502) described another important predictive factor: the finding, by flow cytometric analysis, of an aneuploid cell population in the tumor. This feature was associated with poor outcome.

C-Cell Adenoma

Rare cases diagnosed and reported as C-cell adenoma are found in the literature (527–530). All of these are grossly encapsulated lesions that, with immunostaining or electron microscopy or both, are shown to be C-cell lesions. However, it is best to classify such lesions as encapsulated medullary cancers because such tumors may metastasize (467).

Mixed Follicular and Medullary Carcinoma

These controversial tumors show thyroglobulin and calcitonin immunoreactivity and ultrastructural evidence of differentiation along two cell lines (404,531–543). Some of the series of these tumors may have been confusing, with trapping of follicles at the invading edge of the medullary carcinoma and diffusion of thyroglobulin into the medullary carcinoma, resulting in diagnoses of mixed tumors showing immunostaining with both hormones. Most of these mixed tumors have been diagnosed in the thyroid (502,536–538). However, a few cases of differentiation have been noted in metastatic sites (502,539). Harach and Bergholm (473), LiVolsi (540), and Hedinger et al. (541) suggest caution in making a diagnosis of mixed thyroid carcinoma.

Rare tumors showing medullary and papillary carcinoma have been reported some as composite tumors. These lesions have metastasized as combined lesions (542,543).

C-Cell Hyperplasia

The definition of C-cell hyperplasia is difficult (395, 397,462,544,545). The lower limit of C-cell hyperplasia and the upper limit of normal C-cell mass are not clear. Various studies show C-cell clusters in adults that, taken by themselves, could fit into the category of C-cell hyperplasia. Yet O'Toole et al. (397) and Gibson et al. (395) noted these clusters of C cells at autopsy in apparently endocrinologically normal individuals. Furthermore, the lower limit of medullary carcinoma and upper limit of C-cell hyperplasia are difficult to define. DeLellis and Wolfe (396) state that C-cell hyperplasia ranges from diffuse increase in the cells, to nodules of C-cell-replacing follicles, and once the basement membrane of the follicle is breached, medullary carcinoma should be diagnosed.

However, Carney et al. (446) point out it is not always obvious that the basement membrane has been crossed. Recently, a report from France attempted to define C-cell hyperplasia in terms of numbers of cells per low-power field on a microscopic stage. However, the correlation with serum calcitonin levels was poor (396). Komminuth et al. (462) reported that immunostaining for neural adhesion molecule may differentiate between primary (i.e., preneoplastic C-cell hyperplasia) and secondary forms; the former stain whereas secondary or reactive lesions do not.

In the classic case (41,396,462), the lesion appears as multifocal areas of increased numbers of amphophilic large cells replacing follicular epithelium and also replacing follicles completely forming nodules.

C-cell hyperplasia has been described in hyperparathyroidism, chronic hypercalcemia of other cause, and in residual thyroid tissue following removal of a medullary cancer (sporadic type) (the so-called secondary C-cell hyperplasia) (546–552). C-cell hyperplasia has been reported in Hashimoto's thyroiditis (553) and in the thyroid near nonmedullary carcinoma (552). In addition, one report of medullary carcinoma arising in a thyroiditis gland has been published (554). Because, at least in animals, thyrotropin may stimulate C-cell proliferation, it is possible that C-cell hyperplasia in chronic lymphocytic thyroiditis may be caused by the excess thyrotropin found as a response to the hypothyroid state in these patients.

Anaplastic Thyroid Tumors

Anaplastic or undifferentiated carcinoma of the thyroid has traditionally been divided into two distinct categories: small cell carcinoma, and spindle and giant cell carcinoma (218,229,555–570).

Small cell carcinoma of the thyroid is extremely rare; its existence as an entity at all has been questioned (556,560, 564–570). Numerous electron microscopic and immunohistochemical studies have shown conclusively that many tumors that would have been classified as small cell carcinoma represent either medullary carcinoma (656,560,570), small cell malignant lymphoma (565,566,571–576), or poorly differentiated carcinoma of follicular derivation (insular variant) (556,560,570,574,576,577). In a few cases, especially in series including autopsy results, the small cell carcinoma represents a metastasis to the thyroid from a lung primary (574).

Prognosis

Prognosis for small cell anaplastic tumors varies depending on the subtype involved. Malignant lymphomas of the small cell type, although often of high stage, are indolent tumors, and these patients may survive for many years. On the other hand, small cell medullary carcinomas and insular tumors have significant mortality with distant and regional metastases occurring in 50% to 69% of cases. The 5-year survival rates range from 20% to 35% (570,577), and some patients succumb to tumor after 5 years. However, even these admittedly dismal figures can be appreciated when compared to the miserable survival rates of patients with giant cell carcinomas (<1% at 5 years).

Anaplastic thyroid carcinoma, large cell type, comprises about 3% to 5% of all thyroid tumors and about 10% of malignant ones (181,222,229,555–563,570). This lesion is more frequent in endemic goiter regions of the world (558, 578). Most studies indicate an origin in abnormal thyroid glands in which an apparent transformation of a benign or low-grade lesion has occurred (559,560,562,570,578,579). A history of goiter is found in about 80% of affected patients. Individuals with this tumor are usually elderly (over 50 years of age). A female preponderance is noted (ratio of about 4:1) (181,222,229,555–557,559,561–563,570).

These tumors present as large masses that freely infiltrate extrathyroidal tissues (181,222,229,555–557,559, 561–563,570,578). The tumors appear fleshy and hemorrhagic with necrotic areas. A wide spectrum of patterns is seen. About 20% to 30% show obvious epithelial features, whereas 50% to 60% show spindle or giant cell features or both (556,570,580,581). In all cases, numerous mitoses, often abnormal, are seen (570). Cytologic anaplasia is common. The tumors show marked propensity for invasion.

In the sarcoma-like group, many patterns are seen, including hemangiopericytoma, fibrous histiocytoma, rhabdomyosarcoma, osteoclastoma (222,570,582–587), and angiosarcoma (222,556,561,570).

At the periphery of these tumors, well-differentiated lesions may be found (181,222,556,560,561,570). This may represent adenomatous goiter, an adenomatous nodule (follicular adenoma), or a carcinoma of the well-differentiated type (e.g., papillary, follicular, or Hürthle cell) (555,559,562,578). A few authors have reported cases of dedifferentiated medullary cancers that became anaplastic carcinomas (571,588); the experience of most thyroid pathologists is that this event, if it occurs, is very rare (556,560,570).

Electron microscopic and immunohistologic studies have indicated that almost all anaplastic thyroid tumors are indeed epithelial in nature. The cells contain many cytoplasmic organelles and dense bodies similar to those found in follicular epithelium (570,589–593). Immunohistologic studies suggest that many of these tumors contain keratin; a few stain positively for thyroglobulin (556,560,570,580) but only in areas that abut preexisting thyroid or low-grade thyroid tumor. This probably represents a diffusion phenomenon rather than actual production of thyroid hormone by the tumor cells (556,560,570).

Rarely, anaplastic thyroid cancers can be paucicellular. They are composed of fibrous tissue with few tumor cells. These lesions can be underdiagnosed as well-differentiated fibromatoses or Riedel's disease. A clue in the diagnosis is that the cells entrapped in the fibrous tissue are often cytologically bizarre (594).

Thyroid Sarcoma

Sarcomas of the thyroid are very, very rare. Fibrosarcomas, schwannomas, osteosarcomas, and chondrosarcomas have all been described (558,595–599). In many of these reports, however, modern immunologic or ultrastructural studies are lacking; it is therefore possible that some of these tumors represented anaplastic epithelial tumors (570).

The one truly well-documented sarcoma that does arise in the thyroid is the angiosarcoma or hemangioendothelioma (600–606). This lesion has been most commonly described from the Alpine regions of Europe. Clinically, the affected patients resemble those with anaplastic carcinoma: they are older individuals, with long histories of goiter and recent growth. The gross appearance is that of a hemorrhagic and partially cystic mass. Microscopically, they resemble angiosarcoma of soft tissue (601–606), with interanastomosing vascular channels lined by pleomorphic malignant cells. Immunologic studies clinch the diagnosis: thus both factor VIII-related antigen and *Ulex* lectin can be localized to the tumor cells (605,606).

Carcinosarcoma

Tumors classified as carcinosarcomas are unusual. Most such tumors represent anaplastic carcinomas with mesenchymal metaplasias, usually cartilage or bone (570,607). Carcinosarcoma of the thyroid was reviewed by Donnell et al. (608), who identified 14 acceptable cases including one of their own. Of these 14 cases, 5 had carcinoma associated with fibrosarcoma, 7 had osteosarcoma, and 3 showed osteo- and chondrosarcoma. The patients reported in the literature share clinical and prognostic features with anaplastic carcinomas in general (i.e., they are elderly individuals with fast-growing, rapidly fatal malignancies) (608).

Lymphocytic Lesions Affecting the Thyroid

Malignant Lymphoma

Malignant lymphoma may involve the thyroid as part of systemic lymphoma (secondary lymphoma) or it may arise primarily in the thyroid. About 20% of patients who died of generalized malignant lymphoma showed thyroid involvement at autopsy (328). Rarely is thyroid replacement extensive enough to produce clinical hypothyroidism (609).

Of all thyroid malignancies, 1% to 3.5% are malignant lymphomas (610,611). Primary malignant lymphoma of the thyroid usually arises in an immunologically abnormal gland, usually one affected by chronic lymphocytic thyroiditis (88,609–628). Clinically, thyroid lymphoma affects women more frequently than men (a ratio of from 2.5 to 8.4, to 1). Most patients are elderly (ages 50 to 80). The mass, often arising in patients with goiter, is rapidly growing and may extend outside the gland. The presence of abnormal thyroid function, usually hypothyroidism, has been documented historically in a minority of reported cases (609,613,614,620,628). In most of these cases, hypothyroidism is caused by preexisting chronic thyroiditis. An immunologically abnormal tissue produces the background for lymphoma development. However, primary thyroid lymphoma is rare; Fujimoto et al. (610) found that 3.7% of the thyroid malignancies in their institution were malignant lymphomas. When this is compared to the incidence of thyroiditis, which (depending on the definition used and the population studied) can range from 5% to 54% of the population, the rarity of lymphoma can be appreciated (609,613,614,625,629–631). Hence, it is important not to view autoimmune thyroiditis as a premalignant condition (630,631). Ben-Ezra et al. (632) found no evidence of monoclonality in the lymphoid infiltrate of glands involved in Hashimoto's thyroiditis. The lymphoid tissue present in the thyroid has been considered part of the mucosa-associated lymphoid tissue (MALT) system; lesions of similar MALTs might be expected to occur in patients with primary thyroid lymphoma. Anscombe and Wright (613), in their series of 76 thyroid lymphomas, noted gastrointestinal involvement histologically in five, and clinically in an additional two, patients (total, 10% of their series).

Grossly, most thyroid lymphomas appear as large fleshy tan or gray masses often extending outside the thyroid capsule. Infiltration of the residual thyroid tissue may be seen. The nontumoral thyroid may show the gross appearance of lymphatic thyroiditis, although the findings often depend on the amount of thyroid tissue uninvolved by the tumor (609,613,614,618,625). The microscopic appearance of thyroid lymphomas resembles lymphoma occurring in other sites. The gamut of small, intermediate, and large cell lesions are found; sometimes nodular areas are noted, although a diffuse pattern is more common. The most common histologic subtype is large cell diffuse malignant lymphoma (616,625). Some tumors demonstrate a plasmacytoid appearance; others show features of immunoblastic sarcoma (633). Immunophenotyping studies indicate that most thyroid lymphomas are of B-cell lineage, although a few of these lesions have been T-cell tumors.

The tumors often disclose areas of zonal necrosis. Infiltration of surrounding thyroid is seen. It is common to see infiltration of lymphocytes into residual thyroid follicles; sometimes the malignant cells replace the follicular epithelium (613,625). Invasion beyond the thyroid itself, into surrounding strap muscles and soft tissue, is seen in

50% to 60% of cases (613,616,625). Vascular invasion is common (25% of cases) (625).

A common histologic finding in the MALT lymphomas is the lymphatoepithelial lesion; in the thyroid, this consists of thyroid follicles stuffed with neoplastic lymphoid cells that sometimes partially or totally replace the follicular epithelium.

Treatment for thyroid lymphoma depends upon the staging results. If the disease is widespread, chemotherapy is the choice; on the other hand, if the tumor is localized to the gland only and/or the regional lymph nodes, radiotherapy with or without adjuvant chemotherapy appears warranted (634–637). The prognosis for localized thyroid lymphoma is excellent. Over 50% of affected patients survive 10 years. In recently reported series, survival rates have improved for localized thyroid lymphoma; Tennvall et al. (635) noted a 77% survival rate.

Other Hematopoietic Lesions

Up to 2.6% of patients with multiple myeloma show thyroid involvement (638,639). Extramedullary plasma cell tumors have been reported to occur in the thyroid (633,640–646). Microscopically, the lesion consists of sheets of mature plasma cells replacing thyroid. Capsular extension and/or penetration can be seen (640,643). In at least three cases, areas of the tumor showed histologic evidence of large cell lymphoma (640,641,646).

Other lesions that may rarely involve the thyroid include chronic leukemias (647), Hodgkin's disease (229,625,648), mycosis fungoides (649), chloroma (650), and histiocytoses (651–653).

Unusual Thyroid Tumors

Clear Cell Tumors

Thyroid tumors with clear cells fall into four groups: primary follicular-derived lesions with clear cells, medullary cancer, parathyroid tumors, and metastatic kidney cancer (287,288,472,655–657).

Follicular cells in the thyroid may undergo a variety of metaplastic changes: squamous, oncocytic, and occasionally clear cell. Thyroid nodules and neoplasms can take on clear cell cytology (287,288,654,655).

Clear cells may be caused by formation of intracytoplasmic vesicles, glycogen accumulation, fat accumulation, or deposition of intracellular thyroglobulin (654,656, 658–659).

Clear cell neoplasms of thyroid follicular cell origin form a spectrum of tumors—some papillary, some follicular, and some anaplastic. Often, oncocytic cells are found in close association with the clear cells. Some clear cell follicular tumors are benign (654), and some of these are distinctive lesions showing signet ring cells, called signet-ring adenomas (660–662).

Rarely, tumors of follicular origin show clear cells because of intracytoplasmic fat accumulation (663–666). In some examples, fat admixed with thyroid follicles are found; these lesions have been termed adenolipomas, thyrolipomas, or hamartomas, and they are benign (665, 667). In a few instances, fat and amyloid have been admixed and formed a thyroid mass (666).

Various authors estimate the occurrence of a true intrathyroidal parathyroid tissue (as distinguished from parathyroid tissue abutting the thyroid capsule) as 0.2% (668–671). On rare occasions, such glands may be affected by hyperplasia or neoplasia; hyperparathyroidism may result (668–671). If the tumor is solid it may exhibit a clear cell cytology and be confused with a primary thyroid neoplasm.

The frequency of solitary renal cancer metastases to the thyroid seems disproportionate to the frequency of kidney carcinoma. It is unclear why this tumor often spreads to the thyroid.

The thyroid metastasis may be the initial manifestation of the kidney neoplasm, or the thyroid metastasis may be solitary and represent the only spread of the disease. In patients with a history of kidney cancer, the time interval between the initial renal neoplasm resection and the thyroid metastasis may be many years (672–680). The histopathologic distinction between a clear cell thyroid tumor and a renal cancer metastasis in the thyroid may be quite difficult. Stains for immunoreactive thyroglobulin, if positive, are very helpful (654).

Metastatic Tumors to the Thyroid

Metastases may reach the thyroid by direct extension from tumors in adjacent structures, by retrograde lymphatic spread, or hematogenously (676).

Carcinomas of the larynx, pharynx, trachea, and esophagus may invade the thyroid directly (675–677). Often, multiple areas of the gland are involved; distinction from thyroid primary is usually not difficult.

Retrograde extension via lymphatic routes into the thyroid is unusual. In theory, at least, any tumor involving cervical lymph nodes could extend into the thyroid by this mechanism.

Hematogenous metastases to the thyroid vary according to tumor type (672,673,675,676). Virtually any malignant tumor may metastasize to the thyroid; some of these may resemble primary lesions (674). From the viewpoint of the clinician and the surgical pathologist, the possibility that a solitary mass in the thyroid may represent a metastasis needs to be considered when the histology is unusual for a thyroid primary. Some patients may have a history of cancer elsewhere, but this is not always the case. In surgical series, carcinomas of the kidney and colon and melanoma are most commonly found (672,673,675,678–680); the incidence of these tumor types in thyroid metastases is disproportionate to the frequency of occurrence of these tumors. Grossly, such lesions are often solitary, circumscribed masses; their appearance may be quite compatible with that of a primary tumor. Histologically, the neoplasm may also be a single nodule. Resemblance to colonic adenocarcinoma, breast cancer, or pigmented melanoma reassures the pathologist that this is a metastasis. However, clear cell carcinoma of the kidney as noted above may present a problem (672,674,678–680).

Unusual Tumors

Insular carcinoma (577) consists of a small cell tumor of follicular histogenesis (thyroglobulin positive) that may contain small solid nests, microfollicles, and occasionally papillae. Necrosis is common and the viable tumor cells may be arranged around blood vessels in a peritheliomatous pattern (577). This tumor may also contain zones of dense collagen reminiscent of amyloid. For this reason, some of these tumors may have been diagnosed as medullary carcinomas; however, thyroglobulin is present and calcitonin is not. These lesions probably all represent poorly differentiated papillary or mixed papillary follicular or pure follicular neoplasms; in fact many examples contain zones with cells having ground-glass nuclei. In addition, well-documented anecdotal cases of insular differentiation found in recurrences or metastases of classical papillary or true follicular carcinoma are recorded (229). The prognosis of these tumors is intermediate between well-differentiated follicular-derived tumors (papillary and follicular) and anaplastic tumors; local recurrences and metastases are common (65% or greater). Both nodal and hematogenous metastases are seen. The insular lesions have a 5-year survival rate of about 20% (577,681).

Thymoma

On rare occasions, thymic tissue may be located intrathyroidally (682–685). Rarely, thymomas may arise in these thymic rests (683–685). Tumors that are believed related to thymic or branchial rests in the thyroid include the CASTLE tumor (carcinoma showing thymus-like differentiation) and the SETTLE lesion (spindle and epithelial thymus-like tumor) (686). The Castle tumor is a carcinoma sharing a histologic appearance to lymphoepithelial carcinoma of the nasopharynx. Although some cases had been classified as anaplastic carcinoma, these tumors have a 50% survival rate at 5 years. The SETTLE tumor is a lesion of childhood which is an indolent malignancy; survivals of 20 or more years are known. Because of the combined spindle and epithelial pattern such lesions demonstrate, they have been misclassified as medullary carcinoma or teratoma.

Paraganglioma: Hyalinizing Trabecular Adenoma

Lesions of the thyroid that display the histologic appearance of paraganglioma have been described; their histologic pattern has been compared with some patterns seen in medullary carcinoma (see previous section). Such tumors have been variously termed paraganglioma, hyalinizing trabecular adenoma (687), and paragangliomic-like adenoma of the thyroid (PLAT) (688). Those lesions that by immunostaining are shown to contain calcitonin are appropriately classified as medullary cancer; the others, which contain thyroglobulin, are follicular lesions and most of those reported have been benign (687,688); a few malignant examples are documented (689). It is this writer's view that paragangliomas of the thyroid represent a peculiar variant of follicular lesion that may, like all follicular-derived lesions, show benign and malignant examples.

Teratomas

Clinically, the teratomas in neonates or infants under the age of 1 year present as huge midline neck masses. Often, these tumors measure 10 cm or more (690–695). About 35% of these pregnancies were associated with polyhydramnios (690,692). A significant number of cases reported in series and reviews have been identified in stillborns (690). Grossly, most of these tumors are predominantly or partially cystic. Histologically, the teratomas in newborns and young infants have contained elements of all three germ layers and have been benign. There does not appear to be an increased association of congenital abnormalities in these children.

Teratomas of the thyroid in adults differ from those in newborns because they are more frequently malignant (693–695). It seems likely that these lesions conform to immature teratomas or malignant germ cell neoplasms arising in teratomas, as can occur in the gonads.

Other Mesenchymal Lesions

Isolated cases of hemangioma (696), neurilemmoma (697,698), schwannoma (699), and leiomyoma (697) of the thyroid have been reported.

Squamous Cell Lesions

Squamous cells can be identified in the thyroid in a variety of conditions including developmental rests, inflammatory processes, and neoplasms. Thymic remnants (22,700,701), remnants of the thyroglossal duct (1), and ultimobranchial body rests (solid cell rests) (1,4,6,22, 702,703) can be identified in some carefully sectioned thyroids.

Metaplastic Squamous Lesion of the Thyroid

Inflammatory or destructive processes associated with reparative phenomena can give rise to squamous cells in the thyroid. It is believed that most of these represent metaplasia of follicular epithelium.

Squamous metaplasia is rare in benign adenomatous nodules but may be seen in those that have been aspirated or biopsied (370).

Squamous or squamoid areas can be found focally in about 16% to 40% of ordinary papillary cancers (181,229,704). Franssila (174) did not note any prognostic significance to this finding. As noted above, this unusual variant of papillary carcinoma is characterized by diffuse, often bilateral, involvement of the thyroid by a papillary tumor with many psammoma bodies and prominent squamous metaplasia (175,282,285).

Mucoepidermoid carcinoma is a rare but distinctive variant of thyroid carcinoma, first described as an entity by Rhatigan et al. in 1977 (705). These authors could not prove a histogenesis for this tumor, but they postulated an origin from intrathyroidal ectopic salivary gland rests.

Mucoepidermoid carcinoma of thyroid origin is composed of solid masses of squamoid cells and mucin-producing cells, sometimes forming glands (706–708). The nuclei may on occasion show a ground-glass appearance, and psammoma bodies may be found. Although some authors consider this lesion to be a variant of papillary carcinoma, absence of thyroglobulin or thyroxine by immunostaining and biochemical analysis makes a follicular histogenesis unlikely (706). Some authors (706,708,709) suggested origin from vestiges of ultimobranchial body (solid cell nests); others disagree, assuming mucoepidermoid carcinoma is a variant of papillary cancer (710).

The prognosis of thyroid mucoepidermoid carcinoma is quite good. Of the six cases reported, five patients are alive without disease after therapy at intervals of 18 months to 11 years; one of these five patients developed nodal metastases (706). One of the patients reported by Franssila et al. (706) died of recurrent neck tumor at 13 months.

A variant of mucoepidermoid carcinoma is the *sclerosing mucoepidermoid carcinoma with eosinophilia*, which occurs in the background of chronic fibrosing lymphocytic thyroiditis (711). These tumors, even those which extend beyond the thyroid capsule, behave in a benign fashion on short-term follow-up.

Primary *squamous cell carcinoma* of the thyroid is very rare. In the Huang and Assor review (712), only 54 cases were accepted. Simpson and Carruthers (713) recorded eight new cases. Thyroid squamous cancer occurs in elderly patients who have histories of goiter (712–715). The tumors resemble squamous carcinomas of other organs and range from well- to poorly differentiated lesions, with or without keratinization. Origin in abnormal thyroids is common and as such these tumors clinically and pathologically share features with anaplastic thyroid cancers (570). The prognosis is also similar; these tumors are radioresistant and often rapidly fatal.

Far more common than the primary tumors, metastatic squamous cell carcinoma can involve the thyroid (701,712). Direct extension from laryngeal or esophageal primaries are probably encountered most often. Hematogenous metastases from lung or other primary sites also occur (the latter are often noted at autopsy; thyroid dysfunction is rare). Metastatic squamous cell carcinomas usually present grossly and microscopically as multiple nodules.

Thyroid Tumors in Unusual Locations

Lingual Thyroid

Although clinically significant, lingual thyroid is an unusual disorder (8,716); microscopic remnants of thyroid tissue have been described in 9.8% of tongues examined at autopsy (7).

Grossly, lingual thyroid appears as a mass at the base of the tongue. Histologic examination discloses normal-appearing thyroid follicles interdigitating with skeletal muscle fibers (8,716).

Rare cases of thyroid carcinoma arising in lingual thyroid are recorded (717,718). Of the 25 cases reported in the literature, only ten have documented recurrences of tumor, metastases, or death caused by tumor; the others either have no significant follow-up recorded or have behaved in a clinically benign fashion (718). Most of the tumors were primarily treated surgically.

Carcinoma Arising in Association with Thyroglossal Duct

Neoplasms arising in association with the thyroglossal duct might be expected to be squamous carcinomas, but these are extremely rare (14,719–729); indeed, most tumors occurring in this setting have been thyroid carcinomas and most are described as papillary or mixed papillary and follicular (14,719–725). Nussbaum et al. (726) described one case of anaplastic carcinoma apparently arising in thyroglossal duct remnants. Medullary carcinoma has not been described; because the parafollicular cells are not found in the median thyroid, this is not unexpected (14).

Thyroglossal duct–associated carcinoma is rare and comprises fewer than 1% of all thyroid cancers; almost 200 cases have been documented in the English literature

(14,719–729). The sex ratio favors females (1.5:1); this is interesting because benign thyroglossal cysts are more common in males. Most patients are adults, although a few cases have been diagnosed in children under age 10 (14,722). The symptoms consist of a midline neck swelling; the mass has been noted by the patient for from days to many years. Most of the tumors measure between 2 and 3 cm, although lesions as large as 12 cm have been reported (14,719–729).

The clinical presentation of thyroglossal duct carcinoma is identical to that of benign thyroglossal duct cysts (i.e., a swelling in the anterior neck). Grossly, the lesions are usually cystic, but portions of the cyst may be occupied by solid or even obviously papillary tissue (14, 722–725). Microscopically, the most common tumor type is papillary carcinoma, which makes up about 95% of thyroglossal duct carcinomas.

Rare cases of squamous or epidermoid carcinoma have been reported (726,727); these probably are the only tumors that arise from the duct itself (i.e., the lining epithelium).

Therapy is similar to that for benign thyroglossal duct cyst (i.e., the Sistrunk procedure), which involves removal *en bloc* of the cyst and the hyoid bone (14, 722–726).

When the diagnosis of thyroglossal cyst–associated thyroid cancer is made, the question of its origin arises. Does this tumor represent a metastasis from a primary lesion in the gland, or is the primary site in the region of the cyst? In only 5 of about 50 cases in which the thyroid was examined pathologically were areas of papillary carcinoma found in the gland (14,719–729). Most authors studying this problem conclude that the thyroglossal carcinoma is a primary tumor arising in remnants of thyroid associated with the duct; in those few cases where intrathyroidal tumor has been found, this was considered a separate primary (14,722).

The behavior of thyroglossal duct–associated papillary carcinoma resembles that of thyroid papillary cancer in general. Metastases to lymph nodes have been documented in 15 cases (14,30,719–729). Only rarely do patients die as a result of tumor (723).

Intratracheal and Intralaryngeal Thyroid Carcinomas

Malignant tumors arising in thyroid tissue located within the trachea or larynx are very rare (717,730,731). Dowling et al. (730) reported five carcinomas and two sarcomas.

Mediastinal Thyroid Carcinoma

Thyroid carcinoma apparently arising within substernal or retrosternal goiters has been reported, although most mediastinal goiters are benign. Often, this thyroid tissue is connected to the main gland in the neck. However, the mass lesion is present in the mediastinal location. A case of papillary carcinoma and one of malignant lymphoma in retrosternal goiter were documented by deSouza and Smith (732) in their review of goiter in this site. Mediastinal Hürthle cell carcinoma was reported by Mishriki et al. (733).

Thyroid Cytology

It has become the practice in many large centers that the initial and only approach to the patient with a thyroid nodule is a needle aspiration biopsy (734–739) (see also Chapter 7). FNA biopsy generates a cytologic sample. The use of larger bore needles (14 to 18 gauge, Tru-cut, Vim-Silverman) yields tissue samples that are processed in a routine manner for generating histologic slides. Either of these techniques can be useful in diagnosing thyroid lesions and/or in providing guidance as to which nodules should be surgically removed (734–745).

Fine-needle aspiration biopsy is associated with virtually no mortality and minimal morbidity, and it has never been proven to result in needle-track seeding. The diagnostic accuracy of this test is excellent for papillary, anaplastic, and (less so) medullary carcinomas; however, in this writer's opinion, FNA biopsy provides limited information regarding follicular neoplasms because the periphery of the lesion (i.e., the presence or absence of invasion) cannot be assessed.

On the other hand, the larger bore needle biopsy can be associated with a greater although acceptable morbidity (usually bleeding) (738); on rare occasions, needle-track seeding of cancer has been documented. In many cases, because the sample obtained is larger than with FNA biopsy, diagnosis can be rendered more readily; on occasion, because the larger cutting needle can sample the nodule capsule, evidence of invasion may be identified and the diagnosis of follicular carcinoma may rarely be made (746).

Fine-needle aspiration is discussed in detail in other chapters in this book (Chapter 7, 22, and 29). It should be emphasized that in the modern era, the first approach to an isolated or dominant nodule in the thyroid should be an FNA. In papillary, medullary, anaplastic, and some lymphoid lesions, FNA can be a diagnostic and cost-effective method of planning appropriate surgery or other therapy. FNA is a screening technique for follicular lesions, allowing in many instances the distinction between nodules of goiter and those that may be neoplastic, and thus candidates for surgical removal and histologic evaluation. In the group of follicular nodules, the FNA is not diagnostic in defining benign from malignant tumors, because the diagnostic foci are at the capsule of the lesion which is not sampled by FNA.

Frozen Section Diagnosis and the Thyroid

Before the advent of fine-needle biopsy, the method most used in diagnosis of thyroid nodules was intraoperative frozen section. The nodule or preferably the thyroid lobe was excised and a representative portion (preferably encompassing the nodule–capsule–thyroid interface) was prepared for frozen section and intraoperative interpretation by a pathologist. In those cases in which the diagnosis of papillary, medullary, or anaplastic cancer was given, appropriate surgery was immediately undertaken.

Even with frozen section, however, despite recommendation of sampling two or even four different areas, the diagnosis of follicular carcinoma was notoriously difficult (747). In many cases, the diagnosis rendered was "follicular lesion—diagnosis deferred to permanent sections."

Several studies have evaluated frozen section and FNA diagnostic results for thyroid nodules (747–752). Although frozen section diagnosis may be specific (90% to 97%), it is not sensitive (60%). In addition, deferred diagnoses at frozen section do nothing to alter the operative procedure or to guide the surgeon. Hamburger and Hamburger (749) analyzed 359 patients who had FNA and also intraoperative frozen sections of thyroid nodules; the frozen section results influenced the surgical approach in only three cases (<1%).

Also, in the era of cost containment, it does not seem justified to perform frozen sections for the intraoperative diagnosis of thyroid nodules; this is even more true if a preoperative FNA has been performed with malignant or suspicious results.

It is our practice (350,351) to not perform intraoperative frozen sections on those primary thyroid nodules in which the FNA diagnosis of follicular or Hürthle cell neoplasm was rendered. The majority of these lesions are benign (85% in our series) and those that are malignant are usually minimal carcinomas. In those cases in which an FNA diagnosis of suspect follicular variant of papillary carcinoma is given, we do both an intraoperative cytologic preparation and a frozen section. If appropriate nuclear features are seen, or sclerosis or psammoma bodies are identified, a definite diagnosis of papillary carcinoma is given and therapy for that lesion is undertaken.

REFERENCES

1. Sugiyama S. The embryology of the human thyroid gland including ultimobranchial body and others related. *Adv Anat Embryol Cell Biol* 1970;44(H2):6–110.
2. Janzer RC, Weber E, Hedinger C. The relation between solid cell nests and C-cells of the thyroid gland. *Cell Tissue Res* 1979;197:295–312.
3. Sugiyama S. Histological studies of the human thyroid gland observed from the viewpoint of its postnatal development. *Adv Anat Embryol Cell Biol* 1967;39(H3):7–72.
4. Harach HR. Solid cell nests of the human thyroid in early stages of postnatal life. *Acta Anat (Basel)* 1986;127:262–264.
5. Harach HR. Solid cell nests of the thyroid. *J Pathol* 1988;155:191–200.
6. Yamaoka Y. Solid cell nests (SCN) in the human thyroid gland. *Acta Pathol Jpn* 1973;23:493–506.
7. Baughman RA. Lingual thyroid and lingual thyroglossal tract remnants. *Oral Surg Oral Med Oral Pathol* 1972;34:781–798.
8. Neinas FW, Gorman CA, Devine KD, Woolner LB. Lingual thyroid. Clinical characteristics of 15 cases. *Ann Intern Med* 1973;79:205–210.
9. Reaume CE, Sofie VL. Lingual thyroid. *Oral Surg Oral Med Oral Pathol* 1978;45:841–845.
10. Strickland AL, Macfie JA, Vanwyk JJ, French FS. Ectopic thyroid glands simulating thyroglossal duct cysts. *JAMA* 1969;208:307–310.
11. Allard RHB. The thyroglossal cyst. *Head Neck Surg* 1982;5:134–140.
12. Larochelle D, Arcand P, Belzile M, Gagnon NB. Ectopic thyroid tissue—a review of the literature. *J Otolaryngol* 1979;8:523–530.
13. Noyek AM, Friedberg J. Thyroglossal duct and ectopic thyroid disorders. *Otolaryngol Clin North Am* 1981;14:187–201.
14. LiVolsi VA, Perzin KH, Savetsky L. Carcinoma arising in median ectopic thyroid (including thyroglossal duct tissue). *Cancer* 1974;34:1301–1315.
15. Bone RC, Biller HF, Irwin TM. Intralaryngotracheal thyroid. *Ann Otol Rhinol Laryngol* 1972;81:424–428.
16. Donegan JO, Wood MD. Intratracheal thyroid—a familial occurrence. *Laryngoscope* 1985;95:6–8.
17. Myers EN, Pantangco IP. Intratracheal thyroid. *Laryngoscope* 1975;85:1833–1840.
18. De Andrade MA. A review of 128 cases of post mediastinal goiter. *World J Surg* 1977;1:789–797.
19. de Sauza FM, Smith PE. Retrosternal goiter. *J Otolaryngol* 1983;12:393–396.
20. Kantelip B, Lusson JR, deRiberolles C, Lamaison D, Bailly P. Intracardiac ectopic thyroid. *Hum Pathol* 1986;17:1293–1296.
21. Pollice L, Caneso G. Struma cordis. *Arch Pathol Lab Med* 1986;110:452–453.
22. Carpenter GF, Emery JL. Inclusions in the human thyroid. *J Anat* 1976;122:77–89.
23. Weller GL. Development of the thyroid, parathyroid and thymus glands in man. *Contrib Embryol Carneg Inst* 1933;141:93–140.
24. Finkle HI, Goldman RL. Heterotopic cartilage in the thyroid. *Arch Pathol Lab Med* 1973;95:48–49.
25. Gardner WR. Unusual relationships between thyroid gland and skeletal muscle in infants. *Cancer* 1956;6:681–691.
26. Moses DC, Thompson NW, Nishiyama RH, Sisson JC. Ectopic thyroid tissue in the neck. *Cancer* 1976;38:361–365.
27. Block MA, Wylie JA, Patton RB, Miller JM. Does benign thyroid tissue occur in the lateral part of the neck? *Am J Surg* 1966;112:476–481.
28. Rubenfeld S, Joseph UA, Schwartz MR, Weber SC, Jhingran SG. Ectopic thyroid in the right carotid triangle. *Arch Otolaryngol Head Neck Surg* 1988;114:913–915.
29. Butler JJ, Tulinius H, Ibanez ML, Ballantyne AJ, Clark RL. Significance of thyroid tissue in lymph nodes associated with carcinoma of the head, neck or lung. *Cancer* 1967;20:103–112.
30. Gerard-Marchant R. Thyroid follicle inclusions in cervical lymph nodes. *Arch Pathol Lab Med* 1964;77:637–643.
31. Ibrahim NBN, Milewski PJ, Gillett R, Temple JG. Benign thyroid inclusions within cervical lymph nodes. *Aust N Z J Surg* 1981;51:188–189.
32. Meyer JS, Steinberg LS. Microscopically benign thyroid follicles in cervical lymph nodes. *Cancer* 1969;24:302–311.
33. Roth L. Inclusions of nonneoplastic thyroid tissue within cervical lymph nodes. *Cancer* 1965;18:105–111.
34. Hegedus L, Perrild H, Poulsen LR, Andersen JR, Holm B, Schnohr P, Jensen G, Hansen JM. The determination of thyroid volume by ultrasound and its relationship to body weight, age and sex in normal subjects. *J Clin Endocrinol Metab* 1983;56:260–263.
35. Pankow BG, Michalak J, McGee MK. Adult human thyroid weight. *Health Phys* 1985;49:1097–1103.
36. Vander JB, Gaston EA, Dawber TR. The significance of nontoxic nodules. *Ann Intern Med* 1968;69:537–540.
37. Burch HB. Evaluation and management of the solid thyroid nodule. *Endocrinol Metab Clin North Am* 1995;24:663–710.
38. Brown RA, Al-Moussa M, Beck JS. Histometry of normal thyroid in man. *J Clin Pathol* 1986;39:475–482.

39. Reid JD, Choi CH, Oldroyd NO. Calcium oxalate crystals in the thyroid: their identification, prevalence, origin and possible significance. *Am J Clin Pathol* 1987;87:443–454.
40. DeLellis RA, Nunnemacher G, Wolfe HJ. C-cell hyperplasia: an ultrastructural analysis. *Lab Invest* 1978;36:237–248.
41. Hazard JB. The C-cells (parafollicular cells) of the thyroid gland and medullary thyroid carcinoma. *Am J Pathol* 1977;88:214–249.
42. Leitz H. C-cells: source of calcitonin. *Curr Top Pathol* 1971;55: 109–146.
43. LiVolsi VA. Calcitonin: the hormone and its significance. *Progr Surg Pathol* 1980;1:71–103.
44. Gould VE, Johannessen JV, Sobrinho-Simoes M. The thyroid gland. In: Johannessen JV, ed. *Electron microscopy in human medicine*, vol 10. Endocrine organs. New York: McGraw-Hill, 1981;29–107.
45. Heimann P. Ultrastructure of human thyroid. *Acta Endocrinol (Copenh)* 1966;53(suppl 110):5–102.
46. Hazard JB. Thyroiditis: a review. *Am J Clin Pathol* 1955;25:289–298, 399–442.
47. Berger SA, Zonszein J, Villamena P, Mittman R. Infectious diseases of the thyroid gland. *Rev Infect Dis* 1983;5:108–122.
48. Dan M, Garcia A, von Westrap C. Primary actinomycosis of the thyroid mimicking carcinoma. *J Otolaryngol* 1984;13:109–112.
49. Kakuda K, Kanokogi M, Mitsunobu M, et al. Acute mycotic thyroiditis. *Acta Pathol Jpn* 1983;33:147–151.
50. Loeb JM, Livermore BM, Wofsy D. Coccidioidomycosis of the thyroid. *Ann Intern Med* 1979;91:409–411.
51. Szporn AH, Tepper S, Watson CW. Disseminated cryptococcosis presenting as thyroiditis. *Acta Cytol* 1985;29:449–453.
52. Goldfarb H, Schifrin D, Graig FA. Thyroiditis caused by tuberculous abscess of the thyroid gland. *Am J Med* 1965;38:825–828.
53. Gutman LT, Handwerger S, Zwadyk P, Abramowski CR, Rodgers BM. Thyroiditis due to *Mycobacterium chelonei*. *Am Rev Respir Dis* 1974;110:807–809.
54. Laird SM. Gumma of the thyroid gland. *Br J Vener Dis* 1945;21: 162–165.
55. Leelachaikul P, Chuahirun S. Cysticercosis of the thyroid gland in severe cerebral cysticercosis: report of a case. *J Med Assoc Thai* 1977;60:405–410.
56. Frank TS, LiVolsi VA, Connor AM. Cytomegalovirus infection of the thyroid in immunocompromised adults. *Yale J Biol Med* 1987;60:1–8.
57. Gallant JE, Enriquez RE, Cohen KL, Hammers LW. Pneumocystis carinii thyroiditis. *Am J Med* 1988;84:303–306.
58. Takai SIK, Miyauchi A, Matsuzuka F, Kuma K, Kosaki G. Internal fistula as a route of infection in acute suppurative thyroiditis. *Lancet* 1979;1:751–752.
59. Bastenie PA, Bonnyns M, Neve P. Subacute and chronic granulomatous thyroiditis. In: Bastenie PA, Ermans AM, eds. *Thyroiditis and thyroid function: clinical, morphological and physiological studies*. Oxford: Pergamon Press, 1972;69–97.
60. Greene JN. Subacute thyroiditis. *Am J Med* 1971;51:97–108.
61. Lindsay S, Dailey ME. Granulomatous or giant cell thyroiditis. *Surg Gynecol Obstet* 1954;98:197–212.
62. Volpe R. Thyroiditis: current views of pathogenesis. *Med Clin North Am* 1975;59:1163–1175.
63. Volpe R. Subacute (deQuervain's) thyroiditis. *Bailliers Clin Endocrinol Metab* 1979;8:81–95.
64. Volpe R. The pathology of thyroiditis. *Hum Pathol* 1978;9:429–438.
65. Woolner LB, McConahey WB, Beahrs OH. Granulomatous thyroiditis (deQuervain's thyroiditis). *J Clin Endocrinol Metab* 1957;17: 1202–1221.
66. Bliddal H, Bech K, Feldt-Rasmussen U, Hoier-Madsen M, Thomsen B, Nielsen H. Humoral antoimmune manifestation in subacute thyroiditis. *Allergy* 1985;40:599–604.
67. Strakosch CR, Joyner D, Wall JR. Thyroid stimulating antibodies in patients with subacute thyroiditis. *J Clin Endocrinol Metab* 1978;46: 345–348.
68. Eylan E, Zmucky R, Sheba C. Mumps virus and subacute thyroiditis—evidence of a causal association. *Lancet* 1957;1:1062–1063.
69. DePauw BE, deRooy HAM. DeQuervain's subacute thyroiditis: a report of 14 cases and a review of the literature. *Neth J Med* 1975;18: 70–78.
70. Fennell JS, Tomkin GH. Sub-acute thyroiditis and hepatitis in a case of infectious mononucleosis. *Postgrad Med J* 1978;54:351–352.
71. Goldman J, Bochna AJ, Becker FO. St. Louis encephalitis and subacute thyroiditis. *Ann Intern Med* 1977;87:250.
72. Meachim G, Young MH. DeQuervain's subacute granulomatous thyroiditis: histological identification and incidence. *J Clin Pathol* 1963;16:189–199.
73. Carney JA, Moore SB, Northcutt RC, Woolner LB, Stillwell GK. Palpation thyroiditis (multifocal granulomatous thyroiditis). *Am J Clin Pathol* 1975;64:639–647.
74. Lloyd RV, Johnson TL, Blaivas M, Sisson JC, Wilson BS. Detection of HLA-DR antigens in paraffin-embedded thyroid epithelial cells with a monoclonal antibody. *Am J Pathol* 1985;120:106–111.
75. Volpe R. The immunoregulatory disturbance in autoimmune thyroid disease. *Autoimmunity* 1988;2:55–72.
76. Davies TF, Piccinini LA. Intrathyroidal MHC Class II antigen expression and thyroid autoimmunity. *Endocrinol Metab Clin North Am* 1987;16:247–268.
77. DeBernardo E, Davies TF. Antigen presentation in human autoimmune thyroid disease. *Exp Cell Biol* 1986;54:155–162.
78. Hanafusa T, Pujol-Borrell R, Chiovato L, Russell RCG, Doniach D, Bottazzo GF. Aberrant expression of HLA-DR antigen on thyrocytes in Graves' disease: relevance to autoimmunity. *Lancet* 1983;2: 1111–1115.
79. Kong YM, Bagnasco M, Canonica GW. How do T cells mediate autoimmune thyroiditis? *Immunol Today* 1986;7:337–339.
80. Martin A, Matsuoka N, Concepcion ES, Davies TF. Endogenous antigen presentation by autoantigen-transfected Epstein-Barr virus lymphoblastoid cells: T cell receptor N-region hydrophobicity relates to thyroid antigen recognition. *Autoimmunity* 1995;21:223–230.
81. Lucas-Martin A, Foz-Sala M, Todd I, Bottazzo GF, Pujol-Borrell R. Occurrence of thyrocyte HLA class II expression in a wide variety of thyroid diseases: relationship with lymphocytic infiltration and thyroid autoantibodies. *J Clin Endocrinol Metab* 1988;66:367–375.
82. Matsunaga M, Eguchi K, Fukuda T, et al. Class II histocompatibility complex antigen expression and cellular interactions in thyroid glands of Graves' disease. *J Clin Endocrinol Metab* 1986;62:723–728.
83. Volpe R. Immunoregulation in autoimmune thyroid disease. *N Engl J Med* 1987;316:44–45.
84. Weetman AP, McGregor AM. Autoimmune thyroid disease: developments in our understanding. *Endocr Rev* 1984;5:309–355.
85. Rapoport B. Autoimmune mechanisms in thyroid disease. In: Green WL, ed. *The thyroid*. New York: Elsevier, 1987;47–106.
86. Harland WA, Frantz VK. Clinicopathologic study of 261 surgical cases of so-called "thyroiditis." *J Clin Endocrinol Metab* 1956;11: 1433–1437.
87. Lindsay S, Dailey ME, Friedlander J, Yee G, Soley MH. Chronic thyroiditis: a clinical and pathological study of 354 patients. *J Clin Endocrinol Metab* 1952;12:1578–1600.
88. Woolner LB, McConahey WM, Beahrs OH. Struma lymphatosa (Hashimoto's thyroiditis) and related disorders. *J Clin Endocrinol Metab* 1959;19:53–83.
89. Harach HR, Williams ED. Fibrous thyroiditis—an immunopathological study. *Histopathology* 1983;7:739–751.
90. Katz SM, Vickery AL. The fibrous variant of Hashimoto's thyroiditis. *Hum Pathol* 1974;5:161–170.
91. Totterman TH, Andersson LC, Hayry P. Evidence for thyroid antigen-reactive T lymphocytes infiltrating the thyroid gland in Graves' disease. *Clin Endocrinol (Oxf)* 1979;11:59–68.
92. Gordin A, Lamberg B-A. Natural course of symptomless autoimmune thyroiditis. *Lancet* 1975;2:1234–1238.
93. Check JH, Avellino J. Painless thyroiditis and transient thyrotoxicosis after Graves' disease. *JAMA* 1980;244:1361.
94. Dahlberg PA, Jansson R. Different aetiologies in post-partum thyroiditis? *Acta Endocrinol (Copenh)* 1983;104:195–200.
95. Fein HG, Goldman JM, Weintraub BD. Postpartum lymphocytic thyroiditis in American women: a spectrum of thyroid dysfunction. *Am J Obstet Gynecol* 1980;138:504–510.
96. Jansson R, Bernander S, Karlsson A, Levin K, Nilsson G. Autoimmune thyroid dysfunction in the postpartum period. *J Clin Endocrinol Metab* 1984;58:681–687.
97. Mizukami Y, Michigishi T, Hashimoto T, et al. Silent thyroiditis: a histologic and immunohistochemical study. *Hum Pathol* 1988;19: 423–431.
98. Tachi J, Amino N, Tamaki H, Aozasa M, Iwatani Y, Miyai I. Long term follow-up and HLA association in patients with postpartum thyroiditis. *J Clin Endocrinol Metab* 1988;66:480–484.
99. Vargas MT, Briones-Urbina R, Gladman D, Papsin FR, Walfish PG. Antithyroid microsomal autoantibodies and HLS-DR 5 are associated

100. Woolf PD. Transient painless thyroiditis with hyperthyroidism: a variant of lymphocytic thyroiditis? *Endocr Rev* 1980;1:411–420.
101. Jansson R, Totterman TH, Sallstrom J, Dahlberg PA. Intrathyroidal and circulating lymphocyte subsets in different stages of autoimmune postpartum thyroiditis. *J Clin Endocrinol Metab* 1984;58:942–946.
102. LiVolsi VA. The pathology of autoimmune thyroiditis. *Thyroid* 1994;4:333–339.
103. Harris M, Palmer MK. The structure of the human thyroid in relation to aging and focal thyroiditis. *J Pathol* 1980;130:99–104.
104. Harris M, Summerell JM, Swan AV. The prevalence of focal thyroiditis in Jamaican adults. *J Pathol* 1973;110:309–317.
105. Kurashima C, Hirokawa K. Focal lymphocytic infiltration of thyroids in elderly people. *Surv Synth Pathol Res* 1985;4:457–466.
106. Weaver DK, Batsakis JG, Nishiyama RH. Relationship of iodine to "lymphocytic goiter." *Arch Surg* 1969;98:183–185.
107. Williams ED, Doniach I. The postmortem incidence of focal thyroiditis. *J Pathol Bacteriol* 1962;83:255–264.
108. Inoue M, Taketani N, Sato T, Nakayima H. High incidence of chronic lymphocytic thyroiditis in apparently healthy school children: epidemiological and clinical study. *Endocrinol Jpn* 1975;22:483–489.
109. Gossage AAR, Munro DS. The pathogenesis of Graves' disease. *Clin Endocrinol Metab* 1985;14:299–330.
110. Grubeck-Loebenstein D, Derfler K, Kassal H, et al. Immunological features of nonimmunogenic hyperthyroidism. *J Clin Endocrinol Metab* 1985;60:150–155.
111. Studer H, Peter HJ, Gerber H. Toxic nodular goitre. *Clin Endocrinol Metab* 1985;14:351–372.
112. Shopsin B, Shenkman L, Blum M, Hollander CS. Iodine and lithium-induced hypothyroidism. *Am J Med* 1973;55:695–699.
113. Perrild H, Madsen A, Hansen R. Irreversible myxedema after lithium carbonate. *Br Med J (Clin Res Ed)* 1978;1:1108–1109.
114. Alves LE, Rose EP, Cahill TB. Amiodarone and the thyroid. *Ann Intern Med* 1985;102:412.
115. Amico JA, Richardson V, Alpert B, Klein I. Clinical and chemical assessment of thyroid function during therapy with amiodarone. *Arch Intern Med* 1984;144:487–490.
116. Gammage MD, Franklyn JA. Amiodarone and the thyroid. *Q J Med* 1987;238:83–86.
117. Gudbjornsson B, Kristinsson A, Geirsson G, Hreidarsson AB. Painful autoimmune thyroiditis occurring on amiodarone therapy. *Acta Med Scand* 1987;221:219–220.
118. Hawthorne GC, Campbell NPS, Geddes JS, et al. Amiodarone-induced hypothyroidism. *Arch Intern Med* 1985;145:1016–1019.
119. Martino E, Aghini-Lombardi F, Mariotti S, et al. Amiodarone-induced hypothyroidism. *Clin Endocrinol (Oxf)* 1987;26:227–237.
120. Rabinowe SL, Larsen PR, Antman EM, et al. Amiodarone therapy and autoimmune thyroid disease. *Am J Med* 1986;81:53–57.
121. Smyrk TC, Goellner Jr, Brennan MD, Carney JA. Pathology of the thyroid in amiodarone associated thyrotoxicosis. *Am J Surg Pathol* 1987;11:197–204.
122. Atkins MB, Mier JW, Parkinson DR, Gould JA, Berkman EM, Kaplan MM. Hypothyroidism after treatment with interleukin-2 and lymphokine-activated killer cells. *N Engl J Med* 1988;318:1557–1563.
123. Meijer S, Hausman R. Occlusive phlebitis, a diagnostic feature in Riedel's thyroiditis. *Virchows Arch [A]* 1978;377:339–349.
124. Wold LE, Weiland LH. Tumefactive fibro-inflammatory lesions of the head and neck. *Am J Surg Pathol* 1983;7:477–482.
125. Woolner LB, McConahey WM, Beahrs OH. Invasive fibrous thyroiditis (Riedel's struma). *J Clin Endocrinol Metab* 1957;17:201–220.
126. Schwaegerle SM, Bauer TW, Esselstyn CB. Riedel's thyroiditis. *Am J Clin Pathol* 1988;90:715–722.
127. Comings DE, Skubi KB, van Eyes J, Motulsky AG. Familial multifocal fibrosclerosis. *Ann Intern Med* 1967;66:884–892.
128. Bartholomew LG, Cain JC, Woolner LB, Utz DC, Ferris DO. Sclerosing cholangitis. Its possible association with Riedel's struma and fibrous retroperitonitis. *N Engl J Med* 1963;269:8–12.
129. Coopersmith NH, Appelman HD. Multifocal fibrosclerosis with subcutaneous involvement. *Am J Clin Pathol* 1971;55:369–376.
130. Hellstrom HR, Perez-Stable EC. Retroperitoneal fibrosis with disseminated vasculitis and intrahepatic sclerosing cholangitis. *Am J Med* 1966;46:184–187.
131. Meyer S, Hausman R. Occlusive phlebitis in multifocal fibrosclerosis. *Am J Clin Pathol* 1976;65:274–283.
132. Nielsen HK. Multifocal idiopathic fibrosclerosis. *Acta Med Scand* 1980;208:119–123.
133. Olsen KD, DeSanto LW, Wold LE, Weiland LH. Tumefactive fibroinflammatory lesions of the head and neck. *Laryngoscope* 1986;96:940–944.
134. Raphael HA, Beahrs DH, Woolner LB, Scholz DA. Riedel's struma associated with fibrous mediastinitis. *Mayo Clin Proc* 1966;41:375–382.
135. Mitchinson MJ. Retroperitoneal fibrosis revisited. *Arch Pathol Lab Med* 1986;110:784–786.
136. Constine LS, Donaldson SS, McDougall IR, Cox RS, Link MP, Kaplan HS. Thyroid dysfunction after radiotherapy in children with Hodgkin's disease. *Cancer* 1984;55:878–883.
137. Glennon JA, Gordon ES, Swain CT. Hypothyroidism after low-dose 131-1 treatment of hyperthyroidism. *Ann Intern Med* 1972;76:721–723.
138. Shafer RB, Nuttall FQ, Pollak K, Kuisk H. Thyroid function after radiation and surgery for head and neck cancer. *Arch Intern Med* 1975;135:843–846.
139. Zohar Y, Tovim RB, Laurian N, Laurian L. Thyroid function following radiation and surgical therapy in head and neck malignancy. *Head Neck Surg* 1984;6:948–952.
140. Bhatia S, Robison LL, Oberlin O, Greenberg M, Bunin G, Fossati-Bellani F, Meadows AT. Breast cancer and other second neoplasms after childhood Hodgkin's disease. *N Engl J Med* 1996;334:745–751.
141. Kennedy JS, Thomson JA. The changes in the thyroid gland after irradiation with 131-I or partial thyroidectomy for thyrotoxicosis. *J Pathol* 1974;112:65–81.
142. Komorowski RA, Hanson GA. Morphologic changes in the thyroid following low-dose childhood radiation. *Arch Pathol Lab Med* 1977;101:36–39.
143. Valdiserri RO, Borochovitz D. Histologic changes in previously irradiated thyroid glands. *Arch Pathol Lab Med* 1980;104:150–152.
144. Lindsay S, Dailey ME, Jones MD. Histologic effects of various types of ionizing radiation on normal and hyperplastic human thyroid glands. *J Clin Endocrinol Metab* 1954;14:1179–1219.
145. Spitalnik PR, Strauss FH. Patterns of human thyroid parenchymal reaction following low-dose childhood irradiation. *Cancer* 1978;41:1098–1105.
146. Arean VM, Klein RE. Amyloid goiter; review of the literature and report of a case. *Am J Clin Pathol* 1961;36:341–355.
147. James PD. Amyloid goitre. *J Clin Pathol* 1972;25:683–688.
148. Kennedy JS, Thomson JA, Buchanan WM. Amyloid in the thyroid. *Q J Med* 1972;43:127–143.
149. Rich MW. Hypothyroidism in association with systemic amyloidosis. *Head Neck* 1995;17:343–345.
150. Gordon MB, Klein I, Dekker A, Rodnan GP, Medsger TA. Thyroid disease in progressive systemic sclerosis: increased frequency of glandular fibrosis and hypothyroidism. *Ann Intern Med* 1981;95:431–435.
151. Nicholson D, White S, Lipson A, Jacobs RP, Borenstein DG. Progressive systemic sclerosis and Graves' disease. *Arch Intern Med* 1986;146:2350–2352.
152. Ward JA, Mendeloff J, Coberly JC. Hyperthyroidism followed by scleroderma. *JAMA* 1977;237:1123.
153. Campbell PM, LeRoy EC. Pathogenesis of systemic sclerosis: a vascular hypothesis. *Semin Arthritis Rheum* 1975;4:351–368.
154. Cappell DF, Hutchison HE, Jowett MD. Transfusional siderosis: the effects of excessive iron deposits on the tissues. *J Pathol Bacteriol* 1957;74:245–264.
155. Alexander CB, Herrara GA, Jaffe K, Yu H. Black thyroid. Clinical manifestations, ultrastructural findings and possible mechanisms. *Hum Pathol* 1985;16:72–78.
156. Attwood HD, Dennett X. A black thyroid and minocycline treatment. *Br Med J [Clin Res]* 1976;2:1109–1110.
157. Billano RA, Ward WQ, Little WP. Minocycline and black thyroid. *JAMA* 1983;249:1887–1888.
158. Gordon G, Sparano BM, Kramer AW, Kelly RG, Iatropoulos MJ. Thyroid gland pigmentation and minocycline therapy. *Am J Pathol* 1984;117:98–109.
159. Landas SK, Schelper RL, Tio FO, Turner JW, Moore KC, Bennett-Gray J. Black thyroid syndrome: exaggeration of a normal process? *Am J Clin Pathol* 1986;85:411–418.
160. Medeiros LJ, Federman M, Silverman ML, Balogh K. Black thyroid associated with minocycline therapy. *Arch Pathol Lab Med* 1984;108:268–269.

161. Ohaki Y, Misugi K, Hasegawa H. "Black thyroid" associated with minocycline therapy. *Acta Pathol Jpn* 1986;36:1367–1375.
162. Reid JD. The black thyroid associated with minocycline therapy. *Am J Clin Pathol* 1983;79:739–746.
163. Saul SH, Dekker A, Lee RE, Breitfeld V. The black thyroid: its relation to minocycline use in man. *Arch Pathol Lab Med* 1983;107:173–177.
164. Wajda KJ, Wilson MS, Lucas J, Marsh WL. Fine needle aspiration cytologic findings in the black thyroid syndrome. *Acta Cytol* 1988;32:862–865.
165. Silverberg E, Lubera J. Cancer statistics. *CA* 1986;36:9–25.
166. Young JL, Percy CL, Asire AJ, eds. Surveillance epidemiology and end results: incidence and mortality data, 1973–1977. *Natl Cancer Inst Monogr* 1981;57:1–1082.
167. Williams ED, Doniach I, Bjarnson O, Michie W. Thyroid cancer in an iodide rich area. *Cancer* 1977;39:215–222.
168. Cuello C, Correa P, Eisenberg H. Geographic pathology of thyroid carcinoma. *Cancer* 1969;23:230–238.
169. Harach HR, Escalante DA, Onativia A, Outes JL, Day ES, Williams ED. Thyroid carcinoma and thyroiditis in an endemic goitre region before and after iodine prophylaxis. *Acta Endocrinol (Copenh)* 1985;108:55–60.
170. Hofstadter F. Frequency and morphology of malignant tumours of the thyroid before and after the introduction of iodine prophylaxis. *Virchows Arch [A]* 1980;385:263–270.
171. Wahner HW, Cuello C, Correa P, Uribe LF, Gaitan E. Incidence of thyroid carcinoma in an endemic goiter area, Cali, Columbia. *Am J Med* 1966;40:58–72.
172. Fukunaga FH, Yatani R. Geographic pathology of occult thyroid carcinomas. *Cancer* 1975;36:1095–1099.
173. Carcangiu ML, Zampi G, Rosai J. Papillary thyroid carcinoma. A study of its many morphologic expressions and clinical correlates. *Pathol Annu* 1985;20(pt 1):1–44.
174. Franssila KO. Value of histologic classification of thyroid cancer. *APMIS Suppl* 1971;225:5–76.
175. Vickery AL, Carcangiu M, Johannessen JV, Sobrinho-Simoes M. Papillary carcinoma. *Semin Diagn Pathol* 1985;2:90–100.
176. Woolner LB, Beahrs OH, Black BM, McConahey WM, Keating FR. Classification and prognosis of thyroid carcinoma: a study of 885 cases observed in a thirty year period. *Am Surg* 1961;102:354–387.
177. Beaugie JM, Brown CL, Doniach I, Richardson JE. Primary malignant tumours of the thyroid: the relationship between histological classification and clinical behaviour. *Br J Surg* 1976;63:173–181.
178. Hawk WA, Hazard JB. The many appearances of papillary carcinoma of the thyroid. *Cleveland Clin Q* 1976;43:207–216.
179. Hirabayashi RN, Lindsay S. Carcinoma of the thyroid gland: a statistical study of 390 patients. *J Clin Endocrinol Metab* 1961;21:1596–1610.
180. McConahey WM, Hay ID, Woolner LB, van Heerden JA, Taylor WF. Papillary thyroid cancer treated at the Mayo Clinic, 1946 through 1970: initial manifestations, pathologic findings, therapy and outcome. *Mayo Clin Proc* 1986;61:978–996.
181. Woolner LB. Thyroid carcinoma: pathologic classification with data on prognosis. *Semin Nucl Med* 1971;1:481–502.
182. Mazzaferri EL. Papillary thyroid carcinoma: factors influencing prognosis and current therapy. *Semin Oncol* 1987;14:315–332.
183. Mazzaferri EL, Young RL, Oertel JE, Kemmerer WT, Page CP. Papillary thyroid carcinoma: the impact of therapy in 576 patients. *Medicine (Baltimore)* 1980;56:171–196.
184. Mills SE, Allen MS. Congenital occult papillary carcinoma of the thyroid gland. *Hum Pathol* 1986;17:1179–1181.
185. Franssila KO. Is the differentiation between papillary and follicular thyroid carcinoma valid? *Cancer* 1973;32:853–858.
186. Franssila KO. Prognosis in thyroid carcinoma. *Cancer* 1975;36:1138–1146.
187. Ain K. Papillary thyroid carcinoma. *Endocrinol Metab Clin North Am* 1995;24:711–760.
188. Mazzaferri EL, Jhiang SM. Longterm impact of initial surgical and medical therapy on papillary and follicular thyroid cancer. *Am J Med* 1994;97:418–428.
189. Favus MJ, Schneider AB, Stachura ME. Thyroid cancer occurring as a late consequence of head and neck irradiation. *N Engl J Med* 1976;294:1019–1022.
190. Nikiforov Y, Gnepp DR. Pediatric thyroid cancer after the Chernobyl disaster. *Cancer* 1994;74:748–759.
191. Kaplan MM, Garnick MB, Gelber R. Risk factors for thyroid abnormalities after neck irradiation for childhood cancer. *Am J Med* 1983;74:272–280.
192. Reteloff S, Harrison J, Karanfilski BT. Continuing occurrence of thyroid carcinoma after irradiation to the neck in infancy and childhood. *N Engl J Med* 1975;292:171–175.
193. Block MA, Miller MJ, Horn R. Carcinoma of the thyroid after external radiation to the neck in adults. *Am J Surg* 1969;118:764–768.
194. Samaan NA, Schultz PN, Ordonez NG, Hickey RC, Johnston DA. A comparison of thyroid carcinoma in those who have and have not had head and neck irradiation in childhood. *J Clin Endocrinol Metab* 1987;64:219–223.
195. Farbota LM, Calandra DB, Lawrence AM, Paloyan E. Thyroid carcinoma in Graves' disease. *Surgery* 1985;98:1148–1152.
196. Olen E, Klinck GH. Thyroid carcinoma occurring in Graves' disease. *Arch Intern Med* 1966;117:432–435.
197. Shapiro SJ, Friedman NB, Perzik SL, Catz B. Incidence of thyroid carcinoma in Graves' disease. *Cancer* 1970;26:1261–1270.
198. Vickery AL. Thyroid papillary carcinoma. Pathological and philosophical controversies. *Am J Surg Pathol* 1983;7:797–807.
199. Strauss M, Laurian N, Antebi E. Coexistent carcinoma of the thyroid gland and Hashimoto's thyroiditis. *Surg Gynecol Obstet* 1983;157:228–232.
200. LiVolsi VA, Feind CR. Parathyroid adenoma and nonmedullary thyroid carcinoma. *Cancer* 1976;38:1391–1393.
201. Petro AB, Hardy JD. The association of parathyroid adenoma and non-medullary cancer of the thyroid. *Ann Surg* 1975;181:118–124.
202. Prinz RA, Barbato AL, Braithwaite SS, Brooks MH, Lawrence AM, Paloyan E. Prior irradiation and the development of coexistent differentiated thyroid cancer and hyperparathyroidism. *Cancer* 1982;439:874–877.
203. Naruse T, Koike A, Kanemitsu T, Kato K. Minimal thyroid carcinoma: a report of nine cases discovered by cervical lymph node metastases. *Jpn J Surg* 1984;14:118–121.
204. Arellano L, Ibaarra A. Occult carcinoma of the thyroid gland. *Pathol Res Pract* 1984;179:88–91.
205. Bondeson L, Ljungberg O. Occult papillary thyroid carcinoma in the young and the aged. *Cancer* 1984;53:1790–1792.
206. Hubert JP, Kiernan PD, Beahrs OH, McConahey WM, Woolner LB. Occult papillary carcinoma of the thyroid. *Arch Surg* 1980;115:394–398.
207. Gikas PW, Labow SS, DiGiulio W, Finger JE. Occult metastasis from occult papillary carcinoma of the thyroid. *Cancer* 1967;20:2100–2104.
208. Lissak B, Vannetsel JM, Galloudec N, et al. Solitary skin metastasis as the presenting feature of differentiated thyroid microcarcinoma. *J Endocrinol Invest* 1995;18:813–816.
209. Harach HR, Franssila KO, Wasenius V. Occult papillary carcinoma of the thyroid: a "normal" finding in Finland. A systematic autopsy study. *Cancer* 1985;56:531–538.
210. Bocker W, Schroder S, Dralle H. Minimal thyroid neoplasia. *Recent Results Cancer Res* 1988;106:131–138.
211. Patchefsky AS, Keller IB, Mansfield CM. Solitary vertebral column metastasis from occult sclerosing carcinoma of the thyroid gland. *Am J Clin Pathol* 1970;53:596–601.
212. Hammer M, Wortsman J, Folse R. Cancer in cystic lesions of the thyroid. *Arch Surg* 1982;117:1020–1023.
213. Ruiz-Velasco R, Waisman J, van Herle A. Cystic papillary carcinoma of the thyroid gland. *Acta Cytol* 1978;22:38–42.
214. Schroder S, Pfannschmidt N, Bocker W, Muller HW, DeHeer K. Histopathologic types and clinical behaviour of occult papillary carcinoma of the thyroid. *Pathol Res Pract* 1984;179:81–87.
215. Evans HL. Encapsulated papillary neoplasms of the thyroid: a study of 14 cases followed for a minimum of 10 years. *Am J Surg Pathol* 1987;11:592–597.
216. Klinck GH, Winship T. Psammoma bodies and thyroid cancer. *Cancer* 1959;12:656–662.
217. Batsakis JG, Nishiyama RH, Rich CR. Microlithiasis (calcospherites) and carcinoma of the thyroid gland. *Arch Pathol Lab Med* 1960;69:493–498.
218. Meissner WA, Warren S. *Tumors of the thyroid gland.* AFIP fascicle 4, 2nd series. Washington, DC: Armed Forces Institute of Pathology, 1969.
219. Johannessen JV, Sobrinho-Simoes M. The origin and significance of thyroid psammoma bodies. *Lab Invest* 1980;43:287–296.

220. Dugan JM, Atkinson BF, Avitable A, Schimmel M, LiVolsi VA. Psammoma bodies in fine needle aspirate of the thyroid in lymphocytic thyroiditis. *Acta Cytol* 1987;31:330–334.
221. Patchefsky AS, Hoch WS. Psammoma bodies in diffuse toxic goiter. *Am J Clin Pathol* 1972;57:551–556.
222. Meissner WA, Adler A. Papillary carcinoma of the thyroid: a study of the pathology of two hundred twenty-six cases. *Arch Pathol Lab Med* 1958;66:518–525.
223. Rosai J, Zampi G, Carcangiu M. Papillary carcinoma of the thyroid. *Am J Surg Pathol* 1983;7:809–817.
224. Hapke MR, Dehner LP. The optically clear nucleus: a reliable sign of papillary carcinoma of the thyroid? *Am J Surg Pathol* 1979;3:31–38.
225. Deligeorgi-Politi H. Nuclear crease as a cytodiagnostic feature of papillary thyroid carcinoma in fine-needle aspiration biopsies. *Diagn Cytopathol* 1987;3:307–310.
226. Chan JKC, Saw D. The grooved nucleus: a useful diagnostic criterion of 24 papillary carcinoma of the thyroid. *Am J Surg Pathol* 1986;10:672–679.
227. Shurbaji MS, Gupta PK, Frost JK. Nuclear grooves: a useful criterion in the cytopathologic diagnosis of papillary thyroid carcinoma. *Diagn Cytopathol* 1988;4:91–94.
228. Scopa Cd, Melachrinou M, Saradopoulou C, Merino MJ. The significance of the grooved nucleus in thyroid lesions. *Mod Pathol* 1993;6:691–696.
229. Rosai J, Carcangiu ML, DeLellis RA. *Tumors of the thyroid gland.* AFIP fascicle 5, 3rd series. Washington, DC: Armed Forces Institute of Pathology, 1992.
230. Pontius KI, Hawk WA. Loss of microsomal antigen in follicular and papillary carcinoma of the thyroid: an immunofluorescence and electron-microscopic study. *Am J Clin Pathol* 1980;74:620–629.
231. Matsubayashi S, Kawai K, Matsumoto Y, et al. The correlation between papillary thyroid carcinoma and lymphocytic infiltration in the thyroid gland. *J Clin Endocrinol Metab* 1995;80:3421–3424.
232. Iida F, Yonekura M, Miyakawa M. Study of intraglandular dissemination of thyroid cancer. *Cancer* 1969;24:764–771.
233. Russell WO, Ibanez M, Clark R, White EC. Thyroid carcinoma. Classification, intraglandular dissemination and clinicopathological study based upon whole organ sections of 80 thyroid glands. *Cancer* 1963;16:1425.
234. Hicks DG, LiVolsi VA, Neidich JA, Puck JM, Kant JA. Solitary follicular nodules of the thyroid are clonal proliferations. *Am J Pathol* 1990;137:553–562.
235. Namba H, Matsuo K, Fagin JA. Clonal composition of benign and malignant human thyroid tumors. *J Clin Invest* 1990;86:120–125.
236. Clark OH. Total thyroidectomy: the treatment of choice for patients with differentiated thyroid cancer. *Ann Surg* 1982;196:361–370.
237. Crile G, Antunez AR, Esselstyn CB, Hawk WA, Skillern PG. The advantages of subtotal thyroidectomy and suppression of TSH in the primary treatment of papillary carcinoma of the thyroid. *Cancer* 1985;55:2691–2697.
238. Samaan NA, Maheshwari YK, Nader S, et al. Impact of therapy for differentiated carcinoma of the thyroid: an analysis of 706 cases. *J Clin Endocrinol Metab* 1983;56:1131–1138.
239. Schroder DM, Chambers A, France CJ. Operative strategy for thyroid cancer: is total thyroidectomy worth the price? *Cancer* 1986;58:2320–2328.
240. Vickery AL, Wang CA, Walker AM. Treatment of intrathyroidal papillary carcinoma of the thyroid. *Cancer* 1987;60:2587–2595.
241. Tollefsen HR, Shah JP, Huvos AG. Papillary carcinoma of the thyroid: recurrence in the thyroid gland after initial surgical treatment. *Am J Surg* 1972;124:468–472.
242. Cohn KH, Backdahl M, Forsslund G, et al. Biologic considerations and operative strategy in papillary thyroid carcinoma: arguments against the routine performance of total thyroidectomy. *Surgery* 1984;96:957–970.
243. Cody HS, Shah JP. Locally invasive, well differentiated thyroid cancer: 22 years' experience at Memorial Sloan-Kettering Cancer Center. *Am J Surg* 1981;142:480–483.
244. Tsumori T, Nakao K, Miyata M, et al. Clinicopathologic study of thyroid carcinoma infiltrating the trachea. *Cancer* 1985;56:2843–2848.
245. Tscholl-Ducommun J, Hedinger C. Papillary thyroid carcinoma. Morphology and prognosis. *Virchows Arch [A]* 1982;396:19–39.
246. Hay ID. Nodal metastases from papillary thyroid carcinoma. *Lancet* 1986;2:1283–1284.
247. Noguchi S, Noguchi A, Murakami N. Papillary carcinoma of the thyroid. II. Value of prophylactic lymph node dissection. *Cancer* 1970;26:1061–1064.
248. Maceri DH, Babyak J, Ossakow SJ. Lateral neck mass: sole presenting sign of metastatic thyroid cancer. *Arch Otolaryngol Head Neck Surg* 1986;112:47–49.
249. Yaremchuk K, Goldman ME. Transformation of papillary carcinoma. *Ear Nose Throat J* 1985;64:54–55.
250. Hoie J, Stenwig, AE, Kullman G, Lindegaard M. Distant metastases in papillary thyroid cancer. A review of 91 patients. *Cancer* 1988;61:1–6.
251. Ruegemer JJ, Hay ID, Bergstrilh EJ, Ryan JJ, Offord KP, Gorman CA. Distant metastases in differentiated thyroid carcinoma: a multivariate analysis of prognostic variables. *J Clin Endocrinol Metab* 1988;67:501–508.
253. Hay ID. Papillary thyroid carcinoma. *Endocrinol Metab Clin North Am* 1990;19 545–576.
254. Beaumont A, Othman SB, Fragu P. The fine structure of papillary carcinoma of the thyroid. *Histopathology* 1981;5:377–388.
255. Johannessen JV, Gould VE, Jao W. The fine structure of human thyroid cancer. *Hum Pathol* 1978;9:385–400.
256. Johannessen JV, Sobrinho-Simoes M. Papillary carcinoma of the human thyroid gland. *Prog Surg Pathol* 1980;1:111–128.
257. Permanetter W, Nathrath WBJ, Lohrs U. Immunohistochemical analysis of thyroglobulin and keratin in benign and malignant thyroid tumours. *Virchows Arch [A]* 1982;398:221–228.
258. Wilson NW. Pambakian H, Richardson TC, Stokoe MR, Makin CA, Heyderman E. Epithelial markers in thyroid carcinoma. An immunoperoxidase study. *Histopathology* 1986;10:815–829.
259. Buley ID, Gatter KC, Heryet A, Mason DY. Expression of intermediate filament proteins in normal and diseased thyroid glands. *J Clin Pathol* 1987.40:136–142.
260. Dockhorn-Dworniczak B, Franke WW, Schroder S, Czernobilsky B, Gould VE, Bocker W. Patterns of expression of cytoskeletal proteins in human thyroid gland and thyroid carcinomas. *Differentiation* 1987;35:53–71.
261. Henzen-Logmans SC, Mullink H, Ramaekers FCS, Tadema T, Meijer CJLM. Expression of cytokeratins and vimentin in epithelial cells of normal and pathological thyroid tissue. *Virchows Arch [A]* 1987;410:347–354.
262. Raphael SJ, Apel RL, Asa SL. Detection of high molecular weight cytokeratins in neoplastic and nonneoplastic thyroid tumors using microwave antigen retrieval. *Mod Pathol* 1995;8:870–872.
263. Joensuu H, Klemi P, Ereola E, Tuominen J. Influence of cellular DNA content on survival in differentiated thyroid cancer. *Cancer* 1986;58:2462–2467.
264. Johannessen JV, Sobrinho-Simoes M, Lindmo T, Tangen KO, Kaalhus O, Brennhovd IO. Anomalous papillary carcinoma of the thyroid. *Cancer* 1983;51:1462–1467.
265. Johannessen JV, Sobrinho-Simoes M, Tangen KO, Lindmo T. A flow cytometric DNA analysis of papillary thyroid carcinoma. *Lab Invest* 1981;45:336–344.
266. Cohn KH, Backdahl M, Forsslund G, et al. Prognostic value of nuclear DNA content in papillary thyroid carcinoma. *World J Surg* 1984;8:474–480.
267. Simpson WJ, McKinney SE, Carruthers JS, Gospodarowicz MK, Sutcliffe SB, Panzarrela T. Papillary and follicular thyroid cancer: prognostic factors in 1578 patients. *Am J Med* 1987;83:479–488.
268. Simpson W, Panzarella T, Carruthers JS, Gospodarowicz MK, Sutcliffe SB. Papillary and follicular thyroid cancer: impact of treatment in 1578 patients. *Int J Radiat Oncol Biol Phys* 1988;14:1063–1075.
269. Tollefsen HR, DeCosse JJ, Hutter RVP. Papillary carcinoma of the thyroid: a clinical and pathological study of 70 fatal cases. *Cancer* 1964;17:1035–1044.
270. Torres J, Volpato RD, Power EG, et al. Thyroid cancer: survival in 148 cases followed for 10 years or more. *Cancer* 1985;56:2298–2304.
271. Tubiana M, Schkumberger M, Rougier P, LaPlanche A, Benhamou E, Gardet P, Caillou B, Travagli JP, Parmentier C. Longterm results and prognostic factors in patients with differentiated thyroid carcinoma. *Cancer* 1985;55:794–804.
272. Ibanez ML, Russell WO, Albores-Saavedra J, Lampertico P, White EC, Clark RL. Thyroid carcinoma—biologic behavior and mortality: postmortem findings in 42 cases including 27 in which the disease was fatal. *Cancer* 1966;19:1039–1052.

273. Carcangiu ML, Zampi G, Pupi A, Rosai J. Papillary carcinoma of the thyroid. A clinicopathologic study of 244 cases treated at the University of Florence, Italy. *Cancer* 1985;55:805–828.
274. De Groot LJ. Longterm impact of initial and surgical therapy on papillary and follicular thyroid cancer. *Am J Med* 1994;97:499–500.
275. Chen KTK, Rosai J. Follicular variant of thyroid papillary carcinoma: a clinicopathologic study of six cases. *Am J Surg Pathol* 1977;1:123–130.
276. Tielens ET, Sherman SI, Hruban RH, et al. Follicular variant of papillary thyroid carcinoma: a clinicopathologic study. *Cancer* 1994;73:424–431.
277. Johnson TL, Lloyd RV, Thompson NW, Beierwaltes WH, Sisson JC. Prognostic implications of the tall cell variant of papillary thyroid carcinoma. *Am J Surg Pathol* 1988;12:22–27.
278. Evans HL. Columnar cell carcinoma of the thyroid: a report of two cases of an aggressive variant of thyroid carcinoma. *Am J Clin Pathol* 1986;85:77–80.
279. Sobrinho-Simoes M, Nesland JM, Johannessen JV. Columnar cell carcinoma: another variant of poorly differentiated carcinoma of the thyroid. *Am J Clin Pathol* 1988;89:264–267.
280. Gartner EM, Davidson M, Wenig B. The columnar cell variant of thyroid papillary carcinoma. *Am J Surg Pathol* 1995;19:940–947.
281. Chan JKC, Tsui MS, Tse CH. Diffuse sclerosing variant of papillary carcinoma of the thyroid: a histological and immunohistochemical study of three cases. *Histopathology* 1987;11:191–202.
282. Carcangiu ML, Bianchi S. Diffuse sclerosing papillary carcinoma: clinicopathologic study of 15 cases. *Am J Surg Pathol* 1989;13:1041–1048.
283. Fujimoto Y, Obara T, Ito Y, et al. Diffuse sclerosing variant of papillary carcinoma of the thyroid: clinical importance, surgical treatment and follow-up study. *Cancer* 1990;66:2306–2314.
284. Soares J, Limbert E, Sobrinho-Simoes M. Diffuse sclerosing variant of papillary thyroid carcinoma: a clinicopathologic study of 10 cases. *Pathol Res Pract* 1989;185:200–210.
285. Schroder S, Bocker W, Dralle H, Kortman KB, Stern C. The encapsulated papillary carcinoma of the thyroid. A morphologic subtype of the papillary thyroid carcinoma. *Cancer* 1984;54:90–93.
286. Variakojis D, Getz ML, Paloyan E, Strauss FH. Papillary clear cell carcinoma of the thyroid. *Hum Pathol* 1975;6:384–390.
287. Dickersin GR, Vickery AL, Smith SB. Papillary carcinoma of the thyroid, oxyphil cell type, "clear cell" variant. *Am J Surg Pathol* 1980;4:501–509.
288. Beckner ME, Heffess CS, Oertel JE. Oxyphilic papillary thyroid carcinomas. *Am J Clin Pathol* 1995;103:280–287.
289. Apel RL, Asa SL, LiVolsi VA. Papillary Hürthle cell carcinoma with lymphocytic stroma: "Warthin-like" tumor of the thyroid. *Am J Surg Pathol* 1995;19:810–814.
290. Farid NR, Zou M, Shi Y. Genetics of follicular thyroid cancer. *Endocrinol Metab Clin North Am* 1995;24:865–883.
291. Mizukami Y, Michigishi T, Nonomura A, et al. Autonomously functioning (hot) nodule of the thyroid gland. A clinical and histopathologic study of 17 cases. *Am J Clin Pathol* 1994;101:29–35.
292. Lever EG, Medeiros-Neto GA, DeGroot LJ. Inherited disorders of thyroid metabolism. *Endocr Rev* 1983;4:213–239.
293. Batsakis JG, Nishiyama RH, Schmidt RW. "Sporadic goiter syndrome": a clinicopathologic analysis. *Am J Clin Pathol* 1963;30:241–251.
294. Kennedy JS. The pathology of dyshormonogenetic goitre. *J Pathol* 1969;99:251–264.
295. Moore GH. The thyroid in sporadic goitrous cretinism. *Arch Pathol Lab Med* 1962;74:35–58.
296. Smith JF. The pathology of the thyroid in the syndrome of sporadic goitre and congenital deafness. *Q J Med* 1960;29:297–303.
297. Cooper DS, Axelrod L, DeGroot LJ, Vickery AL, Maloof F. Congenital goiter and the development of metastatic follicular carcinoma with evidence for a leak of nonhormonal iodide: clinical, pathological, kinetic and biochemical studies and a review of the literature. *J Clin Endocrinol Metab* 1981;52:294–303.
298. Vickery AL. The diagnosis of malignancy in dyshormonogenetic goitre. *Clin Endocrinol Metab* 1981;10:317–335.
299. Bech K. Immunological aspects of Graves' disease and importance of thyroid stimulating immunoglobulins. *Acta Endocrinol (Copenh)* 1983;103(suppl 254):1–40.
300. Burman KD, Baker JR. Immune mechanisms in Graves' disease. *Endocr Rev* 1985;6:183–223.
301. Farid NR. Immunogenetics of autoimmune thyroid disorders. *Endocrinol Metab Clin North Am* 1987;16:229–245.
302. Schicha H, Emrich D, Schreivogel I. Hyperthyroidism due to Graves' disease and due to autonomous goiter. *J Endocrinol Invest* 1985;8:399–497.
303. Stenszky V, Kozma L, Balazs C, Rochlitz S, Bear JC, Farid NR. The genetics of Graves' disease: HLA and disease susceptibility. *J Clin Endocrinol Metab* 1985;61:735–740.
304. Spjut HJ, Warren WD, Ackerman LV. Clinical-pathologic study of 76 cases of recurrent Graves' disease, toxic (nonexophthalmic) goiter, and nontoxic goiter. *Am J Clin Pathol* 1957;27:367–392.
305. Furmaniak J, Nakajima Y, Hashim FA, et al. The TSH receptor: structure and interaction with autoantibodies in thyroid disease. *Acta Endocrinol (Copenh)* 1987;(suppl 281):157–165.
306. Chang DCS, Wheeler MH, Woodcock JP, et al. The effect of preoperative Lugol's iodine on thyroid blood flow in patients with Graves' hyperthyroidism. *Surgery* 1987;102:1055–1061.
307. Hamburger JI. The autonomously functioning thyroid nodule: Goetsch's disease. *Endocr Rev* 1987;8:439–447.
308. McKenzie JM. Hyperthyroidism caused by thyroid adenomata. *J Clin Endocrinol Metab* 1966;26:779–781.
309. Cerietty JM, Listwasn WJ. Hyperthyroidism due to functioning metastatic thyroid carcinoma. *JAMA* 1979;242:269–270.
310. Hamburger JI. Solitary autonomously functioning thyroid lesions. *Am J Med* 1975;58:740–748.
311. Hamburger JI. The autonomously functioning thyroid adenoma. *N Engl J Med* 1983;309:1312–1313.
312. Hamilton CR, Maloof F. Unusual types of hyperthyroidism. *Medicine (Baltimore)* 1973;52:195–214.
313. Al-Moussa M, Beck JS. Histometry of thyroids containing few and multiple nodules. *J Clin Pathol* 1986;39:483–488.
314. Beckers C. Thyroid nodules. *Clin Endocrinol Metab* 1979;8:181–192.
315. DeHaven JW, Sherwin RS. The thyroid nodule: approach to diagnosis and therapy. *Conn Med* 1979;43:761–767.
316. Mortensen JD, Woolner LB, Bennett WA. Gross and microscopic findings in clinically normal thyroid glands. *J Clin Endocrinol Metab* 1955;15:1270–1280.
317. Kraiem Z, Glaser B, Yigla M, Pauker J, Sadeh O, Sheinfeld M. Toxic multinodular goiter: a variant of autoimmune hyperthyroidism. *J Clin Endocrinol Metab* 1987;65:659–664.
318. Brown RS, Jackson IMD, Pohl SL, Reichlin S. Do thyroid stimulating immunoglobulins cause nontoxic and toxic multinodular goiter? *Lancet* 1978;1:904–906.
319. Peter HJ, Gerber H, Studer H, Smeds S. Pathogenesis of heterogeneity in human multinodular goiter. *J Clin Invest* 1985;76:1992–2002.
320. Peter HJ, Studer H, Forster R, Gerber H. The pathogenesis of "hot" and "cold" follicles in multinodular goiters. *J Clin Endocrinol Metab* 1982;55:941–946.
321. Peter HJ, Studer H, Groscurth P. Autonomous growth, but not autonomous function in embryonic human thyroids: a clue to understanding autonomous goiter growth? *J Clin Endocrinol Metab* 1988;66:968–973.
322. Ramelli F, Studer H, Bruggisser D. Pathogenesis of thyroid nodules in multinodular goiter. *Am J Pathol* 1982;109:215–223.
323. Studer H. Growth control and follicular cell neoplasia. In: Medeiros-Neto G, Gaitan E, eds. *Frontiers in thyroidology*, vol 1. New York: Plenum, 1986;131–137.
324. Studer H, Hunziker HR, Ruchti C. Morphologic and functional substrate of thyrotoxicosis caused by nodular goiters. *Am J Med* 1978;65:227–234.
325. Studer H, Peter HJ, Gerber H. Morphologic and functional changes in developing goiters. In: Hall R, Kobberling J, eds. *Thyroid disorders associated with iodine deficiency and excess*. New York: Raven Press, 1987;229–241.
326. Studer H, Ramelli F. Simple goiter and its variants: euthyroid and hyperthyroid. *Endocr Rev* 1982;3:40–61.
327. Apel RL, Ezzat S, Bapat BV, et al. Clonality of thyroid nodules in sporadic goiter. *Diagn Mol Pathol* 1995;4:113–121.
328. Meissner WA. Surgical pathology. In: Sedgwick CE, ed. *Surgery of the thyroid gland*. Philadelphia: WB Saunders, 1974;24–40.
329. Joensuu H, Klemi P, Eerola E. DNA aneuploidy in follicular adenomas of the thyroid gland. *Am J Pathol* 1987;124:373–376.
330. Hazard JB, Kenyon R. Atypical adenoma of the thyroid. *Arch Pathol Lab Med* 1954;58:554–563.
331. Franssila KO, Ackerman LV, Brown CL, Hedinger CE. Follicular carcinoma. *Semin Diagn Pathol* 1985;2:101–122.

332. Kahn N, Perzin KH. Follicular carcinoma of the thyroid: an evaluation of the histologic criteria used for diagnosis. *Pathol Annu* 1983;18(part 1):221–253.
333. Lang W, Georgii G, Stauch G, Kienzie E. The differentiation of atypical adenomas and encapsulated follicular carcinomas in the thyroid gland. *Virchows Arch [A]* 1980;385:125–141.
334. Lang W, Georgii G. Minimal invasive cancer in the thyroid. *Clin Oncol* 1982;1:527–537.
335. Williams ED. Pathology and natural history. In: Duncan W, ed. *Thyroid cancer.* Berlin: Springer-Verlag, 1980;47–55.
336. LiVolsi VA, Asa SL. The demise of follicular carcinoma of the thyroid. *Thyroid* 1994;4:233–235.
337. Harach HR, Jasani B, Williams ED. Factor VIII as a marker of endothelial cells in follicular carcinoma of the thyroid. *J Clin Pathol* 1977;36:1050–1054.
338. Evans HL. Follicular neoplasms of the thyroid. *Cancer* 1984;54:535–540.
339. Schmidt RJ, Wang CA. Encapsulated follicular carcinoma of the thyroid: diagnosis, treatment and results. *Surgery* 1986;100:1068–1076.
340. Schroder S, Baisch H, Rehpenning W, et al. Morphologie und Prognose des follicularen Schilddrusencarcinoms—Eine klinisch-pathologische und DNS-cytometrische Untersuchung an 95 Tumoren. *Langenbecks Arch Chir* 1987;370:3–24.
341. Lang W, Choritz H, Hundeshagen H. Risk factors in follicular thyroid carcinomas. A retrospective followup study covering a 14 year period with emphasis on morphological findings. *Am J Surg Pathol* 1986;10:246–255.
342. Grebe SKG, Hay ID. Follicular thyroid cancer. *Endocrinol Metab Clin North Am* 1995;24:761–801.
343. Cady B, Sedgwick CE, Meissner WA, Bookwalter JR, Romagosa V, Werber J. Changing clinical pathologic, therapeutic and survival patterns in differentiated thyroid carcinoma. *Ann Surg* 1976;184:541–553.
344. Cady B, Rossi R, Silverman M, Wood M. Further evidence of the validity of risk group definition in differentiated thyroid carcinoma. *Surgery* 1985;98:1171–1178.
345. Crile G, Pontius KI, Hawk WA. Factors influencing the survival of patients with follicular carcinoma of the thyroid gland. *Surg Gynecol Obstet* 1985;160:409–412.
346. Tollefson HR, Shah JP, Huvos AG. Follicular carcinoma of the thyroid. *Am J Surg* 1973;126:523–528.
347. Silverberg SG, Hutter RVP, Foote FW. Fatal carcinoma of the thyroid: histology, metastases and causes of death. *Cancer* 1970;25:792–802.
348. Yamashina M. Follicular neoplasms of the thyroid: total circumferential evaluation of the fibrous capsule. *Am J Surg Pathol* 1992;16:392–400.
349. Meissner WA. Follicular carcinoma of the thyroid; frozen section diagnosis. *Am J Surg Pathol* 1977;1:171–175.
350. Bronner MP, Hamilton RH, LiVolsi VA. Utility of frozen section analysis in follicular lesions of the thyroid. *Endocr Pathol* 1994;5:154–161.
351. Chen H, Nicols TL, Udelsman R. Follicular lesions of the thyroid: Does frozen section evaluation alter operative management? *Ann Surg* 1995;222:101–106.
352. van Heerden JA, Hay ID, Goellner JR, et al. Follicular thyroid carcinoma with capsular invasion alone: a nonthreatening malignancy. *Surgery* 1992;112:1130–1138.
353. Schroder S, Pfannschmidt N, Dralle H, Arps H, Bocker W. The encapsulated follicular carcinoma of the thyroid. *Virchows Arch [A]* 1984;402:259–273.
354. Iida F. The fate and surgical significance of adenoma of the thyroid gland. *Surg Gynecol Obstet* 1973;136:536–540.
355. Johannessen JV, Sobrinho-Simoes M, Lindmo T, Tangen KO. The diagnostic value of flow cytometric DNA measurements in selected disorders of the human thyroid. *Am J Clin Pathol* 1982;77:20–25.
356. Friedman NB. Cellular involution in thyroid gland; significance of Hürthle cells in myxedema, exhaustion atrophy, Hashimoto's disease and reaction to irradiation, thiouracil therapy and subtotal resection. *J Clin Endocrinol Metab* 1949;9:874–882.
357. Feldman PS, Horvath E, Kovacs K. Ultrastructure of three Hürthle cell tumors of the thyroid. *Cancer* 1972;30:1279–1285.
358. Nesland JM, Sobrinho-Simoes MA, Holm R, Sambade MC, Johannessen JV. Hürthle cell lesions of the thyroid: a combined study using transmission electron microscopy, scanning electron microscopy and immunocytochemistry. *Ultrastruct Pathol* 1985;8:269–290.
359. Tremblay G. Histochemical study of cytochrome oxidase and adenosine triphosphatase in Askanazy cells (Hürthle cells) of the human thyroid. *Lab Invest* 1962;11:514–517.
360. Tremblay G, Pearse AGE. Histochemistry of oxidative enzyme systems in the human thyroid with special reference to Askanazy cells. *J Pathol Bacteriol* 1960;80:353–358.
361. Kendall CH, McCluskey E, Naylor J. Oxyphil cells in thyroid disease: a uniform change? *J Clin Pathol* 1986;39:908–912.
362. LiVolsi VA, LoGerfo P. *Thyroiditis.* Boca Raton: CRC Press, 1981.
363. Bronner MP, Clevenger CV, Edmonds PR, Lowell DM, McFarland MM, LiVolsi VA. Flow cytometric analysis of DNA content in Hürthle cell adenomas and carcinomas of the thyroid. *Am J Clin Pathol* 1988;89:764–769.
364. Bondeson L, Bondeson AG, Ljungberg O, Tibblin S. Oxyphil tumors of the thyroid. Followup of 42 surgical cases. *Ann Surg* 1981;194:677–680.
365. Gundry SR, Burney RE, Thompson NW, Lloyd R. Total thyroidectomy for Hürthle cell neoplasm of the thyroid. *Arch Surg* 1983;118:529–532.
366. Thompson NW, Dunn EL, Batsakis JG, Nishiyama RH. Hürthle cell lesions of the thyroid gland. *Surg Gynecol Obstet* 1974;139:555–560.
367. Bronner MP, LiVolsi VA. Oxyphilic (Askanazy/Hürthle cell) tumors of the thyroid: microscopic features predict biologic behavior. *Surg Pathol* 1988;1:137–150.
368. Tollefson HR, Shah JP, Huvos AG. Hürthle cell carcinoma of the thyroid. *Am J Surg* 1975;130:390–394.
369. Watson RG, Brennan MD, Goellner JR, van Heerden JA, McConahey WM, Taylor WF. Invasive Hürthle cell carcinoma of the thyroid: natural history and management. *Mayo Clin Proc* 1984;59:851–855.
370. Heimann P, Ljunggren JG, Lowhagen T, Hjern B. Oxyphilic adenoma of the human thyroid: a morphological and biochemical study. *Cancer* 1973;31:246–254.
371. Kini SR, Miller JM, Abrash MP, Gaba A, Johnson T. Post fine needle aspiration biopsy infarction in thyroid nodules [abstr]. *Mod Pathol* 1988;1:48A.
372. LiVolsi Va, Merino MJ. Worrisome histologic alterations following FNA thyroid. *Pathol Annu* 1994;29(pt 2):99–120.
373. Bondeson L, Bondeson AG, Ljungberg O. Treatment of Hürthle cell neoplasms of the thyroid [letter]. *Arch Surg* 1983;118:1453.
374. Gonzalez-Campora R, Herrero-Zapatero A, Lerma E, Sanchez F, Galera H. Hürthle cell and mitochondrion-rich cell tumors: a clinicopathologic study. *Cancer* 1986;57:1154–1163.
375. Heppe H, Armin A, Calandra DB, Lawrence AM, Paloyan E. Hürthle cell tumors of the thyroid gland. *Surgery* 1985;98:1162–1165.
376. Rosen IB, Luk S, Katz I. Hürthle cell tumor behavior: dilemma and resolution. *Surgery* 1985;98:777–783.
377. Bondeson L, Azavedo E, Bondeson AG, Caspersson T, Ljungberg O. Nuclear DNA content and behavior of oxyphil thyroid tumors. *Cancer* 1986;58:672–675.
378. Galera-Davidson H, Bibbo M, Bartels PH, Dytch HE, Puls JH, Wied GL. Correlation between automated DNA ploidy measurements of Hürthle cell tumors and their histopathologic and clinical features. *Anal Quant Cytol Histol* 1986;8:158–167.
379. Gardner LW. Hürthle cell tumors of the thyroid. *Arch Pathol* 1955;59:372–381.
380. El-Naggar AK, Batsakis JH, Luna MA, Hickey RC. Hürthle cell tumors of the thyroid: a flow cytometric DNA analysis. *Arch Otolaryngol Head Neck Surg* 1988;114:520–521.
381. McLeod MK, Thompson NW, Hudson JL. Flow cytometric measurements of nuclear DNA and ploidy analysis in Hürthle cell neoplasms of the thyroid. *Arch Surg* 1988;123:849–854.
382. Flint A, Davenport RD, Lloyd RV, Beckwith AL, Thompson NW. Cytophotometric measurements of Hürthle cell tumors of the thyroid gland: correlation with pathologic features and clinical behavior. *Cancer* 1988;61:110–113.
383. Carcangiu M, Bianchi S, Savino D, et al. Follicular Hürthle cell neoplasms of the thyroid gland. A study of 153 cases. *Cancer* 1991;68:1944–1953.
384. Flint A, Lloyd RV. Hürthle cell neoplasms of the thyroid gland. *Pathol Annu* 1990;25(pt 2):37–52.
385. Hazard JB, Hawk WA, Crile G. Medullary (solid) carcinoma of the thyroid: a clinicopathologic entity. *J Clin Endocrinol Metab* 1959;19:152–161.
386. Horn RC. Carcinoma of the thyroid. Description of a distinctive morphological variant and report of seven cases. *Cancer* 1951;4:697–707.

387. Williams ED. Histogenesis of medullary carcinoma of the thyroid. *J Clin Pathol* 1966;19:114–118.
388. Godwin MC. Complex IV in the dog with special emphasis on the relation of the ultimobranchial body to the interfollicular cells in the postnatal glands. *Am J Anat* 1937;60:299–339.
389. Pearse AGE. Common cytochemical and ultrastructural characteristics of cells producing polypeptide hormones (the APUD series) and their relevance to thyroid and ultimobranchial C cells and calcitonin. *Proc R Soc Lond [Biol]* 1968;170:71–80.
390. Pearse AGE, Polak JM. Cytochemical evidence for the neural crest origin of mammalian ultimobranchial C cells. *Histochemie* 1976;27:96–102.
391. Wolfe HJ, DeLellis RA, Voelkel EF, Tashjian AH. Distribution of calcitonin containing cells in the normal neonatal human thyroid gland: a correlation of morphology with peptide content. *J Clin Endocrinol Metab* 1975;41:1076–1081.
392. Wolfe HJ, Voelkel EF, Tashjian AH. Distribution of calcitonin containing cells in the normal adult human thyroid gland: a correlation of morphology and peptide content. *J Clin Endocrinol Metab* 1974;38:688–694.
393. Roediger WEW. The oxyphil and C cells of the human thyroid gland. *Cancer* 1975;36:1758–1770.
394. McMillan PJ, Hooker WM, Deftos LJ. Distribution of calcitonin containing cells in the human thyroid. *Am J Anat* 1974;140:73–80.
395. Gibson WCH, Peng TC, Croker BP. C cell nodules in adult human thyroid: a common autopsy finding. *Am J Clin Pathol* 1980;73:347–351.
396. DeLellis RA, Wolfe HJ. Pathobiology of the human calcitonin (C) cell: a review. *Pathol Annu* 1981;16(pt 2):25–52.
397. O'Toole K, Fenoglio-Preiser C, Pushparaj N. Endocrine changes associated with the human aging process. III. Effect of age on the number of calcitonin immunoreactive cells in the thyroid gland. *Hum Pathol* 1985;16:991–1000.
398. Lips CJM, Landsvater RM, Hoppener JWM, et al. Clinical screening as compared with DNA analysis in families with multiple endocrine neoplasia type 2A. *N Engl J Med* 1994;331:828–835.
399. Mulligan LM, Eng C, Healey CS, et al. Specific mutations of the RET protooncogene are related to disease phenotype in MEN 2A and FMTC. *Nat Genet* 1994;6:70–74.
400. Xing S, Smanik PA, Oglesbee MJ, et al. Characterization of ret oncogene activation in MEN 2 inherited cancer syndromes. *J Clin Endocrinol Metab* 1996;137:1512–1519.
401. Hofstra RMW, Landsvater RM, Ceccherini I, et al. A mutation in the RET protooncogene associated with multiple endocrine neoplasia type 2B and sporadic medullary thyroid carcinoma. *Nature* 1994;367:375–376.
402. Gagel RF. ret Protooncogene mutations and endocrine neoplasia—a story intertwined with neural crest differentiation. *J Clin Endocrinol Metab* 1996;137:1509–1511.
403. Wohlik N, Cote GJ, Evans DB, et al. Application of genetic screening information to the management of medullary thyroid carcinoma and multiple endocrine neoplasia type 2. *Endocrinol Metab Clin North Am* 1996;25:1–25.
404. Hill CS, Ibanez ML, Samaan NA, Ahearn MF, Clark RL. Medullary (solid) carcinoma of the thyroid gland: an analysis of the M.D. Anderson Hospital experience with patients with the tumor, its special features and its histogenesis. *Medicine (Baltimore)* 1973;52:141–171.
405. Deftos LJ. *Medullary thyroid carcinoma*. Basel: Karger, 1983.
406. Dunn EL, Nishiyama RH, Thompson NW. Medullary carcinoma of the thyroid gland. *Surgery* 1973;73:848–858.
407. Freeman D. Medullary carcinoma of the thyroid gland. A clinicopathological study of 33 patients. *Arch Pathol Lab Med* 1965;80:575–582.
408. Gonzalez-Licea A, Hartman WH, Yardley JH. Medullary carcinoma of the thyroid gland. *Am J Clin Pathol* 1968;49:512–520.
409. Gordon PR, Huvos AG, Strong EW. Medullary carcinoma of the thyroid. *Cancer* 1973;31:915–924.
410. Hillyard CJ, Evans IMA, Hill PA, Taylor S. Familial medullary thyroid carcinoma. *Lancet* 1978;1:1009–1011.
411. Ibanez ML, Cole VW, Russell WO, Clark RL. Solid carcinoma of the thyroid gland: analysis of 53 cases. *Cancer* 1967;20:706–723.
412. Keynes WM, Till AS. Medullary carcinoma of the thyroid. *Q J Med* 1971;159:443–456.
413. Khairi MRS, Dexter RN, Burzynski NJ, Johnston CC. Mucosal neuroma, pheochromocytoma and medullary thyroid carcinoma: multiple endocrine neoplasia type 3. *Medicine (Baltimore)* 1975;54:89–112.
414. Sizemore GW. Medullary carcinoma of the thyroid gland. *Semin Oncol* 1987;14:306–314.
415. Steiner AL, Goodman AD, Powers SR. Study of a kindred with pheochromocytoma, medullary thyroid carcinoma, hyperparathyroidism and Cushing's disease: multiple endocrine neoplasia type 2. *Medicine (Baltimore)* 1968;47:371–409.
416. Tashjian AH, Melvin KEW. Medullary carcinoma of the thyroid gland. *N Engl J Med* 1968;279:279–283.
417. Williams ED. A review of 17 cases of carcinoma of the thyroid and pheochromocytoma. *J Clin Pathol* 1965;18:288–292.
418. Graze K, Spiler IJ, Tashjian AH, et al. Natural history of familial medullary thyroid carcinoma. Effect of a program of early diagnosis. *N Engl J Med* 1978;299:980–985.
419. Kakudo K, Miyauchi A, Ogihara T, et al. Medullary carcinoma of the thyroid with ectopic ACTH syndrome. *Acta Pathol Jpn* 1982;32:793–800.
420. Melvin KEW, Tashjian AH, Cassidy CE, Givens JR. Cushing's syndrome caused by ACTH and calcitonin secreting medullary carcinoma of the thyroid. *Metabolism* 1972;19:831–838.
421. Szijj I, Csapo Z, Laslo FA, Kovacs K. Medullary cancer of the thyroid gland associated with hypercorticism. *Cancer* 1969;24:167–173.
422. Williams ED, Karim SMM, Sandler M. Prostaglandin secretion by medullary carcinoma of the thyroid: a possible cause of the associated diarrhea. *Lancet* 1968;1:22–23.
423. Williams ED, Morales AM, Horn RC. Thyroid carcinoma and Cushing's syndrome. *J Clin Pathol* 1968;21:129–135.
424. Sipple JH. The association of pheochromocytoma with carcinoma of the thyroid gland. *Am J Med* 1961;31:163–166.
425. Bigner SH, Cox EB, Mendelsohn G, Baylin SB, Wells SA, Eggleston JC. Medullary carcinoma of the thyroid in the multiple endocrine neoplasia II. A syndrome. *Am J Surg Pathol* 1981;5:459–472.
426. Catalona WJ, Engelman K, Ketcham AS, Hammond WG. Familial medullary thyroid carcinoma, pheochromocytoma and parathyroid adenoma (Sipple's syndrome). *Cancer* 1971;28:1245–1254.
427. Huang SN, McLeish WA. Pheochromocytoma and medullary carcinoma of the thyroid. *Cancer* 1968;21:302–311.
428. Jansson S, Hansson G, Salander H, Stenstrom G, Tisell LE. Prevalence of C cell hyperplasia and medullary thyroid carcinoma in a consecutive series of pheochromocytoma patients. *World J Surg* 1984;8:493–500.
429. Ljungberg O, Cederquist E, Von Studnitz E. Medullary thyroid carcinoma and pheochromocytomas: A familial chromaffinosis. *Br Med J (Clin Res Ed)* 1967;1:279–281.
430. Melvin KEW, Tashjian AH, Miller HH. Studies in familial medullary thyroid carcinoma. *Recent Prog Horm Res* 1972;28:399–470.
431. Ram MD, Rao KN, Brown L. Hypercalcitoninemia, pheochromocytoma and C cell hyperplasia. A new variant of Sipple's syndrome. *JAMA* 1978;239:2155–2156.
432. Sarosi G, Doe RP. Familial occurrence of parathyroid adenomas, pheochromocytoma, and medullary carcinoma of the thyroid with amyloid stroma (Sipple's syndrome). *Ann Intern Med* 1968;68:1305–1308.
433. Schimke RN. Multiple endocrine adenomatosis syndromes. *Adv Intern Med* 1976;21:249–265.
434. Schimke RN, Hartman WH. Familial amyloid producing medullary thyroid carcinoma and pheochromocytoma: a distinct genetic entity. *Ann Intern Med* 1965;63:1027–1039.
435. Schimke RN, Hartman WH, Prout TE, Rimoin DL. Syndrome of bilateral pheochromocytoma, medullary thyroid carcinoma and multiple neuromas. *N Engl J Med* 1968;279:1–17.
436. Baylin SB, Hsu SH, Gann DS, Smallridge RC, Wells SA. Inherited medullary thyroid carcinoma: a final monoclonal mutation in one of multiple clones of susceptible cells. *Science* 1978;199:429–431.
437. Mathew CGP, Chin KS, Easton DF, et al. A linked genetic marker for multiple endocrine neoplasia type 2A on chromosome 10. *Nature* 1987;328:527–528.
438. Simpson NE. Genetic studies of multiple endocrine neoplasia type 2 syndromes. *Henry Ford Hosp Med J* 1984;32:273–276.
439. Simpson NE, Kidd KK, Goodfellow PJ, et al. Assignment of multiple endocrine neoplasia type 2A to chromosome 10 by linkage. *Nature* 1987;328:528–529.
440. Bartlett RD, Myall RWT, Bean LR, Mandelstam P. A neuroendocrine syndrome: mucosal neuromas, pheochromocytoma and medullary thyroid carcinoma. *Oral Surg Oral Med Oral Pathol* 1971;31:206–220.

441. Brown RS, Colle E, Tashjian AH. The syndrome of multiple mucosal neuromas and medullary thyroid carcinoma in childhood. *J Pediatr* 1975;86:77–83.
442. Carney JA, Hales AB. Alimentary tract manifestations of multiple endocrine neoplasia, type 2b. *Mayo Clin Proc* 1977;52:543–548.
443. DeLellis RA, Wolfe HJ, Gagel RF, et al. Adrenal medullary hyperplasia. *Am J Pathol* 1976;83:177–190.
444. Carney JA, Roth SI, Heath H, Sizemore GW, Hales AB. The parathyroid glands in multiple endocrine neoplasia, type 2b. *Am J Pathol* 1980;99:387–398.
445. Carney JA, Hales AB, Pearse AGE, Perry HO, Sizemore GW. Abnormal cutaneous innervation in multiple endocrine neoplasia, type 2b. *Ann Intern Med* 1981;94:262–263.
446. Carney JA, Sizemore GW, Hales AB. Multiple endocrine neoplasia, type 2b. *Pathobiol Annu* 1978;8:105–153.
447. Carney JA, Sizemore GW, Sheps SG. Adrenal medullary disease in multiple endocrine neoplasia, type 2. *Am J Clin Pathol* 1976;66:279–290.
448. Carney JA, Sizemore GW, Tyce GM. Bilateral adrenal medullary hyperplasia in multiple endocrine neoplasia, type 2; The precursor of bilateral pheochromocytoma. *Mayo Clin Proc* 1975;50:3–10.
449. Cunliffe WJ, Hudgson P, Fulthorpe JJ, et al. A calcitonin secreting medullary thyroid carcinoma associated with mucosal neuromas, Marfanoid features, myopathy, and pigmentation. *Am J Med* 1970;48:120–126.
450. Forsman PJ, Jenkins ME. Medullary carcinoma of the thyroid with Marfan-like habitus. *Pediatrics* 1973;52:188–191.
451. Gorlin RJ, Sedano HO, Vickers RA, Corvaniko S. Multiple mucosal neuromas, pheochromocytoma and medullary carcinoma of the thyroid. A syndrome. *Cancer* 1968;22:293–299.
452. Kullberg BJ, Nieuwenhuijzen-Kruseman AC. Multiple endocrine neoplasia type 2b with a good prognosis. *Arch Intern Med* 1987;147:1125–1127.
453. Norman T, Ontnes B. Intestinal ganglioneuromatosis, diarrhea and medullary thyroid carcinoma. *Scand J Gastroenterol* 1969;4:553–559.
454. Vasen HFA, Nieuwenhuijzen-Kruseman AC, Berkel H, et al. Multiple endocrine neoplasia syndrome type 2: the value of screening and central registration. *Am J Med* 1987;83:847–852.
455. Wells SA, Ontjes DA. Multiple endocrine neoplasia type II. *Annu Rev Med* 1976;27:263–268.
456. Whittle TS, Goodwin MN. Intestinal ganglioneuromatosis with the mucosal neuromamedullary thyroid carcinoma-pheochromocytoma syndrome. *Am J Gastroenterol* 1976;65:249–257.
457. Williams ED, Pollock DJ. Multiple mucosal neuromata with endocrine tumors: a syndrome allied to von Recklinghausen's disease. *J Pathol Bacteriol* 1966;91:71–80.
458. Deschryver-Keckemeti K, Clouse RE, Goldstein MN, Gersell D, O'Neal L. Intestinal ganglioneuromatosis. A manifestation of overproduction of nerve growth factor? *N Engl J Med* 1983;308:635–639.
459. Bigazzi M, Revoltella R, Casciano S, Vigneti E. High level of nerve growth factor in the serum of a patient with medullary carcinoma of the thyroid gland. *Clin Endocrinol (Oxf)* 1977;6:105–111.
460. Ekblom M, Valimaki M, Pelkonen R, Jansson R, Sivula A, Franssila KO. Familial and sporadic medullary thyroid carcinoma: clinical and immunohistological findings. *Q J Med* 1987;247:899–910.
461. Emmertsen K, Erno H, Henriques U, Schroder HD. C cells for differentiation between familial and sporadic medullary thyroid carcinoma. *Dan Med Bull* 1983;30:353–356.
462. Komminoth P, Roth J, Saremaslani P, et al. Polysialic acid of the neural cell adhesion molecule in the human thyroid: a marker for medullary thyroid carcinoma and primary C cell hyperplasia. *Am J Surg Pathol* 1994;18:399–411.
463. Romei C, Elisei R, Pinchera A, et al. Somatic mutations of the *ret* protooncogene in sporadic medullary thyroid carcinoma are not restricted to exon 16 and are associated with tumor recurrence. *J Clin Endocrinol Metab* 1996;81:1619–1622.
464. Marsh DJ, Learoyd DL, Andrew SD, et al. Somatic mutations in the RET protooncogene in sporadic medullary thyroid carcinoma. *Clin Endocrinol* 1996;44:249–257.
465. Kini SR, Miller JM, Hamburger JI, Smith J. Cytopathologic features of medullary carcinoma of the thyroid. *Arch Pathol Lab Med* 1984;108:156–159.
466. Saad MF, Ordonez NG, Rashid RK, et al. Medullary carcinoma of the thyroid. A study of the clinical feature and prognostic factors in 161 patients. *Medicine (Baltimore)* 1984;63:319–342.
467. Mendelsohn G, Oertel JE. Encapsulated medullary thyroid carcinoma [abstr]. *Lab Invest* 1981;44:43A.
468. Kakudo K, Miyauchi A, Takai S, Katayama S, Kuma K, Kitamura H. C cell carcinoma of the thyroid: papillary type. *Acta Pathol Jpn* 1979;29:653–659.
469. Albores-Saavedra J, LiVolsi VA, Williams ED. Medullary carcinoma. *Semin Diagn Pathol* 1985;2:137–150.
470. Harach HR, Williams ED. Glandular (tubular and follicular) variants of medullary carcinoma of the thyroid. *Histopathology* 1983;7:83–97.
471. Kakudo K, Miyauchi A, Ogihara T, et al. Medullary carcinoma of the thyroid: giant cell type. *Arch Pathol Lab Med* 1978;102:445–447.
472. Landon G, Ordonez NG. Clear cell variant of medullary carcinoma of the thyroid. *Hum Pathol* 1985;16:844–847.
473. Harach HR, Bergholm U. Medullary (C cell) carcinoma of the thyroid with features of follicular oxyphilic tumours. *Histopathology* 1988;13:645–656.
474. Dominquez-Malagon H, Delgado-Chavez R, Torres-Najera M, Gould E, Albores-Saavedra J. Oxyphil and squamous variants of medullary thyroid carcinoma. *Cancer* 1989;63:1183–1188.
475. Birkenhager JC, Upton GV, Seldenrath HJ, Krieger DT, Tashjian AH. Medullary thyroid carcinoma: ectopic production of peptides with ACTH-like, corticotropin-releasing factor-like and prolactin production-stimulating activities. *Acta Endocrinol (Copenh)* 1976;83:280–292.
476. Deftos LJ, Bone HG, Parthemore JG, Burton DW. Immunohistological studies of medullary thyroid carcinoma and C cell hyperplasia. *J Clin Endocrinol Metab* 1980;51:857–862.
477. Goltzman D, Huang SN, Browne C, Solomon S. Adrenocorticotropin and calcitonin in medullary thyroid carcinoma: frequency of occurrence and localization in the same cell type by immunocytochemistry. *J Clin Endocrinol Metab* 1979;49:364–370.
478. Ghatei MA, Springall DR, Nicholl CG, Polak JM, Bloom SR. Gastrin releasing peptide like immunoreactivity in medullary thyroid carcinoma. *Am J Clin Pathol* 1985;84:581–586.
479. Edbrooke MR, Parker D, McVey JH, et al. Expression of the human calcitonin/CGRP gene in lung and thyroid carcinoma. *EMBO J* 1977;4:939–940.
480. Bethge N, Ahuja S, Diel F. Occurrence of calcitonin, somatostatin-like immunoreactivity and carcinoembryonic antigen in two sisters suffering from familial thyroid medullary carcinoma. *Exp Clin Endocrinol* 1986;88:365–372.
481. Capella C, Bordi C, Monga G, et al. Multiple endocrine cell types in thyroid medullary carcinoma. Evidence for calcitonin, somatostatin, ACTH, 5HT, and small granule cells. *Virchows Arch [A]* 1978;377:111–128.
482. Golouh R, Us-Krasovec M, Auersperg M, Jancar J, Bondi A, Eusebi V. Amphicrine-composite calcitonin and mucin producing carcinoma of the thyroid. *Ultrastruct Pathol* 1985;8:197–206.
483. Skranbanek P, Cannon D, Dempsey J, Kirrane J, Neligan M, Powell D. Substance P in medullary carcinoma of the thyroid. *Experientia* 1979;35:1259–1260.
484. Wurzel HM, Kourides IA, Brooks JSJ. Medullary carcinomas of the thyroid contain immunoreactive human chorionic gonadotropin alpha subunit. *Horm Metab Res* 1984;16:677.
485. Busnardo B, Girelli ME, Simoni N, Nacamulli D, Busetto E. Nonparallel patterns of calcitonin and carcinoembryonic antigen in the followup of medullary thyroid carcinoma. *Cancer* 1984;53:278–285.
486. Busnardo B, Girelli ME, Simoni N, Nacamulli D, Busetto E. Nonparallel patterns of calcitonin and carcinoembryonic antigen in the follow up of medullary thyroid carcinoma. *Cancer* 1984;53:278–285.
487. Baylin SB, Beaven MA, Engelman K, Sjoerdsma A. Elevated histaminase activity in medullary carcinoma of the thyroid gland. *N Engl J Med* 1972;283:1239–1244.
488. Fernandes BF, Bedard YC, Rosen I. Mucus producing medullary cell carcinoma of the thyroid gland. *Am J Clin Pathol* 1982;78:536–540.
489. Zaatari GS, Saigo PE, Huvos AG. Mucin production in medullary carcinoma of the thyroid. *Arch Pathol Lab Med* 1983;107:70–74.
490. Marcus J, Dise CA, LiVolsi VA. Melanin production in a medullary thyroid carcinoma. *Cancer* 1982;49:2518–2526.
491. Kimura N, Ishioka K, Miura Y, et al. Melanin producing medullary thyroid carcinoma with glandular differentiation. *Acta Cytol* 1989;33:61–66.

492. Eng HL, Chen WJ. Melanin producing medullary carcinoma of the thyroid gland. *Arch Pathol Lab Med* 1989;113:377–380.
493. Krisch K, Krisch I, Horvat G, Neuhold N, Ulrich W. The value of immunohistochemistry in medullary thyroid carcinoma: a systematic study of 30 cases. *Histopathology* 1985;9:1077–1090.
494. Sikri KL, Varndell IM, Hamid QA, et al. Medullary carcinoma of the thyroid. An immunocytochemical and histochemical study of 25 cases using eight separate markers. *Cancer* 1985;56:2481–2491.
495. Lippman SM, Mendelsohn G, Trump DL, Wells SA, Baylin SB. The prognostic and biological significance of cellular heterogeneity in medullary thyroid carcinoma. A study of calcitonin, L-DOPA decarboxylase and histaminase. *J Clin Endocrinol Metab* 1982;54:233–240.
496. Rougier P, Calmettes C, LaPlanche A, et al. The value of calcitonin and carcinoembryonic antigen in the treatment and management of nonfamilial medullary thyroid carcinoma. *Cancer* 1983;51:855–862.
497. Rougier P, Parmentier C, LaPlanche A, et al. Medullary thyroid carcinoma: prognostic factors and treatment. *Int J Radiat Oncol Biol Phys* 1983;9:161–169.
498. Ruppert JM, Eggleston JC, DeBustros A, Baylin SB. Disseminated calcitonin poor medullary thyroid carcinoma in a patient with calcitonin rich primary tumor. *Am J Surg Pathol* 1986;10:513–518.
499. Saad MF, Fritsche HA, Samaan NA. Diagnostic and prognostic values of carcinoembryonic antigen in medullary carcinoma of the thyroid. *J Clin Endocrinol Metab* 1984;58:889–894.
500. Saad MF, Ordonez NG, Guido JJ, Samaan NA. The prognostic value of calcitonin immunostaining in medullary carcinoma of the thyroid. *J Clin Endocrinol Metab* 1984;59:850–856.
501. Schroder S, Bocker W, Baisch H, et al. Prognostic factors in medullary thyroid carcinomas: survival in relation to age, sex, stage, histology, immunocytochemistry and DNA content. *Cancer* 1988;61:806–816.
502. Uribe M, Grimes M, Fenoglio-Preiser CM, Feind C. Medullary carcinoma of the thyroid gland: clinical, pathological and immunohistochemical features with review of the literature. *Am J Surg Pathol* 1985;9:577–594.
503. Cooper CW, Schwesinger WH, Mahgoub AM, Ontjes DA. Thyrocalcitonin: stimulation of secretion by pentagastrin. *Science* 1971;172:1238–1240.
504. Graze K, Spiler IJ, Tashjian AH, et al. Natural history of familial medullary thyroid carcinoma. *N Engl J Med* 1978;299:980–985.
505. Kakudo K, Carney JA, Sizemore GW. Medullary carcinoma of the thyroid. Biologic behavior of the sporadic and familial neoplasm. *Cancer* 1985;55:2818–2821.
506. Melvin KEW, Miller HH, Tashjian AH. Early diagnosis of medullary carcinoma of the thyroid by means of calcitonin assay. *N Engl J Med* 1971;285:1115–1120.
507. Norton JA, Doppmann JLO, Brennan MF. Localization and resection of clinically inapparent medullary carcinoma of the thyroid. *Surgery* 1980;87:616–622.
508. Ponder BAJ. Screening for familial medullary thyroid carcinoma: a review. *J R Soc Med* 1984;77:585–594.
509. Ponder BAJ, Finer N, Coffey R. Family screening in medullary thyroid carcinoma presenting without a family history. *Q J Med* 1988;252:299–308.
510. Ponder BAJ, Ponder MA, Coffey R, et al. Risk estimation and screening in families of patients with medullary thyroid carcinoma. *Lancet* 1988;1:397–400.
511. Samaan NA, Schultz PN, Hickey RC. Medullary thyroid carcinoma: prognosis of familial versus sporadic disease and the role of radiotherapy. *J Clin Endocrinol Metab* 1988;67:801–805.
512. Starling JR, Harris C, Granner DK. Diagnosis of occult familial medullary carcinoma of the thyroid using pentagastrin. *Arch Surg* 1978;113:241–243.
513. Tashjian AH, Howland BG, Melvin KEW, Hill CS. Immunoassay of human calcitonin. Clinical measurement relation to serum calcium and studies in patients with medullary carcinoma. *N Engl J Med* 1970;283:890–895.
514. Tashjian AH, Wolfe HJ, Voelkel EF. Human calcitonin: immunologic assay, cytologic localization and studies on medullary carcinoma. *Am J Med* 1974;56:840–849.
515. Wells SA, Baylin SB, Gann DS, et al. Medullary thyroid carcinoma: relationship of method of diagnosis to pathologic staging. *Ann Surg* 1978;188:377–383.
516. Wells SA, Baylin SB, Johnsrude IS, et al. Thyroid venous catherization in the early diagnosis of familial medullary thyroid carcinoma. *Ann Surg* 1982;196:505–510.
517. Wells SA, Baylin SB, Leight GS, Dale JK, Dilley WG, Farndon JR. The importance of early diagnosis in patients with hereditary medullary thyroid carcinoma. *Ann Surg* 1982;195:595–599.
518. Wells SA, Haagensen DE, Linehan WM, Farrell RE, Dilley WG. The detection of elevated plasma levels of carcinoembryonic antigen in patients with suspected or established medullary thyroid carcinoma. *Cancer* 1978;42:1498–1503.
519. Wells SA, Ontjes DA, Cooper CW, et al. The early diagnosis of medullary carcinoma of the thyroid gland in patients with multiple endocrine neoplasia type II. *Ann Surg* 1975;182:362–370.
520. Kaufman FR, Roe TF Isaacs H, Weitzman JJ. Metastatic medullary carcinoma in young children with mucosal neuroma syndrome. *Pediatrics* 1982;70:263–267.
521. Norton JA, Froome BA, Farrell RE, Wells SA. Multiple endocrine neoplasia type IIb: the most aggressive form of medullary thyroid carcinoma. *Surg Clin North Am* 1979;59:109–118.
522. Ibanez ML. Medullary carcinoma of the thyroid gland. *Pathol Annu* 1974;9:263–290.
523. Williams ED, Brown CL, Doniach I. Pathological and clinical findings in a series of 67 cases of medullary carcinoma of the thyroid. *J Clin Pathol* 1966;19:103–113.
524. DeLellis RA, Rule AH, Spiler I, Nathanson L, Tashjian AH, Wolfe HJ. Calcitonin and carcinoembryonic antigen as tumor markers in medullary thyroid carcinoma. *Am J Clin Pathol* 1978;70:587–594.
525. Trump DL, Mendelsohn G, Baylin SB. Discordance between plasma calcitonin and tumor cell mass in medullary thyroid carcinoma. *N Engl J Med* 1984;301:253–254.
526. Mendelsohn G, Wells SA, Baylin SB. Relationship of tissue carcinoembryonic antigen and calcitonin to tumor virulence in medullary thyroid carcinoma. An immunohistochemical study in early, localized and virulent disseminated stages of disease. *Cancer* 1984;54:657–662.
527. Beshid M. C cell adenoma of the human thyroid gland. *Oncology* 1979;36:19–22.
528. Beshid M, Lorenc R, Rosciszewska A. A thyroid C cell adenoma in man. *J Pathol* 1971;103:343–346.
529. Kodama T, Okamoto T, Fujimoto Y, et al. C cell adenoma of the thyroid: a rare but distinct clinical entity. *Surgery* 1988;104:997–1003.
530. Kodama T, Tamura M, Kanaji Y, et al. A case of calcitonin producing adenoma of the thyroid. *Endocrinol Jpn* 1984;31:63–70.
531. Bussolati G, Monga G. Medullary carcinoma of the thyroid with atypical patterns. *Cancer* 1979;44:1769–1777.
532. Hales M, Rosenau W, Okerlund MD, Galante M. Carcinoma of the thyroid with a mixed medullary and follicular pattern. *Cancer* 1982;50:1352–1359.
533. Ljungberg O, Bondeson L, Bondeson AG. Differentiated thyroid carcinoma, intermediate type: a new tumor entity with features of follicular and parafollicular cell carcinoma. *Hum Pathol* 1984;15:218–228.
534. Polliack A, Freund U. Mixed papillary and follicular carcinoma of the thyroid gland with stromal amyloid. *Am J Clin Pathol* 1970;53:592–597.
535. Valenta LJ, Michel-Bechet M, Mattson JC, Singer FR. Microfollicular thyroid carcinoma with amyloid rich stroma resembling the medullary carcinoma of the thyroid (MCT). *Cancer* 1977;39:1573–1586.
536. Holm R, Sobrinho-Simoes M, Nesland JM, Sambade C, Johannessen JV. Medullary carcinoma of the thyroid gland with thyroglobulin immunoreactivity. A special entity? *Lab Invest* 1987;57:258–268.
537. Holm R, Sobrinho-Simoes M, Nesland JM, Johannessen JV. Concurrent production of calcitonin and thyroglobulin by the same neoplastic cells. *Ultrastruct Pathol* 1987;10:241–251.
538. Ogawa H, Kino I, Arai T. Mixed medullary-follicular carcinoma of the thyroid. *Acta Pathol Jpn* 1989;39:67–72.
539. Pfaltz M, Hedinger CE, Muhlethaler JP. Mixed medullary and follicular carcinoma of the thyroid. *Virchows Arch [A]* 1983;400:53–59.
540. LiVolsi VA. Mixed thyroid tumors: a real entity? *Lab Invest* 1987;57:237–239.
541. Hedinger C, Williams ED, Sobin LH. The WHO histological classification of thyroid tumors: a commentary on the second edition. *Cancer* 1989;63:908–911.
542. Albores-Saavedra J, Gorraz de la Mora T, de la Torre-Rendon F, Gould E. Mixed medullary-papillary carcinoma of the thyroid. *Hum Pathol* 1990;21:1151–1155.
543. Apel RL, Alpert LC, Rizzo A, et al. A metastasizing composite carcinoma of the thyroid with distinct medullary and papillary components. *Arch Pathol Lab Med* 1994;118:1143–1147.
544. Lips CJM, Leo JR, Berends MJH, et al. Thyroid C cell hyperplasia

and micronodules in close relatives of MEN-2A patients: pitfalls in early diagnosis and reevaluation of criteria for surgery. *Henry Ford Hosp Med J* 1987;35:133–138.
545. Williams ED. C cell hyperplasia. *Bull Cancer (Paris)* 1984;71:122–124.
546. Broulik PD, Hradec E, Pacovsky V. Calcitonin activity of the thyroid gland in primary hyperparathyroidism. *Acta Endocrinol (Copenh)* 1978;89:122–125.
547. LiVolsi VA, Feind CR. Incidental medullary thyroid carcinoma in sporadic hyperparathyroidism. *Am J Clin Pathol* 1979;71:595–599.
548. LiVolsi VA, Feind CR, LoGerfo P, Tashjian AH. Demonstration by immunoperoxidase staining of hyperplasia of parafollicular cells in the thyroid gland in hyperparathyroidism. *J Clin Endocrinol Metab* 1973;37:550–559.
549. Ljungberg O, Dymling JF. Pathogenesis of C cell neoplasia in thyroid gland: C cell proliferation in a case of chronic hypercalcemia. *APMIS* 1972;80:577–588.
550. Tashjian AH, Voelkel EF. Decreased thyrocalcitonin in thyroid glands from patients with hyperparathyroidism. *J Clin Endocrinol Metab* 1967;27:1353–1357.
551. Ulbright TM, Kraus FT, O'Neal LW. C cell hyperplasia developing in residual thyroid following resection for sporadic medullary carcinoma. *Cancer* 1981;48:2076–2079.
552. Albores-Saavedra J, Monforte H, Nadji M, Morales AR. C-cell hyperplasia in thyroid tissue adjacent to follicular cell tumors. *Hum Pathol* 1988;19:795–799.
553. Libbey NP, Nowakowski KJ, Tucci JR. C cell hyperplasia of the thyroid in a patient with goitrous hypothyroidism and Hashimoto's thyroiditis. *Am J Surg Pathol* 1989;13:71–77.
554. Weiss LM, Weinberg DS, Warhol MJ. Medullary carcinoma arising in a thyroid with Hashimoto's disease. *Am J Clin Pathol* 1983;80:534–538.
555. Aldinger KA, Samaan NA, Ibanez M, Hill CS. Anaplastic carcinoma of the thyroid: a review of 84 cases of spindle and giant cell carcinoma of the thyroid. *Cancer* 1978;41:2267–2275.
556. Carcangiu ML, Steeper T, Zampi G, Rosai J. Anaplastic thyroid carcinoma: a study of 70 cases. *Am J Clin Pathol* 1985;83:135–158.
557. Hayashi Y, Tokuoka S. Anaplastic carcinoma of the thyroid gland. *Acta Pathol Jpn* 1979;29:119–133.
558. Hedinger CE. Sarcoma of the thyroid gland. In: Hedinger CE, ed. *Thyroid cancer.* Heidelberg: Springer-Verlag, 1969;47.
559. Hutter RVP, Tollefsen HR, DeCosse JJ, Foote FW, Frazell EL. Spindle and giant cell metaplasia in papillary carcinomata of the thyroid. *Am J Surg* 1965;110:660–668.
560. LiVolsi VA, Brooks JJ, Arendash-Durand B. Anaplastic thyroid tumors: immunohistology. *Am J Clin Pathol* 1987;87:434–442.
561. Nel CJC, van Heerden JA, Goellner JR, et al. Anaplastic carcinoma of the thyroid: a clinicopathologic study of 82 cases. *Mayo Clin Proc* 1985;60:51–58.
562. Nishiyama RH, Dunn EL, Thompson WW. Anaplastic spindle cell and giant cell tumors of the thyroid gland. *Cancer* 1971;30:113–127.
563. Rafla S. Anaplastic tumors of the thyroid. *Cancer* 1969;23:668–677.
564. Walt AJ, Woolner LB, Black MB. Small cell malignant lesions of the thyroid gland. *J Clin Endocrinol Metab* 1957;17:45–60.
565. Buckwalter JA, Meredith LK. Small cell carcinoma of the thyroid gland of youth. *Pediatrics* 1955;15:317–321.
566. Cameron RG, Seemayer TA, Wang NS, Ahmed MN, Tabah EJ. Small cell malignant tumors of the thyroid: a light and electron microscopic study. *Hum Pathol* 1975;6:731–740.
567. Luna MA, Mackay B, Hill CS, Hussey DH, Hickey RC. Malignant small cell tumor of the thyroid. *Ultrastruct Pathol* 1980;1:265–270.
568. Meissner WA, Phillips MJ. Diffuse small cell carcinoma of the thyroid. *Arch Pathol* 1962;74:291–297.
569. Rayfield EJ, Nishiyama RH, Sisson JC. Small cell tumors of the thyroid: a clinicopathologic study. *Cancer* 1971;28:1023–1030.
570. Rosai J, Saxen EA, Woolner L. Undifferentiated and poorly differentiated carcinoma. *Semin Diagn Pathol* 1985;2:123–136.
571. Mambo NC, Irwin SM. Anaplastic small cell neoplasms of the thyroid: an immunoperoxidase study. *Hum Pathol* 1984;15:55–60.
572. Myskow MW, Krajewski AS, Dewar EA, Milfar EP, McLaren K, Febre JW. The role of immunoperoxidase techniques on paraffin embedded tissue in determining the histogenesis of undifferentiated thyroid neoplasms. *Clin Endocrinol (Oxf)* 1986;243:335–341.
573. Ralfkiaer N, Gatter KC, Alcock C, Heryet A, Ralfkiaer E, Mason DY. The value of immunocytochemical methods in the differential diagnosis of anaplastic thyroid tumours. *Br J Cancer* 1985;52:167–170.
574. Schmid KW, Kröll M, Hofstädter F, Ladurner D. Small cell carcinoma of the thyroid. A reclassification of cases originally diagnosed as small cell carcinoma of the thyroid. *Pathol Res Pract* 1986;181:540–543.
575. Tobler A, Maurer R, Hedinger CE. Undifferentiated thyroid tumors of diffuse small cell type. Histological and immunohistochemical evidence of their lymphomatous nature. *Virchows Arch [A]* 1984;404:117–126.
576. Burt AD, Kerr DJ, Brown IL, Boyle P. Lymphoid and epithelial markers in small cell anaplastic thyroid tumours. *J Clin Pathol* 1985;38:893–896.
577. Carcangiu ML, Zampi G, Rosai J. Poorly differentiated ("insular") thyroid carcinoma. *Am J Surg Pathol* 1984;8:655–668.
578. Kapp DS, LiVolsi VA, Sanders MM. Anaplastic carcinoma following well-differentiated thyroid cancer: etiological considerations. *Yale J Biol Med* 1982;55:521–528.
579. Moore JH, Bacharach B, Choi HY. Anaplastic transformation of metastatic follicular carcinoma of the thyroid. *J Surg Oncol* 1985;29:216–221.
580. Wilson NW, Pambakian H, Richardson TC, Stokoe MR, Makin CA, Heyderman E. Epithelial markers in thyroid carcinoma: an immunoperoxidase study. *Histopathology* 1986;10:815–829.
581. Hurlimann J, Gardiol D, Scazziga B. Immunohistology of anaplastic thyroid carcinoma. A study of 43 cases. *Histopathology* 1987;11:567–580.
582. Cibull ML, Gray GF. Ultrastructure of osteoclastoma-like giant cell tumor of thyroid. *Am J Surg Pathol* 1978;2:401–405.
583. Esmaili HJ, Hafez GR, Warner TFCS. Anaplastic carcinoma of the thyroid with osteoclastoma-like giant cells. *Cancer* 1983;52:2122–2128.
584. Gubetta L. Undifferentiated carcinoma of the thyroid with spindle cells and giant cells of osteoclastic aspects. *Pathologica* 1983;68:271–276.
585. Hashimoto F, Koga S, Watanabe H, Enjoji M. Undifferentiated carcinoma of the thyroid gland with osteoclast-like giant cells. *Acta Pathol Jpn* 1980;30:323–334.
586. Kobayashi S, Yamadori I, Ohmori M, Kurokawa T, Umeda M. Anaplastic carcinoma of the thyroid with osteoclast-like giant cells. *Acta Pathol Jpn* 1987;37:807–815.
587. Silverberg SG, DeGiorgi LS. Osteoclastoma-like giant cell tumor of the thyroid. *Cancer* 1973;31:621–625.
588. Mendelsohn G, Bigner SH, Eggleston JC, Baylin SB, Wells SA. Anaplastic variants of medullary thyroid carcinoma. *Am J Surg Pathol* 1980;4:333–341.
589. Fisher ER, Gregorio R, Shoemaker R, Howat B, Hubay C. The derivation of so-called giant cell and spindle cell undifferentiated thyroid neoplasm. *Am J Clin Pathol* 1974;61:680–689.
590. Gaal JM, Horvath E, Kovacs K. Ultrastructure of two cases of anaplastic giant cell tumor of the human thyroid gland. *Cancer* 1975;35:1273–1279.
591. Graham H, Daniel C. Ultrastructure of anaplastic carcinoma of the thyroid. *Am J Clin Pathol* 1974;61:690–696.
592. Jao W, Gould VE. Ultrastructure of anaplastic (spindle and giant cell) carcinoma of the thyroid. *Cancer* 1975;35:1280–1292.
593. Newland JR, Mackay B, Hill CS, Hickey RC. Anaplastic thyroid carcinoma: an ultrastructural study of 10 cases. *Ultrastruct Pathol* 1981;2:121–129.
594. Wan SK, Chan JKC, Tang SK. Paucicellular variant of anaplastic thyroid carcinoma. *Am J Clin Pathol* 1996;105:388–393.
595. Livingstone DJ, Sandison AT. Osteogenic sarcoma of thyroid. *Br J Surg* 1962;50:291–293.
596. Roberts C. Sarcomata of the thyroid gland: a report of 2 cases. *J Pathol Bacteriol* 1968;95:537–540.
597. Shin W-Y, Afalion B, Hotchkiss E, Schenkman R, Berkman J. Ultrastructure of a primary fibrosarcoma of the human thyroid gland. *Cancer* 1979;44:584–591.
598. Syrjänen KJ. An osteogenic sarcoma of the thyroid gland (Report of a case and survey of the literature). *Neoplasm* 1979;26:623–628.
599. Tamada A, Makimoto K, Tasaka Y, Nakamoto Y, Iwasaki H. Yamabe H. Radiation-induced fibrosarcoma of the thyroid. *J Laryngol Otol* 1984;98:1063–1066.
600. Chan YF, Ma L, Boey J, Young H. Angiosarcoma of the thyroid. An immunohistochemical and ultrastructural study of a case in a Chinese patient. *Cancer* 1986;57:2381–2388.

601. Chesky VE, Dreese WC, Hellwig CA. Hemangioendothelioma of the thyroid. *J Clin Endocrinol Metab* 1953;13:801–808.
602. Eckert F, Schmid U, Gloor F, Hedinger Chr E. Evidence of vascular differentiation in anaplastic tumours of the thyroid—an immunohistological study. *Virchows Arch [A]* 1986;412:203–215.
603. Egloff B. The hemangioendothelioma of the thyroid. *Virchows Arch [A]* 1983;400:119–142.
604. Pfaltz M, Hedinger C, Saremaslani P, Egloff B. Malignant hemangioendothelioma of the thyroid and factor VIII-related antigen. *Virchows Arch [A]* 1983;401:177–184.
605. Ruchti C, Gerber HA, Schaffner T. Factor VIII-related antigen in malignant hemangioendothelioma of the thyroid: additional evidence for the endothelial origin of this tumor. *Am J Clin Pathol* 1984;82:474–477.
606. Tanda F, Massarelli G, Bosincu L, Cossu A. Angiosarcoma of the thyroid: a light, electron microscopic and immunohistological study. *Hum Pathol* 1988;19:742–745.
607. Arean VM, Schildecker WW. Carcinosarcoma of the thyroid gland: report of two cases. *South Med J* 1964;57:446–451.
608. Donnell CA, Pollock WJ, Sybers WA. Thyroid carcinosarcoma. *Arch Pathol Lab Med* 1987;111:1169–1172.
609. Woolner LB, McConahey WM, Beahrs OH. Primary malignant lymphoma of the thyroid. Review of forty-six cases. *Am J Surg* 1966;111:502–523.
610. Fujimoto Y, Suzuki H, Abe K, Brooks JR. Autoantibodies in malignant lymphoma of the thyroid gland. *N Engl J Med* 1967;276:380–383.
611. Schwarze EW, Papadimitriou CS. Non-Hodgkin's lymphoma of the thyroid. *Pathol Res Pract* 1980;167:346–362.
612. Allevato PA, Kini SR, Rebuck JW, Miller JM, Hamburger JI. Signet ring cell lymphoma of the thyroid: a case report. *Hum Pathol* 1985;16:1066–1068.
613. Anscombe AM, Wright DH. Primary malignant lymphoma of the thyroid—a tumour of mucosa-associated lymphoid tissue: review of seventy-six cases. *Histopathology* 1985;9:81–97.
614. Aozasa K, Inoue A, Tajima K, Miyauchi A, Matsuzuka F, Kuma K. Malignant lymphomas of the thyroid gland. Analysis of 79 patients with emphasis on histologic prognostic factors. *Cancer* 1986;58:100–104.
615. Aozasa K, Inoue A, Yoshimura H, et al. Intermediate lymphocytic lymphoma of the thyroid. An immunologic and immunohistologic study. *Cancer* 1986;57:1762–1767.
616. Burke JS, Butler JJ, Fuller LM. Malignant lymphomas of the thyroid. *Cancer* 1977;39:1587–1602.
617. Chak LY, Hoppe RT, Burke JS, Kaplan HS. Non-Hodgkin's lymphoma presenting as thyroid enlargement. *Cancer* 1981;48:2712–2716.
618. Compagno J, Oertel JE. Malignant lymphoma and other lymphoproliferative disorders of the thyroid gland: a clinicopathologic study of 245 cases. *Am J Clin Pathol* 1980;74:1–11.
619. Grimley RP, Oates GD. The natural history of malignant thyroid lymphomas. *Br J Surg* 1980;67:475–477.
620. Hamburger JI, Miller JM, Kini SR. Lymphoma of the thyroid. *Ann Intern Med* 1983;99:685–693.
621. Hermann R, Vannineuse A, DeSloover C. Malignant lymphomas and undifferentiated small cell carcinoma of the thyroid: a clinicopathologic review in light of the Kiel classification of malignant lymphomas. *Histopathology* 1978;2:201–213.
622. Hyjek E, Isaacson PG. Primary B cell lymphoma of the thyroid and its relationship to Hashimoto's thyroiditis. *Hum Pathol* 1988;19:1315–1326.
623. Kapadia SB, Dekker A, Cheng VS, Desai U, Watson CG. Malignant lymphoma of the thyroid gland: a clinicopathologic study. *Head Neck Surg* 1982;4:270–280.
624. Maurer R, Taylor CR, Terry R. Non-Hodgkin lymphomas of the thyroid. A clinicopathological review of 29 cases applying the Lukes-Collins classification and an immunoperoxidase method. *Virchows Arch [A]* 1979;383:293–317.
625. Oertel JE, Heffess CS. Lymphoma of the thyroid and related disorders. *Semin Oncol* 1987;14:333–342.
626. Sirota DK, Segal RL. Primary lymphomas of the thyroid gland. *JAMA* 1979;242:1743–1746.
627. Williams ED. Malignant lymphoma of the thyroid. *Clin Endocrinol Metab* 1981;10:379–389.
628. Noguchi M, Mori N, Kojima M, Ono T. A case report of malignant lymphoma with Hashimoto's thyroiditis. *Am J Clin Pathol* 1985;83:650–655.
629. Mitchell JD, Kirkham N, Mackin D. Focal lymphocytic thyroiditis in Southampton. *J Pathol* 1984;144:269–273.
630. Crile G. Struma lymphomatosa and carcinoma of the thyroid. *Surg Gynecol Obstet* 1978;147:350–352.
631. Crile G, Hazard JB. Incidence of cancer in struma lymphomatosa. *Surg Gynecol Obstet* 1962;115:101–103.
632. Ben-Ezra J, Wu A, Sheibani K. Hashimoto's thyroiditis lacks detectable clonal immunoglobin and T cell receptor gene rearrangements. *Hum Pathol* 1988;19:1444–1448.
633. Shaw RC, Smith FB. Plasmacytoma of the thyroid gland. *Arch Surg* 1940;40:646–657.
634. Rasbach DA, Mondschein MS, Harris NL, Kaufman DS, Wang CA. Malignant lymphoma of the thyroid gland: a clinical and pathologic study of twenty cases. *Surgery* 1985;98:1166–1170.
635. Tennvall J, Cavallin-Stahl E, Akerman M. Primary localized non-Hodgkin's lymphoma of the thyroid: a retrospective clinicopathological review. *Eur J Surg Oncol* 1987;13:297–302.
636. Tupchong L, Hughes F, Harmer CL. Primary lymphoma of the thyroid: clinical features, prognostic factors, and results of treatment. *Int J Radiat Oncol Biol Phys* 1986;12:1813–1821.
637. Vigliotti A, Kong JS, Fuller LM, Velasquez WS. Thyroid lymphomas stages IE and IIE: comparative results for radiotherapy only, combination chemotherapy only, and multimodality therapy. *Int J Radiat Oncol Biol Phys* 1986;12:1807–1812.
638. Kapadia SB. Multiple myeloma: a clinicopathologic study of 62 consecutively autopsied cases. *Medicine (Baltimore)* 1980;59:380–392.
639. Kapadia SB, Desai U, Cheng VA. Extramedullary plasmacytoma of the head and neck: a clinicopathologic study of 20 cases. *Medicine (Baltimore)* 1982;61:317–329.
640. Aozasa K, Inoue A, Yoshimura H, Miyauchi A, Matsuzuka F, Kuma K. Plasmacytoma of the thyroid gland. *Cancer* 1986;58:105–110.
641. Buss DH, Marshall RB, Holleman IK, Myers RT. Malignant lymphoma of the thyroid gland with plasma cell differentiation (plasmacytoma). *Cancer* 1980;46:2671–2675.
642. Macpherson TA, Dekker A, Kapadia SB. Thyroid gland plasma cell neoplasms (plasmacytoma). *Arch Pathol Lab Med* 1981;105:570–572.
643. More JRS, Dawson DW, Ralston AJ, Craig ISLA. Plasmacytoma of the thyroid. *J Clin Pathol* 1968;21:661–667.
644. Otto S, Peter I, Vegh S, Juhos E, Besznyak I. Gamma chain heavy chain disease with primary thyroid plasmacytoma. *Arch Pathol Lab Med* 1986;110:893–896.
645. Aozasa K, Inoue A, Katagiri SA, Matsuzuka F, Katayama S, Yonezawa T. Plasmacytoma and follicular lymphoma in a case of Hashimoto's thyroiditis. *Histopathology* 1986;10:735–740.
646. Shimaoka K, Gailani S, Tsukada Y. Plasma cell neoplasm involving the thyroid. *Cancer* 1978;41:1140–1146.
647. Naylor B. Secondary lymphoblastomatous involvement of the thyroid gland. *Arch Pathol* 1959;67:432–438.
648. Feigin GA, Buss DH, Paschal B, Woodruff RD, Myers RT. Hodgkin's disease manifested as a thyroid nodule. *Hum Pathol* 1982;13:774–776.
649. Rappaport H, Thomas LB. Mycosis fungoides: the pathology of extracutaneous involvement. *Cancer* 1974;34:1198–1229.
650. Neiman RS, Barcos M, Berard C, et al. Granulocytic sarcoma: a clinicopathologic study of 61 biopsied cases. *Cancer* 1981;48:1426–1437.
651. Coode PE, Shaikh MU. Histiocytosis X of the thyroid masquerading as thyroid carcinoma. *Hum Pathol* 1988;19:239–241.
652. Teja K, Sabio H, Langsdon DR, Johanson AJ. Involvement of the thyroid gland in histiocytosis X. *Hum Pathol* 1981;12:1137–1139.
653. Larkin DFP, Dervan PA, Munnelly J, Finucane J. Sinus histiocytosis with massive lymphadenopathy simulating subacute thyroiditis. *Hum Pathol* 1986;17:321–324.
654. Carcangiu ML, Sibley RK, Rosai J. Clear cell change in primary thyroid tumors. *Am J Surg Pathol* 1985;9:705–722.
655. Civantis F, Albores-Saavedra J, Nadji M, Morales AR. Clear cell variant of thyroid carcinoma. *Am J Surg Pathol* 1984;8:187–192.
656. Schroder S, Bocker WL. Clear cell carcinoma of thyroid gland: a clinicopathological study of 13 cases. *Histopathology* 1986;10:75–89.
657. Segal K, Har-el G, Avidor K, Shvero J, Lubin E, Sidi J. Clear cell carcinoma of the thyroid gland. *Head Neck Surg* 1986;8:313–319.
658. Valenta LJ, Michel-Bechet M. Electron microscopy of clear cell thyroid tumors. *Arch Pathol Lab Med* 1977;101:140–144.

659. Fisher ER, Kim WS. Primary clear cell thyroid carcinoma with squamous features. *Cancer* 1977;39:2497–2502.
660. Schroder S, Bocker W. Signet ring cell thyroid tumors: a follicle cell tumor with arrest of folliculogenesis. *Am J Surg Pathol* 1985;9: 619–629.
661. Mendelsohn G. Signet ring cell simulating microfollicular adenoma of the thyroid. *Am J Surg Pathol* 1984;8:705–708.
662. Gherardi G. Signet ring cell "mucinous" thyroid adenoma: a follicle cell tumour with abnormal accumulation of thyroglobulin and a peculiar histochemical profile. *Histopathology* 1987;11:317–326.
663. Schroder S, Bocker W, Husselmann H, Dralle H. Adenolipoma (thyrolipoma) of the thyroid gland: report of two cases and review of the literature. *Virchows Arch [A]* 1984;404:99–103.
664. Schroder S, Husselmann H, Bocker W. Lipid rich adenoma of the thyroid gland. Report of a peculiar thyroid tumor. *Virchows Arch [A]* 1984;404:105–108.
665. Simha MR, Doctor VM. Adenolipomatosis of the thyroid gland. *Indian J Cancer* 1983;20:215–217.
666. Fuller RH. Hamartomatous adiposity with superimposed amyloidosis of thyroid gland. *J Laryngol Otol* 1963;77:92–93.
667. Trites AEW. Thyrolipoma, thymolipoma and pharyngeal lipoma: a syndrome. *Can Med Assoc J* 1966;95:1254–1259.
668. Akerstrom G, Malmaeus J, Bergstrom R. Surgical anatomy of human parathyroid glands. *Surgery* 1984;95:14–21.
669. Goodman ML, Egdahl RH, Kemp A, Carey LC. Hyperparathyroidism from intrathyroid parathyroid adenomas. *Arch Pathol* 1969;87: 418–422.
670. Spiegel AM, Marx SJ, Doppman JL, et al. Intrathyroidal parathyroid adenoma or hyperplasia: an occasionally overlooked cause of surgical failure in primary hyperparathyroidism. *JAMA* 1975;234: 1029–1033.
671. Tolstedt GE, Cammock EE, Bell JW. Hyperparathyroidism associated with intrathyroidal parathyroid glands. *Am J Surg* 1960;100: 757–760.
672. Elliot RHE, Frantz VK. Metastatic carcinoma masquerading as primary thyroid cancer: a report of authors' 14 cases. *Ann Surg* 1960; 151:551–561.
673. Ivy HK. Cancer metastatic to the thyroid: A diagnostic problem. *Mayo Clin Proc* 1984;59:856–859.
674. Green LK, Ro JY, Mackay B, Ayala AG, Luna MA. Renal cell carcinoma metastatic to the thyroid. *Cancer* 1989;63:1810–1815.
675. McCabe DP, Farrar WB, Petkov TM, Finkelmeier W, O'Dwyer P, James A. Clinical and pathologic correlations in disease metastatic to the thyroid. *Am J Surg* 1985;150:519–523.
676. Gowing NFC. The pathology and natural history of thyroid tumours. In: Smithers D, ed. Tumours of the thyroid gland. Edinburgh: ES Livingstone, 1970;103–129.
677. Harrison DFN. Thyroid gland in the management of laryngopharyngeal cancer. *Arch Otolaryngol* 1973;97:301–302.
678. Czech JM, Lichtor TR, Carney JA, van Heerden JA. Neoplasms metastatic to the thyroid gland. *Surg Gynecol Obstet* 1982;155: 503–505.
679. Harcourt-Webster JN. Secondary neoplasm of the thyroid presenting as a goitre. *J Clin Pathol* 1965;18:282–287.
680. Shima H, Mori H, Takahashi M, Nakamura S, Miura K, Tarao M. A case of renal cell carcinoma of solitarily metastasized to thyroid 20 years after the resection of primary tumor. *Pathol Res Pract* 1985; 179:666–670.
681. Flynn SD, Forman BH, Stewart AF, Kinder BK. Poorly differentiated ("insular") carcinoma of the thyroid: an aggressive subset of differentiated thyroid neoplasms. *Surgery* 1988;104:963–970.
682. Martin JME, Randhawa G, Temple WJ. Cervical thymoma. *Arch Pathol Lab Med* 1986;110:354–357.
683. Asa SL, Dardick I, Van Nostrand P, Bailey DJ, Gullane P. Primary thyroid thymoma: a distinct clinicopathologic entity. *Hum Pathol* 1988; 19:1463–1467.
684. Miyauchi A, Kuma K, Matsuzuka F, et al. Intrathyroidal epithelial thymoma: an entity distinct from squamous cell carcinoma of the thyroid. *World J Surg* 1985;9:128–135.
685. Neill J. Intrathyroidal thymoma. *Am J Surg Pathol* 1986;10:660–661.
686. Vhan JKC, Rosai J. Tumors of the neck showing thymic or related branchial pouch differentiation: a unifying concept. *Hum Pathol* 1991;22:349–367.
687. Carney JA, Ryan J, Goellner JR. Hyalinizing trabecular adenoma of the thyroid gland. *Am J Surg Pathol* 1987;11:583–591.
688. Bronner M, LiVolsi VA, Jennings T. Paraganglioma-like adenomas of the thyroid *Surg Pathol* 1988;1:383–389.
689. Sambade C, Franssila K, Cameselle-Teijeiro J, et al. Hyalinizing trabecular adenoma: a misnomer for a peculiar tumor of the thyroid gland. *Endocr Pathol* 1991;2:83–91.
690. Hajdu SI, Faruque AA, Hajdu EO, Morgan WS. Teratoma of the neck in infants. *Am J Dis Child* 1966;111:412–416.
691. Newstedt JR, Shirkey HC. Teratoma of the thyroid region. *Am J Dis Child* 1964;107:88–95.
692. Fisher JE, Cooney DR, Voorhees ML, Jewett TC. Teratoma of thyroid gland in infancy: review of the literature and two case reports. *J Surg Oncol* 1982;21:135–140.
693. Hajdu SI, Hajdu EO. Malignant teratoma of the neck. *Arch Pathol* 1967;83:567–570.
694. Buckley N, Burch WM, Leight GS. Malignant teratoma of the thyroid gland in an adult: a case report and a review of the literature. *Surgery* 1986;100:932–937.
695. Kimler SC, Muth WF. Primary malignant teratoma of the thyroid. Case report and literature review of cervical teratomas in adults. *Cancer* 1978;42:311–317.
696. Pickleman JR, Lee JF, Straus FH, Paloyan E. Thyroid hemangioma. *Am J Surg* 1975;129:331–336.
697. Andrion A, Bellis D, Delsedime L, Bussolati G, Mazzucco G. Leiomyoma and neurilemoma: report of two unusual non-epithelial tumours of the thyroid gland. *Virchows Arch [A]* 1988;413:367–372.
698. Delaney WE, Fry KE. Neurilemoma of the thyroid gland. *Ann Surg* 1964;160:1014–1016.
699. Goldstein J, Tovi F, Sidi J. Primary schwannoma of the thyroid gland. *Int Surg* 1982;67:433–434.
700. Harcourt-Webster JN. Squamous epithelium in the human thyroid gland. *J Clin Pathol* 1966;19:384–388.
701. LiVolsi VA, Merino MJ. Squamous cells in the human thyroid gland. *Am J Surg Pathol* 1978;2:133–140.
702. Autelitano F, Santeusanio G, Tondo UD, Costantino AM, Renda F, Autelitano M. Immunohistochemical study of solid cell nests of the thyroid gland found from an autopsy study. *Cancer* 1987;59:477–483.
703. Nadig J, Weber E, Hedinger C. C cells in vestiges of the ultimobranchial body in human thyroid glands. *Virchows Arch [B]* 1978;27: 189–191.
704. Klinck GH, Menk KF. Squamous cells in the human thyroid. *Milit Surg* 1951;109:406–414.
705. Rhatigan RM, Roque JL, Bucher RL. Mucoepidermoid carcinoma of the thyroid gland. *Cancer* 1977;39:210–214.
706. Franssila KO, Harach HR, Wasenius VM. Mucoepidermoid carcinoma of the thyroid. *Histopathology* 1984;8:847–860.
707. Harach HR. A study on the relationship between solid cell nests and mucoepidermoid carcinoma of the thyroid. *Histopathology* 1985;9: 195–207.
708. Mizukami Y, Matsubara F, Hashimoto T, et al. Primary mucoepidermoid carcinoma in the thyroid gland. *Cancer* 1984;53:1741–1745.
709. Wenig BM, Adair CF, Heffess CS. Primary mucoepidermoid carcinoma of the thyroid gland. *Human Pathol* 1995;26:1099–1108.
710. Viciana MJ, Galera-Davidson H, Martin-Lacave I, Segura DI, Loizaga JM. Papillary carcinoma of the thyroid with mucoepidermoid differentiation. *Arch Pathol Lab Med* 1996;120:397–398.
711. Chan JKC, Albores-Saavedra J, Battifora H, et al. Sclerosing mucoepidermoid carcinoma of the thyroid with eosinophilia. *Am J Surg* 1991;15:438–448.
712. Huang TY, Assor D. Primary squamous cell carcinoma of the thyroid gland: a report of four cases. *Am J Clin Pathol* 1971;55:93–98.
713. Simpson WJ, Carruthers J. Squamous cell carcinoma of the thyroid gland. *Am J Surg* 1988;156:44–46.
714. Budd DC, Fink DL, Rashti MY, Woo TH. Squamous cell carcinoma of the thyroid. *J Med Soc N J* 1982;79:838–840.
715. Saito K, Kuratomi Y, Yamamoto K, et al. Primary squamous cell carcinoma of the thyroid associated with marked leucocytosis and hypercalcemia. *Cancer* 1981;48:2080–2083.
716. Monroe JB, Fahey D. Lingual thyroid: case report and review of the literature. *Arch Otolaryngol* 1975;101:574–576.
717. Fih J, Moore RM. Ectopic thyroid tissue and ectopic thyroid carcinoma. *Ann Surg* 1963;157:212–222.
718. Potdar GG, Desai PB. Carcinoma of the lingual thyroid. *Laryngoscope* 1971;81:427–429.
719. Judd ES. Thyroglossal duct cysts and sinuses. *Surg Clin North Am* 1963;43:1023–1032.

720. Mobini J, Krouse TB, Klinghoffer JF. Squamous cell carcinoma arising in a thyroglossal duct cyst. *Am Surg* 1974;40:290–294.
721. Shepard GH, Rosenfeld G. Carcinoma of thyroglossal duct remnants. *Am J Surg* 1968;115:125–130.
722. Jaques DA, Chambers RG, Oertel JE. Thyroglossal tract carcinoma: a review of the literature and addition of eighteen cases. *Am J Surg* 1970;120:439–446.
723. Joseph TJ, Komorowski RA. Thyroglossal duct carcinoma. *Hum Pathol* 1975;6:717–729.
724. Kristensen S, Juul A, Moesner J. Thyroglossal cyst carcinoma. *J Laryngol Otol* 1984;98:1277–1280.
725. Liu AHF, Littler ER. Thyroid carcinoma originating in thyroglossal cyst. *Am Surg* 1970;36:546–548.
726. Nussbaum M, Buchwald RP, Ribner A, Mori K, Litwins J. Anaplastic carcinoma arising from median ectopic thyroid (thyroglossal duct remnants). *Cancer* 1981;48:2724–2728.
727. White IL, Talbert WM. Squamous cell carcinoma arising in thyroglossal duct remnant cyst epithelium. *Otolaryngol Head Neck Surg* 1982;90:25–31.
728. Roses DF, Snively SL, Phelps RG, Cohen N, Bloom M. Carcinoma of the thyroglossal duct. *Am J Surg* 1983;145:266–269.
729. Choy FJ, Ward R, Richardson R. Carcinoma of the thyroglossal duct. *Am J Surg* 1964;108:361–369.
730. Dowling EA, Johnson IM, Collier FCD, Dillard RA. Intratracheal goiter: a clinicopathologic review. *Ann Surg* 1962;156:258–267.
731. Waggoner LG. Intralaryngeal intratracheal thyroid. *Ann Otol Rhino Laryngol* 1958;67:61–71.
732. deSouza FM, Smith PE. Retrosternal goiter. *J Otolaryngol* 1983;12:393–396.
733. Mishriki YY, Lane BP, Lozowski MS, Epstein H. Hürthle cell tumor arising in the mediastinal ectopic thyroid and diagnosed by fine needle aspiration. *Acta Cytol* 1983;27:188–192.
734. Miller JM, Hamburger JI, Kini SR. The impact of needle biopsy on the preoperative diagnosis of thyroid nodules. *Henry Ford Hosp Med J* 1980;28:145–148.
735. Silverman JF, West LR, Larkin EW, et al. The role of fine needle aspiration biopsy in the rapid diagnosis and management of thyroid neoplasm. *Cancer* 1986;57:1164–1170.
736. Ashcraft MW, van Herle AJ. Management of the thyroid nodule: Scanning techniques, thyroid suppressive therapy and fine needle aspiration. *Head Neck Surg* 1981;3:297–322.
737. Blum M. The diagnosis of the thyroid nodule using aspiration biopsy and cytology. *Arch Intern Med* 1984;144:1140–1142.
738. Boey J, Hsu C, Collins RJ, Wong J. A prospective controlled study of fine needle aspiration and Tru-cut needle biopsy of dominant thyroid nodules. *World J Surg* 1984;8:458–465.
739. Boey J, Hsu C, Wong J, Ong GB. Fine needle aspiration versus drill needle biopsy of thyroid nodules: a controlled clinical trial. *Surgery* 1982;91:611–615.
740. Esselstyn CB, Crile G. Evaluation of various types of needle biopsies of the thyroid. *World J Surg* 1984;8:452–457.
741. Griffies WS, Donegan E, Abel ME. The role of fine needle aspiration in the management of the thyroid nodule. *Laryngoscope* 1985;95:1103–1106.
742. Hamberger B, Gharib H, Melton LJ, Goellner JR, Zinsmeister AR. Fine needle aspiration biopsy of thyroid nodules: impact on thyroid practice and cost of care. *Am J Med* 1982;73:381–384.
743. Hawkins F, Bellido D, Bernal C, et al. Fine needle aspiration biopsy in the diagnosis of thyroid cancer and thyroid diseases. *Cancer* 1987;59:1206–1209.
744. Rojeski MT, Gharib H. Nodular thyroid disease. *N Engl J Med* 1985;313:428–436.
745. Silverman JF, West RL, Finley JL, et al. Fine needle aspiration versus large needle biopsy or cutting needle biopsy in evaluation of thyroid nodules. *Diagn Cytopathol* 1986;2:25–30.
746. Miller JM, Kini SR, Hamburger JI. *Needle biopsy of the thyroid.* New York: Praeger, 1983.
747. Kraemer BB. Frozen section and the thyroid. *Semin Diagn Pathol* 1987;4:169–189.
748. Bugis SP, Young JEM, Archibald SD, Chen VSM. Diagnostic accuracy of fine needle aspiration biopsy versus frozen section in solitary thyroid nodules. *Am J Surg* 1986;152:411–416.
749. Hamburger JI, Hamburger SW. Declining role of frozen section in surgical planning for thyroid nodules. *Surgery* 1985;98:307–312.
750. Keller MP, Crabbe MM, Norwood SH. Accuracy and significance of fine needle aspiration and frozen section in determining the extent of thyroid resection. *Surgery* 1987;101:632–635.
751. Bronner MP, Hamilton R, LiVolsi VA. Utility of frozen section analysis on follicular lesions of the thyroid. *Endocrine Pathol* 1994;5:154–161.
752. Chen H, Nicol TL, Udelsman R. Follicular lesions of the thyroid: Does frozen section evaluation alter operating management? *Annals Surg* 1995;222:101–106.

CHAPTER 7

Fine-Needle Biopsy of the Thyroid

Michael M. Kaplan and Joel I. Hamburger

The problem of appropriate management of thyroid nodules arises because only about 5% of clinically evident thyroid nodules are malignant (1,2), but the proper treatment—surgical thyroidectomy—of the small number of malignant nodules involves discomfort, some risk of more serious morbidity, and considerable expense. The problem is accentuated when many small thyroid nodules are discovered in the course of neck imaging studies done for unrelated conditions, such as carotid Doppler testing or CT or MRI imaging for dysphagia, neck pain, or cervical spine disease. Such incidental findings in the thyroid are unlikely to be malignant even when they are palpable, and impalpable lesions smaller than 1 cm have a very low risk of being clinically significant cancers (3–5), but their discovery generally prompts further evaluation. Fine-needle biopsy (FNB) of the thyroid is the procedure of choice to determine which thyroid nodules carry enough risk of malignancy to justify surgical removal, and which nodules are so likely to be benign that observation is the preferred treatment (see Chapters 6, 22, and 29 for other discussions of FNB).

Prior to the use of needle biopsy, management decisions about thyroid nodules were based on clinical and noninvasive laboratory investigations. Clinical findings suggesting cancer (6) are rapid nodule enlargement, a firm to hard irregular nodule, vocal cord paralysis, adjacent enlarged cervical lymph nodes, family history of medullary carcinoma, distant metastases, and prior radiation therapy. However, most of these findings are not conclusive. Some hard nodules are benign calcified lesions, with an eggshell radiographic pattern of calcification, not to be confused with the scattered fine calcifications of some papillary carcinomas (Fig. 1). A history of hoarseness rarely turns out to be from vocal cord paralysis. Nodules in young people under 20, particularly young men, are more often malignant than those in middle-aged women, as are nodules in men over age 60 (6). Hypothyroidism, especially from Hashimoto's thyroiditis, suggests that a nodular goiter is benign, but it does not exclude coexistent cancer. Figure 2 shows a 70-year-old woman whose progressively enlarging thyroid had

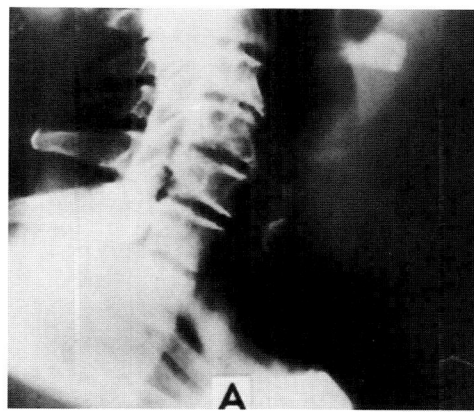
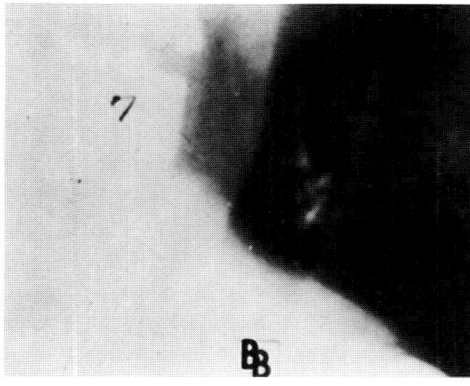

FIG. 1. A: A ring-like calcified shell is seen in the anterior neck. **B:** Irregular calcification is visible in a papillary carcinoma.

M. M. Kaplan: Departments of Medicine and Nuclear Medicine, William Beaumont Hospital, West Bloomfield, Michigan 48074.
J. I. Hamburger: West Bloomfield, Michigan 48034.

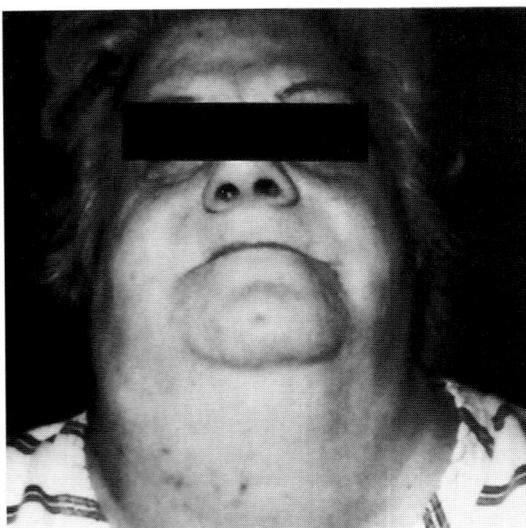

FIG. 2. Massive neck swelling in an elderly woman with lymphoma of the thyroid.

nearly filled her neck. She was mildly hypothyroid and had strongly positive antithyroid antibody titers. Needle biopsy showed both Hashimoto's thyroiditis and lymphoma of the thyroid [which commonly arises in a background of Hashimoto's thyroiditis (7), although only a small minority of patients with Hashimoto's thyroiditis ever develop lymphomas]. Although a nodule that is seen to be hypofunctioning on pertechnetate or radioiodine thyroid imaging might be a thyroid cancer, 80% to 90% of hypofunctioning nodules are benign.

When thyroid nodule patients were selected for surgery on the basis of the foregoing clinical-laboratory evaluation, about half of them had operations and about 75% of the operations were unnecessary, resulting only in the removal of a benign nodule (8). The advent of FNB has changed the situation dramatically. When selection is based on FNB, it is possible to reduce the proportion of patients having operations to less than 20%, and more than 50% of the excised lesions are malignant (9). The clinical and economic implications of this change are obvious.

The only palpable nodular thyroid lesions for which we consider FNB unnecessary are those that have increased radioactive iodine uptake, relative to the rest of the thyroid, on iodine-123 scintigraphy. These are autonomously functioning adenomas or functioning hyperplastic nodules that have a very low risk of malignancy but may produce suspicious FNB cytology results (10). Fewer than 15 cases have been reported in which such a hyperfunctioning thyroid nodule was a follicular or papillary carcinoma, although a few other cases have been described in which a tiny carcinoma appeared to be embedded in the hot nodule or to be located adjacent to it (11,12). However, it is advisable to biopsy hypofunctioning areas within functioning nodules.

Because the chances of malignancy in nodules with cystic components or in discrete nodules within multinodular goiters do not appear to be much different from the chances in apparently solitary nodules (6,13–16), ultrasound does not provide useful information about the nature of a nodule, and these types of lesions should be evaluated by FNB. Similarly, the chances of cancer in a nodule in a thyroid gland exposed to irradiation is not much different from the risk in the absence of x-ray exposure, and the reliability of FNB results is as good for those nodules as for others (17,18).

Credit is owed to European, especially Scandinavian, physicians for the early trials of FNB that showed it was possible to make reliable diagnoses from rather minute amounts of cytologic material (19–23). Although their early data were reported in the 1950s and 1960s, it was not until the 1970s that North American clinicians became motivated to try FNB (24–27), and not until the late 1980s that fears about frequent false-negative results were shown to be unfounded. By now, the advantages of thyroid FNB have been confirmed by numerous investigators, its successful application in the community setting has been demonstrated (28,29), and its central role in the evaluation of thyroid nodules has been repeatedly reviewed (2,3,30,31).

FINE-NEEDLE BIOPSY TECHNIQUE

To achieve the best results with thyroid FNB, it is necessary to employ the best technique.

The patient is placed in the recumbent position with the head extended over a pillow placed under the shoulders. This brings the thyroid nodule into an anterior position in the neck. FNB is not, strictly speaking, a sterile procedure, but it is a clean procedure; the neck is cleansed with alcohol and gloves are worn by the physician. We recommend local anesthesia with 1% lidocaine, because multiple aspirations are performed and the anesthesia provides reasonable patient comfort. Also, without anesthesia the involuntary cervical muscular contraction

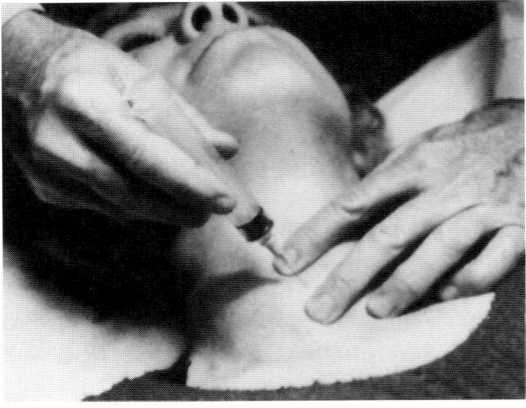

FIG. 3. Fine-needle biopsy technique. The needle is inserted in a direction roughly perpendicular to the anterior surface of the neck at the medial edge of the nodule.

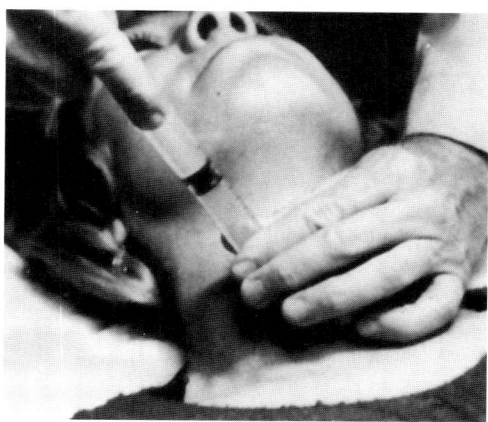

FIG. 4. Fine-needle biopsy technique. Suction is applied and the needle is moved in an in-and-out direction through a 1- to 2-mm depth of the nodule until the specimen appears in the hub of the needle.

in response to the needling can cause loss of finger contact with small nodules, with a corresponding loss of the precision of needle placement. Figures 3 to 5 illustrate the basic steps in the FNB procedure.

Although various sizes of needles have been recommended for FNB, the best all-purpose needle is a 25-gauge, 1½-inch-long needle. Larger needles tend to induce excessive bleeding and prevent the acquisition of suitable specimens. Finer needles are too flexible for accurate placement. The needle is attached to a 10-mL disposable syringe. The next question is where to insert the needle. Although it is tempting to insert the needle into the center of the nodule, this is not a good spot, because nodules commonly undergo spontaneous degeneration, and that process is most likely to originate centrally. Areas of degeneration are least likely to contain useful material for cytologic evaluation. The larger the nodule, the more likely there will be central degeneration. A better FNB technique is circumferential sampling at the periphery of the nodule, where viable thyroid parenchyma is nearly always present. The potential drawback to peripheral sampling is missing the nodule and sampling adjacent normal tissue. With experience, this is more a theoretical than a practical problem, especially because peripheral sampling is most important in larger nodules for which it is simpler. For nodules smaller than 1.5 cm, it may be impractical to do anything other than insert the needle into the center of the nodule.

Once the needle is inserted into the nodule, it is necessary to induce some disruption of the tissue to dislodge a specimen for aspiration into the needle. Merely applying suction is adequate for loosely organized vascular lesions. As soon as blood-tinged fluid appears in the hub of the needle, suction is released. If aspiration alone does not produce a specimen, one should maintain suction and move the needle in and out through 1 to 3 mm of nodule tissue repetitively until material appears in the hub of the needle (32). On rare occasions, even that maneuver will fail to dislodge a specimen, as in very dense papillary carcinomas. For these cases, a combined in-and-out movement plus rotation of the needle within the nodule through 360° will allow the sharp bevel of the needle to sever a specimen for aspiration. Using a larger needle also may be effective, but it is simpler to use one needle size for nearly all patients, and adjust the movement of the needle to the individual nodule's physical characteristics.

Once the specimen has been obtained, suction is released before the needle is withdrawn from the nodule. Otherwise, the specimen will be aspirated into the barrel of the syringe where it is much more difficult to recover. The needle is then detached from the syringe, and 3 to 4 mL of air is taken into the syringe and forced out through the reattached needle to express the specimen on to a glass slide. Some prefer to introduce air into the syringe before performing the aspiration, to avoid detaching the needle, thereby minimizing the chances of the operator's being contaminated by the patient's blood. However, if too much air is taken in, the effectiveness of the suction is diminished.

Some operators use a syringe holder, but we find that this device makes it more difficult to manipulate the needle. Recently, a nonsuction technique was advocated for FNA sampling of lesions in various organs, including the thyroid (33). In this technique, for which 25-gauge, 1½-inch needles are still satisfactory, the needle is held in a "pencil grip," moved in and out over 2 to 3 mm, and rotated between the fingers, and then kept still for 5 to 10 seconds, to allow the freed cells to flow into the needle by capillary action. It is easy to see when material enters the hub of the needle. If this method does not produce enough material, or if cyst fluid needs to be aspirated, suction is used. One of us (MMK) has begun using the nonsuction technique for many nodules, finding after about 300 cases that the absence of a syringe allows more precise needle placement for small nodules, and results in

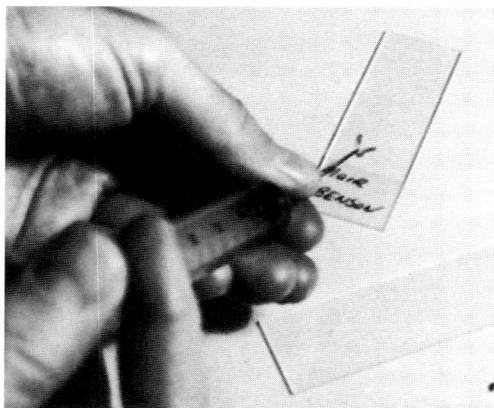

FIG. 5. Fine-needle biopsy technique. The small drop of fluid, expressed onto a glass slide, illustrates optimal FNB specimen size.

a smaller fraction of specimens being diluted by excessive blood (or containing only blood).

The ideal FNB specimen consists of one drop of red-orange fluid. Specimens that are more voluminous or consist of thin, pale to greenish-brown degeneration fluid are less likely to contain adequate numbers of cells for diagnostic purposes. Some physicians have described methods for concentrating specimens that are too diluted with blood (32,34), but it is simpler and quicker just to discard the specimen and take another one, if local anesthesia is used.

The specimens are smeared on a slide and immediately fixed with the fixative preferred by the cytopathologist who will be reading them. It is essential to avoid air drying for best results with the Papanicolaou stain, the stain preferred by pathologists in North America. We find that the best method for smearing the specimen is to place a second slide flat on top of the slide containing the specimen. The specimen is compressed between the two slides by the index finger, and the top slide is slid lengthwise off the bottom slide, producing an evenly distributed smear.

ADEQUACY OF FNB SAMPLING

Fundamental to the use of FNB is an understanding of the difference between the amount of cytologic material needed to exclude malignancy with reasonable confidence and that required to affirm a diagnosis of malignancy. A few cancer cells may be perfectly adequate to make a diagnosis of malignancy. However, a similar number of benign cells would be totally inadequate to exclude cancer. Virtually all thyroid glands contain benign thyroid epithelial cells, whether or not there is also a cancer. It is relatively easy to aspirate some of these benign cells if the needle is misplaced. Also, some malignant tumors are highly pleomorphic, with some areas composed of cells indistinguishable from normal and other areas composed of suspicious or frankly malignant cells. Hence, more stringent criteria are necessary to exclude cancer than to confirm it.

How much cellular material is adequate for a thyroid FNB? In 1979, in an effort to avoid the false-negative diagnoses made from our first 1000 FNBs (34), we established the following criteria: to perform a minimum of six separate aspirations from different portions of each nodule, and to require that there be at least six clusters of benign cells on each of at least two aspirates from different sites. Although some of our errors had been the result of inexperience, others were directly attributable to making diagnoses of "benign" on the basis of inadequate cytologic material, especially a few clusters of benign-appearing cells on a single slide. Evaluation of a second 1000 patients showed that these criteria for adequacy led to the near elimination of false-negative diagnoses (35), a level of performance confirmed in a more recent series in which the FNB diagnoses were made by a different cytopathologist using the same criteria (9).

These criteria have not been widely accepted. There seems to be great reluctance on the part of many physicians to perform six aspirations, probably because many do not employ local anesthesia. Some say that the injection obscures the nodule and makes the FNB more difficult, but a moment's gentle massage readily disperses the fluid. A survey of reports on FNB showed that many physicians employed only one to four aspirations, with all series reporting false-negative diagnoses (36–44). Cytologic diagnoses rendered despite inadequate sampling continued to represent a significant percentage of such cases.

To test this point further, one of us (JIH) selected six cases of thyroid cancers for which sparsely cellular FNB specimens contained too few cells to exclude malignancy, along with 14 benign cases, to be reviewed by collaborating pathologists from four major medical centers that were actively using FNB. Of 24 possible false-negative diagnoses (six cases, each read at four institutions), six false-negative diagnoses were made on the specimens that failed our criteria for adequacy (45). That experience suggests that even at major medical centers, cytopathologists had been making FNB diagnoses of "benign" despite inadequate numbers of benign cells. In contrast, 72 of 73 consecutive patients who had operations in spite of FNB diagnoses of benign by our criteria had benign nodules. Thus, even though the criteria we advocate for exclusion of malignancy will not be effective in all cases, they appear to avoid most false-negative diagnoses.

How many FNB aspirates are necessary to obtain at least six clusters of cells on at least two smears from aspirates at different sites? To answer this question, 100 consecutive patients, for whom six to ten aspirates were taken and whose specimens had adequate cells to fulfill our criteria, were evaluated. The slides were numbered sequentially and the numbers of cell clusters present were reported for each slide (only one slide having been prepared from each aspiration). For 77% of the patients, four aspirations would have been enough to provide at least two slides with six cell-clusters each. However, for 23% of the patients, five to eight aspirations were necessary. None of the patients who had ten aspirations needed more than eight. Hence, obtaining one to four aspirations carries a substantial risk of inadequate sampling, and the common practice of taking one to two aspirates and making a diagnosis of benign disease on the basis of a few clusters of benign cells is to be condemned. If the FNB is performed in a location where immediate cytologic evaluation can be done, then it may be practical and advantageous to perform only three or four aspirations and have the slides checked for cellularity. More aspirations can then be taken only when necessary.

The complications of thyroid FNB are rare and generally mild. Occasionally there is a local hematoma, which is usually immediately evident, and for which application of an ice pack for 30 to 60 minutes is helpful. Rarely, the entire thyroid or the pre-thyroid soft tissue swells acutely

(46,47); this swelling resolves spontaneously in 24 to 48 hours or less. One of our patients had mild pain radiating from the biopsy site to the ear, which lasted for several months. We are aware of only one case of tumor seeding of the needle tract from thyroid FNBs (48).

MANAGEMENT OF THYROID NODULES BASED ON FNB FINDINGS

Fine-needle biopsy diagnoses of definite malignancy are highly reliable (about 2% to 5% false positive rate) when made by an experienced pathologist, and recommendations for surgery can be made accordingly. A benign diagnosis is equally reliable, assuming adequate specimens, and justifies a recommendation for observation, unless the firmness of the nodule, its size, its rate of growth, or evidence of vocal cord paralysis increases the level of suspicion enough to warrant surgical removal. There are also occasional special situations in which surgery is advisable regardless of a benign FNB diagnosis, such as a pertechnetate or radioiodine imaging study showing uptake in cervical lymph nodes, or a family history of medullary thyroid carcinoma.

Diagnoses of "suspected" malignancy are less specific, indicating about a 25% to 75% chance of cancer, depending on the specific findings, but they carry a high enough risk of cancer to justify the recommendation for operation (2,3,30,31,49).

The FNB diagnoses of follicular adenoma, microfollicular adenoma, cellular adenoma, or Hürthle cell tumor, with no specific findings (such as nuclear atypia) of malignancy, indicate approximately a 5% to 10% chance of thyroid cancer in our patient population. Most of these malignancies are low-grade tumors with minimal capsular or vascular invasion, and they have a low probability of causing either important morbidity or mortality in the near future if they are not promptly excised. However, if left *in situ* for years, they may behave more aggressively (50). Unfortunately, there is inadequate information about the safe duration of observation for low-risk nodules. The approach that we take for tumors with these FNB diagnoses is to recommend surgery for young healthy patients and observation for older or infirm patients or for those who prefer the risks of observation to those of operation. Obviously, this approach presupposes a full and frank discussion of the risks and benefits of the alternative management strategies with both the patient and the primary physician.

The final nonspecific diagnosis is of small numbers of (seemingly benign) cells that are too few to exclude malignancy. This finding adds nothing to the management implications that can be derived from the standard clinical evaluation. It is almost the same as if no biopsy had been done, especially if the FNB specimens are acellular. If there are some benign cells, then the usefulness of the information depends on how many cells are present and the size of the nodule. For larger nodules, which are more often pleomorphic, one would want more cells on more slides. For nodules of 1 cm or smaller, it may be more difficult to obtain many cells, but it is more likely that any cells that are obtained are representative, especially if there are cells on several slides. For example, two to three clusters of benign cells on three slides might be more reassuring than six to nine clusters on a single slide that might have been obtained from adjacent normal tissue if the needle had been misplaced.

When the cytologic material is inadequate for exclusion of malignancy, the next step is to repeat the FNB. About half the time a satisfactory specimen will be obtained on the repeat procedure (44). If not, a few more benign-appearing cell clusters are sometimes obtained. The more often even limited numbers of benign cells are obtained, with no malignant or suspicious cells, the more likely it is that one is dealing with a benign nodule. The failure to obtain adequate FNB specimens, even when the procedure is repeated and multiple aspirates are taken, is usually because extensive degeneration or fibrosis limits the available number of follicular cells, or because the nodule is small and deep-seated and difficult to localize. In that case, the FNB can be performed with real-time ultrasound guidance (51–53).

If repeated FNB procedures fail to provide enough cytologic material for confidence in the exclusion of a malignant nodule, one may either continue to observe, with or without administering thyroid hormone, or advise operation. This decision will depend on other clinical findings and the patient's preference. In every case, the patient should be informed of the relative risks of observation versus operation and encouraged to participate in the final decision.

FOLLOW-UP OF NODULES FOR WHICH OBSERVATION IS ADVISED

It is our practice to administer thyroxine to all patients who show evidence of hypothyroidism, and to euthyroid patients under 50 or 60 years of age unless there is a history of heart disease or suspicion, from the combination of serum TSH and scintigraphy, that autonomous thyroid function is present. The usefulness of thyroid hormone treatment is controversial. The studies suggesting that it is ineffective are flawed in some respects, whereas the studies suggesting benefit for some nodules have different limitations (54). Experience in a nonblinded series of solid cold nodules showed that 28 of 100 decreased in size by 50% or more during thyroxine therapy, whereas only 4 of 51 untreated patients had a similar response (55). More recent studies have reported 37% to 39% response rates, with much lower percentages of untreated patients showing spontaneous shrinkage (54–56). Perhaps equally important is the detection of growth of a nodule in spite of thyroxine therapy. This finding requires further investigation. Hemorrhage, inflammation, and unappreciated autonomous function are more common causes of enlargement than cancer. Imaging while the patient is taking thyroxine will immediately expose autonomous function. Otherwise, repeat FNB will usually clarify the differential diagnosis. We also advise a repeat FNB for nodules that persist without a change in size after about a year of thyroxine therapy. Six of 236 such patients who initially had benign FNB studies had evidence of malignancy on a repeat FNB (57).

RELIANCE OF FNB FOR PLANNING THE EXTENT OF A THYROID OPERATION

Once the decision to operate is made, regardless of the reason, it is essential to design an operation of appropriate extent for the disease at hand. If the nodule is benign, a simple lobectomy, with or without removal of the isthmus, will be adequate to eliminate the lesion and confirm the diagnosis. If the nodule is a minimal cancer (i.e., a unifocal, minimally invasive, well-differentiated papillary or follicular carcinoma smaller than 1 to 1.5 cm, not associated with metastases) and there are no contralateral abnormalities suggesting other foci of cancer, many physicians would also accept lobectomy–isthmectomy as an adequate operation. For larger or more invasive tumors, many physicians prefer a total, or near-total, thyroidectomy to remove any tumor in the contralateral lobe, to reduce the chances of clinically evident cancer recurrence, and to create conditions favorable for ^{131}I scanning and/or therapy.

The conventional approach to decision making in these cases is to perform an initial lobectomy–isthmectomy and then rely on the findings on frozen section. Unfortunately, this strategy often leads to suboptimal treatment. Because most thyroid nodules are benign lesions, for which safer, limited operations are adequate, many pathologists prefer to have the surgeon stop short of the extended cancer operation if there is doubt, and report that there is no definite malignancy or defer a diagnosis until permanent sections are evaluated. Completion surgery can be done a few days later for the small number of patients with malignant lesions. Although this practice serves to reduce the number of needlessly aggressive operations, it subjects some patients to two operations rather than one. Furthermore, under these circumstances, the patient goes under anesthesia not knowing what operation is going to be performed, placing an extra burden on the surgeon to ensure that informed consent has been obtained for several contingencies.

Can FNB data provide a better option for surgical planning? Although each institution must answer this question for itself, there is evidence in favor of placing reliance upon FNB. The purpose of this discussion is not to downgrade frozen section studies or to promote FNB, but to emphasize that knowledge of the relative reliability of FNB and frozen section studies allows the clinician to offer the most reasonable advice on surgical planning. The recommendations suitable for our practice, in which about 500 FNB diagnoses are made annually by very experienced cytopathologists, may not be suitable for an institution where 25 to 50 FNB thyroid diagnoses are made annually.

In our experience, the FNB diagnosis of definite thyroid cancer is correct about 98% of the time (although the type of carcinoma is not always correctly identified by FNB), whereas frozen section is not quite as reliable in these cases (58,59). Therefore, a cancer operation is appropriate, regardless of the frozen section result, for an FNB result unequivocally positive for malignancy. Similarly, we find unequivocal FNB diagnoses of benign disease (nodular goiter or Hashimoto's thyroiditis, with adequate specimens) to be accurate about 98% of the time. Even in the population of patients who come to surgery for reasons other than the biopsy results (e.g., nodule size or growth rate), frozen section was reliable, but no better than FNB, because of deferred diagnoses in a few cases. Thus, for patients with benign FNB diagnoses, a limited operation, usually lobectomy, seems appropriate, and frozen section is unnecessary. Several other investigators agree that the extent of surgery can be based on highly confident FNB results, rather than frozen section findings (60–62).

The situation is more complex when the FNB result is inconclusive, either because the diagnosis is ambiguous (e.g., Hürthle cell tumor, follicular adenoma, or suspected carcinoma) or the FNB specimens are inadequate. In these cases, frozen section examination is certainly appropriate. Unfortunately, our experience is that very few frozen section diagnoses are sufficiently conclusive or suspicious to change the operative strategy that could be formulated from the FNB results (58,59). Faced with these facts, the patient and surgeon can discuss the extent of surgery in advance, and the patient can express a preference, if he or she wishes. In our experience, many patients perceive the prospect of a second operation to be a greater threat than an operation that may be unnecessarily extensive.

In other special situations, frozen section is still very useful. If an operation is being performed for a low-risk nodule, and a nodule elsewhere in the thyroid is discovered that had not been detected preoperatively, a frozen section diagnosis, if positive, may appropriately alter the surgical plan. The exact surgical procedure can also be guided by frozen section evaluation of lymph nodes, parathyroid glands, or tumor invasion into fat and muscle (60). Otherwise, most frozen sections can be eliminated once reasonable FNB skills have been acquired. This not only will save pathology costs, but it will also reduce the costs for operating room and anesthesia time.

There are other reasons for preoperative FNB evaluation of thyroid nodules, even when they are highly suspicious on clinical grounds. FNB findings can eliminate unnecessary surgery for certain malignancies such as lymphoma, anaplastic thyroid carcinoma, or carcinoma metastatic to the thyroid, and they can direct the patient's evaluation or therapy in the appropriate direction. FNB may identify patients with medullary thyroid carcinoma who should have preoperative calcitonin and carcinoembryonic antigen tests, evaluation for pheochromocytoma, and, possibly, genetic screening.

USES OF THYROID FNB IN CONDITIONS OTHER THAN NODULES

Fine-needle biopsy can be used to evaluate diffusely enlarged thyroid glands (see Fig. 2) or lobes, if other tests do not establish the cause of the abnormality. The areas of concern are surveyed by FNB sampling of six to eight sites using the same technique as for nodules. The results help distinguish antibody-negative Hashimoto's thyroiditis, lymphoma, and diffuse multifocal carcinoma from the more common simple goiter. If suppurative thyroiditis is suspected, FNB provides material for Gram stain and culture. FNB has been used to diagnose *Pneumocystis carinii* thyroiditis in patients with the acquired immune deficiency syndrome (63).

Two types of nodules can be eliminated by FNB-based methods. First, purely cystic nodules can sometimes be evacuated completely, although about half will reaccumulate fluid and need to be reaspirated (64). The usual recommendation is that reappearance of a cystic nodule after three aspirations is an indication for surgical removal, because the cyst fluid rarely contains diagnostically useful material. Any solid remnant left after removal of cyst fluid should have FNB evaluation. Second, some groups have ablated solid, autonomously functioning thyroid nodules by repeated injection of ethanol into the lesion under ultrasound guidance (65). The efficacy and safety of this procedure have not yet been tested in enough patients to provide guidelines for its appropriate use, and, in many settings in the United States, there might be problems in reimbursement for repeated use of ultrasound facilities.

In the research setting, FNB has been used to obtain enough thyroid tissue to detect mutations in the thyroid-stimulating hormone (TSH) receptor gene, using reverse transcriptase–polymerase chain reaction amplification (66).

REFERENCES

1. Caruso D, Mazzaferri EL. Fine needle aspiration biopsy in the management of thyroid nodules. *Endocrinologist* 1991;1:194–202.
2. Gharib H, Goellner JR. Fine-needle aspiration biopsy of the thyroid: an appraisal. *Ann Intern Med* 1993;118:282–289.
3. Mazzaferri EL. Management of a solitary thyroid nodule. *N Engl J Med* 1993;328:553–559.
4. Ezzat S, Sarti DA, Cain DR, Braunstein GD. Thyroid incidentalomas. Prevalence by palpation and ultrasonography. *Arch Intern Med* 1994;154:1838–1840.
5. Tan GH, Gharib H, Reading CC. Solitary thyroid nodule. Comparison between palpation and ultrasonography. *Arch Intern Med* 1995;155:2418–2423.
6. Belfiore A, La Rosa G, La Porta G, et al. Cancer risk in patients with cold thyroid nodules: relevance of iodine intake, sex, age, and multinodularity. *Am J Med* 1992;93:363–369.
7. Hamburger JI, Miller JM, Kini SR. Lymphoma of the thyroid. *Ann Intern Med* 1983;99:685–693.
8. Hamburger JI. Clinical exercises in internal medicine, vol 1: thyroid disease. Philadelphia: WB Saunders, 1978;221.
9. Hamburger JI, Husain M. Semiquantitative criteria for fine-needle biopsy diagnosis: reduced false-negative diagnoses. *Diagn Cytopathol* 1988;4:14–17.
10. Walfish PG, Strawbridge HTG, Rosen IB. Management implications from routine needle biopsy of hyperfunctioning thyroid nodules. *Surgery* 1985 98:1179–1183.
11. Rubenfeld S, Wheeler TM. Thyroid cancer presenting as a hot thyroid nodule: report of a case and review of the literature. *Thyroidology* 1988;1:61–68
12. Hamburger JI. The autonomously functioning thyroid nodule: Goetsch's disease. *Endocr Rev* 1987;8:439–447.
13. Hammer M, Wortsman J, Folse R. Cancer in cystic lesions of the thyroid. *Arch Surg* 1982;117:1020–1023.
14. de los Santos ET, Keyhani-Rofagha S, Cunningham JJ, Mazzaferri EL. Cystic thyroid nodules. The dilemma of malignant lesions. *Arch Intern Med* 1990;150:1422–1427.
15. McColl A, Jarosz H, Lawrence AM, Paloyan E. The incidence of thyroid carcinoma in solitary cold nodules and in multinodular goiters. *Surgery* 1986;100:1128–1132.
16. Franklyn JA, Daykin J, Young J, Oates GD, Sheppard MC. Fine needle aspiration cytology in diffuse or multinodular goitre compared with solitary thyroid nodules. *Br Med J* 1993;307:240.
17. Rosen IB, Palmer JA, Bain J, Strawbridge H, Walfish PG. Efficacy of needle biopsy in postradiation thyroid disease. *Surgery* 1983;94:1002–1007.
18. Pretorius HT, Katikineni M, Kinsella TJ, et al. Thyroid nodules after high-dose external radiotherapy. Fine-needle aspiration cytology in diagnosis and management. *JAMA* 1982;247:3217–3220.
19. Söderström N. Puncture of goiters for aspiration biopsy. A preliminary report. *Acta Med Scand* 1952;144:235–244.
20. Persson PS. Cytodiagnosis of thyroiditis. A comparative study of cytological, histological, immunological and clinical findings in thyroiditis, particularly in diffuse lymphoid thyroiditis. *Acta Med Scand* 1967;483(suppl):7–25.
21. Einhorn J, Franzen S. Thin-needle biopsy in the diagnosis of thyroid disease. *Acta Radiol* 1962;58:321–336.
22. Galvan G. Thin needle aspiration biopsy and cytological examination of hypofunctional "cold" thyroid nodules in routine clinical work. *Clin Nucl Med* 1977;2:413–421.
23. Löwhagen T, Sprenger E. Cytologic presentation of thyroid tumors in aspiration biopsy smear. *Acta Cytol* 1974;18:192–197.
24. Crockford PM, Bain GO. Fine-needle aspiration biopsy of the thyroid. *Can Med Assoc J* 1974;110:1029–1032.
25. Walfish PG, Hazani E, Strawbridge HTG, et al. Combined ultrasound and needle aspiration cytology in the assessment and management of hypofunctioning thyroid nodule. *Ann Intern Med* 1977;87:270–274.
26. Frable WJ. Thin-needle aspiration biopsy. A personal experience with 469 cases. *Am J Clin Pathol* 1976;65:168–182.
27. Gershengorn MC McClung MR, Chu EW, et al. Fine-needle aspiration cytology in the preoperative diagnosis of thyroid nodules. *Ann Intern Med* 1977;87:265–269.
28. Dwarakanathan AA, Ryan WG, Staren ED, Martirano M, Economou SG. Fine-needle aspiration biopsy of the thyroid. Diagnostic accuracy when performing a moderate number of such procedures. *Arch Intern Med* 1989;149:2007–2009.
29. Pepper GM, Zwickler D, Rosen Y. Fine-needle aspiration biopsy of the thyroid nodule. Results of a start-up project in a general teaching hospital setting. *Arch Intern Med* 1989;149:594–596.
30. Hamburger JI. Diagnosis of thyroid nodules by fine needle biopsy: use and abuse. *J Clin Endocrinol Metab* 1994;79:335–339.
31. Ridgway EC. Clinician's evaluation of a solitary thyroid nodule. *J Clin Endocrinol Metab* 1992;74:231–235.
32. Löwhagen T, Willems JS, Lundell G, et al. Aspiration biopsy cytology in diagnosis of thyroid cancer. *World J Surg* 1981;5:61–73.

33. Santos JE, Leiman G. Nonaspiration fine needle cytology: application of a new technique to nodular thyroid disease. *Acta Cytol* 1988;32:353–356.
34. Hamburger JI, Miller JM, Kini SR. *Clinical-pathological diagnosis of thyroid nodules handbook and atlas*. Southfield, MI: Private publication, 1979;79.
35. Miller JM, Kini SR, Hamburger JI. *Needle biopsy of the thyroid*. New York: Praeger, 1983;1–27.
36. Hall TL, Layfield LJ, Philippe A, Rosenthal DL. Sources of diagnostic error in fine needle aspiration of the thyroid. *Cancer* 1988; 63:718–725.
37. Anderson JB, Webb AJ. Fine-needle aspiration biopsy and the diagnosis of thyroid cancer. *Br J Surg* 1987;74:292–296.
38. Ramacciotti CE, Pretorius HT, Chu EW, et al. Diagnostic accuracy and use of aspiration biopsy in the management of thyroid nodules. *Arch Intern Med* 1984;144:1169–1173.
39. Schwartz AE, Nieburgs HE, Davies TF, et al. The place of fine needle biopsy in the diagnosis of nodules of the thyroid. *Surg Gynecol Obstet* 1982;155:54–58.
40. Suen KC, Quenville NF. Fine needle aspiration biopsy of the thyroid gland: a study of 304 cases. *J Clin Pathol* 1983;36:1036–1045.
41. Hamaker RC, Singer MI, DeRossi RV, et al. Role of needle biopsy in thyroid nodules. *Arch Otolaryngol* 1983;109:225–228.
42. Boey J, Hsu C, Colling RJ, et al. A prospective controlled study of fine-needle aspiration and tru-cut needle biopsy of dominant thyroid nodules. *World J Surg* 1984;8:458–465.
43. Hawkins F, Bellido D, Bernal C, et al. Fine needle aspiration biopsy in the diagnosis of thyroid cancer and thyroid disease. *Cancer* 1987;59: 1206–1209.
44. Goellner JR, Gharib H, Grant CS. Fine needle aspiration cytology of the thyroid, 1980 to 1986. *Acta Ctyol* 1987;31:587–590.
45. Hamburger JI, Husain M, Nishiyama R, Nunes C, Solomon D. Increasing the accuracy of fine-needle biopsy for thyroid nodules. *Arch Pathol Lab Med* 1989;113:1035–1041.
46. Haas SN. Acute thyroid swelling after needle biopsy of the thyroid. *N Engl J Med* 1982;307:1349.
47. Velkeniers B, Noppen M, Vanhaelst L. Delayed swelling of prethyroid soft tissue after fine needle aspiration biopsy. *J Endocrinol Invest* 1988;11:225.
48. Hales MS, Hsu FS. Needle tract implantation of papillary carcinoma of the thyroid following aspiration biopsy. *Acta Cytol* 1990;34:801–804.
49. McHenry CR, Walfish PG, Rosen IB. Non-diagnostic fine needle aspiration biopsy: a dilemma in management of nodular thyroid disease. *Am Surg* 1993;59:415–419.
50. Mazzaferri EL, Jhiang SM. Long-term impact of initial surgical amd medical therapy on papillary and follicular thyroid cancer. *Am J Med* 1994;97:418–428.
51. Cochand-Priollet B, Guillausseau P-J, Chagnon S, et al. The diagnostic value of fine-needle aspiration biopsy under ultrasonography in nonfunctional thyroid nodules: a prospective study comparing cytologic and histologic findings. *Am J Med* 1994;97:152–157.
52. Gharib H. Fine-needle aspiration was sensitive for nonfunctional thyroid nodules. *ACP J Club* 1995;122 (Suppl 1):20
53. Sanchez RB, van Sonnenberg E, D'Agostino HB, et al. Ultrasound guided biopsy of nonpalpable and difficult to palpate thyroid masses. *J Am Coll Surg* 1994;178:33–37.
54. Blum M. Why do clinicians continue to debate the use of levothyroxine in the diagnosis and management of thyroid nodules? *Ann Intern Med* 1995;122:653–64.
55. Hamburger JI, Husain M. Fine needle biopsy: extended observations In: *Diagnostic methods in thyroidology*. New York: Springer-Verlag, 1989;221–249.
56. La Rosa GL, Lupo L, Giuffrida D, Gullo D, Vigneri R, Belfiore A. Levothyroxine and potassium iodide are both effective in treating benign solitary cold nodules of the thyroid. *Ann Int Med* 1995;122:1–8.
57. Hamburger JI. Consistency of sequential needle biopsy findings for thyroid nodules. Management implications. *Arch Intern Med* 1987; 147:97–99.
58. Hamburger JI, Hamburger SW. Declining role of frozen section in surgical planning for thyroid nodules. *Surgery* 1985;98:307–312.
59. Hamburger JI, Husain M. Contribution of intraoperative pathology evaluation to surgical management of thyroid nodules. *Endocrinol Metab Clin North Am* 1990;19:509–522.
60. LiVolsi VA. Surgical pathology of the thyroid. Philadelphia: WB Saunders, 1990;367.
61. Kopald KH, Layfield LJ, Mohrmann R, Foshag LJ, Giuliano AE. Clarifying the role of fine-needle aspiration cytologic evaluation and frozen section examination in the operative management of thyroid cancer. *Arch Surg* 1989;124:1201–1205.
62. Keller MP, Crabbe MM, Norwood SH. Accuracy and significance of fine-needle aspiration and frozen section in determining the extent of thyroid resection. *Surgery* 1987;101:632–637.
63. Guttler R, Singer P. *Pneumocystis carinii* thyroiditis. Report of three cases and review of the literature. *Arch Intern Med* 1993;153:393–396.
64. Lee J-K, Tai F-T, Lin H-D, Chou Y-H, Kaplan MM, Ching K-N. Treatment of recurrent thyroid cysts by injection of tetracycline or minocycline. *Arch Intern Med* 1989;149:599–601.
65. Papini E. Panunzi C, Pacella CM, et al. Percutaneous ultrasound-guided ethanol injection: a new treatment of toxic autonomously functioning thyroid nodules? *J Clin Endocrinol Metab* 1993;76:411–416.
66. Porcellini A, Ciullo I, Laviola L, Amabile, G, Fenzi G, Avvedimentao V. Novel mutation of thyrotropin receptor gene in thyroid hyperfunctioning adenomas. *J Clin Endocrinol Metab* 1994;79:335–338.

CHAPTER 8

Uptake Tests, Thyroid and Whole Body Imaging with Isotopes

George A. Wilson and Robert E. O'Mara

The use of radiopharmaceuticals in the evaluation of thyroid disease can be divided into two broad categories: those procedures that are used primarily to evaluate the *function* of the gland, and the imaging procedures that evaluate the *anatomy* of the gland. The radioactive iodine uptake test has been used extensively for years to evaluate the function of the thyroid gland. More recently, there has been a decrease in the number of these procedures because of the availability of reliable methods for the assay of thyroid and thyroid-stimulating hormones. Radioiodine uptake tests, however, remain useful for differentiating the various causes of thyroid dysfunction present, for example, in silent thyroiditis, where the 24-hour iodine uptake is low compared to the elevated assay of thyroid hormone (1–6). The radioiodine uptake frequently serves as the basis for the dose of radioactive iodine to be used in the treatment of hyperthyroidism. Images of the thyroid delineate the functional anatomy of the gland. Such images establish the nature and location of the functional abnormality, as in thyroiditis, and may serve as a guide for biopsy of the gland. One of the most common uses of imaging is to ascertain the amount of function within a nodule. This determination has a direct bearing on the type of pathology present in the nodule. A special technique utilizing total body images performed with radioiodine may help define the extent of metastasis from thyroid carcinoma (7). Single photon emission computed tomography (SPECT) imaging has not proven helpful in this area.

G. A. Wilson (Deceased): Former Associate Professor of Radiology, University of Rochester School of Medicine and Dentistry, Rochester, New York 14642.
R. E. O'Mara: University of Rochester School of Medicine and Dentistry; Chief, Division of Nuclear Medicine, Strong Memorial Hospital, Rochester, New York 14642.

However, as better collimators, even pinhole, are developed for SPECT, better localization and detection of smaller lesions may result.

RADIOPHARMACEUTICALS

Five different radioisotopes have been used in the evaluation of thyroid disease: iodine-131, iodine-123, iodine-125, technetium-99m (Tc-99m), and thallium-201. Currently, only two of the isotopes of iodine are used in a clinical setting, I-123 and I-131. I-125 is no longer used because its emissions are too low in energy for optimal detection and because of the high radiation dose associated with its 60-day half-life. Tc-99m pertechnetate, with its 6-hr half-life, is used primarily for thyroid imaging. Thallium-201 has special characteristics and uses that will be described later. Table 1 outlines the characteristics of the various radiopharmaceuticals used in the evaluation of the thyroid (8,9).

Iodine-131

Sodium I-131 is obtained as a by-product from a nuclear reaction and has been used for thyroid uptake and imaging studies for many decades. I-131 decays by emission of a beta particle that has a maximum energy of 806 keV. Its principal gamma emission is 364 keV. The physical half-life is 8.05 days, resulting in a biologic half-life much greater than that of I-123. This results in a relatively high radiation dose to the thyroid, largely from the energetic beta particles and the prolonged biologic half-life. This isotope is used primarily for uptake studies, in doses of less than 10 µCi (370 kBq) administered orally. It has limited use as an imaging agent primarily because of the large radiation dose per millicurie. In addition,

TABLE 1. *Characteristics of radioisotopes used in thyroid evaluation*

	Iodine-123	Iodine-125	Iodine-131	Tc-99m pertechnetate
Physical half-life	13.0 hr	60.2 days	8.06 days	6.03 hr
Mode of decay	Electron capture	Electron capture	Beta minus	Isomeric transition
Principal energy	159 keV	35 keV	364 keV	140 keV
Radiation dose (rads/mCi)				
Total body	0.027	0.29	0.47	0.014
Thyroid 5% uptake	2.4	140	260	—
15% uptake	7.5	450	800	0.13[a]
24% uptake	13.0	790	1300	—
Uptake dose	20 µCi (740 kBq)		5–10 µCi (180–370 kBq)	
Imaging dose	150–400 µCi (550–14,800 kBq)		50–100 µCi (1850–3700 kBq)	5–10 mCi (185–370 MBq)

[a]Not calculated on percent thyroid uptake

modern gamma cameras are less efficient in detecting the higher energy 364 keV proton than the lower energies of Tc-99m pertechnetate or I-123.

As a result of the increased thyroid-to-background ratios that are obtainable with iodine, relatively small foci of ectopic hypofunctioning thyroid tissue may be detected when imaging with iodine. Iodine-131 is especially valuable in the detection of foci of functioning ectopic thyroid tissue located in the mediastinum or abdomen, and it is used in evaluating the extent and location of functioning thyroid carcinoma in preparation for therapeutic administration.

Iodine-123

Iodine-123 is a cyclotron product with a physical half-life of 13.3 hr. It decays by electron capture and has no beta particle associated with it. Its principal gamma energy is 150 keV, which occurs in 83% of the disintegrations. In addition, gamma energies of 440 and 525 keV are present. This isotope is suitable for both thyroid uptake studies and for imaging (10). The absorbed radiation dose to the thyroid on a per millicurie basis of radioactivity is roughly 1/100 that of I-131. The usual oral dose administered for imaging purposes is in the range of 100 to 400 µCi (3750 to 15,000 kBq). Doses in this range permit imaging with a standard gamma camera fitted with a pinhole collimator. Images may be obtained between 8 and 24 hr after radioiodine administration. I-123 is not only trapped but is organified by the thyroid and may be used in studies requiring physiologic intervention. The biologically effective half-life in the thyroid is reduced when compared with I-131. For this reason, I-123 is a good agent for performing uptake and imaging studies (11–14). To date, however, it is not widely used because its cost is high, its short shelf life requires prior scheduling of patients with at least 24-hr notice, and there is possible contamination with an impurity, iodine-124. However, new methods of production have resulted in a much purer product.

Tc-99m Pertechnetate

The most widely used radiopharmaceutical for imaging the thyroid is Tc-99m sodium pertechnetate. This radiopharmaceutical is inexpensive and readily available in nuclear medicine units. This has allowed the development of "one-stop" evaluation, in which a patient may be seen in the clinical setting, receive the scan shortly thereafter, and return to the clinical setting for further decision making. We have used this combined approach with our Endocrinology Department in a joint clinic for several years with great success. It has a single gamma energy of 140 keV. It decays by electron capture, has no beta emissions, and a physical half-life of 6 hr. The technetium pertechnetate ion is trapped by the thyroid but is not organified; therefore, the effective biologic half-life in the thyroid is quite short. The absorbed radiation dose to the thyroid on a millicurie per millicurie basis is approximately 1/6000 that of I-131. Intravenous doses from 5 to 10 mCi (185 to 370 MBq) of Tc-99m pertechnetate are frequently used for imaging. This results in a high count rate that permits multiple different projections to be obtained, without undue patient discomfort, using a gamma camera equipped with a pinhole collimator. Tc-99m is not ideal for imaging ectopic thyroid tissue located deep within the body, because of its lower energy and the higher body background associated with it. Adequate images may be obtained, on occasion, as a result of the increased photon flux that is generated as a result of the larger radiopharmaceutical dose (15). With the doses administered for thyroid imaging, it is possible to obtain flow images and assess the perfusion to the thyroid gland and any nodules present. As the pertechnetate ion is trapped but not organified, it is useful in evaluating the anatomy of a gland in the patient who may have a low iodine uptake, be on antithyroid medications, or have a congenital organification defect (16).

Thallium-201

Thallium-201, in the form of thallous chloride, is a cyclotron product used for thyroid imaging. Thallium decays by electron capture and emits principally mercury x-rays of 135 and 167 keV. It has a physical half-life of 72 hr. Unlike the aforementioned radiophamaceuticals, thallium is neither actively trapped nor organified, depending on a poorly defined mechanism (possibly perfusion alone) for its incorporation into the thyroid. The exact mechanism has not been clearly defined, but it may permit imaging of the thyroid when there is a large-body iodine pool, or in a hypofunctioning gland when iodine or technetium will not produce a satisfactory image (17–22). Its use today has been primarily for the detection of extrathyroidal metastasis from thyroid carcinoma (23–25). The exact value of this radiopharmaceutical in the evaluation of thyroid disease remains to be delineated.

INSTRUMENTATION

Iodine Uptake

The radioactive iodine uptake test is usually performed with a probe in conjunction with a neck phantom. The probe generally consists of a sodium iodide crystal 2 inches in diameter and approximately 2 inches thick, encased in a flat-field collimator and coupled to a single or multichannel analyzer with a scaler. The neck phantom, a solid cylinder usually of clear plastic with multiple chambers that simulates the position of the thyroid in the neck, is used to determine the amount of activity in the administered dose or in an aliquot of the administered dose. The readily available standard international Atomic Energy Agency neck phantom has been carefully developed to provide a reasonable simulation of the average neck geometry. With the use of a standard neck phantom, differences in thyroid uptake values between different laboratories may be minimized. As a result of the different energies between I-123 and I-131, different uptake values may be obtained with each isotope (26). This variation may be more marked with I-123 because of its lower energy. The counting rates will vary with the square of the distance from the radioactive source to the probe (27). Optimal distance for each laboratory should be determined and then adhered to rigorously. Minor errors in distance measurement will have a great effect on the uptake determination value.

Imaging

Two devices are used for thyroid imaging: the rectilinear scanner and the scintillation camera.

Rectilinear Scanner

The rectilinear scanner consists of sodium iodide crystal with a focused collimator, preferably with a focal length of 3 inches. The crystal and collimator are moved back and forth over the thyroid, indexing at the end of each pass. The amount of activity found in any one location is recorded on film at a corresponding location, resulting in an image. Its principal advantage is that it produces a life-sized image of the thyroid and permits precise localization of thyroidal and extrathyroidal anatomy and pathology (Fig. 1). It does have several limitations. The sensitivity is greatly reduced compared with the scintillation camera, and the longer imaging time frequently results in motion artifacts owing to patient movement. In an attempt to place the thyroid in a single plane so that the focused collimator may produce an optimum image, extension of the neck is required, producing sufficient patient discomfort that obtaining images in children and in the elderly is quite difficult. Oblique and lateral views are difficult or impossible to obtain because of shoulder anatomy and the focal length of the collimator. Perfusion images are impossible to obtain. For these reasons, these devices are rarely used at this time.

Scintillation Camera

The scintillation camera offers several advantages in imaging the thyroid. Two types of collimation are used. A parallel-hole, low-energy collimator is used for perfusion

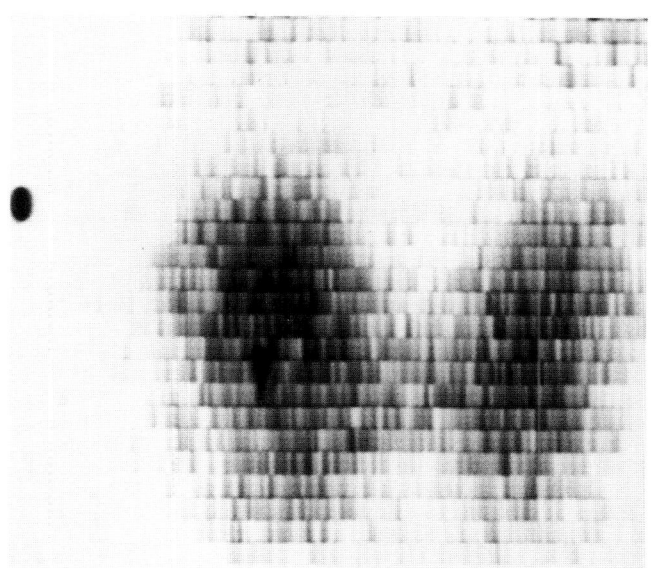

FIG. 1. Rectilinear scan performed with Tc-99m pertechnetate in 46-year-old woman, demonstrating mild asymmetry of the thyroid.

studies performed with Tc-99m pertechnetate and for evaluating ectopic tissues with either I-123 or pertechnetate. Perfusion studies are performed using Tc-99m pertechnetate, with serial images obtained at 2- to 5-sec intervals after the intravenous injection of pertechnetate as a bolus (Fig. 2A). The gamma camera should be centered over the neck and upper thorax. The pinhole collimator has higher resolution than the parallel hole collimator and is widely used to define the anatomy of the thyroid gland, especially small nodules (28–32). The pinhole collimator enables thyroid lesion of 4 mm or larger to be detected on pertechnetate images. The scintillation camera offers the advantage of oblique views that are easily obtained (33,34) (see Fig. 2B). The imaging time is much shorter than with the rectilinear scanner. Therefore, patient motion is usually less of a problem. Localization of anatomic or pathologic sites is somewhat difficult with a pinhole collimator; however, this may be accomplished by using a weak source of radioactivity to mark the anatomic landmarks. Such marking must be done with great care because of the possibility of parallax errors. These errors may be minimized by carefully placing the pinhole over the center of the lesion to be marked. When using imaging I-131 for the detection of thyroid metastasis, a medium energy parallel hole collimator is used, and images of the total body or spot views of the head, neck, chest, and abdomen are obtained.

Patient Preparation

Normal thyroid physiology is utilized to localize the radiotracer in the thyroid. Factors that cause abnormalities in the thyroid physiology will affect both the uptake and the thyroid images. In certain situations, deliberate modification of thyroid physiology prior to the study may be desirable; those techniques will be described later.

One of the most common alterations in thyroid physiology is a result of the administration of exogenous thyroid preparations (35,36). This results in the lower turnover of thyroidal iodine with an abnormal decrease in the radioiodine uptake and a decrease in the amount of the radioactive tracer localized in the thyroid, with subsequent degradation of the image. The time required for recovery of the hypothalamic–pituitary–thyroid axis depends in part on the duration of administration of exogenous thyroid. For prolonged periods of administration, it may take as long as 6 weeks off the exogenous thyroid for the hypothalamic–pituitary–thyroid axis to recover. If the exogenous administration has been for only a short period of time, recovery may be in 1 to 2 weeks. The type of exogenous thyroid administered also influences the recovery period. Patients who have been receiving thyroxine with its 8-day biologic half-life will require a longer period of time than those receiving triiodothyronine, which clears much more rapidly from the system owing to its 1-day biologic half-life. Another major factor that influences the rate of incorporation of iodine into the thyroid gland is the size of the total body iodine pool. If this pool has been expanded as a result of diet or ingestion of medications containing large amounts of iodine, such as saturated solution of potassium iodide (SSKI) or Lugol's solution, 2- to 4-week periods of abstinence from the ingestion of these preparations may be required.

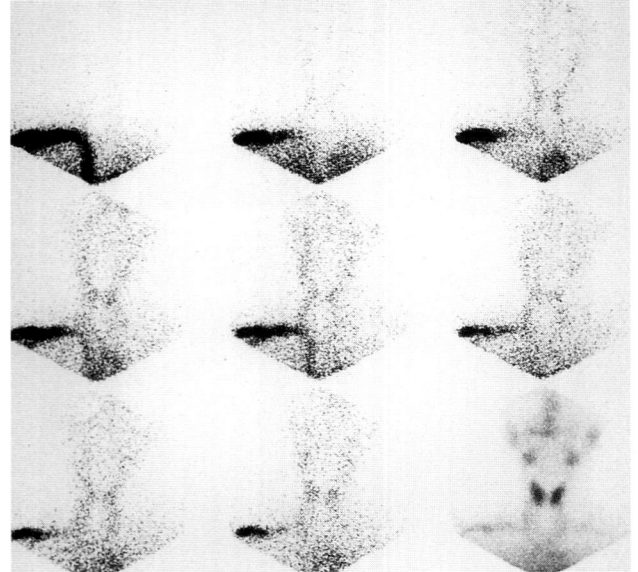
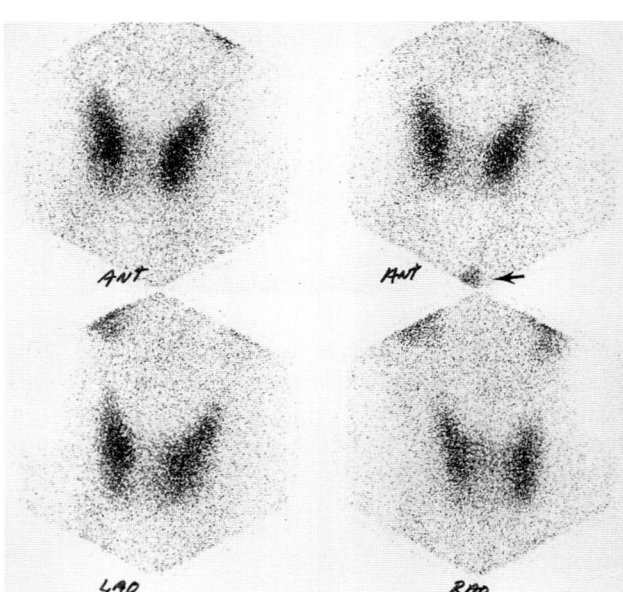

FIG. 2. A: Normal perfusion images performed with 5 mCi Tc-99m pertechnetate in 22-year-old woman. **B:** Normal images of the thyroid including anterior (ANT) image with sternal marker *(arrow)*, and left (LAO) and right anterior oblique (RAO) views.

Many common radiographic procedures utilize contrast materials containing iodinated compounds that will add to the body iodine pool. The water-soluble contrast materials used primarily for computed tomography (CT) and intravenous pyelograms will have a significant effect lasting up to 4 to 6 weeks. The fat-soluble contrast agent used in gallbladder images may have an effect lasting up to 12 weeks. The oil-based contrast agents frequently used in myelography and bronchography may interfere with normal thyroid physiology for up to 1 year. The degree to which these iodine containing compounds interfere with an accurate diagnosis of the thyroid physiology varies in part with the individual. In patients who are hyperthyroid, the iodine pool turns over more rapidly, and these patients may have a shorter recovery time and may demonstrate elevated 24-hr iodine uptakes even in the presence of an expanded body iodine pool. Such uptakes, although not a true indicator of the extent of the disease, may be used to confirm the diagnosis of hyperthyroidism.

THYROID UPTAKE DETERMINATION

The thyroid uptake test is a quantitative evaluation of the function of the thyroid. It measures the factors involved in the incorporation of iodine into the gland, including the trapping mechanism and the organification process. Accurate evaluations of these functions can be performed only by measuring the kinetics of iodine. Both I-131 and I-123 are used for this purpose (10). Five to 10 Ci (180 to 370 kBq) of I-131 or 20 Ci (740 kBq) of I-123 given orally are usually sufficient and will provide adequate statistics at 24 hr (37). If imaging with these radiopharmaceuticals is contemplated, then larger doses are usually administered, as discussed below. Room background counts are determined; then the dose to be administered or a known aliquot of the dose is placed in the neck phantom and counted with the thyroid uptake probe at the predetermined optimal distance. The dose is then administered to the patient. At the appropriate time, usually at 24 hr, the patient is placed on the table and the neck is counted. Careful attention must be paid to maintaining the correct distance from the probe to the neck (Fig. 3). This distance must be the same as that used to calibrate the dose in the neck phantom. Background counts may be determined by placing the probe over the thigh or placing a heavy lead shield between the thyroid and the probe.

In situations where a rapid turnover of iodine may be suspected, uptake determinations should be obtained at 4, 8, and 24 hr. In most conditions, a 24-hr uptake value is sufficient for establishing a diagnosis. The percentage uptake is then calculated by the following formula: neck counts divided by administered counts times 100, where neck counts are equal to gross counts per min, divided by the neck counts per min (minus thigh or lead shield background counts per min). Administered counts are equal to gross counts per min in neck phantom minus room background counts per min, multiplied by the appropriate decay factor. If I-131 has been used, with its 8-day half-life, no decay factor is necessary for readings up to 6 hr. At 24 hr, a decay factor of 0.9177 is used. When I-123 is used, appropriate decay factors must be used after 2 hr.

Uptake Interpretation

The normal range of radioiodine must be established for each individual laboratory, as minor differences in the methodology of obtaining the uptake may bias the range. In addition, there are regional differences in dietary habits and iodine ingestion that may produce a considerable range of normal values (38). This procedure is not reliable in establishing the diagnosis of hypothyroidism; low values

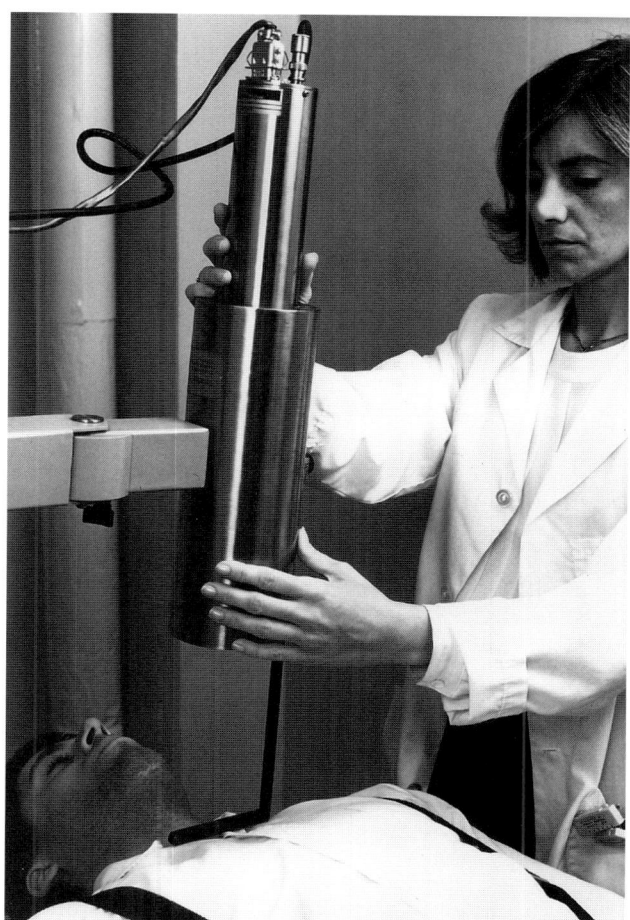

FIG. 3. Technician placing uptake probe at optimal distance from the patient's thyroid. Distance is maintained by use of the bar attached to the probe, which has been preset at the optimal distance. After proper placement, a series of 1-minute counts are obtained.

may be seen in patients with primary or secondary hypothyroidism as well as in patients with a large iodine pool. Patients receiving exogenous thyroid and patients in certain phases of subacute or chronic thyroiditis may have low uptake values. Elevated uptake values 2 to 3 times the normal range are typically seen in Graves' disease and may be present in toxic multinodular goiter; however, toxic multinodular goiter values are frequently only mildly elevated (39). Occasionally, increased uptake may be seen in patients with Hashimoto's disease, where the increase in thyroid stimulating hormone (TSH) results in increased uptake (40). In iodine deficiency, the iodine uptake value is increased as a normal physiologic response to conserve iodine. Patients who have been on antithyroid medications usually have a low value that is increased for several days after withdrawal of the medication (35).

Imaging with Iodine

Imaging of the thyroid may take place 24 hr after the oral administration of 50 to 100 µCi (1850 to 3700 kBq) of I-131, or 8 to 24 hr after the administration of 150 to 400 µCi (5550 to 14,800 kBq) of I-123. Imaging may be performed either with a rectilinear scan or a gamma camera. For rectilinear scanning, an information density of approximately 100,000 counts per square centimeter should be obtained. An anterior view with the neck extended and the focused collimator 3 inches from the gland is obtained. Anatomic markings are placed on the scan as indicated. Oblique and lateral views are difficult to obtain, as the anatomy of the shoulder interferes with maintaining the correct collimator-to-thyroid distance. The rectilinear scan does offer the advantage of providing a one-to-one anatomic size ratio, permitting accurate localization of clinically detected lesions within the thyroid.

Gamma camera imaging is performed using a pinhole collimator. Images containing 50,000 to 100,000 counts are obtained (Fig. 4). Multiple views must be obtained including both the right and left anterior oblique views. This allows visualization of the posterior aspect of both lobes. Anatomic markers may be added as indicated. In our laboratory, we frequently mark the suprasternal notch, especially when looking for a substernal thyroid. If a superior mediastinal mass detected on chest x-ray is suspected of being a substernal thyroid, then the patient should be imaged in the same upright position that was used when the x-ray was obtained. In many patients, the thyroid is quite mobile, and when the patient is recumbent with the neck extended, the thyroid will rise out of the substernal area and into the neck.

Tc-99m Pertechnetate Imaging

Thyroid imaging is usually performed 15 to 20 min after the injection of 5 to 10 mCi (185 to 370 MBq) of Tc-

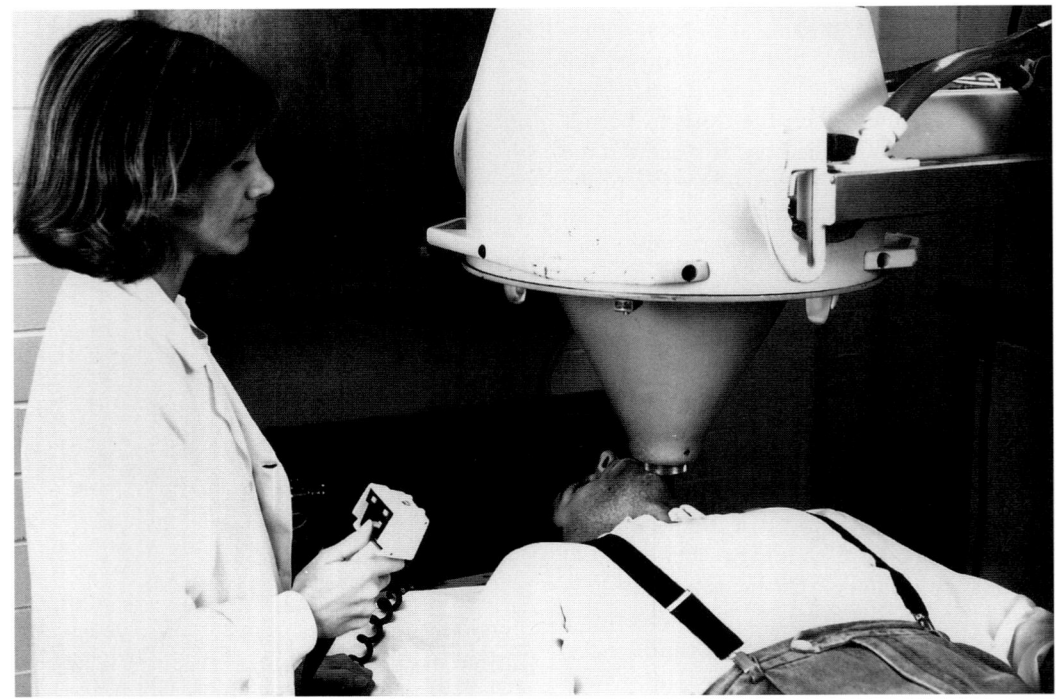

FIG. 4. Patient being imaged with gamma camera equipped with pinhole collimator. Magnification factor will vary with the distance of the pinhole from the patient.

99m pertechnetate. Imaging may be performed with the rectilinear scanner in much the same fashion as with iodine imaging (41–43). With the increase of photon flux from the larger radioactive dose permissible with the use of technetium pertechnetate, the image time is much shorter. With a gamma camera equipped with a high sensitivity or all-purpose parallel hole collimator, a flow study can be performed after a bolus injection of 5 mCi (185 MBq) of Tc-99m pertechnetate. Serial images over the anterior neck are obtained at 3- to 5-sec intervals. Upon completion of the perfusion study, a static image of 250,000 to 500,000 counts including the neck, salivary glands, and upper thorax should be obtained. This is useful for evaluating the relative ratio of uptake between the thyroid and salivary glands, and it serves as a crude indicator of thyroid function (44–46). With the use of a pinhole collimator, images containing 150,000 to 200,000 counts, and multiple images including anterior and both right and left anterior obliques are obtained. Marks may be placed to demarcate anatomic locations or clinically detectable abnormalities. Care must be taken to place the pinhole collimator directly over the lesion, as parallax errors may be introduced (47). In those patients where ectopic thyroid tissue is suspected, the images should be obtained with the parallel hole collimator. Activity outside the thyroid gland may be detected and may be caused by isotope in swallowed saliva within the esophagus. This may be eliminated if the patient swallows a glass of water before imaging, and it should project posterior to the thyroid when evaluated on the oblique projections. A pyramidal lobe may be present and is usually seen as a linear area on the medial aspect of the left lobe of the thyroid. Activity may be seen in the lower portion of the thyroglossal duct under the influence of stimulating immunoglobulins (Fig. 5) (48). Extrathyroidal activity has been noted rarely in lymph nodes with differentiated thyroid carcinoma (Fig. 6). Thyroid metastasis is not usually detectable in a patient with a normal functioning thyroid gland (49).

PHARMACOLOGIC INTERVENTION

The thyroid uptake tests and images may be manipulated by the addition of different drugs to study different parameters of thyroid function. Most of these interfere with the hypothalamic–pituitary–thyroid axis and are used to better define certain functional states. However, with the development of better chemical and laboratory tests [e.g., second and third generation TSH assays, thyrotropin-releasing hormone (TRH) stimulation tests] not involving radioactivity, these procedures are performed only in selected, difficult cases today.

Thyroid Suppression Test

This procedure is used to determine if autonomy is present within the thyroid (50,51). To evaluate the whole gland, a 24-hr radioiodine uptake test is performed, after which triiodothyronine (T_3) is administered daily for 7 days (or L-thyroxine in a single large (2–3 mg) dose], and a repeat 24-hr radioiodine uptake is obtained. In a normal suppression, the radioiodine uptake value should be decreased by at least 50% from the baseline. The patient should be carefully monitored during the administration of the triiodothyronine if autonomy is present, as the patient may develop symptoms of hyperthyroidism. This is especially dangerous in older individuals; thus, careful monitoring of the patient is necessary. Imaging following suppression is used to determine if autonomy is present in a functioning nodule. Again, there should be a drop in the 24-hr uptake as well as in the amount of activity noted in the nodule on the image. If the nodule is suppressible, imaging with radioiodine should demonstrate an overall decrease in the amount of activity in the entire thyroid compared with the baseline image. Nonsuppressible nodules will demonstrate no significant change from the baseline image. In most cases, the change of function within the nodule will also be reflected on the pertechnetate scan, because the trapping mechanism is under the influence of TSH.

The usual daily dose of T_3 is 75 µg administered in divided doses; larger doses may be administered to assure adequate suppression, but this carries an increased risk of side effects. A modification of this procedure may be per-

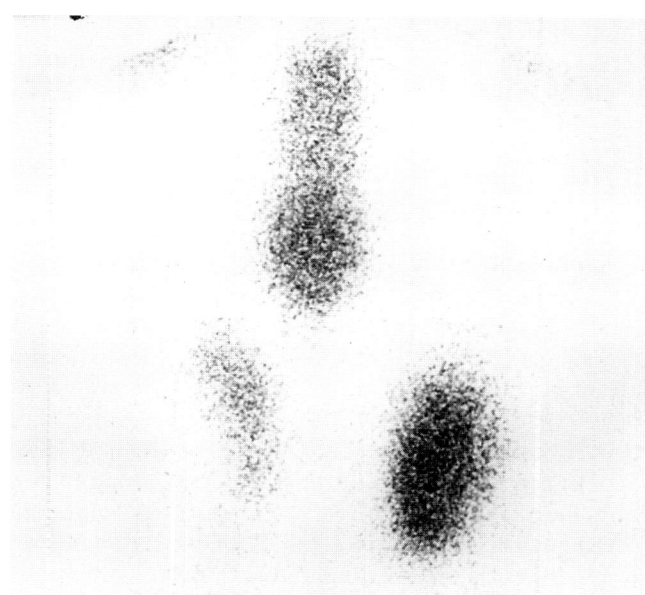

FIG. 5. This 35-year-old woman with a history of hyperthyroidism was treated with surgery 5 years previously and now returns with symptoms of hyperthyroidism. The pertechnetate image demonstrates postoperative changes in the right lobe, with a normal left lobe and a large thyroglossal duct remnant superior to the thyroid. Activity did not change after ingestion of bread and water.

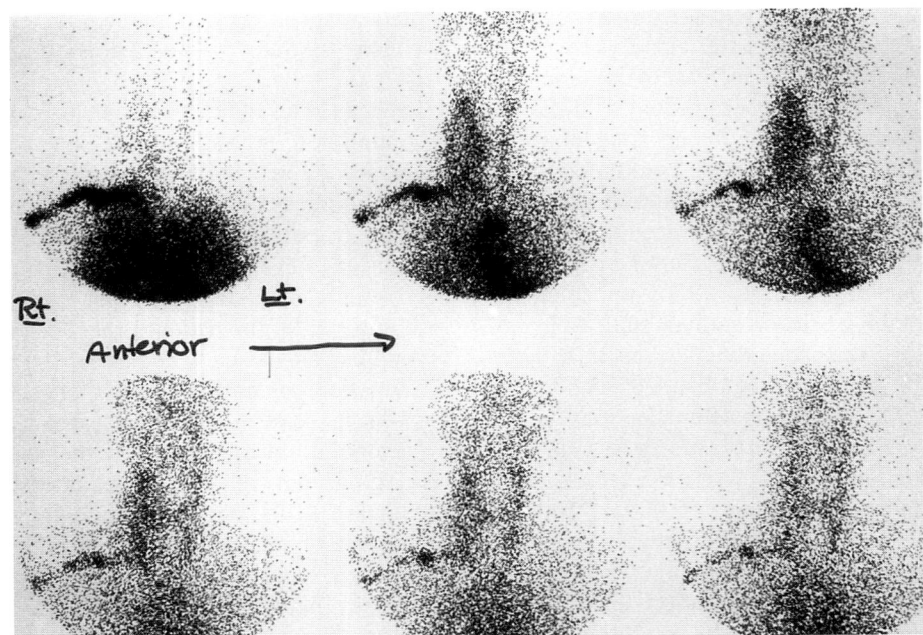

FIG. 6. A: A 37-year-old woman with fullness and discomfort on the right side of her neck. On palpation, no nodules were felt, but there was a fullness to the right side of the neck. Thyroid study was performed with pertechnetate and demonstrated increased perfusion to the right side of the neck.

formed to determine if adequate suppression is being achieved in individuals who are on long-term therapy with thyroid medication, as is used for the treatment of multinodular goiters. The suppression test may also be performed using determination of TSH and/or TRH serum values, thereby avoiding even the minimal radiation exposure to the patient. As a result, the thyroid suppression test is rarely performed except to assess nodule suppressibility or effect of long-term thyroid hormone replacement therapy.

Thyroid Stimulation Test

This procedure is used to stimulate incorporation of the radionuclide into suppressed thyroid tissue. This is useful in patients with suspected substernal thyroids and other ectopic tissues that may be hypofunctioning. It is quite valuable in differentiating the patient with a functioning nodule and suppression of the remaining thyroid from the patient with Graves' disease in a single lobe and agenesis of the remaining lobe (52). This differentiation is important, as the two conditions are treated differently. The procedure involves the administration of exogenous TSH, which increases the trapping and organification mechanisms, resulting in increased uptake of the radionuclide in the thyroid tissue. Intramuscular or subcutaneous injection of 5 to 10 units of bovine TSH are administered daily for 3 days. Then the uptake and imaging procedures are performed under careful supervision, as they require the injection of a foreign protein and a hypersensitivity reaction to the protein is possible (53). The coming availability of human TSH will obviously avoid this problem.

Perchlorate Discharge Test

This procedure is used to evaluate disorders in thyroid hormone synthesis where organification of the iodine is reduced, resulting in increases of unbound thyroidal iodine (54). Potassium perchlorate acts as a competitive inhibitor of iodide within the gland and results in a discharge of unbound iodide from the gland. The iodine that has been organified and bound is not affected by the perchlorate, and the level of bound iodine in the gland remains constant. The procedure requires an iodine uptake test to be performed 2 hr after the administration of the radioiodine. Immediately after the 2-hr uptake determination is complete, 600 to 1000 mg of potassium perchlorate is administered orally, and a second uptake measurement is obtained 1 hr later. A decrease in the uptake value by 5% or more is considered indicative of an organification defect.

IMAGING THYROID CARCINOMA

The well-differentiated thyroid carcinomas commonly retain sufficient amounts of their enzyme pathways to allow them to trap and organify iodine. The majority of tu-

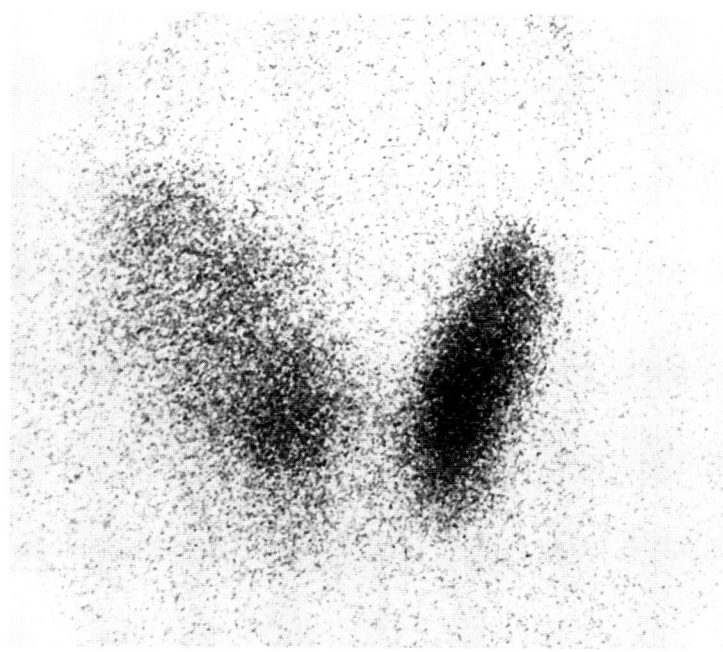

FIG. 6. B: Decreased activity demonstrated in the upper pole of the right lobe of the thyroid. At surgery, there was a mixed papillary follicular carcinoma involving the right lobe of the thyroid with metastasis to the right cervical lymph nodes.

mors are not capable of performing this function as well as normal thyroid tissue, but enough of the function may remain to allow for imaging and treatment of well-differentiated carcinomas. This capability to metabolize iodine is almost completely lost in medullary and anaplastic types of thyroid carcinomas. The amount of radioiodine picked up by the well-differentiated carcinoma can be maximized by reducing the stable iodine pool and increasing the TSH level to 5 to 10 times normal levels. Avoidance of diagnostic procedures requiring contrast material and medications containing iodine or thyroid are essential to obtain adequate images. In addition, diets low in iodine have been recommended to further reduce the stable iodine pool (55). The TSH level is maximized by reducing the amount of thyroid hormone present. This is accomplished after thyroidectomy by ablation of any remnants left after surgery with radioactive iodine and withdrawal of any supplementary thyroid hormone (36,56,57). The patient who is on supplemental thyroid hormone consisting of thyroxine must have the medication withdrawn for at least 6 weeks to produce a satisfactory rise in the TSH; for the first 3 weeks, the shorter-acting T_3 preparations may be substituted to aid in maintaining the patient in a euthyroid state (58,59). However, withdrawal of these preparations should be for at least 2 to 3 weeks to allow the TSH level to rise. If necessary, the patient may be maintained on replacement hormone and an artificial rise in TSH produced by a 3-day course of bovine TSH injections with the same care and concerns as described earlier. Again, the advent of human TSH may do away with the necessity of making the patient hypothyroid. In the patient who has had total thyroidectomy, 2 to 10 mCi (74 to 370 MBq) of I-131 is administered orally, and imaging takes place 48 to 72 hr after ingestion of the iodine (60) (Fig. 7). Again, I-123 can be substituted for I-131, but this is rarely done because the shorter half-life results in higher background activity when imaging is performed 24 hours later. A rough estimate of the amount of uptake and size of the residual or metastatic activity should be performed. This assists in the calculation of the therapeutic dose of I-131 to be administered. Size can also be estimated, if necessary, with other imaging modalities such as ultrasound, CT, or magnetic resonance imaging (MRI). Total body images including the head, neck, chest, and abdomen are obtained. Normal activity may be seen in the nasal area, stomach, and bladder (see Fig. 7). If a therapeutic dose of radioiodine is administered, imaging should be performed 72 to 120 hr later.

The ability to pick up metastasis on the image appears to be related in part to the amount of radioiodine administered (61,62). Therefore, more metastases, if present, may be detected with the larger therapeutic dose. Recently the specter of "stunned" function of metastases following a diagnostic dose in the range of 5 to 10 mCi has been raised (63,64). This may prevent adequate uptake of the therapeutic dose. The authors have never seen this phenomenon in evaluation of over 450 thyroid cancer patients and do not think it is a real concern. This procedure is quite specific for this type of carcinoma, although other malignancies, including pulmonary adenocarcinoma, undifferentiated large-cell bronchogenic carcinoma, papillary meningiomas, and disseminated gastric adenocarcinoma, have been reported to concentrate io-

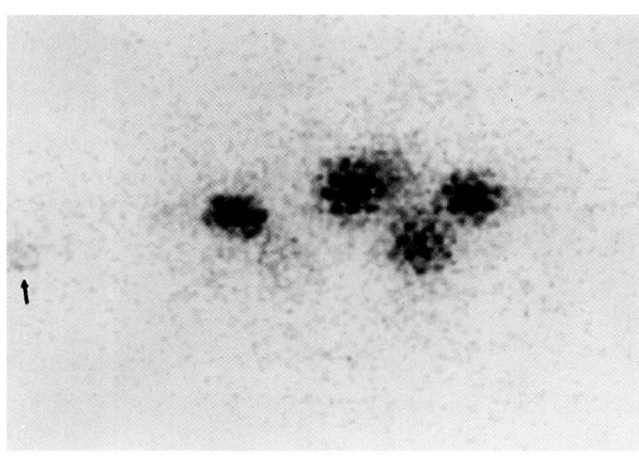

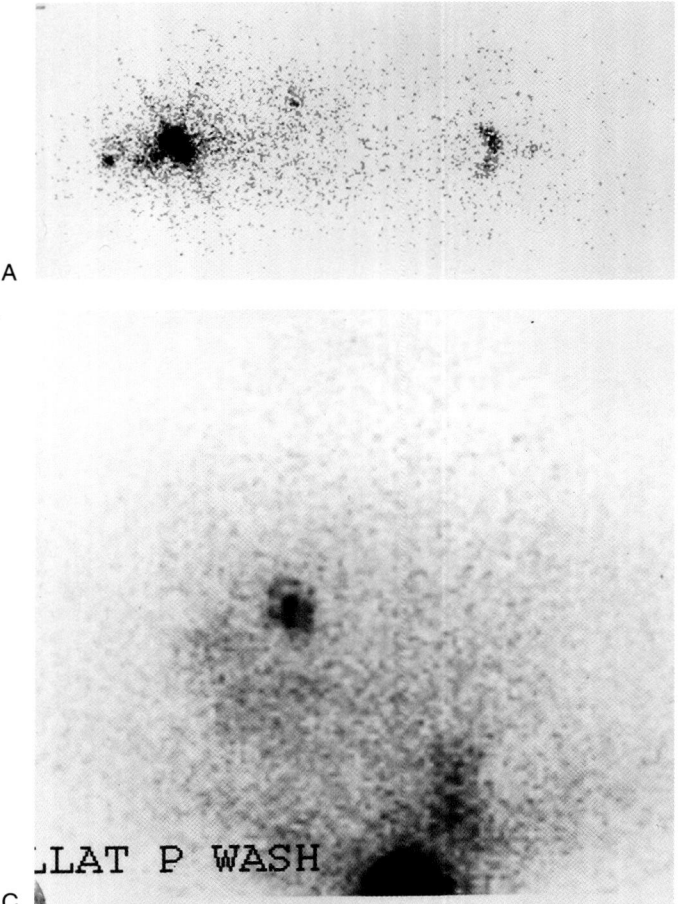

FIG. 7. Total body (**A**) spot views of neck (**B**) and lateral view (**C**) of upper neck and skull obtained after the oral administration of 5 mCi of I-131 to a 61-year-old man who had a total thyroidectomy for carcinoma of the thyroid 6 weeks ago. Note the intense activity in the thyroid bed and nodal regions in the neck. Note also at the very top of (B), the faint lesion to the right of midline *(arrow)*, which in C is shown to be retro-orbital soft-tissue uptake. This last figure was performed after washing the scalp to make sure there was no skin or hair contamination. These lesions were successfully treated with therapeutic doses of I-131.

dine to a lesser degree (65–68). The finding of diffuse liver uptake in a patient with sufficient functioning thyroid tissue does not necessarily indicate metastases in the liver. The liver serves as a site of detoxification of the various iodinated tyrosines and the uptake in the liver may represent metabolism of these compounds by the liver.

Image Interpretation

The images represent an anatomic localization of thyroid physiology. One of the most common indications for thyroid imaging is the assessment of the degree of function in a thyroid nodule. Nodules within the thyroid may be classified into many different categories. They may be hypo- or hyperfunctioning, single or multiple, and they may represent benign or malignant disease. Single nodules that are hypofunctioning on static imaging carry a 10% to 20% possibility of being malignant (69,70). However, nodules that are hypofunctioning on static imaging but are euperfused or hyperperfused (71,72) in relation to the rest of the gland on the flow study carry a nearly 40% possibility of being malignant (Fig. 8). Hypoperfused nodules are rarely malignant.

Iodine and pertechnetate produce similar images in most physiologic states (73). A few malignant lesions may retain sufficient trapping to produce a relatively normal image with technetium pertechnetate but will have limited ability to organify iodine; thus, on iodine scans there will be a defect at the site of the nodule. Carcinoma of the thyroid is present in approximately 40% to 70% of those nodules demonstrating this type of disparate imaging (44,74–76).

Nodules that have normal function without suppression of the remainder of the gland on pertechnetate image should be re-imaged with I-123. If they do suppress the rest of the gland, they are rarely malignant. Hypofunction on the iodine image should carry a high suspicion of malignancy. Benign adenomas show the same pattern of activity as malignant lesions, and thus, there are no distinguishing imaging characteristics that are capable of separating benign from malignant lesions (Fig. 9). Benign adenomas may demonstrate an abnormal 24-hr radioiodine uptake; however, on both technetium and radioiodine images there is usually decreased activity at the site of the nodule. The multinodular gland usually can be detected clinically by palpation, but in some cases the

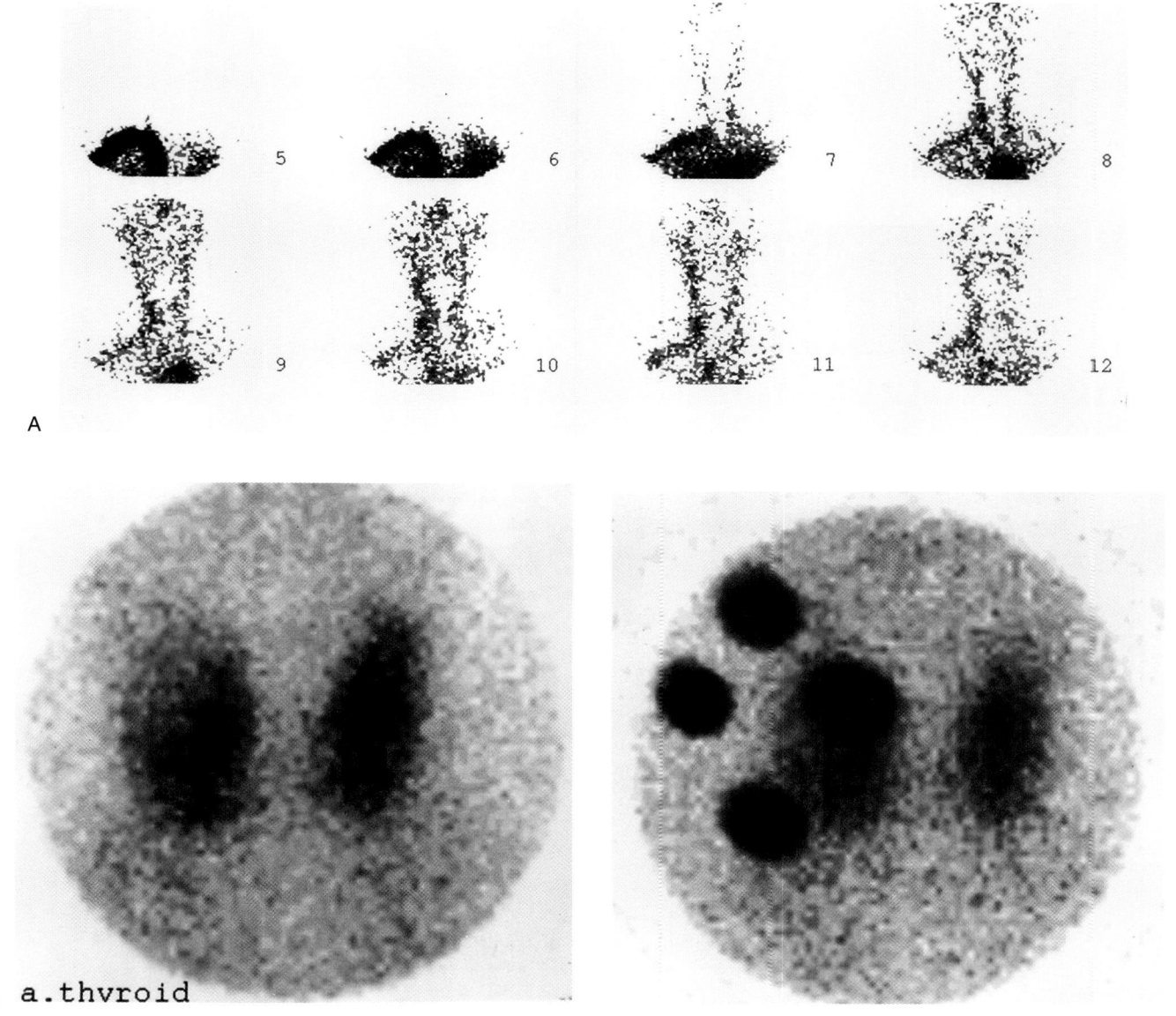

FIG. 8. A: Anterior perfusion scans every 3 seconds in duration in a 48-year-old woman with a palpable nodule in the right upper lobe of the thyroid. Note the slight increase in perfusion to this area. **B:** Hypofunctioning nodule involving the superior lateral portion of the right lobe. **C:** Similar view with external radioactive markers placed over the palpated nodule. It is always important to confirm with such marking techniques that the palpated nodule in the scanning position corresponds to the lesion denoted on the scan.

nodules may not be obvious. Nodules larger than 0.4 cm should be readily detectable with pertechnetate imaging performed with a gamma camera equipped with a pinhole collimator (Fig. 10). The incidence of carcinoma is markedly reduced in the gland with multiple nodules.

The hyperfunctioning nodule may have a normal or an elevated 24-hr radioiodine uptake that will reflect whether the patient is euthyroid or hyperthyroid. Such hyperfunctioning nodules will show hyperperfusion on the technetium perfusion scan. Hyperfunctioning nodules can suppress the remainder of the thyroid. At times, the remainder of the gland can be seen by simply covering the hyperfunctioning nodule with a lead shield and repeating the images. This results in the counts forming the image coming only from the suppressed forming portion of the gland (Fig. 11). If this technical trick does not work, then a course of TSH with a repeat scan may be necessary, if felt to be clinically indicated. When the non-involved thyroid is visualized, the nodule is assumed to be producing insufficient thyroid hormone to suppress the TSH axis. In cases of hyperthyroidism secondary to an autonomous functioning nodule, the TSH thyroid axis

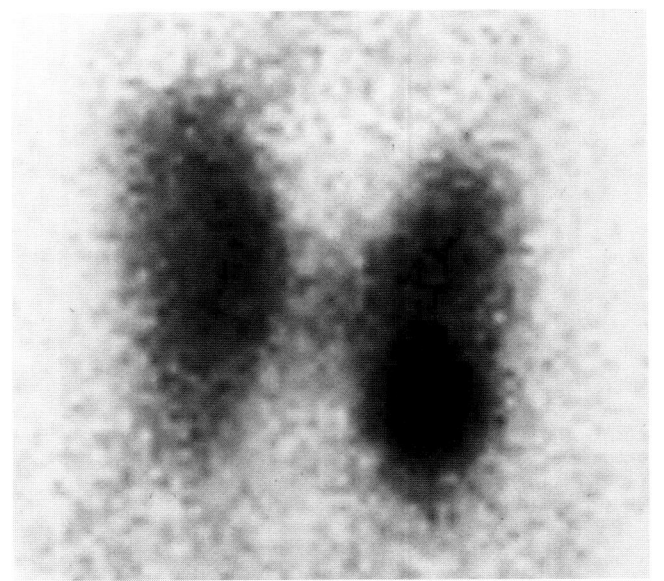
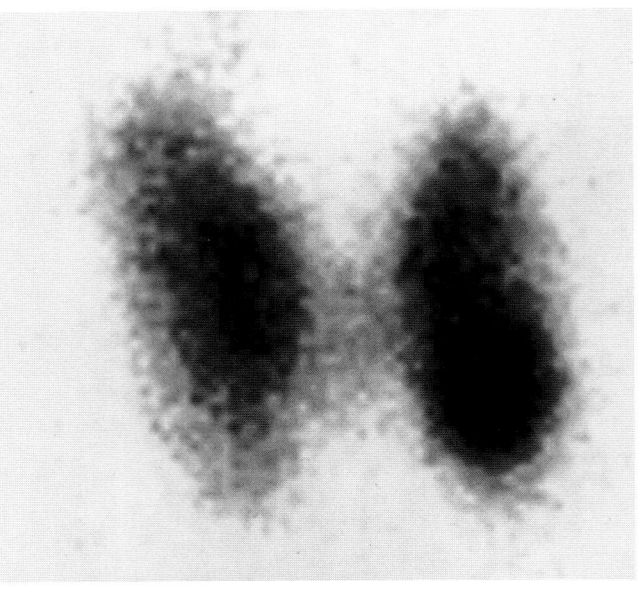

FIG. 9. Anterior views of the neck performed using Tc-99m pertechnetate **(A)** and I-123 **(B)** in a 43-year-old woman with a palpable nodule in the lower pole of the left lobe. This is a functioning nodule on pertechnetate scanning without suppression of the rest of the gland. The iodine study, performed the next day, shows similar findings. This is an example of nondisparate imaging indicating that the lesion can both trap and organify the agents and therefore is benign.

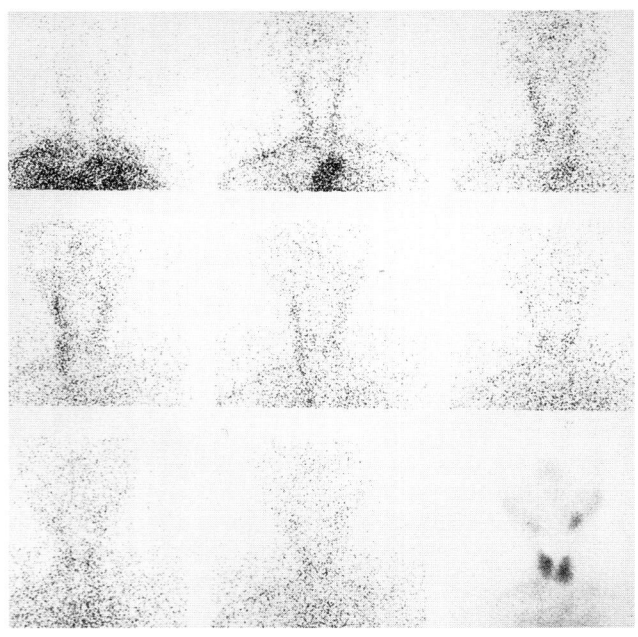
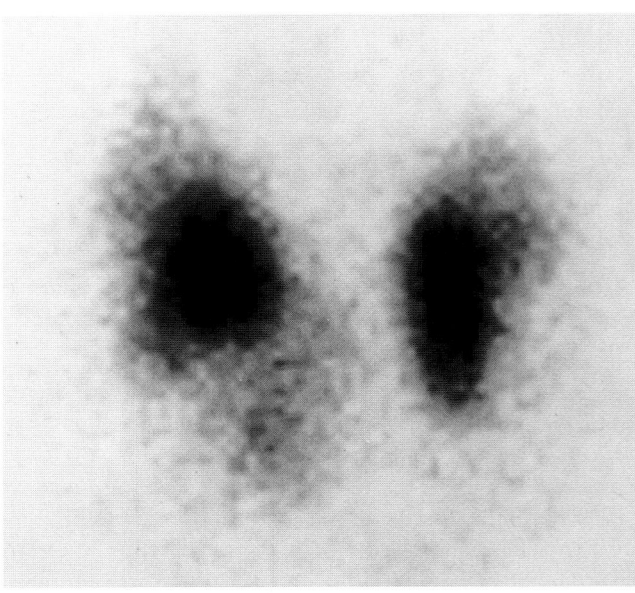

FIG. 10. A: Pertechnetate perfusion images in a 45-year-old woman who was felt to have a multinodular gland clinically; note the uneven perfusion to the gland. **B:** Anterior view of the gland revealing multiple areas of decreased and increased function consistent with typical multinodular goiter.

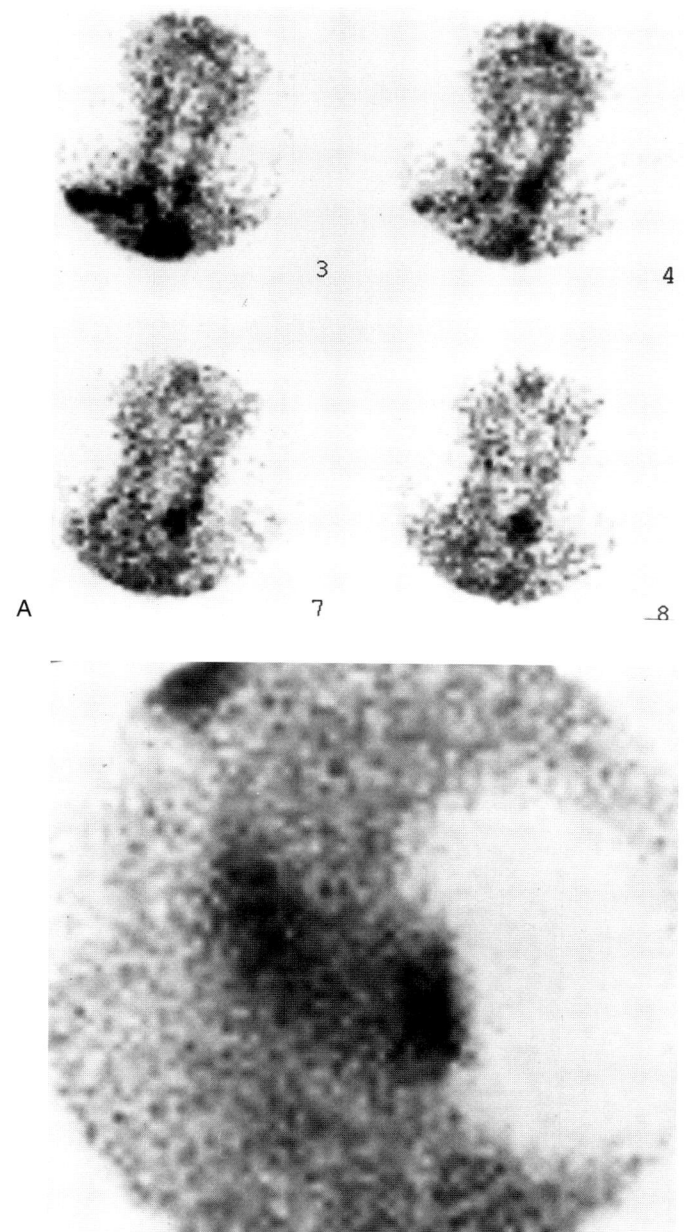

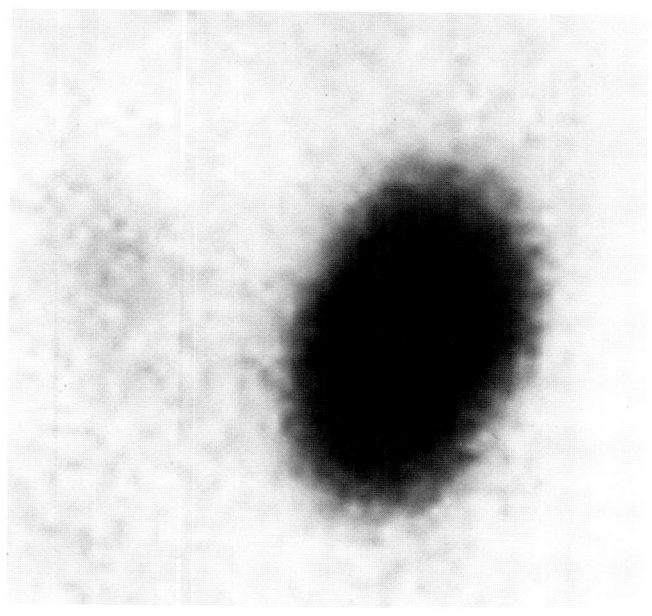

FIG. 11. A: Pertechnetate perfusion images in a 27-year-old woman who was felt to be normal clinically except for a palpable left-side nodule. These demonstrate focus hyperperfusion to a large left-side nodule. **B:** Delayed static imaging showing a large functioning nodule with apparent suppression of the rest of the gland. **C:** Repeat static view with the nodule partially covered by a lead shield (large blank area) demonstrating rest of gland to have residual function and only partial suppression.

will be suppressed and visualization of the remainder of the gland is impaired (77) (Fig. 12). If the remainder of the thyroid is not identified on imaging after TSH stimulation, then dysembryogenesis of a lobe of the thyroid should be suspected rather than a functioning nodule with suppression of the normal thyroid (53).

The role of radioisotopic imaging must be balanced in each institution with the availability of other imaging modalities and diagnostic approaches. Ultrasonography is a benign procedure that involves no radiation to the patient. It can give quite good morphologic information about the size and structure of the gland and any nodules that may be present. The use of complex scans to include Doppler flow studies may allow assessment of blood flow to nodules in certain cases. It may also be used to direct localization of needle biopsy in selected cases, especially those with small nodules. Although CT and MRI can also be used to evaluate the structure of the gland, the high cost and complexity of these procedures curtails their usefulness in most patients. X-ray fluorescent imaging of the thyroid can provide accurate information about the distribution of stable iodine within the gland. The emission image can assess the size and shape of the gland, and the presence and iodine content of nodules, and it allows

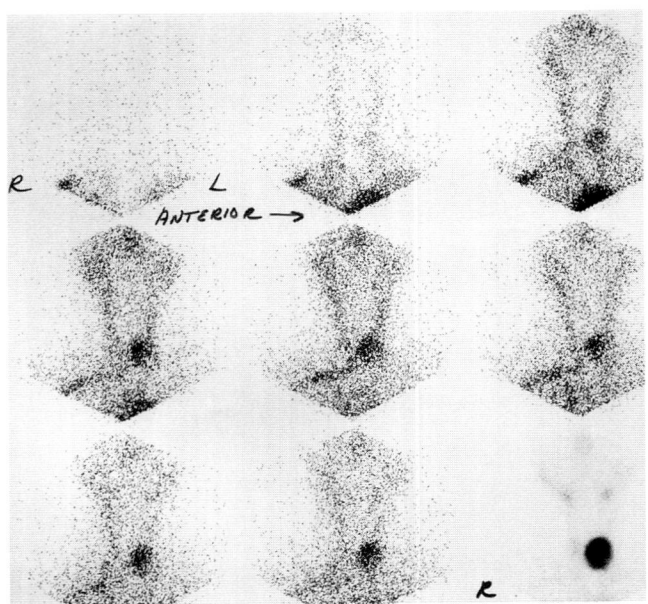

FIG. 12. A 40-year-old woman with clinical and chemical hyperthyroid status and a palpable nodule in the lower portion of the left neck. The 24-hr iodine uptake was 32%. Perfusion images demonstrate increased focal perfusion to the nodule with increased trapping and abnormal thyroid to salivary gland ratio. The remainder of the gland was not able to be visualized by any means and the nodular activity was nonsuppressible. These findings are typical of a toxic, nonsuppressible hyperfunctioning nodule.

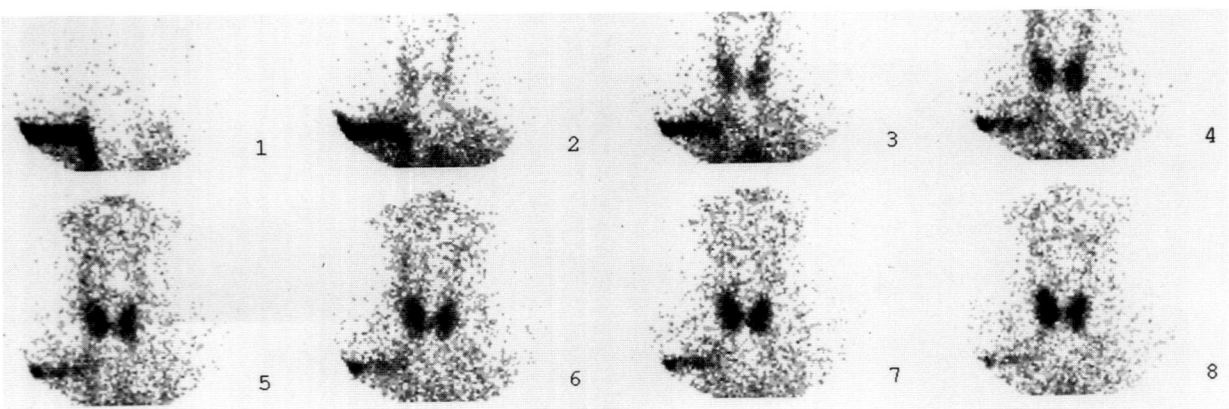

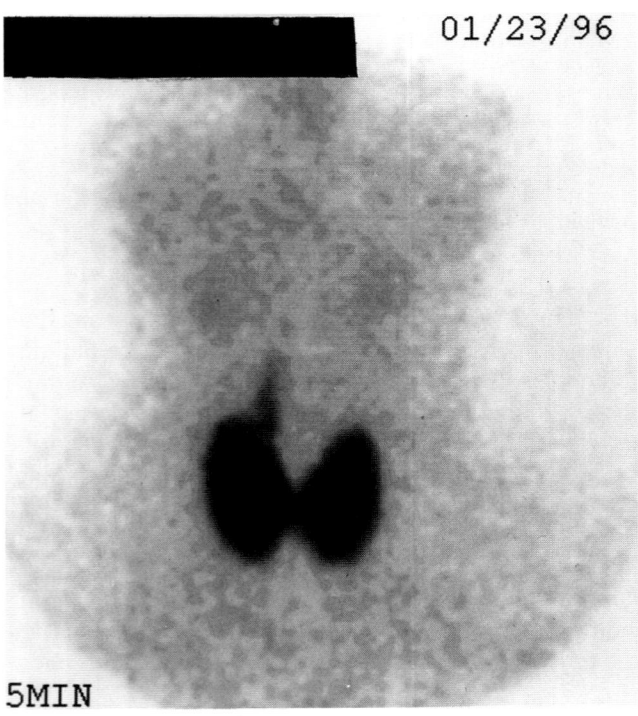

FIG. 13. A: Anterior pertechnetate perfusion images of a 31-year-old woman with symptoms of hypothyroidism. Note the marked increase in both time and amount of perfusion of the gland. **B:** Anterior image at 5 min, demonstrating the increased activity in the enlarged goiter. The thyroid-to-salivary-gland ratio is markedly abnormal, with the salivary glands not visible. A 24-hr radioactive iodine uptake was 78%.

for assessment of thyroid function. As with CT and MRI, the specialized equipment and high procedure cost prevent widespread use.

In addition, at some institutions, fine-needle aspiration (FNA) may be carried out on all nodules. Although it is a simple procedure with few complications, it requires accurate cytopathologic interpretation and it is costly, especially when performed on all nodules. At our institution, charges for procedures increase in the following order: scintigraphic study, ultrasound, CT, MRI, FNA. As a result, we prefer to select patients for needle biopsy based on cost and clinical factors.

HYPO- AND HYPERTHYROIDISM

In patients with hypothyroidism, the 24-hr uptake of radioactive iodine is suppressed. In most cases, the technetium image obtained will be of inferior quality, with a relatively large amount of background present. Iodine images are degraded even more in quality and require a prolonged period of time to obtain adequate statistics for the image.

In patients with hyperthyroidism, the 24-hr uptake is usually elevated. Some patients with rapid turnover of their iodine pool in the gland may have a normal 24-hr uptake value; however, uptake values obtained at 2 to 12 hr will be elevated. The flow study performed with pertechnetate usually demonstrates increased perfusion to the gland (Fig. 13). The immediate image that includes the salivary glands may serve as a crude indicator of the function of the gland. Images of patients with hyperthyroidism usually demonstrate an increase in the thyroid-to-salivary-gland ratio over the normal 1:1 ratio. Normal to mildly elevated 24-hr iodine uptakes with normal perfusion and intensity on the image, or even hypointensity on the image, are not uncommonly seen in patients with large toxic multinodular goiters (39) (Fig. 14).

Acute Thyroiditis

In acute thyroiditis, uptake is usually within normal limits or low; however, the image will demonstrate areas of decreased activity that correspond to the areas of acute inflammation or abscess formation. This defect is present on both technetium and iodine imaging.

Subacute Thyroiditis

Subacute thyroiditis may demonstrate a normal or depressed 24-hr uptake depending upon when in the stage of the disease the activity is sampled. Initially, the uptake

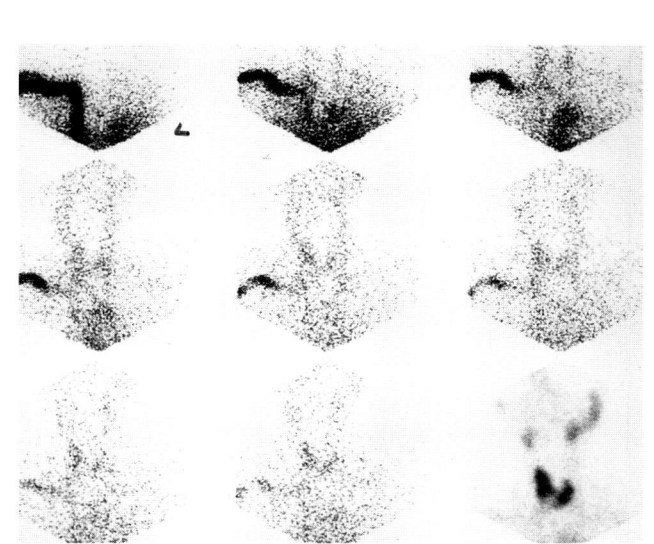
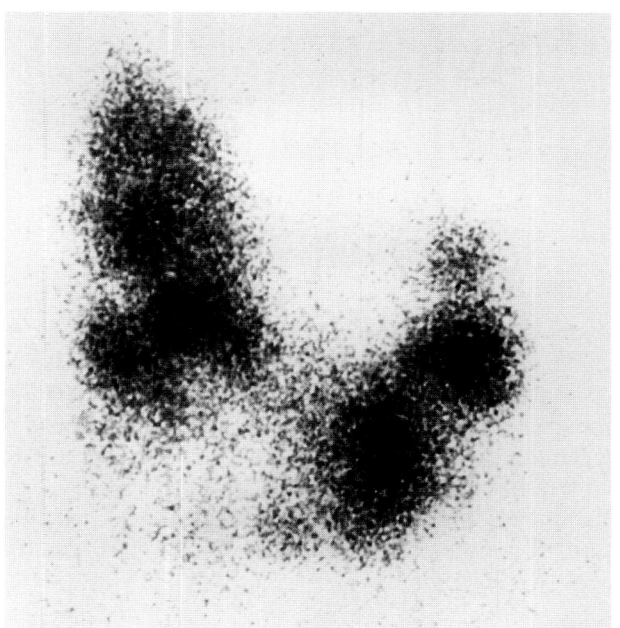

FIG. 14. A: Anterior pertechnetate perfusion imaging demonstrating slight increased perfusion to the thyroid gland. Note the 5-min image in the lower right-hand portion demonstrating slight increase in the thyroid-to-salivary ratio. **B:** Pinhole images demonstrating marked irregularity and multiple areas of nodules in both lobes. The 24-hr uptake was 35%, consistent with a toxic multinodular goiter. It can be difficult at times to discern toxic multinodular goiters from scan alone, because the irregular uptake and perfusion patterns may not be strikingly abnormal as they are in Graves' disease.

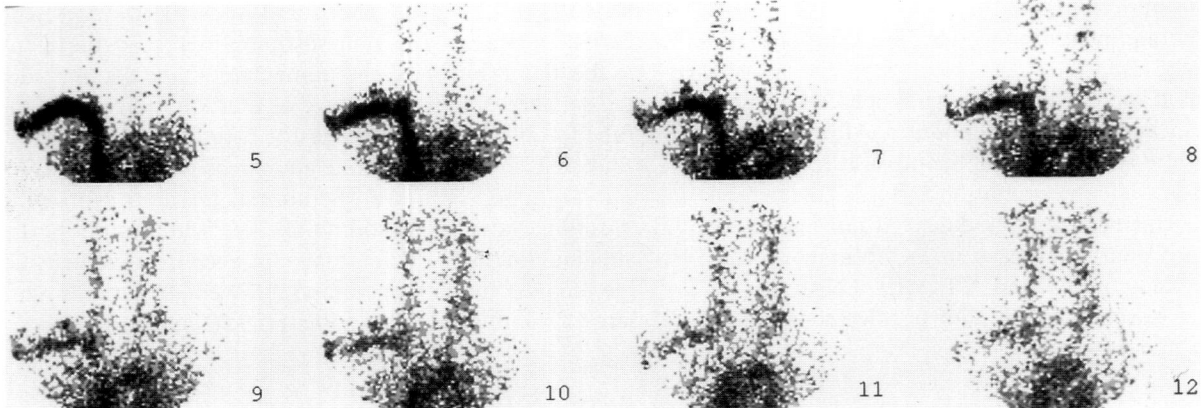

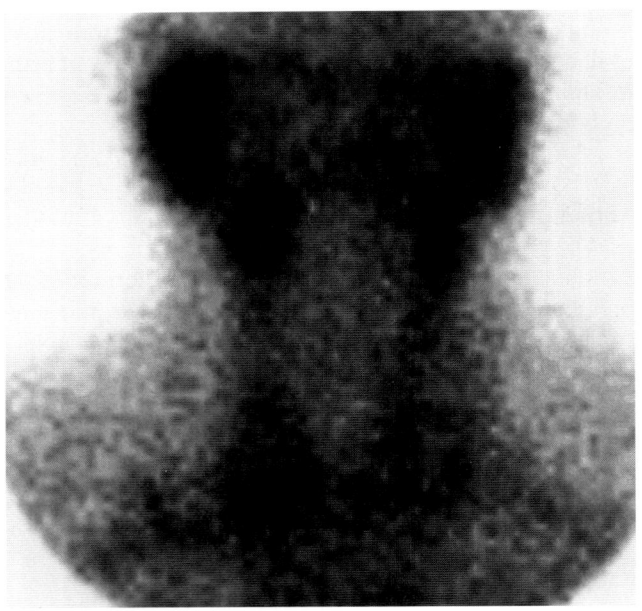

FIG. 15. A: Anterior pertechnetate perfusion images at 3-sec intervals, demonstrating decreased perfusion both in time and amount to a clinically enlarged gland by palpation. **B:** Delayed pinhole images in the anterior projection demonstrating marked nonvisualization of the gland. The 24-hr radioactive iodine uptake was 1.2%. These findings in the typical clinical picture and blood values are consistent with subacute thyroiditis.

remains normal and then becomes depressed, slowly returning to normal as the inflammation subsides. Perfusion frequently is increased reflecting the inflammation; however, the images may be of poor quality because of interference with the normal metabolic activity of the gland, resulting in a low uptake as well (Fig. 15). As the inflammatory process subsides, both uptake and imaging return to normal. This may take anywhere from a few weeks to a few months.

Hashimoto's Thyroiditis

Hashimoto's thyroiditis is one of the most common causes of hypofunctioning thyroid disease, with depression of the 24-hr iodine uptakes. The images in patients with Hashimoto's disease usually are of poor quality because of the depressed thyroid metabolism; however, in patients with thyrotoxicosis, the uptake may be elevated and have an appearance similar to those with Graves' disease. Some patients with Hashimoto's thyroiditis may demonstrate mild asymmetry or focal areas of decreased activity that are usually irregular in shape and are not associated with any clinically detectable nodularity (Fig. 16). The activity pattern can aid in the localization of the pathology for FNA.

Lymphomas in the thyroid commonly have a normal 24-hr radioiodine uptake. Large glands with areas of irregularly decreased activity noted on the image without a palpable nodule are suggestive of a lymphoma (78). The activity distribution pattern is again useful in defining the area for biopsy.

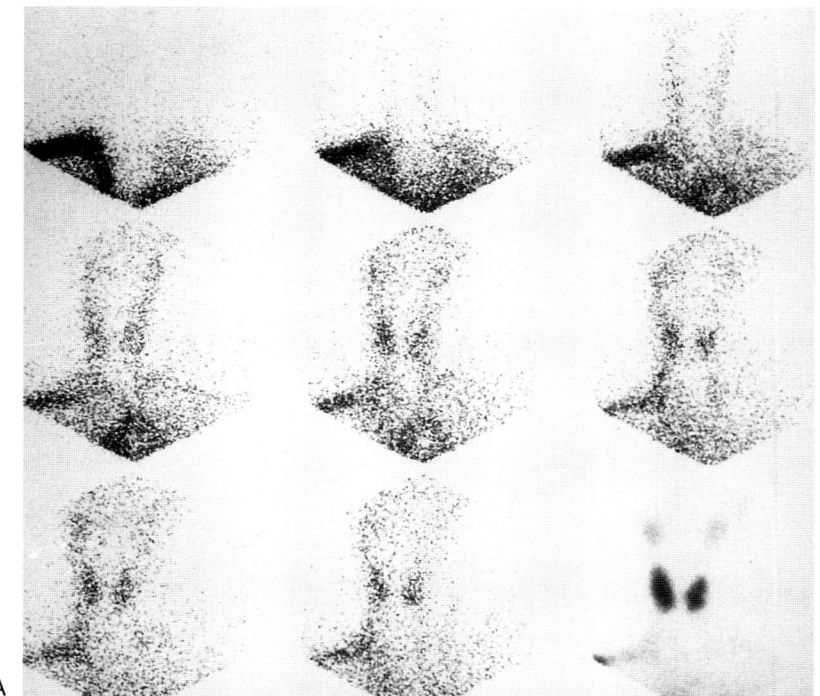

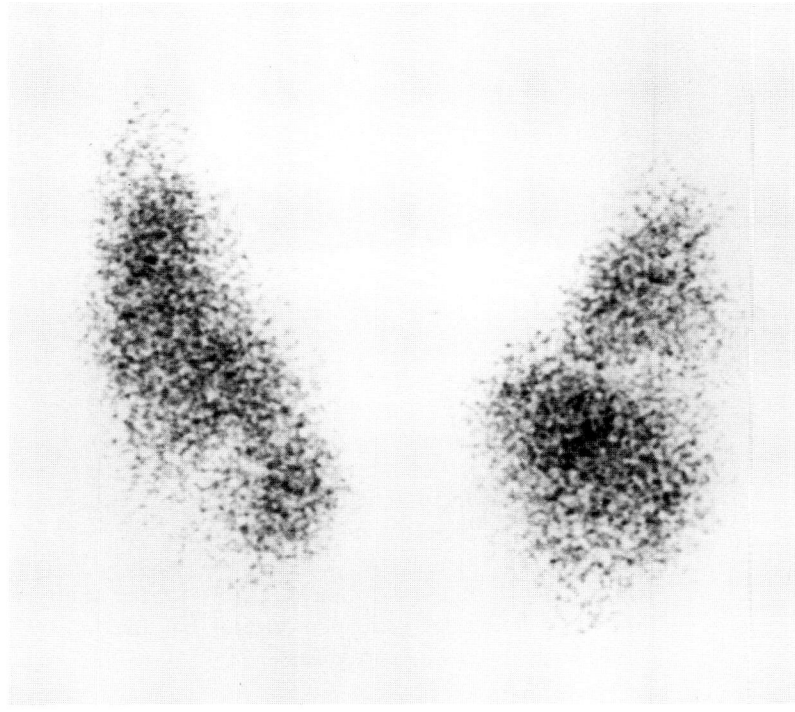

FIG. 16. A 15-year-old girl with a 2-year history of goiter and normal thyroid function tests who recently developed symptoms of hypothyroidism. Perfusion study **(A)** demonstrates increased perfusion to an enlarged gland with a multinodular pattern on pinhole image **(B)**. Her T_4 was 0.2, with a TSH titer of >100 and a thyroid antibody titer >1 to 5100, establishing a diagnosis of Hashimoto's thyroiditis. The patient responded well to replacement therapy.

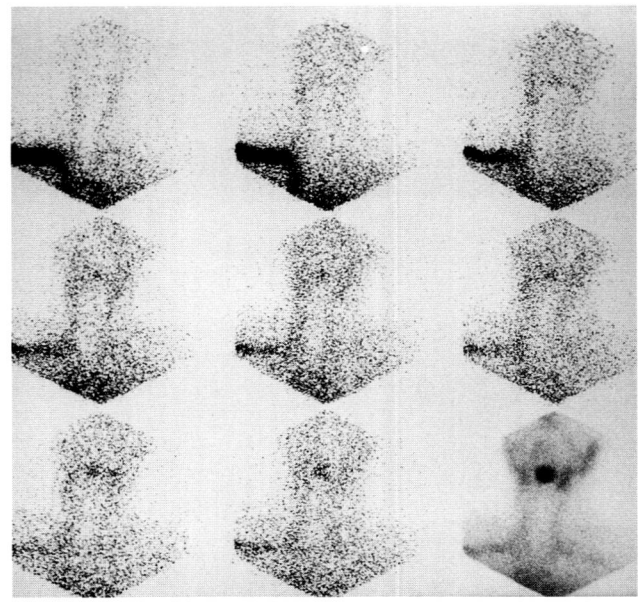 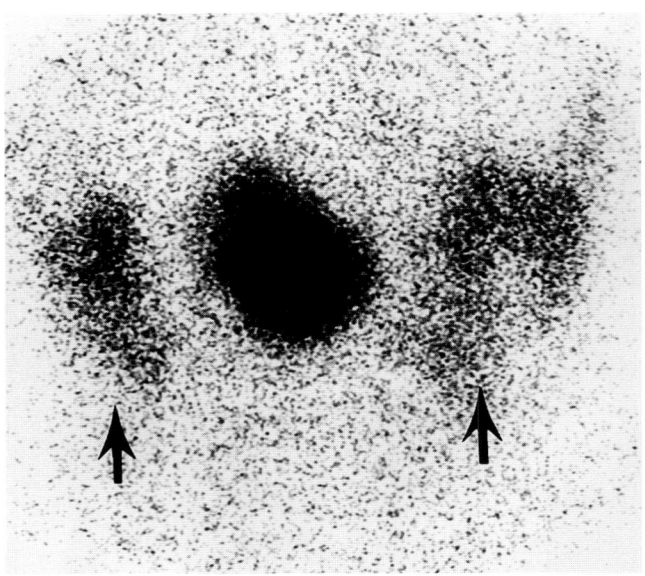

FIG. 17. A 29-year-old woman who was noted to have a midline external neck mass on routine physical examination. Clinical diagnosis was thyroglossal duct cyst. Pertechnetate thyroid study demonstrates perfusion **(A)** to the mass with trapping ability. There is no evidence of functioning thyroid tissue in the normal thyroid bed on images of the neck **(B)**. *Arrows* point to the salivary glands. This represents an ectopic thyroid in a euthyroid individual.

Cysts

Cysts within the thyroid are clinically detectable as nodules. Usually the consistency is not as firm as a solid nodule, and the finding may be confirmed by ultrasound. Cysts usually are associated with a normal 24-hr radioiodine uptake. The cyst demonstrates absent perfusion to the area of the cyst on perfusion image, and an absence of activity in the area on both the technetium and the iodine image.

Congenital Lesions

There are two broad categories of congenital lesions of the thyroid. Dyshormonogenesis occurs where there is a defect in the metabolic chain resulting in a decreased ability to produce thyroid hormone. Dysembryogenesis results in failure of the thyroid to form properly and migrate from the base of the tongue (Fig. 17) to its final resting place in the neck. In ectopic thyroids, the 24-hr radioiodine uptake is frequently unreliable because of interfering anatomic structures or because of misplacement of the probe as a result of the ectopia. Functioning ectopic thyroid tissue can be demonstrated with either pertechnetate or iodine (79,80), although iodine with its low background is preferred for areas other than the neck (81–83). 123-Iodine should be used because the overwhelming majority of these patients are children or young adults. Functioning tissue can be demonstrated at the base of the tongue and the upper portion of neck and, if migration has been excessive, in the mediastinum. Images are helpful in the differentiation of neck masses by separating functioning thyroid tissue from other etiologies. Thyroglossal duct cysts may be present along the route of migration of the thyroid and, with the exception of those cases in which there may be excessive TSH stimulation, are not visualized on either pertechnetate or iodine imaging (48).

Dyshormonogenesis may be suspected when serum levels of T_3 and T_4 are depressed with excessive levels of TSH. A hyperstimulated gland that may be ectopic may be visualized on pertechnetate imaging when the thyroid trapping mechanism remains intact (Fig. 18). Since these patients have a defect in the synthesis of thyroid hormone, the iodine images are of poor quality. In most cases, iodine imaging is not necessary for the diagnosis and may not be desirable, considering that many of these patients being studied are infants.

CONCLUSION

The radionuclide studies described are helpful in defining both the function of the thyroid gland and the anatomy and location of the pathology within the gland. These studies may be used not only to confirm clinical diagnosis, but also to localize areas of pathology for biopsy and to evaluate therapy. The usefulness of the studies is maximized by the correct choice of the proper

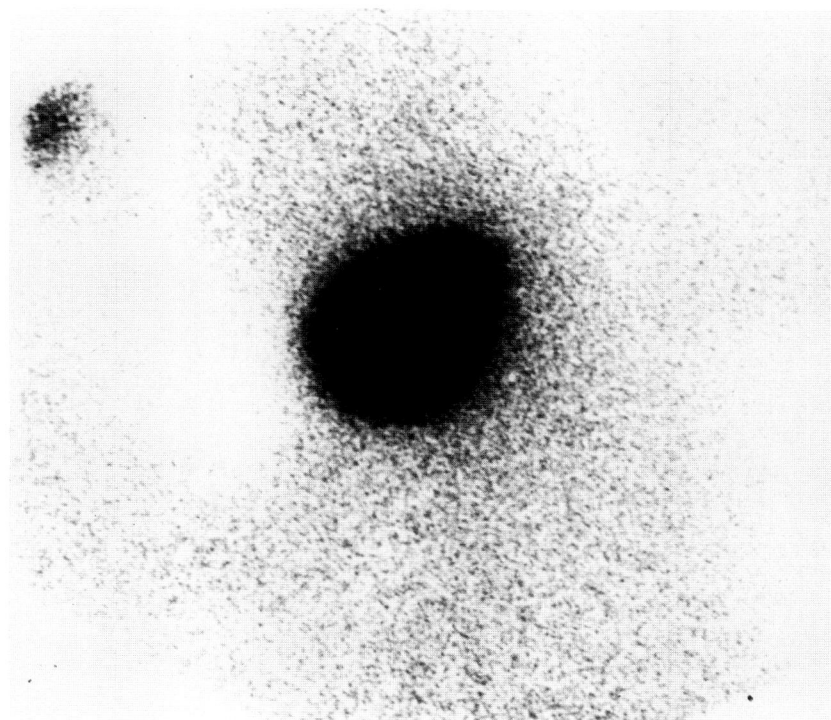

FIG. 18. A 15-day-old female infant who is on thyroid screening had a TSH elevated above 200 units and a depressed T_4 of less than 4. Pertechnetate imaging demonstrates an enlarged gland with increased trapping and a normal background. Presumptive diagnosis is an organification defect.

study, which can only be accomplished by a thorough understanding of the thyroid physiology and pathophysiology, so that the proper functional and imaging procedure may be selected.

ACKNOWLEDGMENT

This revision is dedicated to the memory of George A. Wilson, M.D.—friend, co-worker, physician, scientist, and family man. We miss him.

We would like to express our appreciation and thanks to Mrs. Marilyn Phillips and Mrs. Anne Kirchoff, without whose patience and effort this revision could not have been accomplished.

REFERENCES

1. Hamburger JI. Subacute thyroiditis: diagnostic difficulties and simple treatment. *J Nucl Med* 1974;15:81–89.
2. Gluck FB, Nusynowitz ML, Plymate S. Chronic lymphocytic thyroiditis, thyrotoxicosis, and low radioactive iodine uptake: report of four cases. *N Engl J Med* 1975;293:624–628.
3. Woolf PD. Painless thyroiditis as a cause of hyperthyroidism: subacute or chronic lymphocytic? *Arch Intern Med* 1978;138:26–27.
4. Dorfman SG, Cooperman MT, Nelson RL, et al. Painless thyroiditis and transient hyperthyroidism without goiter. *Ann Intern Med* 1977;86:24–28.
5. Teixeira VL, Romaldini JH, Rodrigues HF, et al. Thyroid function during the spontaneous course of subacute thyroiditis. *J Nucl Med* 1985;256:457–460.
6. Bartels PC, Boer RO. Subacute thyroiditis (de Quervain) presenting as a painless "cold" nodule. *J Nucl Med* 1987;28:1488–1490.
7. Pupi A, Castagnoli A, Morotti A. Prognostic value of the 131-I whole body scan in postsurgical therapy for differentiated thyroid cancer. *Cancer* 1983;52:439–441.
8. MIRD dose estimate report no. 5. Summary of current radiation dose estimates to humans from I-123, I-124, I-125, I-126, I-130, I-131 and I-132 as sodium iodide. *J Nucl Med* 1975;16:857–860.
9. MIRD dose estimate report no. 8. Summary of current radiation dose estimates to normal humans from Tc-99m as sodium pertechnetate. *J Nucl Med* 1976;17:74–77.
10. Hooper PL, Turner JR, Conway MJ, et al. Thyroid uptake of I-123 in normal population. *Arch Intern Med* 1980;140:757–758.
11. Baker GA, Lum DJ, Smith EM, et al. Significance of radiocontaminates in I-123 for dosimetry and scintillation camera imaging. *J Nucl Med* 1976;17:740–743.
12. Hughes JA, Williams CC, Thomas SR, et al. Potential errors caused by variable radionuclide purity of I-123. *J Nucl Med Technol* 1979;7:167–170.
13. Paras P, Hamilton DR, Evans C, et al. Iodine-123 assay using a radionuclide calibrator. *Int J Nucl Med Biol* 1983;10:111–115.
14. Chervu S, Chervu LR, Goodwin PN, et al. Thyroid uptake measurements with I-123: problems and pitfalls (concise communication). *J Nucl Med* 1982;23:667–670.
15. Strauss HW, Hurley PJ, Wagner HN Jr. Advantges of 99m-Tc pertechnetate for thyroid scanning patients with decreased radioiodine uptake. *Radiology* 1970;97:307–310.
16. Price DA, Ehrlich RM, Walfish PG. Congenital hypothyroidism. Clinical and laboratory characteristics of infants detected by neonatal screening. *Arch Dis Child* 1981;56:845–851.
17. Tonami N, Bunko H, Michigishi T, et al. Clinical applications of Tl-201 scintigraphy in patients with cold thyroid nodules. *Clin Nucl Med* 1978;3:217–221.
18. Hisada K, Norhisa T, Miyamae T, et al. Clinical evaluation of tumor imaging with Tl-201 chloride. *Radiology* 1978;129:497–500.
19. Ichiya Y, Nakashima T, Gunasekera R, et al. Coexistence of a nonfunctioning thyroid nodule in Plummer's disease demonstrated by thallium-201 imaging. *Clin Nucl Med* 1988;13:117–119.
20. Tennvall J, Palmer J, Biorklund FA, et al. Kinetics of Tl-201 uptake in adenomas and well-differentiated carcinomas of the thyroid: a double isotope investigation with Tc-99m and Tl-201. *Acta Radiol Oncol* 1984;23:55–59.

21. Brendel AJ, Guyot M, Jeandot R, et al. Thallium-201 imaging in the follow-up of differentiated thyroid carcinoma. *J Nucl Med* 1988;29: 1515–1520.
22. Corstens F, Huymans D, Kloppenborg P, et al. Thallium-201 scintigraphy of the suppressed thyroid: an alternative for iodine-123 scanning after TSH stimulation. *J Nucl Med* 1988;29:1360–1363.
23. Tonami N, Hisada K. Tl-201 scintigraphy in postoperative detection of thyroid cancer: a comparative study with I-131. *Radiology* 1980;136: 461–464.
24. Hoefnagel CA, Delprat CC, Marcuse HR, et al. Role of thallium-201 total-body scintigraphy in follow up of thyroid carcinoma. *J Nucl Med* 1986;27:1854–1857.
25. Arnstein NB, Juni JE, Sisson JC, et al. Recurrent medullary carcinoma of the thyroid demonstrated by thallium-201 scintigraphy. *J Nucl Med* 1986;27:1564–1568.
26. Martin PM, Rollo FD. Estimation of thyroid depth and correction for I-123 uptake measurements. *J Nucl Med* 1977;18:919–924.
27. Hine GI, Williams JB. Thyroid radioiodine uptake measurements. In: Hine GJ, ed. *Instrumentation in nuclear medicine*, vol. 1. New York: Academic Press, 1967;327–350.
28. Ryo UY, Arnold J, Colman M, et al. Thyroid scintigram: sensitivity with sodium pertechnetate Tc-99m and gamma camera with pinhole collimator. *JAMA* 1976;235:1235–1238.
29. Favus MF, Schneider AB, Stachura ME, et al. Thyroid cancer occurring as a late consequence of head-and-neck irradiation: evaluation of 1056 patients. *N Engl J Med* 1976;294:1019–1025.
30. Maxon JR, Saenger EL, Thomas SR, et al. Clinically important radiation-associated thyroid disease. *JAMA* 1980;244:1802–1805.
31. Cicerio G, Grohman LA, Bekerman C, et al. Scintigraphic thyroid abnormalities after radiation: a controlled study with Tc-99m pertechnetate scanning. *Ann Intern Med* 1982;97:55–58.
32. Pinsky SM, Ryo UV. Technique and utility of thyroid scans. In: DeGroot L, Frohman LA, Kaplan EL, Refetoff S, eds. *Radiation-associated thyroid carcinoma*. New York: Grune & Stratton, 1977;297–785.
33. Karelitz JR, Richards JB. Necessity of oblique views in evaluating the functional status of a thyroid nodule. *J Nucl Med* 1974;15:782–785.
34. Blum M, Goldman AB. Improved diagnostic of "nondelineated" thyroid nodules by oblique scintillation scanning and echography. *J Nucl Med* 1975;16:713–715.
35. Grayson RR. Factors which influence the radioactive iodine thyroidal uptake test. *Am J Med* 1960;28:397–415.
36. Krugman LC, Hershman JM, Chopra U, et al. Patterns of recovery of the hypothalmic-pituitary-thyroid axis in patients taken off chronic thyroid therapy. *J Clin Endocrinol Metab* 1975;41:70–80.
37. Floyd JL, Rose PR, Brochert RD, et al. Thyroid uptake and imaging with iodine-123 standard. *J Nucl Med* 1984;26:884–887.
38. Robertson JS, Norlan NG, Wahner HW, et al. Thyroid radioiodine uptakes and scans in euthyroid patients. *Mayo Clin Proc* 1975;50:79–84.
39. Hamburger JI, Hamburger SW. Diagnosis and management of large toxic multinodular goiters. *J Nucl Med* 1985;26:888–892.
40. Fisher DA, Oddie TH, Johnson DE, et al. The diagnosis of Hashimoto's thyroiditis. *J Clin Endocrinol Metab* 1975;40:795–801.
41. Atkins HL, Klipper JR, Lambrecht RM, et al. A comparison of technetium-99m and iodine-123 for thyroid imaging. *Am J Roentgenol* 1973;117:195–201.
42. Arnold JE, Pinsky S. Comparison of Tc-99m and I-123 for thyroid imaging. *J Nucl Med* 1976;17:261–267.
43. Ryo UY, Vaidya P, Schneider AB, et al. Thyroid imaging agents: a comparison of I-123 and Tc-99m pertechnetate. *Radiology* 1983;148: 819–822.
44. Hurley PJ, Maisey MN, Natarajan TK, et al. A computerized system for rapid evaluation of thyroid function. *J Clin Endocrinol Metab* 1972;34: 354–360.
45. Schneider PB. Simple, rapid thyroid function testing with Tc-99m pertechnetate thyroid uptake ratio and neck/thigh ratio. *Am J Roentgenol* 1979;132:249–253.
46. Sucupiara MS, Camargo EE, Nickoloff EL, et al. The role of Tc-99m pertechnetate uptake in the evaluation of thyroid function. Work in progress. *Int J Nucl Med Biol* 1983;10:29–33.
47. McKitrick WL, Park HM, Kosegi JE. Parallax error in pinhole thyroid scintigraphy: a critical consideration in the evaluation of substernal goiters. *J Nucl Med* 1985;26:418–420.
48. Fuerstein IM, Harbert JC. Hypertrophied thyroid tissue in a thyroglossal duct remnant. *Clin Nucl Med* 1986;11:135.
49. Bouvier JF, You E, Peau JY, et al. Diffuse uptake of technetium-99m pertechnetate in a patient with metastases from thyroid carcinoma. *Clin Nucl Med* 1986;11:728–729.
50. Burke G. The triiodothyronine suppression test. *Am J Med* 1967;42: 600–608.
51. Blum M, Seltzer TF, Campbell CC, et al. Evaluation of euthyroid solitary autonomous nodule of the thyroid gland: importance of scintillation scanning and thyrotropin-releasing hormone testing. *JAMA* 1982; 247:1991–1993.
52. Burman KD, Adler RA, Wartofsky L. Hemiagenesis of the thyroid gland. *Am J Med* 1975;58:143–146.
53. Kirshmanurthy GT. Human reaction to bovine TSH (concise communication). *J Nucl Med* 1978;19:284–286.
54. Baschieri L, Benedetti E, DeLuca F, et al. Evaluation and limitations of the perchlorate test in the study of thyroid function. *J Clin Endocrinol Metab* 1963;23:786–791.
55. Lakshamana M, Schaffer A, Robbins J, et al. A simplified low iodine diet in I-131 scanning and therapy of thyroid cancer. *Clin Nucl Med* 1988;13:866–868.
56. Beierwaltes WH. The treatment of thyroid carcinoma with radioactive iodine. *Semin Nucl Med* 1978;8:79–103.
57. Leeper RD, Katsutaro S. Treatment of metastatic thyroid cancer. *Clin Endocrinol Metab* 1980;9:383–404.
58. Goldman JM, Line BR, Aamodt RL, et al. Influence of triiodothyronine withdrawal time on I-131 uptake post-thyroidectomy for thyroid cancer. *J Clin Endocrinol Metab* 1980;50:734–739.
59. Schneider AB, Line BR, Goldman JM, et al. Sequential serum thyroglobulin determinations, I-131 scans, and I-131 uptakes after triiodothyronine withdrawal in patients with thyroid cancer. *J Clin Endocrinol Metab* 1981;53:1199–1206.
60. Arnstein NB, Carey JE, Spaulding SA, et al. Determination of iodine-131 diagnostic dose for imaging metastatic thyroid cancer. *J Nucl Med* 1986;20:1764–1769.
61. Halpern SE, Preisman R, Hagan PL. Scanning dose and the detection of thyroid metastases. *J Nucl Med* 1979;20:1099–1100.
62. Nemee J, Rohling S, Zamrazil V, et al. Comparison of the distribution of diagnostic and thyroablative I-131 in the evaluation of differentiated thyroid cancers. *J Nucl Med* 1979;20:92–97.
63. Jeevannram RK, Shah DH, Sharma SM, Ganatra RD. Influence of initial large dose on subsequent uptake of therapeutic radioiodine in thyroid cancer patients. *Nucl Med Biol* 1986;13:277–279.
64. Park HM, Perkins OW, Edmonson JW, Schnute RP, Manatunga A. Influence of diagnostic radioiodine on the uptake of ablative dose of iodine-131. *Thyroid* 1994;4:49–54.
65. Fernandez-Ulloa M, Maxon HR, Mehta S, et al. Iodine-131 uptake by primary lung adenocarcinoma: misinterpretation of I-131 scan. *JAMA* 1976;236:857–858.
66. Preisman RA, Halpern SE, Shishido R, et al. Uptake of I-131 by a papillary meningioma. *Am J Roentgenol* 1977;129:349–350.
67. Acosta J, Chitkara R, Khan F, et al. Radioactive iodine uptake by a large cell undifferentiated bronchogenic carcinoma. *Clin Nucl Med* 1983;7:368–369.
68. Sing-Yung W, Kollin J, Coodley E, et al. I-131 total body scan: localization of disseminated gastric adenocarcinoma. Case report and survey of literature. *J Nucl Med* 1984;25:1204–1209.
69. Ashcraft MW, Van Herle AJ. Management of thyroid nodules II: scanning techniques, thyroid suppressive therapy, and fine needle aspiration. *Head Neck Surg* 1981;3:297–322.
70. Molitch ME, Bec JR, Dreisman M, et al. The cold thyroid nodule: an analysis of diagnostic and therapeutic options. *Endocr Rev* 1984;5: 185–199.
71. Moe R, Frankel S, Chacko A. Radionuclide thyroid angiograph: surgical correlation. *Arch Otolaryngol* 1984;110:717–723.
72. Kleiger PS, Wilson GA, Greenspan B. The usefulness of the dynamic phase in pertechnetate thyroid imaging for solitary hypofunctioning images. *Clin Nucl Med* 1989;17:617–622.
73. Ryo UY, Stachura ME, Schneider AB, et al. Significance of extrathyroidal uptake of Tc-99m and I-123 in the thyroid scan (concise communication). *J Nucl Med* 1981;22:1039–1042.
74. Shambaugh GE III, Quinn JL, Oyasu R, et al. Disparate thyroid imaging: combined with sodium pertechnetate Tc-99m and radioactive iodine. *JAMA* 1974;228:886–869.
75. Szonyi G, Bowers P, Allwright S, et al. A comparative study of Tc-99m and I-131 in thyroid scanning. *Eur J Nucl Med* 1982;7:444–446.

76. Thrall JH, Burman KD, Wartofsky L, et al. Discordant imaging of a thyroid nodule with I-131 and Tc-99m: concordance of I-131 and fluorescent scans. *Radiology* 1978;128:705–706.
77. Fawcett DH, Winsett MZ, Yudt WM, et al. Hyperthyroidism and the single lobe. *Clin Nucl Med* 1987;12:57–59.
78. Hamburger JI, Miller JM, Kini SR. Lymphoma of the thyroid. *Ann Intern Med* 1983;99:685–693.
79. Park HM, Tarver RD, Siddiqui AR, et al. Efficacy of thyroid scintigraphy in the diagnosis of intrathoracic goiter. *Am J Roentgenol* 1987;148:527–529.
80. Prakas R, Lakshmipathi N, Jena A, et al. Hyperthyroidism caused by a toxic intrathoracic goiter with a normal sized cervical thyroid gland. *J Nucl Med* 1986;27:1423–1427.
81. Woodruff JD, Rauh JT, Markley RI. Ovarian struma. *Obstet Gynecol* 1966;27:194–201.
82. Kempers RD, Dockerty MB, Hoffman DL, et al. Struma ovariascitic, hyperthyroid, and asymptomatic syndromes. *Ann Intern Med* 1970;72:883–893.
83. Yeh EL, Meade RC, Ruetz PP. Radionuclide study of struma ovarii. *J Nucl Med* 1973;14:118–121.

CHAPTER 9

Diagnostic Imaging of the Thyroid Gland

Arnold M. Noyek, David M. Finkelstein, Ian J. Witterick, and Joel C. Kirsh

The thyroid gland, with its superficial position in the neck, is accessible to clinical examination and fine-needle aspiration. Our current concepts of the anatomy and physiology of the thyroid gland, the development of new imaging modalities, and the refinement of established modalities enable the contemporary thyroid surgeon to select from a wide range of diagnostic imaging techniques in the diagnosis and treatment of thyroid disease. The clinician/surgeon must have a grasp of the strengths and limitations of the various imaging techniques, so that intelligent, cost-effective decisions can be made. This chapter focuses primarily on the imaging assessment of surgical disease, relying heavily on illustrations.

Diagnostic information derived from imaging data can be classified as either quantitative or qualitative. Quantitative information identifies anatomic parameters such as shape, size, location, and relationship to surrounding structures. Qualitative information identifies the biologic activity or functional nature of the disease. Both quantitative and qualitative details are obtained in the imaging assessment of thyroid disorders, especially in defining extent of disease pre- and posttreatment and in identifying a specific diagnosis to direct further intervention (1). A single study may provide quantitative information (as in the ultrasound of a thyroid nodule), qualitative information (as in the radionuclide study of thyroid nodule function), or both [as in the computed tomography (CT) assessment of thyroid malignancy invading the airway]. "Routine" studies provide only routine information; every meaningful study should be sensitively tailored to solve a specific clinical problem.

The challenge for clinician and imager is to choose, in consultation, the appropriate imaging modalities that will yield the maximal meaningful diagnostic data with minimal risk and expense. With careful technique, and good communication between clinician and imager, most thyroid disorders can be investigated to provide an effective description of the extent of disease (i.e., size: focal, multifocal, or diffuse), the physiology involved (i.e., a "hot" versus a "warm," "cool," or "cold" nodule), and the involvement of surrounding structures (e.g., airway, lymph nodes). Imaging techniques rarely provide "tissue" diagnosis with 100% accuracy, which highlights the integral relationship imaging has to medicine and surgery. Imaging data can and should be used to direct further investigation (e.g., the ultrasound-guided fine-needle aspiration), and treatment (e.g., total thyroidectomy versus a lesser procedure).

Thus, imagers are teammates with surgeons, pathologists, and other caregivers. Advances in the technology used to image the thyroid gland are exciting and create substantial, new opportunities for professional development in this ever-changing field. For the purpose of organization, thyroid imaging can be conveniently divided into modalities as follows:

1. conventional imaging
2. diagnostic ultrasound
3. computed tomography
4. magnetic resonance imaging
5. radionuclide imaging
6. angiography

INDEX TO THYROID IMAGING FIGURES IN THIS CHAPTER

There are a large number of figures in this chapter, and many have multiple illustrations. To allow the reader easy

---

A. M. Noyek: Department of Otolaryngology, University of Toronto, Mount Sinai Hospital, Toronto, Ontario, Canada M5G 1X5.

D. M. Finkelstein: Department of Surgery, Division of Otolaryngology, York County Hospital, Newmarket, Ontario, Canada, L3Y 5G8.

I. J. Witterick: Department of Otolaryngology, University of Toronto, Mount Sinai Hospital, Toronto, Ontario, Canada M5G 1X5.

J. C. Kirsh: Department of Diagnostic Imaging, The Credit Valley Hospital, Mississauga, Ontario, Canada, L5M 2N1.

access and better understanding, the following index lists the figures by clinical/pathologic context and imaging modality. All figures appear at the end of the chapter.

Normal Thyroid

Fig. 1. Normal transverse ultrasound of the thyroid gland and adjacent anatomy; ultrasound.
Fig. 2. Normal radionuclide thyroid scans; pertechnetate scan, I-123 scan.
Fig. 3. Pyramidal lobe; pertechnetate scan.
Fig. 4. Esophageal pertechnetate simulates thyroid abnormality; pertechnetate scan.

Ectopic Thyroid

Fig. 5. Lingual thyroid; conventional, pertechnetate scan.
Fig. 6. Radionuclide findings in lingual thyroid; pertechnetate scan.
Fig. 7. Thyroglossal duct cyst; ultrasound.
Fig. 8. Huge thyroglossal duct cyst; CT.
Fig. 9. Thyroglossal duct cyst with functioning thyroglossal duct remnant tissue; pertechnetate scan.
Fig. 10. Superior mediastinal thyroid cyst; CT.
Fig. 11. Enormous retrosternal multinodular goiter; conventional, CT, pertechnetate scan, digital subtraction angiogram (DSA).

Thyroid (Benign), Cysts

Fig. 12. Thyroid cyst pre- and postaspiration; the role of ultrasound; ultrasound.
Fig. 13. Hemorrhagic cyst; magnetic resonance (MR). Thyroid (Benign), Calcification.
Fig. 14. Calcified solid nodule; conventional, ultrasound.
Fig. 15. Calcified solid nodule; ultrasound.
Fig. 16. Calcified thyroid nodule without ultrasound entry; conventional, ultrasound.
Fig. 17. Dense but incompletely calcified thyroid nodule allowing ultrasound entry; ultrasound.

Thyroid (Benign), Solid

Fig. 18. Huge goiter with calcific nodule and displacement of trachea and esophagus; conventional.
Fig. 19. Small follicular adenoma and the limit of resolution of radionuclide scan; pertechnetate scan.
Fig. 20. Follicular adenoma and the role of ultrasound-guided fine-needle aspiration; pertechnetate scan, ultrasound.
Fig. 21. Large follicular adenoma, with small colloid nodule in opposite lobe upper pole; ultrasound.
Fig. 22. Large follicular adenoma; conventional, CT.
Fig. 23. Large degenerating follicular adenoma (cold nodule), and contralateral false-functioning follicular adenoma (false, hot nodule); pertechnetate scan, I-123 scan, ultrasound.
Fig. 24. Follicular adenoma and parathyroid adenoma; ultrasound.
Fig. 25. Follicular adenoma with cystic changes and hemorrhage; MR.
Fig. 26. Extrinsic mass (parathyroid adenoma) simulates intrinsic cold nodule; pertechnetate scan.

Thyroid (Benign), Functioning

Fig. 27. Two hot or functioning thyroid nodules, with comparison of radionuclide imaging studies; pertechnetate scan, I-131 scan, I-123 scan.
Fig. 28. Functioning nodule; I-123 scan, ultrasound.
Fig. 29. Functioning thyroid nodule; pertechnetate scan, I-123 scan.
Fig. 30. False-functioning thyroid nodule; pertechnetate scan, I-123 scan.

Malignant Thyroid Tumors; Imaging the Primary Tumor and Direct Extension

Fig. 31. Tracheal invasion by carcinoma of the thyroid; conventional.
Fig. 32. Anaplastic carcinoma of thyroid gland with intralaryngeal and intratracheal extension; pertechnetate scan, conventional.
Fig. 33. Medullary carcinoma of the thyroid; pertechnetate scan.
Fig. 34. Papillary carcinoma involving the isthmus; pertechnetate scan, ultrasound.
Fig. 35. Thyroid cyst with papillary carcinoma; ultrasound.
Fig. 36. Papillary carcinoma; MR.
Fig. 37. Papillary carcinoma with extracapsular extension; MR.
Fig. 38. Sclerosing papillary carcinoma with recurrent laryngeal nerve involvement; pertechnetate scan, ultrasound, MR.
Fig. 39. Follicular adenocarcinoma with retrosubclavian extension; pertechnetate scan, CT, digital subtraction angiogram.
Fig. 40. Histiocytic lymphoma; pertechnetate scan, CT, conventional.
Fig. 41. Anaplastic carcinoma of the thyroid gland with posterior extension; CT, MR.
Fig. 42. Carcinoma thyroid with tracheal invasion; MR.

Thyroid Carcinoma and Metastases

Fig. 43. Mixed papillary-follicular carcinoma with metastases to recurrent laryngeal lymph nodes; ultrasound.

Fig. 44. Occult papillary carcinoma of the thyroid presenting with a "cystic" lateral neck mass; pertechnetate scan, ultrasound, CT.

Fig. 45. Papillary carcinoma with cervical and superior mediastinal lymph node metastases; pertechnetate scan, ultrasound, CT.

Fig. 46. Impalpable metastatic carcinoma in middle deep cervical lymph node; MR.

Fig. 47. Metastatic thyroid carcinoma in lymph node; MR.

Fig. 48. Follicular adenocarcinoma of the thyroid gland with metastases; pertechnetate scan, I-131 scan, bone scan, conventional.

Fig. 49. Bony metastases; bone scan, conventional.

CONVENTIONAL IMAGING

Radiographs produced by conventional x-ray techniques are a simple, inexpensive, and widely available means to obtain selective information about thyroid dysfunction. Their use is limited to identifying two radiographic signs: (a) airway and esophageal displacement and/or invasion secondary to a thyroid soft-tissue mass, and (b) calcification within the thyroid or a thyroid-associated soft-tissue mass [anteroposterior (AP) and lateral neck radiographs].

The pattern of such calcification (coarse or fine; ringlike, irregular, or psammomatous) can suggest a diagnosis. For example, psammomatous calcifications may indicate a papillary thyroid carcinoma. Hence, conventional radiographs may suggest additional, more definitive imaging techniques. Clearly, however, conventional radiographs are not commonly used or suggested as a first-line test. Indeed, many of the signs discussed above are seen incidentally on conventional chest or cervical spine images.

ULTRASONOGRAPHY

Ultrasonography has a unique and valuable role in imaging the thyroid gland. It extends the palpating fingers of the clinician to provide excellent and reproducible anatomic images that are safe, comfortable for the patient, and moderate in cost (Fig. 1). The role of ultrasonography has evolved to provide important data in many clinical scenarios: to confirm or deny the presence of a questionable or difficult-to-palpate lesion; to accurately determine thyroid volume (2); to screen for occult disease in the "at risk" (i.e., previously irradiated) neck; to determine whether a palpated nodule is part of a focal, multifocal, or diffuse disease, and whether that nodule is solid, cystic, or calcified; to demonstrate properties of the contour of a nodule; to follow the size of a nodule over time (i.e., after suppression); to guide fine-needle aspiration (especially for posteriorly placed nodules) (3); to image lymph nodes and the thyroid bed after excision for malignancy (4–7); and to evaluate ectopic thyroid tissue (i.e., thyroglossal duct cysts) (Fig. 7).

The advent of "small parts" transducers (i.e., at 7.5 or 10 MHz) allows for excellent resolution of small nodules (down to a measurement of 3.0 mm for certain solid nodules or cysts) (8,9) much more reliably than clinical palpation or radionuclide studies. However, a major drawback of ultrasound is that, despite its high sensitivity in detecting lesions, it has a low tissue specificity and cannot be used to definitely differentiate benign from malignant disease (see later) (10–12).

Indications

Thyroid Volume

Palpation is relatively inaccurate for assessing thyroid volume (13). Various volume calculations may be applied using two-dimensional ultrasound measurements (14,15). The estimation of thyroid volume is of value in following patients with Graves' disease and is especially useful in titrating the dose of radioiodine for therapy (16). In addition, volume estimation is useful in assessing the response of diffuse nontoxic goiter to thyroid hormone (17), for screening for thyroid enlargement in pre-term infants (18) and in pregnancy (1), and in nationwide surveys (19). Yokoyama et al. (16) compared volume estimated by ultrasonic scanning (using a 7.5-MHz annular array transducer) to the actual weights of specimens removed at surgery and found excellent agreement between the two. Indeed, they calculated correlation coefficients as high as 0.99. Hence, ultrasonography should be considered the imaging modality of choice when assessing thyroid volume

Thyroid Nodules

The most common indication for thyroid ultrasonography is as a screening study for patients with a thyroid nodule (20). Recently, the continued practice of scanning these patients has elicited a lively and sometimes polarized debate in the literature. Current opinion has shifted in the last few years to accommodate the experience of many different workers in the field.

Thyroid nodules are relatively common and thyroid cancer is relatively uncommon. There is a high prevalence of clinically undetected nodular disease in the general population. Brander et al. (21) found thyroid echo abnormalities in 69 of 253 (27.3%) randomly selected adults with no clinical evidence of thyroid disease in an area of Finland where goiter was not endemic. The challenge clinicians face is to deduce which nodules have a high probability of being malignant (22).

The rationale for performing ultrasonography in the past was essentially based on two possibilities. First, ultrasound can be used to assess the remainder of a gland in which a solitary nodule has been palpated; the study may find other nodules in up to 50% of cases, or might suggest that the palpable nodule was part of a multinodular goiter (23–25) (Fig. 21). Second, ultrasonography can be used in the evaluation of solitary nodules that appear "cold" on radionuclide scanning, and differentiate solid from cystic lesions (12) (Figs. 12,14,15,23). Purely cystic lesions, less than 4.0 cm in diameter, have a very low incidence of malignancy (1% to 2%), whereas solid nodules are malignant in 12.5% to 32% of cases (23,26). This second possibility has been vigorously challenged in the last few years. Simeone and coworkers (27) studied 550 patients with thyroid nodules and found only one that they considered purely cystic; they felt that almost all thyroid cysts contained some old blood or tissue and suggested that this commonly occurred from degeneration of follicular adenomas. Another group described a higher incidence (12%) of malignancy in cystic lesions than had previously been reported (28). This was confirmed by Al Sayer et al. (8) who reported a higher incidence (33%) of malignancy in cystic lesions brought to the operating room.

There is some observer variation in ultrasound assessment of the thyroid gland. Jarlov et al. (29) found "moderate agreement" between observers evaluating solitary thyroid nodules by ultrasound. The observer agreement ranged from 0.80 to 0.91 and the kappa statistic ranged from 0.55 to 0.60. Furthermore, ultrasound does not necessarily detect all of the nodules found by the pathologist; some of these undetected nodules are malignant (30,31). Witterick et al. (30) compared palpation and ultrasound findings with the final pathology in 50 total-thyroidectomy specimens. Palpation and ultrasound detected only 24% and 43% respectively of the nodules identified by the pathologist. However, the expectation of detecting these nodules was not high because the median diameter of undetected nodules was less than 0.3 cm. In addition, the relevance of detecting small occult or multifocal papillary carcinomas is questioned, as their biologic significance is not known.

Many sonographic characteristics have been examined in detail to see if they provided clues to a nodule's underlying pathology. Some of the more carefully studied examples include the presence of a "halo" (a hypoechoic band) surrounding the nodule; the presence of cystic components; the presence of calcifications (Figs. 14–17); hypoechogenicity; the presence of heterogeneity within the internal echo pattern; an irregular or indistinct border; and massive extrathyroidal extension (32) (Fig. 38). Other than the last example (a rare but reliable sign of malignancy), these characteristics cannot be considered to be definitive in their demonstration of either the benign (i.e., a halo), or malignant (i.e., fine calcifications) character of a nodule. Common sense would dictate, however, that a lesion with many of the characteristics suggestive of malignancy (fine calcifications, an irregular border, solid) should be viewed with suspicion.

It has been suggested that color Doppler sonography may be a useful tool for differentiating malignant from benign disease on the basis of the hypervascular nature of malignant nodules. Unfortunately, several studies have shown this to be an unreliable indicator of malignancy (33,34). In addition, color Doppler has not been found to be useful in distinguishing thyroid gland from parathyroid gland (35).

Many groups now advocate needle biopsy aspiration for cytology in the evaluation of suspicious nodules (8,28,36). This has caused some to question the relevance of ultrasonographic findings (37). Fine-needle aspiration biopsy is considered by many clinicians to be the single most precise method for selecting patients for surgery (22). Interestingly, though, this emphasis has displayed a new use for ultrasound: to guide difficult biopsies (i.e., from small or posteriorly placed nodules) (8,9,38,39) (Fig. 12). Ultrasound guidance has also been used by some to guide the percutaneous injection of ethanol as treatment for both functioning (40) and nonfunctioning (41) nodules.

Other uses for ultrasound include the demonstration of normal thyroid gland in its usual expected anatomic location (or lack thereof). For example, in the assessment of thyroglossal duct abnormalities, ultrasound may obviate the need for the relatively more invasive nuclear scan in identifying the presence or absence of a normally positioned thyroid gland (42). Others have noted the efficacy of diagnosing lymphomas of the thyroid (43) and evaluating congenital hypothyroidism (44). Echographic patterns have been found to have prognostic significance in patients with Graves' disease (45). In addition, with the use of a small parts apparatus, ultrasound is now considered by many the method of choice in screening for small tumor recurrences or metastatic lymph nodes in the thyroid bed postthyroidectomy, or in the neck (4–7,46) (Figs. 43–45).

COMPUTED TOMOGRAPHY

Computed tomographic scanning has an important role to play in the diagnosis and staging of thyroid disorders. Although CT is generally not used as a "first line" imaging modality in this field, it can provide valuable data detailing extrathyroid tumor extension and/or invasion, and it is particularly effective in imaging disease in the superior mediastinum and regional cervical lymph nodes. A comparison of the strengths and weaknesses of CT and MR modalities will be presented at the end of the section on MR (see later).

General Principles

The thyroid has complex anatomic relationships with many structures in the neck; previous reviews give an excellent summary of these (47,48). The gland itself is readily identified on CT, having a denser appearance than the surrounding soft-tissue structures (23). Indeed, normal thyroid tissue has a CT number between 70 and 120 Hounsfield units (49), which is said to be a result of the gland's intrinsic high iodine content (50).

After the injection of intravenous contrast, the thyroid will enhance proportionately to the surrounding soft-tissue structures and hence will still appear denser than its surroundings (51). As one might predict, hypothyroid patients and those taking thyroid hormone supplements may have a lower density than normal controls (23). Also, as subjects age, the gland tends to store less iodine and hence appears less dense and less homogeneous (48). It is important to remember that a relatively large amount of an iodine-containing contrast agent may be used. These organic compounds partially deiodinate *in vivo* and can affect thyroid function for weeks to come (52,53). Contrast given for CT imaging too close to the time of I-131 treatment (e.g., for treatment of well-differentiated carcinoma) can affect the subsequent uptake of I-131 by residual local, regional, or metastatic disease.

Congenital Lesions

Computed tomography can be used to identify thyroglossal duct cysts and remnant thyroid within them, lingual thyroids, and other aberrant thyroid tissues (48,54), although radionuclide scanning is often used in some of these situations. On contrast-enhanced CT scans, these tissues, like a normal thyroid gland, will appear as high-attenuation masses. CT is particularly useful in defining the relationship of a thyroglossal duct cyst, or remnant thyroid, to the hyoid bone and base of tongue, two structures that are of obvious importance to surgical planning (48) (Fig. 8).

Thyroid Masses

A CT scan can provide precise and detailed information regarding the size, shape, location, and internal structure (solid versus cystic) of a thyroid mass; further, it can determine whether a mass is solitary or part of a multinodular process (23,48) (Fig. 22). It should be stressed that characteristics of an individual mass cannot be used to infer a histopathologic diagnosis, as there is too wide an overlap between benign and malignant lesions with respect to easily reproducible CT findings (such as solid versus cystic, relative density, and border contour) (23).

Computed tomography can, however, provide important clues to aid in diagnosis, and is unsurpassed in assessing the extent and invasion pathways of malignant disease. It has been suggested that malignant lesions have a more irregular border than do benign lesions (23). Further, the presence of certain ancillary findings may make a lesion highly suspicious for malignancy; these include the following:

1. The loss of integrity of the fascial planes between the thyroid and the adjacent muscles indicates muscle infiltration by tumor (23).
2. A CT scan can easily show destruction, infiltration, or displacement of the larynx, trachea, esophagus, common carotid artery, or internal jugular vein (23,48,55) (Fig. 39).
3. CT scans can reliably demonstrate retrosternal or retrotracheal extension of thyroid tumor and therefore can forewarn a surgeon about the need for a more radical surgical approach (i.e., a median sternotomy) (55) (Fig. 41).
4. CT can be used to assess both palpable and impalpable cervical and distant adenopathy (Fig. 45). CT can accurately assess size, location, and relationship to contiguous structures, and thus it can help stage the extent of disease and help the surgeon plan the extent of the operation, as the decision to perform various types of neck dissection is based on the presence and localization of metastatic nodes (23).
5. A CT scan can reliably locate both local and distant (e.g., lung, liver, brain) metastatic deposits (23,55).

Computed tomographic scanning can be useful in other situations not directly involved with evaluating a thyroid mass per se, but which bear upon the localization of malignant thyroid disease. CT can be used to evaluate a lower neck mass of unknown origin, and it can demonstrate a thyroid origin of some of these masses (48) (Fig. 44). Also, a baseline CT can be obtained 3 to 4 months after thyroidectomy, and then serial scans can be used to monitor tumor recurrences in the thyroid bed (55).

The CT scan also plays an important role in the preoperative assessment of large goiters (Fig. 11). As is the case with thyroid malignancies, CT can be used to assess compression of surrounding structures and mediastinal extension of disease (56). Bashist et al. (57) list six CT findings in intrathoracic disease: continuity with the cervical gland; well-defined borders; punctate coarse or ringlike calcifications; nonhomogeneous density, with well-defined low-density areas; attenuation values at least 15 HU greater than the surrounding muscles, which rise to at least 25 HU after the injection of contrast; and "cradling" of the goiter by the brachiocephalic vessels high in the mediastinum, with extension behind the great vessels to the paratracheal or retrotracheal areas.

MAGNETIC RESONANCE IMAGING

Rarely in the history of diagnostic imaging has a new technology been embraced with the enthusiasm that has been accorded to MR. Like CT, MR is a valuable "second line" imaging modality that is useful in defining extrathyroidal disease extension, and it is particularly good at defining relationships between a mass and surrounding vascular structures. In addition, MR can be used to examine regional lymph nodes and the morphology of intra- and extrathyroidal tumor.

Although the physics underlying MR transcends the space available here, a short summary of MR terminology is in order. When a strong magnetic field is applied to tissues, the protons or hydrogen nuclei tend to line up with a longitudinal magnetic vector as a result of an inherent magnetic moment being present from nuclear spin. When a radiofrequency pulse is then applied at 90 degrees to the magnetic force, the protons will "tip" into either a transverse or perpendicular configuration; however, this higher energy state cannot be maintained, and the protons soon realign with the magnetic force when the radiofrequency pulse is terminated (9). The realignment process causes the nuclei to emit radio waves at the same frequency of the initial radiofrequency pulse. This is the magnetic resonance signal. Hence, nuclear magnetic resonance is the spontaneous emission of energy in the form of radio signals by previously excited nuclei.

The period of time during which the nuclei liberate energy as they realign into their original position within the applied magnetic field is the relaxation period. The energy so liberated is detected by a radiofrequency receiver coil.

The T1 relaxation time is an exponential rate proportional to the time required for the magnetized nuclei to realign along the original axis of the static magnetic field. The T2 relaxation time is an exponential rate dependent on the loss of coherence among spins. Proton density (the number of protons per unit volume) has a direct linear relationship to the overall intensity of the emitted MR signal. Hence, tissues with a greater proton density (e.g., fat) demonstrate more intensity, whereas those with less proton density (e.g., compact bone) show less intensity. The time taken to degenerate from the high energy state to the normal configuration (T1), is called the longitudinal, thermal, or spin lattice time and appears to be specific for different tissues. In contrast, the T2 image is obtained by measuring the time protons remain resonating in phase after there is a rapid reduction of the proton's spin (9).

Normal Thyroid

Normal thyroid is reported to have a medium intensity on T1-weighted images, with a signal lower than surrounding fat and higher than the adjacent strap muscles (58). On T2-weighted images, the thyroid appears markedly more signal intense (brighter) than the strap muscles, more so than on T1-weighted images (59–61). Generally, the gland appears homogeneous on T1 images and usually homogeneous on T2 images; however, some normals are reported to have nonhomogeneous T2-weighted images (58).

Diffuse Parenchymal Disease

Different studies have noted the correlation between the increased signal intensity on both T1- and T2-weighted images and active Graves' disease (58,59). Charkes et al. (59) showed that the ratio of thyroid to muscle signal intensity was linearly related to both the serum thyroxine and the 24-hr radioactive iodine uptake. Noma et al. (60) have noted similar intensity findings and demonstrated the hypervascularity of Graves' disease on MR. They suggest that this finding can be used to differentiate Graves' from Hashimoto's disease.

In general, MR findings in thyroiditis are not specific; there is frequently increased glandular volume and signal inhomogeneity (62). In the three patients with subacute thyroiditis studied by Otsuka et al. (63), T1-weighted images showed regions with slightly increased intensity and irregular margins, whereas T2-weighted images showed markedly increased intensity at the same sites. Follow-up MR in two of the patients after the active phase of thyroiditis was over showed reversal of these findings.

Nodules

As would be expected, MR can show, in exquisite detail, the characteristics of single or multiple thyroid nodules (58,60,64) (Fig. 25). In particular, the use of a surface coil as a receiver element with a 1.5-tesla (T) unit, gives images with excellent resolution of small anatomic structures (60). MR is very precise in assessing thyroid volume in large multinodular goiters, making it potentially useful for monitoring nonsurgical treatment (65). As discussed above, ultrasound is also an excellent method to assess thyroid volume and is less expensive than MR.

Magnetic resonance can distinguish the size, shape, border contour, and location of a nodule, and it can demonstrate impingement upon contiguous structures (Figs. 38,41,42). However, as is the case with ultrasound and CT, the MR characteristics of a nodule can only hint at, but cannot prove, underlying histopathology (Figs. 36,37). In particular, both adenomas and carcinomas tend to have higher T2-weighted image intensities than surrounding normal thyroid tissue (58); however, there tends to be a large spectrum of intensities. T1-weighted images of nodules also show a wide variety of signal intensities, but high T1-intensities can be demonstrated when there has been hemorrhage or colloid degeneration of a nodule (58) (Figs. 13,25). One study of 77 patients with thyroid nodules found adenomas were always hyperintense on T2-weighted images but had variable signal intensity on T1-weighted images (65). The exception was Hürthle cell adenomas, which were hyperintense on both T1- and T2-weighted sequences. In some cases, MR can demonstrate pseudocapsules and capsular invasion.

Magnetic resonance (especially T1-weighted images) shows the interface between tumor and muscle in greater detail than CT (66). Because fibrous tissue has a short T2-weighted relaxation time (and a correspondingly low T2-weighted signal intensity), it has been suggested that T2-weighted images postoperatively may be a sensitive method to monitor recurrences (58,65). In addition, because of the superb soft-tissue definition, MR is an excellent method to image lingual thyroids (67,68).

Magnetic resonance, like CT, can be used to detect lymphadenopathy in the neck. Lymph nodes as small as 3.0 mm in diameter can be detected, although the distinction between malignant and reactive glands cannot be definitively made by MR (60).

COMPUTED TOMOGRAPHY VERSUS MAGNETIC RESONANCE

The roles of CT and MR in the evaluation of thyroid disease, which have been detailed by Friedman et al. (55), are remarkably similar: to determine the location of a nodule and its impingement on or invasion of contiguous structures; to evaluate substernal or retrotracheal extension of a nodule or goiter; to detect regional metastatic disease and lymphadenopathy; and to monitor local recurrence. What are the advantages and disadvantages, then, of each modality?

Computed tomographic scans are widely available, familiar to most radiologists, and less expensive than MR. In addition, they show calcifications better than MR. However, CT is prone to streak artifact caused by motion, and beam hardening (60), and it may need contrast enhancement for delineation of vascular structures.

Magnetic resonance provides exquisite soft-tissue detail and an unsurpassed view of tumor–muscle interface. Further, it can be used without intravenous contrast and does not expose the patient to ionizing radiation (69). In addition, MR can provide direct coronal images and can demonstrate the neck, cervicothoracic junction, and superior mediastinum on just one or two images (58). MR is excellent for vascular imaging: flowing blood creates a signal void. However, MR is expensive, needs special housing units, and is not widely available in some locales. Some patients cannot bear the claustrophobic conditions in the MR suite, and others cannot have an MR because of indwelling metal prostheses.

Either CT or MR will provide the necessary information a clinician needs to further direct diagnostic and/or therapeutic procedures. There is no clear superiority of one technique over another in thyroid imaging.

RADIONUCLIDE IMAGING

Radionuclide imaging remains a first-line modality in the investigation of many thyroid disorders. This is the only imaging modality that provides physiologic as well as anatomic data, and hence it provides valuable information to direct further studies, treatment, and follow-up (55,70–72). Radionuclide scanning is useful in diverse clinical situations (73,74). This imaging modality can be used in the investigation of diffuse hyperfunctioning glands, focal areas of both hyper- and hypofunction within a gland, ectopic function (e.g., lingual thyroid), and extension of a thyroid mass into the superior mediastinum. In addition, radiopharmaceuticals can be used in the treatment of cancer and Graves' disease, and as a screening study for metastatic deposits.

Common Radionuclides Useful in Thyroid Imaging

Technetium-99m Pertechnetate

Technetium-99m (Tc-99m) pertechnetate, a radionuclide imaging agent, is the most widely used biologic tracer in thyroid scintigraphy, and it is particularly useful as a screening examination. It is inexpensive, widely available, has a short (approximately 1-hr) test time, and delivers a low dose of radiation to the patient (9,55,71). Tc-99m pertechnetate scans can discern a variety of lesions, with a resolution approaching 5.0 mm under favorable conditions. Pertechnetate is trapped by the thyroid gland but is not organified; hence, only a radioiodide scan can show the true physiologic status of the patient's gland. This accounts for the occasional discordance seen between Tc-99m pertechnetate and radioiodide scans (see later) (70). Also, the target-to-background ratio is less favorable in Tc-99m pertechnetate scans than in radioiodide scans, and this may lead to errors of interpretation, especially around the base of the tongue (70).

Iodine-123

The radionuclide iodine-123 (I-123) provides a true physiologic picture of the thyroid tissue being scanned. Moreover, it has a favorable half-life (13.2 hr), which allows for relatively rapid scanning after an oral dose, and it gives a scan with excellent resolution and minimal background (9,55). I-123 produces no particulate emissions and hence delivers an acceptable radiation dose to the patient (75). Disadvantages of I-123 include high cost, minimal shelf life, and occasional radionuclide contaminants (70); however, in recent years, the cost of I-123 has become less prohibitive, and it has become more readily available. Its advantages far outweigh its disadvantages and it remains an excellent definitive choice for physiologic thyroid imaging.

Iodide-131

Iodide-131 (I-131), a beta-emitter, played an important role in the historical developments of thyroid radionuclide imaging (71). It is relatively inexpensive, but it also delivers high-energy gamma photons to the patient, as well as beta-emissions. Further, the high-energy gamma photons tend to be poorly resolved by the gamma camera and, thus, I-131 studies tend to have poor resolution. These factors make I-131 a poor choice for use as an imaging agent, but it maintains an important role in routine quantitative assessment of radioactive iodine uptake (RAIU). This isotope still finds use in the treatment of Graves' disease and toxic adenoma and in the detection and treatment of well-differentiated thyroid cancer.

Clinical Uses

Diffuse Disorders

Radionuclide imaging has been used to delineate the thyroid gland in cases of hyperthyroidism, in conjunction with clinical and biochemical examination. In Graves' disease, the stimulatory immunoglobulins induce hormonogenesis in the gland; hence, both increased trapping and organification are noted (70). Thus, there is a diffuse increased uptake on both Tc-99m pertechnetate and radioiodide studies (70,76). In contrast, toxic multinodular goiter presents as focal areas of increased uptake on both Tc-99m and radioiodide scans, with the intervening tissue being cold or nonfunctioning as a result of feedback suppression (76). Interestingly, in the Jod-Basedow phenomenon, when a patient has unwittingly or purposefully ingested large amounts of iodine, the gland has a very low uptake of all radionuclides, having been saturated by the exogenous source (70).

Radionuclide scans find less use in hypothyroidism. Hashimoto's thyroiditis may present on scans in any number of ways, with diffuse or focal areas of increased or decreased uptake; indeed, Ramtoola et al. (77) have termed such scans "the great mimic" for their protean presentations.

Congenital Disorders

Technetium-99m pertechnetate or iodine scanning can be used to detect ectopic thyroid tissue, as may be found in thyroglossal duct cysts and lingual thyroids (Figs. 5,6,9). In addition, scanning identifies whether a normally positioned and functioning thyroid gland is present.

The Thyroid Nodule

There is controversy as to whether thyroid scanning is required at all in the initial investigation of nodular thyroid disease (55,78). Conventionally, thyroid nodules are classified at imaging with respect to the relative amount of activity present. The four functional categories include: hot/hyperfunctional (nodule concentrates more radionuclide than the normal portions of the gland); warm/functional/nondelineated (nodule concentrates radionuclide equally as well as the normal portions of the gland); cool/hypofunctional (nodule concentrates some radionuclide but less than normal portions of the gland); and cold/nonfunctional (no concentration of radionuclide by the nodule) (73). Warm, cool, and cold nodules should all be considered cold in subsequent management of the patient.

Technetium-99m pertechnetate is readily available, making it the initial imaging agent for many centers. When a Tc-99m pertechnetate scan reveals no abnormality or a cool/cold nodule, usually no further radionuclide study is indicated. Cold nodules are usually nonfunctional neoplasms or cysts. They carry a risk of malignancy ranging from 1.5% to 38.1%, depending on the series (71). A reasonable estimate would be that between 10% and 20% of cold nodules prove to be malignant (9,71). Hypofunctioning isthmic nodules may be missed, unless suspected on palpation, because there is normally little visible uptake in the isthmus. Palpation of the thyroid by the nuclear physician is essential for accurate correlative imaging (73).

Warm or hot nodules on Tc-99m pertechnetate scanning should be reinvestigated with I-123 to assess the physiologic status of the nodule (7,26). Some well-differentiated thyroid carcinomas retain the ability to trap pertechnetate, and hence may be warm or hot on Tc-99m pertechnetate scans (72). The vast majority of these malignancies will prove to be cold on I-123 scanning (Fig. 30). These discordant nodules should be considered cold in the subsequent management of the patient. Rare reports have been cited in which a malignant nodule is hot on both Tc-99m and radioiodine scans (79,80). Hot nodules are more commonly adenomas [either thyroid-stimulating-hormone (TSH)-dependent or autonomous], or a toxic solitary nodule (70) (Figs. 20,27,29).

Iodine-131 has an important role to play in the management of well-differentiated (papillary and follicular) thyroid carcinoma. Medullary and anaplastic thyroid carcinoma rarely concentrate I-131. After total thyroidectomy for well-differentiated thyroid carcinoma, I-131 scanning may be used to assess for local, regional, and distant metastases (81). Patients should be off thyroid medication for a sufficient period prior to the study to elevate TSH levels and increase the uptake of I-131 into any residual functioning thyroid tissue. A diet low in iodine prior to the scan is also of benefit. The scan may be performed after administration of a tracer dose or after an ablative dose of I-131. For scanning alone, 2 to 5 millicuries (mCi) of I-131 is given p.o., and whole-body imaging is performed approximately 72 hours later (Fig. 48). If residual functioning thyroid tissue is identified, a treatment dose (e.g., 30 to 149 mCi) of I-131 is generally given. Alternatively, some clinicians routinely give these patients a treatment dose of I-131 and perform whole-body imaging approximately 7 days later (81). See Chapter 31 for a more detailed discussion.

Investigational Radionuclides

Numerous radionuclides are being studied that may prove useful in the diagnosis and treatment of thyroid disorders. Other radiopharmaceuticals such as Tc-99m-sestamibi and thallium-201 (Tl-201) have been studied with the hope of differentiating benign from malignant nodular disease. Tl-201 has proven to be well incorporated into lesions that are cold on Tc-99m scan (55) and for visualizing solitary autonomous nodules after TSH stimulation (82). One report contends that by combining the information from both early and delayed Tl-201 images, differentiation between benign and malignant cold nodules is feasible (83). Others have attempted to label monoclonal antibodies against thyroglobulin with radionuclides (84). Unfortunately, no radiopharmaceutical has achieved sufficient sensitivity or specificity in differentiating benign from malignant nodular disease to alter current clinical practice (85,86).

Several agents have been used in the attempt to image medullary thyroid carcinoma (MTC) in either its primary focus or metastases (87). These include Tl-201 (88), Tc-99m pentavalent dimercaptosuccinic acid [Tc-99m (V) DMSA] (89,90), 131-I-metaiodobenzyl guanidine (I-131-M MIBG) (91), Tc-99m sestamibi (92), somatostatin receptors (93–95) and indium-111-labeled monoclonal antibodies to carcinoembryonic antigen (97–100). Although there has been some very promising progress made with these agents, further study and clinical trials are required to confirm their diagnostic efficacy.

ANGIOGRAPHY

Regional angiography, with or without digital subtraction, plays a small but specialized role in the evaluation of thyroid disease. As would be expected, the major use for this modality is the delineation of the vascular relations surrounding and/or involving a thyroid mass, as well as examining disease extension into the mediastinum (Figs. 11,39). However, Morita (101) was able to correctly differentiate benign from malignant nodules 94.7% of the time by examining the morphologic character of the feeding vessel, the margin of the tumor blush, and the density of the tumor blush with contrast. Further clinical trials are required to fully assess these findings. The role of magnetic resonance angiography has not yet been defined.

POSITRON EMISSION TOMOGRAPHY

Relatively few centers have the resources or expertise to perform positron emission tomography (PET) of thyroid masses. Adler and Bloom (102) studied nine patients with thyroid nodules prior to surgical excision with PET after administration of [^{18}F]-2-deoxy-2-fluoro-D-glucose (FDG). Three patients had papillary cancers and the remainder had benign disease (four follicular adenomas, two multinodular goiters with dominant nodules). Increased FDG uptake was seen in the three cancers and four of the six benign nodules. The mean dose/uptake ratio (DUR) for the three cancers was significantly higher than for the benign nodules. Further research is required to fully assess this technology in the differentiation of benign from malignant disease.

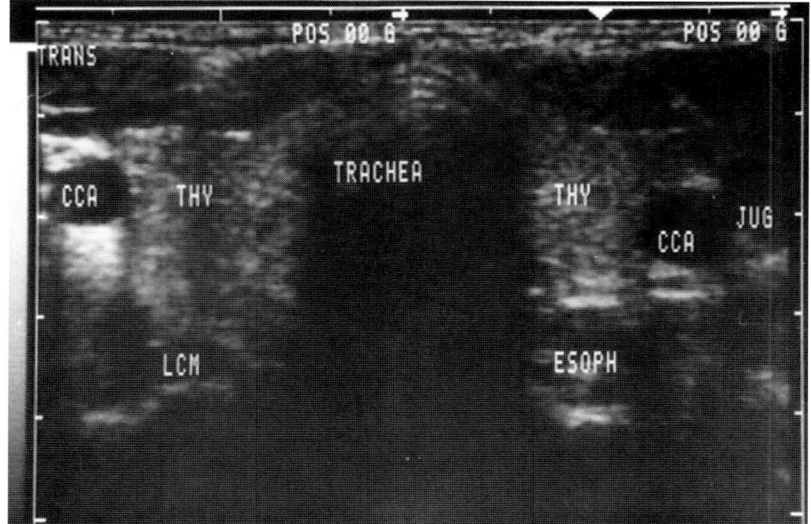

FIG. 1. Normal transverse ultrasound of the thyroid gland and adjacent anatomy. The impedance characteristics of the thyroid gland allow its imaging in relation to other structures. The overlying strap muscles are easily identified. THY, normal right and left thyroid lobes; ESOPH, esophagus (it lies, as anticipated, just to the left of the midline); LCM, longus colli muscle; CCA, right and left common carotid arteries; JUG, left internal jugular vein.

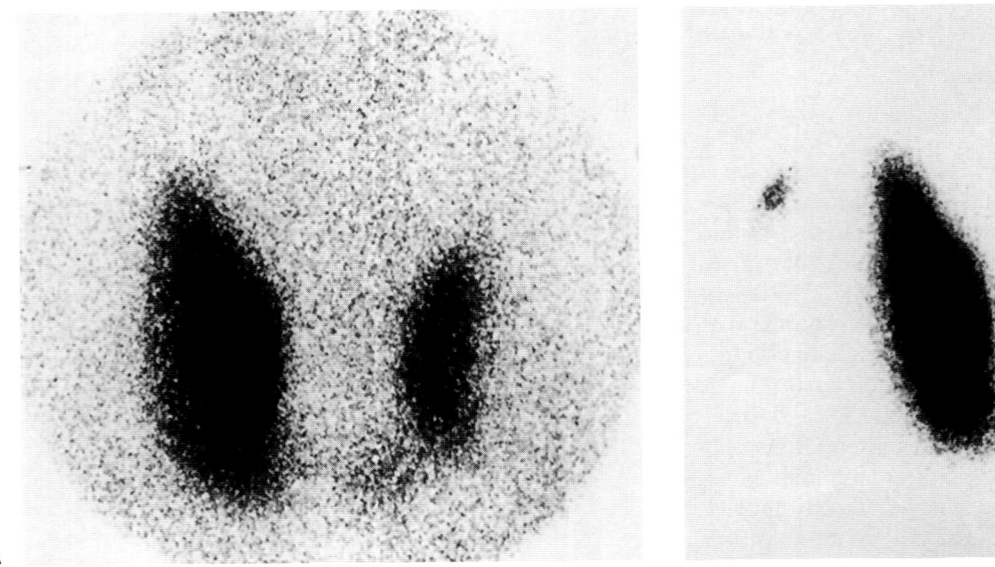

FIG. 2. Normal radionuclide thyroid scans. **A:** A sodium pertechnetate Tc-99m thyroid scan demonstrates a normal thyroid gland in a 45-year-old man. The right lobe is larger than the left. The isthmus is poorly visualized, a common finding resulting from minimally functioning tissue in the plane of the image. There is considerable background noise. **B:** An I-123 scan identifies the identical structural features, and the image is much clearer. (From ref. 103, with permission.)

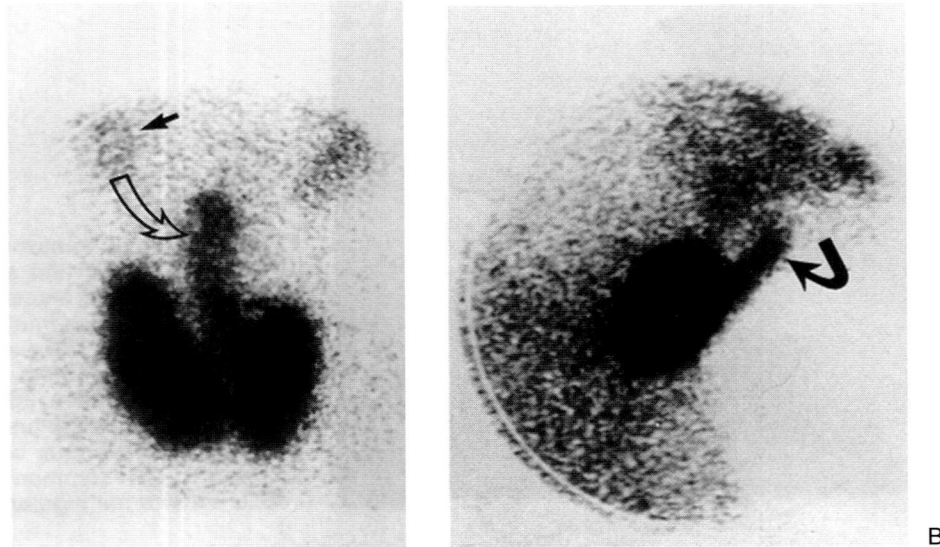

FIG. 3. Pyramidal lobe. **A:** An anterior view of a pertechnetate thyroid scan demonstrates normal trapping of the anion by the right and left thyroid lobes; the right lobe is slightly bigger than the left. A midline pyramidal lobe extends superiorly *(hollow, curved arrow)*. There is radionuclide accumulation in the right submandibular gland *(small arrow)*. **B:** A lateral view identifies the pyramidal lobe *(curved arrow)* on the same study. (From ref. 103, with permission.)

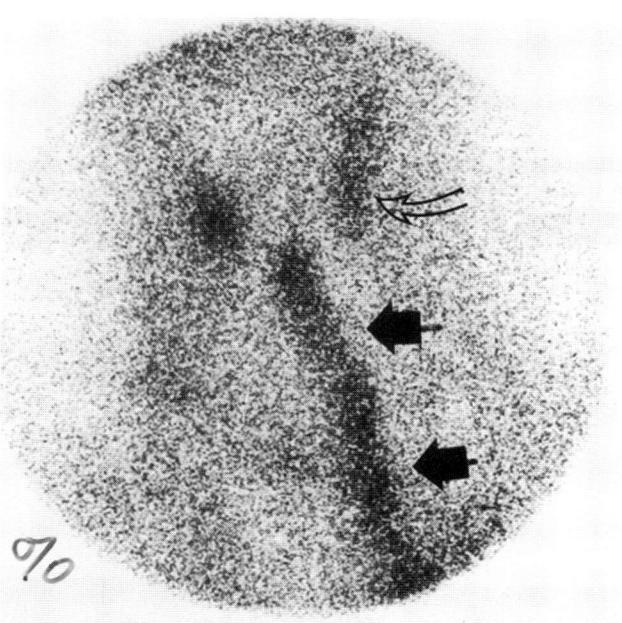

FIG. 4. Esophageal pertechnetate simulates thyroid abnormality. An anterior view of a sodium pertechnetate Tc-99m thyroid scan demonstrates a long, somewhat vertically oriented area of radionuclide uptake *(solid arrows)* in thyroid location. The *curved arrow* indicates the left submandibular gland in this anterior view. The remainder of the thyroid gland is suppressed in this patient who is taking exogenous thyroid hormone. After a drink of water, the esophagus was washed out and the pertechnetate-contaminated saliva swallowed. (From ref. 103, with permission.)

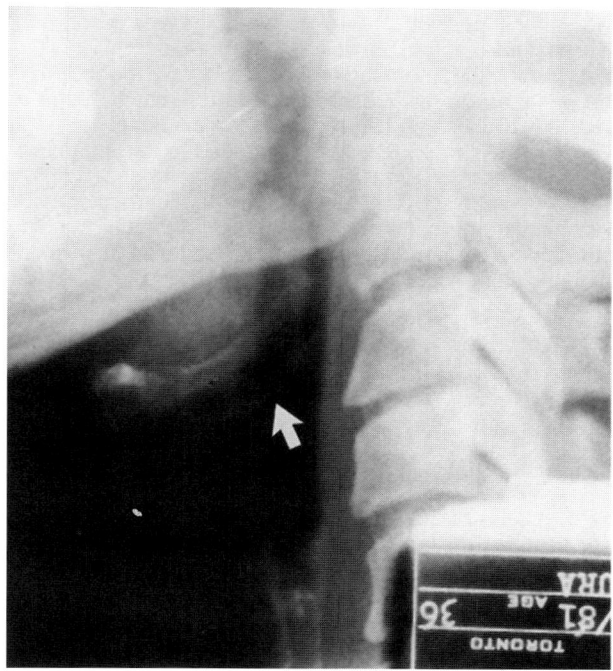
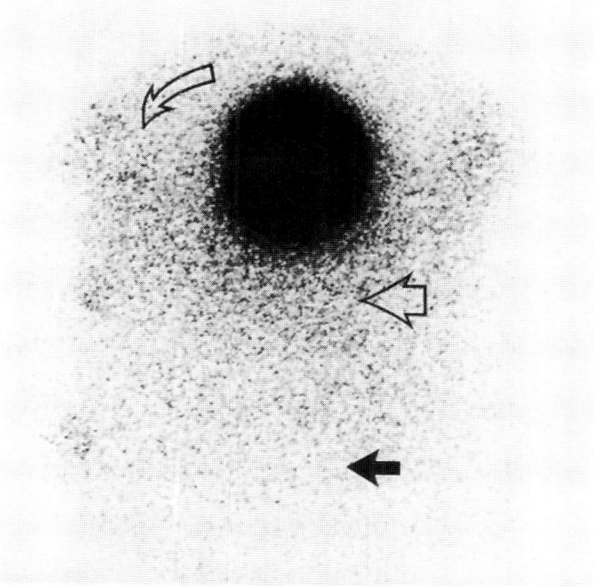

FIG. 5. Lingual thyroid. A: A conventional lateral soft-tissue radiograph demonstrates a smooth mass in the region of the base of the tongue that depresses the epiglottis inferiorly *(arrow)*. B: An anterior view of a pertechnetate scan demonstrates the intense anterior midline activity resulting from trapping of the pertechnetate anion within a midline lingual thyroid gland. The *hollow curved arrow* indicates the region of the right submandibular gland. The *hollow straight arrow* indicates the level of the hyoid bone. The *solid arrow* indicates the anticipated level of the thyroid gland; there is no function at this level as there is no thyroid gland present in normal position. The patient is a 36-year-old woman with a complaint of a lump in the throat. (Part A from ref. 103, with permission.)

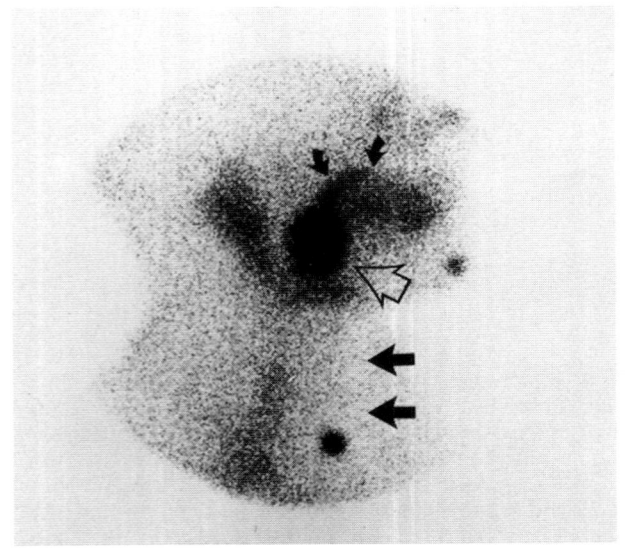
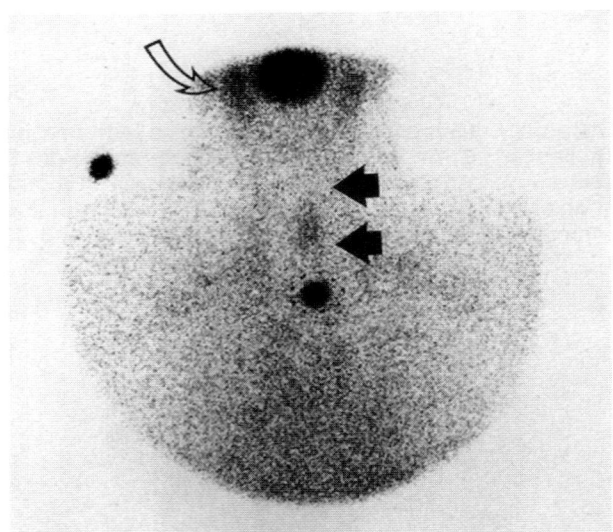
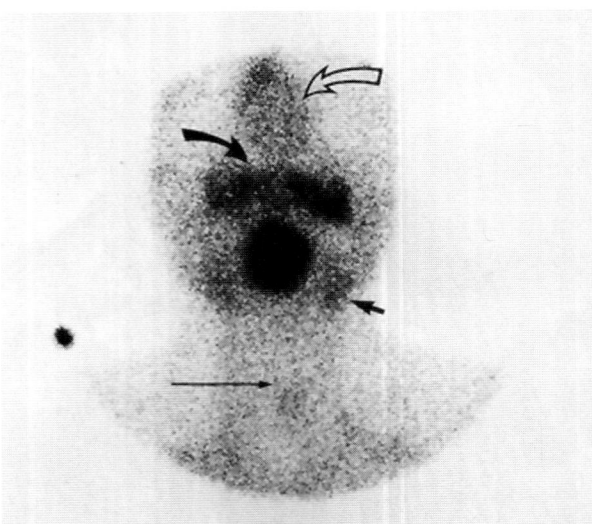

FIG. 6. Radionuclide findings in lingual thyroid. **A:** A lateral view of a pertechnetate scan indicates a mass in the base of the tongue *(hollow arrow)* that traps pertechnetate. The dorsal surface of the tongue is seen *(curved arrows)* as it is covered with hot saliva excreted from the salivary glands. There is no thyroid in the normal anticipated location on this lateral view *(heavy black arrows)*. There is a marker on the chin and in the suprasternal notch. **B:** An anterior view of the thyroid region, with the neck in extension, demonstrates the mass in the base of the tongue at the level of the submandibular glands; the *hollow arrow* indicates the right submandibular gland. There is no thyroid tissue in anticipated cervical position *(heavy arrows)*. There is a hot marker in the suprasternal notch, as well as a right marker. **C:** Following a sialagogue, the submandibular glands are still imaged, but most of the radionuclide has cleared into the oral cavity *(solid curved arrow)*. There is also pertechnetate within the nasal cavity *(hollow curved arrow)*. The *short arrow* indicates the left submandibular gland. The *long thin arrow* demonstrates the absence of function in the plane of the anticipated location of the thyroid gland. A positive pertechnetate scan in the diagnosis of lingual thyroid does not need to be confirmed by radioactive iodine scan. The findings are usually quite specific.

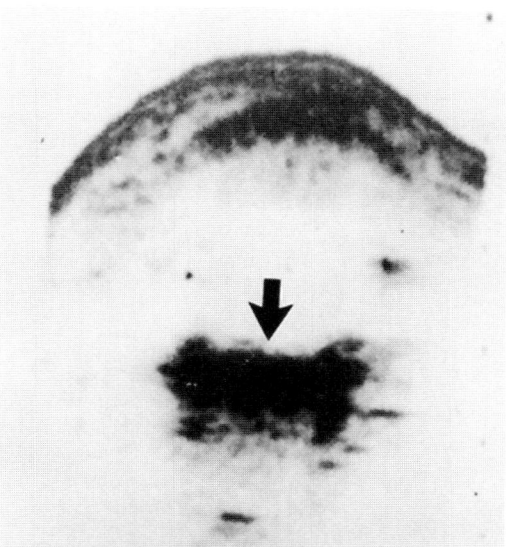

FIG. 7. Thyroglossal duct cyst. A transverse ultrasound examination identifies a relatively sonolucent lesion in infrahyoid position. The occasional internal echoes reflect inspissated debris within a thyroglossal duct cyst. The *arrow* indicates the strong back wall definition resulting from through-transmission of sound in this 27-year-old woman.

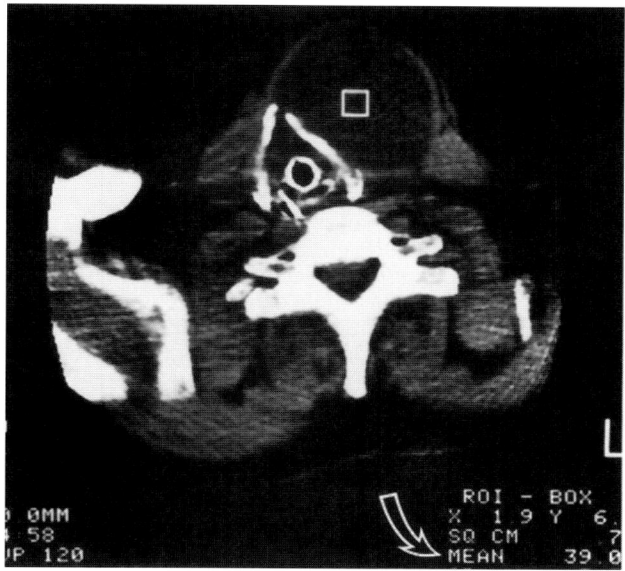

FIG. 8. Huge thyroglossal duct cyst. An axial computed tomography (CT) cut demonstrates a huge, reduced-density cystic lesion *(cursor)* occupying the bulk of the anterior midline cervical structures and displacing the larynx to the right. An endotracheal tube has been positioned in this patient, who presented in coma with a cerebrovascular accident. The attenuation reading of the lesion *(curved arrow)* indicates a density of 39 Hounsfield units; this is above water density but less than usual thyroid density. (From ref. 103, with permission.)

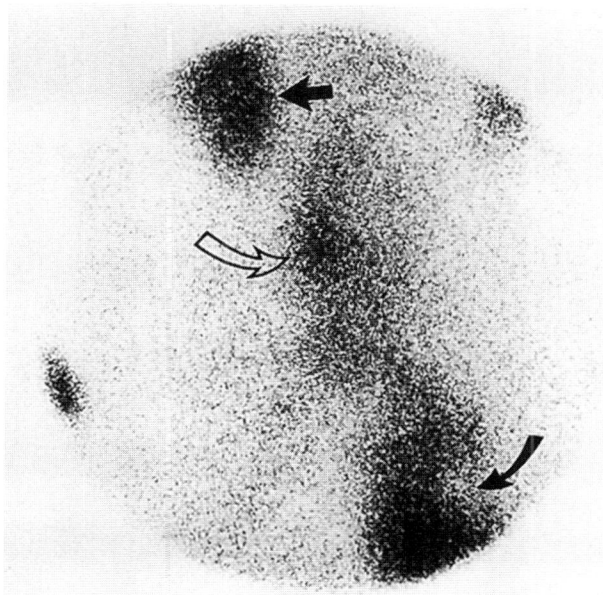

FIG. 9. Thyroglossal duct cyst with functioning thyroglossal duct remnant tissue. An anterior view of a sodium pertechnetate thyroid scan demonstrates a midline functioning lesion in a thyroglossal duct cyst at the level of the hyoid bone *(open curved arrow)*. The gamma camera is centered about the hyoid region. The *upper solid arrow* indicates the right submandibular gland and its accumulation of pertechnetate. The *solid curved arrow* demonstrates a cold (hypofunctioning) defect within the left thyroid lobe. No right thyroid lobe is seen. (From ref. 103, with permission.)

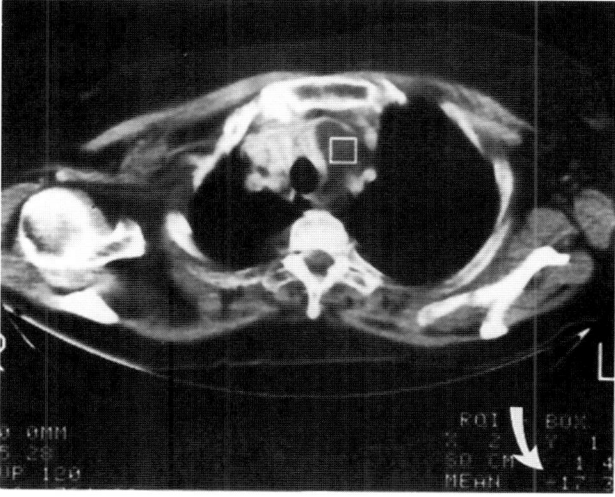

FIG. 10. Superior mediastinal thyroid cyst. An 88-year-old woman presented with a left recurrent laryngeal paralysis. An axial CT scan at the level of the superior mediastinum demonstrates a cystic lesion *(square region-of-interest cursor)*. It has a mean density *(arrow)* of -17 Hounsfield units, compatible with a cyst. The lesion was removed by a transcervical approach, relieving the patient's recurrent laryngeal paralysis within 3 months.

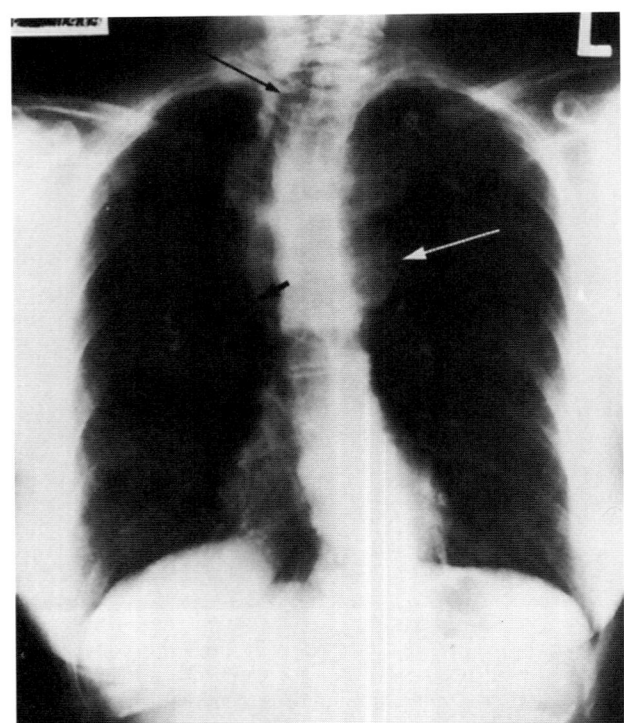
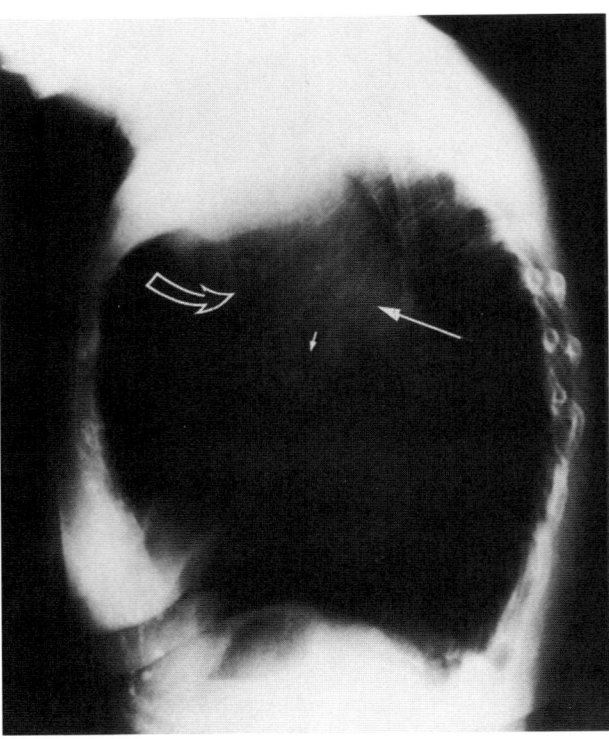

FIG. 11. Enormous retrosternal multinodular goiter. **A:** A posteroanterior (PA) film of the chest identifies the trachea at the level of the thoracic inlet *(long thin black arrow)* and the deformation of the trachea just above the carina *(short black arrow)*. The superior mediastinum is occupied by a soft-tissue mass in relation to the aortic arch *(white arrow)*. **B:** A lateral view of the chest demonstrates the mass *(long white arrow)* and its relationship to the trachea *(hollow curved arrow)*, and the left main bronchus inferiorly *(tiny arrow)*. **C:** An axial CT cut demonstrates diminished density *(black arrow)* within a large mediastinal mass. The trachea is deformed and pushed to the right *(white arrow)*. The left common carotid artery is identified by the *hollow arrow*. **D:** A lower CT cut identifies the trachea *(curved white arrow)*, and the aortic arch *(straight black arrow)*. The two *tiny white arrows* indicate calcification laterally, and the *curved black arrow* demonstrates calcification medially in the wall of the aorta. The *long white arrow* indicates the relationship to the esophagus. The variably reduced density within the mass is typical of multinodular goiter. **E:** A pertechnetate thyroid scan has a large marker positioned in the suprasternal notch; the inferior margin of the marker is indicated by the *thin black arrow*. The *hollow arrow* indicates the reduced uptake of the left thyroid lobe. The *heavier long arrow* indicates reduced uptake in the right thyroid lobe. The *short wide arrow* indicates the superior mediastinal extension of this mass, and also confirms its thyroid origin. **F:** A digital subtraction angiogram (DSA) injected via the superior vena cava *(curved arrow)* demonstrates the arch of the aorta *(hollow arrow)* and the carotid vessels on each side, which are splayed apart by the thyroid mass. The *long straight arrow* indicates the superior thyroid artery on the right, and the two *short straight arrows* demonstrate a large inferior thyroid artery supplying the mass. There are no parasitic vessels to the mass in the mediastinum. The patient is a 72-year-old woman presenting with an increasing history of stridor over 3 years.

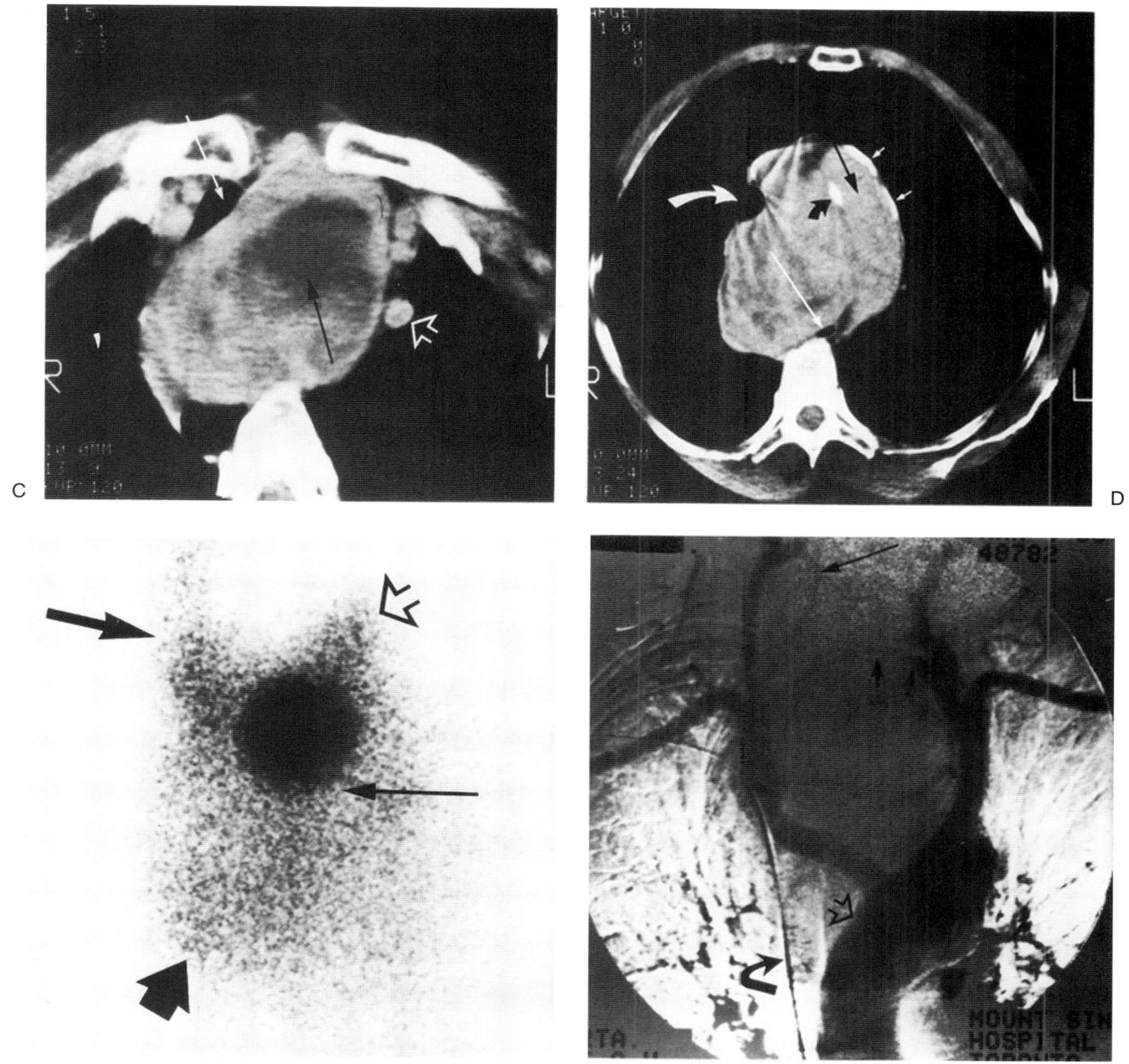

FIG. 11. Continued.

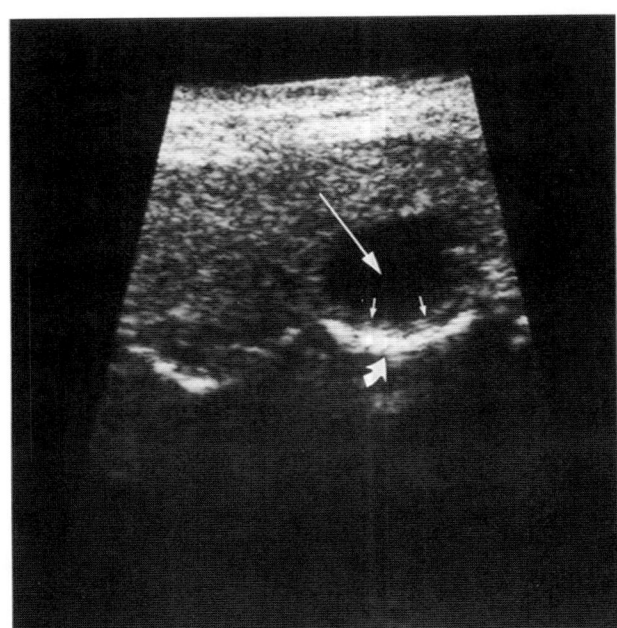
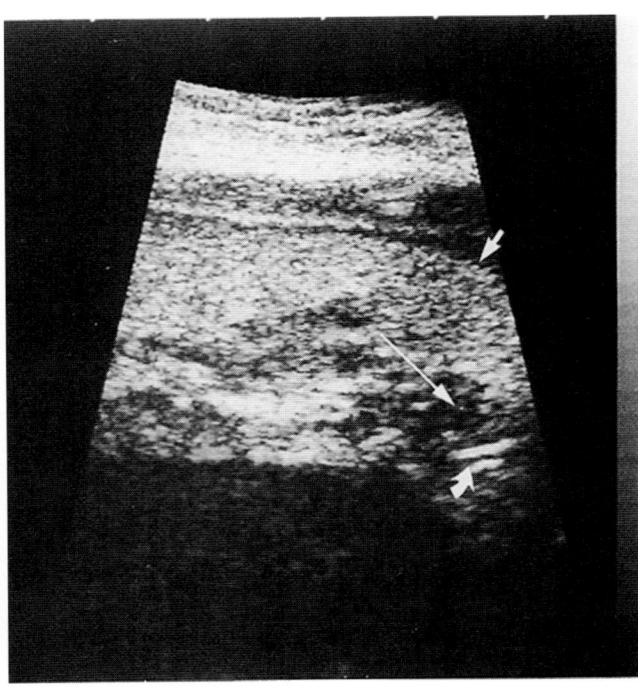

FIG. 12. Thyroid cyst pre- and postaspiration. **A:** A sagittal (longitudinal) ultrasound reveals a cyst *(long arrow)* posteriorly positioned toward the lower pole of the left thyroid lobe. The intrathyroidal nature of this sonolucent lesion is identified by the rim of residual posteriorly marginating thyroid gland *(tiny arrows)*. The adjacent longus colli muscle *(heavy curved arrow)* is identified. **B:** The dates have been left on the images. Six weeks after aspiration, the cyst has disappeared *(long arrow)*. The longus colli muscle is again identified in the same position by the *curved arrow.* The *small straight arrow* indicates the anteroinferior aspect of the thyroid gland in the region of the lower pole. This is well defined against the overlying strap muscle. Ultrasound is useful in the aspiration of cysts and in their follow-up.

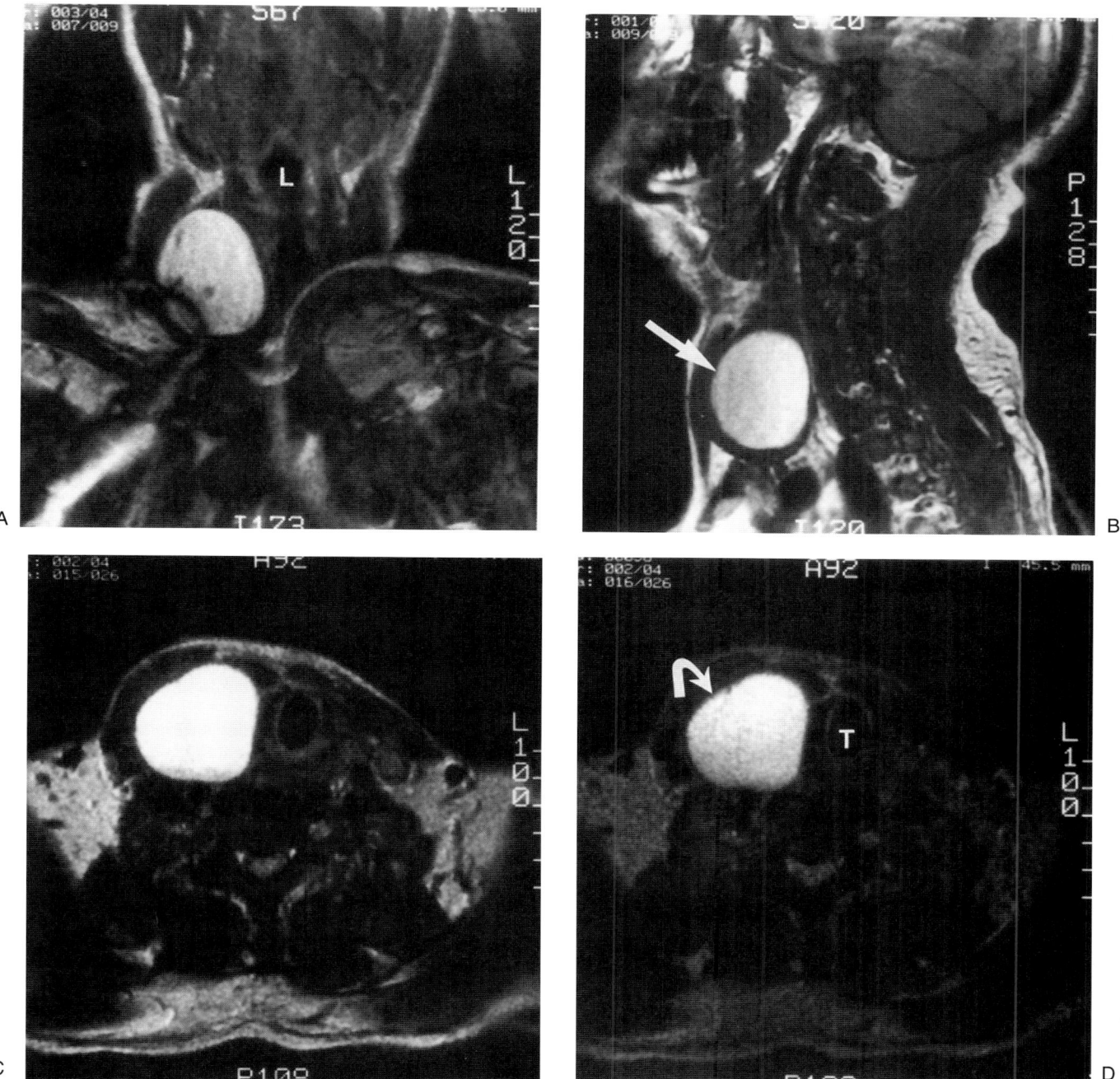

FIG. 13. Hemorrhagic cyst. **A:** A coronal T1-weighted magnetic resonance (MR) image in a spin-echo imaging sequence identifies a bright signal emanating from a large, smoothly outlined mass in the right thyroid lobe. TR = 600, TE = 20. **B:** A sagittal T1-weighted image demonstrates the morphology of the mass *(arrow)*. **C:** An axial proton-density MR image (TR = 2000, TE = 35) demonstrates the extremely bright signal emanating from the cystic lesion. **D:** An axial T2-weighted image (TR = 2000, TE = 70) demonstrates the same anatomic level as in C. The cystic lesion does not lose its signal, and thus a high protein content is indicated. (Courtesy of Dr. Walter Kucharczyk and the Toronto MR Centre, University of Toronto, Toronto, Ontario, Canada.)

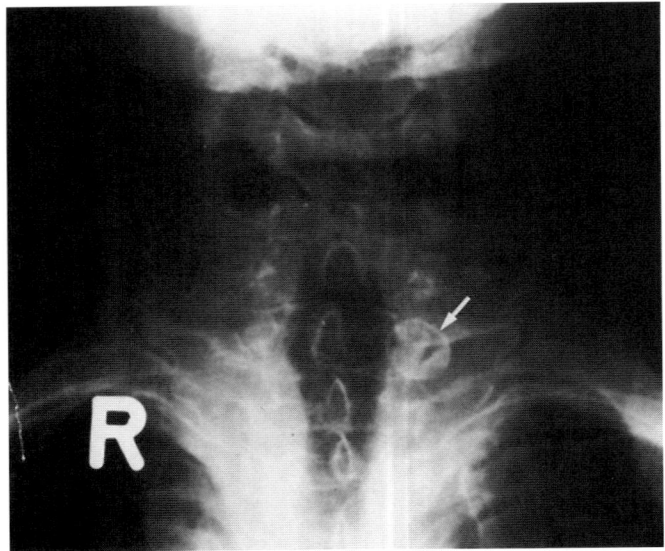

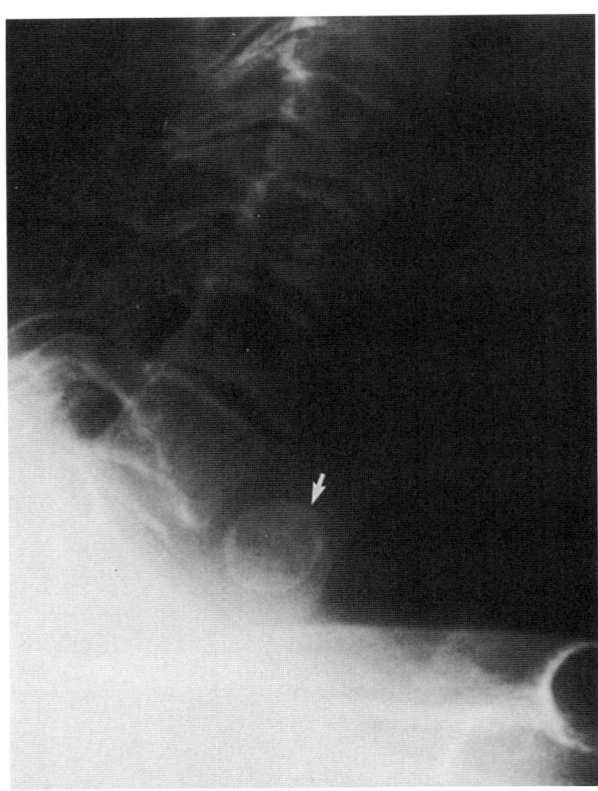

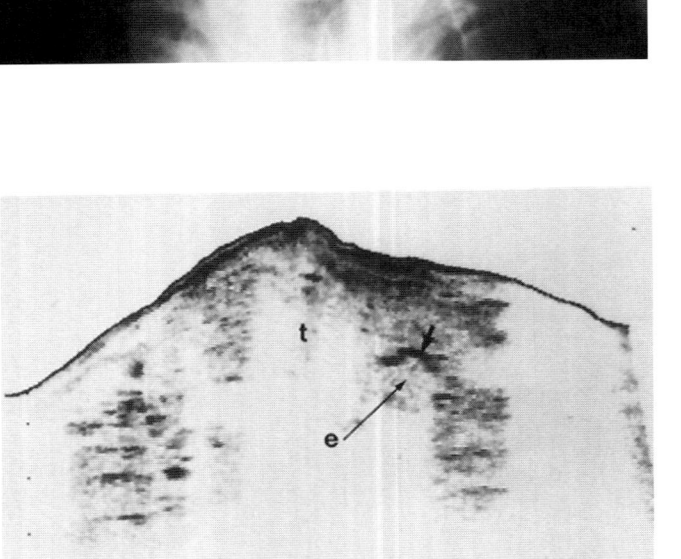

FIG. 14. Calcified solid nodule. **A:** A conventional AP x-ray defines a circumscribed calcified mass in the plane of the left thyroid lobe *(arrow)*. **B:** A soft-tissue lateral radiograph of the neck identifies the morphology and location *(arrow)* of the lesion as well. This was presumed to be a calcified colloid nodule in a 70-year-old woman. **C:** A transverse ultrasound examination allows definition of a solid (echogenic) lesion (e), posteriorly positioned in the left thyroid lobe. There is sufficient calcification to define the anterior surface of the nodule *(arrow)*; however, sound entry permits adequate diagnostic imaging of this solid nodule as well. t, trachea. (From ref. 103, with permission.)

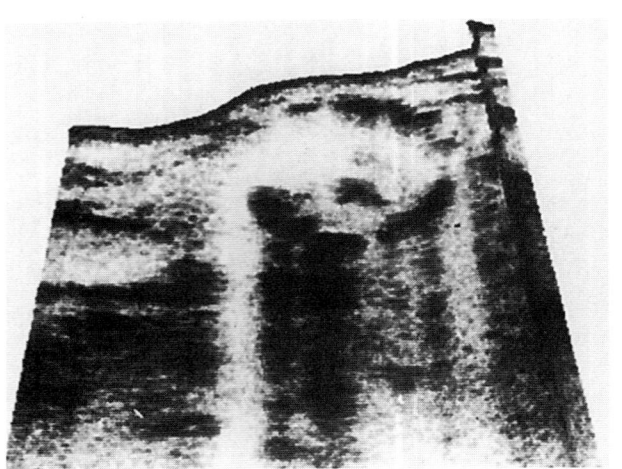

FIG. 15. Calcified solid nodule. A longitudinal ultrasound demonstrates a large lesion of mixed echogenicity with dense calcification anteriorly and posteriorly. A shadowing effect is noted in this mixed solid-cystic lesion. Solid-cystic lesions are considered solid with cystic degeneration. Cystic lesions are fluid filled; extremely sonolucent homogeneous solid masses may occasionally simulate cyst if there are no stromal interfaces and blood vessels to cause sound transmission changes owing to altered acoustic impedance.

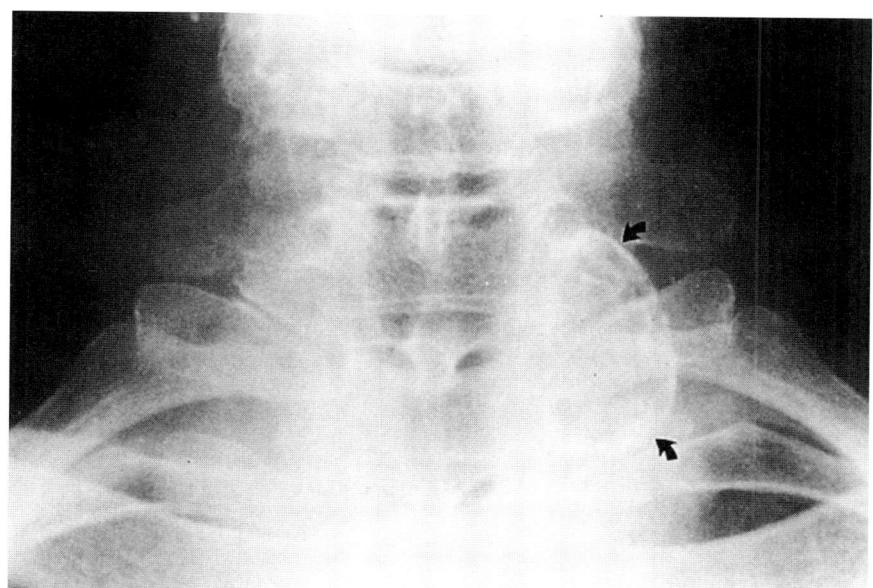

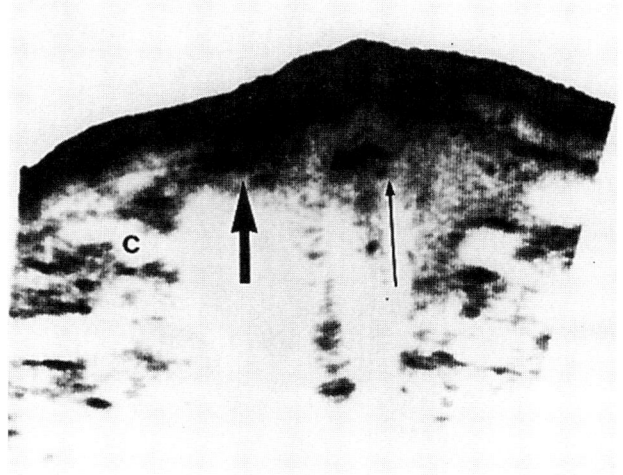

FIG. 16. Calcified thyroid nodule without ultrasound entry. **A:** An AP x-ray demonstrates a large calcified nodule *(arrows)* in the plane of the left thyroid lobe. **B:** The morphology of the nodule is further defined by a transverse ultrasound. The *heavy arrow* indicates the anterior aspect of the nodule, which is densely calcified; thus, sound waves do not penetrate the lesion and do not permit its definition as either solid or cystic. The *thin arrow* indicates the anterior wall of the trachea. C, left common carotid artery. Note that this is an older reversed image in which the patient's left is on the reader's left rather than the contemporary orientation of patient's left on reader's right. (From ref. 103, with permission.)

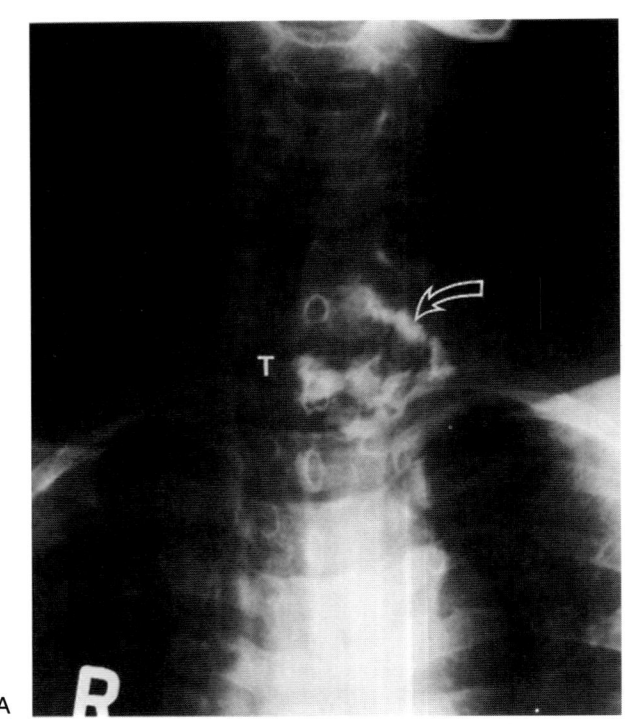
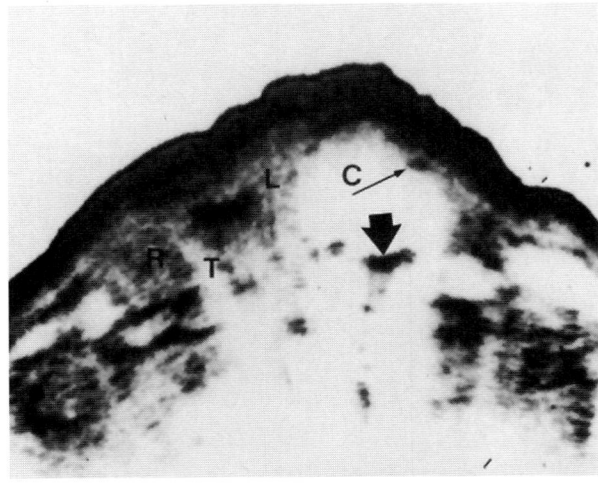
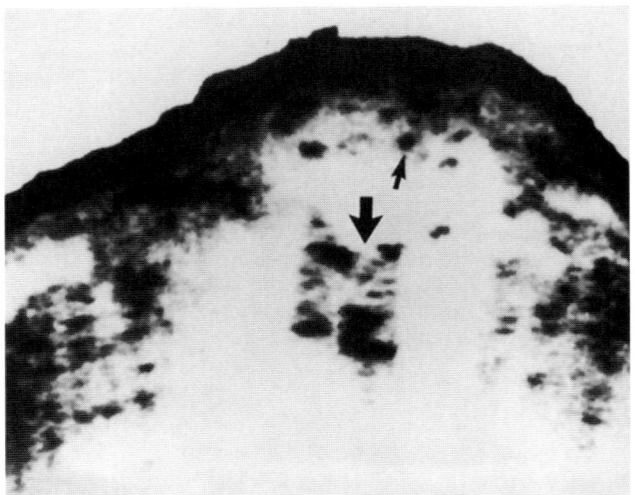

FIG. 17. Dense but incompletely calcified thyroid nodule allowing ultrasound entry. **A:** An AP radiograph demonstrates a dense but irregularly calcified mass in the plane of the left lobe of the thyroid gland *(arrow)*. The marginal calcifications appear coarse and irregular. T, displaced trachea to right. **B:** A transverse thyroid ultrasound demonstrates a large sonolucent cyst (C) occupying most of the left thyroid lobe (L). An area of dense anterior calcification is indicated by the *long thin arrow.* Sound transmitted through the cyst indicates a strong back wall image *(heavy arrow)*, a typical ultrasound finding. T, trachea; R, right thyroid lobe. **C:** A further transverse ultrasound image, somewhat more inferiorly, demonstrates the increased size of the cyst. There are multiple clumps of coarse anterior calcification *(small arrow)*, and sound penetration indicates the calcified back wall of the lesion *(heavy arrow)*. Calcification is irregular in this area as well. Note the shadowing effect resulting from the reflection of anterior dense calcifications. (From ref. 103, with permission.)

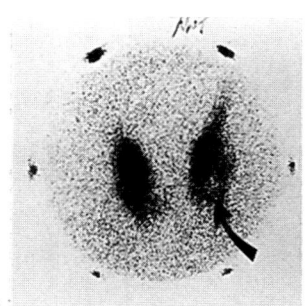
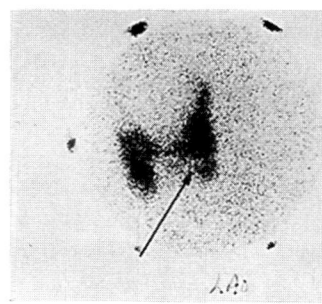
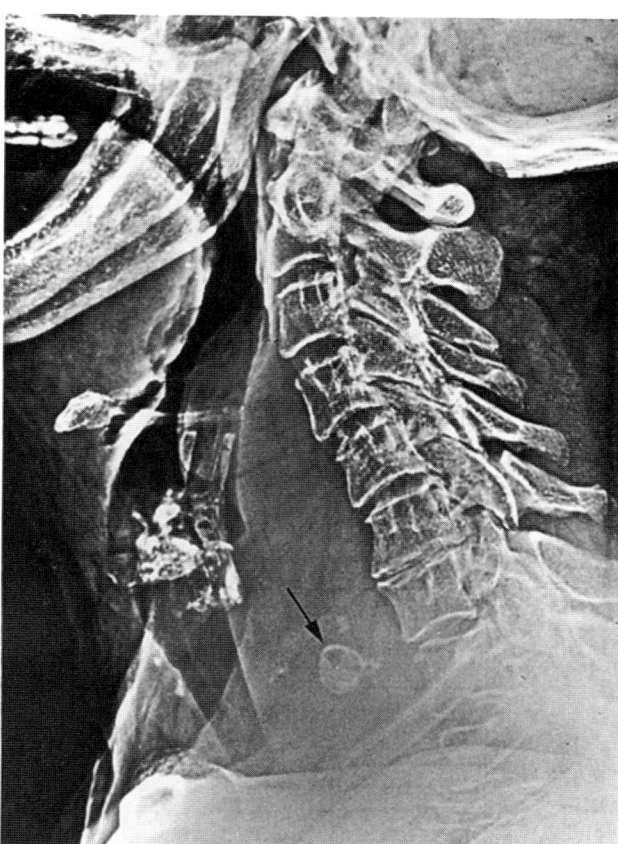

FIG. 18. Huge goiter with calcific nodule and displacement of trachea and esophagus. A lateral xeroradiograph demonstrates a calcific nodule *(arrow)* within a large soft-tissue mass displacing the trachea anteriorly; the posterior wall in the trachea is compressed somewhat. There are other foci of calcification within the thyroid gland in this large, multinodular goiter in an elderly woman presenting with dysphagia. (From ref. 103, with permission.)

FIG. 19. Small follicular adenoma and the limit of resolution of radionuclide scan. **A:** An anterior view of a pertechnetate scan demonstrates a small area of hypofunction *(arrow)* within the lower pole of the left thyroid lobe caused by an 8.0-mm follicular adenoma. **B:** A left anterior oblique view better defines this small lesion and its position *(arrow)*. The resolution of radionuclide studies is generally in the range of 0.5 cm to 1.0 cm for hypofunctioning lesions. (From ref. 103, with permission.)

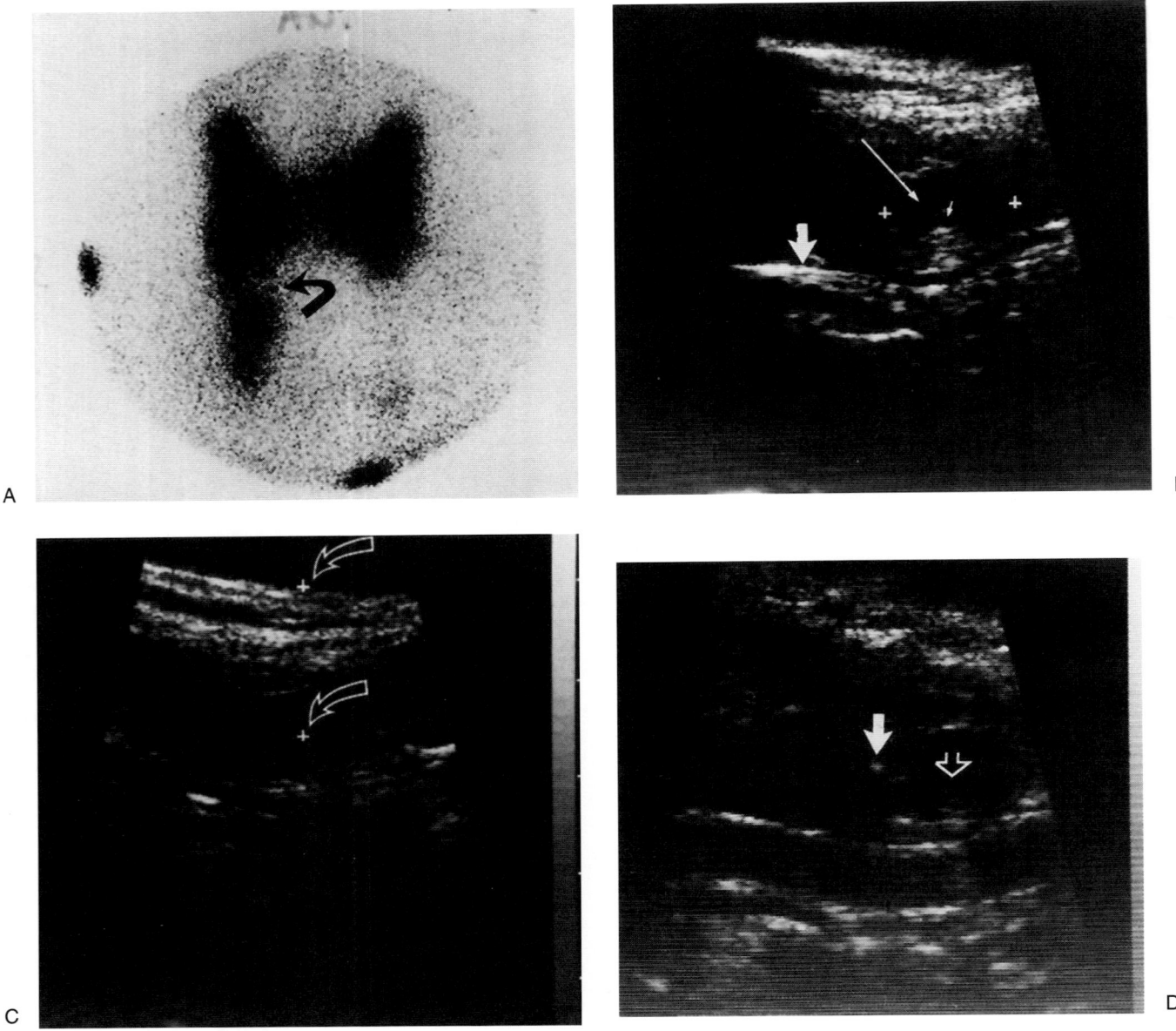

FIG. 20. Follicular adenoma and the role of ultrasound-guided fine-needle aspiration. **A:** A small, cold defect *(curved arrow)* is noted on pertechnetate scan on this 51-year-old woman who has received radiation to the head and neck for acne as a teenager. The right thyroid lobe is quite elongated. **B:** A longitudinal ultrasound identifies a sonolucent lesion *(long thin arrow)* within the lower pole of the right thyroid lobe, posteriorly. The lesion measures *(between cursors)* 1.28 cm in longitudinal dimension. The *heavy arrow* indicates the longus colli muscle. However, there is a posteriorly positioned mass *(tiny arrow)* projecting into the "cyst." **C:** On the same study, the imager measures the distance from the skin surface to the top of the mass *(cursors, curved arrows)*. The distance is 1.52 cm, and this allows the imager to identify the depth at which the ultrasound-guided needle will enter the lesion. **D:** An ultrasound image identifies the position of the mass *(hollow arrow)* as the needle tip *(solid arrow)* approaches it. This proved to be a follicular adenoma.

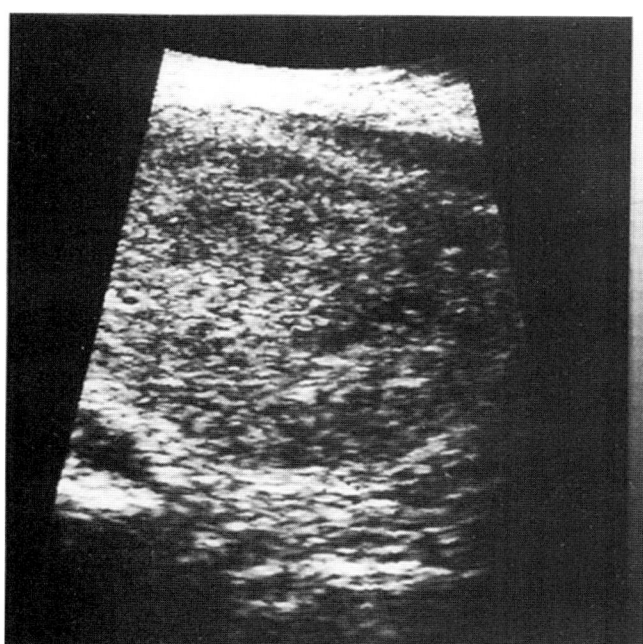 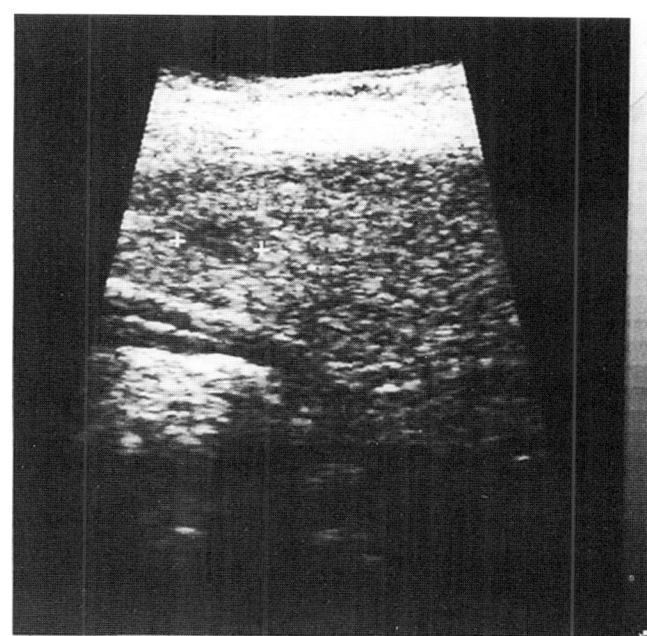

FIG. 21. Large follicular adenoma, with small colloid nodule in opposite lobe, upper pole. **A:** A longitudinal ultrasound demonstrates a large follicular adenoma with areas of mixed echogenicity. Lesion is well marginated and some characteristics of the halo sign are present. This follicular adenoma occupies almost the entire length of the left thyroid lobe. **B:** A longitudinal ultrasound of the right thyroid lobe demonstrates normal thyroid structure except for the presence of a solid lesion with somewhat reduced echogenicity measuring 0.68 cm *(cursors)*. This proved to be a colloid nodule.

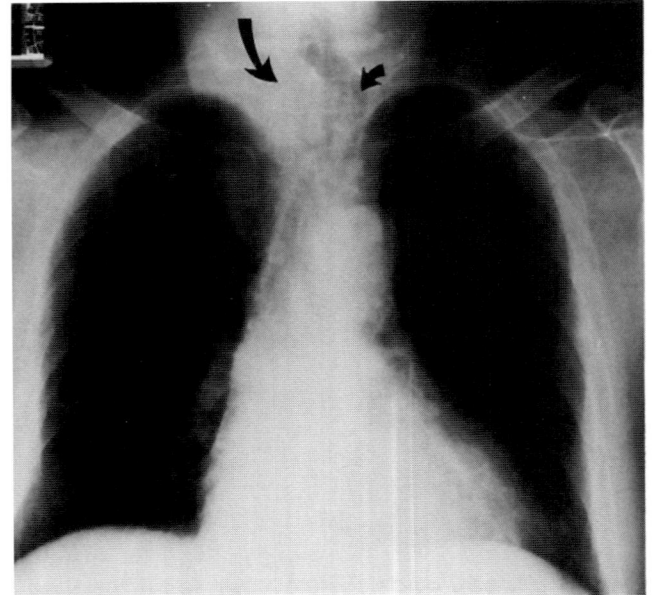
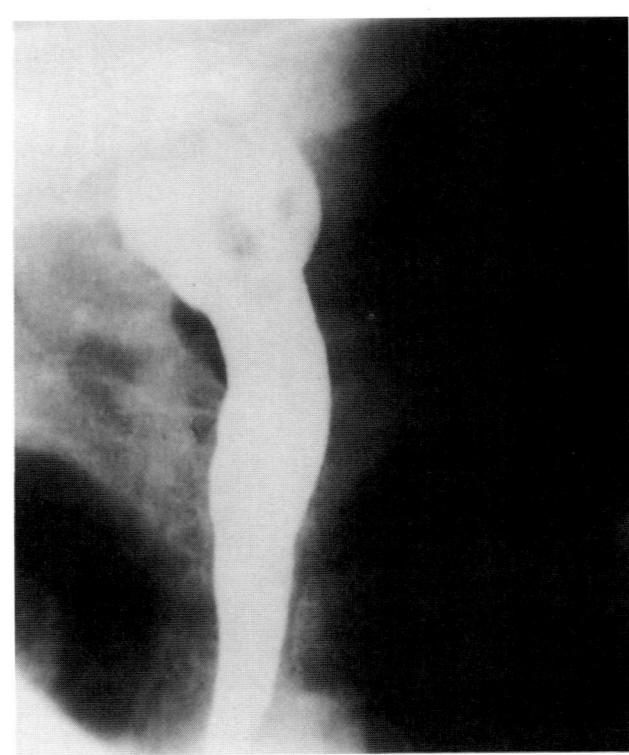
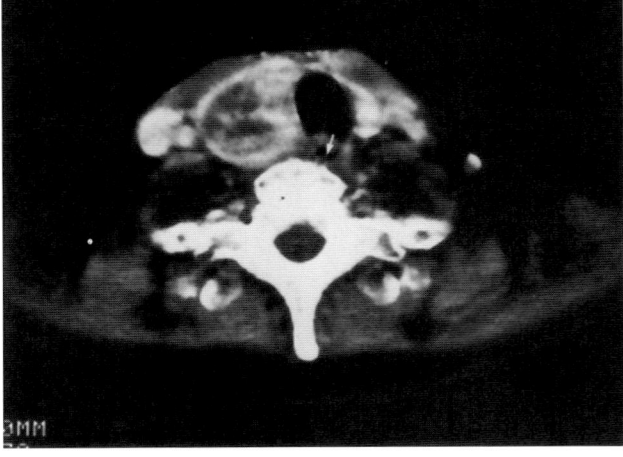

FIG. 22. Large follicular adenoma. **A:** A PA chest film demonstrates a soft-tissue mass *(large curved arrow)* indenting the trachea and pushing it to the left of the midline at the level of the thoracic inlet. The *short curved arrow* indicates the left lateral margin of the tracheal outline. **B:** A barium esophagram demonstrates indentation of the esophagus at the level of the thoracic inlet. **C:** An axial CT scan demonstrates a large, smoothly outlined thyroid mass with a clearly defined, contrast-enhanced rim. The trachea is pushed to the left of the midline, as is the esophagus *(short arrow)*. There is also some calcification within the right thyroid lobe in this 76-year-old man.

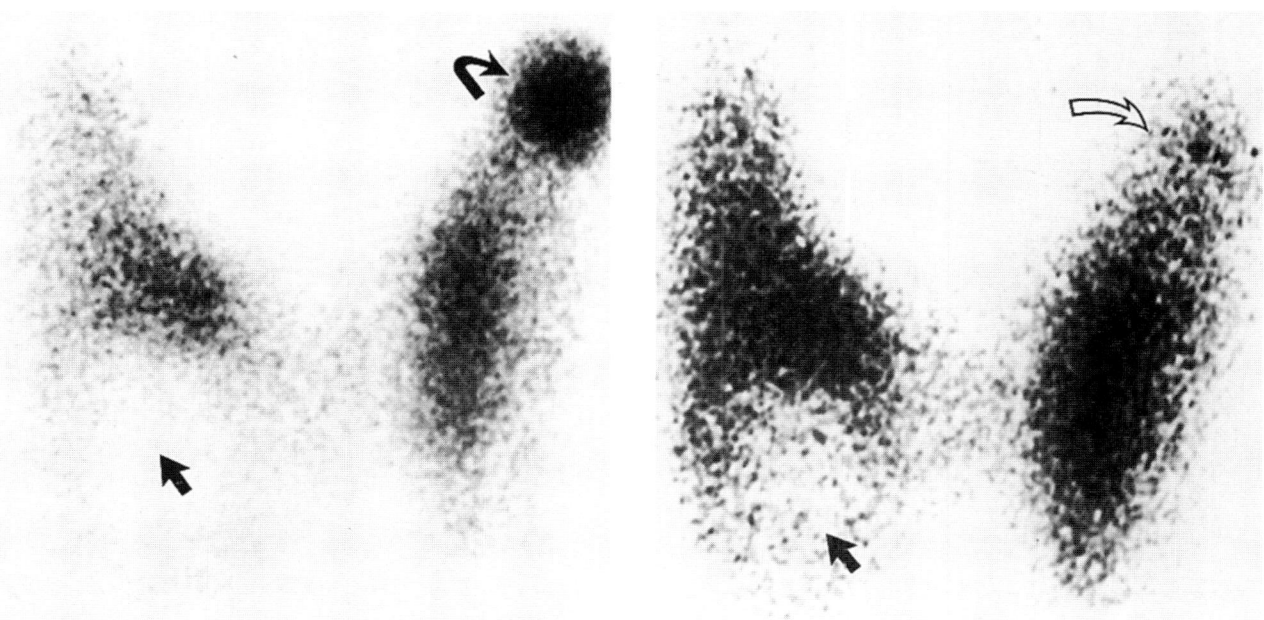

FIG. 23. Large degenerating follicular adenoma (cold nodule), and contralateral false-functioning follicular adenoma (false hot nodule). **A:** A pertechnetate scan in anterior display demonstrates a cold nodule occupying the lower pole of the right thyroid lobe *(straight arrow)*, and an area of increased uptake involving the uppermost portion of the left thyroid lobe *(curved arrow)*. **B:** An I-123 scan confirms the presence of a cold nodule in the right lower pole *(straight arrow)* and further demonstrates isofunction in the apex of the left upper pole *(curved arrow)*. An I-123 scan is always required whenever increased uptake is identified on pertechnetate scan; the radioiodine will confirm or deny the true function of hormonogenesis. **C:** A transverse ultrasound of the right thyroid lobe demonstrates a circumscribed lesion *(cursors)* with a halo, measuring 2.2 cm × 1.6 cm in this plane. The hypoechoic center portion *(white arrow)* suggests degeneration and cystic change. Black arrow indicates anterior tracheal cartilage. V, right internal jugular vein; A, right common carotid artery; T, trachea. **D:** A longitudinal ultrasound of the right thyroid lobe demonstrates morphology *(cursors)* similar to C in the lower portion of the thyroid lobe. The *short curved arrow* indicates cystic degeneration. The *long curved arrow* indicates the inferior limit of lower pole. **E:** A transverse ultrasound of the left thyroid lobe, at the level of the superior pole and larynx (L), demonstrates a nodule *(cursors)*. a, left common carotid artery; v, left internal jugular vein; M, muscle. **F:** A longitudinal ultrasound of the left thyroid lobe identifies the reduced echogenicity of the mass and its margins *(cursors)* within the upper portion of the thyroid lobe. The *arrow* is the lower pole. The patient is a 30-year-old woman found to have a thyroid mass on routine physical examination.

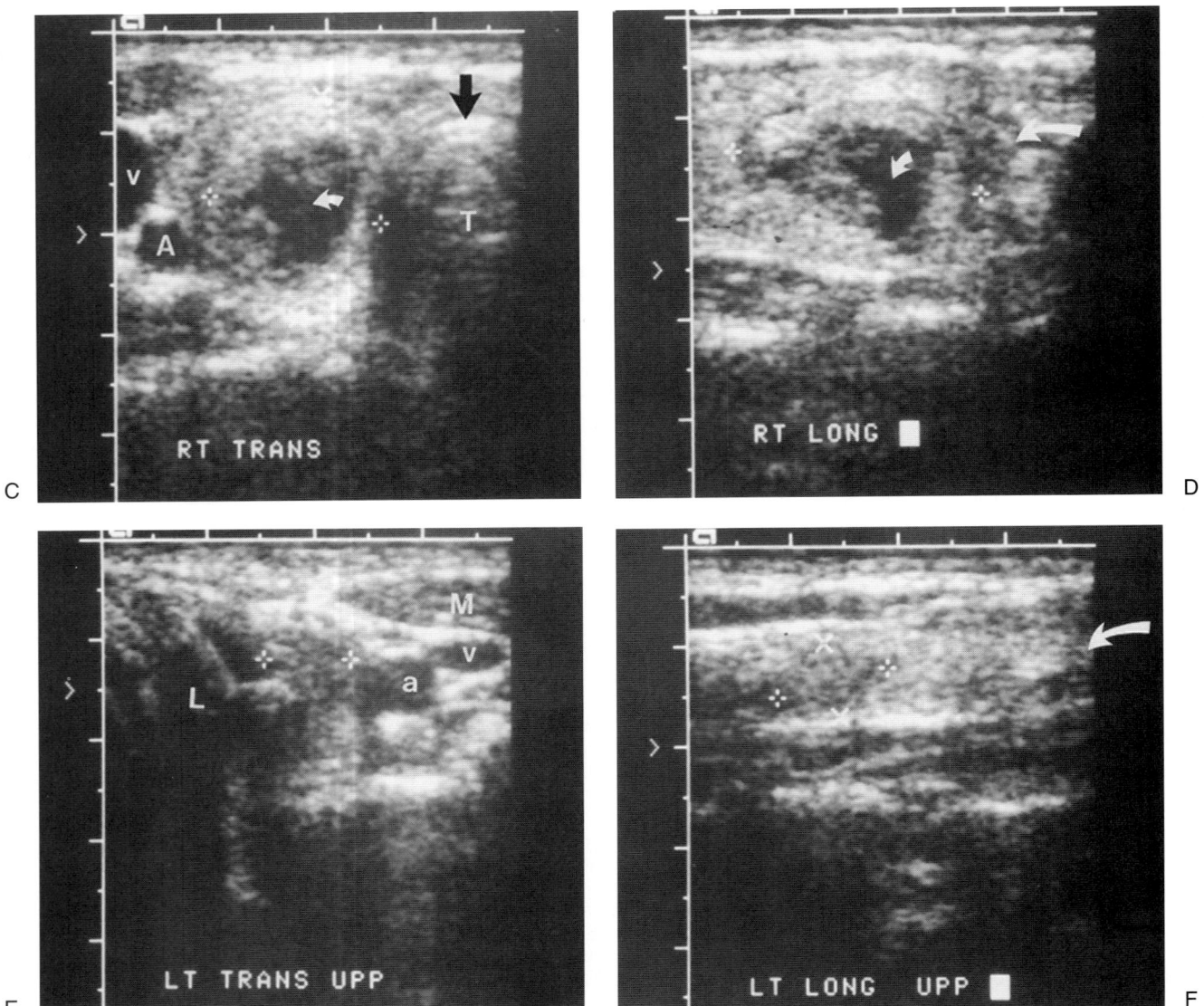

FIG. 23. *Continued.*

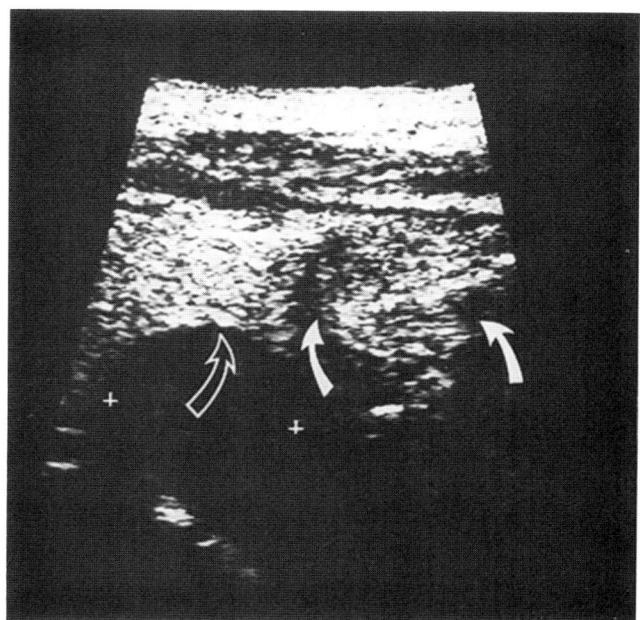

FIG. 24. Follicular adenoma and parathyroid adenoma. A longitudinal ultrasound of the left thyroid lobe identifies a mass lesion inferiorly; the *curved solid arrows* indicate a halo around this follicular adenoma. Posteriorly and superiorly, a hypoechoic mass measuring 1.5 cm impresses the thyroid lobe from behind *(curved open arrow)*. This imaging sign indicates the extrinsic origin of the sonolucent mass; its hypoechoic appearance is entirely compatible with a parathyroid adenoma in this patient with primary hyperparathyroidism as well as a palpable thyroid nodule.

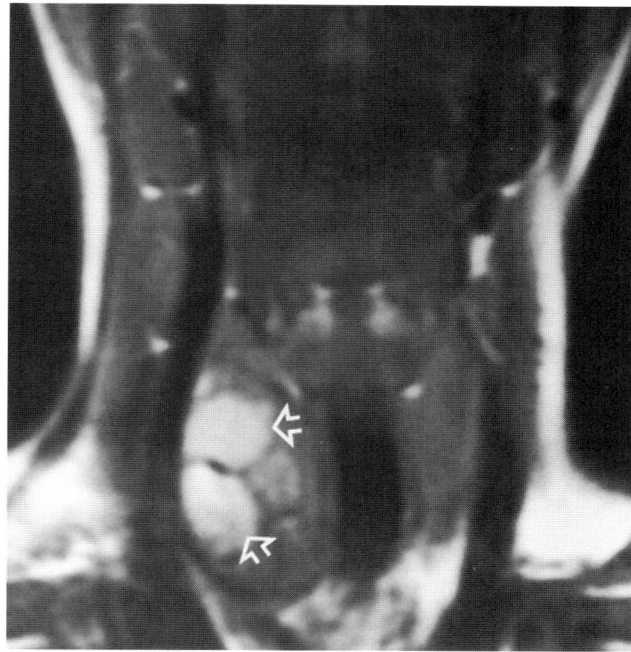

A

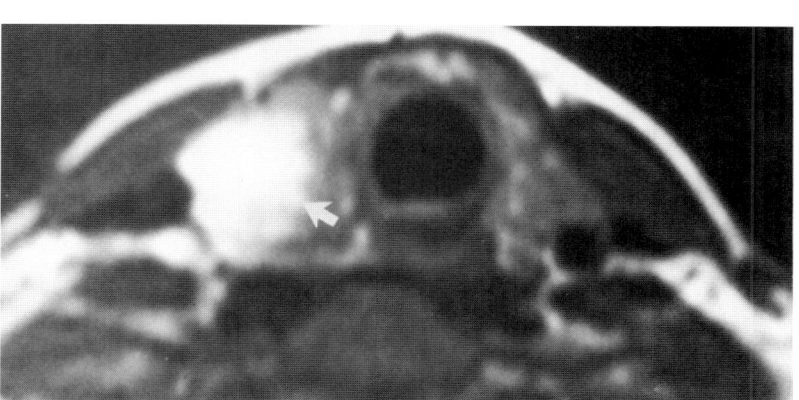

B

FIG. 25. Follicular adenoma with cystic changes and hemorrhage. **A:** A coronal T1-weighted image identifies a follicular adenoma involving the right thyroid lobe with areas of cystic change and hemorrhage *(arrows)*. **B:** A T2-weighted MR image identifies the same abnormalities *(arrow)*. (Courtesy of Dr. Mahmood Mafee, Professor of Radiology, Director MR Center, University of Illinois, Chicago, Illinois.)

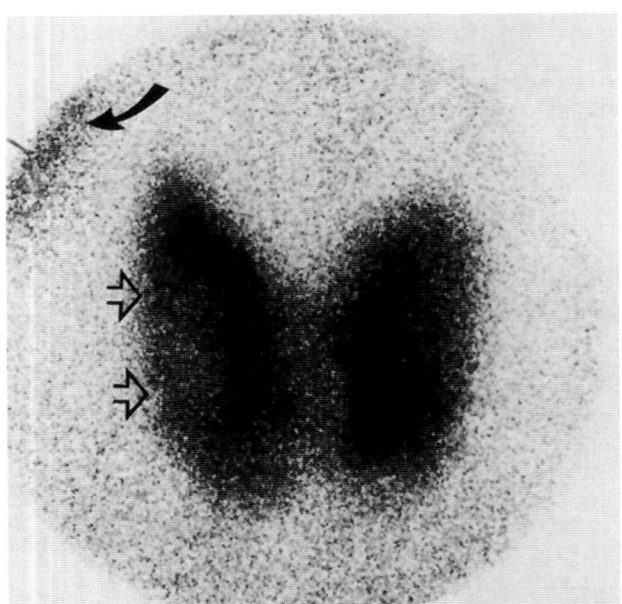

FIG. 26. Extrinsic mass (parathyroid adenoma) simulates intrinsic cold nodule. An anterior view of a sodium pertechnetate scan identifies a relatively large photon-deficient area *(between hollow arrows)*, presumably a result of hypofunction within the right thyroid lobe in its midportion. The appearance is actually owing to a reduction in functioning thyroid tissue in the plane of the image caused by the presence of an extremely large parathyroid adenoma—a very rare cause of this imaging sign. The *curved arrow* indicates a right side marker. (From ref. 103, with permission.)

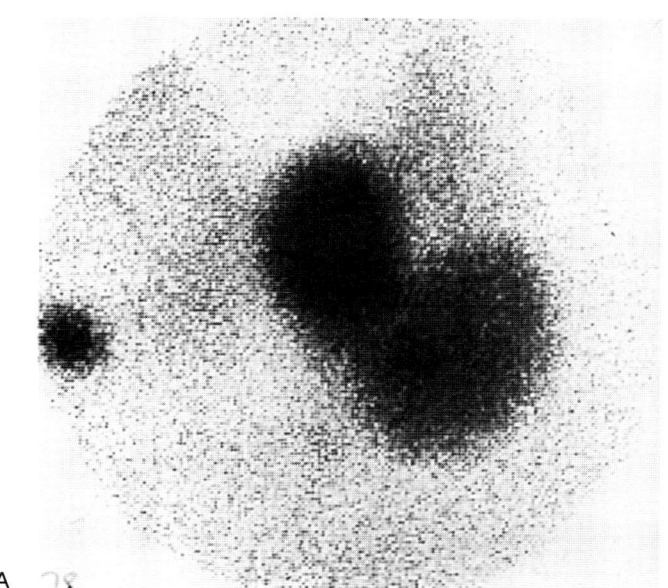
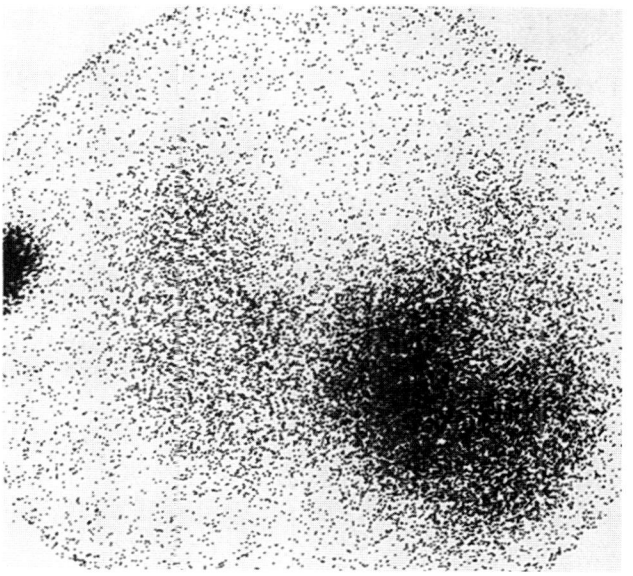
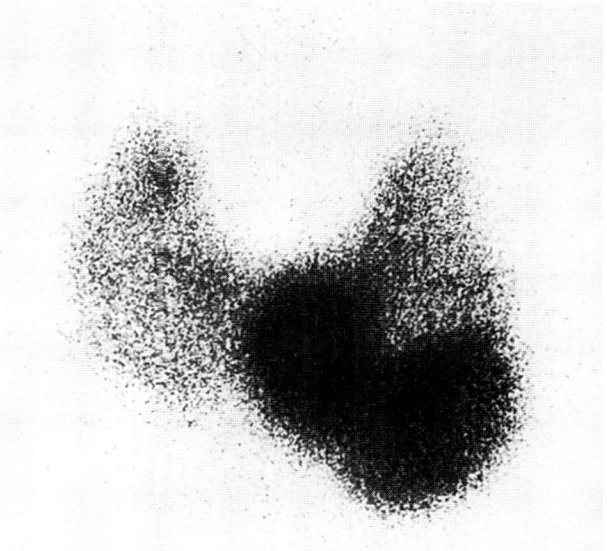

FIG. 27. Two hot or functioning thyroid nodules, with comparison of radionuclide imaging studies. **A:** A sodium pertechnetate Tc-99m thyroid scan. The two nodules trap the radionuclide and there is some imaging of the remainder of the normal thyroid gland. Note the significant background noise. **B:** An I-131 scan (1 year later) shows incorporation of the radioiodine by the two hot nodules. The I-131 scan should not be used for routine diagnosis, only for the management of the patient with known thyroid carcinoma. **C:** An I-123 thyroid scan (2 years later) shows the best resolution and morphologic definition, and demonstrates the distribution of hormonogenesis of the organified radioactive iodine within the thyroid gland. (From ref. 103, with permission.)

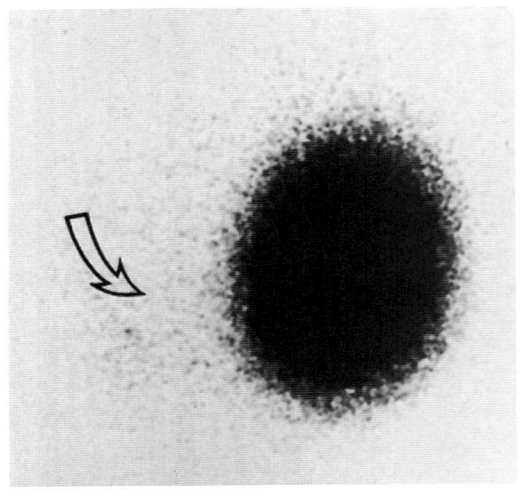

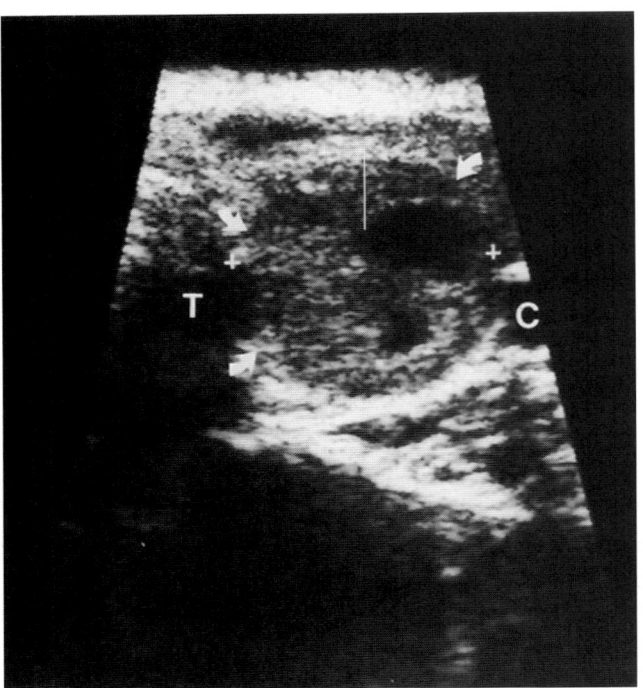

FIG. 28. Functioning nodule. **A:** An I-123 scan demonstrates the true function of a large mass occupying the left thyroid lobe. There is almost no uptake by the right lobe *(arrow)*. **B:** A 7.5-MHz transverse ultrasound demonstrates a discrete thyroid nodule *(cursors)* with areas of reduced echogenicity within it. The mixed solid–cystic lesion has a very benign discrete appearance *(arrows)*. T, trachea; C, left common carotid artery.

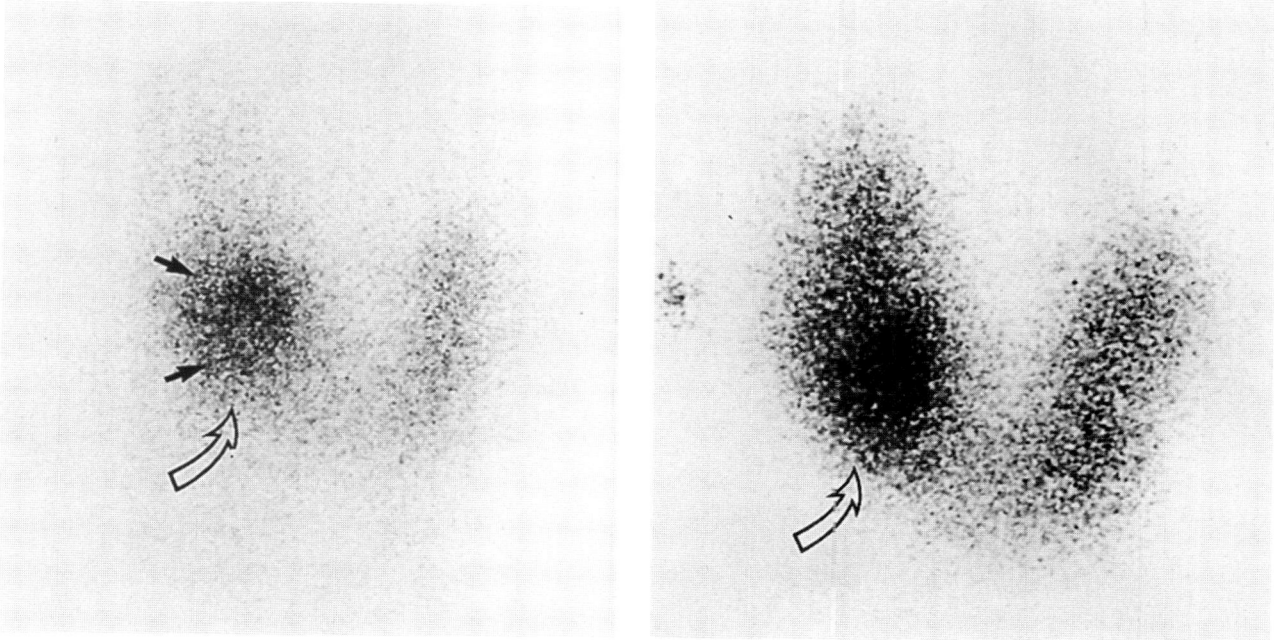

FIG. 29. Functioning thyroid nodule. **A:** An anterior view of a pertechnetate scan identifies an area of increased uptake *(between solid arrows)* involving the midportion of the right thyroid lobe, toward the lower pole *(curved arrow)*. **B:** This apparent function must be confirmed or denied by I-123 scan, which will demonstrate hormonogenesis. This anterior view of the subsequent I-123 scan verifies this "true" function *(arrow)*. It also better identifies thyroid morphology. It should be remembered that the pertechnetate scan provides only an approximation of thyroid function because of pertechnetate trapping. Pertechnetate is trapped by the thyroid gland, as is iodide, but pertechnetate is not organified.

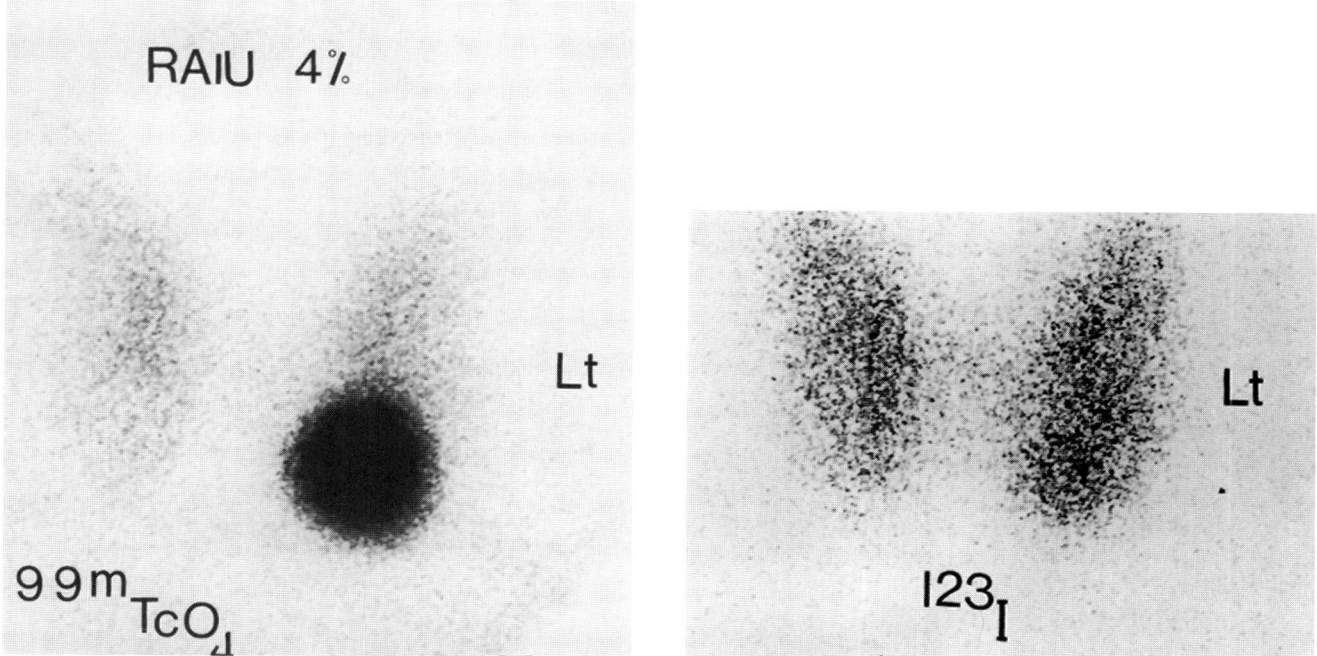

FIG. 30. "False" functioning thyroid nodule. **A:** A pertechnetate thyroid scan demonstrates a discrete focus of increased radionuclide uptake corresponding to a palpable mass in a 16-year-old girl who has a follicular adenoma. The remainder of the thyroid gland is not well imaged. **B:** An I-123 scan demonstrates the false function of this nodule; there is no incorporation of radioactive iodine in the plane of the image.

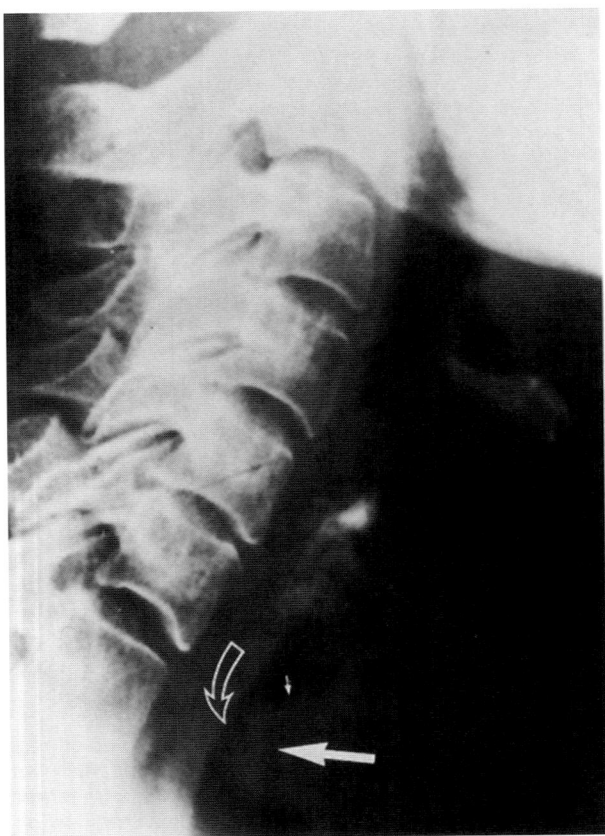

FIG. 31. Tracheal invasion by carcinoma of the thyroid. A soft-tissue lateral radiograph demonstrates the AP dimension of a lobulated soft-tissue mass within the trachea; it originates anteriorly *(heavy arrow)* from the thyroid gland and almost completely occludes the airway. There is a small, residual air space posteriorly *(curved arrow)* in this patient presenting with stridor and a thyroid mass. The *tiny arrow* indicates the superior surface of this intratracheal mass. (From ref. 103, with permission.)

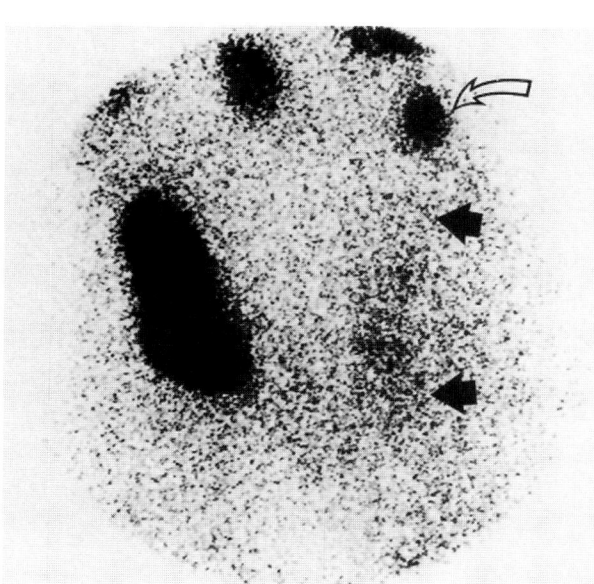
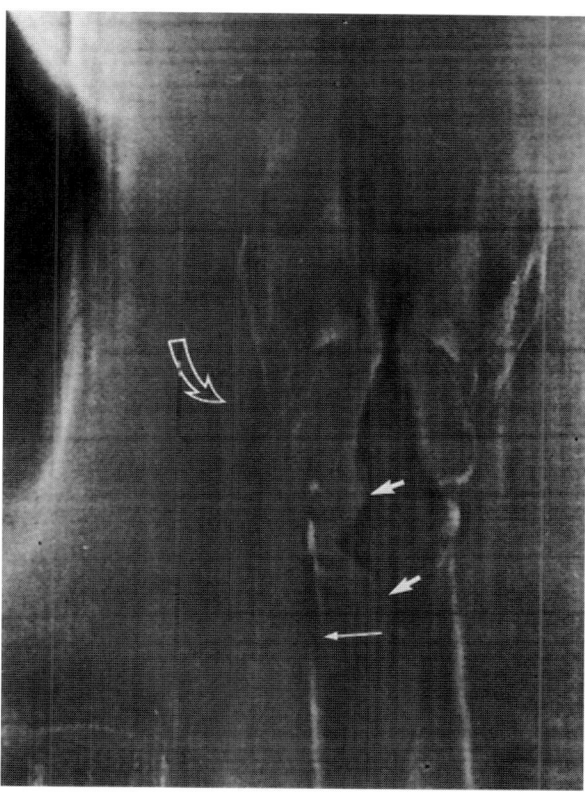

FIG. 32. Anaplastic carcinoma of thyroid gland with intralaryngeal and intratracheal extension. **A:** An anterior view of a pertechnetate thyroid scan demonstrates enlargement of the left thyroid lobe with almost no detectable uptake *(between heavy arrows)*. The right thyroid lobe appears uninvolved on radionuclide scan. The *hollow curved arrow* demonstrates the left submandibular gland. **B:** An anteroposterior xerotomograph (xeroradiograph image is reversed right to left) demonstrates a soft-tissue density in the region of the left thyroid lobe *(hollow arrow)*, which displaces and extends into the larynx *(upper short arrow)* and trachea *(lower short arrow)*, as a bilobulated soft-tissue mass. There is obvious cartilage destruction of the trachea *(long thin arrow)*, as well as the nferolateral aspect of the cricoid cartilage *(at the level of the upper short arrow)*. (From ref. 103, with permission.)

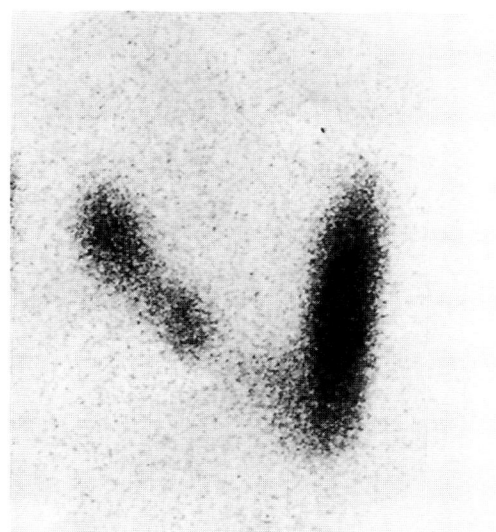
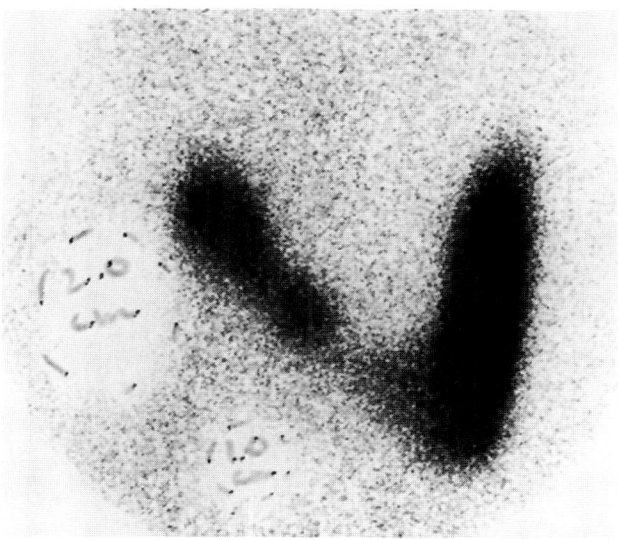

FIG. 33. Medullary carcinoma of the thyroid. **A:** An anterior view of a pertechnetate thyroid scan demonstrates involvement of the right thyroid lobe by medullary carcinoma. **B:** The morphologic radionuclide findings are correlated with the position of cold markers. Routine examination of the patient's neck by the nuclear physician at the time of the scan is essential for accurate interpretation. "Hot" or "cold" markers are placed over suspicious areas found by palpation and correlated with the scan findings. (From ref. 103, with permission.)

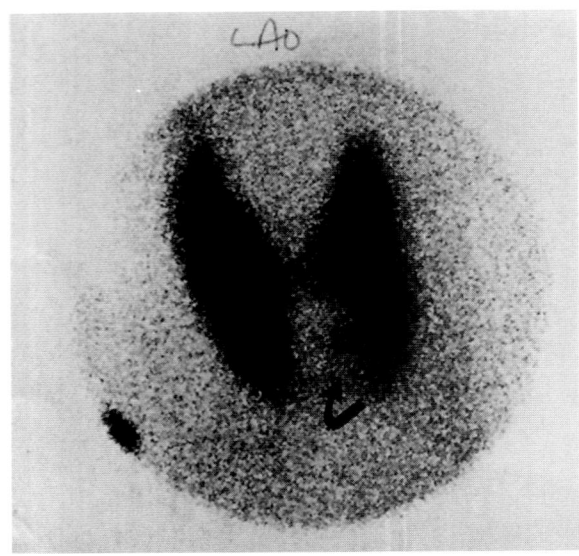
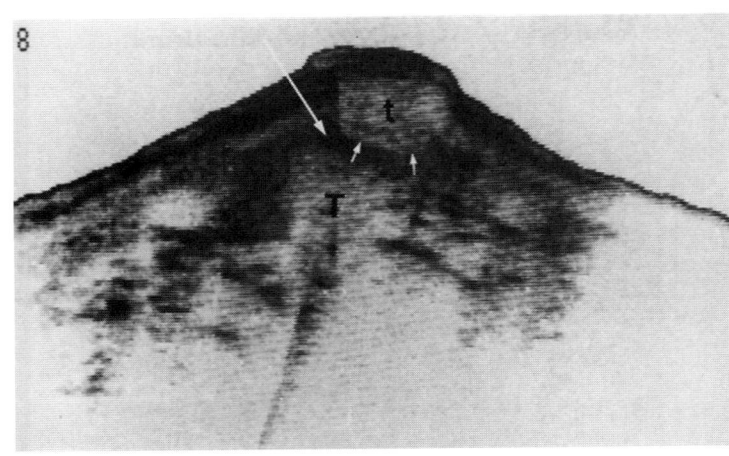

FIG. 34. Papillary carcinoma involving the isthmus. **A:** A pertechnetate scan in left anterior oblique display identifies a cold nodule involving the isthmus at the junction with the left thyroid lobe *(curved arrow)*. **B:** A transverse (axial) ultrasound examination clearly defines the relatively superficial position of the solid tumor mass (t). It originates in the isthmus *(long arrow)* just to the left of the midline. The posterior surface of the tumor is indicated by the two *tiny arrows*. The tumor elevates the external surface of the isthmus and left thyroid lobe, producing a strongly projecting echogenic tumor mass. The patient is a 29-year-old woman. T, trachea. (From ref. 103, with permission.)

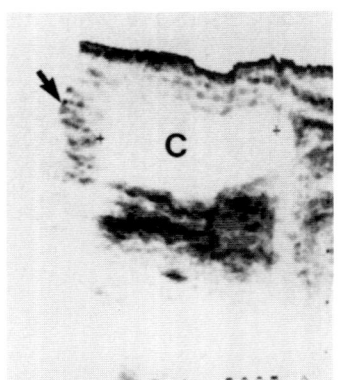
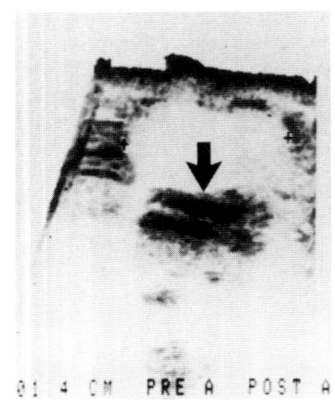
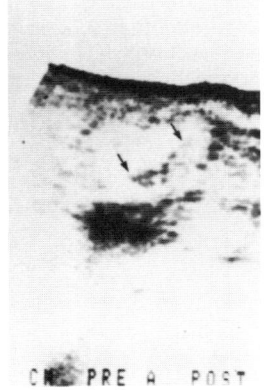

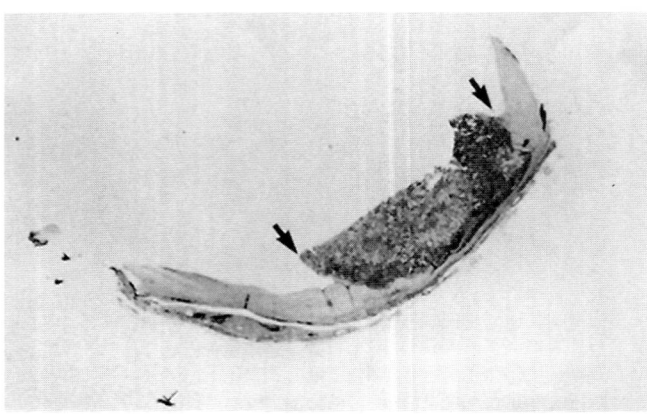

FIG. 35. Thyroid cyst with papillary carcinoma. **A:** A longitudinal (sagittal) ultrasound examination of the right thyroid lobe demonstrates a sonolucent lesion (C) occupying almost the entire right thyroid lobe. A small portion of the intact superior pole is still identified *(arrow)*. **B:** A further longitudinal ultrasound image identifies the sharp back wall *(heavy arrow)* resulting from through-transmission of sound in the cyst. **C:** An additional ultrasound image identifies a semilunar echogenic solid lesion *(between tiny arrows)* within the cyst. **D:** A low-power photomicrograph of the thyroid cyst, oriented in the same position as the longitudinal ultrasound section in C, demonstrates an elevated focus of papillary carcinoma *(between arrows)* arising from the cyst wall. (From ref. 103, with permission.)

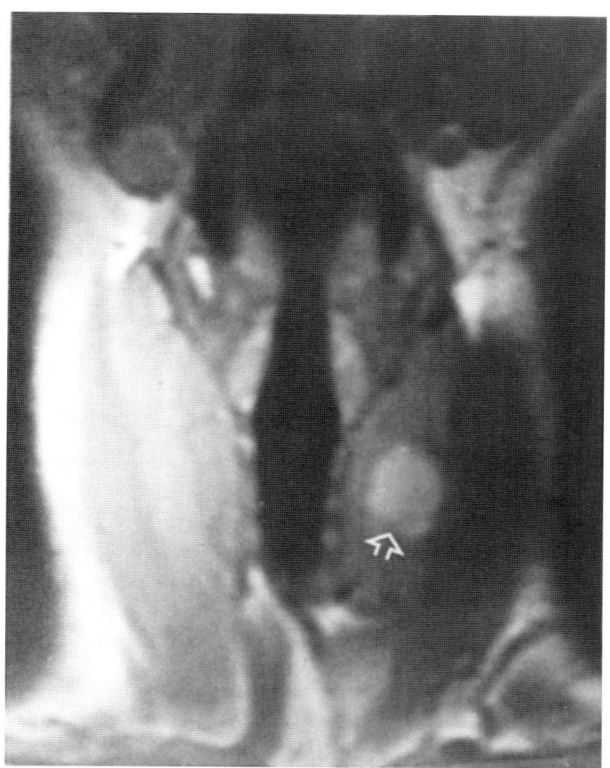

FIG. 36. Papillary carcinoma. A coronal proton-density MR image identifies a papillary carcinoma of the thyroid *(arrow)*; its intrathyroidal location is evident, as well as its relationship to the trachea and larynx. (Courtesy of Dr. Mahmood Mafee, Professor of Radiology, Director, MR Center, University of Illinois, Chicago, Illinois.)

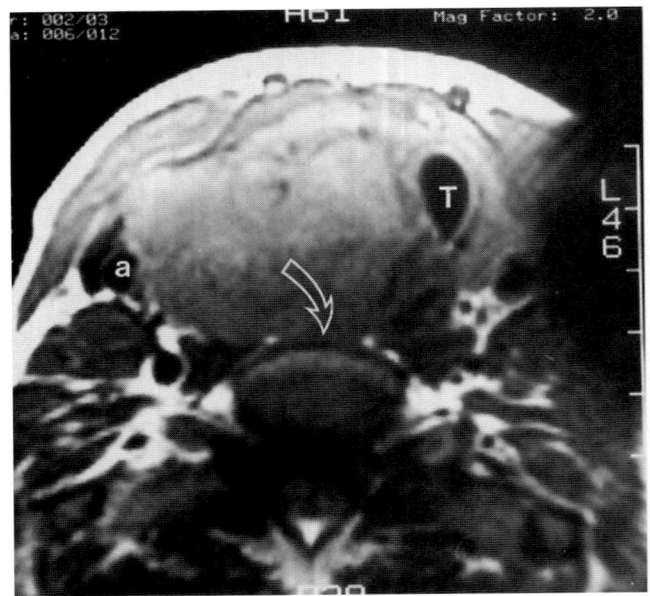
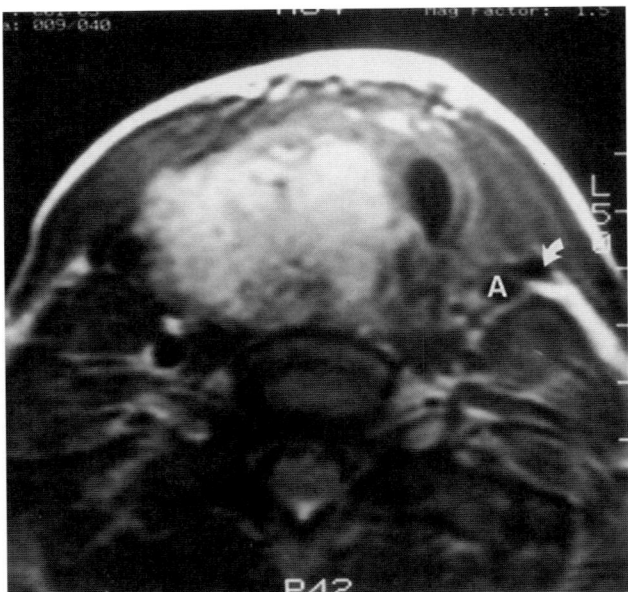
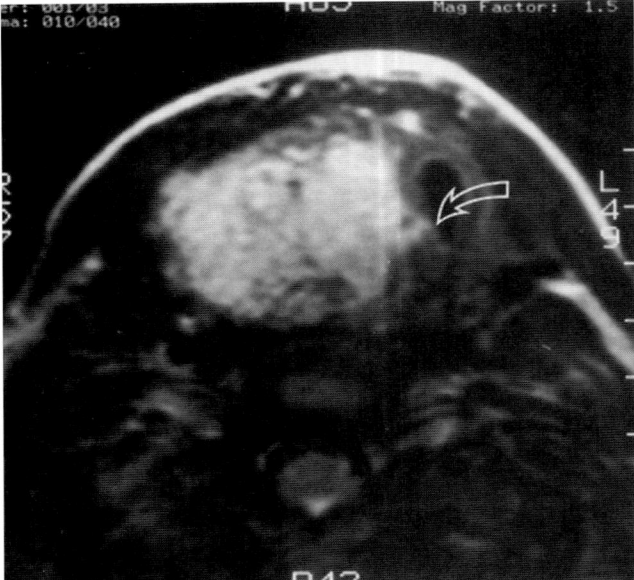

FIG. 37. Papillary carcinoma with extracapsular extension. **A:** A T1-weighted image in a spin-echo sequence (TR = 600, TE = 20), demonstrates a huge mass occupying the thyroid lobe and extending posteriorly *(arrow)*. The T1-weighted image is characterized by a short TR and a short TE. T, displaced trachea; A, right common carotid artery. **B:** A proton-density image at the same level in the same sequence is characterized by a long TR and a short TE. The mass is identified by the bright signal. The *arrow* indicates the left internal jugular vein. A, left common carotid artery. **C:** A T2-weighted image in the same spin-echo sequence is characterized by a long TR and a long TE. Paratracheal invasion is evident *(arrow)* in this 29-year-old woman who presents with a papillary carcinoma and a right recurrent laryngeal nerve paralysis. (Courtesy of Dr. Walter Kucharczyk and the Toronto MR Centre, University of Toronto, Toronto, Ontario, Canada.)

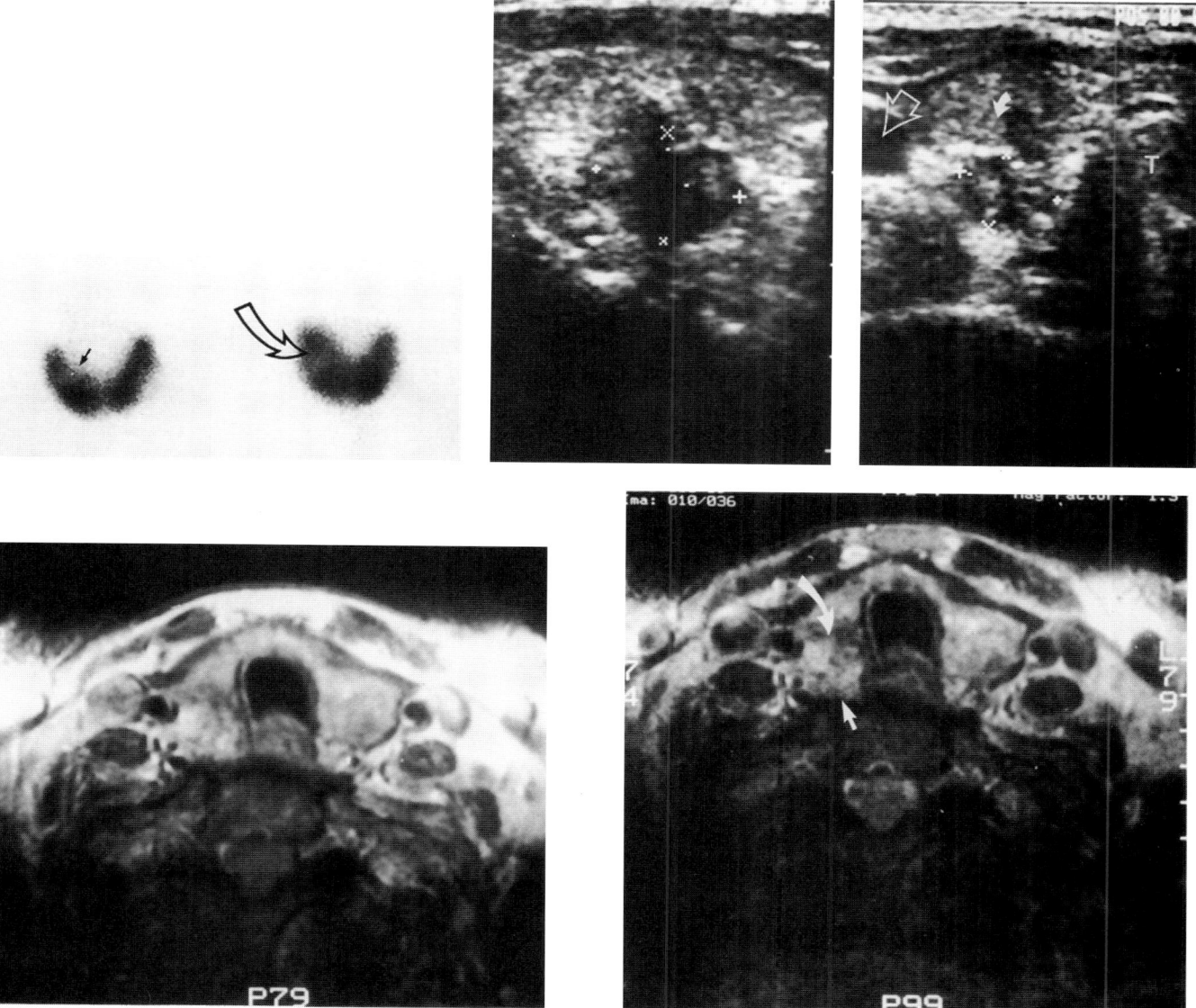

FIG. 38. Sclerosing papillary carcinoma with recurrent laryngeal nerve involvement. **A:** A pertechnetate thyroid scan demonstrates a small area of decreased uptake *(tiny arrow)* on anterior view. This corresponds to a posteriorly positioned mass that is difficult to palpate. On the right anterior oblique image the cold defect is better defined *(hollow arrow)*. **B:** A longitudinal high-resolution ultrasound identifies the 1.6 × 1.2 cm mass *(cursors)*. There is calcification and a hypoechoic center noted within the right thyroid lobe. **C:** A transverse ultrasound demonstrates the posterior position of this papillary carcinoma within the right thyroid lobe. The *curved arrow* indicates the noninvolved anterior portion of the lobe. The tumor is identified by *cursors;* there are areas of calcification associated with it. The *hollow arrow* demonstrates the adjacent right common carotid artery. T, trachea. **D:** A proton density axial MR image demonstrates the posteriorly positioned carcinoma, extending into the region of the right recurrent laryngeal nerve. This image matches the ultrasound image in C. **E:** A T2-weighted image at the same level as D identifies the tumor *(arrows)* by the presence of increased signal because of its increased fluid content. The *curved arrow* demonstrates the anterior margin of the tumor. The *straight arrow* indicates its posterior extension where it involves the recurrent laryngeal nerve. The patient is a 65-year-old man presenting with a 3-month history of hoarseness and a right recurrent laryngeal nerve paralysis clinically.

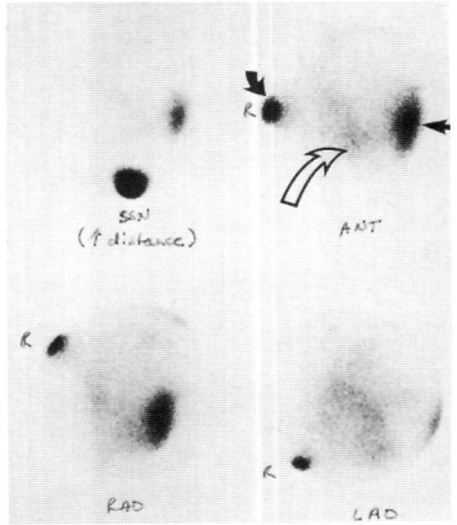
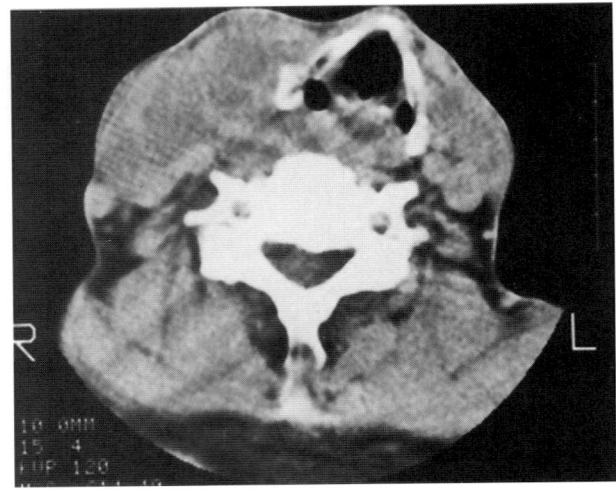
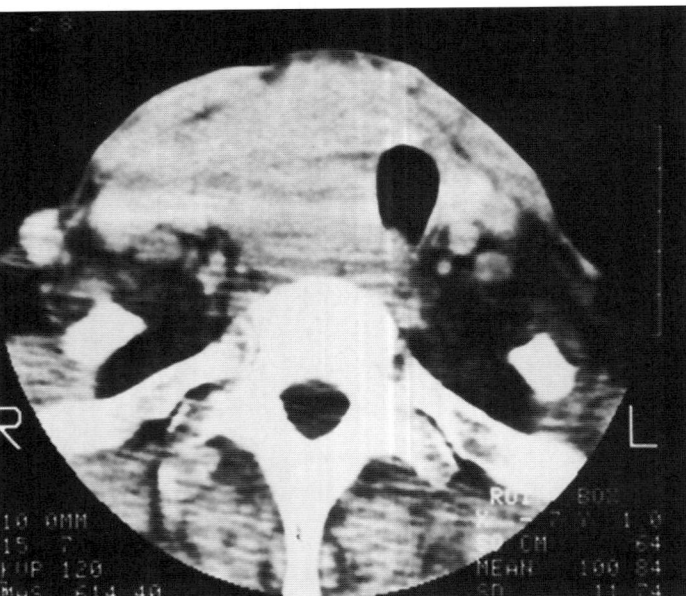
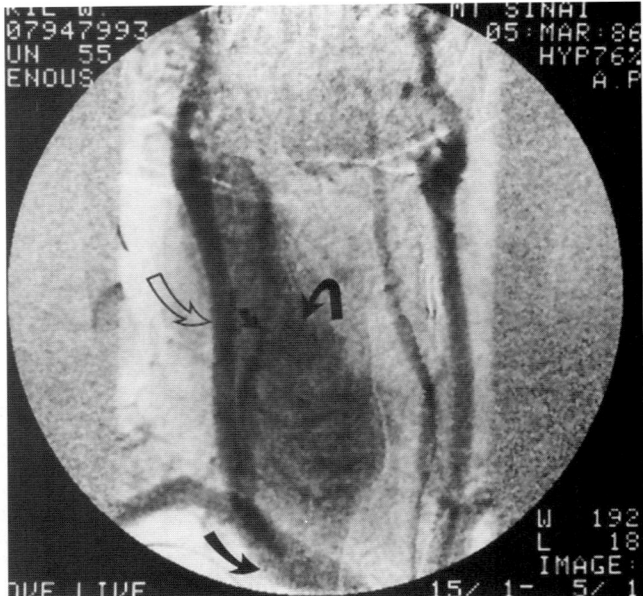

FIG. 39. Follicular adenocarcinoma with retrosubclavian extension. **A:** A pertechnetate thyroid scan demonstrates hypofunction of the entire right thyroid lobe *(hollow arrow)* on this patient with a huge palpable mass. The *straight arrow* indicates the still functioning small left lobe. The *curved solid arrow* demonstrates a right marker. **B:** A CT scan at the level of the larynx demonstrates the mass and laryngeal displacement. **C:** A CT scan 4.0 cm inferiorly demonstrates the tracheal and superior mediastinal relationship in axial display. With contrast enhancement, the relationship of the tumor mass to the right common carotid artery is uncertain. **D:** A digital subtraction angiogram, carried out via the intravenous route, demonstrates the vascular blush *(solid large recurved arrow)* of a follicular adenocarcinoma. The right common carotid artery *(hollow arrow)* is uninvolved. The right vertebral artery is identified by the *short curved black arrow.* Extension below and behind the right subclavian artery is identified by the *lower black curved arrow.* The patient is a 77-year-old man presenting with a large neck mass and a right recurrent laryngeal nerve paralysis.

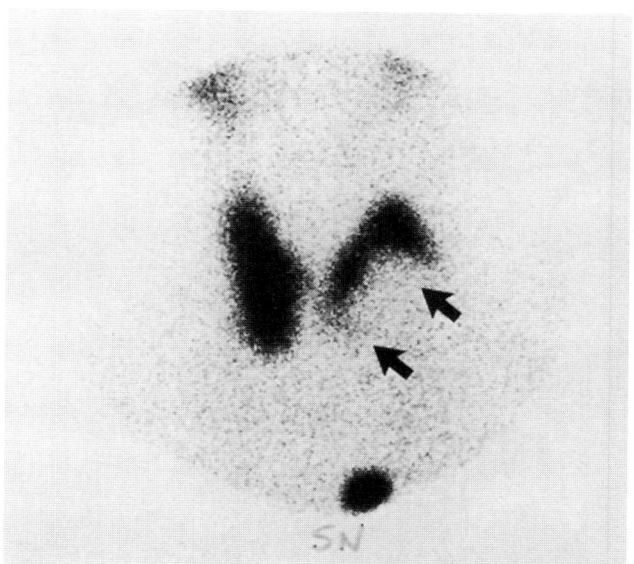
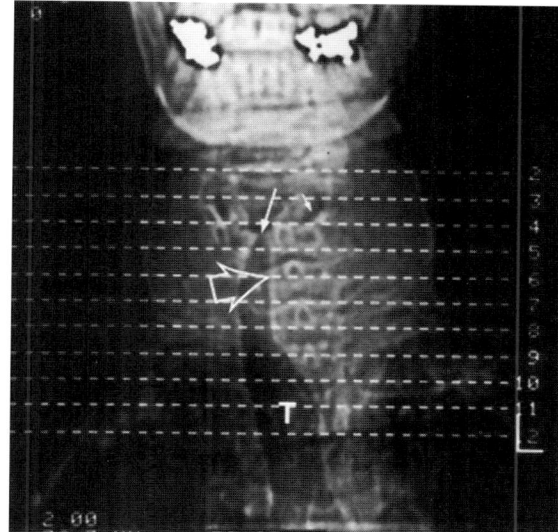
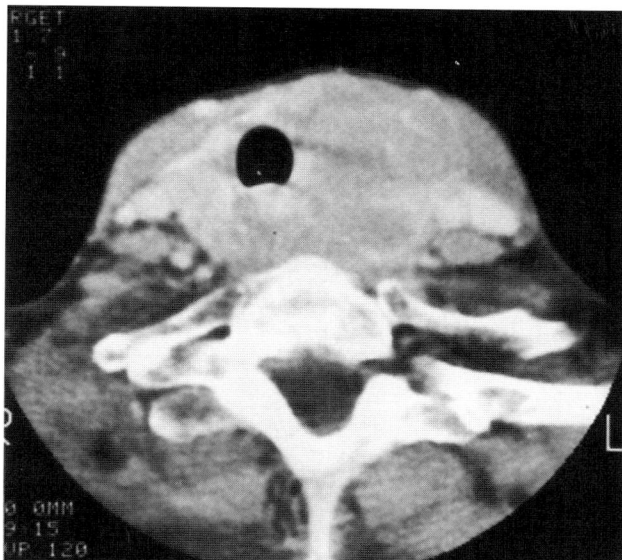
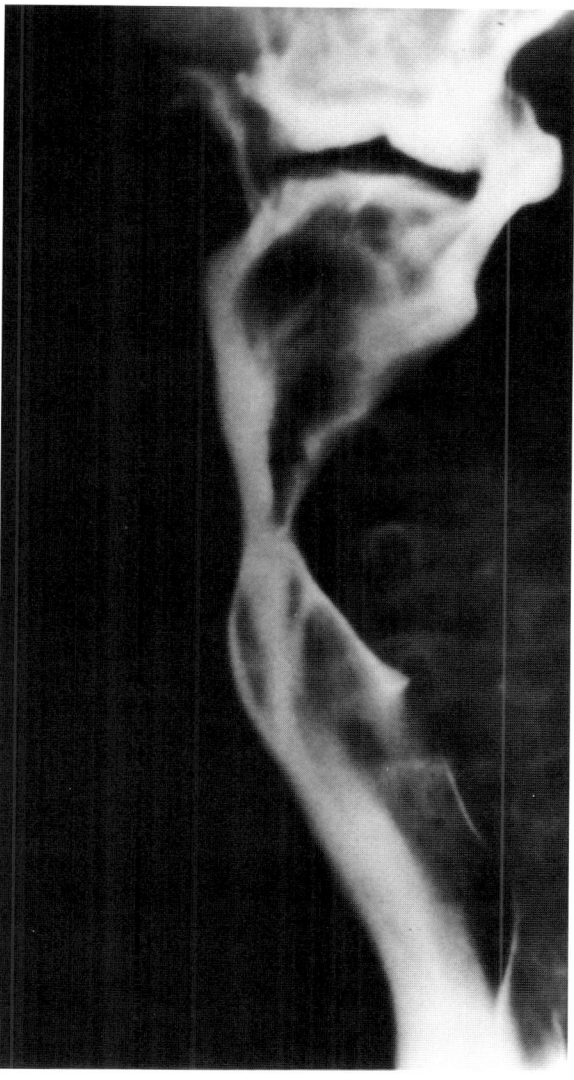

FIG. 40. Histiocytic lymphoma. **A:** An anterior view of a pertechnetate thyroid scan demonstrates a large, cold defect *(arrows)* occupying most of the inferolateral aspect of the left thyroid lobe. **B:** An AP preliminary scout image in an axial CT series demonstrates a huge mass in the plane of the left thyroid lobe deforming the larynx from the subglottis *(hollow arrow)*, down to the upper trachea (T). The *long thin arrow* indicates the level of the glottis; the *tiny arrow* indicates the air-containing left pyriform sinus. **C:** A huge, irregular mass circumscribes the trachea on the left and posteriorly. The mass has an intrinsic lobulated appearance, with areas of increased density. **D:** A barium esophagram demonstrates esophageal displacement in this 73-year-old woman. (Courtesy of Dr. Jeremy L. Freeman, Mount Sinai Hospital, Toronto, Ontario, Canada.).

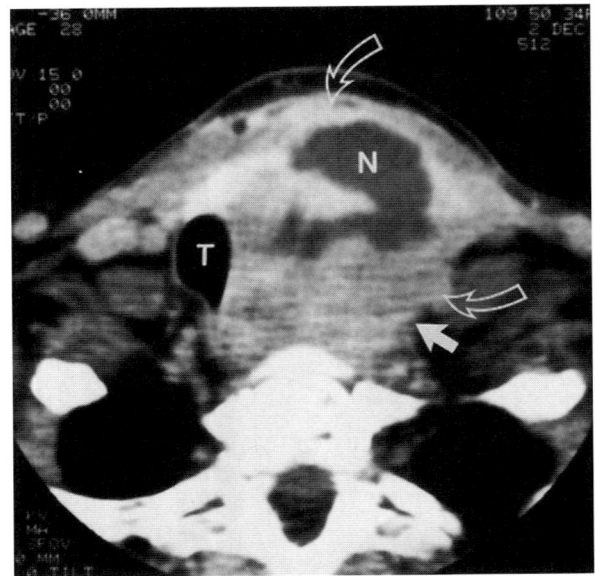

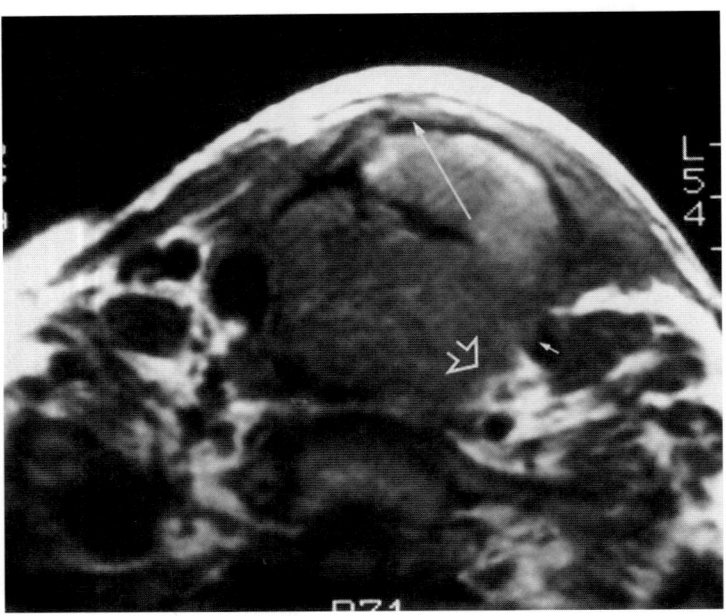

FIG. 41. Anaplastic carcinoma of the thyroid gland with posterior extension. **A:** A CT scan demonstrates the varying density of an anaplastic carcinoma that infiltrates widely. There is necrosis anteriorly (N). There appears to be a capsule anteriorly in the midline *(anterior hollow arrow)*, but there is obvious extension posteriorly *(solid arrow)* and posterolaterally *(lower curved arrow)*. The trachea is displaced to the right (T). Vascular involvement cannot be assessed. **B:** An axial T1-weighted spin-echo MR image matches the CT scan above. The region of the false capsule is indicated by the *long arrow*. The posterolateral extension of the tumor infiltrate is indicated by the *hollow arrow*. The relationship of the tumor mass to the left common carotid artery is identified by the *tiny white arrow*. (Courtesy of Dr. Walter Kucharczyk and the Toronto MR Centre, University of Toronto, Toronto, Ontario, Canada.)

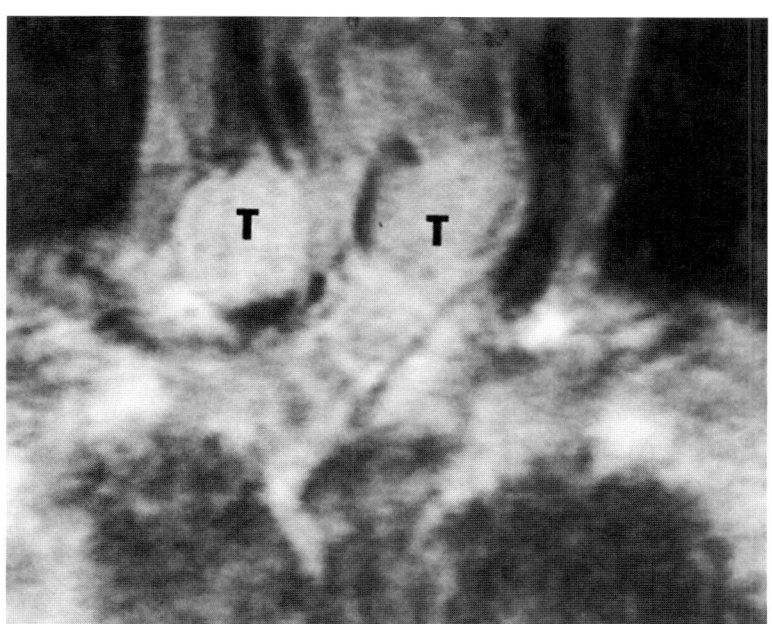

FIG. 42. Carcinoma of the thyroid with tracheal invasion. A coronal MR image (proton density) identifies a carcinoma (T,T) invading the trachea. (Courtesy of Dr. Mahmood Mafee, Professor of Radiology, Director, MR Center, University of Illinois, Chicago, Illinois.)

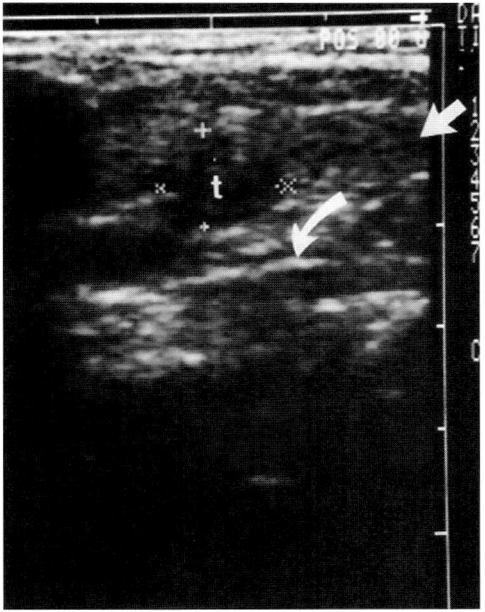
A

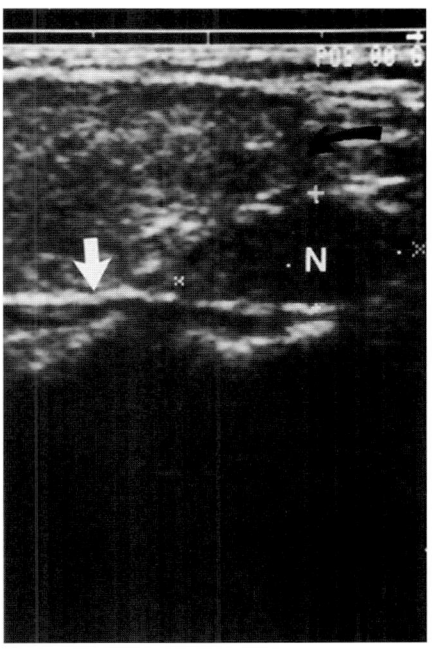
B

FIG. 43. Mixed papillary-follicular carcinoma with metastases to recurrent laryngeal lymph nodes. **A:** A sagittal ultrasound of the right thyroid lobe demonstrates a 1.0 cm × 1.1 cm slightly irregular somewhat hypoechoic solid mass *(cursors)* within the midportion of the right thyroid lobe. The inferior aspect of the right thyroid lobe is indicated by the *straight white arrow*. This proved to be a mixed papillary-follicular carcinoma at total thyroidectomy and regional lymph node dissection. The *curved arrow* indicates the longus colli muscle. t, thyroid tumor. **B:** A sagittal ultrasound demonstrates the lower portion of the right thyroid lobe and its relationship to a hypoechoic, somewhat irregular mass. This proved to be a metastatic lymph node measuring 2.2 cm × 1.1 cm. Its position is also compatible with that of a parathyroid adenoma, but here it represents paratracheal and pararecurrent laryngeal nerve lymph nodes. The *curved black arrow* indicates the inferior aspect of the lower pole of the right thyroid lobe. The longus colli muscle is indicated by the *white arrow*. The patient is a 34-year-old woman. N, metastatic lymph node.

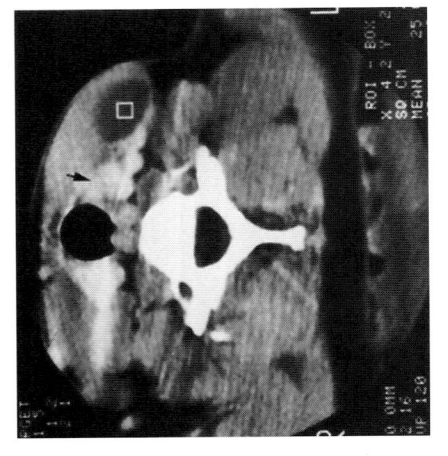
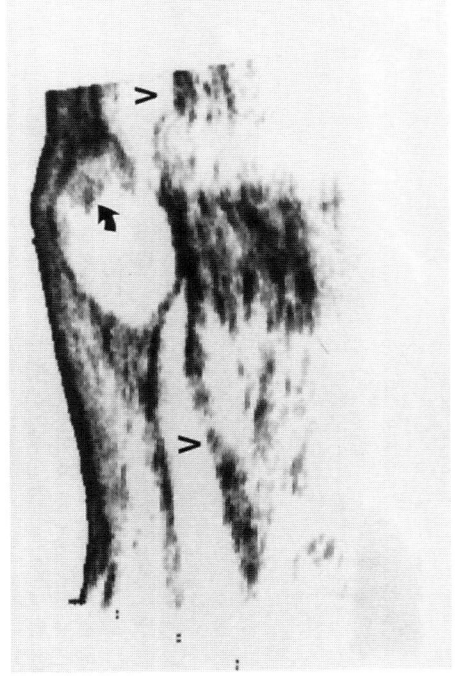
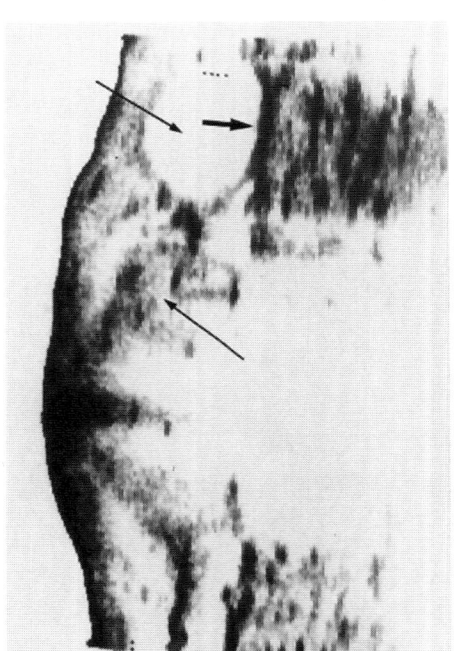
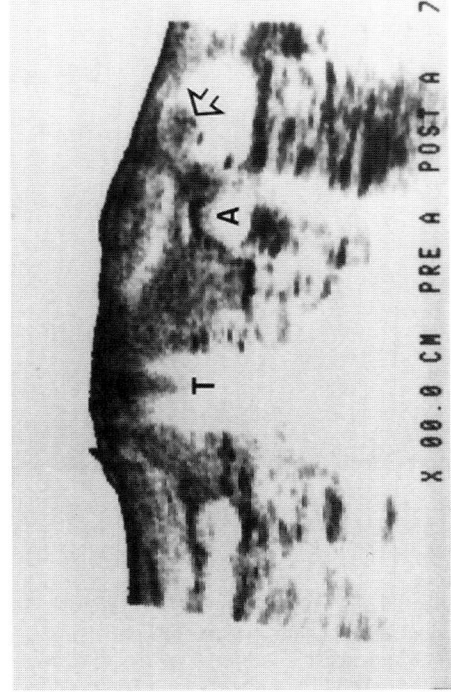
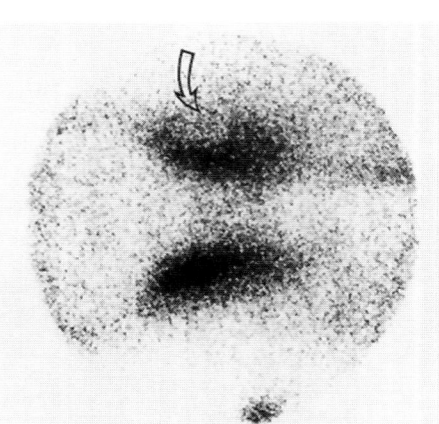

FIG. 44. Occult papillary carcinoma of the thyroid presenting with a "cystic" lateral neck mass. **A:** A pertechnetate radionuclide scan identifies a cold area superolaterally in the left thyroid lobe *(arrow)* in this 26-year-old man presenting with what appeared to be a branchial cleft cyst deep to the sternomastoid muscle at the level of the thyroid gland. No thyroid lesion was palpable. **B:** A transverse ultrasound demonstrates a lateral neck cyst. The *laterally located oblique arrow* indicates a relatively large sonolucent lesion. The *straight short arrow* indicates the strong back wall image of this apparent cyst. The *medially located oblique arrow* demonstrates some enlargement of the left thyroid lobe, but no specific lesion is identified. **C:** An axial CT image at the same level as the preceding ultrasound image in B indicates a cystic lesion in the lateral neck *(square cursor)* deep to the sternomastoid muscle. The "cyst" has a mean density of 25 HU. The *black arrow* indicates an inhomogeneous area within the left thyroid lobe; the thyroid finding is equivocal. **D:** A transverse ultrasound image just below B demonstrates enlargement of the left thyroid lobe without discrete intrathyroid morphologic change. The cyst at this level, however, contains a small anteriorly positioned echogenic focus *(hollow arrow).* T, trachea; A, adjacent left common carotid artery. **E:** A longitudinal ultrasound identifies a sonolucent cystic lesion with a small echogenic projection *(curved arrow)* anteroinferiorly. The patient's feet are to the reader's right. The lateral neck "cyst" proved to be cystic necrosis in an inferior deep cervical lymph node resulting from metastatic papillary carcinoma of the thyroid gland. The primary papillary carcinoma focus was in the left thyroid lobe, and no other lymph nodes were positive on functional neck dissection, which accompanied near-total thyroidectomy. V,V, compressed internal jugular vein.

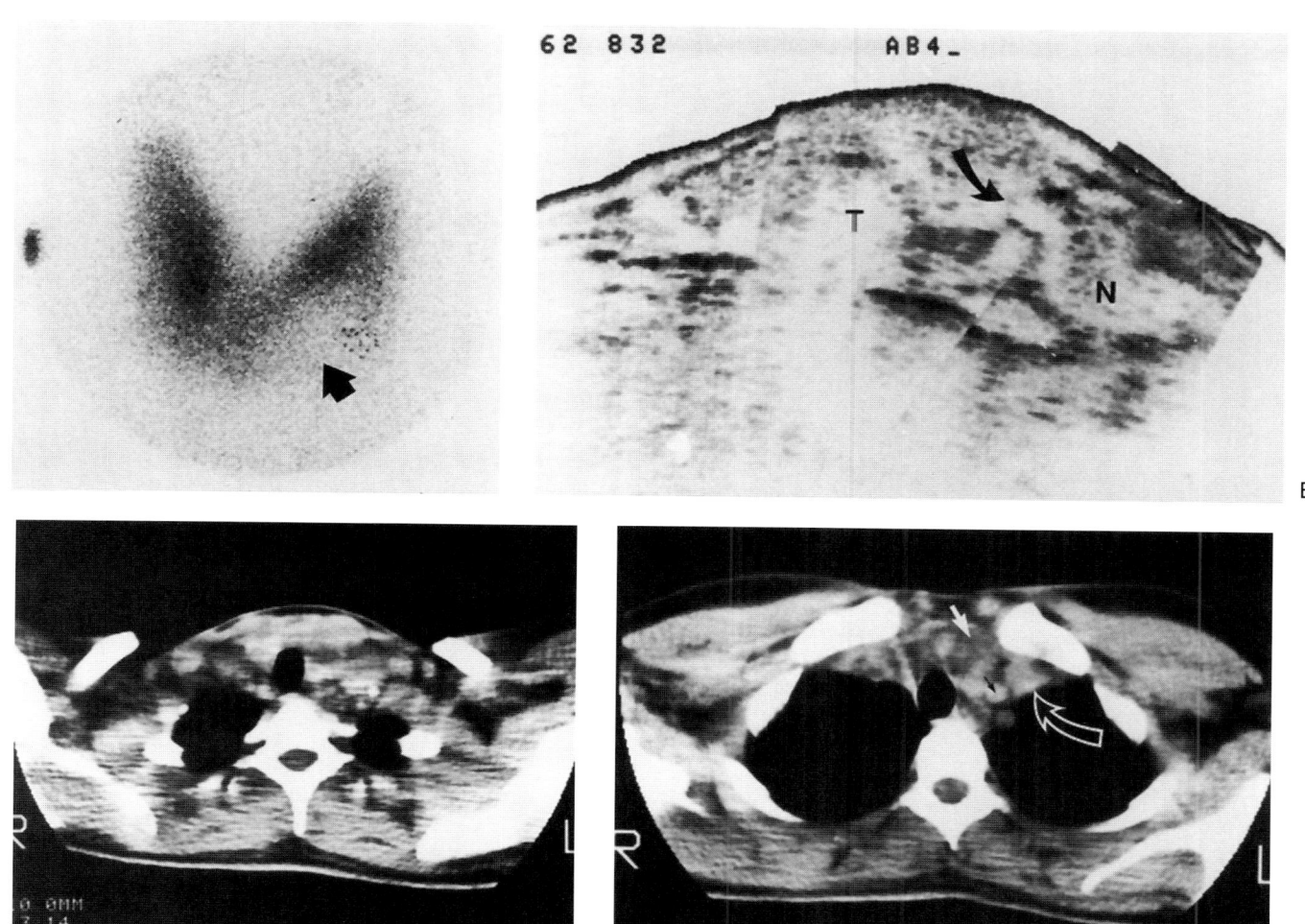

FIG. 45. Papillary carcinoma with cervical and superior mediastinal lymph node metastases. **A:** A pertechnetate thyroid scan demonstrates a large cold defect *(arrow)* in this 22-year-old woman with a mass in the left thyroid lobe. **B:** A transverse 5.0-MHz ultrasound demonstrates irregularity and enlargement of the left thyroid lobe. Tumor extends laterally and posteriorly *(arrow)*. T, trachea; N, mass of deep cervical metastatic lymph nodes in relation to left carotid sheath. **C:** An axial CT scan at the level of the thoracic inlet demonstrates the dimensions of this left thyroid mass and adjacent lymph nodes. **D:** Superior mediastinal lymph nodes are identified *(curved arrow)* in relation to the adjacent mediastinal extension of the thyroid tumor, which has an area of irregularly reduced density within it, presumably a result of tumor necrosis. Lymph nodes are seen in relation to the great vessels *(tiny black arrow)*. The thyroid tumor itself extends into the superior mediastinum *(solid white arrow)*. (Courtesy of Dr. Jeremy L. Freeman, Mount Sinai Hospital, Toronto, Ontario, Canada.)

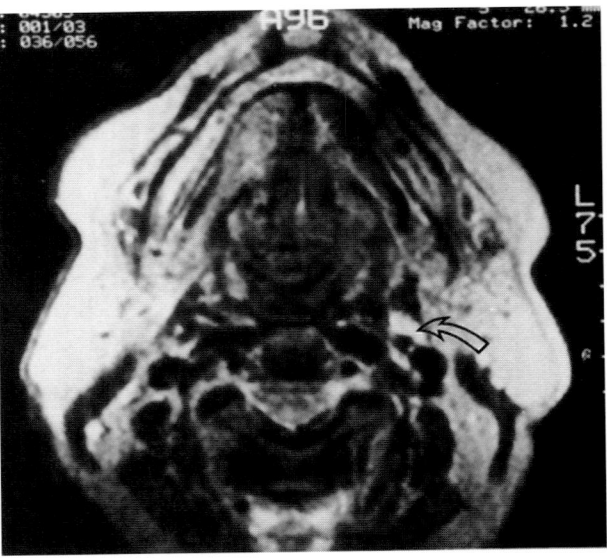

FIG. 46. Impalpable metastatic carcinoma in middle deep cervical lymph node. **A:** A T1-weighted spin-echo pulse sequence image, at the level of the tongue, identifies a 1.0-cm node *(arrow)* in relation to the carotid sheath. The TR is 700; the TE is 20. **B:** A T2-weighted image at the same level identifies the bright signal from this 1.0 cm metastatic lymph node *(arrow)* which was impalpable. (Courtesy of Dr. Walter Kucharczyk and the Toronto MR Centre, University of Toronto, Toronto, Ontario, Canada.)

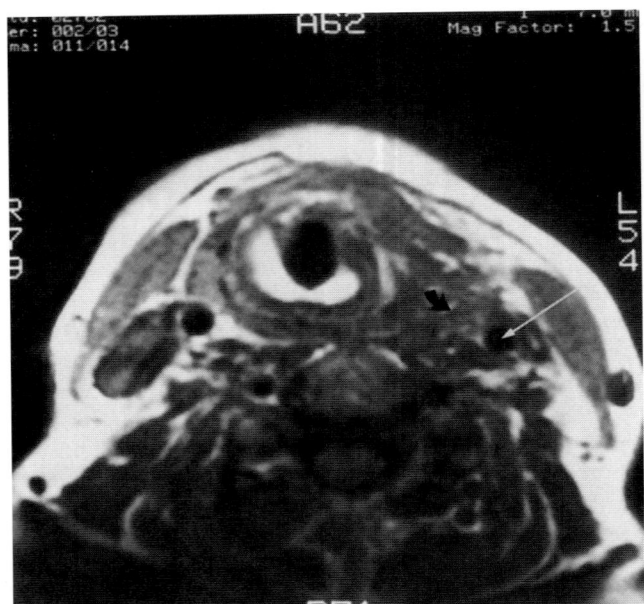
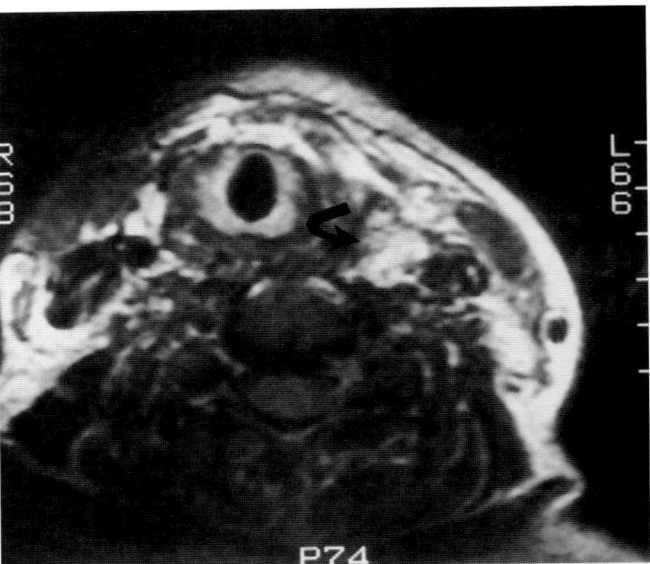

FIG. 47. Metastatic thyroid carcinoma in lymph node. **A:** A spin-echo pulse sequence MR, T1-weighted, with a TR of 700 and TE of 20, demonstrates a mass *(black arrow)* between the displaced left common carotid artery *(white arrow)* and the larynx. **B:** A T2-weighted image, in axial display at the same level, with a TR of 2500 and a TE of 80, demonstrates the bright signal emanating from metastatic thyroid carcinoma to a lower deep cervical lymph node *(black arrow)*. (Courtesy of Dr. Walter Kucharczyk and the Toronto MR Centre, University of Toronto, Toronto, Ontario, Canada.)

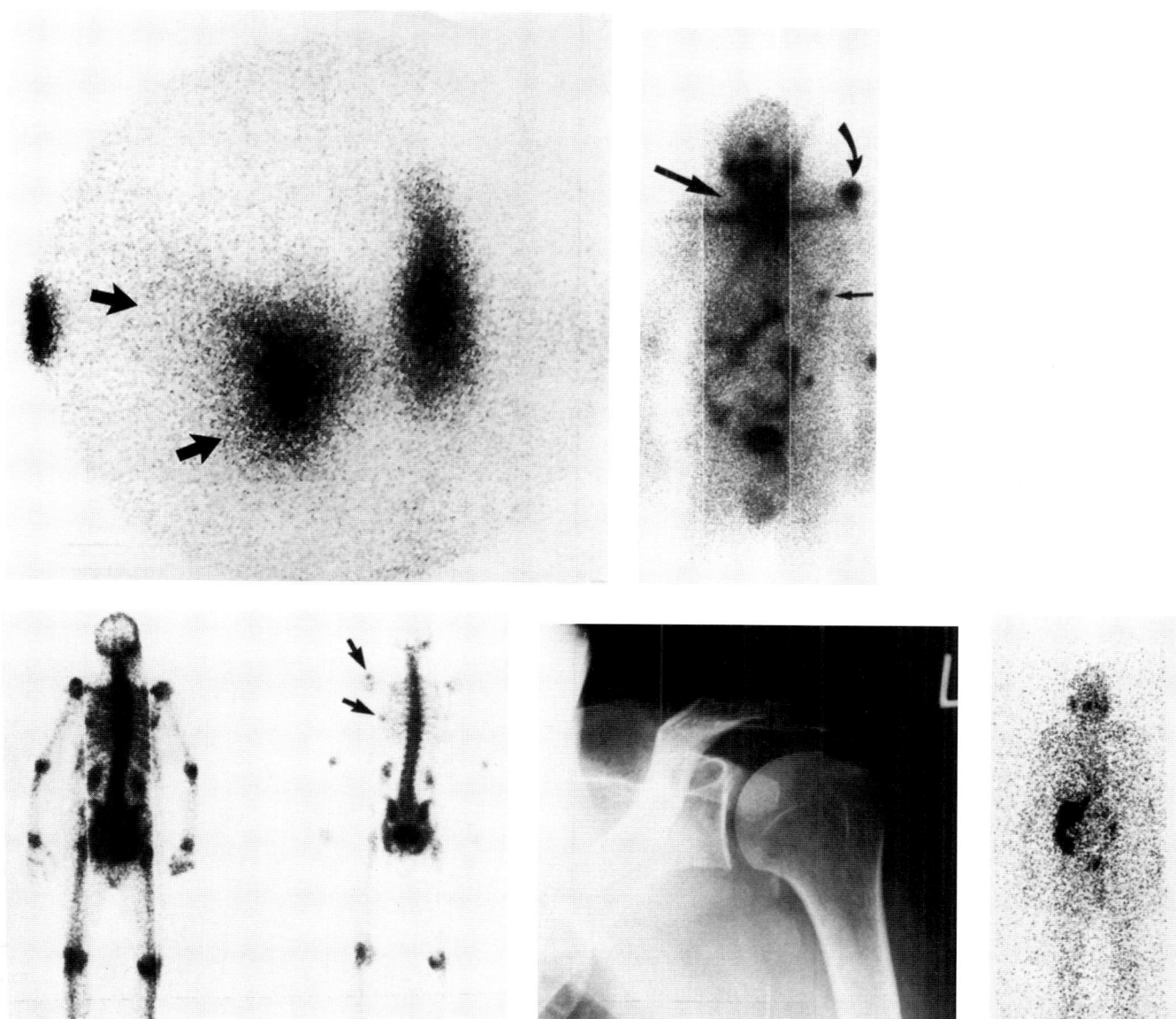

FIG. 48. Follicular adenocarcinoma of the thyroid gland with metastases. **A:** A pertechnetate thyroid scan demonstrates a large, cold defect occupying the lateral portion of the right thyroid lobe *(arrows)* which is substantially enlarged. **B:** The patient was treated with subtotal thyroidectomy and postoperative sodium iodide (I-131) was given therapeutically. An anterior image of a whole-body scan demonstrates the intense uptake of residual thyroid gland *(heavy arrow)*. This is termed the thyroid star, and it is an artifact related to penetration of the collimator septa by the high energy photons of the I-131 concentrated in the thyroid bed. Functioning metastases are evident in the left shoulder *(curved arrow)* and the left rib cage *(small horizontal arrow)*. **C:** Posterior whole-body bone scan views (methylene diphosphonate) identify the osteoblastic reaction of the two bony metastases in the left shoulder and rib cage *(arrows)*. The I-131 identifies the metastases; the bone scan identifies the bony reaction about the metastases. **D:** A plain film examination of the left humerus identifies minimal morphologic changes; the physiologic radionuclide images are much more revealing. **E:** Six months after I-131 treatment, the metastases have resolved. The I-131 scan in diagnostic dose, in whole-body display, indicates no residual thyroid gland uptake. There is the usual oral activity resulting from radionuclide-contaminated saliva and the usual gut activity resulting from gastric and colonic excretion of iodine. (From ref. 103, with permission.)

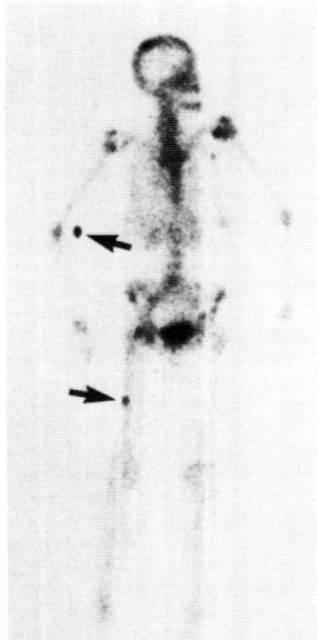

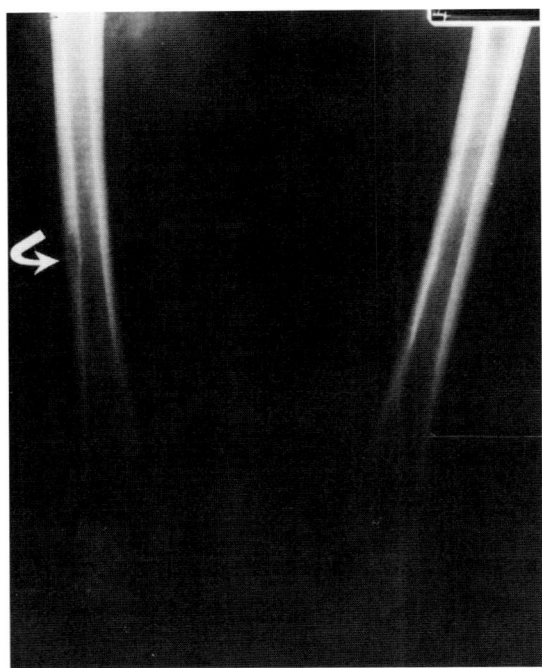

FIG. 49. Bony metastases. **A:** A whole-body methylene diphosphonate (MDP) bone scan indicates bony metastases in several areas, including the right midfemur *(lower arrow)*. There are other areas of skeletal uptake, but no bone lesions were identified on conventional radiographs except for B. The *upper arrow* indicates an area of interstitial injection of the radioactive tracer in the antecubital fossa on the right. This is a whole body image; focal region-of-interest views are now used with current wide-field-of-view gamma cameras. **B:** Comparative views of both femurs indicates bony involvement of the midfemoral cortex *(curved arrow)* on the right. Bone scan changes precede morphologic changes on conventional x-rays.

ACKNOWLEDGMENT

This work was supported by The Saul A. Silverman Family Foundation, Toronto, Ontario, Canada as an Isabel Silverman Canada-International Scientific Exchange Program (CISEPO) project.

REFERENCES

1. Torizuka T, Kasagi K, Hatabu H, et al. Clinical diagnostic potentials of thyroid ultrasonography and scintigraphy: an evaluation. *Endocr J* 1993; 40:329–336.
2. Nelson M, Wickus GG, Caplan RH, Beguin EA. Thyroid gland size in pregnancy—an ultrasound and clinical study. *J Reprod Med* 1987;32: 888–890.
3. Baatenburg de Jong RJ, Rongen RJ. Ultrasound of the head and neck. *ORL J* 1993;55:250–257.
4. Sutton RT, Reading CC, Charboneau JW, James EM, Grant CS, Hay ID. US-guided biopsy of neck masses in postoperative management of patients with thyroid cancer. *Radiology* 1988;168:769–772.
5. Simeone JF, Daniels GH, Hall DH, et al. Sonography in the follow up of 100 patients with thyroid cancer. *AJR* 1987;148:45–49.
6. Gorman B, Charboneau JW, James EM, et al. Medullary thyroid carcinoma: role of high-resolution US. *Radiology* 1987;162:147–150.
7. Frank K, Raue F, Lorenz D, Herfarth C, Ziegler R. Importance of ultrasound examination for the follow-up of medullary thyroid carcinoma: comparison with other localization methods. *Henry Ford Hosp Med J* 1987;35:122–123.
8. Al Sayer HM, Bayliss AP, Krukowski ZH, Matheson NA. The limitation of ultrasound in thyroid swellings. *J R Coll Surg Edinb* 1986;31:27–31.
9. Smith O, Noyek AM. Advances in imaging, scanning and intervention. In: Gray RF, Rutka JA, eds. *Recent advances in otolaryngology* (6). New York: Churchill Livingstone, 1988;49–71.
10. Lu C, Chang TC, Hsiao YL, Kuo MS. Ultrasonographic findings of papillary thyroid carcinoma and their relation to pathologic changes. *J Formosan Med Assoc* 1994;93:933–938.
11. Garretti L, Cassinis MC, Cesarani F, Drogo M, Papotti M, Ragona R. The reliability of echotomographic diagnosis in assessing thyroid lesion. A comparison with cytology and histology. *Radiologia Medica* 1994;88:598–605.
12. Tramalloni J, Leehardt L. Echography of the thyroid nodules. What the clinician is waiting for. *J Radiol* 1994;75:187–190.
13. Vitti P, Martino E, Aghini-Lombardi, et al. Thyroid volume measurement by ultrasound in children as a tool for the assessment of mild iodine deficiency. *J Clin Endocrinol Metab* 1994;79:600–603.
14. Szebeni A, Beleznay E. New simple method for thyroid volume determination by ultrasonography. *J Clin Ultrasound* 1992;20:329–337.
15. Chanoine JP, Toppet V, Lagasse R, Spehl M, Delange F. Determination of thyroid volume by ultrasound from the neonatal period to late adolescence. *Eur J Pediatr* 1991;150:395–399.
16. Yokoyama N, Nagayama Y, Kakezono F, et al. Determination of the volume of the thyroid gland by a high resolution ultrasonic scanner. *J Nucl Med* 1986;9:1475–1479.
17. Perrild H, Hansen JM, Hegedii L, et al. Triiodothyronine and thyroxine treatment of diffuse non-toxic goiter evaluated by ultrasonic scanning. *Acta Endocrinol (Copenh)* 1982;100:382–387.
18. Ares S, Pastor I, Quero J, Morreale de Escobar G. Thyroid gland volume as measured by ultrasonography in preterm infants. *Acta Paediatr* 1995;84:58–62.
19. Golkowski F, Szybinski Z, Huszno B, Stanuch H, Zarnecki A. Ultrasound measurement of thyroid volume in the nation-wide epidemiologic survey on iodine deficiency in Poland. *Endokrynologia Polska* 1993;44:351–358.
20. McIvor NP, Freeman JL, Salem S. Ultrasonography of the thyroid and parathyroid glands. *ORL J* 1993;55:303–308.
21. Brander A, Viikinkoski P, Nickels J, Kivisaari L. Thyroid gland: US screening in a random adult population. *Radiology* 1991;181:683–687.
22. Ross DS. Evaluation of the thyroid nodule. *J Nucl Med* 1991;32: 2181–2192.
23. McShane DP, Freeman JL, Noyek AM, Steinhardt MI. A review of conventional and CT imaging in the evaluation of thyroid malignancies. *J Otolaryngol* 1987;16:1–9.
24. Vander JB, Gaston EA, Dawber TR. The significance of nontoxic thyroid nodules. *Ann Intern Med* 1968;69:537–540.
25. Brander A, Viikinkoski P, Tuuhea J, Voutilainen L, Kivisaari L. Clinical versus ultrasound examination of the thyroid gland in common clinical practice. *J Clin Ultrasound* 1992;20:37–42.
26. Miskin M, Rosen IB, Walfish PG. Ultrasonography of the thyroid gland. *Radiol Clin North Am* 1975;13:475–492.
27. Simeone JF, Daniels GH, Mueller PR, et al. High resolution real-time sonography of the thyroid. *Radiology* 1982;145:431–435.
28. Rosen IB, Wallace C, Strawbridge HG, Walfish PG. Re-evaluation of needle aspiration cytology in detection of thyroid cancer. *Surgery* 1981;90:747–756.
29. Jarlov AE, Nygard B, Hegedus L, Karstrup S, Hansen JM. Observer variation in ultrasound assessment of the thyroid gland. *Br J Radiol* 1993;66:625–627.
30. Witterick IJ, Abel SM, Noyek AM, Freeman JL, Chapnik JS. Nonpalpable occult and metastatic papillary thyroid carcinoma. *Laryngoscope* 1993;103:149–155.
31. Price R, Horvath K, Moore FD Jr. Surgery for solitary thyroid nodules: assessment of methods to select patients at low risk for unsuspected malignancy in the unaffected lobe and the possible utility of preoperative thyroid ultrasound. *Thyroid* 1993;3:87–92.
32. Mann WJ. *Ultraschall im kopf-hals-Bereich.* Berlin: Springer-Verlag, 1984.
33. Clark KJ, Cronan JJ, Scola FH. Color Doppler sonography: anatomic and physiologic assessment of the thyroid. *J Clin Ultrasound* 1995; 23:215–223.
34. Hubsch P, Niederle B, Barton P, et al. Color-coded Doppler sonography of the thyroid: an advance in carcinoma diagnosis? *ROFO* 1992; 156:125–129.
35. Gooding GA, Clark OH. Use of Doppler imaging in the distinction between thyroid and parathyroid lesions. *Am J Surg* 1992;164:51–56.
36. McLaughlin SJ, Gray JG, Marshall T. Aspiration cytology and ultrasonography of cold thyroid nodules. *Aust NZ J Surg* 1986;56: 331–334.
37. Reading CC, Gorman CA. Thyroid imaging techniques. *Clin Lab Med* 1993;13:711–724.
38. Goldfinger M, Rothberg R, Stoll S. Sonographic guidance of thyroid needle biopsy. *J Can Assoc Radiol* 1986;37:186–188.
39. Boland GW, Lee MJ, Mueller PR, Mayo-Smith W, Dawson SL, Simeone JF. Efficacy of sonographically guided biopsy of thyroid masses and cervical lymph nodes. *Am J Roentgenol* 1993;161:1053–1056.
40. Ozdemir H, Ilgit ET, Yucel C, et al. Treatment of autonomous thyroid nodules: safety and efficacy of sonographically guided percutaneous injection of ethanol. *Am J Roentgenol* 1994;163:929–932.
41. Goletti O, Monzani F, Lenziardi M, et al. Cold thyroid nodules: a new application of percutaneous ethanol injection treatment. *J Clin Ultrasound* 1994;22:175–178.
42. Lim-Dunham JE, Feinstein KA, Yousefzadeh DK, Ben-Ami T. Sonographic demonstration of a normal thyroid gland excludes ectopic thyroid in patients with thyroglossal duct cyst. *Am J Roentgenol* 1995;164: 1489–1491.
43. Parulekar SG, Kazman RA. Primary malignant lymphoma of the thyroid: sonographic appearance. *J Clin Ultrasound* 1986;14:60–62.
44. Ueda D, Mitamura R, Suzuki N, Yano K, Okuno A. Sonographic imaging of the thyroid gland in congenital hypothyroidism. *Pediatric Radiol* 1992;22:102–105.
45. Vitti P, Rago T, Mancusi F, et al. Thyroid hypoechogenic pattern at ultrasonography as a tool for predicting recurrence of hyperthyroidism after medical treatment in patients with Graves' disease. *Acta Endocrinol* 1992;126:128–131.
46. Tovi F, Barki Y, Zirkin H. Ultrasonic diagnosis of a metastatic cyst lymph node. *Ann Otol Rhinol Laryngol* 1987;96:716–717.
47. Reede DL. Imaging modalities for the evaluation of neck pathology. In: Valvassori GE, Mafee MF, eds. *Otolaryngol Clin North Am* 1988;21: 495–511.
48. Syenave P. Surgical pathology of the thyroid gland—diagnostic contribution of computed tomography. *Acta Otorhinolaryngol Belg* 1987;41: 677–684.
49. Swartz JD, Korsvik H, Saluk PH, Popky GL. High resolution computed tomography, Part 1: soft tissue of the neck. *Head Neck Surg* 1984;7: 73–80.
50. Wolf BS, Nakagawa H, Yeh HC. Visualization of the thyroid gland with computed tomography. *Radiology* 1977;123:368.
51. Silverman PM, Newman GE, Korobkin M, Workman JB, Moore AV,

Coleman RE. Computed tomography in the evaluation of thyroid disease. *AJR* 1984;141:897–902.
52. Surks MI, Sievert R. Drugs and thyroid function. *N Engl J Med* 1995; 333:1688–1694.
53. Shih WJ, Magoun S, Lahr B. Demonstratable photopenic lesion on Tc-99m pertechnetate thyroid imaging after recent contrast radiographic procedure. *Clin Nucl Med* 1994;19:181–183.
54. Shah HR, Boyd CM, Williamson M, Angtuaco T, Suen JY, Eudy SI. Lingual thyroid: unusual appearance on computed tomography. *Comput Med Imaging Graph* 1988;12:263–266.
55. Friedman M, Toriumi DM, Mafee MF. Diagnostic imaging techniques in thyroid cancer. *Am J Surg* 1988;155:215–223.
56. Cohen O, Herskovitz P, Shindell B, Leiba S, Hadar H. Pitfalls in the follow-up of cervical and mediastinal goitres: role of CT imaging. *J Laryngol Otol* 1992;106:65–70.
57. Bashist B, Ellis K, Gold RP. Computed tomography of intrathoracic goiters. *AJR* 1983;140:455–460.
58. Higgins CB, McNamara MT, Fisher MR, Clark OH. MR imaging of the thyroid. *AJR* 1986;145:1255–1261.
59. Charkes ND, Maurer AH, Siegel JA, Radecki PD, Malmud LS. MR imaging in thyroid disorders: correlation of signal intensity with Graves' disease activity. *Radiology* 1987;164:491–494.
60. Noma S, Nishimura K, Togashi K, et al. Thyroid gland: MR imaging. *Radiology* 1987;164:495–499.
61. Mountz JM, Glazer GM, Dmuchowski C, Sisson JC. MR imaging of the thyroid: comparison with scintigraphy in the normal and diseased gland. *J Comput Assist Tomogr* 1987;11:612–619.
62. Huysmans DA, de Haas MM, van den Broek WJ, et al. Magnetic resonance imaging for volume estimation of large multinodular goitres: a comparison with scintigraphy. *Br J Radiol* 1994;67:519–523.
63. Otsuka N, Nagai K, Morita K, et al. Magnetic resonance imaging of subacute thyroiditis. *Radiat Med* 1994;12:273–276.
64. Gefter WB, Spritzer CE, Eisenberg B, et al. Thyroid imaging with high field strength surface-coil MR. *Radiology* 1987; 164:483–490.
65. Beomonte Zobel B, Cardone G, Tella S, et al. Magnetic resonance in the diagnosis of thyroid diseases. *Radiol Med* 1992;84:36–42.
66. Glazer HS, Niemeyer JH, Balfe DM, et al. Neck neoplasms: MR imaging. 1. Initial evaluation. *Radiology* 1986;160:343–348.
67. Declerck S, Casselman JW, Depondt M, Vandevoorde P. Lingual thyroid imaging. *J Belge Radiol* 1993;76:241–242.
68. Guneri A, Ceryan K, Igci E, Kovanlikaya A. Lingual thyroid: the diagnostic value of magnetic resonance imaging. *J Laryngol Otol* 1991; 105:493–495.
69. Jacobson HG, ed. Topics in radiology-magnetic resonance imaging of the head and neck: present status and future potential. *JAMA* 1988; 260:3313–3326.
70. Chevigne-Brancart M, Baudoux A, Salamon E. Thyroid imaging using 99m TC, 123I and 131I. *Acta Otorhinolaryngol Belg* 1987;41: 637–648.
71. Beckers C. Trends in thyroid imaging. *Horm Res* 1987;26:28–32.
72. Clarke SEM. Radionuclide imaging in thyroid cancer. *Nucl Med Commun* 1988;9:79–84.
73. Noyek AM, Witterick IJ, Kirsh JC. Radionuclide imaging in otolaryngology-head and neck surgery. *Arch Otolaryngol Head Neck Surg* 1991;117:372–378.
74. Price DC. Radioisotopic evaluation of the thyroid and the parathyroids. *Radiol Clin North Am* 1993;31:991–1015.
75. Freitas JE, Gross MD, Ripley S, Shapiro B. Radionuclide diagnosis and therapy of thyroid cancer. *Semin Nucl Med* 1985;15:106–131.
76. Fogelman I, Cooke SG, Maisey MN. The role of thyroid scanning in hyperthyroidism. *Eur J Nucl Med* 1986;11:397–440.
77. Ramtoola S, Maisey MN, Clarke SEM, Fogelman I. The thyroid scan in Hashimoto's thyroiditis: the great mimic. *Nucl Med Commun* 1988; 9:639–645.
78. Gordon DL, Wagner R, Dillehay GL, et al. The effect of fine-needle aspiration biopsy on the thyroid scan. *Clin Nucl Med* 1993;18: 495–497.
79. Sandler MP, Fellmeth B, Salhany KE, Patton JA. Thyroid carcinoma masquerading as a solitary benign hyperfunctioning nodule. *Clin Nucl Med* 1988;13:410–415.
80. Katagiri M, Suzuki S, Sadahiro S, et al. Accumulation of Iodine-131 and Technetium-99m pertechnetate in thyroid carcinoma. *Clin Nucl Med* 1988;13:276–279.
81. Pacini F, Lippi F, Formica N, et al. Therapeutic doses of Iodine-131 reveal undiagnosed metastases in thyroid cancer patients with detectable serum thyroglobulin levels. *J Nucl Med* 1987;28: 1888–1891.
82. Corstens F, Huysmans D, Kloppenborg P. Thallium-201 scintigraphy of the suppressed thyroid: an alternative for Iodine-123 scanning after TSH stimulation. *J Nucl Med* 1988;29:1360–1363.
83. el-Desouki M. Tl-201 thyroid imaging in differentiating benign from malignant thyroid nodules. *Clin Nucl Med* 1991;16:425–430.
84. Fischer M, Hoffmann UJ, Kohnlein W, Skutta D. Radioimmunoscintigraphy with anti-thyroglobulin monoclonal antibodies. *Nuklearmedizin* 1986;25:232–234.
85. Wei JP, Burke GJ. Characterization of the neoplastic potential of solitary solid thyroid lesions with Tc-99m-pertechnetate and Tc-99m-sestamibi scanning. *Ann Surg Oncol* 1995;2:233–237.
86. Foldes I, Levay A, Stotz G. Comparative scanning of thyroid nodules with technetium-99m pertechnetate and technetium-99m methoxyisobutylisonitrile. *Eur J Nucl Med* 1993;20:330–333.
87. Hoefnagel CA, Delprat CC, Zanin D, Van Der Schoot JB. New radionuclide tracers for the diagnosis and therapy of medullary thyroid carcinoma. *Clin Nucl Med* 1988;13:159–165.
88. Bigsby RJ, Lepp EK, Litwin DE, Wilkinson AA, Matte GG. Technetium 99m pentavalent dimercaptosuccinic acid and thallium 201 in detecting recurrent medullary carcinoma of the thyroid. *Can J Surg* 1992;35:388–392.
89. Clarke SEM, Lazarus C, Mistry R, Maisey MN. The role of technetium-99m pentavalent DMSA in the management of patients with medullary carcinoma of the thyroid. *Br J Radiol* 1987;60: 1089–1092.
90. Udelsman R, Ball D, Baylin SB, Wong CY, Osterman FA Jr, Sostre S. Preoperative localization of occult medullary carcinoma of the thyroid gland with single-photon emission tomography dimercaptosuccinic acid. *Surgery* 1993;114:1083–1089.
91. Itoh H, Sugie K, Toyooka S, et al. Detection of metastatic medullary thyroid cancer with 131 I MIBG scans in Sipple's syndrome. *Eur J Nucl Med* 1986;11:502–504.
92. Lebouthillier G, Morais J, Picard M, Picard D, Chartrand R, D'Amour P. Tc-99m sestamibi and other agents in the detection of metastatic medullary carcinoma of the thyroid. *Clin Nucl Med* 1993; 18:657–661.
93. Biersack HJ, Briele B, Hotze AL, et al. The role of nuclear medicine in oncology. *Ann Nucl Med* 1992;6:131–136.
94. Dorr U, Wurstlin S, Frank-Raue K, et al. Somatostatin receptor scintigraphy and magnetic resonance imaging in recurrent medullary thyroid carcinoma: a comparative study. *Horm Metabol Res* 1993;27(suppl):48–55.
95. Dorr U, Sautter-Bihl ML, Bihl H. The contribution of somatostatin receptor scintigraphy to the diagnosis of recurrent medullary carcinoma of the thyroid. *Semin Oncol* 1994;21:42–45.
96. Krenning EP, Kwekkeboom DJ, Oei HY, et al. Somatostatin receptor scintigraphy in carcinoids, gastrinomas and Cushing's syndrome. *Digestion* 1994;55(suppl):54–59.
97. Edington HD, Watson CG, Levine G, et al. Radioimmunoimaging of metastatic medullary carcinoma of the thyroid gland using an indium-111-labeled monoclonal antibody to CEA. *Surgery* 1988;104: 1004–1010.
98. Vuillez JP, Peltier P, Caravel JP, Chetanneau A, Saccavini JC, Chatal JF. Immunoscintigraphy using 111In-labeled F(ab′)2 fragments of anticarcinoembryonic antigen monoclonal antibody for detecting recurrences of medullary thyroid carcinoma. *J Clin Endocrinol Metab* 1992;74:157–163.
99. O'Byrne KJ, Hamilton D, Robinson I, Sweeney E, Freyne PJ, Cullen MJ. Imaging of medullary carcinoma of the thyroid using 111In-labelled anti-CEA monoclonal antibody fragments. *Nucl Med Commun* 1992;13:142–148.
100. Peltier P, Curtet C, Chatal JF, et al. Radioimmunodetection of medullary thyroid cancer using a bispecific anti-CEA/anti-indium-DTPA antibody and an indium-111-labeled DTPA dimer. *J Nucl Med* 1993;34:1267–1273.
101. Morita Y. Selective thyroid angiography: techniques, diagnosis and indications. *Hokkaido J Med Sci* 1993;68:251–264.
102. Adler LP, Bloom AD. Positron emission tomography of thyroid masses. *Thyroid* 1993;3:195–200.
103. Noyek AM, Greyson ND, Steinhardt MI, et al. Thyroid tumor imaging. *Arch Otolaryngol* 1983;109:205–224.

CHAPTER 10

Molecular Basis of Thyroid Disease

Donald L. St. Germain

Recent advances in molecular biology have led to unprecedented insights into the mechanisms of hormone action and the pathophysiology of endocrine diseases. In particular, the explosion of knowledge in the areas of gene regulation, cell signalling mechanisms, and oncogenesis has increased our information concerning the cellular effects of thyroid hormones and thyrotropin (TSH), the biochemical basis of thyroid hormone resistance syndromes, and the pathogenesis of nodular goiter, Graves' disease, and thyroid cancer. Such studies have also provided powerful new experimental methods and reagents for use in both the clinical and research laboratories. In addition, unexpected aspects of thyroid physiology, such as the critical role that selenium plays in thyroid hormone metabolism, have been discovered recently.

In this section of *Thyroid Disease*, these and other selected topics relevant to the study of the thyroid axis will be reviewed. This initial chapter will cover basic concepts of molecular biology as they relate to thyroid hormone action and metabolism, the signalling pathways utilized by TSH and thyrotropin-releasing hormone (TRH), and oncogenesis. Subsequent chapters discuss these topics and their clinical relevance in greater detail. For convenience, a glossary is provided at the end of this section of the text.

REGULATION OF GENE EXPRESSION

The Central Paradigm of Cell Biology

The central paradigm of cellular and molecular biology (Fig. 1) holds that the genetic information that determines protein structure is encoded in the double-stranded DNA in the cell's nucleus (1). The synthesis of a particular protein is thus initiated in this cellular compartment. Using a process termed transcription, the region of DNA that codes for the protein of interest is used as a template for the synthesis of a single-stranded messenger RNA (mRNA) molecule. The mRNA carries this genetic information into the cytoplasm, where it associates with specialized organelles called ribosomes. Here the mRNA is itself used as a template to direct translation, the process of amino acid polymerization that results in the synthesis of a specific protein. The proteins so produced then serve a variety of functions within the cell.

The human genome is composed of 3 billion nucleotides, the "building blocks" of DNA, and it is estimated to contain 60,000 to 70,000 protein-encoding genes (2). Of note, all cells (excluding germ cells) contain a complete copy of the genomic DNA, yet in any given cell at a particular time, only a fraction of these genes, perhaps 10,000, are being transcribed for protein synthesis. Some genes, so called house-keeping genes, code for proteins that are expressed in all cells. These genes may number approximately 2500 (2). However, each cell type also expresses a unique subset of proteins that determine that particular cell's structure and function: thyroid cells express thyroglobulin, thyrotrophs in the anterior pituitary gland synthesize and secrete the protein subunits of TSH, and neurons in the paraventricular nuclei express and process the precursor protein for TRH.

The complement of proteins being synthesized by a cell is a dynamic process. Genes are frequently turned on and off, or their transcriptional activity modified, in response to intracellular and extracellular stimuli such as stress, injury, hormones, growth factors, and nutritional status (3,4). Some of the most complex and dramatic examples of coordinated alterations in gene expression take place during the developmental period as pluripotential cells take on more differentiated phenotypes (5). Oncogenesis likewise involves an alteration in expression of one or more key genes that code for proteins that regulate the cell's replicative machinery (6).

D. L. St. Germain: Departments of Medicine and Physiology, Dartmouth Medical School, Lebanon, New Hampshire 03756.

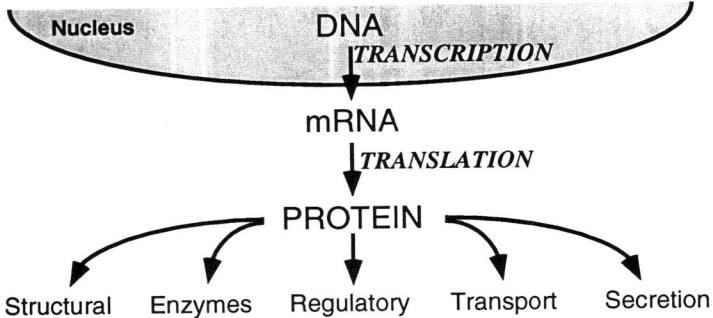

FIG. 1. The central paradigm of cell and molecular biology wherein information dictating the amino acid sequence and hence the structure of the cell's proteins is encoded in the DNA.

Thus, the processes that regulate the timing of gene expression, as well as its level of activity, are critical to cellular function and the overall health of the organism (7). One of the great triumphs of molecular biology has been the insight it has provided into the mechanisms of transcriptional control (7). With this has come the realization that the processes controlling gene expression are some of the most ancient and highly conserved in biology; many of the components of the regulatory machinery are interchangeable between such diverse species as yeast and humans (8).

Structural Organization of a Gene

Knowledge of the structural organization of a gene (Fig. 2) is crucial to an understanding of its function and regulation. Each gene is composed of a central core, termed the transcription unit, which serves as the template for mRNA synthesis (7). Surrounding this core unit are upstream and downstream regions. The DNA within the transcription unit is divided into regions termed exons and introns. Although the entire transcription unit is initially transcribed to form a large precursor RNA molecule, various processing steps occur prior to export of the RNA from the nucleus (7). Splicing results in the removal of the intronic sequences, and then the joining together of the exonic sequences to form the "mature" mRNA molecule. The mRNA is usually further modified by the addition of a string of adenosines to the 3' end of the molecule to make a poly(A) tail. This may function to stabilize the mRNA molecule. Contained within a contiguous stretch of the mature mRNA is the coding region for the protein (7). This consists of the triplet nucleotide sequences of the genetic code that determine the protein's amino acid sequence.

Each gene's transcription unit may extend for tens of thousands of nucleotides along the chromosome. The length is dependent on the size of the protein encoded by the gene and the number and size of the interspersed introns. The function(s) of the introns remains uncertain.

Whereas sequences within the transcription unit determine the structure of the gene's protein product, it is the sequences in the upstream region of the gene, termed the promoter/enhancer region, that regulate the timing and the amount of gene transcription that occurs (7). The importance of this region was hinted at over 20 years ago when the β-globin gene was isolated and compared in normal individuals and those with β-thalassemia. It was soon noted that a deficiency of β-globin protein and mRNA could result from the presence of a single base mutation in the upstream region of the gene (9).

The Promoter Region and the Basal Transcriptional Apparatus

In discussing the structural features of the promoter region (Fig. 3), a numbering system for designating location is useful. The nucleotide where transcription begins is by

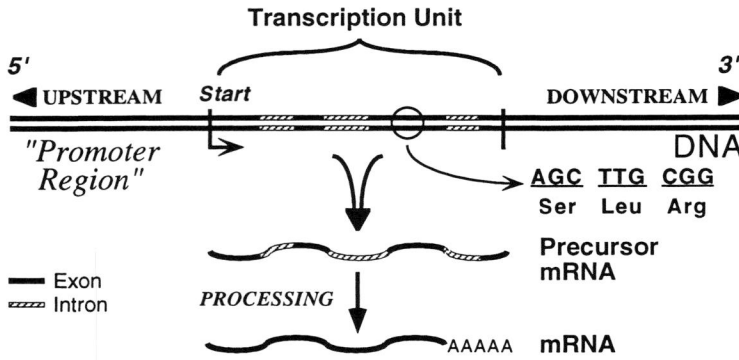

FIG. 2. Structural organization of a gene. The protein-encoding transcription unit is flanked by upstream and downstream regions of the DNA. Sequences dictating regulatory control are typically found in the upstream "promoter" region.

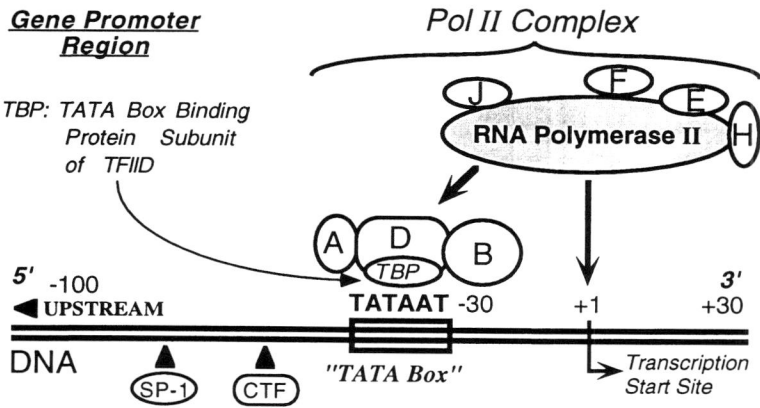

FIG. 3. The promoter region and the basal transcriptional apparatus composed of the RNA polymerase II complexed to several other proteins that serve to regulate transcription.

convention assigned +1. Nucleotides toward the 3' (downstream) direction are designated with progressively larger positive numbers, whereas nucleotides upstream in the promoter region are assigned negative numbers. The promoter typically encompasses approximately the first 100 nucleotides upstream from the transcriptional start site (nucleotides −1 to −100) and includes in most genes a region of DNA rich in adenosine (A) and thymidine (T) nucleotides termed a TATA box. Most commonly this sequence reads TATAAT (7). This short stretch of DNA is critical for transcriptional control, because it serves as the binding site, or anchor, for the assemblage of the large complex of proteins that constitutes the basal transcriptional apparatus (10,11). An essential component of this complex is the RNA polymerase II (pol II), the enzyme that synthesizes the mRNA using the DNA of the transcription unit as a template. In addition to pol II, the general transcriptional apparatus (also termed the pol II complex) includes at least eight protein cofactors (12). These are termed general transcription factors. The general transcription factor IID (TFIID) is composed of several subunits, one of which, the TATA box binding protein (TBP), is the factor that recognizes and binds to the TATAAT sequence (13). This results, remarkably, in a sharp 90° bend and unwinding of the DNA (8,14) and triggers the binding of another cofactor, TFIIB, which stabilizes the TBP–DNA interaction (8,15). Pol II is then recruited to the site along with the other cofactors. Thus, TBP binding to DNA initiates assembly of the pol II complex.

TFIIB and TFIID also appear to be important in the regulation of gene transcription by hormones. Several nuclear hormone receptors, including those for thyroid hormone, make contact with the basal transcriptional apparatus through direct interactions with these pol II cofactors (16–21). Other proteins in the transcriptional complex subserve additional critical functions, such as unwinding and separation of the DNA strands and DNA repair (12).

Located upstream from the TATA box are binding sites for additional proteins that interact with the pol II complex (22). These include the CAAT transcription factor (CTF), so called because of the DNA sequence (CCAAT) to which it binds, and stimulatory protein 1 (SP-1), which binds to a GC-rich region of DNA. These proteins stabilize the basal transcriptional apparatus and thereby enhance the rate of gene expression. In genes whose promoter regions lack a TATA box, TBP is still an essential component of the basal transcriptional apparatus. In such cases, SP-1 and CAAT binding proteins are of particular importance in assigning the start site of transcription (12).

Transcription Factors and Response Elements

The interactions of TBP, CAAT, and SP-1 proteins with the DNA promoter region illustrate the paradigm of the molecular mechanisms that underlie transcriptional control—namely, that gene expression is regulated by proteins that bind to specific short regions of DNA and then interact directly or indirectly via protein–protein interactions with components of the basal transcriptional apparatus (22). Such interactions can serve to influence the rate of transcription in either a positive or a negative fashion (23). As in the case of the TBP, the binding of these regulatory proteins results in bending of the DNA, which may facilitate critical protein–protein interactions (24–26). These DNA binding proteins are collectively referred to as transcription factors (trans factors) and the specific DNA elements to which they bind are termed response elements (cis elements) (Fig. 4). Thus, the TATAAT sequence is a response element for the TBP protein of the TFDII complex. As a general rule, each transcription factor recognizes only a single DNA sequence as a high-affinity response element. However, there are many examples where multiple transcription factors bind to the same DNA sequence (see later).

Most of these protein–DNA interactions occur upstream of the promoter, in the area referred to as the enhancer region (27). Literally dozens of protein–DNA and protein–protein interactions may be occurring in the promoter and enhancer regions of actively transcribed genes. The transcription factors involved may be ubiquitous, such as SP-1, or they may be specialized in the sense that

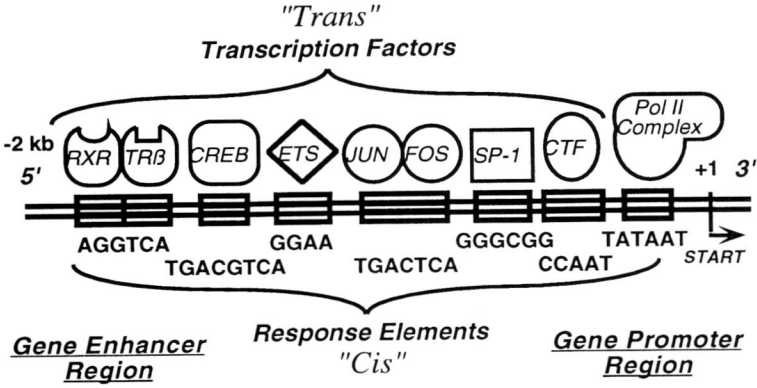

FIG. 4. Transcription factors and response elements. The binding of proteins to specific DNA sequences (termed response elements) within the promoter and enhancer regions is critical to the regulation of transcription. The transcription factors, once bound to DNA, interact with the pol II complex either via direct or indirect protein–protein interactions.

they are dependent on the particular cell type, the nutritional or developmental state of the cell, the stage of the cell cycle, or factors external to the cell such as hormones or growth factors. Note that the promoter–enhancer region of any given gene contains response elements for only a subset of transcription factors. In a sense, this complement of response elements constitutes a second genetic code, which, instead of dictating amino acid sequence as in the case of the coding region of the gene, determines what factors are involved in regulating the gene's level of expression. Because the promoter region sequences for any given gene are inherent to the genome and thus invariant from cell to cell, the ultimate arbiter of expression of a particular gene becomes the specific set of transcription factors being expressed and regulated in the cell.

The Steroid/Thyroid Hormone Nuclear Receptor Superfamily

In the past decade, hundreds of transcription factors have been identified (4). Although some of these are constitutively (inherently) active in either stimulating or repressing transcription, others require alterations in their structure in order to bind to their response element or interact with other proteins to effect gene expression. Common mechanisms of structural alteration include the phosphorylation or dephosphorylation of transcription factors in response to signals from elsewhere in the cell (such as those induced by the binding of growth factors to cell surface receptors) (28), or the binding of a small ligand to the protein such as occurs when thyroid hormone binds to its nuclear receptor (4). Indeed one of the largest classes of transcription factors is that of the nuclear receptor superfamily, which now includes over 150 members (Fig. 5) (29).

The concept that steroid hormones and other small lipophilic compounds such as thyroid hormone interacted with nuclear proteins to directly affect gene expression developed over 30 years ago when the availability of radiolabeled ligands allowed for the first time the demonstration of the presence of high-affinity binding sites for these compounds in the cell nucleus (30). Although the existence of these proteins could clearly be demonstrated, their low abundance made traditional purification schemes problematic. In the mid 1980s, however, molecular techniques allowed the identification of complementary DNAs (cDNAs) for the glucocorticoid (31), estrogen (32), and thyroid hormone receptors (33,34) (GR, ER, TR, respectively). [cDNAs are the DNA equivalent of an mRNA in that they contain the genetic coding sequence for a protein (35). Their isolation and characterization by DNA sequencing provides both important structural in-

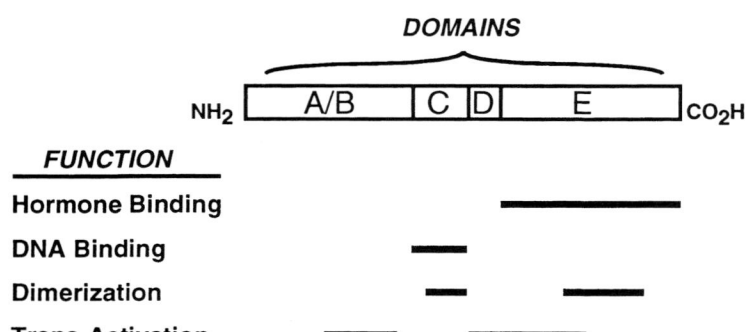

FIG. 5. Structural features of the steroid/thyroid hormone nuclear receptor superfamily members. Domains associated with hormone binding, DNA binding, dimerization, and activation functions are depicted.

formation about a protein and a powerful experimental reagent that can be used for studying gene expression and protein structure and function.]

As deduced from their cDNA sequences, GR, ER, and TR were found to share certain structural features, particularly in the central region of the molecules that form the DNA-binding domain (30,36). Here, two zinc ions are complexed to stretches of amino acids that resemble the fingers of a glove. These proteins are thus referred to as zinc-finger transcription factors. Since the initial isolation of the steroid and thyroid hormone receptors, molecular cloning techniques have been used to isolate cDNAs for many other transcription factors that share these structural features. These include the nuclear receptors for vitamin D (VDR), vitamin A (retinoic acid receptor, RAR) and one of its metabolites 9-cis retinoic acid (RXR), and the other classic steroid hormones (testosterone, progesterone, aldosterone) (30).

All of these proteins have a modular structure (see Fig. 5), in that they are composed of several discrete domains, each of which subserves one or more specific receptor functions (37). Thus, the hormone (ligand) binding domain is located in the carboxy-terminal half of the protein and is quite variable in its structure from receptor to receptor. This is not unexpected, given that different ligands bind in this region. The central core of the receptor contains the DNA-binding zinc fingers, which are similar in overall structure for all the receptors. However, differences in a few amino acid residues in this region are present between receptors, and it is these subtle differences that determine the specific DNA sequence that the receptor recognizes as its response element. Other regions of the protein are involved in the interactions of the receptor with other transcription factors (dimerization domain) or are important for communicating either directly or indirectly with the pol II complex to regulate transcriptional activity (transactivation domains). For example, a short region of the amino-terminus in the thyroid hormone receptor has recently been demonstrated to be important for interacting with TFIIB (18). Specific regions of the steroid hormone receptors also bind to chaperones termed heat shock proteins, which are involved in segregating the receptor between the nuclear and cytoplasmic compartments as ligand binds or dissociates (37). However, most of these transcription factors, including thyroid hormone receptors, appear to maintain a strictly nuclear location.

As additional members of the steroid/thyroid hormone superfamily were isolated, it became apparent that there were many more transcription factors in this class than there were traditional hormones that might serve as ligands (29). Thus, the majority of these proteins are termed orphan receptors, because activating ligands have not been identified; many may be constitutively active as transcription factors and not require a ligand interaction. However, the search for ligands for these orphans has resulted in the recognition that 9-cis retinoic acid (38,39) and long-chain fatty acids (40) can serve as activating ligands for specific nuclear receptors [the RXR and peroxisome proliferator activating receptor (PPAR), respectively]. Additional novel observations about the regulatory role of small molecules are likely to be made by further study of the orphan receptors and their functions (29). Indeed, recent studies in mice, using a genetic technique termed homologous recombination that results in inactivation or a deficiency of a given protein (so called knockout mice), have demonstrated essential roles for several of the orphan receptors (41).

MOLECULAR ASPECTS OF THYROID HORMONE ACTION

Thyroid Hormone Receptors

The TRs (Fig. 6) are nuclear transcription factors whose activities are regulated by the binding of 3,5,3′-triiodothyronine (T_3) to a hydrophobic pocket in the ligand-binding domain of the protein (42). Like many members of the nuclear receptor superfamily, TRs are present in several different isoforms which differ somewhat in their structure (43). These different forms of the TR are coded from two separate genes. The *TRα* gene, located on chromosome 17,

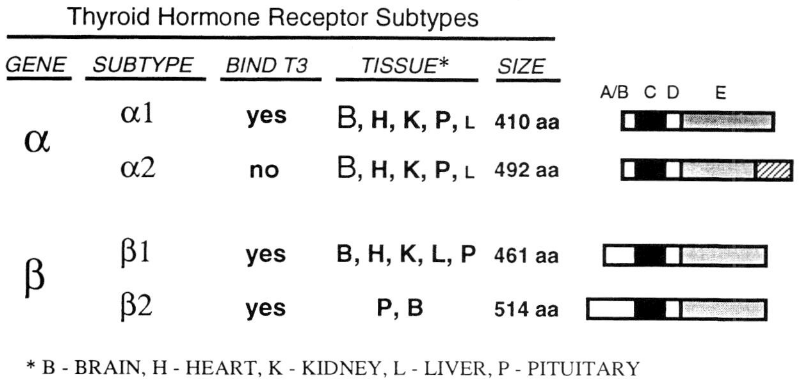

Thyroid Hormone Receptor Subtypes

GENE	SUBTYPE	BIND T3	TISSUE*	SIZE
α	α1	yes	B, H, K, P, L	410 aa
	α2	no	B, H, K, P, L	492 aa
β	β1	yes	B, H, K, L, P	461 aa
	β2	yes	P, B	514 aa

* B - BRAIN, H - HEART, K - KIDNEY, L - LIVER, P - PITUITARY

FIG. 6. Different types and subtypes of the nuclear thyroid hormone receptors. Multiple receptor subtypes are derived from two receptor genes via the use of alternative splicing (in the case of the α receptors) or the use of alternative promoters (for the β-receptor subtypes).

gives rise to at least three different isoforms (designated TRα$_1$, α$_2$, and α$_3$). These are derived by a process termed alternative splicing, wherein different exons from the downstream portion of the transcription unit are linked together at the time of mRNA processing (44). The TRα$_1$ isoform is expressed in numerous tissues (45) and binds T$_3$ with high affinity (46). The TRα$_2$ and TRα$_3$ isoforms differ in that the distal part of the ligand-binding domains at the carboxy-terminus has been replaced by larger amino acid sequences coded by a separate exon. This substitution alters the ligand-binding domain such that the TRα$_2$ and TRα$_3$ proteins are not able to bind T$_3$ (46). Thus, they are not true receptors in that their activities are not regulated by ligand binding. Rather, the TRα$_2$ appears to act as a constitutive repressor, and it is able to block T$_3$-mediated transcriptional activity (47) by competing with activated TRs for DNA binding sites, (48) or through other, as yet undefined, mechanisms (49). A fourth TR-related isoform, termed Rev-ErbAα, is also coded by the TRα gene, but the template used is the DNA strand opposite to that used to code the other TRα isoforms (50–52). Rev-ErbAα also fails to bind T$_3$, and it currently carries the status of an orphan receptor (50,51). Its role in thyroid hormone action and transcriptional regulation is uncertain.

Two additional TR isoforms, the TRβ$_1$ and TRβ$_2$, are coded by a second gene located on chromosome 3—the *TRβ* gene (43). The isoforms from this gene arise not through alternative splicing mechanisms, but rather from the use of different promoter regions of this gene which alter the choice of upstream exons used to code the amino-terminus of the protein. TRβ$_1$ is expressed in many tissues (45). In the brain it is developmentally regulated, being highest during late gestation and in the early neonatal period, when the brain appears to be most sensitive to the effects of thyroid hormones (45). TRβ$_2$ expression appears to be limited primarily to the brain and anterior pituitary gland (53).

A question of considerable interest is, Why are there so many isoforms of the TR? Most tissues express more than one isoform (45), suggesting that they may serve different regulatory roles in the cell. Proving this thesis has been difficult. The *in vitro* properties of the three major T$_3$-binding isoforms (TRα$_1$, TRβ$_1$, and TRβ$_2$) are remarkably similar in terms of their DNA and hormone-binding properties, although the β isoforms do have a higher binding affinity for triac than the TRα$_1$ (46). Such similar binding affinities are not surprising, given the amino acid sequence similarity in the DNA and ligand-binding domains of the TR isoforms (43). However, recent studies have demonstrated potentially important functional differences between the various isoforms (54), as for example, when T$_3$ and glucocorticoids are both involved in regulating the same gene (e.g., growth hormone) (55). This suggests that the isoforms may differ in their interactions with other proteins involved in transcriptional regulation.

Thyroid Hormone Receptor Response Elements

The DNA sequences that comprise the response elements for the nuclear receptors are surprisingly short and few in number (Fig. 7A) (56). The steroid hormone receptors (other than ER) bind optimally to the sequence AGAACA, whereas, for TR, ER, VDR, RAR, RXR, and several of the orphan receptors, the analogous sequence is AGGTCA (37). These sequences are referred to as *core consensus half-sites*—terms that refer to several features of these response elements: (a) that nucleotides adjacent to the AGGTCA sequence may influence receptor binding affinity (57,58), hence AGGTCA forms a core sequence; (b) that in some response elements, other nucleotides may be used in the core sequence (59), hence AGGTCA represents a consensus sequence; and (c) that the response elements in many natural (native) promoters consist of two closely spaced repeats of the core sequence, thereby allowing both the receptor protein and its dimerization partner to bind to a separate core sequence; hence the term half-site sequence (56).

The spacing and orientation of the core half-sites dictate which specific receptors bind to a given response element (see Fig. 7B) (29). The TR response element (TRE) may be composed of a single, monomeric half-site, in which case the octomer TAAGGTCA has been demonstrated to be the optimal sequence for binding of a monomeric TR (58). Alternatively, the TRE may be composed of two half-sites fashioned into one of several configurations: (a) a direct repeat with the core sequences oriented in the same direction; (b) a palindrome, also termed an inverted repeat; or (c) an inverted palindrome, also termed an everted repeat (29). The spacing of the half-sites is a critical determinant of receptor binding specificity (see Fig. 7C). Thus, an inverted repeat where the half sites are adjacent to each other serves as a TRE or an RAR response element. If the inverted half-sites are separated by three nucleotides of any sequence, however, then the region becomes an ER response element such that an ER homodimer is attracted to the site. The spacing of direct repeats is also important (see Fig. 7C). TR regulation occurs primarily at direct repeats separated by four nucleotides (DR$_4$), because this configuration provides for the optimal binding of TR and its dimerization partner (see later) (29). Direct repeats with other spacings between the half-sites serve as optimal response elements for other nuclear receptor hormones and their partners (e.g., DR$_3$ for VDR dimers, DR$_5$ for RAR dimers) (29).

The structure of the nuclear receptor response elements found in native promoter regions are generally more complex than the idealized sequences discussed above (56). Nonetheless, these rules for half-site orientation and spacing provide useful guidelines for sorting out promoter region architecture.

As illustrated in Figure 7D, native response elements may contain more than two half-sites with the sequence

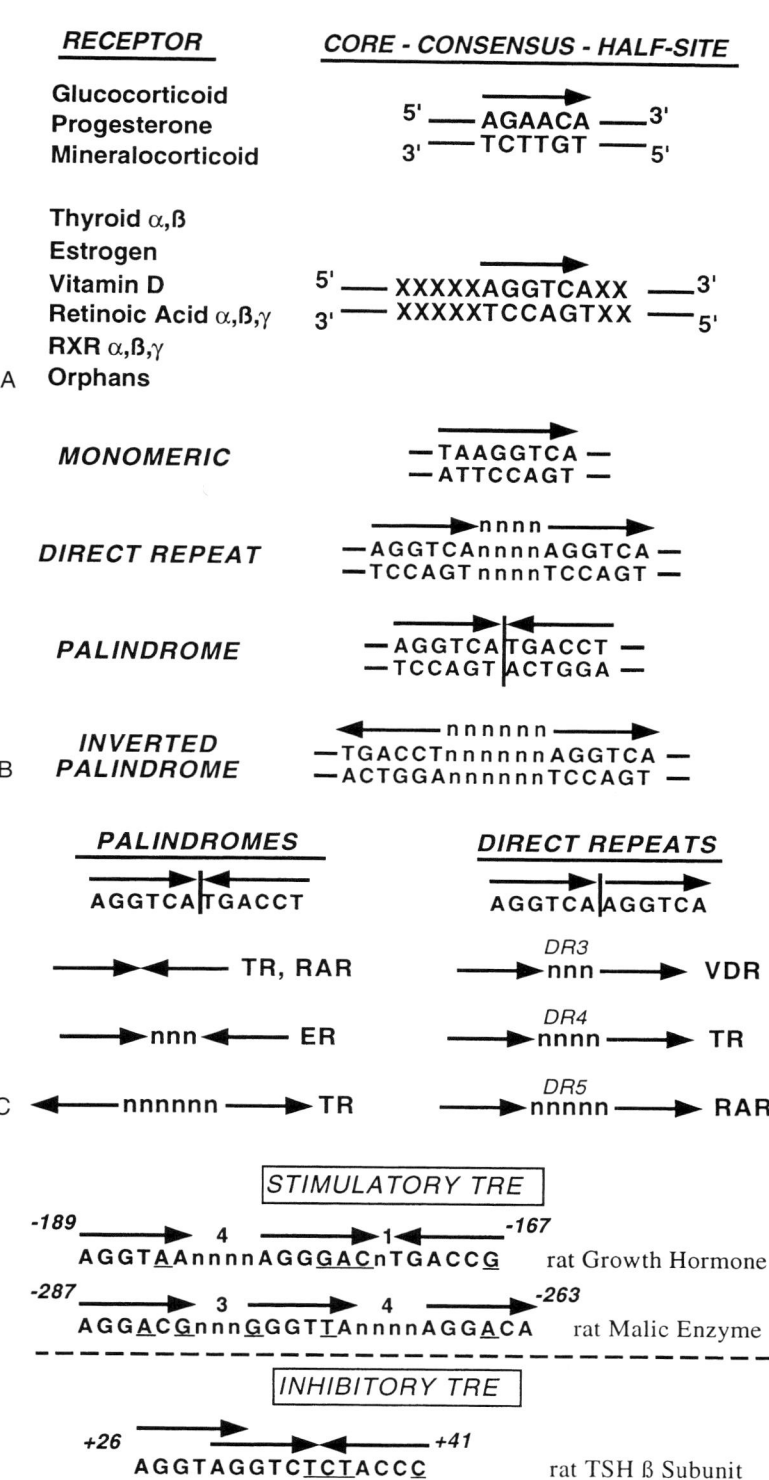

FIG. 7. Receptor response elements. **A:** The core, consensus, half-site sequences for the glucocorticoid- and thyroid hormone-related subgroups of receptors. **B,C:** Differing arrangements of the consensus half-site into thyroid hormone response elements. **D:** The sequence of some native stimulatory and inhibitory thyroid hormone response elements.

of each deviating to some extent from the AGGTCA consensus. The most inviolate nucleotides are the two Gs at positions 2 and 3 of the hexamer; these appear to be required for TR recognition. Some degree of "wobble" in the nucleotides used at the other positions (as indicated by underlining in Fig. 7D) is relatively common (56). The significance of this remains uncertain, although it may in some cases diminish receptor binding affinity. Additional complexity in native response elements occurs when two or more response elements for different transcription factors are contiguous or overlap. Such arrangements may allow for complex interactions between the regulatory proteins.

Thyroid hormones can regulate gene transcription in either a positive (stimulatory) or negative (inhibitory) fashion (60). Indeed, one of the best characterized physiologic effects of T_3 is the suppression of TSH synthesis, which involves TR-mediated inhibition of both *TSH*α (61) and *TSH*β (62) gene transcription. What determines whether transcription of a gene is stimulated or inhibited by thyroid hormones? The location and the architecture of the TRE appear to be important factors (60). Whereas stimulatory TREs usually lie in the enhancer region some distance from the transcriptional start site [e.g., -167 to -189 in the rat growth hormone gene (see Fig. 7D)], negative response elements often are found much closer to the start site, or actually in the transcription unit itself (e.g., $+26$ to $+41$ in the rat *TSH*β subunit gene). Such a location may allow for a direct inhibitory interaction of the TR with the pol II complex, or result in steric hindrance of the complex's assembly or progression along the DNA as transcription proceeds. A second feature of inhibitory TREs is that they often make use of single half-sites or utilize multiple half-sites in very compact arrangements (56).

All of the native TREs defined to date differ significantly in their structure, and this has made it difficult to determine the functional significance of these differing patterns (56). Presumably, they allow for greater diversity or flexibility in the regulatory response to thyroid hormone and other transcription regulators.

TRIPs, TRAPs, and TRUPs: Thyroid Hormone Receptor Binding Proteins

A characteristic of the TRs and other nuclear receptors is their proclivity to bind to themselves and to other nuclear proteins (63). This feature is essential to their functioning as transcriptional regulators. Although a TR may bind as a monomer to certain response elements (64), more commonly TRs appear to function as dimers complexed with other DNA binding proteins—either another TR (forming a homodimer) or one of the other members of the receptor superfamily (to form a heterodimer) (65). Such dimerization partners have been referred to generically as TRAPs—thyroid receptor auxiliary proteins (66). It is now clear that the most important TRAPs are the RXR subfamily of nuclear receptors (29,67,68). Heterodimers of TR and RXR have significantly greater binding affinity for certain TREs, and they are more effective than TR alone at stimulating transcription in many *in vitro* assay systems (69). Both of these consequences likely result from specific conformational changes in the receptor induced by the dimerization process (29).

RXR is now recognized as a universal heterodimerization partner; in addition to TR, it complexes with RAR, VDR, and several orphan receptors (29). The exact properties of RXR that make it useful to subserve this role are uncertain. These RXR heterodimers bind to the direct repeat response elements described above in a very specific orientation—namely, with the VDR, TR, or RAR component bound to the downstream (or 3′) half-site. Thus the RXR's heterodimerization partner (e.g., TR) is closest, in terms of nucleotide distance, to the transcriptional start site and the pol II complex. The dimerization partner also dictates the hormonal specificity for transactivation.

As the concepts of transcriptional regulation evolved, it became apparent that transcription factors must somehow interact with the basal transcriptional apparatus in order to affect gene expression. In some cases, such interactions may be direct and facilitated by the bending of DNA that occurs with transcription factor binding (24,25). Thus, in experimental assay systems, TRs and other receptors have been demonstrated to bind directly to TFIIB (18,20) and TBP (21). In many cases, however, this becomes more problematic as the transcription factors may be bound to response elements located hundreds or thousands of nucleotides upstream from the transcriptional start site. Because of this, it was postulated that accessory, or adaptor, proteins exist to act as a bridge between the pol II complex and the bound transcription factors (63). Recently, such proteins that interact with members of the nuclear receptor superfamily have been identified (70). They are referred to as co-activators or co-repressors, depending on whether they mediate stimulatory or inhibitory effects of the receptor complex on gene expression. For example, a protein named steroid receptor coactivator-1 (SRC-1) has been identified and demonstrated to enhance the stimulatory activity of several members of the steroid hormone receptor family, including TRs (71). Another protein, designated thyroid hormone intermediary protein-1 (TRIP-1), may subserve a similar function (72), whereas N-CoR (nuclear receptor co-repressor) (73) and SMRT (silencing mediator for retinoid and thyroid hormone receptors) (74) mediate repressive effects of receptor complexes. These adaptor proteins thus represent another class of thyroid hormone receptor binding proteins. They differ from the previously defined TRAPs, however, in that they are not themselves DNA-binding transcription factors but are involved only in protein–protein interactions.

Adding an additional layer of complexity to this regulatory system are proteins that have been demonstrated to inhibit receptor function by binding to the receptor and impairing its ability to bind to DNA. One such recently identified protein has been called TRUP—thyroid hormone receptor uncoupling protein (75).

The Role of T_3 and Other Ligands in Thyroid Hormone Receptor Function

Recent crystallographic data have dramatically demonstrated that T_3, upon binding to the TR, becomes entirely buried within the ligand-binding domain and actually forms part of the hydrophobic core of this globular protein (Fig. 8) (42). A similar phenomenon has been demonstrated for the binding of retinoic acid to RAR, suggesting that this is a common structural feature of members of the steroid/thyroid hormone receptor superfamily (76). This binding results in critical conformational changes in the receptor that influence its ability to regulate transcription. Activation of transcription by ligand-binding to a TR complex may involve several mechanisms, including the disruption of local chromatin structure (77), the dissociation of corepressor proteins from the receptor, and the binding of coactivators as new binding interfaces become available. Indeed, it is these conformation changes in the various domains of the protein that are the biochemical basis of the receptor's function. Other steroid and thyroid hormone binding proteins, such as those present in the plasma, do not undergo changes in conformation: ligand enters and exits from a static binding pocket (42).

Unlike the steroid hormone receptors, TRs can bind to response elements as homodimers in the unliganded state and act as constitutive repressors (78). This effect is particularly potent when receptor binding occurs at a response element located downstream (3') to the TATA box (78). Under such circumstances, TR binding may inhibit the formation of the pol II complex by direct interactions with TBP (21,79). Unliganded TRs have also been observed to stimulate transcription in certain cell types (80) or under selected circumstances. For example, on genes whose expression is normally inhibited by thyroid hormone (e.g., the *TSHβ* and *TRH* genes), unliganded TRs may activate promoter activity (81–83). Thus, an unliganded TR is not inactive or inert, but rather it may be actively involved in transcriptional regulation. This situation is reminiscent, in some respects, to the TRα$_2$ isoform, which has important functional effects in spite of its inability to bind T$_3$ (47).

Ligand binding to the receptor can also change its DNA-binding properties. T$_3$ greatly enhances the binding of monomeric TR to DNA (84). In contrast, TR homodimers appear to dissociate from their DNA response elements, thereby relieving basal repression (85), whereas the TR/RXR heterodimer continues to bind to DNA and mediate transcriptional activation as described (86).

Because many of the regulatory effects of TRs on transcription appear to be mediated by TR/RXR heterodimers, the RXR ligand 9-cis RA could potentially influence thyroid hormone action. Recent studies demonstrate that the interactions of the TR/RXR with its ligands are complex. Because regions of the ligand-binding domain are involved in the dimerization process, formation of the heteroduplex may alter the receptors' abilities to bind their hormones (87). This appears to be the case when the TR/RXR binds to a DR$_4$ response element; 9-cis RA binding to RXR is inhibited, whereas T$_3$ binding affinity is maintained (87). Indeed, the binding of T$_3$ to the TR component of the heterodimer complex appears to essentially eliminate the ability of RXR to bind its ligand. Thus, the TR/RXR heterodimer functions primarily as a T$_3$-regulated transcription factor complex on this particular TRE. On other response elements (e.g., some inverted palindromes and complex response elements), both ligands appear to be necessary for efficient activation of transcription (88,89). Such disparate findings reinforce the concept that the configuration of the TRE can influence the functional characteristics of the receptor complex, presumably by inducing different conformational states (90). The importance of the TRE configuration and location was noted previously when discussing negative response elements.

Mutant Thyroid Hormone Receptors

Mutations in the genes that code for the nuclear receptors can have significant functional, and hence clinical, consequences (Fig. 9). This is perhaps most dramatically demonstrated in the testicular feminization syndrome, where a mutation in the gene coding for the testosterone

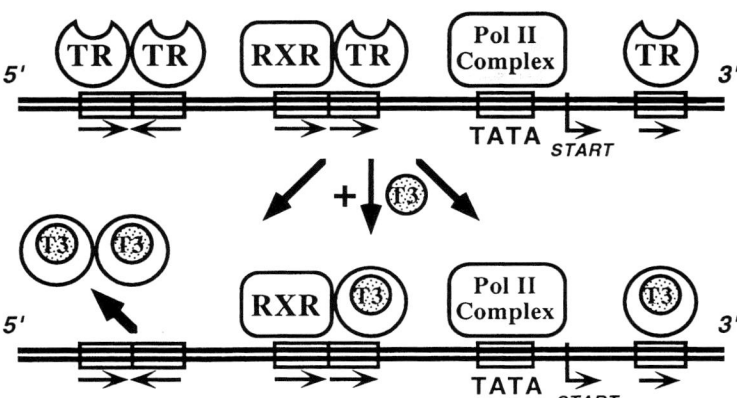

FIG. 8. The role of T$_3$ in thyroid hormone receptor function. Depending on the receptor configuration, T$_3$ may induce dissociation of receptors from DNA, or enhance DNA binding and induce transactivation.

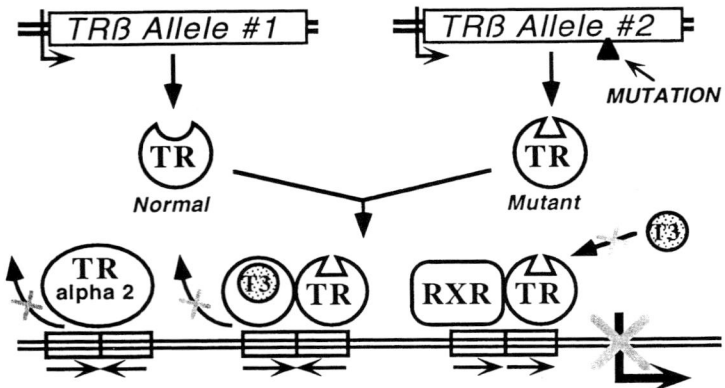

FIG. 9. Mutant thyroid hormone receptors. Mutations within the hormone-binding domain of the *TR* can induce abnormal receptor function and thus resistance to the effects of TH.

receptor results in the expression of a nonfunctional receptor protein (91). As a result, genetic males with this mutation are unable to respond to androgens and remain completely feminized, in spite of high circulating testosterone levels. Analogous mutations in the *TRβ* gene have been reported in a number of families, and these result in the syndrome of resistance to thyroid hormones (92). This is characterized by variable signs and symptoms of hypothyroidism occurring in spite of high circulating T_4 and T_3 levels (93). In the vast majority of families with the thyroid hormone resistance syndrome, the phenotype is inherited in an autosomal dominant pattern and involves a mutation in the ligand-binding domain of only one of the two *TRβ* alleles. Mutant receptors from this allele are unable to bind T_3, or bind the ligand with a lower than normal affinity. Affected individuals, however, do have one normal *TRβ* and two normal *TRα* alleles, which code for functional receptors. The question thus arises as to why these individuals are resistant to T_3. The answer derives from the mutant receptors' continued ability to form homo- and heterodimers and to bind normally to DNA response elements (94,95). Thus, in tissues that express significant amounts of the *TRβ* isoforms, the mutant receptors may form homo- and heterodimers that bind to DNA. Because the mutant receptors bind ligand poorly, these homodimers do not dissociate from the DNA and thus continue to mediate transcriptional repression in the presence of normal or even elevated T_3 levels (96). In contrast, the lack of T_3 binding to the mutant TR in the TR/RXR heterodimer means that this complex cannot be activated to stimulate transcription. Thus, the mutant receptors have the capacity to block the actions of the normal TRs. Such effects are termed a dominant negative mutation, and they explain the autosomal dominant mode of inheritance. The extent to which these inhibitory effects occur depends on a number of factors, including the nature of the mutant protein, the relative amounts of mutant versus normal receptors expressed in the cell, the structure of the TRE present in the promoter region of the gene in question, and the concentration of T_3 in the nucleus (96,97).

Additional insights into the clinical consequences and molecular pathogenesis of thyroid hormone resistance syndromes are presented in Chapter 12.

The Molecular Mechanism of Thyroid Hormone Action: Summary

Figure 10 shows in schematic fashion the promoter/enhancer region of a gene and illustrates some of the potential molecular interactions that may be involved in

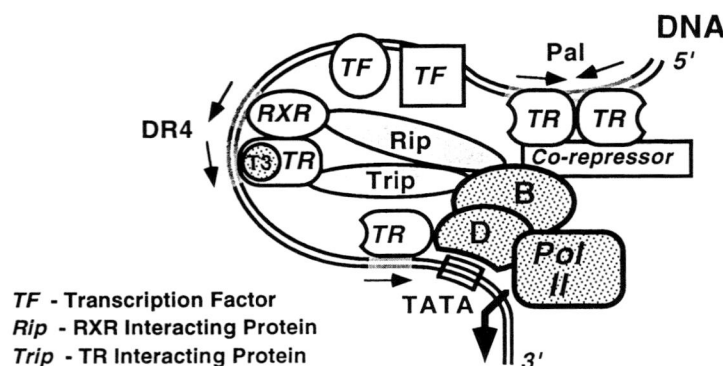

FIG. 10. A diagrammatic summary of selected aspects of the molecular mechanism of TH action.

TABLE 1. *The complexity of thyroid hormone action*

Gene	Isoforms	Type binding	Response elements	TRAPS	Other factors	Ligands	Misc.
α	α1, α2, α3, Rev-ErbAα	Monomeric	Palindromic	RXRα	TFIIB		
			Inverted palindrome	RXRβ	TFIID		
				RXRγ	Co-activators	±T3	
		Homodimer	Direct repeats 0–6		Co-inhibitors		
				RARα	GR/ER		
			Natural + resp element	RARβ	Pit-1		± PO4
β	β1, β2, β mutants	Heterodimer		RARγ	AP-1		
					TRUPS	± 9-cis RA	
			Natural + resp element	COUP	Nuclear matrix		
				PPAR	Chromatin		
			Complex resp element	Vit DR	v-erb A		

the regulation of gene transcription by thyroid hormone and its receptors. An unliganded TR homodimer is shown binding to a palindromic TRE and exerting suppressive effects on the pol II complex via a corepressor adaptor molecule. Elsewhere, a liganded TR/RXR heterodimer interacts with TFBII via coactivators for TR (TRIP) and RXR (RIP). In addition, an unliganded TR monomer is shown interacting directly with TFDII. Additional interactions between TR complexes and other transcription factors could be illustrated.

Table 1 is a summary of the factors involved in the molecular mechanisms of thyroid hormone action. Some entries in the table, such as the phosphorylation state of the TR (98), the role of a TR-related viral oncogene termed v-*erb* A (99–101), and interactions between TRs and other transcription factor complexes such as Pit-1 (102) and AP-1 (81,103), have not been formally discussed, but they may be of considerable importance in selected circumstances. Although it is obvious that our knowledge in this field has expanded greatly over the past decade, there is still much more to learn before a comprehensive picture of the complex events that regulate gene expression emerges.

SIGNALLING CASCADES FROM THE CELL SURFACE

Transmembrane Receptors

The enormous insights garnered during the past decade into the nuclear events controlling gene expression have been matched by an explosion of information related to signalling cascades that originate from the cell surface (Fig. 11). Such knowledge is relevant not only to an understanding of the mechanisms of action of hormones such as TSH and TRH, but also to the cellular processes involved in cell growth and oncogenesis (104,105).

Cells are constantly interacting with their immediate surroundings through cell surface receptors. These large molecules, many of which are composed of several subunits, traverse the plasma membrane. The extracellular domains function not unlike the ligand-binding domain of members of the nuclear steroid receptor family. By recognizing and binding one or more specific ligands, the extracellular region initiates conformation changes in other portions of the receptor complex, such as the cytoplasmic domain. This triggers a cascade of second mes-

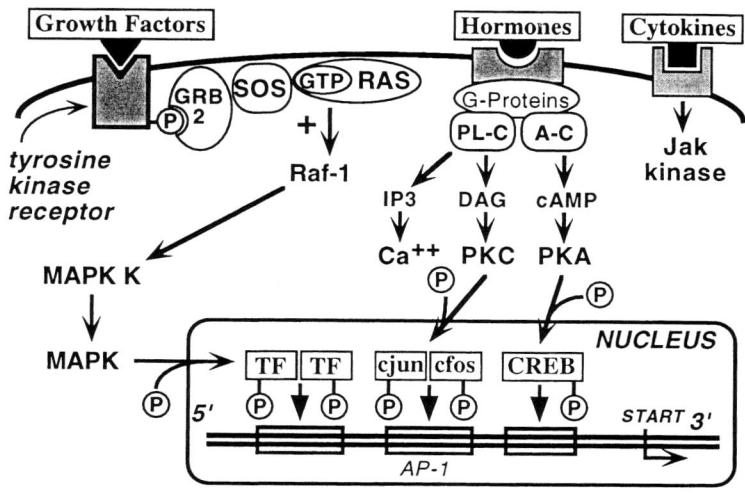

FIG. 11. Signalling cascades from the cell surface. Factors interacting with cell surface receptors, such as hormones, growth factors, or cytokines, induce second messenger systems which, among other effects, can influence gene transcription by altering the activity of transcription factors through phosphorylation and dephosphorylation mechanisms. (See text for definitions and additional details.)

senger systems (with the receptor ligand being the first messenger) within the cell, which mediate the effects of the ligand–receptor complex, including effects in the nucleus on transcriptional regulation (106).

Such receptors interact with a wide range of ligands that include all of the classic peptide hormones, catecholamines, other neurotransmitters, growth factors, products from immune cells such as cytokines and interferons, and extracellular matrix proteins (105,107–110). Cell surface receptors are also important constituents of the visual and olfactory pathways (111). This diverse range of ligands has recently been extended further by the discovery that the mechanism used by parathyroid and renal cells to sense the extracellular calcium concentration is, in fact, a transmembrane receptor. These calcium sensors manifest structural similarities to the receptors for catecholamines and certain peptide hormones, and they utilize the same intracellular pathways to propagate their physiologic signals (112,113).

G-Protein-Mediated Second Messenger Systems

The prototypical second messenger molecule is cyclic AMP (cAMP), a small nucleotide first proposed by Sutherland in 1965 to be an important intracellular mediator of the actions of epinephrine (114). The level of cAMP in the cell is dependent on its rate of synthesis by adenylate cyclase and its rate of hydrolysis by phosphodiesterases. The activities of both these enzymes can be either stimulated or inhibited by ligands binding to various cell surface receptors (105).

Typically, adenylate cyclase is coupled to (associated with) large receptors that traverse the plasma membrane exactly seven times (115,116). The receptors for both TSH and TRH are in this structural category (117,118), although signalling from the TRH receptor does not appear to involve cAMP (see later) (119). In the case of receptors for small hormones, such as the catecholamines and TRH, the transmembrane segments form a core into which the ligand completely or partially binds (120). For receptors of this class that recognize larger ligands, such as TSH, an extended extracellular tail composed of the amino-terminus of the protein is configured into a hormone-binding site (121). The carboxy-terminus of the receptor, which is intracellular in location, as well as portions of the cytoplasmic loops that are formed as the protein weaves its way through the plasma membrane, are the structural portions of the receptor that physically interact with the second messenger-generating systems (116). This entails contact initially between the receptor and "G-proteins," so named because they bind and are activated by the small cytoplasmic nucleotide guanosine triphosphate (GTP). These G-proteins serve as intermediate transducers in a fashion entirely analogous to the adapter proteins involved in regulating gene transcription; they bridge the gap between the ligand-activated receptor and the enzyme complex [pol II for nuclear receptors, adenylate cyclase (A-C) for cell surface receptors] that will ultimately carry out the physiologic effect (122). And just as nuclear adaptor proteins can be coactivators or co-repressors, G-proteins can be stimulatory or inhibitory on cAMP production (122) or other second messenger systems.

An increase in the cellular cAMP level activates protein kinase A (PKA) (105). The active subunit of this enzyme diffuses freely within the cell, where it selectively phosphorylates various proteins, thus initiating physiologic effects (123). In the nucleus, PKA phosphorylates a specific transcription factor, termed cAMP response-element-binding protein (CREB) (124). Phosphorylation of CREB is analogous to T_3 binding to the TR: it alters the protein's conformation and enhances its activity and binding to a specific cAMP response element (consensus DNA sequence, TGACGTCA). Rates of transcription of specific genes are then altered through the interactions of CREB with adaptor proteins [e.g., CREB binding protein (CBP)] and directly with TFBII and TFDII (17,124).

In addition to linking receptors to adenylate cyclase, G-proteins may couple to another second messenger system that regulates both the intracellular calcium concentration and the activity of a second important kinase—protein kinase C (PKC) (125). The proximate events in this signalling cascade involve the G-protein activation of phospholipase C (PL-C), which hydrolyzes the breakdown of phosphatidylinositol bisphosphate (PIP2) to inositol triphosphate (IP3) and diacylglycerol (DAG). IP3 in turn stimulates a rapid and transient increase in intracellular free Ca^{2+} by inducing its release from intracellular stores. This is then followed by a sustained increase in cellular Ca^{2+} levels mediated by an influx of the ion through specific membrane calcium channels (126). DAG, in turn, activates PKC, which, like PKA, phosphorylates a number of specific target proteins within the cell (125). These include the transcription factors *c-fos* and *c-jun*, which form a heterodimer termed the AP-1 transcription factor complex. The AP-1 complex is an important regulator of cellular proliferation (127).

Which signalling pathways are utilized appears to be determined by the particular G-proteins present in the receptor complex (122). The TSH receptor may utilize both the cAMP and the Ca^{2+}/PKC pathways (117), whereas the TRH receptor appears to be coupled only to the latter system; cellular adenylate cyclase activity is unaltered by TRH binding (119).

Mutations in the genes coding the G-proteins, or the receptors to which they couple, may result in clinical disease (128–130). As discussed in Chapter 11, both activating and inactivating mutations of the TSH receptor have been identified (131). Activating mutations that occur in the germline will be present in all thyroid follicular cells and thus cause an inherited, autosomal dominant form of nonautoimmune hyperthyroidism associated with a diffuse goiter (132,133). If the mutation occurs after conception (a somatic mutation), then the follicular cell expressing the activated receptor will: (a) oversecrete thyroid hormones, and (b) realize a growth advantage over the other thyrocytes. This results clinically in a sporadic toxic adenoma (134). Activating mutations of the TSH receptor have also been implicated in the pathogenesis of thyroid cancer (135). In addition, the extracellular nature of portions of these proteins makes them a potential target for the immune system, as occurs in Graves' disease (130,136).

Non-G-Protein-Mediated Second Messenger Systems

A number of cell surface receptors do not couple to G-proteins, but rather initiate their own signalling cascades (105). These include the receptors for insulin, growth factors, and several cytokines, all of which possess inherent tyrosine kinase or serine/threonine kinase activity (107, 108,137). Ligand binding activates the enzymatic activity of the receptor, which in turn leads to a series of phosphorylation events in the cell, resulting in numerous physiologic effects (138). In many cases, activated signalling pathways link the events at the cell surface with the nuclear machinery that controls gene expression and cellular proliferation (106). For example, insulin and various growth factor receptors are coupled to the Ras/mitogen-activated protein kinase (MAPK) signalling pathway (139–142), whereas cytokine receptors activate a Jak kinase pathway (143,144). The delineation of these pathways during the past decade represents a milestone in medical research and has provided key insights into the mechanisms of hormone action and oncogenesis (145).

The complexity of the signalling mechanisms arising from receptors located at the cell surface is almost overwhelming. Not only is each pathway complicated in its own right, with the involvement of multiple transduction proteins, ligands, and enzymes, but components of these pathways clearly interact, thus providing for a seemingly Byzantine network of regulatory processes. For example, elevations of cAMP inhibit growth in some cells by preventing Ras from binding to Raf-1 and activating the MAP kinase cascade (146). Additional levels of "cross-talk" between these effector systems appear to be important in the mediation of TSH action in thyroid cells (147).

Additional information on the structure and function of the TSH receptor is found in Chapter 11.

ONCOGENESIS

Molecular Pathogenesis of Neoplasia

Neoplasia results from cellular proliferation that is either inopportunely timed or inappropriately regulated. Thus, the factors that control the orderly events of cell division, termed the cell cycle, become critical determinants of a cell's oncogenic potential (148,149). Many of the factors discussed above impact on a cell's proliferative state (150). For example, growth factors act through the various signalling cascades originating from the cell surface to alter the expression and/or activity of transcription factors involved in cell cycle regulation (104,151). Under normal circumstances, these complex processes are tightly controlled by a system of checks and balances. However, alterations in one or more components of these regulatory pathways can result in inappropriate cell proliferation (152).

Transformation of a normal cell to a neoplastic phenotype involves alterations in the genetic makeup of the cell (6,153). Two fundamentally different mechanisms are involved. The first involves the activation, or "gain in function," of a gene product that is capable of stimulating cell proliferation (e.g., *Ras*), but which normally does so only under very controlled circumstances (145). Often, this results from a mutation within the coding region of the gene, such that the protein product synthesized is constitutively active, and not subject to normal regulatory processes (154). Cellular proliferation is thus stimulated. Such genes are referred to as proto-oncogenes in their normal, native state, and as oncogenes when they have become mutated and code for a constitutively active protein product. Not all oncogenes code for structurally abnormal proteins, however. In some cases, the genetic alteration in the proto-oncogene involves the promoter region, rather than the transcription unit (155). In such cases, inappropriately high levels of a structurally normal protein product are expressed and stimulate cell proliferation. In general, an activating mutation in only one of the two alleles of a proto-oncogene is sufficient to influence a cell's proliferative state. Thus, oncogenes are expressed in a dominant pattern in cells (6).

Numerous classes of oncogenes have been discovered that can contribute to the neoplastic phenotype (Fig. 12). These include growth factors, tyrosine kinase receptors, G-proteins such as *Ras*, cellular kinases, cell cycle–regulating transcription factors, and proteins such as *bcl-2* that serve to protect cells from programmed cell death, or apoptosis (145) For example, the oncogene most directly implicated in both papillary and medullary thyroid carcinoma, *ret/PTC*, is a transmembrane protein with tyrosine kinase activity (156,157). To date, about 70 oncogenes have been identified, although less than half have been implicated in human cancers (158).

The second mechanism involved in abnormal cellular proliferation arises from inactivating mutations in genes that normally serve to limit cell proliferation (159). Such genes are termed tumor suppressor genes, and normally they are involved in such critical cellular processes as coordinating progression through the cell cycle (retinoblastoma protein, *pRb*), halting proliferation in the case of

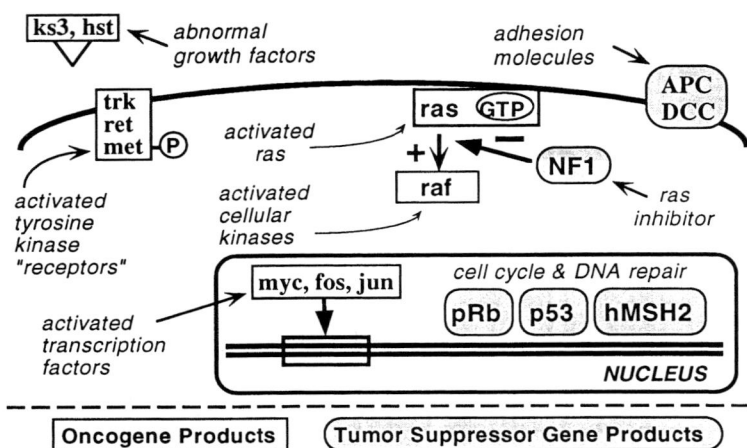

FIG. 12. Molecular principles of oncogenesis based on the concepts of oncogene and tumor suppressor gene products. (See text for definitions and additional details.)

DNA damage (*p53*), DNA repair (h*MSH2*), or cell adhesion *(APC, DCC)* (6,153,160,161). In general, a single functional copy of a tumor suppressor gene is sufficient to provide normal physiologic effects. Thus, both alleles of a tumor suppressor gene must be inactivated in order for cell proliferation to go unchecked. This may occur by mutations that result in an inactive protein product and/or by chromosomal alterations that result in gene deletions (6). The fundamental difference in the function of oncogenes and tumor suppressor genes is easily demonstrated in the research laboratory. The injection of an oncogene into a normal cell induces uncontrolled proliferation and a cancerous phenotype, whereas the injection of a tumor suppressor gene will halt this progression.

The progression from a normal cell to a cancer cell generally involves the accumulation of several genetic abnormalities that involve both oncogene activation and tumor suppressor gene inactivation (6,153). The two most common abnormalities detected in a broad range of human cancers are *p53* mutations (both alleles being inactivated in 50% of cancers) and Ras activations (30%). However, certain tumor types are highly associated with specific oncogenes or tumor suppressor genes. For example, abnormalities in the ret/PTC oncogene are found in 90% of cases of the multiple endocrine neoplasia type II syndrome (156), and both alleles of *pRb* are inactivated in the tumors of essentially all patients with childhood retinoblastoma (159).

Additional details concerning the molecular pathogenesis of thyroid neoplasms are found in Chapter 13.

MOLECULAR ASPECTS OF THYROID HORMONE METABOLISM

Iodothyronine Deiodinases: Expression, Function, and Regulation

As discussed in Chapter 3, deiodination is the predominant mechanism by which thyroid hormones are metabolized (162). Although the thyroid gland expresses the type I deiodinase (DI), which converts T_4 to T_3 (163,164), the majority of deiodination occurs in extrathyroidal tissues. Three deiodinases have been identified that differ in their catalytic activities, tissue distribution, sensitivity to inhibitors such as propylthiouracil, and mechanisms of regulation (165). Because of these factors, they appear to subserve different physiologic roles.

The DI is highly expressed in the liver and kidney, where it mediates both the outer ring deiodination of T_4 to T_3, and the inner ring metabolism of T_3-sulfate and T_4-sulfate to inactive compounds (166). Thus the DI can serve as both an activating and an inactivating deiodinase, and its exact physiologic role remains somewhat uncertain.

The type II deiodinase (DII) functions solely as an outer ring enzyme and is of importance in the conversion of T_4 to T_3 in the brain (167), anterior pituitary gland (168), and brown fat (169). Its presence in the fetal and neonatal brain is of particular importance to ensure an adequate supply of T_3 for this organ during critical periods of development (170–172). In the adult human brain, DII mRNA expression is widespread, being highest in the neocortex, hippocampus, and putamen, with lesser levels in the cerebellum, brainstem, and spinal cord (173). This pattern of expression largely parallels that of the TRs and reinforces the importance of the DII in the regulation of thyroid hormone action in this tissue (174,175).

The type III deiodinase (DIII) functions primarily to inactivate T_4 and T_3 by inner ring deiodination (176). DIII is the predominant isoform expressed in the placenta and during early development in many fetal tissues (177,178). It may function to ensure that the developing embryo is not exposed prematurely to adult levels of active thyroid hormone, a situation that has been shown to result in the untimely termination of cellular proliferation in the maturing brain (179,180).

An important feature of the deiodinases is their response to alterations in thyroid status (165). Most dramatic is the inverse relationship between DII activity and circulating thyroid hormone levels; activity is elevated several-fold in the hypothyroid state, seemingly to maximize T_3 production when T_4 is in limited supply (181, 182). Hyperthyroidism results in a rapid decline in DII activity in all tissues where it is expressed. These responses in the central nervous system account in large part for the relative stability of T_3 levels in this tissue over a broad range of circulating thyroid hormone concentrations (183,184). The mechanisms involved in DII regulation by thyroid hormones involve both alterations in the rate of enzyme synthesis and inactivation by posttranslational processes (173,185–187). DI and DIII activities are also responsive to thyroid hormone, both being increased in the hyperthyroid state (188). In the case of DIII, this may be an adaptive measure that results in increased T_3 degradation (172).

Structural Features of the Deiodinases

The deiodinases are intracellular, membrane-bound proteins located in the endoplasmic reticulum and/or plasma membrane (189–191). They have proven difficult to purify, hence until recently, little was known about their structure and biochemical properties. However, molecular cloning techniques have now succeeded in identifying cDNAs for all three deiodinases from multiple species, including humans (173,192–197). A comparison of the predicted protein structure of the three rat deiodinase isoforms is shown in Figure 13. All are approximately 30 kDa in molecular mass, and all contain the rare amino acid selenocysteine at the catalytic core (198). The amino acid homology between the three proteins in this region is quite high (80% identity); however, in other regions, the homology is considerably less. Overall, about 25% of the amino acids are identical in the three isoforms.

The presence of selenocysteine in these enzymes is critically important to their catalytic activity; the substitution of the sulfur-containing amino acid cysteine in place of selenocysteine markedly decreases the catalytic efficiency of the enzyme (193,195,197,199). This likely results from the fact that selenocysteine is ionized at physiologic pH (pI 5.5) and is thus a much more potent nucleophile than cysteine (Fig. 14). In addition to selenocysteine, other structural features shared by the three proteins are two essential histidine residues and a hydrophobic domain in the amino-terminus, which likely functions as a membrane-spanning domain (200,201).

Incorporation of Selenocysteine

The importance of selenocysteine to the function of the deiodinases and a limited number of other cellular selenoproteins (e.g., glutathione peroxidase, GPx) has prompted considerable interest in the mechanism by which this amino acid is incorporated into the structure of proteins. Much of our knowledge concerning this process is derived from studies performed in bacteria, which also synthesize a limited number of selenoproteins (202).

In both bacteria and eukaryotic cells, selenocysteine is incorporated into proteins at the time of translation (203) (Fig. 15); its presence does not result from posttranslational modification. A specific transfer RNA in the cell is charged with selenocysteine and donates this amino acid during the translation process (204). In the mRNA, the triplet UGA codes for selenocysteine (205) Under most circumstances, however, UGA functions as a "stop" codon. What then signals the ribosome and the translational apparatus to "read through" the UGA codon and incorporate selenocysteine rather than terminate translation? The answer lies in the primary sequence and secondary structure of the 3'-untranslated region of the mRNA molecules that code for selenoproteins (206, 207). A stem-loop structure in this region of the mRNA, termed a selenocysteine insertion sequence (SECIS), interacts with a specific translation factor (Sel B) to facilitate selenocysteine incorporation during protein synthesis (206). The importance of the SECIS to translation of the deiodinases can be demonstrated experimentally. If this portion of the 3'-untranslated region is removed from the mRNA, then translation is terminated at the UGA codon, and a truncated, nonfunctional protein results (208,209).

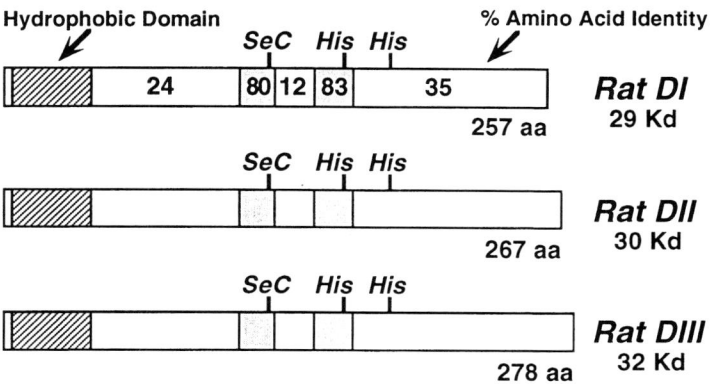

FIG. 13. Structural comparison of the three deiodinase isoforms as deduced from their cDNA sequences. Selenocysteine is present at the active site of all three enzymes and is critical for catalytic activity. Highly conserved domains of the proteins are present in the region of the selenocysteine and one of two essential histidine residues. The hydrophobic domain likely represents a membrane-spanning region.

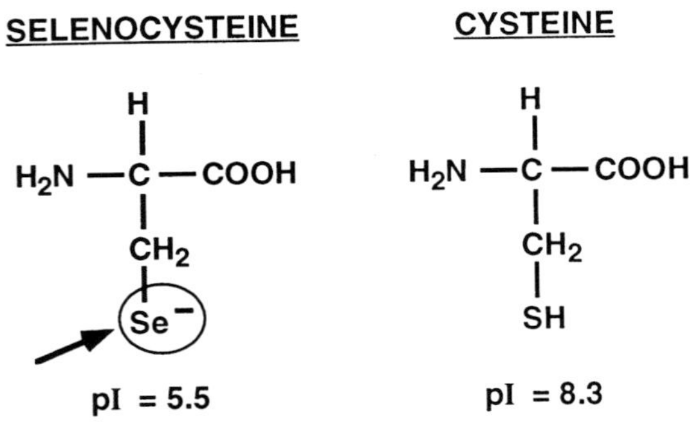

SELENOCYSTEINE

$H_2N-\overset{\overset{\displaystyle H}{|}}{\underset{\underset{\displaystyle Se^-}{|}}{\underset{\displaystyle CH_2}{C}}}-COOH$

pI = 5.5

CYSTEINE

$H_2N-\overset{\overset{\displaystyle H}{|}}{\underset{\underset{\displaystyle SH}{|}}{\underset{\displaystyle CH_2}{C}}}-COOH$

pI = 8.3

FIG. 14. Comparison of the structure of selenocysteine and cysteine.

Effects of Selenium Deficiency on Thyroid Hormone Metabolism

Given the essential role of selenium in deiodination, one would expect nutritional selenium deficiency to result in profound changes in thyroid hormone metabolism. However, with the levels of selenium deficiency that can be achieved in laboratory rodents, the alterations in circulating thyroid hormone levels are surprisingly modest; although serum T_4 levels are increased approximately 40%, T_3 and TSH levels are largely unchanged (210,211). In this animal model system, the principal deiodinase activities affected by selenium deficiency are those in the liver, kidney, and brown fat—tissues that appear predisposed to selenium deficiency (212,213). Thus, DI protein and activity levels are diminished by greater than 90% in the liver and kidney (214), whereas DII activity is low in brown fat and is relatively unresponsive to the stimulatory effects of cold exposure (215). This decrease in extrathyroidal DI activity results in decreased T_4 clearance, hence the elevated serum T_4 levels. Although T_3 production is compromised in this situation, this is offset by diminished clearance of T_3 in the form of T_3-sulfate, and by continued secretion of T_3 from the thyroid gland (216). Hence, T_3 levels remain largely unchanged.

Other organs, such as the thyroid gland, brain, placenta, and endocrine organs, appear much more resistant to selenium deficiency, and deiodinase activities in these tissues are maintained at essentially normal levels (217–219). Another factor serves to maintain deiodinase activity under these circumstances. Cells appear to prioritize the expression of selenoproteins when their selenium supplies are compromised, with the synthesis of deiodinases taking precedence over other selenoproteins such as GPx (220). The molecular basis for this selectivity is uncertain.

Although it seems likely that a more severe degree of selenium deficiency than that readily achieved in rodent model systems would have profound effects on the thyroid hormone metabolism, it is uncertain if such a level of deficiency is ever achieved in humans. However, thyroid function in severe iodine deficiency may be compromised by concurrent selenium deficiency (221). This may result from enhanced oxidative damage to the thyroid gland, secondary to decreased GPx activity (222).

SUMMARY AND FUTURE DIRECTIONS

The last decade has clearly seen tremendous advances in our understanding of the fundamental mechanisms by which the hormones of the thyroid axis function. Insights into the molecular mechanisms of thyroid hormone action are shown to be particularly fascinating, but at the same time they are shown to be bewilderingly complex. Although we have learned much about the receptor–ligand, receptor–DNA, and protein–protein interactions that appear to be involved in the regulation of gene expression, the sequence of events occurring *in vivo* on native promoter elements remains largely unexplored because of a lack of suitable experimental techniques. However, it seems likely that continued progress in this field, and the others touched upon in this chapter, will provide further insights into the pathophysiologic processes that underlie thyroid disease and perhaps assist in the development of better therapeutic strategies.

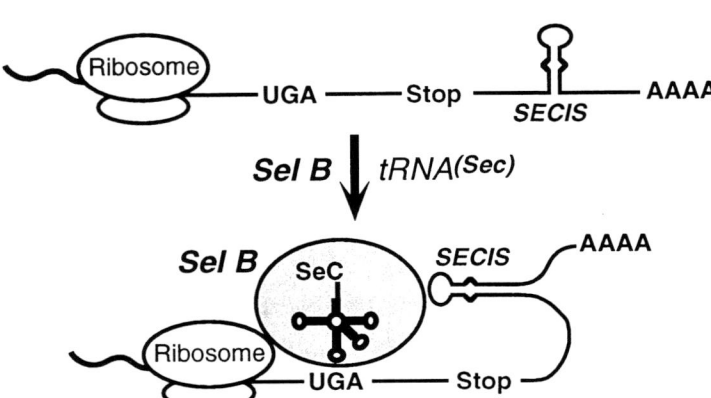

FIG. 15. The likely molecular mechanism whereby selenocysteine is incorporated into proteins during translation. The sel B protein appears to interact with a stem loop structure in the 3'-untranslated region of the mRNA to prevent termination of translation at the UGA codon and insertion of selenocysteine. (From ref. 206.)

ACKNOWLEDGMENT

The work presented in this chapter was supported by the National Institutes of Health in the form of grants DK-42271 and HD-09020.

REFERENCES

1. Lewin B. *Genes V*, 5th ed. Oxford: Oxford University Press, 1994.
2. Fields C, Adams M, White O, Venter JC. How many genes in the human genome? *Nat Genet* 1994;7:345–346.
3. Mager WH, De Kruijff AJ. Stress-induced transcriptional activation. *Microbiol Rev* 1995;59:506–531.
4. Papavassiliou AG. Transcription factors. *N Engl J Med* 1995;332:45–47.
5. Russo VEA. *Development: the molecular genetic approach.* New York: Springer-Verlag, 1992.
6. Goddard AD, Solomon E. Genetic aspects of cancer. *Adv Hum Genet* 1993;21:321–376.
7. Rosenthal N. Regulation of gene expression. *N Engl J Med* 1994;331:931–933.
8. Strul K. Duality of TBP, the universal transcription factor. *Science* 1994;263:1103–1104.
9. Kazazian HHJ. The thalassemia syndromes: molecular basis and prenatal diagnosis in 1990. *Semin Hematol* 1990;27:209–228.
10. Roberts SGE, Green MR. The basic transcriptional machinery. In: Karin M, ed. *Gene expression: general and cell-type-specific.* Boston: Birkäuser, 1993;1–24.
11. Buratowski S. The basics of basal transcription by RNA polymerase II. *Cell* 1994;77:1–3.
12. Maldonado E, Reinberg D. News on initiation and elongation of transcription by RNA polymerase II. *Curr Opin Cell Biol* 1995;7:352–361.
13. Goodrich JA, Tijian R. TBP-TAF complexes: selectivity factors for eukaryotic transcription. *Curr Opin Cell Biol* 1004;6:403–409.
14. Kim Y, Geiger JH, Hahn S, Sigler PB. Crystal structure of a yeast TBP/TATA-box complex. *Nature* 1993;365:512–520.
15. Choy B, Green MR. Eukaryotic activators function during multiple steps of preinitiation complex assembly. *Nature* 1993;366:531–536.
16. Ing NH, Beekman JM, Tsai SY, Tsai M-J, O'Mallet BW. Members of the steroid hormone receptor superfamily interact with TFIIB (S300-II). *J Biol Chem* 1992;267:17617–17623.
17. Xing L, Gopal VK, Quinn PG. cAMP response element-binding protein (CREB) interacts with transcription factors IIB and IID. *J Biol Chem* 1995;270:17448–17493.
18. Hadzic E, Desai-Yajnik V, Helmer E, et al. A 10-amino-acid sequence in the N-terminal A/B domain of thyroid hormone receptor alpha is essential for the transcriptional activation and interaction with general transcription factor TFIIB. *Mol Cell Biol* 1995;15:4507–4517.
19. Petty KJ. Tissue and cell-specific distribution of proteins that interact with the human thyroid hormone receptor-β. *Mol Cell Endocrinol* 1995;108:131–142.
20. Baniahmad A, Ha I, Reinberg S, Tsai S, Tsai M-J, O'Malley BW. Interaction of the human thyroid receptor β with the transcriptional factor TFIIB may mediate target gene derepression and activation by thyroid hormone. *Proc Natl Acad Sci USA* 1993;90:8832–8836.
21. Fondell JD, Brunel F, Hisatake K, Roeder RG. Unliganded thyroid hormone receptor α can target TATA-binding protein for transcriptional repression. *Mol Cell Biol* 1996;16:281–287.
22. Mitchell PJ, Tjian R. Transcriptional regulation in mammalian cells by sequence-specific DNA binding proteins. *Science* 1989;245:371–378.
23. Cowell IG. Repression versus activation in the control of gene transcription. *Trends Biochem Sci* 1994;19:38–42.
24. Tjian R, Maniatis T. Transcriptional activation: a complex puzzle with few easy pieces. *Cell* 1994;77:5–8.
25. Ansari AZ, Brader JE, O'Halloran TV. DNA-bend modulation in a repressor-to-activator switching mechanism. *Nature* 1995;374:371–375.
26. Grosschedl R. Higher-order nucleoprotein complexes in transcription: analogies with site-specific recombination. *Curr Opin Cell Biol* 1995;7:362–370.
27. Polyanovsky OL, Stepchenko AG. Eukaryotic transcription factors. *Bioessays* 1990;12:205–210.
28. Weigel NL. Receptor phosphorylation. In: Tsai M-J, O'Malley BW, eds. *Molecular biology unit: mechanism of steroid hormone regulation of gene transcription.* Austin, TX: RG Landes, 1994;93–110.
29. Mangelsdorf DJ, Evans RM. The RXR heterodimers and orphan receptors. *Cell* 1995;83:841–850.
30. Mangelsdorf DJ, Thummel C, Beato M, et al. The nuclear receptor superfamily: the second decade. *Cell* 1995;83:835–839.
31. Hollenberg SM, Weinberger C, Ong ES, et al. Primary structure and expression of a functional human glucocorticoid receptor cDNA. *Nature* 1985;318:635–641.
32. Green S, Walter P, Kumar V, et al. Human oestrogen receptor cDNA: sequence, expression and homology to v-erb-A. *Nature* 1986;320:134–139.
33. Sap J, Muñoz A, Damm K, et al. The c-erb-A protein is a high-affinity receptor for thyroid hormone. *Nature* 1986;324:635–640.
34. Weinberger C, Thompson CC, Ong ES, Lebo R, Gruol DJ, Evans RM. The c-erb-A gene encodes a thyroid hormone receptor. *Nature* 1986;324:641–646.
35. Rosenthal N. Stalking the gene—DNA libraries. *N Engl J Med* 1994;331:599–600.
36. Schwabe JWR, Rhodes D. Beyond zinc fingers: steroid hormone receptors have a novel structural motif for DNA recognition. *Trends Biochem Sci* 1991;16:291–296.
37. Tsai MJ, O'Malley BW. Molecular mechanisms of action of steroid/thyroid receptor superfamily members. *Ann Rev Biochem* 1994;63:451–486.
38. Levin AA, Sturzenbecker LJ, Kazmer S, et al. 9-cis retinoic acid stereoisomer binds and activates the nuclear receptor RXR alpha. *Nature* 1992;355:359–361.
39. Heyman RA, Mangelsdorf DJ, Dyck JA, et al. 9-cis retinoic acid is a high affinity ligand for the retinoid X receptor. *Cell* 1992;68:397–406.
40. Keller H, Dreyer C, Medin J, Ozato K, Wahli W. Fatty acids and retinoids control lipid metabolism through activation of peroxisome proliferator-activated receptor-retinoid X receptor heterodimers. *Proc Natl Acad Sci USA* 1993;90:2160–2164.
41. Kastner P, Mark M, Chambon P. Nonsteroid nuclear receptors: what are genetic studies telling us about their role in real life? *Cell* 1995;83:859–869.
42. Wagner RL, Apriletti JW, McGrath ME, West BL, Baxter JD, Fleterick RJ. A structural role for hormone in the thyroid hormone receptor. *Nature* 1995;378:690–697.
43. Lazar MA. Thyroid hormone receptors: multiple forms, multiple possibilities. *Endocr Rev* 1993;14:184–193.
44. McKeown M. Alternative mRNA splicing. *Ann Rev Cell Biol* 1992;8:155–155.
45. Strait KA, Schwartz HL, Perez-Castillo A, Oppenheimer JH. Relationship of c-erbA mRNA content to tissue triiodothyronine nuclear binding capacity and function in developing and adult rats. *J Biol Chem* 1990;265:10514–10521.
46. Schueler PA, Schwartz HL, Strait KA, Mariash CN, Oppenheimer JH. Binding of 3,5 3'-triiodothyronine (T3) and its analogs to the in vitro translational products of c-erbA protooncogenes: differences in the affinity of the α- and β-forms for the acetic acid analog and failure of the human testis and kidney α-2 products to bind T3. *Mol Endocrinol* 1990;4:227–234.
47. Koenig RJ, Lazar MA, Hodin RA, et al. Inhibition of thyroid hormone action by a non-hormone binding c-erbA protein generated by alternative mRNA splicing. *Nature* 1989;337:659–661.
48. Katz D, Lazar MA. Dominant negative activity of an endogenous thyroid hormone receptor variant (α2) is due to competition for binding sites on target genes. *J Biol Chem* 1993;268:20904–20910.
49. Liu R-T, Suzuki S, Miyamoto Y, Takeda T, Ozata M, DeGroot LJ. The dominant negative effect of thyroid hormone receptor splicing variant α2 does not require binding to a thyroid response element. *Mol Endocrinol* 1995;9:86–95.
50. Lazar MA, Hodin RA, Darling DS, Chin WW. A novel member of the thyroid/steroid hormone receptor family is encoded by the opposite strand of the rat c-erbAα transcription unit. *Mol Cell Biol* 1989;9:1128–1136.
51. Lazar MA, Jones KE, Chin WW. Isolation of a cDNA encoding human Rev-erbAα: transcription from the non-coding DNA strand of a thyroid hormone receptor gene results in a related protein that does not bind thyroid hormone. *DNA Cell Biol* 1990;9:77–83.
52. Miyajima N, Horiuchi R, Shibuya Y, et al. Two erbA homologs encoding proteins with different T3 binding capacities are transcribed

from opposite DNA strands of the same genetic locus. *Cell* 1989;57: 31–39.
53. Lechan RM, Qi Y, Berrodin TJ, et al. Immunocytochemical delineation of thyroid hormone receptor beta 2-like immunoreactivity in the rat central nervous system. *Endocrinology* 1993;132:2461–2469.
54. Hollenberg AN, Monden T, Wondisford FE. Ligand-independent and -dependent functions of thyroid hormone receptor isoforms depend upon their distinct amino termini. *J Biol Chem* 1995;270:14278–14280.
55. Spanjaard RA, Nguyen VP, Chin WW. Repression of glucocorticoid receptor-mediated transcriptional activation by unliganded thyroid hormone receptor (TR) is TR isoform-specific. *Endocrinology* 1995; 136:5084–5092.
56. Williams GR, Brent GA. Thyroid hormone response elements. In: Weintraub BD, ed. *Molecular endocrinology: basic concepts and clinical correlations.* New York: Raven Press, 1995;217–239.
57. Kim H-S, Crone DE, Sprung CN, et al. Positive and negative thyroid hormone response elements are composed of strong and weak half-sites 10 nucleotides in length. *Mol Endocrinol* 1992;6:1489–1501.
58. Katz RW, Koenig RJ. Nonbiased identification of DNA sequences that bind thyroid hormone receptor alpha 1 with high affinity. *J Biol Chem* 1993;268:19392–19397.
59. Brent GA, Harney JW, Chen Y, Warne RL, Moore DD, Larsen PR. Mutations of the rat growth hormone promoter which increase and decrease response to thyroid hormone define a consensus thyroid hormone response element. *Mol Endocrinol* 1989;3:1996–2004.
60. Brent GA, Williams GR, Harney JW, et al. Effects of varying the position of thyroid hormone response elements within the rat growth hormone promoter: implications for positive and negative regulation by 3,5,3′-triiodothyronine. *Mol Endocrinol* 1991;5:542–548.
61. Chatterjee VKK, Lee J-K, Rentoumis A, Jameson JL. Negative regulation of the thyroid-stimulating hormone α gene by thyroid hormone: receptor interaction adjacent to the TATA box. *Proc Natl Acad Sci USA* 1989;86:9114–9118.
62. Bodenner DL, Mroczynski MA, Weintraub BD, Radovick S, Wondisford FE. A detailed functional and structural analysis of a major thyroid hormone inhibitory element in the human thyrotropin beta-subunit gene. *J Biol Chem* 1991;266:21666–21673.
63. Martin KJ. The interactions of transcription factors with their adaptors, coactivators and accessory proteins. *Bioessays* 1991;13:499–503.
64. Katz RW, Koenig RJ. Specificity and mechanism of thyroid hormone induction from an octamer response element. *J Biol Chem* 1994;269: 18915–18920.
65. Zhang XK, Pfahl M. Regulation of retinoid and thyroid hormone action through homodimeric and heterodimers receptors. *Trends Endocrinol Metab* 1993;4:10–16.
66. Rosen ED, O'Donnell AL, Koenig RJ. Protein-protein interactions involving erbA superfamily receptors: through the TRAPdoor. *Mol Cell Endocrinol* 1991;78:C83–C88.
67. Bugge TH, Pohl J, Lonnoy O, et al. RXR alpha, a promiscuous partner of retinoic acid and thyroid hormone receptors. *EMBO J* 1992;11: 1409–1418.
68. Hsu JH, Zavacki AM, Harney JW, Brent GA. Retinoid-X receptor (RXR) differentially augments thyroid hormone response in cell lines as a function of the response element and endogenous RXR content. *Endocrinology* 1995;136:421–430.
69. Yu VC, Delsert C, Anderson B, et al. RXR beta: a co-regulator that enhances the binding of retinoic acid, thyroid hormone, and vitamin D receptors to their cognate response elements. *Cell* 1991;67:1251–1266.
70. Lee JW, Choi H, Gyuris J, Brent R, Moore DD. Two classes of proteins dependent on either the presence or absence of thyroid hormone for interaction with the thyroid hormone receptor. *Mol Endocrinol* 1995;9:243–254.
71. Oñate S, Tsai SY, Tsai M-J, O'Malley BW. Sequence and characterization of a coactivator for the steroid hormone receptor superfamily. *Science* 1995;270:1354–1357.
72. Lee JW, Ryan F, Swaffield JC, Johnston SA, Moore DD. Interaction of thyroid-hormone receptor with a conserved transcriptional mediator. *Nature* 1995;374:91–94.
73. Hörlein AJ, Naar AM, Heinzel T, et al. Ligand-independent repression by the thyroid hormone receptor mediated by a nuclear receptor co-repressor. *Nature* 1995;377:397–404.
74. Chen JD, Evans RM. A transcriptional co-repressor that interacts with nuclear thyroid hormone receptors. *Nature* 1995;377:454–457.
75. Burris TP, Nawaz Z, Tsai MJ, O'Malley BW. A nuclear hormone receptor-associated protein that inhibits transactivation by the thyroid hormone and retinoic acid receptors. *Proc Natl Acad Sci USA* 1995; 92:9525–9529.
76. Renaud J-P, Rochel N, Ruff M, et al. Crystal structure of the RAR-γ ligand-binding domain bound to all-*trans* retinoic acid. *Nature* 1995; 378:681–689.
77. Wong J, Shi Y-B, Wolffe AP. A role for nucleosome assembly in both silencing and activation of the *Xenopus* TRβ A gene by the thyroid hormone receptor. *Genes Dev* 1995;9:2696–2711.
78. Piedrafita FJ, Bendik I, Ortiz MA, Pfahl M. Thyroid hormone receptor homodimers can function as ligand-sensitive repressors. *Mol Endocrinol* 1995;9:563–578.
79. Fondell JD, Roy AL, Roeder RG. Unliganded thyroid hormone receptor inhibits formation of a functional preinitiation complex: implications for active repression. *Genes Dev* 1993;7:1400–1410.
80. Helmer EB, Raaka BM, Samuels HH. Hormone-dependent and -independent transcriptional activation by thyroid hormone receptors are mediated by different mechanisms. *Endocrinology* 1996;137:390–399.
81. Wondisford FE, Steinfelder HJ, Nations M, Radovick S. AP-1 antagonizes thyroid hormone receptor action on the thyrotropin beta-subunit gene. *J Biol Chem* 1993;268:2749–2754.
82. Feng P, Li Q-L, Satoh T, Wilber JF. Ligand (T3) dependent and independent effects of thyroid hormone receptors upon human TRH gene transcription in neuroblastoma cells. *Biochem Biophys Res Commun* 1994;200:171–177.
83. Hollenberg AN, Monden T, Flynn TR, Boers M-E, Cohen O, Wondisford FE. The human thyrotropin-releasing hormone gene is regulated by thyroid hormones through two distinct classes of negative thyroid hormone response elements. *Mol Endocrinol* 1995;9:540–550.
84. Ribeiro RCJ, Kushner PJ, Apriletti JW, West BL, Baxter JD. Thyroid hormone alters *in vitro* DNA binding of monomers and dimers of thyroid hormone receptors. *Mol Endocrinol* 1992;6:1142–1152.
85. Yen PM, Darling DS, Carter RL, Forgione M, Umeda PK, Chin WW. Triiodothyronine (T3) decreases binding to DNA by T3-receptor homodimers but not receptor-auxiliary protein heterodimers. *J Biol Chem* 1992;267:3565–3568.
86. Yen PM, Sugawara A, Chin WW. Triiodothyronine (T3) differentially affects T3-receptor/retinoic acid receptor and T3-receptor/retinoid X receptor heterodimer binding to DNA. *J Biol Chem* 1992;267: 23248–23252.
87. Forman BM, Umesono K, Chen J, Evans RM. Unique response pathways are established by allosteric interactions among nuclear hormone receptors. *Cell* 1995;81:541–550.
88. Rosen ED, O'Donnell AL, Koenig RJ. Ligand-dependent synergy of thyroid hormone and retinoid X receptors. *J Biol Chem* 1992;267: 22010–22013.
89. Schräder M, Carlberg C. Thyroid hormone and retinoic acid receptors from heterodimers with retinoid X receptors on direct repeats, palindromes, and inverted palindromes. *DNA Cell Biol* 1994;13:333–341.
90. Force WR, Tillman JB, Sprung CN, Spindler SR. Homodimer and heterodimer DNA binding and transcriptional responsiveness to triiodothyronine (T3) and 9-cis-retinoic acid are determined by the number and order of high affinity half-sites in a T3 response element. *J Biol Chem* 1994;269:8863–8871.
91. Quigley CA, De Bellis A, Marschke KB, el-Awady MK, Wilson EM, French FS. Androgen receptor defects: historical, clinical, and molecular perspectives. *Endocr Rev* 1995;16:271–321.
92. Refetoff S, Weiss RE, Usala S. The syndromes of resistance to thyroid hormones. *Endocr Rev* 1993;14:348–399.
93. Beck-Peccoz P, Chatterjee VK. The variable clinical phenotype in thyroid hormone resistance syndrome. *Thyroid* 1994;4:225–232.
94. Jameson JL. Mechanisms by which thyroid hormone receptor mutations cause clinical syndromes of resistance to thyroid hormone. *Thyroid* 1994;4:485–492.
95. Yen PM, Chin WW. Molecular mechanisms of dominant negative activity by nuclear hormone receptors. *Mol Endocrinol* 1994;8: 1450–1454.
96. Zhu X-G, Yu C-L, McPhie P, Wong R, Cheng S-Y. Understanding the molecular mechanism of dominant negative action of mutant thyroid hormone $β_1$-receptors: the important role of the wild-type/mutant receptor heterodimer. *Endocrinology* 1996;137:712–721.
97. Zavacki AM, Harney JW, Brent GA, Larsen PR. Dominant negative inhibition by mutant thyroid hormone receptors is thyroid hormone response element and receptor isoform specific. *Mol Endocrinol* 1993;7:1319–1330.
98. Sugawara A, Yen PM, Apriletti JW, et al. Phosphorylation selectively

increases triiodothyronine receptor homodimer binding to DNA. *J Biol Chem* 1994;269:433–437.
99. Schroeder C, Gibson L, Zenke M, Beug H. Modulation of normal erythroid differentiation by the endogenous thyroid hormone and retinoic acid receptors: a possible target for v-erbA oncogene action. *Oncogene* 1992;7:217–227.
100. Sharif M, Privalsky ML. v-erbA oncogene function in neoplasia correlates with its ability to repress retinoic acid receptor action. *Cell* 1991;66:885–893.
101. Barlow C, Meister B, Lardelli M, Lendahl U, Vennstrom B. Thyroid abnormalities and hepatocellular carcinoma in mice transgenic for v-erbA. *EMBO J* 1994;13:4241–4250.
102. Sanchez-Pacheco A, Palomino T, Aranda A. Negative regulation of expression of the pituitary-specific transcription factor GHF-1/Pit-1 by thyroid hormones through interference with promoter enhancer elements. *Mol Cell Biol* 1995;15:6322–6330.
103. Lopez G, Schaufele F, Webb P, Holloway J, Baxter J, Kushner PJ. Positive and negative modulation of jun action by thyroid hormone receptor at a unique AP1 site. *Mol Cell Biol* 1993;13:3042–3049.
104. Cross M, Dexter TM. Growth factors in development, transformation, and tumorigenesis. *Cell* 1991;64:271–280.
105. Davis JRE, Bidley SP, Tomlinson S. Signal transduction in endocrine tissues. *Clin Endocrinol* 1992;36:437–449.
106. Karin M. Signal transduction from the cell surface to nucleus in development and disease. *FASEB J* 1992;6:2581–2590.
107. Ihle JN. Cytokine receptor signalling. *Nature* 1995;377:591–594.
108. Massagué J. Receptors for the TGF-β family. *Cell* 1992;69:1067–1070.
109. Collins S, Caron MG, Lefkowitz RJ. From ligand binding to gene expression: new insights into the regulation of G-protein coupled receptors. *Trends Biochem Sci* 1992;17:37–39.
110. Segre GV, Goldring SR. Receptors for secretin, calcitonin, parathyroid hormone (PTH)/PTH-related peptide, vasoactive intestinal peptide, glucagonlike peptide 1, growth hormone releasing hormone, and glucagon belong to a newly discovered G-protein-linked receptor family. *Trends Endocrinol Metab* 1993;4:309–314.
111. Menini A. Cyclic nucleotide-gated channels in visual and olfactory transduction. *Biophys Chem* 1995;55:185–196.
112. Brown EM, Gamba G, Riccardi D, et al. Cloning and characterization of an extracellular Ca(2+)-sensing receptor from bovine parathyroid. *Nature* 1993;366:575–580.
113. Riccardi D, Park J, Lee WS, Gamba G, Brown EM, Hebert SC. Cloning and functional expression of a rat kidney extracellular calcium/polyvalent cation-sensing receptor. *Proc Natl Acad Sci USA* 1995;92:131–135.
114. Sutherland EW, Oye I, Butcher RW. The action of epinephrine and the role of the adenylyl cyclase system in hormone action. *Recent Prog Horm Res* 1965;21:623–646.
115. Collins S, Lohse MJ, O'Dowd B, Caron MG, Lefkowitz RJ. Structure and regulation of G protein-coupled receptors: the β2-adrenergic receptor as a model. *Vitam Horm* 1991;46:1–39.
116. Baldwin JM. Structure and function of receptors coupled to G proteins. *Curr Opin Cell Biol* 1994;6:180–190.
117. Kohn LD, Shimura H, Shimura Y, et al. The thyrotropin receptor. *Vitamins Horm* 1995;50:287–384.
118. Straub RE, Frech GC, Joho RH, Gershengorn MC. Expression cloning of a cDNA encoding the mouse pituitary thyrotropin-releasing hormone receptor. *Proc Natl Acad Sci USA* 1990;87:9514–9518.
119. Lee TW, Anderson LA, Eidne KA, Milligan G. Comparison of the signalling properties of the long and short isoforms of the rat thyrotropin-releasing-hormone receptor following expression in rat 1 fibroblasts. *Biochem J* 1995;310:291–298.
120. Han B, Tashjian AHJ. Identification of Asn289 as a ligand binding site in the rat thyrotropin-releasing hormone (THR) receptor as determined by complementary modifications in the ligand and receptor: a new model for THR binding. *Biochemistry* 1995;34:13412–13422.
121. Combarnous Y. Molecular basis of the specificity of binding of glycoprotein hormones to their receptors. *Endocr Rev* 1992;13:670–689.
122. Simon MI, Strathmann MP, Gautam N. Diversity of G proteins in signal transduction. *Science* 1991;252:802–808.
123. Meinkoth JL, Ji L, Taylor SS, Feramisco JR. Dynamics of the distribution of cyclic AMP-dependent protein kinase in living cells. *Proc Natl Acad Sci USA* 1990;87:9595–9599.
124. Lalli E, Sassone-Corsi P. Signal transduction and gene regulation: the nuclear response to cAMP. *J Biol Chem* 1994;269:17359–17362.
125. Berridge MJ, Irvine RF. Inositol phosphates and cell signalling. *Nature* 1989;341:197–205.
126. Shupnik MA, Weck J, Hinkle PM. Thyrotropin (TSH)-releasing hormone stimulates TSHβ promoter activity by two distinct mechanisms involving calcium influx through L type Ca^{2+} channels and protein kinase C. *Mol Endocrinol* 1996;10:90–99.
127. Pestell RG, Jameson JL. Transcriptional regulation of endocrine genes by second-messenger signaling pathways. In: Weintraub BD, ed. *Molecular endocrinology: basic concepts and clinical correlations.* New York: Raven Press, 1995;59–76.
128. Landis CA, Masters SB, Spada A, Pace A, Bourne HR, Vallar L. GTPase inhibiting mutations activate the α chain of G_s and stimulate adenylate cyclase in human pituitary tumours. *Nature* 1989;340:692–696.
129. Liri T, Herzmark P, Nakamoto JM, Van Dop C, Bourne HR. Rapid GDP release from $G_{s\alpha}$ in patients with gain and loss of endocrine function. *Nature* 1994;371:164–168.
130. Pearce SHS, Trump D. G-protein-coupled receptors in endocrine disease. *Q J Med* 1995;88:3–8.
131. Stein SA, Oates EL, Hall CR, et al. Identification of a point mutation in the thyrotropin receptor of the hyt/hyt hypothyroid mouse. *Mol Endocrinol* 1994;8:129–138.
132. Duprez L, Parma J, Van Sande J, et al. Germline mutations in the thyrotropin receptor gene cause non-autoimmune autosomal dominant hyperthyroidism. *Nat Genet* 1994;7:396–401.
133. Kopp P, van Sande J, Parma J, et al. Congenital hyperthyroidism caused by a mutation in the thyrotropin-receptor gene. *N Engl J Med* 1995;332:150–154.
134. Parma J, Duprez L, Van Sande J, et al. Somatic mutations in the thyrotropin receptor gene cause hyperfunctiong thyroid adenomas. *Nature* 1993;365:649–651.
135. Russo D, Arturi F, Schlumberger M, et al. Activating mutations of the TSH receptor in differentiated thyroid carcinomas. *Oncogene* 1995;11:1907–1911.
136. Nagayama Y, Rapaport B. The thyrotropin receptor 25 years after its discovery: new insights after its molecular cloning. *Mol Endocrinol* 1992;6:145–156
137. Ullrich A, Schlessinger J. Signal transduction by receptors with tyrosine kinase activity. *Cell* 1990;61:203–212.
138. Daly C, Reich NC. Receptor to nucleus signaling via tyrosine phosphorylation of the p91 transcription factor. *Trends Endocrinol Metab* 1994;5:159–164
139. Cobb MH, Goldsmith EJ. How MAP kinases are regulated. *J Biol Chem* 1995;270:14843–14846.
140. Satoh T, Nakafuku M, Kaziro Y. Function of ras as a molecular switch in signal transduction. *J Biol Chem* 1992;267:24149–24152.
141. Liu J-J, Choa J-R, Jiang M-C, Ng S-Y, Ten JJ-Y, Yang-Yen H-F. Ras transformation results in an elevated level of cyclin D1 and acceleration of G_1 progression in NIH 3T3 cells. *Mol Cell Biol* 1995;15:3654–3663.
142. Karin M. The regulation of AP-1 activity by mitogen-activated protein kinases. *J Biol Chem* 1995;270:16483–16486.
143. Shuai K, Ziemiecki A, Wilks AF, et al. Polypeptide signaling to the nucleus through tyrosine phosphorylation of Jak and Stat proteins. *Nature* 1993;366:580–583.
144. Silvennoinen O, Ihle JN, Schlessinger J, Levy DE. Interferon-induced nuclear signalling by Jak protein tyrosine kinases. *Nature* 1993;366 (583–585).
145. Krontiris TG. Oncogenes. *N Engl J Med* 1995;333:303–306.
146. Malarkey K, Belham CM, Paul A, et al. The regulation of tyrosine kinase signalling pathways by growth factor and G-protein-coupled receptors. *Biochem J* 1995;309:361–375.
147. Kupperman E, Wofford D, Wen W, Meinkoth JL. Ras inhibits thyroglobulin expression but not cyclic adenosine monophosphate-mediated signaling in Wistar rat thyrocytes. *Endocrinology* 1996;137:96–104.
148. Hartwell LH, Kastan MB. Cell cycle and cancer. *Science* 1994;266:1821–1828.
149. Müller R. Transcriptional regulation during the mammalian cell cycle. *Trends Genet* 1995;11:173–178.
150. Karp JE, Broder S. Molecular foundations of cancer: new targets for intervention. *Nature Med* 1995;1:309–320.
151. Wilks AF. Protein tyrosine kinase growth factor receptors and their ligands in development, differentiation, and cancer. *Adv Cancer Res* 1993;60:43–73.

152. Bishop JM. Molecular themes in oncogenesis. *Cell* 1991;64:235–248.
153. Bodmer W, Bishop T, Karran P. Genetic steps in colorectal cancer. *Nat Genet* 1994;6:217–219.
154. Cantley LC, Auger KR, Carpenter C, et al. Oncogenes and signal transduction. *Cell* 1991;64:281–302.
155. Rabbitts TH. Chromosomal translocations in human cancer. *Nature* 1994;372:143–149.
156. Hofstra RMW, Landsvater RM, Ceccherinl I, et al. A mutation in the RET protooncogene associated with the multiple endocrine neoplasia type 2B and sporadic medullary thyroid carcinoma. *Nature* 1994;367:375–376.
157. Jhiang SM, Sagartz JE, Tong Q, et al. Targeted expression of the ret/PTC1 oncogene induces papillary thyroid carcinomas. *Endocrinology* 1996;137:375–378.
158. Marx J. Oncogenes reach a milestone. *Science* 1994;266:1942–1944.
159. Weinberg R. Tumor supressor genes. *Neuron* 1993;11:191–196.
160. Cox LS, Lane DP. Tumor suppressors, kinases and clamps: how p53 regulates the cell cycle in response to DNA damage. *Bioessays* 1995;17:501–508.
161. Picksley SM, Lane DP. p53 and Rb: their cellular roles. *Curr Opin Cell Biol* 1994;6:853–858.
162. Engler D, Burger AG. The deiodination of the iodothyronines and their derivatives in man. *Endocr Rev* 1984;5:151–184.
163. Ishii H, Inada M, Tanaka K, et al. Triiodothyronine generation from thyroxine in human thyroid: enhanced conversion in Graves' thyroid tissue. *J Clin Endocrinol Metab* 1981;52:1211–1217.
164. Erickson VJ, Cavalieri RR, Rosenberg LL. Thyroxine 5′-deiodinase of rat thyroid, but not liver, is dependent on thyrotropin. *Endocrinology* 1982;111:434–440.
165. St. Germain DL. Iodothyronine deiodinases. *Trends Endocrinol Metab* 1994;5:36–42.
166. Moreno M, Berry MJ, Horst C, et al. Activation and inactivation of thyroid hormone by type I iodothyronine deiodinase. *FEBS Lett* 1994;344:143–146.
167. Visser TJ, Leonard JL, Kaplan MM, Larsen PR. Kinetic evidence suggesting two mechanisms for iodothyronine 5′-deiodination in rat cerebral cortex. *Proc Natl Acad Sci USA* 1982;79:5080–5084.
168. Visser TJ, Kaplan MM, Leonard JL, Larsen PR. Evidence for two pathways of iodothyronine 5′-deiodination in rat pituitary that differ in kinetics, propylthiouracil sensitivity, and response to hypothyroidism. *J Clin Invest* 1983;71:992–1002.
169. Leonard JL, Mellen SA, Larsen PR. Thyroxine 5′-deiodinase activity in brown adipose tissue. *Endocrinology* 1983;112:1153–1155.
170. Calvo R, Obregón MJ, Ruiz de Ona C, Escobar del Rey F, de Escobar GM. Congenital hypothyroidism, as studied in rats: crucial role of maternal thyroxine but not 3,5,3′-triiodothyronine in the protection of the fetal brain. *J Clin Invest* 1990;85:889–899.
171. Obregon MJ, Ruiz de Ona C, Calvo R, Escobar del Rey F, Morreale de Escobar G. Outer ring iodothyronine deiodinases and thyroid hormone economy: responses to iodine deficiency in the rat fetus and neonate. *Endocrinology* 1991;129:2663–2673.
172. Silva JE, Matthews PS. Production rates and turnover of triiodothyronine in rat-developing cerebral cortex and cerebellum: responses to hypothyroidism. *J Clin Invest* 1984;74:1035–1049.
173. Croteau W, Davey JC, Galton VA, St. Germain DL. Cloning of the mammalian type II iodothyronine deiodinase: a selenoprotein differentially expressed and regulated in the human brain and other tissues. *J Clin Invest* 1996;98:405–417.
174. Mellström B, Naranjo JR, Santos A, Gonzalez AM, Bernal J. Independent expression of the α and β c-erbA genes in developing rat brain. *Mol Endocrinol* 1991;5:1339–1350.
175. Bradley DJ, Towle HC, Young WS. Spatial and temporal expression of α- and β-thyroid hormone receptor mRNAs, including the β2-subtype, in the developing mammalian nervous system. *J Neurosci* 1992;12:2286–2302.
176. St. Germain DL. Biochemical study of type III iodothyronine deiodinase. In: Wu S-Y, Visser TJ, eds. *Thyroid hormone metabolism: molecular biology and alternative pathways*. Ann Arbor: CRC Press, 1994;45–66.
177. Wu S, Fisher DA, Polk D, Chopra I. Maturation of thyroid hormone metabolism. In: Wu S, ed. *Thyroid hormone metabolism, regulation and clinical implications*. Boston: Blackwell Scientific, 1991;293–320.
178. Huang T, Chopra IJ, Boado R, Solomon DH, Chua Teco GN. Thyroxine inner ring monodeiodinating activity in fetal tissues of the rat. *Pediatr Res* 1988;23:196–199.
179. Nunez J. Effects of thyroid hormones during brain differentiation. *Mol Cell Endocrinol* 1984;37:125–132.
180. Pasquini JM, Adamo AM. Thyroid hormones and the central nervous system. *Dev Neurosci* 1994;16:1–8.
181. St. Germain DL, Galton VA. Comparative study of pituitary-thyroid hormone economy in fasting and hypothyroid rats. *J Clin Invest* 1985;75:679–688.
182. Silva JE, Leonard JL. Regulation of rat cerebrocortical and adenohypophyseal type II 5′-deiodinase by thyroxine, triiodothyronine, and reverse triiodothyronine. *Endocrinology* 1985;116:1627–1635.
183. Escobar-Morreale H, Obregón MJ, Escobar del Rey F, Morreale de Escobar G. Replacement therapy for hypothyroidism with thyroxine alone does not ensure euthyroidism in all tissues, as studied in thyroidectomized rats. *J Clin Invest* 1995;96:2828–2838.
184. van Doorn J, Roelfsema F, van der Heide D. Conversion of thyroxine to 3,5,3′-triiodothyronine in several rat tissues in vivo: the effect of hypothyroidism. *Acta Endocrinol* 1986;113:59–64.
185. St. Germain DL. The effects and interactions of substrates, inhibitors, and the cellular thiol-disulfide balance on the regulation of type II iodothyronine 5′-deiodinase. *Endocrinology* 1988;122:1860–1868.
186. Leonard JL, Silva JE, Kaplan MM, Mellen SA, Visser TJ, Larsen PR. Acute posttranscriptional regulation of cerebrocortical and pituitary iodothyronine 5′-deiodinases by thyroid hormone. *Endocrinology* 1984;114:998–1004.
187. Halperin Y, Shapiro LE, Surks MI. Down-regulation of type II L-thyroxine, 5′-monodeiodinase in cultured GC cells: different pathways of regulation by L-triiodothyronine and 3,3′,5′-triiodo-L-thyronine. *Endocrinology* 1994;135:1464–1469.
188. Leonard JL. Biochemical basis of thyroid hormone deiodination. In: Wu S, ed. *Thyroid hormone metabolism: regulation and clinical implications*. Boston: Blackwell Scientific, 1991;1–28.
189. Courtin F, Pelletier G, Walker P. Subcellular localization of thyroxine 5′-deiodinase activity in bovine anterior pituitary. *Endocrinology* 1985;117:2527–2533.
190. Leonard JL, Ekenbarger DM, Frank SJ, Farwell AP, Koehrle J. Localization of type I iodothyronine 5′-deiodinase to the basolateral plasma membrane in renal cortical epithelial cells. *J Biol Chem* 1991;266:11262–11269.
191. Kaplan MM. Changes in the particulate subcellular component of hepatic thyroxine-5′-monodeiodinase in hyperthyroid and hypothyroid rats. *Endocrinology* 1979;105:548–554.
192. St. Germain DL, Dittrich W, Morganelli CM, Cryns V. Molecular cloning by hybrid arrest of translation in *Xenopus laevis* oocytes: identification of a cDNA encoding the type I iodothyronine 5′-deiodinase from rat liver. *J Biol Chem* 1990;265:20087–20090.
193. Berry MJ, Banu L, Larsen PR. Type I iodothyronine deiodinase is a selenocysteine-containing enzyme. *Nature* 1991;349:438–440.
194. Mandel SJ, Berry MJ, Kieffer JD, Harney JW, Warne RL, Larsen PR. Cloning and in vitro expression of the human selenoprotein, type I iodothyronine deiodinase. *J Clin Endocrinol Metab* 1992;75:1133–1139.
195. St. Germain DL, Schwartzman R, Croteau W, et al. A thyroid hormone regulated gene in *Xenopus laevis* encodes a type III iodothyronine 5-deiodinase. *Proc Natl Acad Sci USA* 1994;91:11282.
196. Croteau W, Whittemore SL, Schneider MJ, St. Germain DL. Cloning and expression of a cDNA for a mammalian type III iodothyronine deiodinase. *J Biol Chem* 1995;270:16569–16575.
197. Davey JC, Becker KB, Schneider MJ, St. Germain DL, Galton VA. Cloning of a cDNA for the type II iodothyronine deiodinase. *J Biol Chem* 1995;270:26786–26789.
198. Böck A, Forchhammer K, Heider J, et al. Selenocysteine: the 21st amino acid. *Mol Microbiol* 1991;5:515–520.
199. Berry MJ, Maia AL, Kieffer JD, Harney JW, Larsen PR. Substitution of cysteine for selenocysteine in type I iodothyronine deiodinase reduces the catalytic efficiency of the protein but enhances its translation. *Endocrinology* 1992;131:1848–1852.
200. Toyoda N, Berry MJ, Harney JW, Larsen PR. Topological analysis of the integral membrane protein, type 1 iodothyronine deiodinase (D1). *J Biol Chem* 1995;270:12310–12318.
201. Berry M. Identification of essential histidine residues in rat type I iodothyronine deiodinase. *J Biol Chem* 1992;267:18055–18059.

202. Stadtman TC. Biosynthesis and function of selenocysteine-containing enzymes. *J Biol Chem* 1991;266:16257–16260.
203. Stadtman TC. Selenium biochemistry. *Ann Rev Biochem* 1990;59:111–127.
204. Lee BJ, Worland JN, Davis JN, Stadtman TC, Hatfield D. Identification of a selenocysteyl-tRNA(Ser) in mammalian cells that recognizes the nonsense codon, UGA. *J Biol Chem* 1989;264:9724–9727.
205. Böck A, Forchhammer K, Heidler J, Baron C. Selenoprotein synthesis: an expansion of the genetic code. *Trends Biochem Sci* 1991;16:463–467.
206. Berry MJ, Banu L, Harney JW, Larsen PR. Functional characterization of the eukaryotic SECIS elements which direct selenocysteine insertion at UGA codons. *EMBO J* 1993;12:3315–3322.
207. Shen Q, Leonard JL, Newburger PE. Structure and function of the selenium translation element in the 3′-untranslated region of human cellular glutathione peroxidase mRNA. *RNA* 1995;1:519–525.
208. Berry MJ, Banu L, Chen Y, et al. Recognition of UGA as a selenocysteine codon in type I deiodinase requires sequences in the 3′ untranslated region. *Nature* 1991;353:273–276.
209. Berry MJ, Harney JW, Ohama T, Hatfield DL. Selenocysteine insertion or termination: factors affecting codon fate and complementary anticodon:codon mutations. *Nucleic Acids Res* 1994;22:3753–3759.
210. Arthur JR, Nicol F, Hutchinson AR, Beckett GJ. The effects of selenium depletion and repletion on the metabolism of thyroid hormones in the rat. *J Inorg Biochem* 1990;9:101–108.
211. Chanoine J, Safran M, Farwell AP, et al. Effects of selenium deficiency on thyroid hormone economy in rats. *Endocrinology* 1992;131:1787–1792.
212. Beckett GJ, Beddows SE, Morrice PC, Nicol F, Arthur JR. Inhibition of hepatic deiodination of thyroxine is caused by selenium deficiency in rats. *Biochem J* 1987;248:443–447.
213. Beckett GJ, MacDougal DA, Nicol F, Arthur JR. Inhibition of types I and II iodothyronine deiodinase activity in rat liver, kidney and brain produced by selenium deficiency. *Biochem J* 1989;259:887–892.
214. DePalo D, Kinlaw WB, Zhao C, Engelberg-Kulka H, St. Germain DL. Effect of selenium deficiency on type I 5′-deiodinase. *J Biol Chem* 1994;269:16223–16228.
215. Arthur JR, Nicol F, Beckett GJ, Trayhurn P. Impairment of iodothyronine 5′-deiodinase activity in brown adipose tissue and its acute stimulation by cold in selenium deficiency. *Can J Physiol Pharmacol* 1991;69:782–785.
216. Chanoine J, Braverman LE, Farwell AP, et al. The thyroid gland is a major source of circulating T3 in the rat. *J Clin Invest* 1993;91:2709–2713.
217. Behne D, Hilmert H, Scheid S, Gessner H, Elger W. Evidence for specific selenium target tissues and new biologically important selenoproteins. *Biochim Biophys Acta* 1988;966:12–21.
218. Meinhold H, Campos-Barros A, Walzog B, Köhler R, Müller F, Behne D. Effects of selenium and iodine deficiency on type I, type II, and type III iodothyronine deiodinases and circulating thyroid hormones in the rat. *Exp Clin Endocrinol* 1993;101:87–93.
219. Chanoine J, Alex S, Stone S, et al. Placental 5′-deiodinase activity and fetal thyroid hormone economy are unaffected by selenium deficiency in the rat. *Pediatr Res* 1993;34:288–292.
220. Gross M, Oertel M, Köhrle J. Differential selenium-dependent expression of type I 5′-deiodinase and glutathione peroxidase in the porcine epithelial kidney cell line LLC-PK1. *Biochem J* 1995;306:851–856.
221. Vanderpas JB, Contempré B, Duale NL, et al. Selenium deficiency mitigates hypothyroxinemia in iodine-deficient subjects. *Am J Clin Nutr* 1993;57:271S–275S.
222. Howie AF, Walker SW, Åkesson B, Arthur JR, Beckett GJ. Thyroidal extracellular glutathione peroxidase: a potential regulator of thyroid-hormone synthesis. *Biochem J* 1995;308:713–7171.

GLOSSARY

Agarose gel electrophoresis: a method for separating DNA or RNA molecules by size (see electrophoresis).
Allele: Alternative forms of a gene at a given locus.
Allelic heterogeneity: Similar or identical phenotypes caused by different mutant alleles at the same genetic locus. For example, a variety of different mutations in the thyroid hormone β receptor gene result in the phenotype of thyroid hormone resistance.
Amino acids: The building blocks of proteins. There are 20 common amino acids plus the uncommon amino acid selenocysteine; they are joined together in a strictly ordered "string" that determines the structure and function of each protein.
Antigen: Any molecule that provokes synthesis of an antibody.
Antisense strand (of DNA): The noncoding strand of double-stranded DNA. It is complementary to the mRNA and serves as the template for RNA synthesis.
Antisense RNA: RNA that is complementary to the "sense" messenger RNA. Antisense RNA is derived from a gene constructed in the 3′-5′ (or opposite) orientation.
Apoptosis: The process of programmed cell death that cells undergo in response to certain types of stress or senescence.
Autoradiogram: A method for detecting radioactivity by exposure to x-ray film. Used to localize radioactive probes hybridized to Southern (DNA) or Northern (RNA) blots.
Autosomal disease: A disease encoded by a gene on one of the 22 pairs of autosomes.
Autosome: Any chromosome other than the sex chromosomes.
Bacteriophage (phage): A virus that infects a bacterial cell. A phage consists of a core of genetic material (DNA or RNA) carrying the particle's genetic information, surrounded by a protein coat or capsule. When a phage infects a host cell, the cell machinery that manufactures protein in response to genetically encoded instructions is commandeered by the phage and used to produce offspring phage. The lambda bacteriophage is frequently used as a vector in recombinant gene experiments.
Base pair (bp): In double-stranded DNA, there is complementary hydrogen bonding (adenine–thymine and guanine–cytosine). The hydrogen-bonded residue pair designates 1 bp. This unit is used for measuring the length of pieces of DNA (see DNA).
Carrier: An individual heterozygous for a mutant allele that causes disease only in the homozygous state.
Centimorgan (cM): A unit of genetic distance. Two loci are 1 cM apart if there is a 1% chance of recombination between them in a given meiotic event (see meiosis).
Chromosome: The location of hereditary (genetic) material within the cell. This hereditary material is packaged in the form of a very long, double-stranded molecule of DNA surrounded by and complexed with several different forms of protein. Genes are found arranged in a linear sequence along chromosomes, as is also a large amount of DNA of unknown function.
Chimera: That produced by the joining together of two or more units that are not normally found together. For

example, a chimera of the TSH and FSH receptor could be made by joining together the extracellular hormone-binding domain of the TSH receptor to the transmembrane and cytoplasmic signalling domain of the FSH receptor.

CHO cells: Chinese hamster ovarian cells. A relatively undifferentiated cell line frequently used in molecular biology experiments.

Cis element: A region of a molecule that affects only its own state of activation, as opposed to proteins such as transcription factors, which can influence the activity of other molecules. Usually, this refers to a region of a gene or mRNA that is involved in regulation (e.g., the response elements of the enhancer region are cis-acting elements).

Clone: A group of genetically identical cells or organisms asexually descended from a common ancestor. All cells in the clone have the same genetic material and are exact copies of the original.

Cloning: The generation of a large number of identical DNA fragments.

Co-activator: A protein that binds to transcription factors and conveys a stimulatory signal to the basal transcriptional apparatus.

Coding region: That portion of the mRNA that dictates the amino acid sequence of the protein, and which is thus translated by the ribosome.

Codon: A group of three sequential nucleotides within RNA that codes for a specific amino acid in the corresponding protein. Codons are the "words" of the genetic code (e.g., AUG means methionine, and it also means "start translation here") (see reading frame).

Complementarity: The specific binding of adenine to thymine (or uracil in RNA) and cytosine to guanine on opposite strands of DNA or RNA (see DNA).

Complementary DNA (cDNA): DNA synthesized from a messenger RNA template. cDNA is often used as a probe to help locate a specific gene in DNA.

Compound heterozygote: An individual with two different mutant alleles at a given locus.

Co-repressor: A protein that binds to transcription factors and conveys an inhibitory signal to the basal transcriptional apparatus.

Crossing over: The reciprocal breaking and rejoining of homologous chromosomes in meiotic prophase I that results in exchange of chromosomal segments (see meiosis).

Deiodination: The enzymatic removal of an iodine from either the inner or outer ring of an iodothyronine (e.g., thyroxine) molecule.

Dimerization: The binding together of two (identical or different) transcription factors to form a complex that is involved in transcriptional regulation.

DNA (deoxyribonucleic acid): The molecule containing hereditary information in all but the most primitive organisms (some viruses use RNA). The molecule is double-stranded, with an external "backbone" formed by a chain of alternating phosphate and sugar (deoxyribose) units and an internal ladder-like structure formed by nucleotide base-pairs held together by hydrogen bonds. The nucleotide base-pairs consist of the bases adenine (A), cytosine (C), guanine (G), and thymine (T), whose structures are such that A can hydrogen bond only with T, and C only with G. The sequence of each individual strand can be deduced by knowing that of its partner strand. This complementarity is the key to the information-transmitting capabilities of DNA, and of its ability to be replicated.

DNA polymerase: The enzyme that synthesizes DNA from a complementary DNA template. In the cell, it replicates the DNA strands prior to cell division.

DNA probe: A nucleic acid molecule of known structure and/or function that has been tagged with some tracer substance (e.g., a radioactive isotope) that is used to locate and identify a specific gene or region of a chromosome or portion of the genome. It may also be used to identify a specific mRNA. DNA probes are used for detection on Southern (DNA) and Northern (RNA) blots.

Domain: A region of the amino acid sequence of a protein that can be equated with a particular function, or a corresponding segment of a gene. For example, the members of the steroid/thyroid hormone receptor superfamily have defined regions that bind to specific DNA sequences (i.e., the DNA-binding domain).

Dominant negative: A mutation in a single allele that confers a dominant mode of inheritance as a result of the mutated gene product inactivating the product from the normal allele.

Electrophoresis: A technique used to separate molecules by applying an electrical current that causes them to move through a gel at a rate determined by their size.

Endonuclease: An enzyme that cleaves bonds within a DNA or RNA strand. This contrasts with an exonuclease, which digests the ends of a DNA strand. Endonucleases recognize a specific DNA sequence. For example: GAATTC is the sequence recognized by the restriction endonuclease *Eco*R1. Each enzyme is designated by the organism from which it was obtained (e.g., *Eco*R1 from *E. coli* RY13).

Enhancer: The region of DNA upstream from the promoter. Transcription factors bind to this region and regulate gene transcription.

Enzyme: A functional protein that catalyzes a chemical reaction.

Ethidium bromide: A dye that causes DNA and RNA to become fluorescent. It is used to visualize nucleic acid bands on agarose gels after electrophoresis.

Exon: Sequences within the DNA that are represented (expressed) in the final, mature RNA (see intron).

Expression: The process by which the information contained in DNA is converted into mRNA and protein.

Fos: A proto-oncogene that codes for a transcription factor involved in the control of cellular proliferation. Part of the AP-1 complex.

G-proteins: A family of GTP-binding proteins involved in the coupling of cell surface receptors to intracellular second messenger systems such as those that generate cAMP.

Gene: The portion of a DNA molecule that is sufficient for the expression of a functional polypeptide.

Gene amplification: A process that increases the number of copies of the same gene within a cell. Amplification may be spontaneous or induced.

Genetic engineering: A technique used to modify the genetic information in a living cell, reprogramming it for a desired purpose [such as the production of a protein it would not naturally produce (e.g., insulin production by *E. coli*)].

Genetic locus: A specific position or location on a chromosome.

Genetic marker: A locus whose alleles are readily detectable. It may or may not be part of an expressed gene.

Genetic screening: Testing a population to identify individuals at high risk of having or transmitting a specific genetic disorder.

Genome: The complete DNA sequence of an organism, containing its complete genetic information. The human genome consists of about 60,000 to 70,000 genes, and about 3 billion base pairs (bp) of DNA.

Germline mutation: Mutations that are present in a parent, or that occur during gametogenesis, so that they are inherited through the sex cells.

Haplotype: Genotype of a group of alleles from two or more closely linked loci on one chromosome, usually inherited as a unit (e.g., the HLA complex).

Heterodimer: A complex of two different transcription factors that is involved in transcriptional regulation (e.g., a $TR\beta_1$-RXR heterodimer).

Heterozygote (heterozygous): An individual who has two different alleles at a given locus on a pair of homologous chromosomes.

Homology: Similarity between two distinct genes in their nucleotide sequence.

Homodimer: A complex of two identical transcription factors that is involved in transcriptional regulation (e.g., a $TR\beta_1$ homodimer).

Homozygote (homozygous): An individual who has two identical alleles at a given locus on a pair of homologous chromosomes.

Hot spot: A region of a gene wherein a higher-than-expected frequency of mutations occurs.

Hybridization: Pairing of an RNA and a DNA strand, or of two different DNA strands. Efficient hybridization requires a high degree of complementarity (i.e., homology) of the two strands.

Intron: Sequences within the DNA of a gene that are not represented in the final RNA. They are removed from the precursor RNA within the nucleus, and the remaining pieces of the RNA are spliced together prior to export out of the nucleus.

In situ hybridization: The localization of RNA sequences by hybridization of labeled probes to tissue sections. It is used to identify the regions or cell type in a tissue that expresses a given gene (e.g., expression of the various thyroid hormone receptor isoforms in the central nervous system).

Isoform: A structurally related member of a protein family (e.g., the thyroid hormone receptor family includes, among others, the $TR\alpha_1$ and $TR\beta_1$ isoforms).

Kilobase (kb): One thousand base pairs in a DNA sequence.

Knockout mouse: A mouse strain that has been genetically altered so that a specific gene has been inactivated.

Jun: A proto-oncogene that codes for a transcription factor involved in the control of cellular proliferation. Part of the AP-1 complex.

Library: A collection of pieces of DNA that represent the genes of an organism (like books in a library). The DNA pieces are stored in a form that allows convenient access and screening for specific sequences, and for their replication in bacteria. Libraries may be made from genomic DNA or from cDNA, and they may be expression or nonexpression. In expression libraries, as opposed to nonexpression libraries, the genes are transcribed into RNA, which is then translated into protein by the bacteria. Thus, in expression libraries, the protein is expressed. Genomic libraries contain all the genetic information within the genome of a given organism, whereas a cDNA library contains only that information that is expressed in the particular tissue from which the mRNA used to make the cDNAs was derived.

Ligand: A molecule that binds to a receptor and influences its activity (e.g., T_3 is the ligand for the thyroid hormone receptor).

Ligase: An enzyme that joins fragments of DNA. It is used to form recombinant DNA molecules.

Linkage: Co-inheritance of two or more nonallelic genes because their loci are in close proximity on the same chromosome, so that after meiosis they remain associated more often than the 50% expected for unlinked genes.

Linkage map: A chromosome map showing relative positions of genetic markers of a given species, as determined by linkage analysis; this differs from a gene map generated by a physical analysis of the DNA.

Lod score: A statistical method that tests whether a set of linkage data indicates that two loci are linked or unlinked. The lod score is the base 10 logarithm of the odds favoring linkage. By convention, a lod score of +3 (1:1000 odds) is taken as proof of linkage; a score of −2 (100:1 odds against) indicates no linkage.

MAP kinase: A kinase that is a member of the RAS signalling pathway.

Meiosis: Special type of cell division occurring in germ cells of sexually reproducing organisms, during which the gametes containing the haploid chromosome number are produced from diploid cells. Two meiotic divisions occur: meiosis I and II; reduction in chromosome number takes place during meiosis I.

Messenger RNA (mRNA): An RNA transcribed from the DNA of a gene, forming the template from which a protein is translated.

Missense mutation: A single DNA base substitution resulting in a codon specifying a different amino acid.

Molecular genetics: The study of the nature and biochemistry of the genetic material. It includes the technologies of genetic engineering that involve the direct manipulation of the genetic material itself.

Monoclonal antibodies: Antibodies produced by a single source (clone) of cells that recognize only a single antigen.

Myc: A proto-oncogene that codes for a transcription factor involved in the control of cellular proliferation.

Mutation: Any change that alters the sequence of bases along the DNA, thus changing the genetic material. A mutation may or may not result in clinical disease, depending on the nature of the mutation and its location in the genome.

Northern blot: A technique, analogous to Southern blotting, for detecting RNA fragments by hybridization. The blot reveals the size and abundance of the RNA complementary to the probe used for detection.

Nucleic acid: A DNA or an RNA polymer composed of nucleotide subunits.

Oligonucleotides: Short pieces of single- or double-stranded DNA, frequently 10 to 30 nucleotides in length, that are derived from the sequence of a specific gene of interest. They can be used as probes or as primers in polymerase chain reaction (PCR) or cloning experiments.

Oncogene: A mutated or altered proto-oncogene. When an oncogene is expressed, abnormal cell proliferation and neoplasia occurs.

Orphan receptor: A member of the steroid/thyroid hormone receptor family whose activating ligand is not yet identified.

Palindromic sequence: A nucleotide sequence that reads the same in either direction ("Madam I'm Adam"). Restriction endonuclease recognition sites in DNA are typically palindromes.

Phage: See bacteriophage.

Phenotype: The appearance or characteristics of an organism that result from the interaction between its genotype and the environment.

Plasmid: Independently replicating, extrachromosomal, circular DNA molecules, often bearing antibiotic resistance genes and propagated in bacteria; used in recombinant DNA technology as vectors to carry cloned DNA segments.

Point mutation: Substitution of one nucleotide for another in DNA.

Poly(A)+ tail: A string of adenosine nucleotides found at the 3′ end of most mRNA molecules.

Polymerase chain reaction (PCR): Enzymatic technique for the production of many copies of one DNA sequence in a test tube. Repeated cycles of temperature changes allow sequential denaturation, priming, and strand synthesis steps that result in an exponential production of the desired DNA molecule.

Polymorphism: The occurrence in a population of two or more genetically determined alternative phenotypes at such a frequency that the rarest could not be maintained by recurrent mutation alone. In practice, a genetic locus is considered polymorphic if heterozygotes carrying the allele occur at a frequency greater than 2%.

Primers: Oligonucleotides used in conjunction with a DNA polymerase to initiate DNA synthesis. Used in PCR and various cloning methods.

Probe: A labeled DNA or RNA sequence used to detect the presence of a complementary sequence by molecular hybridization; a reagent capable of recognizing the desired clone in a complex mixture of many DNA or RNA sequences.

Promoter: The region of DNA immediately upstream of the transcriptional start site in a gene. The RNA polymerase II complex binds in this region to initiate transcription.

Protein: A linear polymer of amino acids; proteins are the products of gene expression and are the functional and structural components of cells.

Protein kinase A: A serine/threonine protein kinase whose activity is stimulated by the presence of the second messenger cAMP.

Protein kinase C: A serine/threonine protein kinase whose activity is stimulated by the presence of the second messenger diacylglycerol.

Proto-oncogene: A normal gene that promotes or regulates the proliferative state of a cell.

Ras: A proto-oncogene that codes for a GTP-binding protein integral to several signalling transduction pathways utilized by various cell surface receptor molecules.

Reading frame: The grouping of nucleotides in RNA into triplet codons. Thus, an RNA sequence contains three different reading frames. The "true" reading frame of an RNA sequence is determined by the position of the start codon, AUG. Because this codon also denotes the amino acid methionine, all proteins contain an initial methionine residue (see codon).

Recessive trait: Those conditions that are clinically manifest only in individuals homozygous for the mutant gene (i.e., carrying a double dose of the particular gene).

Recombinant DNA: DNA molecules that have been assembled with the use of restriction enzymes, usually but not always by splicing together fragments from different species.

Recombination: The formation of new combinations of linked genes by crossing over (breaking and rejoining) between their loci.

Replication: The formation of two new strands of DNA from existing DNA, permitting the reproduction of an identical new cell as the result of division.

Response element: A specific sequence of DNA to which a transcription factor binds.

Restriction endonuclease: See restriction enzyme.

Restriction enzyme: An endonuclease that recognizes a specific sequence in DNA and cleaves the DNA strand at that point; used in recombinant DNA technology (see endonuclease).

Restriction fragment length polymorphism (RFLP): A variation in DNA sequence (a mutation or polymorphism) that alters the length of a fragment generated by digestion with a restriction endonuclease. This occurs, for example, when a mutation destroys or creates a restriction enzyme recognition site within the DNA. RFLPs provide convenient markers for linkage analysis.

Ret: A proto-oncogene that encodes a cell surface protein with tyrosine kinase activity. Activating mutations can result in several diseases including medullary carcinoma of the thyroid or thyroid papillary cell carcinoma.

Reverse transcriptase: An enzyme that synthesizes DNA from an RNA template.

Ribonucleic acid (RNA): A polynucleotide consisting of a backbone of alternating phosphate and sugar (ribose) molecules to which are attached the nucleotide bases adenine (A), cytosine (C), guanine (G), and uracil (U) [which replaces the thymine (T) of DNA]. There are several classes of RNA that serve different purposes, including messenger RNA (mRNA), transfer RNA (tRNA), and ribosomal RNA (rRNA).

Ribosomes: The structures that synthesize (translate) the protein encoded by a messenger RNA molecule.

RNA polymerase: The enzyme that synthesizes RNA from a DNA template. RNA polymerase II specifically synthesizes mRNA, whereas other RNA polymerases produce transfer RNAs or ribosomal RNAs.

RT-PCR: A modification of the PCR technique whereby mRNA is used as the starting material to initially synthesize a specific cDNA (using reverse transcriptase and a specific primer), which is then used in the PCR reaction. This represents an extremely sensitive technique to detect specific mRNA molecules in a biologic sample.

RXR: A member of the steroid/thyroid hormone receptor family that binds 9-cis retinoic acid as its ligand. RXRs frequently dimerize with thyroid hormone receptors to regulate transcription.

SECIS: Selenocysteine insertion sequence. A specific region in the 3′-untranslated region of eukaryotic mRNAs that code for selenoproteins. The region is necessary for incorporation of selenocysteine into the protein during translation.

Selenocysteine: An uncommon amino acid whereby the element selenium is substituted for sulfur, resulting in a more highly reactive molecule. Selenocysteine is present at the active site of the deiodinase enzymes.

Somatic mutation: A mutation that occurs in the genetic material of an individual cell after fertilization. It would thus not be inherited by offspring (assuming the cell involved was not a gamete).

Southern blot: Technique designed by Edward Southern for transferring DNA fragments separated by agarose gel electrophoresis to a filter, on which specific DNA fragments can then be detected by their hybridization to labeled probes.

Splicing: The processing of precursor mRNA whereby the introns are excised and the exons joined together to form the mature mRNA.

Stringency: The conditions of hybridization that determine the specificity of binding between two strands of nucleic acid. Increasing the temperature, for example, leads to increased stringency.

TATA box: A specific DNA sequence (TATAAT) found in the promoter region of many genes; it serves to direct the binding of the RNA polymerase II complex to the start site of transcription.

TBP: The TATA box binding protein (see TFIID).

Template: The nucleic acid sequence that is "read" by DNA or RNA polymerases to synthesize a complementary nucleic acid strand.

TFIIB: A transcription factor complex that is associated with the basal transcriptional apparatus and DNA polymerase II.

TFIID: A transcription factor complex that is associated with the basal transcriptional apparatus and DNA polymerase II. A subunit of the TFIID complex, termed the TATA box binding protein (TBP). It binds to the TATAAT sequence in the promoter region to initiate assembly of the basal transcriptional apparatus.

Transactivation: The process whereby an activated transcription factor stimulates transcription.

Transcription: The synthesis of RNA on a DNA template. The information within the DNA is transcribed into multiple RNA copies.

Transcription factor: A protein that binds to a specific sequence of DNA (a response element) in the promoter or enhancer region of a gene and thereby regulates transcriptional activity.

Transcription unit: That part of the gene that encompasses the exonic and intronic regions that will be transcribed into precursor mRNA.

Transfection: The process of forcing cells to take up DNA from the external environment.

Transgenic: A state wherein an organism contains within its germ-line both parental and foreign DNA sequences. The foreign sequences are transmissible to the offspring.

Translation: The synthesis of a polypeptide with an amino acid sequence specified by the codon sequence of a corresponding messenger RNA.

TRAPs: Thyroid hormone receptor auxiliary proteins. A generic term that refers to nuclear proteins that bind to the thyroid hormone receptor to form heterodimers (e.g., RXR).

TTF-1, TTF-2: Thyroid transcription factors 1 and 2. Transcription factors expressed specifically in thyroid follicular cells and involved in the regulation of several thyroid cell–specific proteins such as thyroid peroxidase, thyroglobulin, and the thyrotropin receptor.

Tumor suppressor gene: A gene that encodes a protein that normally restrains cell division, or promotes differentiation, DNA repair, or apoptosis.

Untranslated regions: Those portions of an mRNA that flank (in the 3′ or 5′ direction) the coding region, and thus are not translated into protein.

Vector: A transmission agent; a DNA vector is a self-replicating DNA molecule that transfers, or carries, a piece of DNA from one host to another.

Virus: An infectious agent that requires a host cell in order for it to replicate. It is composed of either RNA or DNA wrapped in a protein coat.

Western blot: A blotting technique, analogous to Southern blotting, for detecting proteins, usually by using antibodies as "probes."

Wild type: The normal or native gene, or gene product.

CHAPTER 11

Molecular Biology of the Thyroid Stimulating Hormone Receptor

Shigenobu Nagataki and Yuji Nagayama

The differentiated functions and proliferation of the thyroid gland are entirely dependent on the pituitary hormone thyrotropin (thyroid stimulating hormone, TSH) (1). TSH mediates its biologic actions through a plasma membrane receptor, the TSH receptor. Therefore, the TSH receptor is an indispensable molecule for preserving the thyroid cell phenotype. Upon TSH binding, the TSH receptor couples to both Gs and Gq proteins, thus stimulating adenylyl cyclase and phospholipase Cβ (PLCβ). This results in increases in the intracellular second messengers cAMP, and diacylglycerol and inositol 1,4,5-triphosphate (IP$_3$), respectively. Most of the TSH effect can be explained by the Gs protein–adenylyl cyclase–cAMP pathway. Stimulation of PLCβ requires higher concentrations of TSH than does the stimulation of adenylyl cyclase (2).

The TSH receptor, like other thyroid specific proteins—thyroglobulin (Tg) and thyroid peroxidase (TPO)—is a major autoantigen in human autoimmune thyroid disease. Thus, thyroid stimulating antibodies (TSAbs) are present in most patients with Graves' disease, and TSH-binding inhibiting immunoglobulins (TBII) occur in a fraction of patients with Hashimoto's thyroiditis or myxedema (3).

For these reasons, an understanding of the relationship between structure and function of the TSH receptor is important from both physiologic and pathophysiologic points of view. Although biochemical studies of the TSH receptor have long been hampered by the paucity (10^3 to 10^4 molecules per cell) and the fragility of the receptor protein, molecular cloning of the TSH receptor cDNA in 1989 (4–6) and the recent rapid spread of molecular biology techniques have led to significant progress in our understanding of molecular biology of the TSH receptor (7–9).

MOLECULAR CLONING OF THE TSH RECEPTOR

Antibody Screening

The TSH receptor protein has never been purified sufficiently for partial amino acid sequence analysis. Attempts to identify the TSH receptor cDNA by screening a thyroid cDNA expression library with IgG from patients with positive anti-TSH receptor autoantibodies, or putative TSH receptor monoclonal antibodies, resulted in isolation of a number of clones. None of these, however, coded for the TSH receptor.

Nucleic Acid Screening

Even before the molecular cloning of the TSH receptor cDNA, it was assumed that this receptor would belong to a superfamily of G protein–coupled receptors with seven transmembrane-spanning regions. Furthermore, the receptors for the pituitary glycoprotein hormones, TSH, lutropin (LH), and follitropin (FSH), were thought likely to be closely related to each other because of their functional similarities and also because of the structural similarities of their ligand hormones.

Based on this assumption, Vassart and his colleagues employed the low stringency polymerase chain reaction (PCR) using thyroid cDNA and genomic DNA as templates and degenerate oligonucleotide primers based on transmembrane regions of known members of the G protein–coupled receptor superfamily. Several cDNAs for new G protein–coupled receptors, including a putative FSH receptor, were cloned (4,10). With this cDNA as a probe, the TSH

S. Nagataki: The First Department of Internal Medicine, Nagasaki University School of Medicine, Nagasaki, 852 Japan.
Y. Nagayama: Department of Pharmacology 1, Nagasaki University School of Medicine, Nagasaki, 852 Japan.

receptor cDNA was successfully obtained by screening a dog thyroid cDNA library (4). Shortly thereafter, the human and rat TSH receptor cDNAs were isolated (5,6,11–13).

PRIMARY STRUCTURE OF THE TSH RECEPTOR

The full-length human TSH receptor cDNA is approximately 4 kilobases (kb) in length and contains a single open reading frame of 2292 base pairs (bp), encoding a protein of 764 amino acids including a 21-amino-acid signal peptide. The amino acid structure of the receptor is shown in Figure 1. The calculated molecular mass is 84.5 kDa. Comparison to other G protein–coupled receptors and hydropathy profile analysis indicates that the amino (N)-terminal half of the receptor encompasses the extracellular domain (397 amino acids after removal of the signal peptide), whereas the carboxyl (C)-terminal region includes the transmembrane and cytoplasmic regions (346 amino acids). Because of their apparently distinct structures and functional properties, these two regions are separately discussed.

Extracellular Domain

The extracellular domain of the glycoprotein hormone receptors are extremely large compared to those of other G protein–coupled receptors, such as adrenergic receptors. In general, the size of the receptor extracellular domains appears to correlate directly with the mass of the respective ligands in this receptor superfamily.

There is very high amino acid homology among the human, dog, and rat TSH receptors in this domain (85% to 90%), whereas the homology is less with other glycoprotein hormone receptors (35% to 45%). The comparison of amino acid homology between the TSH receptor and other glycoprotein hormone receptors is shown in Figure 2. This dissimilarity is particularly apparent at the extreme ends of the extracellular domain (TSH receptor amino acids 1 to 57 and 287 to 404). These relatively unconserved regions among the glycoprotein hormone receptors contain two additional segments or insertions in the TSH receptor (amino acids 38 to 45 and 317 to 366, the solid boxes in Fig. 2). In contrast, the middle region of the extracellular domain (amino acids 58 to 286) has a relatively high degree of amino acid homology and comprises nine leucine-rich repeats (LRRs). LRRs are observed in numerous proteins and are thought to be very important for protein–protein interaction (14). The characteristics of LRRs are high contents of aliphatic amino acids and the periodic pattern of the consensus sequence. The consensus sequence of the LRRs we propose is x-Leu-x-x-Thr-x-x-Leu-Thr-x-Leu-Pro-x-x-Ala-Phe-x-x-Leu-x-x-Leu-x-x-x-Leu (Fig. 3).

The receptor extracellular domain features six potential N-linked glycosylation sites (Asn-x-Ser/Thr, where x is any amino acid except Pro) and 11 cysteines, which form disulfide bridges.

The functional properties of these structural elements are discussed later.

Transmembrane/Cytoplasmic Regions

The structure of the C-terminal half of the TSH receptor is a characteristic of members of the G protein–coupled receptor family and includes seven transmembrane segments linked by three extracellular and three cytoplasmic loops, ending with the C-terminal cytoplasmic tail (see Fig. 1). The homology in this region is 85% to 90% for the TSH receptor among different species, 70% to 75% to the other glycoprotein hormone receptors (see Fig. 2), and 20% to 25% to other members of the G protein–coupled receptor superfamily. Notably, the third cytoplasmic loop and the C-terminal cytoplasmic tail are the least homologous. The transmembrane segments contain several conserved proline residues that are thought to be important for proper insertion of the receptor protein into the plasma membrane (15). The cytoplasmic regions harbor several consensus sequences for phosphorylation sites by protein kinase C and G protein–coupled receptor kinases (GRKs), but not by cAMP-dependent kinase (protein kinase A) (8). TSH-dependent phosphorylation by GRKs may be involved in homologous desensitization of the receptor.

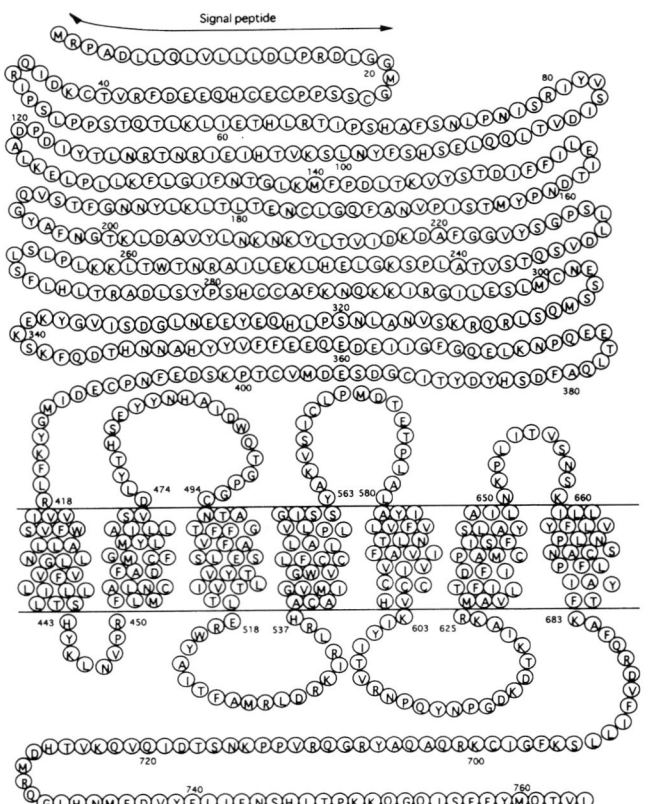

FIG. 1. Amino acid structure of the human TSH receptor.

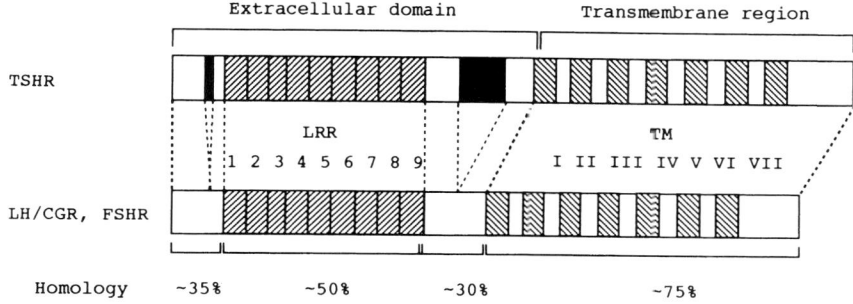

FIG. 2. Comparison of the structures of the TSH receptor and other glycoprotein hormone receptors (LH and FSH receptors). The receptors are divided into subregions according to the homology. The *shaded areas* are leucine-rich repeats 1 to 9 (LRR) and transmembrane segments I to VII (TM). The *solid areas* are the regions unique to the TSH receptor. (Reproduced with permission from ref. 7.)

GENOMIC STRUCTURE OF THE TSH RECEPTOR

The human TSH receptor gene is located on chromosome 14q31 (16,17). The translated region of the gene is coded by ten exons and spans more than 60 kb (18) (Fig. 4). There appear to be at least four alternative polyadenylation sites in the 3'-noncoding region (7). The extracellular domain of the receptor is encoded by the first nine exons and a part of the tenth exon, and the transmembrane/cytoplasmic regions by the rest of the tenth exon. Of interest is that each of exons 2 to 8 corresponds to a LRR. This correspondence between the exons and LRRs is also observed in the LH and FSH receptors (19–21). Because the prototypic gene for G protein–coupled receptors is intronless, these findings suggest common evolutionary events that resulted in the formation of the glycoprotein hormone receptor genes. That is, the glycoprotein hormone receptor genes arose from the integration of multiple genes coding LRR motifs into a prototypic intronless G protein–coupled receptor gene, followed by differentiation into three distinct genes encoding the receptors for TSH, LH, and FSH.

TSH RECEPTOR GENE EXPRESSION

Tissue Distribution of the Receptor mRNA

As it has also been suggested that the TSH receptor plays a role in the pathogenesis of the extrathyroidal manifestations of human autoimmune thyroid disease, particularly pretibial myxedema and ophthalmopathy in Graves' disease, it was of interest to define the tissue distribution of the TSH receptor mRNA. Before the cloning of the receptor cDNA, high-affinity TSH binding had been demonstrated in lymphocytes and in the guinea pig epididymal fat pad as well as the thyroid cells.

The tissue distribution of the TSH receptor mRNA expression has been studied with conventional Northern blot analysis and/or the combination of reverse transcription and PCR (RT-PCR). One should, however, be cautious to interpret the data obtained with RT-PCR, because RT-PCR is an extremely sensitive method by which transcripts for any gene can be detected in any cell type (22). Therefore, it is difficult to answer whether TSH receptor transcripts detected in extrathyroidal tissues by RT-PCR,

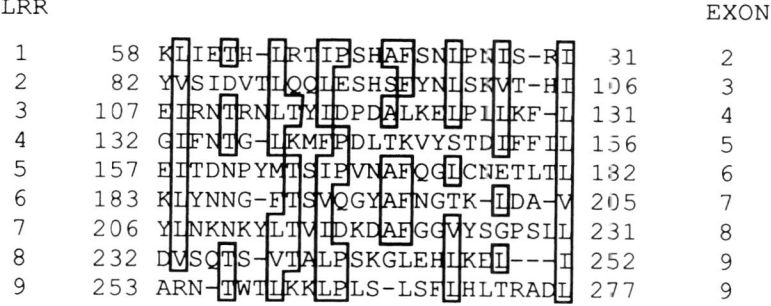

FIG. 3. Leucine-rich periodicity in the TSH receptor extracellular domain. The amino acids conserved at a particular position are boxed. The consensus sequence is shown in the bottom of the figure, where *x* indicates no consensus. (Reproduced with permission from ref. 7.)

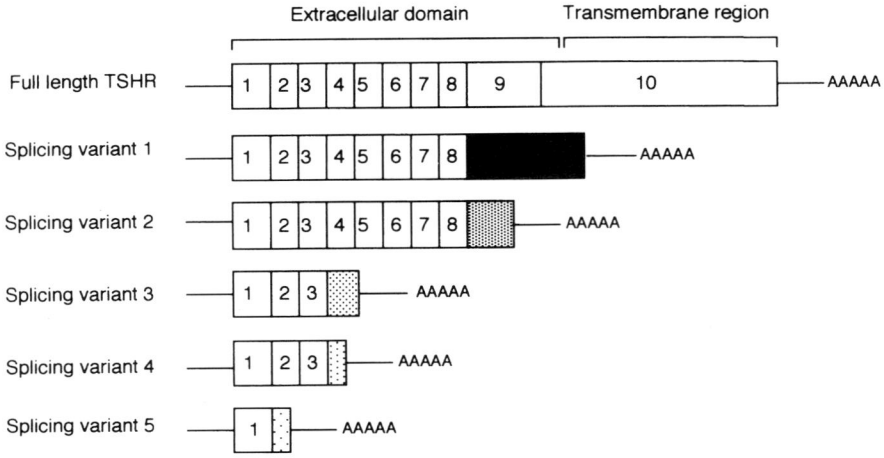

FIG. 4. Schematic representation of the structure of the full-length and truncated TSH receptor cDNAs (28,37,38). *Open boxes* indicate the full-length sequences, and *shaded areas,* unique sequences in each variant. The numberings in the open boxes are number of exons. AAAAA, poly(A) tail.

not by Northern blot, can be translated into protein or are only a result of illegitimate transcription and are of no physiologic significance. More confusingly, different studies using RT-PCR on this subject all demonstrated different results.

Using Northern blot analysis, the expression of the TSH receptor mRNA is clearly detected in adipose tissue as well as in thyroid tissue (23,24). Indeed, the wild-type TSH receptor cDNA was isolated from a fat cell cDNA library (25). Further, TSH stimulates lipolysis in isolated fat cells. Unexpectedly, the message was also detected in cardiac muscle by Northern blot (26), although its functional relevance remains unknown.

As mentioned, RT-PCR yielded controversial data on TSH receptor mRNA expression in lymphocytes, retroorbital tissues, and fibroblasts. Some groups (27,28), but not others (23,29), detected the TSH receptor mRNA in lymphocytes. TSH receptor mRNA was detected in the retro-orbital tissue of the rat, but not of the guinea pig (23,24). In humans, retro-orbital fat appears to express TSH receptor mRNA, but expression in other retro-orbital tissues such as fibroblasts and extraocular muscles remains uncertain (24,27,29–32). Recently, immunofluorescence staining with a polyclonal antibody against a TSH receptor peptide was reported to detect TSH receptor protein in retro-orbital and pretibial fibroblasts (33,34).

Detection by RT-PCR of mRNA coding for only the extracellular region of the receptor has also been reported (35,36).

Alternative Splicing

Northern blot analysis of the TSH receptor in human thyroid tissue shows multiple mRNA transcripts with major bands of approximately 4.6 and 3.9 kb and minor transcripts of 1.8 and 1.2 kb. The two major transcripts likely contain the full-length receptor coding region connected to distinct 3'-noncoding regions that utilize alternative sites for polyadenylation.

Corresponding to the smaller TSH receptor transcripts, five shorter TSH receptor cDNAs have been isolated (28, 37,38) (Fig. 4), all of which appear to be created by alternative splicing. These clones encode various portions of the receptor extracellular domain, but they do not include coding regions for the transmembrane regions. This suggests the possibility that these transcripts encode fragments of the receptor that can be secreted, function as TSH binding proteins, and/or serve as autoantigens. Interestingly, TSH receptor-like immunoreactivity has been identified in peripheral blood (39).

Regulation of the Gene Expression

The regulation of TSH receptor mRNA expression has been studied in primary cultures of human and dog thyroid cells and the rat FRTL5 thyroid cell line. Although there are some conflicting data from these experiments that indicate that the results may be secondary to species specificity or to the inherent difference between cells in primary culture and an established cell line, TSH itself appears to induce a transient increase and then a subsequent decrease in the TSH receptor mRNA levels (12,40, 41). *In vivo,* however, the TSH receptor mRNA level appears to be affected to only a small extent by TSH when compared to the strong inductive effect of TSH on Tg and TPO expression (41). Alteration in the TSH receptor mRNA levels may result from either posttranscriptional nuclear events that influence RNA processing (42), or an increased transcriptional rate as demonstrated in FRTL5 cells (40). In this cell line, insulin, insulin-like growth factor-I (IGF-I), and serum all increase the TSH receptor mRNA transcriptional rate (40).

An inverse relationship between the TSH receptor mRNA levels and the levels of HLA I and II transcripts has been demonstrated in human thyroids (43). Furthermore, the suppression of TSH receptor mRNA levels by interferon-gamma is accompanied by an increase in HLA expression (44). These findings are of interest in terms of the pathogenesis of human autoimmune thyroid disease.

The TSH receptor mRNA levels seem to be lower in thyroid cancers, thyroid cancer cell lines, and experimentally transformed thyroid cells compared to normal thyroid cells (45–51), suggesting that the TSH receptor mRNA levels correlate with the degree of cellular differentiation. Whether the levels of TSH receptor mRNA are useful as predictors of prognosis in thyroid carcinoma has not yet been established.

The 5'-flanking regions of the human and rat TSH receptor genes have been isolated and characterized (18,52). Multiple transcription start sites, a characteristic of "housekeeping" genes, are present, as are a cAMP response element (CRE) and binding sites for a number of transcription factors including AP1, AP2, thyroid-specific transcription factor-1 (TTF-1). This region lacks a TATA box, CCAAT site, or GC box motif. The functional properties of this region have been extensively studied in FRTL5 cells. Approximately the first 200 bp of the 5'-flanking region (referred to as "the minimum promoter region") are sufficient for basal transcriptional activity, tissue specificity, and autoregulations by TSH and insulin/IGF-1 (52,53). The TSH receptor minimum promoter region, however, shows structural differences from those of Tg and TPO (Fig. 5). The 5'-flanking regions of the Tg and TPO genes contain three TTF-1, one TTF-2, and one Pax-8 binding sites, but no CRE (54), whereas the minimum promoter region of the TSH receptor contains two TTF-1 binding sites (−189 to −175/−134 to −116 bp) and a CRE (−139 to −131 bp), but no TTF-2 or Pax-8 binding site.

The CRE appears to function as a constitutive enhancer, with the flanking sequences having a repressive effect on this constitutive enhancer activity (52,53,55). Single-stranded and double-stranded DNA binding proteins can bind to this region (55). Binding of TTF-1 to the upstream TTF-1 binding site in the minimum promoter region and another upstream TTF-1 binding site (−881 to −866 bp) defines thyroid-specific expression and TSH/cAMP-mediated regulation of the receptor (56–58). Such expression can be enhanced by binding of single-stranded DNA binding proteins to the site adjacent to TTF-1 binding site (58,59). Both the TTF-1 binding sites and the CRE are required for the full expression of the TSH receptor gene in the thyroid cells (56,57). TSH increases TSH receptor mRNA levels by stimulating the phosphorylation and binding of TTF-1 in a short time. The mRNA levels then decline with decreasing TTF-1 mRNA levels (57).

Another mechanism for TSH down-regulation of the TSH receptor expression has also been proposed. Thus, TSH-induction of the inducible cAMP early repressor (ICER) isoform of the cAMP response element modulator (CREM) binds to the CRE in the minimal promoter region of the receptor and represses its expression (60). Third TTF-1 binding site (−134 to −116 bp), which is not involved in TSH receptor promoter activity, has been identified as being required for synergistic action of

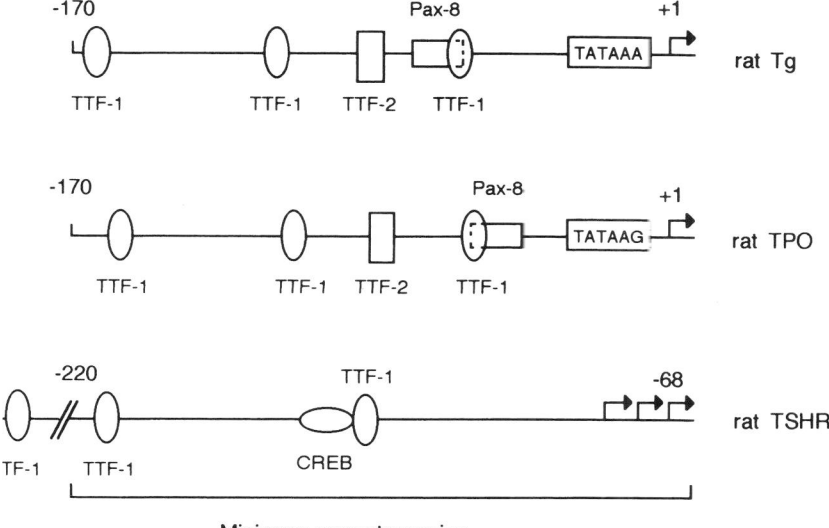

FIG. 5. Structure of rat Tg, TPO, and TSH receptor promoters. Only binding sites for TTF-1, TTF-2, Pax-8, and CRE are shown. Numberings above the promoters indicate the distance from transcription start site for Tg and TPO, and those from the translation initiation codon, for the TSH receptor.

CREB and TTF-1 (61). A short-loop inhibitory effect of thyroid hormone on TSH receptor promoter activity has also been reported (62). Further, an insulin response element (IRE) is identified in the 5′ region flanking the TTF-1 binding site (63).

However, it should be noted here that, in a patient with congenital defective Tg synthesis due to absent TTF-1, the expression level of TSH receptor mRNA is reportedly similar to that in control subjects (64). Further, in transgenic mice expressing the A2 adenosine receptor in the thyroid, a large increase in TSH receptor mRNA levels is observed (65). These data suggest that the data obtained *in vitro* with the FRTL5 cell line may not necessarily be applicable to the *in vivo* situation.

Another interesting aspect concerning the regulation of TSH receptor mRNA expression is that the 1.6-kb 3′-untranslated region (3′-UTR) of the receptor has a destabilizing effect on steady state levels of TSH receptor mRNA *in vitro* (66). The stability of mRNA is in general influenced by binding of trans-acting protein(s) to specific recognition sequence in the 3′-UTR. Thyrotropin receptor mRNA levels may also be regulated at the posttranscriptional level.

STRUCTURE–FUNCTION RELATIONSHIP OF THE TSH RECEPTOR

Protein Expression

The expression of intact, functional, recombinant TSH receptor protein is a requirement for studying the structure–function relationship of the receptor. The TSH receptor has been expressed transiently or permanently in a number of eukaryotic cells such as Chinese hamster ovary (CHO) cells, 293 human embryonal kidney (HEK) cells, COS7 cells, L cells, and myeloma cells. The affinity for TSH to recombinant TSH receptor expressed in these cell lines is essentially identical to that of the native TSH receptor expressed in thyroid tissue, with a dissociation constant (Kd) of approximately 3×10^{-10} M (67). In addition to this high-affinity TSH binding, a low-affinity TSH binding site is also observed, with a Kd of approximately 7×10^{-8} M; the physiologic relevance of this site has long been a matter of debate. The fact that nontransfected cells and even plastic culture plates can bind TSH with low affinity strongly suggests that the low-affinity TSH binding is an artifact.

The specificity of interaction between glycoprotein hormones and their receptors, particularly between the TSH receptor and human choriogonadotropin (hCG), has long been a subject of controversy. For example, *in vitro* studies have demonstrated a wide variation in the ability of thyroid cells to respond to hCG. Although asialo-hCG seems to be able to bind to the TSH receptor (68,69), the physiologic significance of this finding is uncertain because the cross-reactivity between hCG and the TSH receptor appears to depend on the species of the cells and the receptor used, the number of receptors per cell, and carbohydrate variations in hCG (70–76).

In the eukaryotic cell systems described above, the number of receptors expressed per cell is 10- to 100-fold higher than that in native thyroid cells (66), yet insufficient in amount for receptor purification. Thus, several DNA recombinant techniques have been employed to produce large amounts of the purified, functional TSH receptor protein. For example, the TSH receptor has been expressed as a bacterial fusion protein with glutathione S-transferase, maltose-binding protein, or β-galactosidase. These fusion proteins, however, do not appear to be functional; that is, the fusion proteins do not bind to TSH with high affinity. Further, whether autoantibodies bind to the fusion proteins remains in dispute (77–79). Because proteins produced by bacteria in general are not glycosylated and do not contain disulfide bonds, these data are in agreement with data obtained with mutagenesis studies identifying the importance of the carbohydrate side chains and disulfide bonds for receptor function (see later).

The baculovirus system has been employed for production of the full length and the extracellular domain of the TSH receptor (80,81). When the conventional polyhedron promoter is utilized for expression, incomplete or improper carbohydrate compositions of the side chains are observed (82,83). These proteins indeed do not bind TSH with high affinity. With another promoter, the late basic protein promoter, the TSH receptor extracellular domain with complete, mature carbohydrates is expressed (83). Further study, however, will be required to analyze the functional property of this protein. Overall, it is only eukaryotic mammalian cells that can express the intact, fully functional TSH receptor protein.

TSH and Autoantibody Binding Sites

The binding sites for TSH and the anti-TSH receptor autoantibodies have been extensively studied by mutagenesis and with synthetic peptides corresponding to specific portions of the TSH receptor. Unfortunately, many data are unconvincing and substantial amounts of controversy exist. For example, mutagenesis studies (84) revealed that the region including amino acids 317 to 366, one of the unique regions of the TSH receptor extracellular domain, can be deleted without affecting the ability of the receptor to interact with TSH and autoantibodies, whereas peptides corresponding to regions in this domain were reportedly immunogenic (77). Also, mutagenesis and peptide studies yielded conflicting data as to whether the N-terminus of the receptor extracellular domain contains specific binding sites for TSH and autoantibodies (84–88).

Theoretical considerations suggest that data from both types of experiments should be interpreted with caution. Since the binding sites for ligands and antibodies in native proteins are in general nonlinear and require specific conformations, it is uncertain whether peptides can provide definitive information on high-affinity binding for TSH and autoantibodies to the native TSH receptor. On the other hand, mutagenesis studies may also have a serious limitation in that alternations in binding may result from conformational changes induced by mutation, rather than being a direct consequence of the particular amino acid substitution. However, studies with chimeric receptors (homologous substitution) may be by far the most sophisticated approach.

In considering these technical limitations, an acceptable interpretation of the available data may be as follows. First, the high-affinity binding sites for TSH and autoantibodies appear to be situated in the extracellular domain of the receptor. As evidence of this, the TSH receptor extracellular domain connected to either a short hydrophobic peptide or the LH receptor transmembrane/cytoplasmic region retains the ability to bind TSH and TSAb (89,90). The studies with chimeric receptors, furthermore, demonstrate that the binding sites are very likely to span the entire extracellular domain (91–95), suggesting that the binding sites are conformational. Second, the regions involved in the TSH binding site may not be identical to those bound by autoantibodies; studies with chimeric receptors demonstrated that homologous substitutions of the N- and C-termini of the TSH receptor lead to complete or partial loss of TSAb and TBII binding, respectively, whereas high-affinity TSH binding remains unaltered (92,95).

Mutations of two out of the six N-linked glycosylation sites in the extracellular domain of the receptor (amino acids 77 and 113) impair the functional expression of the receptor (96). Mutation of amino acid 77 completely abolishes high-affinity TSH binding, suggesting that the receptor may not be properly inserted into the plasma membrane. This makes it difficult to interpret the data on the significance of the carbohydrate chain at this position in TSH binding. Mutation of amino acid 113 results in partial loss of high-affinity TSH binding, suggesting that the carbohydrate at this site may compose part of the TSH binding site, or it may be important for preserving the TSH receptor's tertiary structure.

There are 11 cysteines in the receptor's extracellular domain and two in the extracellular loops, suggesting the formation of six disulfide bonds with one orphan cysteine. The functional significance of these cysteine residues has also been studied with mutagenesis. Although it is at present unclear which cysteines pair to form disulfide bonds, nine of the 13 residues are reported to be critical for the correct folding of the protein (85,97–99).

A structural model for the TSH receptor–TSH complex has recently been proposed (100) based on crystallization and x-ray diffraction analysis of RNase inhibitor (RI), another protein containing LRRs. For RI, the individual LRRs correspond to an α-β structural unit, with the protein forming a nonglobular, horseshoe shape with the β-sheet exposed. Of note, the binding site for RNase in RI is more extensive than those of typical protease–inhibitor and antibody–antigen complexes (101,102). In the analogous TSH receptor model, the concave surface made up of β-sheets interacts with TSH over widely distributed areas (Fig. 6). This prediction is compatible with the data obtained with the chimeric receptors mentioned previously.

Crystallization and x-ray diffraction analysis of the TSH receptor itself and also TSH receptor–TSH (or –autoantibody) complex is now required for a complete understanding of the structure–function relationship of this protein. In this regard, the purification of the functional TSH receptor is of paramount importance.

Signal Transduction

After TSH binding, the TSH receptor transduces a signal into the cells by coupling to Gs and Gq proteins (103), thereby stimulating the cAMP and inositol phosphate pathways. Unlike other G protein–coupled receptors, in which small ligands bind directly to a "pocket" formed by the seven transmembrane segments, glycoprotein hormones appear to bind to the receptor extracellular domain (see previous). Therefore, the signal must be transduced first from the extracellular domain to the intracellular region of the receptor. The mechanisms by which this occurs is at present unclear.

The regions in the TSH receptor that interact with the G proteins have also been analyzed by site-directed mutagenesis (104–108). Although there are also some conflicting data, the multiple discontinuous regions seem to participate in coupling to G proteins. The C-terminal half of the cytoplasmic tail can be deleted without altering the ability of the receptor to stimulate cAMP production, whereas the N-terminal half of the cytoplasmic tail is implicated in the IP_3 pathway.

The TSH receptor undergoes homologous desensitization after prolonged or repeated TSH stimulation in the thyroid cells. Whether the same phenomenon can be seen in nonthyroidal cells, particularly in CHO cells, is controversial at present (67,109–111). The molecular mechanisms of homologous desensitization have been extensively studied in the β-adrenergic receptor (β-AR). Using 293 HEK cells, data are emerging that the ligand-occupied form of the TSH receptor, like β-AR, is desensitized, presumably by phosphorylation of the receptor by G protein–coupled receptor kinase(s) (GRKs), and subsequent binding of arrestins (112). Of six distinct isoforms of GRKs so far cloned, isoform 5 is a predominant GRK in the thyroid and is likely involved in the TSH receptor desensitization (113).

Internalization

The TSH receptor undergoes TSH-dependent endocytosis and internalization. One consensus sequence for inter-

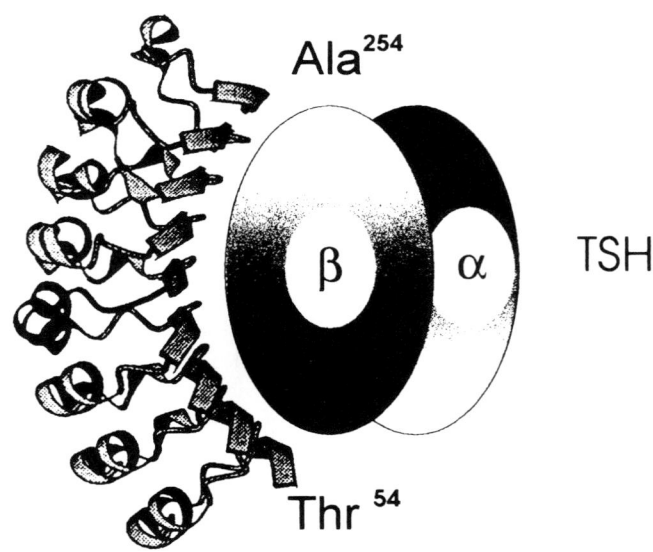

FIG. 6. Putative structure of the TSH receptor extracellular domain containing the leucine-rich repeats, estimated by analogy with the RNAse–RNAse inhibitor complex (101,102). (Reproduced with permission from ref. 100.)

nalization, Asn-Pro-X-X-Tyr (or NPXXY), where X is any amino acid, is situated in the boundary between the seventh transmembrane segment and the C-terminal tail of the TSH receptor. Substitution of Tyr at 678 completely abolishes the cAMP response to TSH stimulation and significantly reduces TSH receptor internalization (114). Further, deletion of the C-terminal half of the receptor's cytoplasmic tail enhances internalization. Thus, internalization appears to be positively and negatively dependent on the NPXXY motif and the cytoplasmic tail, respectively.

Subunit Structure

Before the cloning of the TSH receptor cDNA, considerable controversy existed concerning the TSH receptor subunit structure. The most widely held model was that the receptor was an 80-kDa heterodimer linked by disulfide bonds. That is, a hydrophilic 50-kDa TSH-binding *A* subunit was linked to a membrane-spanning 30kDa *B* subunit (3). However, the apparent molecular mass of the recombinant TSH receptor expressed in eukaryotic cells, as deduced from gel electrophoresis studies, is approximately 100 to 120 kDa, dependent on cells used (82,115–118).

Because the 743-amino-acid polypeptide backbone of the TSH receptor is approximately 84.5 kDa, the remaining (15.5 to 36 kDa) is likely carbohydrate moieties. Pulse-chase studies with transfected cells clearly demonstrate that the approximately 95 kDa high-mannose glycoprotein precursor is processed to the approximately 120 kDa species with mature oligosaccharides, and further to two subunits (82). There is controversy, however, as to whether the site of cleavage is upstream of amino acid residue 317 or downstream of amino acid 366 (115, 117). Enzymatic deglycosylation studies revealed that the deglycosylated *A* subunit is approximately 35 kDa (82), suggesting that the former may be correct.

TSH RECEPTOR AND AUTOIMMUNITY

Humoral Immunity

Anti-TSH receptor autoantibody binding sites have been extensively studied with mutagenesis and synthetic peptides as described. There is amino acid homology and cross-reactivity between the TSH receptor and a retroviral antigen, HIV-1 nef (119). Also reported is that antibodies against *Yersinia enterocolitica* envelope proteins can cross-react with the TSH receptor (120). Although these are intriguing in terms of "antigen mimicry," the data have not yet been fully substantiated.

Whether mutations in the TSH receptor increase its immunogenicity is of interest. Mutation of Pro to Thr at amino acid 52 was identified in a fraction of patients with autoimmune thyroid disease (121), although it may be a fortuitous polymorphism (122). *In vitro* functional analysis revealed that this mutation produces a receptor with enhanced cAMP production, with EC50 being identical to that in the wt-receptor (123), whereas *in vivo* two individuals who are homozygous for Thr at 52 are euthyroid with detectable, normal serum TSH levels in a sensitive

TSH assay (124). It remains to be elucidated, and will be difficult to discern, whether this amino acid alteration enhances the immunogenicity of the receptor.

Although the purification of the TSH receptor has not yet succeeded, the recombinant protein expressed in whole eukaryotic cells and crude membrane preparations have been used for autoantibody analysis (125–132). The sensitivity of these assays is reportedly similar or superior to conventional assays with FRTL5 and porcine or human thyroid cells. However, there are some discrepancies reported between assays using the recombinant human TSH receptor and conventional assays, implying species specificity in anti-TSH receptor autoantibodies. Mutant TSH receptors that react with particular types of antibodies were reported (133,134), which may be useful for dissecting the immune response to this protein.

Cellular Immunity

Several groups have utilized synthetic peptides to analyze T-cell epitopes in peripheral or intrathyroidal lymphocytes from patients with autoimmune thyroid disease (135–140). In two studies (141,142), T-cell lines were established. These studies all demonstrated that T cells from individual patients responded to different sets of peptides, suggesting multiple T-cell epitopes on the TSH receptor protein. The relationship between HLA subtypes and T-cell epitopes are at present unclear, however. Recently, cloning of T cells specific for the TSH receptor has been achieved by using Epstein-Barr virus (EBV)-transformed B-cell lines stably expressing the TSH receptor as autologous antigen-presenting cells (143). Identification of T-cell epitopes in these cells will provide more definite evidence.

It is well known that immunization of susceptible animals with Tg or TPO induces experimental autoimmune thyroiditis (EAT) characterized by intrathyroidal inflammatory cell infiltration and autoantibody production. Immunization with TSH receptor antigen does or does not induce EAT or increased/decreased serum thyroid hormone levels in susceptible mice (144–149). The reasons for these discrepant results are at present unknown, except for differences in methods, such as preparation of antigens, and immunization protocols.

NATURALLY OCCURRING MUTATIONS

Somatic and germline mutations leading to gain of function (constitutive activation) or loss of function have been described in a number of receptors including the TSH receptor.

Gain of Function

The constitutive activating mutations of the α-subunit of the stimulatory G protein (*gsp* mutation) was first identified in growth hormone–secreting pituitary adenomas (150), and then in other functioning endocrine tumors including hyperfunctioning thyroid adenomas (151–153). The discovery of this new type of oncogene suggested that gain-of-function mutations in any step of the adenylyl cyclase–cAMP pathway could be oncogenic. This assumption was confirmed in 1993 by Vassart's group (154), who found somatic point mutations in the third cytoplasmic loop of the TSH receptor in 3 out of 11 autonomously functioning thyroid adenomas. Transfection studies verified that these mutations led to constitutive elevation of intracellular cAMP concentrations, but not IPn. Subsequently, screening for gain-of-function mutations of the TSH receptor in toxic adenomas have been performed by several groups (100,155–160). The studies demonstrate the following: (a) such mutations occur throughout the transmembrane/cytoplasmic regions of the receptor with the third cytoplasmic loop and the sixth transmembrane segment being "hot spots" (Fig. 7), (b) some mutations lead to constitutive elevation of not only cAMP but also IP_3 contents, (c) the incidence of these mutations is very high in Europe (10% to 80%), but extremely low in Japan (~0%), and (d) these mutations are observed not only in benign hyperfunctioning adenomas but also in malignant thyroid carcinomas. Of interest is that the same mutations are also identified in congenital nonautoimmune hyperthyroidism as a germline mutation (161,162).

Importantly, the wild type TSH receptor displays measurable constitutive activity when overexpressed (100, 163). The "noisy" character of the receptor can be observed in some other G protein–coupled receptors, but not in the LH receptor, a close relative of the TSH receptor. Selective pressure that makes the unliganded receptors silent may be insufficient in such receptors.

Some mutations (or polymorphisms) were also identified in the TSH receptor from thyroid carcinomas, the functional significance of which, however, remains unclear (164).

Loss of Function

It is also a reasonable assumption that loss of function mutations in any step of the adenylyl cyclase–cAMP cascade could result in hypothyroidism associated with TSH unresponsiveness. The first report, from Japan, evaluating three such patients with congenital hypothyroidism failed to identify mutations in the TSH receptor–coding region (28). However, a loss-of-function mutation of the TSH receptor was subsequently discovered in a family with congenital hypothyroidism with TSH unresponsiveness in the United States (165). Interestingly, affected siblings have two different mutations in the extracellular domain of the receptor on each allele, indicating inheritance of different inactivating mutations from each parent (compound heterozygotes).

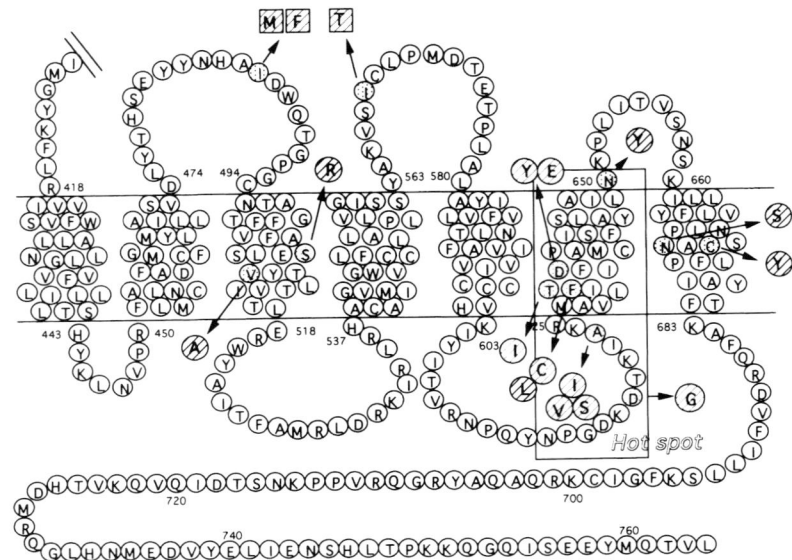

FIG. 7. Amino acid structure of the TSH receptor and localization of gain-of-function mutations (100,154–162). The large N-terminus of the receptor is omitted. "Hot spots" for constitutively activating mutations are *boxed*. *Circles* indicate constitutive activating mutation of cAMP cascade, and *squares*, those of both cAMP and IP pathways.

A loss-of-function mutation is also present in the hyt/hyt congenital hypothyroid mouse (166). In this case, a highly conserved proline residue in the transmembrane segment IV has been replaced by leucine. This results in disruption of high-affinity TSH binding, possibly by interference with insertion of the protein into the plasma membrane.

SUMMARY

The molecular cloning of the TSH receptor has contributed rapid advances in our understanding of the molecular basis for the TSH receptor. We may be closer to understanding how TSH interacts with and activates its receptor, and how the immune system recognizes the receptor to elicit autoimmune thyroid disease. However, we should keep in mind that for complete understanding of the TSH receptor at the molecular level, there are a number of controversial issues that remain to be addressed.

REFERENCES

1. Dumont JE, Lamy F, Roger P, Maenhaut AC. Physiological and pathological regulation of thyroid cell proliferation and differentiation by thyrotropin and other factors. *Physiol Rev* 1992;72:667–697.
2. Van Sande J, Raspe E, Perret J, et al. Thyrotropin activates both the cyclic AMP and the PIP2 cascades in CHO cells expressing the human cDNA of TSH receptor. *Mol Cell Endocrinol* 1991;74:R1–R6.
3. Rees Smith B, McLachlan SM, Furmaniak J. Autoantibodies to the thyrotropin receptor. *Endocr Rev* 1988;9:106–121.
4. Parmentier M, Libert F, Maenhaut C, et al. Molecular cloning of the thyrotropin receptor. *Science* 1989;246:1620–1622.
5. Nagayama Y, Kaufman KD, Seto P, Rapoport B. Molecular cloning, sequence and functional expression of the cDNA for the human thyrotropin receptor. *Biochem Biophys Res Commun* 1989;165:1184–1190.
6. Libert F, Lefort A, Gerard C, et al. Cloning, sequence and expression of the human thyrotropin receptor: evidence for binding of autoantibodies. *Biochem Biophys Res Commun* 1989;165:1250–1255.
7. Nagayama Y, Nagataki S. The thyrotropin receptor; its gene expression and structure-function relationships. *Thyroid Today* 1994;17:1–9.
8. Nagayama Y, Rapoport B. The thyrotropin receptor twenty-five years after its discovery: new insight following its molecular cloning. *Mol Endocrinol* 1992;6:145–156.
9. Vassart G, Dumont JE. The thyrotropin receptor and the regulation of thyrocyte function and growth. *Endocr Rev* 1992;13:596–611.
10. Libert F, Parmentier M, Lefort A, et al. Selective amplification and cloning of four new members of the G protein-coupled receptor family. *Science* 1989;244:569–572.
11. Misrahi M, Loosfelt H, Atger M, Sar S, Guiochon-Mantel A, Milgrom E. Cloning, sequencing and expression of human TSH receptor. *Biochem Biophys Res Commun* 1990;166:394–403.
12. Akamizu T, Ikuyama S, Saji M, et al. Cloning, chromosomal assignment, and regulation of the rat thyrotropin receptor: expression of the gene is regulated by thyrotropin, agents that increase cAMP levels, and thyroid autoantibodies. *Proc Natl Acad Sci USA* 1990;87:5677–5681.
13. Frazier AL, Robbins LS, Stork PJ, Sprengel R, Segaloff DL, Cone RD. Isolation of TSH and LH/CG receptor cDNAs from human thyroid: regulation by tissue-specific splicing. *Mol Endocrinol* 1990;4:1264–1271.
14. Takahashi N, Takahashi Y, Putnam FW. Periodicity of leucine and tandem repetition of a 24-amino acid segment in the primary structure of leucine-rich α2-glycoprotein of human serum. *Proc Natl Acad Sci USA* 1985;82:1906–1910.
15. Brandl CJ, Deber CM. Hypothesis about the function of membrane-buried proline residues in transport proteins. *Proc Natl Acad Sci USA* 1986;83:917–921.
16. Libert F, Passage E, Lefort A, Vassart G, Mattei MG. Localization of human thyrotropin receptor gene to chromosome region 14q31 by in situ hybridization. *Cytogenet Cell Genet* 1990;54:82–83.
17. Rousseau-Merck MF, Misrahi M, Loosfelt H, Atger M, Milgrom E. Assignment of the human thyroid stimulating hormone receptor (TSHR) gene to chromosome 14q31. *Genomics* 1990;8:233–236.
18. Gross B, Misrahi M, Sar S, Milgrom E. Composite structure of the human thyrotropin receptor gene. *Biochem Biophys Res Commun* 1991;177:679–687.
19. Koo YB, Ji I, Slaughter RG, Ji TH. Structure of the luteinizing hor-

mone receptor gene and multiple exons of the coding sequence. *Endocrinology* 1991;128:2297–2308.
20. Tsai-Morris CH, Buczko E, Wang W, Xie X-Z, Dufau ML. Structural organification of the rat luteinizing hormone (LH) receptor gene. *J Biol Chem* 1991;266:11355–11359.
21. Heckert LL, Daley IJ, Griawold MD. Structural organization of the follicle-stimulating hormone receptor gene. *Mol Endocrinol* 1992;6:70–80.
22. Chelly J, Concordet J-P, Kaplan J-C, Kahn A. Illegitimate transcription: transcription of any gene in any cell type. *Proc Natl Acad Sci USA* 1989;86:2617–2621.
23. Roselli-Rehfuss L, Robbins LS, Cone RD. Thyrotropin receptor messenger ribonucleic acid is expressed in most brown and white adipose tissues in the guinea pig. *Endocrinology* 1992;130:1857–1861.
24. Endo T, Ohno M, Kotani S, Gunji K, Onaya T. Thyrotropin receptor in non-thyroid tissues. *Biochem Biophys Res Commun* 1993;190:774–779.
25. Endo T, Ohta K, Haraguchi K, Onaya T. Cloning and functional expression of a thyrotropin receptor cDNA from rat fat cells. *J Biol Chem* 1995;270:10833–10837.
26. Drvota V, Janson A, Norman C, et al. Evidence for the presence of functional thyrotropin receptor in cardiac muscle. *Biochem Biophys Res Commun* 1995;211:426–431.
27. Francis T, Burch HB, Cai W-Y, et al. Lymphocytes express thyrotropin receptor specific mRNA as detected by the PCR technique. *Thyroid* 1991;1:223–228.
28. Takeshita A, Nagayama Y, Yamashita S, et al. Sequence analysis of the thyrotropin (TSH) receptor gene in congenital primary hypothyroidism associated with TSH unresponsiveness. *Thyroid* 1994;4:255–259.
29. Feliciello A, Porcellini A, Ciullo I, Bonavolonta G, Avvedimento EV, Fenzi G. Expression of thyrotropin-receptor mRNA in healthy and Graves' disease retro-orbital tissue. *Lancet* 1993;342:337–338.
30. Paschke R, Elisei R, Vassart G, Ludgate M. Lack of evidence supporting the presence of mRNA for the thyrotropin receptor in extraocular muscle. *J Endocrinol Invest* 1993;16:329–332.
31. Heufelder AE, Dutton CM, Sarkar G, Donovan KA, Bahn RS. Detection of TSH receptor RNA in cultured fibroblasts from patients with Graves ophthalmopathy and pretibial dermopathy. *Thyroid* 1993;3:297–300.
32. Mengistu M, Lukes YG, Nagy EV, et al. TSH receptor gene expression in retroocular fibroblasts. *J Endocrinol Invest* 1994;17:437–441.
33. Burch HB, Sellitti D, Barnes SG, Nagy EV, Bahn RS, Burman KD. Thyrotropin receptor antisera for the detection of immunoreactive protein species in retroocular fibroblasts obtained from patients with Graves' ophthalmopathy. *J Clin Endocrinol Metab* 1994;78:1384–1391.
34. Heufelder AE. Involvement of the orbital fibroblast and TSH receptor in the pathogenesis of Graves' disease. *Thyroid* 1995;5:331–340.
35. Chang T-C, Wu S-L, Hsiao Y-L, et al. TSH and TSH receptor antibody-binding sites in fibroblasts of pretibial myxedema are related to the extracellular domain of entire TSH receptor. *Clin Immunol Immunopath* 1994;71:113–120.
36. Paschke R, Metcalfe A, Alcalde L, Vassart G, Weetman A, Ludgate M. Presence of nonfunctional thyrotropin receptor variant transcripts in retroocular and other tissues. *J Clin Endocrinol Metab* 1994;79:1234–1238.
37. Graves PN, Tomer Y, Davies TF. Cloning and sequencing of a 1.3 kb variant of human thyrotropin receptor mRNA lacking the transmembrane domain. *Biochem Biophys Res Commun* 1992;187:1135–1143.
38. Hunt N, Willey KP, Abend N, et al. Novel splicing variants of the human thyrotropin receptor encode truncated polypeptides without a membrane-spanning domain. *Endocrine* 1995;3:233–240.
39. Murakami M, Miyashita K, Yamada M, Iruuchijima T, Mori M. Characterization of human thyrotropin receptor-related peptide-like immunoreactivity in peripheral blood of Graves' disease. *Biochem Biophys Res Commun* 1992;186:1074–1080.
40. Saji M, Akamizu T, Sanchez M, et al. Regulation of thyrotropin receptor gene expression in rat FRTL5 thyroid cells. *Endocrinology* 1992;130:520–533.
41. Maenhaut C, Brabant G, Vassart G, Dumont JE. In vitro and in vivo regulation of thyrotropin receptor mRNA accumulation levels in dog and human thyroid cells. *J Biol Chem* 1992;267:3000–3007.
42. Huber GK, Conception ES, Graves PN, Davies TF. Positive regulation of human thyrotropin receptor mRNA by thyrotropin. *J Clin Endocrinol Metab* 1991;72:1394–1396.
43. Schuppert F, Reiser M, Scheumann GFW, et al. Expression levels of the thyrotropin receptor gene in autoimmune thyroid disease: coregulation with parameters of thyroid function and inverse relation to major histocompatibility complex classes I and II. *J Clin Endocrinol Metab* 1993 76:1349–1356.
44. Nishikawa T, Yamashita S, Namba H, et al. Interferon-γ inhibition of human thyrotropin receptor gene expression. *J Clin Endocrinol Metab* 1993 77:1084–1089.
45. Berlingieri MT, Akamizu T, Fusco A, et al. Thyrotropin receptor gene expression in oncogene-transfected rat thyroid cells: correlation between transformation, loss of thyrotropin-dependent growth, and loss of thyrotropin receptor gene expression. *Biochem Biophys Res Commun* 1990;173:172–178.
46. Brabant G, Maenhaut C, Kohrle J, et al. Human thyrotropin receptor gene: expression in thyroid tumors and correlation to markers of thyroid differentiation and dedifferentiation. *Mol Cell Endocrinol* 1991;82:R7–R12.
47. Ohta K, Enco T, Onaya T. The mRNA levels of thyrotropin receptor, thyroglobulin and thyroid peroxidase in neoplastic human thyroid tissues. *Biochem Biophys Res Commun* 1991;174:1148–1153.
48. Heldin N-E Cvejic D, Smeds S, Westermark B. Coexpression of functionally active receptors for thyrotropin and platelet-derived growth factor in human thyroid carcinoma cells. *Endocrinology* 1991;129:2187–2193.
49. Ledent C, Dumont JE, Vassart G, Parmentier M. Thyroid adenocarcinomas secondary to tissue-specific expression of simian virus-40 large T-antigen in transgenic mice. *Endocrinology* 1991;129:1391–1401.
50. Shi Y, Zou M, Farid NR. Expression of thyrotropin receptor gene in thyroid carcinomas is associated with a good prognosis. *Clin Endocrinol* 1993;39:269–274.
51. Bronnegard M, Torring O, Boos J, Sylven C, Marcus C, Wallin G. Expression of thyrotropin receptor and thyroid hormone receptor messenger ribonucleic acid in normal, hyperplastic, and neoplastic human thyroid tissue. *J Clin Endocrinol Metab* 1994;79:384–389.
52. Ikuyama S, Niller HH, Shimura H, Akamizu T, Kohn LD. Characterization of the 5′-flanking region of the rat thyrotropin receptor gene. *Mol Endocrinol* 1992;6:793–804.
53. Ikuyama S, Shimura H, Hoeffler JP, Kohn LD. Role of the cyclic adenosine 3′,5′-monophosphate response element in efficient expression of the rat thyrotropin receptor promoter. *Mol Endocrinol* 1992;6:1701–1715.
54. Damante G, Di Lauro R. Thyroid-specific gene expression. *Biochim Biophys Acta* 1994;1218:255–266.
55. Shimura H, Ikuyama S, Shimura Y, Kohn LD. The cAMP response element in the rat thyrotropin receptor promoter. *J Biol Chem* 1993;268:24125–24137.
56. Civitareale D, Castelli MP, Falasca P, Saiardi A. Thyroid transcription factor 1 activates the promoter of the thyrotropin receptor gene. *Mol Endocrinol* 1993;7:1589–1595.
57. Shimura H, Okajima F, Ikuyama S, et al. Thyroid-specific expression and cyclic adenosine 3′,5′-monophosphate autoregulation of the thyrotropin receptor gene involves thyroid transcription factor-1. *Mol Endocrinol* 1994;8:1049–1069.
58. Ohmori M, Shimura H, Shimura Y, Ikuyama S, Kohn LD. Characterization of an up-stream thyroid transcription factor-1 binding site in the thyrotropin receptor promoter. *Endocrinology* 1995;136:269–282.
59. Shimura H, Shimura Y, Ohmori M, Ikuyama S, Kohn LD. Single strand DNA-binding proteins and thyroid transcription factor-1 conjointly regulate thyrotropin receptor gene expression. *Mol Endocrinol* 1995;9:527–539.
60. Lalli E, Sassone-Corsi P. Thyroid-stimulating hormone (TSH)-directed induction of the CERM gene in the thyroid gland participates in the long-term desensitization of the TSH receptor. *Proc Natl Acad Sci USA* 1995;92:9633–9637.
61. Saiardi A, Falasca P, Civitareale D. Synergistic transcriptional activation of the thyrotropin receptor promoter by cyclic AMP-responsive-element-binding protein and thyroid transcription factor 1. *Biochem J* 1995;310:491–496.
62. Saiardi A, Falasca P, Civitareale D. The thyroid hormone inhibits the thyrotropin receptor promoter activity: evidence for a short loop regulation. *Biochem Biophys Res Commun* 1994;205:230–237.
63. Shimura Y, Shimura H, Ohmori M, Ikuyama S, Kohn LD. Identification of a novel insulin-responsive element in the rat thyrotropin receptor promoter. *J Biol Chem* 1994;269:31908–31914.
64. Acebron A, Aza-Blanc P, Rossi DL, Lamas L, Santisteban P. Congen-

ital human thyroglobulin defect due to low expression of the thyroid-specific transcription factor-1. *J Clin Invest* 1995;96:781–785.
65. Ledent C, Dumont JE, Vassart G, Parmentier M. Thyroid expression of an A2 adenosine receptor transgene induces thyroid hyperplasia and hyperthyroidism. *EMBO J* 1992;11:537–542.
66. Kakinuma A, Chazenbalk GD, Filetti S, McLachlan SM, Rapoport B. Both the 5′ and 3′ non-coding regions of the thyrotropin receptor messenger RNA influence the level of receptor protein expression in transfected mammalian cells. *Endocrinology* 1996;137:2664–2669.
67. Chazenbalk GD, Nagayama Y, Kaufman KD, Rapoport B. The functional expression of recombinant human thyrotropin receptors in nonthyroidal eukaryotic cells provides evidence that homologous desensitization to thyrotropin stimulation requires a cell-specific factor. *Endocrinology* 1990;127:1240–1244.
68. Hoermann R, Broexker M, Grossman M, Mann K, Derwahl M. Interaction of human chorionic gonadotropin (hCG) and asialo-hCG with recombinant human thyrotropin receptor. *J Clin Endocrinol Metab* 1994;78:933–938.
69. Yoshimura M, Pekary AE, Pang X-P, Berg L, Goodwin TM, Hershman JM. Thyrotropic activity of basic isoelectric forms of human chorionic gonadotropin extracted from hydatidiform mole tissues. *J Clin Endocrinol Metab* 1994;78:862–866.
70. Yoshimura M, Hershman JM, Pang X-P, Berg L, Pekary AE. Activation of the thyrotropin (TSH) receptor by human chorionic gonadotropin and luteinizing hormone in Chinese hamster ovary cells expressing functional human TSH receptors. *J Clin Endocrinol Metab* 1993;77:1009–1013.
71. Hidaka A, Minegishi T, Kohn LD. Thyrotropin, like luteinizing hormone (LH) and chorionic gonadotropin (CG), increases cAMP and inositol phosphate levels in cells with recombinant human LH/CG receptor. *Biochem Biophys Res Commun* 1993;196:187–195.
72. Gunji K, Endo T, Ohno M, Minegishi T, Onaya T. Recombinant thyrotropin stimulates cAMP formation in CHO-K1 cells expressing recombinant chorionic gonadotropin receptor. *Biochem Biophys Res Commun* 1993;197:1530–1535.
73. Nagayama Y, Yamasaki H, Takeshita A, et al. Thyrotropin binding specificity for the thyrotropin receptor. *J Endocrinol Invest* 1995;18:283–287.
74. Yoshimura M, Pekary AE, Pang X-P, et al. Effect of peptide nicking in the human chorionic gonadotropin α-subunit on stimulation of recombinant human thyroid-stimulating hormone receptors. *Eur J Endocrinol* 1994;130:92–96.
75. Hoermann R, Poertl S, Liss I, Amir SM, Mann K. Variation in the thyrotropic activity of human chorionic gonadotropin in Chinese hamster ovary cells arises form differential expression of the human thyrotropin receptor and microheterogeneity of the hormone. *J Clin Endocrinol Metab* 1995;80:1605–1610.
76. Poertl S, Liss I, Mann K, Hoermann R. Crude urinary human chorionic gonadotropin contains variant forms of HCG with low sialic acid content that exhibit an increased thyrotropic activity in CHO cells expressing the human TSH receptor. *Exp Clin Endocrinol* 1995;103:168–174.
77. Takai O, Desai RK, Seetharamaiah GS, et al. Prokaryotic expression of the thyrotropin receptor and identification of an immunogenic region of the protein using synthetic peptides. *Biochem Biophys Res Commun* 1991;179:319–326.
78. Harfst E, Johnstone AP, Nussey SS. Characterization of the extracellular region of the human thyrotropin receptor expressed as a recombinant protein. *J Mol Endocrinol* 1992;9:227–236.
79. Huang GC, Collison KS, McGregor AM, Banga JP. Expression of a human thyrotropin receptor fragment in *Escherichia coli* and its interaction with the hormone and autoantibodies from patients with Grave's disease. *J Mol Endocrinol* 1992;8:137–144.
80. Huang GC, Page MJ, Nicholson LB, Collison KS, MaGregor AM, Banga JP. The thyrotropin hormone receptor of Graves' disease: overexpression of the extracellular domain in insect cells using recombinant baculovirus, immunoaffinity purification and analysis of autoantibody binding. *J Mol Endocrinol* 1993;10:127–142.
81. Seetharamaiah GS, Desai RK, Dallas JS, Tahara K, Kohn KD, Prabhakar BS. Induction of TSH binding inhibitory immunoglobulins with the extracellular domain of human thyrotropin receptor produced using baculovirus expression system. *Autoimmunity* 1993;14:315–320.
82. Misrahi M, Ghinea N, Sar S, et al. Processing of the precursors of the human thyroid-stimulating hormone receptor in various eukaryotic cells (human thyrocytes, transfected L cells and baculovirus-infected insect cells). *Eur J Biochem* 1994;222:711–719.
83. Chazenbalk GD, Rapoport B. Expression of the extracellular domain of the thyrotropin receptor in the baculovirus system using a promoter active earlier than the polyhedrin promoter. Implications for the expression of functional highly glycosylated proteins. *J Biol Chem* 1995;270:1543–1549.
84. Wadsworth HL, Chazenbalk GD, Nagayama Y, Russo D, Rapoport B. An insertion in the human thyrotropin receptor critical for high affinity hormone binding. *Science* 1990;249;1423–1425.
85. Murakami M, Mori M. Identification of immunogenic regions in human thyrotropin receptor for immunoglobulin G of patients with Graves disease. *Biochem Biophys Res Commun* 1990;171:512–528.
86. Attasi MZ, Manshouri T, Sakata S. Localization and synthesis of the hormone-binding regions of the human thyrotropin receptor. *Proc Natl Acad Sci USA* 1991;88:3613–3617.
87. Mori T, Sugawa H, Piraphatdist T, Inoue D, Enomoto T, Imura H. A synthetic oligonucleotide derived from human thyrotropin receptor sequence binds to Graves immunoglobulin and inhibits thyroid stimulating antibody activity but lacks interaction with TSH. *Biochem Biophys Res Commun* 1991;178:165–172.
88. Nagy EV, Burch HB, Mahoney K, Lukes YG, Morris III JC, Burman KD. Graves IgG recognizes linear epitopes in the human thyrotropin receptor. *Biochem Biophys Res Commun* 1992;188:28–33.
89. Shi Y, Zou M, Parhar RS, Farid NR. High-affinity binding of thyrotropin to the extracellular domain of its receptor transfected in Chinese hamster ovary cells. *Thyroid* 1993;3:129–133.
90. Nagayama Y, Takeshita A, Luo W, Ashizawa K, Yokoyama N, Nagataki S. High affinity binding of thyrotropin (TSH) and thyroid stimulating autoantibodies for the TSH receptor extracellular domain. *Thyroid* 1994;4:155–159.
91. Nagayama Y, Wadsworth HL, Chazenbalk GD, Russo D, Seto P, Rapoport B. Thyrotropin-luteinizing hormone/chorionic gonadotropin receptor extracellular chimeras as probes for thyrotropin receptor function. *Proc Natl Acad Sci USA* 1991;88:902–905.
92. Nagayama Y, Wadsworth HL, Russo D, Chazenbalk GD, Rapoport B. Binding domain of stimulatory and inhibitory thyrotropin (TSH) receptor autoantibodies determined with chimeric TSH-LH/CG receptor. *J Clin Invest* 1991;88:336–340.
93. Nagayama Y, Russo D, Wadsworth HL, Chazenbalk GD, Rapoport B. Eleven amino acids (Lys-201 to Lys-211) and 9 amino acids (Gly-222 to Leu-230) in the human thyrotropin receptor are involved in ligand binding. *J Biol Chem* 1991;266:14926–14930.
94. Nagayama Y, Russo D, Chazenbalk GD, Wadsworth HL, Rapoport B. Extracellular domain chimeras of the TSH and LH/CG receptors reveal the mid-region (amino acids 171-260) to play a vital role in high affinity TSH binding. *Biochem Biophys Res Commun* 1991;173:1150–1156.
95. Tahara K, Ban T, Minegishi T, Kohn LD. Immunoglobulins from Graves disease patients interact with different sites on TSH receptor/LH-CG receptor chimeras than TSH or immunoglobulins from idiopathic myxedema patients. *Biochem Biophys Res Commun* 1991;179:70–77.
96. Russo D, Chazenbalk GD, Nagayama Y, Wadsworth HL, Rapoport B. Site-directed mutagenesis of the human thyrotropin receptor: role of asparagine-linked oligosaccharides in the expression of a functional receptor. *Mol Endocrinol* 1991;5:29–33.
97. Kosugi S, Ban T, Akamizu T, Kohn LD. Site-directed mutagenesis of a portion of the extracellular domain of the rat thyrotropin receptor important in autoimmune thyroid disease and nonhomologous with gonadotropin receptors. *J Biol Chem* 1991;266:19413–19418.
98. Kosugi S, Ban T, Akamizu T, Kohn LD. Identification of separate determinants on the thyrotropin receptor reactive with Graves' thyroid-stimulating antibodies and with thyroid-stimulating blocking antibodies in idiopathic myxedema: these determinants have no homologous sequence on gonadotropin receptors. *Mol Endocrinol* 1992;6:168–180.
99. Kosugi S, Ban T, Akamizu T, Kohn LD. Role of cysteine residues in the extracellular domain and exoplasmic loops of the transmembrane domain of the TSH receptor: effect of mutation to serine on TSH receptor activity and response to thyroid stimulating autoantibodies. *Biochem Biophys Res Commun* 1992;187:887–893.
100. Van Sande J, Parma J, Tonacchera M, Swillens S, Dumont J, Vassart G. Somatic and germline mutations of the TSH receptor gene in thyroid diseases. *J Clin Endocrinol Metab* 1995;80:2577–2585.
101. Kobe B, Deisenhofer J. Crystal structure of porcine ribonuclease inhibitor, a protein with leucine-rich repeats. *Nature* 1993;366:751–756.
102. Kobe B, Deisenhofer J. A structural basis of the interactions between leucine-rich repeats and protein ligands. *Nature* 1995;374:183–186.
103. Allgeier A, Offermanns S, Van Sande J, Spicher K, Schultz G, Du-

mont JE. The thyrotropin receptor activated G-proteins Gs and Gq/11. *J Biol Chem* 1994;269:13733–13735.
104. Chazenbalk GD, Nagayama Y, Russo D, Wadsworth HL, Rapoport B. Functional analysis of the cytoplasmic domains of the human thyrotropin receptor by site-directed mutagenesis. *J Biol Chem* 1990; 165:20970–20975.
105. Kosugi S, Okajima FT, Hidaka A, Shenker A, Kohn LD. Substitutions of different regions of the third cytoplasmic loops of the thyrotropin (TSH) receptor have selective effects on constitutive, TSH-, and TSH receptor autoantibody-stimulated phosphoinosine and 3′,5′-cyclic adenosine monophosphate signal transduction. *Mol Endocrinol* 1993; 7:1009–1020.
106. Kosugi S, Mori T. The first cytoplasmic loop of the thyrotropin receptor is important for phosphoinositide signalling but not for agonist-induced adenylate cyclase activation. *FEBS Lett* 1994;341: 162–166.
107. Kosugi S, Kohn LD, Akamizu T, Mori T. The middle portion in the second cytoplasmic loop of the thyrotropin receptor plays a crucial role in adenylate cyclase activation. *Mol Endocrinol* 1994;8:498–509.
108. Kosugi S, Mori T. The third exoplasmic loop of the thyrotropin receptor is partially involved in signal transduction. *FEBS Lett* 1994; 349:89–92.
109. Tezelman S, Shaver JK, Grossman RF, et al. Desensitization of adenylate cyclase in Chinese hamster ovary cells transfected with human thyroid-stimulating hormone receptor. *Endocrinology* 1994; 134:1561–1569.
110. Heldin N-E, Gustavsson B, Hermansson A, Westermark B. Thyrotropin (TSH)-induced receptor internalization in nonthyroidal cells transfected with a human TSH-receptor complementary deoxyribonucleic acid. *J Clin Endocrinol Metab* 1994;134:2032–2036.
111. Haraguchi K, Saito T, Kanashige M, Endo T, Onaya T. Desensitization of a thyrotropin receptor lacking the cytoplasmic carboxy-terminal region. *J Mol Endocrinol* 1994;13:283–288.
112. Nagayama Y, Chazenbalk GD, Takeshita A, et al. Studies on homologous desensitization of the thyrotropin receptor in 293 human embryonal kidney cells. *Endocrinology* 1994;135:1060–1065.
113. Nagayama Y, Tanaka K, Namba H, et al. Involvement of G-protein coupled receptor kinase 5 in homologous desensitization of the thyrotropin receptor. *J Biol Chem* 1996;271:10143–10148.
114. Shi Y, Zou M, Ahring P, Al-Sedairy ST, Farid NR. Thyrotropin internalization is directed by a highly conserved motif in the seventh transmembrane region of its receptor. *Endocrine* 1995;3:409–413.
115. Ban T, Kosugi S, Kohn LD. Specific antibody to the thyrotropin receptor identifies multiple receptor forms in membranes of cells transfected with wild-type receptor complementary deoxyribonucleic acid: characterization of their relevance to receptor synthesis, processing, structure and function. *Endocrinology* 1992;131:815–829.
116. Russo D, Chazenbalk GD, Nagayama Y, Wadsworth HL, Seto P, Rapoport B. A new structural model for the thyrotropin receptor as determined by covalent crosslinking of thyrotropin to the recombinant receptor in intact cells; evidence for a single polypeptide chain. *Mol Endocrinol* 1991;5:1607–1612.
117. Russo D, Nagayama Y, Chazenbalk GD, Wadsworth HL, Rapoport B. Role of amino acids 261-418 in proteolytic cleavage of the extracellular region of the human thyrotropin receptor. *Endocrinology* 1992; 130:2135–2138.
118. Johnstone AP, Cridland JC, DaCosta CR, Harfst E, Shepherd PS. Monoclonal antibodies that recognize the native human thyrotropin receptor. *Mol Cell Endocrinol* 1994;105:R1–R9.
119. Burch HB, Nagy EV, Lukes YG, Cai WY, Wartofsky L, Burman KD. Nucleotide and amino acid homology between the human thyrotropin receptor and the HIV-1 nef protein: identification and functional analysis. *Biochem Biophys Res Commun* 1991;181:498–505.
120. Luo G, Seetharamaiah GS, Niesel DW, et al. Purification and characterization of *Yersinia enterocolitica* envelope proteins which induce antibodies that react with human thyrotropin receptor. *J Immunol* 1994;152:2555–2561.
121. Cuddihy RM, Dutton CM, Bahn RS. A polymorphism in the extracellular domain of the thyrotropin receptor is highly associated with autoimmune thyroid disease in females. *Thyroid* 1995;5:89–95.
122. Sunthornthepvarakul T, Hayashi Y, Refetoff S. Polymorphism of a variant human thyrotropin receptor (hTSHR) gene. *Thyroid* 1994;4: 147–149.
123. Loos U, Hagner S, Bohr URM, Bogatkewitsch GS, Jakobs KH, Van Koppen CJ. Enhanced cAMP accumulation by the human thyrotropin receptor variant with the Pro52Thr substitution in the extracellular domain. *Eur J Biochem* 1995;232:62–65.
124. Cuddihy RM, Bryant WP, Bahn RS. Normal function in vivo of a homozygotic polymorphism in the human thyrotropin receptor. *Thyroid* 1995;5:255–257.
125. Ludgate M, Perret J, Parmentier M, et al. Use of the recombinant human thyrotropin receptor expressed in mammalian cell lines to assay TSH-R autoantibodies. *Mol Cell Endocrinol* 1990;73:R13–R18.
126. Costagliola S, Swillens S, Niccoli P, Dumont JE, Vassart G. Binding assay for thyrotropin receptor autoantibodies using the recombinant receptor protein. *J Clin Endocrinol Metab* 1992;75:1540–1544.
127. Endo T, Ohmori M, Ikeda M, Anzai E, Onaya T. Heterogeneous responses of recombinant human thyrotropin receptor to immunoglobulins from patients with Grave's disease. *Biochem Biophys Res Commun* 1992;186:1391–1396.
128. Vitti P, Elisei R, Tonacchera M, et al. Detection of thyroid-stimulating antibody using Chinese hamster ovary cells transfected with cloned human thyrotropin receptor. *J Clin Endocrinol Metab* 1993;76: 499–503.
129. Chiovato L, Vitti P, Bendinelli G, et al. Detection of antibodies blocking thyrotropin effect using Chinese hamster ovary cells transfected with the cloned human TSH receptor. *J Endocrinol Invest* 1994;17: 809–816.
130. Murakami M, Miyashita K, Kakizaki S, et al. Clinical usefulness of thyroid-stimulating antibody measurement using Chinese hamster ovary cells expressing human thyrotropin receptors. *Eur J Endocrinol* 1995;133:80–86.
131. Michelangeli VP, Munro DS, Poon CW, Frauman AG, Colman PG. Measurement of thyroid stimulating immunoglobulins in a new cell line transfected with a functional human TSH receptor (JPO9 cells), compared with an assay using FRTL-5 cells. *Clin Endocrinol* 1994; 40:645–652.
132. Matsuba T, Yamada M, Suzuki H, et al. Expression of recombinant human thyrotropin receptor in myeloma cells. *J Biochem* 1995;118: 265–270.
133. Nagayama Y, Rapoport B. Thyroid stimulatory autoantibodies in different patients with autoimmune thyroid disease do not all recognize the same components of the human thyrotropin receptor; selective role of receptor amino acids Ser25-Glu30. *J Clin Endocrinol Metab* 1992;75:1425–1430.
134. Kosugi ST, Akamizu T, Valente W, Kohn LD. Use of thyrotropin receptor (TSHR) mutants to detect stimulating TSHR antibodies in hypothyroid patients with idiopathic myxedema, who have blocking TSHR antibodies. *J Clin Endocrinol Metab* 1993;77:19–24.
135. Tandon N, Freeman MA, Weetman AP. T cell responses to synthetic TSH receptor peptides in Graves' disease. *Clin Exp Immunol* 1992; 89:468–473.
136. Fan J-L, Desai RK, Seetharamaiah GS, Dallas JS, Wagle NM, Prabhakar BS. Heterogeneity in cellular and antibody responses against thyrotropin receptor in patients with Graves' disease detected using synthetic peptides. *J Autoimmunol* 1993;6:799–808.
137. Sakata S, Tanaka S, Okuda K, Miura K, Manshouri T, Atassi MZ. Autoimmune T-cell recognition sites of human thyrotropin receptor in Graves' disease. *Mol Cell Endocrinol* 1993;92:77–82.
138. Okamoto Y, Yamagawa T, Fisfalen M-E, DeGroot LJ. Proliferative responses of peripheral blood mononuclear cells from patients with Graves' disease to synthetic peptides epitopes of human thyrotropin receptor. *Thyroid* 1994;4:37–42.
139. Mukuta T, Yoshikawa N, Arreaza G, et al. Activation of T lymphocyte subsets by synthetic TSH receptor peptides and recombinant glutamate decarboxylase in autoimmune thyroid disease and insulin-dependent diabetes. *J Clin Endocrinol Metab* 1995;80:1264–1272.
140. Nagy EV, Morris JC, Burch HB, Bhatia S, Salata K, Burman KD. Thyrotropin receptor T cell epitopes in autoimmune thyroid disease. *Clin Immunol Immunopath* 1995;75:117–124.
141. Akamizu T, Ueda Y, Hua L, Okuda J, Mori T. Establishment and characterization of an antihuman thyrotropin (TSH) receptor-specific CD4+ T cell line from a patient with Graves' disease: evidence for multiple T cell epitopes on the TSH receptor including the transmembrane domain. *Thyroid* 1995;5:259–264.
142. Soliman M, Kaplan E, Fisfalen M-E, Okamoto Y, DeGroot L. T-cell reactivity to recombinant human thyrotropin receptor extracellular domain and thyroglobulin in patients with autoimmune and nonautoimmune thyroid diseases. *J Clin Endocrinol Metab* 1995;80:206–213.
143. Mullins R, Cohen SBA, Webb LMC, et al. Identification of thyroid

stimulating hormone receptor-specific T cells in Graves' disease thyroid using autoantigen-transfected Epstein-Barr virus-transformed B cell lines. *J Clin Invest* 1995;96:30–37.
144. Costagliola SC, Many MC, Stalmans-Falys M, Tonacchera M, Vassart G, Ludgate M. Recombinant thyrotropin receptor and the induction of autoimmune thyroid disease in BALB/c mice: a new animal model. *Endocrinology* 1994;135:2150–2159.
145. Costagliola S, Alcalde L, Tonacchera M, Ruf J, Vassart G, Ludgate M. Induction of thyrotropin receptor (TSH-R) autoantibodies and thyroiditis in mice immunized with the recombinant TSH-R. *Biochem Biophys Res Commun* 1994;199:1027–1034.
146. Vlase H, Nakashima M, Graves PN, Tomer Y, Morris JC, Davies TF. Defining the major antibody epitopes on the human thyrotropin receptor in immunized mice: evidence for intramolecular epitope spreading. *Endocrinology* 1995;136:4415–4423.
147. Marion S, Braun JM, Ropars A, Kohn LD, Charreire J. Induction of autoimmunity by immunization of mice with human thyrotropin receptor. *Cell Immunol* 1994;158:329–341.
148. Wagle NM, Dallas JS, Seetharamaiah GS, et al. Induction of hyperthyroxinemia in BALB/C but not in several other strains of mice. *Autoimmunity* 1994;18:103–112.
149. Carayanniotis G, Huang GC, Nicholson LB, Scott T, et al. Unaltered thyroid function in mice responding to a highly immunogenic thyrotropin receptor: implications for the establishment of a mouse model for Graves' disease. *Clin Exp Immunol* 1995;99:294–302.
150. Landis CA, Masters SB, Spada A, Pace AM, Bourne HR, Vallar L. GTPase inhibiting mutations activate the alpha chain of Gs and stimulate adenyl cyclase in human pituitary tumors. *Nature* 1989;340:692–696.
151. Lyons J, Landis CA, Harsh G, et al. Two G protein oncogenes in human endocrine tumors. *Science* 1990;249:655–659.
152. O'Sullivan C, Barton CM, Staddon SL, Brown CL, Lemoine NR. Activating point mutations of *gsp* oncogene in human thyroid adenomas. *Mol Carcinogen* 1991;4:345–349.
153. Suarez HG, du Villard JA, Caillou B, et al. *gsp* mutations in human thyroid tumours. *Oncogene* 1991;6:677–679.
154. Parma J, Duprez L, Van Sande J, et al. Somatic mutations in the thyrotropin receptor gene cause hyperfunctioning thyroid adenomas. *Nature* 1993;365:649–665.
155. Porcellini A, Ciullo I, Laviola L, Amabile G, Fenzi G, Avvedimento VE. Novel mutations of thyrotropin receptor gene in thyroid hyperfunctioning adenomas. Rapid identification by fine needle aspiration biopsy. *J Clin Endocrinol Metab* 1994;79:657–661.
156. Takeshita A, Nagayama Y, Yokoyama N, et al. Rarity of oncogenic mutations in the thyrotropin receptor of autonomously functioning thyroid nodules in Japan. *J Clin Endocrinol Metab* 1995;80:2607–2611.
157. Russo D, Arturi F, Wicker R, et al. Genetic alternations in thyroid hyperfunctioning adenomas. *J Clin Endocrinol Metab* 1995;80:1347–1351.
158. Russo D, Arturi F, Schlumberger M, et al. Activating mutations of the TSH receptor in differentiated thyroid carcinomas. *Oncogene* 1995;11:1907–1911.
159. Parma J, Van Sande J, Swillens S, Tonacchera M, Dumont J, Vassart G. Somatic mutations causing constitutive activity of the thyrotropin receptor are the major cause of hyperfunctioning thyroid adenomas: identification of additional mutations activating both the cyclic adenosine 3′,5′-monophosphate and inositol phosphate-Ca^{2+} cascades. *Mol Endocrinol* 1995;9:725–733.
160. Paschke R, Tonacchera M, Van Sande J, Parma J, Vassart G. Identification and functional characterization of two new somatic mutations causing constitutive activation of the thyrotropin receptor in hyperfunctioning autonomous adenomas of the thyroid. *J Clin Endocrinol Metab* 1994;79:1785–1789.
161. Duprez L, Parma J, Van Sande J, et al. Germline mutations in the thyrotropin receptor gene cause non-autoimmune autosomal dominant hyperthyroidism. *Nat Genet* 1994;7:396–401.
162. Kopp P, Van Sande J, Parma J, et al. Congenital hyperthyroidism caused by a mutation in the thyrotropin-receptor gene. *N Engl J Med* 1995;332:150–154.
163. Van Sande J, Swillens S, Gerard C, et al. In Chinese hamster ovary cells dog and human thyrotropin receptors activate both the cyclic AMP and the phosphatidylinositol 4,5-bisphosphate cascades in the presence of thyrotropin and the cyclic AMP cascade in its absence. *Eur J Biochem* 1995;229:338–343.
164. Ohno M, Endo T, Ohta K, Gunji K, Onaya T. Point mutations in the thyrotropin receptor in human thyroid tumors. *Thyroid* 1995;5:97–100.
165. Sunthornthepvarakul T, Gottschalk ME, Hayashi Y, Refetoff S. Resistance to thyrotropin caused by mutations in the thyrotropin-receptor gene. *N Engl J Med* 1995;332:155–160.
166. Stein SA, Oates EL, Hall CR, et al. Identification of a point mutation in the thyrotropin receptor of the hyt/hyt hypothyroid mouse. *Mol Endocrinol* 1994;8:129–138.

CHAPTER 12

Thyroid Hormone Resistance Syndromes

Stephen J. Usala

CLINICAL DEFINITIONS AND PHENOTYPES

In 1967, a bizarre finding in two young deaf-mutes was reported by Refetoff and coworkers (1). These patients had delayed bone ages and stippled epiphyses consistent with juvenile hypothyroidism, but, paradoxically, they had significantly elevated levels of circulating thyroid hormones. It was concluded by the authors that there was a tissue-specific combination of hypothyroidism, euthyroidism, and hyperthyroidism. Because tissues such as bone and brain were judged to lack the appropriate sensitivity to the high levels of thyroid hormone and the patients failed to manifest many of the common symptoms and signs of hyperthyroidism, it was proposed that the Refetoff patients were the first example of thyroid hormone resistance (1,2).

Time has validated this conclusion. The Refetoff patients demonstrated what is now called generalized resistance to thyroid hormone (GRTH), a condition of reduced inhibition by thyroid hormone of thyroid stimulating hormone (TSH) secretion in the pituitary (central resistance) and resistance to thyroid hormone action in peripheral tissues (peripheral resistance) (Fig. 1). The clinical diagnosis of GRTH is made with the following triad: (a) elevated serum levels of free thyroxine (free T_4) and free triiodothyronine (free T_3), (b) "inappropriately normal" TSH level, and (c) peripheral euthyroidism or hypothyroidism (3,4). In a less common variant, selective pituitary resistance to thyroid hormone (PRTH), patients also present with elevated free T_4 and free T_3 and inappropriately normal TSH, but they are symptomatic and have physical signs of hyperthyroidism (5) (see Fig. 1). Finally, one well-documented case of selective peripheral resistance has been reported (6) (see Fig. 1).

As manifested by the Refetoff patients, there are variable degrees of tissue resistance to thyroid hormone. In other examples, patients with GRTH displayed reduced intelligence quotient resulting in part from thyroid hormone resistance in brain, but there was no resistance in the bone compartment (i.e., patients were of normal adult height) (4). Variable tissue resistances are reflected in the different phenotypes of GRTH. However, by definition, patients with generalized resistance lack the clinical stigmata of hyperthyroidism, such as weight loss, heat intolerance, nervousness, and hyperkinesis, and the compensatory elevation of thyroid hormones is such that the patients do not have complaints of hypothyroidism. In 108 kindreds with GRTH, most patients were identified after screening motivated simply by goiter (4,7).

In PRTH, the sensitivity to thyroid hormone is decreased in the pituitary relative to the peripheral tissues. Most patients with this form of resistance have inappropriately normal TSH at elevated levels of free thyroid hormones similar to GRTH. The clinical criterion of hyperthyroidism necessary for the diagnosis of PRTH is frequently a subjective one. Because the phenotypic borders are often not sharp, differentiating selective pituitary from generalized resistance to thyroid hormone can be a problem (8). It may be that selective peripheral resistance to thyroid hormone is more common than reported. The markers of thyroid hormone action in humans, with the exception of TSH levels, lack precision, and consequently patients with selective peripheral resistance may escape diagnosis.

RTH SYNDROMES ARE CAUSED BY β RECEPTOR MUTATIONS

Generalized resistance to thyroid hormone is a genetic disease. Most reported cases belong to families with multiple affected members (4,7). Inspection of the pedigrees reveals that, in all but the original Refetoff kindred, the GRTH trait is transmitted dominantly. The most compelling evidence that GRTH is a disease of the c-*erb*Aβ thyroid hormone receptor gene has come from linkage studies in many

---

S. J. Usala: Texas Technical University Health Sciences Center School of Medicine, Amarillo, Texas 79106.

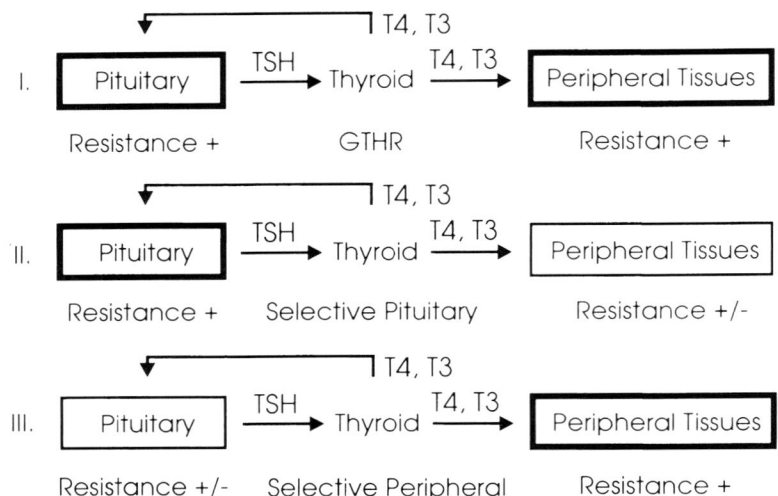

FIG. 1. Three clinical forms of thyroid hormone resistance in humans. I shows blockage of biologic response to thyroxine (T_4) and triiodothyronine (T_3) in the pituitary and peripheral tissues (Resistance +), characteristic of generalized resistance to thyroid hormone (GRTH). II shows selective blockage in the pituitary, characteristic of selective pituitary resistance to thyroid hormone (PRTH). In this case, resistance in the pituitary (Resistance +) is greater than that in peripheral tissues (Resistance +/-). III shows selective blockage at peripheral tissues described in one patient. In this case, resistance is greater in the peripheral tissues (Resistance +) than that in the pituitary (Resistance +/-). Patients with identical mutations in the c-erbAβ thyroid hormone receptor (β receptor) can present clinically with GRTH or PRTH. *Darkened boxes* denote refractoriness to thyroid hormones. (Reprinted with permission from ref. 3.)

unrelated kindreds (4,9–11). Using restriction fragment length polymorphisms (RFLPs) of c-erbAβ, one can test whether a specific c-erbAβ allele segregates or "tracks" with the disease (9). This established linkage between GRTH and the thyroid hormone receptor gene on chromosome 3 (9). Besides *Bam*HI, *Eco*RV, and *Hin*dIII RFLPs for c-erbAβ, dinucleotide repeats have been reported in this gene (12), enabling haplotyping and linkage analysis in almost any kindred. Also, once the mutation in a kindred has been determined in c-erbAβ by direct sequencing, the mutation itself can be used to haplotype a kindred and compute a lod score (10,11). A lod score (logarithm of the odds) gives the probability that a particular gene (e.g., thyroid hormone receptor gene) has segregated with a particular trait (e.g., β thyroid hormone resistance) by chance. For example, a lod score of 3.0 means there was an approximately 1/1000 probability that an observed segregation occurred through chance alone. A lod score of 3.0 or greater is accepted as significant evidence for linkage. Tight linkage with the β thyroid hormone receptor gene (lod score, >3) has been established in GRTH kindreds with diverse phenotypes [kindreds A, D, and WR (refs. 9,10,13, respectively)]. To date there is no published counterexample to linkage between c-erbAβ and GRTH (4,7). Consequently, GRTH can be considered a genetically homogeneous condition. One can speculate that a human α receptor gene mutation has not been identified because such a mutation is lethal or, perhaps, the phenotype is not thyroid hormone resistance.

Numerous mutations in the T_3-binding domain of the c-erbAβ gene have been isolated from different families with GRTH (4,7) (Fig. 2). These mutations exist as single (heterozygous) alleles, except in two homozygous cases,

FIG. 2. Mutations in the c-erbAβ thyroid hormone receptor gene responsible for GTHR. The relative sites of the mutations in the T_3-binding domain of the receptor with the alterations in amino acids are indicated. The last three exons of the β gene comprise amino acids 247 to 295, 296 to 381, and 382 to 461. The relative deficiencies in the T_3-binding affinities of the mutant receptors measured *in vitro* (1.0 = no defect, 0.01 = 100-fold reduction in Ka) are shown (Ka mutant/Ka wild-type). The mean total T_4, total T_3, and thyroid stimulating hormone (TSH) levels for the patients are listed; the results in *brackets* are mean values expressed as a percent of the corresponding mean levels of unaffected family members or the mean value for the laboratory. F100, F102, and F108 had prior (inappropriate) ablative therapy and were on T_3 therapy. F68 values are free T_4 and free T_3 given in picomoles per liter. The T_3-binding domain of c-erbAβ spans amino acids 243 to 461, at the carboxy-terminus. The *black bars* represent areas that interact with thyroid hormone auxiliary proteins (TRAPs) and stabilize TRAP-receptor heterodimers. Some of these regions may stabilize homodimers of c-erbAβ as well. The 349-to-428 region contains heptad repeats *(gray boxes)* with hydrophobic amino acids that form a leucine zipper structure, which is involved in receptor dimerization. Some of these heptads appear to be critical for the dominant negative function of mutant c-erbAβ1 receptors, although other domains may be involved too. (Reprinted with permission from ref. 4.)

FAMILY	CODON	MUTATION	$\frac{K_a \text{ mutant}}{K_a \text{ wild type}}$	SERUM [mean ± SD] (percent of the mean)		
				TT_4 µg/dl	TT_3 ng/dl	TSH µU/ml
F99	310	Met → Thr	--	15.8 ± 3.7 (190)	253 ± 72 (171)	4.7 ± 2.1
F89	317	Ala → Thr	--	28.0 (350)	205 (173)	4.2
F100	317	Ala → Thr	0.22 ± 0.07	--	--	--
F54	320	Arg → Cys	0.49 ± 0.10	15.3 ± 2.3 (180)	246 ± 35 (141)	3.2 ± 1.4
F67	320	Arg → His	0.51 ± 0.29	14.9 ± 1.8 (165)	286 ± 53 (169)	2.2 ± 1.3
F14	332	Gly → Arg	--	22.1	334	7.6
F66	337	Thr deletion	<0.01	17.5 ± 2.5 (198)	238 ± 33 (150)	1.9 ± 0.7
F29	338	Arg → Trp	--	22.0 ± 1.6 (272)	342 ± 89 (224)	2.8 ± 1.9
F106	338	Arg → Trp	--	19.8 ± 2.8 (271)	284 ± 69 (206)	3.6 ± 2.6
F56	340	Gln → His	0.46 ± 0.16	14.6 ± 2.0 (197)	219 ± 49 (133)	3.1 ± 1.3
F44	345	Gly → Arg	<0.03	23.9 ± 2.4 (299)	304 ± 91 (253)	1.8 ± 0.8
F18	345	Gly → Ser	--	19.2 ± 1.5 (247)	218 ± 29 (177)	2.3 ± 1.8
F101	345	Gly → Val	--	17.8 (223)	268 (214)	2.0
F17	345	Gly → Asp	--	22.3 ± 1.3 (262)	423 ± 144 (282)	2.4 ± 1.5
F102	347	Gly → Glu	--	--	--	--
F45	438	Arg → His	0.14 ± 0.21	16.8 ± 3.2 (210)	332 ± 74 (242)	3.8 ± 2.9
F68	438	Arg → His	--	51 ± 5 (255)	11.5 ± 1.1 (230)	1.3 ± 0.7
F103	442	Met → Val	0.17	21.2 (249)	268 (214)	0.7
F107	443	Lys → Glu	0.09	23.0 ± 2.2 (288)	295 ± 57 (246)	2.5 ± 0.9
F108	446	Cys → Stop	--	--	--	--
F104	448	Thr → frame shift	<0.05	15.2 (190)	230 (184)	1.9
F86	451	Phe → Ile	--	14.1	237	1.46
F105	453	Pro → Thr	0.41	15.2	230	1.9
F85	453	Pro → Thr	0.46 ± 0.02	18.4 ± 0.2 (184)	256 ± 16 (157)	1.7 ± 0.9
F27	453	Pro → Ser	--	17.8 (225)	253 (195)	3.3
F22	453	Pro → His	0.16 ± 0.4	20.6 ± 3.1 (286)	247 ± 46 (172)	3.8 ± 2.3
F26	454	Leu → frame shift	--	17.5 ± 3.5 (206)	276 ± 15 (211)	4.5 ± 1.7

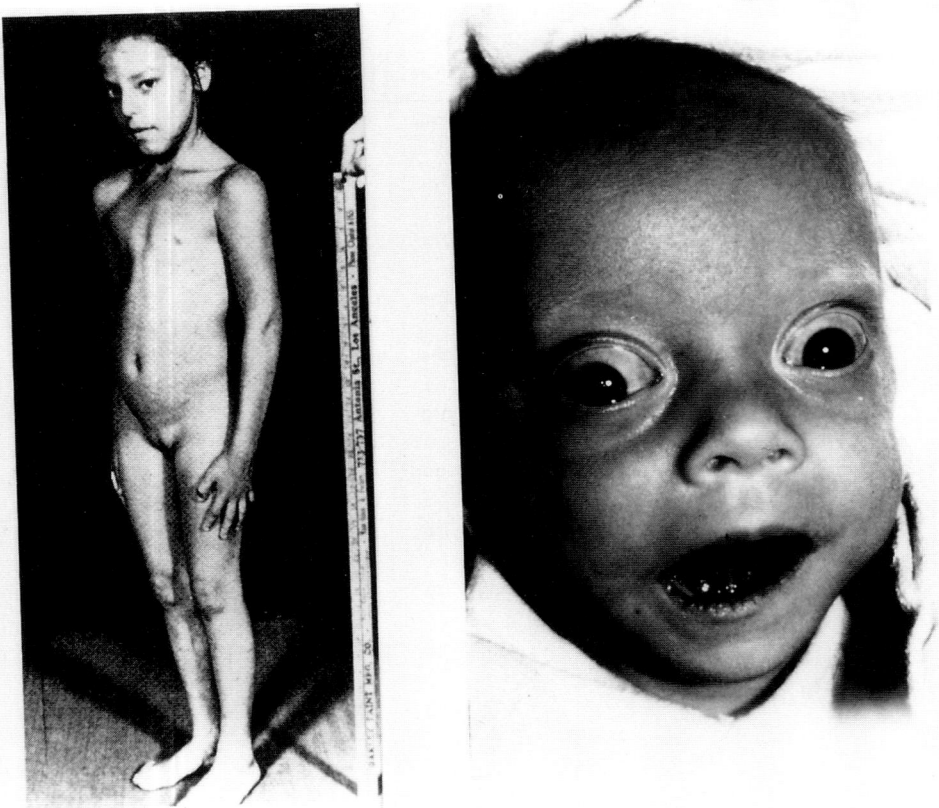

FIG. 3. The Refetoff patient at 8.5 years of age *(left)* and the Bercu patient at 3.5 weeks of age *(right)*. The Refetoff patient has a complete absence of functional β receptors. The Bercu patient was homozygous for a dominant negative β receptor (i.e., S receptor). The Bercu patient had a serum TSH level of 389 mU/L and a total thyroxine of 50.7 g/dL, whereas heterozygous from his kindred, S, had a TSH of 1.9 ± 0.6 mU/L and total thyroxine of 17.0 ± 2.5 g/dL. The Refetoff patient had a serum TSH level of 5.8 mU/L and a total thryoxine of 23.8 g/dL. Heterozygotes of the Refetoff kindred had normal TSH and total thyroxine levels. Normal ranges: TSH, 0.5–4.0 mU/L; total thyroxine, 5.0–11.9 g/dL. (Reprinted with permission from ref. 14.)

the Refetoff and Bercu patients, described later (11,14, 15). Also, with the exception of one mutation (16), all congregate in subregions or "hot spots" of the penultimate and final exons of the β gene (4,7,17). These exons comprise the carboxy-terminal portions of the T_3-binding domain. Certain nucleotides in these exons have a propensity for mutations, and most mutations are located in cytosine/guanine–rich regions (18).

Careful studies of the genetics of different patients with thyroid hormone resistance syndromes have revealed complexities to thyroid hormone action that go beyond the dictum, "one specific mutation—one specific phenotype." Several identical mutations were found in different families with lack of a common ancestor confirmed by genetic analysis; differences in clinical and laboratory findings in unrelated families harboring identical β mutations suggested variability of other factors modulating the resistance phenotype (18). Patients with identical mutations in the β thyroid hormone receptor can present clinically with GRTH or PRTH. For example, patients with an Arg-316-His allele have been described with severe PRTH and mild GRTH (see later) (19–21).

REFETOFF AND BERCU PATIENTS: TWO DIFFERENT HOMOZYGOUS β RECEPTOR MUTANTS

Two human mutants, the Refetoff and Bercu patients, have been elucidated that provide important information on the interrelationships of the α and β receptors in mediating thyroid hormone action in humans (Fig. 3). These human mutants are homozygous for very different abnormalities in the β receptor gene, and they have very different phenotypes.

The resistance syndrome of the Refetoff patients is considerably milder than that of the Bercu patient. Although the original bone radiographs of the Refetoff patients were suggestive of juvenile hypothyroidism, their final adult height was above the parental mean. Furthermore, the intelligence quotients of the Refetoff patients were quite normal when compared with the ranges seen in hearing-impaired individuals (1,2). The Refetoff patients have a major deletion in both β receptor alleles and have only functional α receptor (15). Significantly, the obligate heterozygotes in the Refetoff kindred are phenotypically normal; these heterozygotes have normal TSH and thyroid hormone levels. One can conclude from the Refetoff patients the following: (a) only one β receptor allele is necessary (with two α receptor alleles) for normal thyroid hormone action in humans; (b) most, or at least, life-sustaining thyroid hormone action can be mediated solely through the α receptor; and (c) the heterozygous mutant c-erbAβ alleles in resistant patients act as "dominant negative" genes. This third conclusion is inferred from this kindred because the obligate heterozygotes demonstrate that it is not the loss of function of a β receptor allele that results in thyroid hormone resistance.

The Bercu patient of Kindred S is a complex pattern of hyper- and hypothyroidism resulting from homozygosity of a dominant negative allele (S mutant allele) (11,14). This patient manifested severe pituitary resistance with strikingly elevated TSH levels in the setting of very high free thyroid hormone levels. In addition, there was significant growth and profound bone retardation, suggestive of hypothyroidism. However, this patient was tachycardic and appeared to be hypermetabolic, consistent with hyperthyroidism. The patient was severely mentally retarded, although it is not clear whether this was secondary to hyper- or hypothyroidism or both conditions in distinct regions of the brain. The combination of hyper- and hypothyroid states in the Bercu patient indicates that different tissues are regulated by different contributions, functionally speaking, of β versus α receptors. This can be a result of different relative concentrations of β and α receptors, depending on the tissue; one can also speculate that there are isoform-specific genes that are tissue specific. In addition, the fact that the Bercu patient showed severe inhibition of thyroid hormone action in some tissues relative to the Refetoff patients (e.g., in the bone compartment) suggests that α receptor pathways are inhibited by the mutant S receptor and/or that the S receptor has silencing properties.

MUTANT β RECEPTORS ARE DOMINANT NEGATIVE PROTEINS

The genetics of GRTH indicate that the mutant β receptors antagonize the normal regulation of gene expression by wild-type β and α receptors. The mutant β receptors that have been cloned and synthesized *in vitro* all have compromised T_3-binding affinity (4). The ability of these mutant receptors to increase the level of expression from model gene promoters that are known to be regulated by thyroid hormone has been studied using transient transfection in various cell lines (22,23). These receptors all have diminished ability to transactivate reporter genes in response to T_3, although mutant receptors with significant thyroid hormone–binding affinity can transactivate at superphysiologic concentrations of T_3 in the transient transfection assays (22,23). The dominant negative function of the mutant β receptors can be demonstrated in transient transfection assays; in these studies, mutant β receptor can inhibit activation of T_3-regulated reporter genes by cotransfected normal β receptor (22,23). The α and β receptors influence transcription rate by binding to hexameric DNA sequences (thyroid hormone response elements or TREs) in cognate gene promoters. A consensus hexameric sequence or "half-site," AGGTCA, binds one molecule of receptor, and TREs consist of various configurations of two or more half-sites. These TREs are often "positive," in that binding of T_3-occupied β or α receptors up-regulates gene expression (24). However, some TREs are negative; that is, T_3-occupied receptor represses, and unoccupied receptor transactivates, genes containing negative elements. For example, a negative TRE regulates human TSHβ gene expression and enables repression of serum TSH levels in hyperthyroidism (25). A current model for dominant negative function and the resultant thyroid hormone resistance is based on simple competitive inhibition between a mutant β receptor (or complex thereof) and normal β or α receptor complexes at TREs in cognate gene promoters (4). An alternative model, which does not exclude concurrent competitive inhibition, is "active repression" or silencing where a mutant β receptor complex blocks the transcriptional preinitiation complex and decreases the rate of basal gene expression (26,27). The DNA-binding function of the mutant receptors appears to be required for dominant negative activity (28). It is noteworthy that there are no DNA-binding mutations in the β thyroid hormone receptor gene in man, except for the total deletion of the β alleles in the Refetoff patients, which is not dominant negative. A related member of the hormone receptor gene superfamily, the vitamin D receptor, has been found in man with DNA-binding domain mutations and, as one might expect, these are not dominant negative; vitamin D resistance is transmitted as a recessive trait (29).

The DNA-binding affinity of thyroid hormone receptors is enhanced by receptor dimerization. Thyroid hormone receptors can homodimerize or combine as a heterodimer with other nuclear proteins called TRAPs (thyroid hormone receptor auxiliary proteins) (30). Retinoid X receptors (RXRs) are cellular TRAPs, and, as heterodimers with thyroid hormone receptors, they can increase transcription at specific promoters (31). Thyroid hormone receptor homodimers or receptor-TRAP heterodimers bind to TREs (32). Thyroid hormone induces the dissociation of receptor homodimers from certain TREs and, therefore, it is believed that receptor–RXR heterodimers are the main complex involved in T_3-induced transactivation (33). However, mutant receptors have deficient ability to bind T_3. Consequently, they are not readily dissociated from certain TREs and, thus, competitively inhibit and/or silence gene expression. The properties of receptor heterodimerization and homodimerization are mediated by regions in the ligand-binding domain. A segment of the T_3-binding region (bounded by amino acids 334 to 428 in the β1 receptor) contains a series of heptad repeats that forms a leucine zipper structure that also mediates dimerization activity (34). Most of the heptad repeats in the T_3-binding domain and the concomitant heterodimerization function are probably necessary for dominant negative function. Artificial mutations in the region spanning codons 348 to 437 (which contains eight heptad repeats) produced either weak or no dominant negative effect (35).

Given the convoluted functions of the T_3-binding domain of the thyroid hormone receptor—T_3-binding, dimerization, transactivation, and silencing (active repression)—one can speculate that different mutations affecting these subdomains might variably affect the level of thyroid hormone resistance in patients.

MOLECULAR MECHANISMS OF VARIABLE THYROID HORMONE RESISTANCE

Variability in pituitary and peripheral tissue resistance between patients within a given kindred and between different kindreds has been noted (36). For example, a minority of patients with thyroid hormone resistance demonstrate short stature (4). Also, there is a wide variation in the level of pituitary resistance in patients with GRTH and PRTH: some patients have only mildly elevated levels of free thyroid hormones (19–21, 37), whereas other patients have two- to threefold or higher levels than normal (4,21). The level of thyroid hormone necessary to maintain a normal TSH level is presently the most quantitative measurement of resistance in humans.

The reasons for clinical heterogeneity in thyroid hormone resistance syndromes are complex. There is no correlation between the magnitude of T_3-binding affinity and the level of resistance to thyroid hormone. Three recent explanations have been espoused.

Allelic levels of β1 expression were investigated in a kindred, A, with short stature associated with affected phenotype (38). The kindred A receptor (Pro-453-His) was found to be overexpressed at the level of messenger RNA in fibroblasts from affected children with reduced growth velocity (38). Interestingly, as the ratio of mutant to wild-type β1 receptor mRNA in fibroblasts normalized in one of the affected children with time, the growth velocity also improved. It was proposed that overexpression of the mutant allele in kindred A (85:15, mutant:wild-type β1 receptor mRNA) contributed to reduced linear growth. Heterozygotes from other kindreds without associated short stature have been evaluated, and there were approximately equivalent levels of expression of mutant and wild-type β1 receptor (39,40). Differential allelic expression may be one mechanism that can potentially affect the level of dominant negative activity.

A study of the genotype and level of pituitary resistance of 35 members of a kindred with GRTH suggested that there are multiple genetic factors modulating resistance (41). Thyroid function tests were measured in three groups from this kindred with an Arg-320-His gene mutation: (a) heterozygotes for the mutant allele, (b) homozygotes for the normal allele who were first-degree relatives, and (c) homozygotes for the normal allele who were relatives by marriage. Interestingly, the free thyroxine, total thyroxine, and total triiodothyronine were significantly greater for the "related" normals than the "unrelated" normals, indicating another gene in addition to the mutant Arg-320-His allele contributing to the level of pituitary resistance.

Finally, homodimerization function may also modulate the dominant negative strength of certain human mutant β receptors and the level of thyroid hormone resistance. An Arg-316-His mutation was reported in two patients from a kindred G-H who were clinically euthyroid. These patients not only had normal TSH levels, but they also had normal free thyroxine and total T_3 levels (19). In addition to having no evidence of significant pituitary resistance, the patients were clinically normal and had no manifestations of hypothyroidism. Furthermore, two other kindreds with Arg-316-His have been found, and their thyroid hormone levels were generally only mildly elevated and sometimes overlapped the high normal ranges in affected members (20,21).

This was a bizarre finding, given that the Arg-316-His receptor had very reduced T_3-binding function and was predicted to be a strong dominant negative protein. It was determined that the Arg-316-His receptor formed homodimers very poorly on certain TREs, which may explain its relatively weak dominant negative activity (32). Two separate laboratories have documented that the Arg-316-His receptor has relatively low dominant negative function in transient transfection assays (18,19).

PRTH AND TREATMENT CONSIDERATIONS

Pituitary resistance to thyroid hormone, as mentioned previously, results from mutations in the β receptor gene. Identical mutations have been found in different patients classified with GRTH and PRTH (4,8,21); this clinical discrepancy may result, in part, from the difficulty in accurately discriminating PRTH from GRTH. Patients with nervousness and tachycardia as their only thyrotoxic symptom and sign have been variously scored as having PRTH or GRTH. Other genetic or acquired factors alluded to previously may modify the effects of mutant β receptors. A striking example of this putative genetic factor(s) can be seen in the proband of kindred G-H, who presented at 12.5 years of age with markedly elevated free thyroxine and severe PRTH; she harbored the Arg-316-His allele, as did her normal father and half-sister.

The clinical distinction of GRTH versus PRTH does have a bearing on treatment. The vast majority of patients with GRTH have normal TSH levels and require no medical therapy; that is, exogenous thyroid hormone or antithyroid medications should generally be avoided. In cases of GRTH where the patient has received inappropriate radio-iodine ablation or thyroidectomy, thyroid hormone should be given. However, for unclear reasons, it is sometimes impossible to completely normalize the TSH in these patients without rendering them clinically hyperthyroid; it may be necessary to maintain a thyroid hormone replacement dose that keeps the patient clinically euthyroid with an elevated TSH.

Therapy for PRTH has included β-blockers such as inderal, bromocriptine, methimazole or propylthiouracil, 3,5,3′-triiodothyroacetic acid (triac), somatostatin, and thyroidectomy (42–44). The proband of kindred G-H with severe PRTH has been treated for years with methimazole without evidence of pituitary hyperplasia (42). In many patients with PRTH, where the symptoms and signs are mild, there is a tendency for the clinical hyperthyroidism to remit; these patients can often be followed without antithyroid medication (8).

ATTENTION DEFICIT HYPERACTIVITY DISORDER AND THYROID HORMONE RESISTANCE SYNDROMES

Attention deficit hyperactivity disorder (ADHD) is commonly found in patients with thyroid hormone resistance syndromes (45). Indicative of learning disabilities, discrepancies often exist between achievement and visual–motor development scores compared with intelligence quotients (37). In a recent study of 49 affected (GRTH) and 55 unaffected members of kindreds, 50% of affected adults met the criteria for ADHD and 70% of affected children were diagnosed with ADHD (45). However, the converse study, which examined 277 children with ADHD, found no thyroid hormone resistance, although there was a 5.4% prevalence of other thyroid abnormalities (46). Thus, thyroid hormone resistance syndromes are a very rare cause of ADHD, although perhaps TSH and free thyroxine measurements are advisable in children with ADHD given the high prevalence of other thyroid diseases (46).

ACKNOWLEDGMENT

This review was supported by DHHS-PHS grant DK42807 and a grant from the Knoll Pharmaceutical Company Thyroid Research Advisory Council.

REFERENCES

1. Refetoff S, DeWind LT, DeGroot LJ. Familial syndrome combining deaf-mutism, stippled epiphyses, goiter, and abnormally high PBI: possible target organ refractoriness to thyroid hormone. *J Clin Endocrinol Metab* 1967;27:279–294.
2. Refetoff S, DeGroot LJ, Bernard B, DeWind LT. Studies of a sibship with apparent hereditary resistance to the intracellular action of thyroid hormone. *Metabolism* 1972;21:723–756.
3. Usala SJ, Weintraub BD. Familial thyroid hormone resistance: clinical and molecular studies. In: Mazzaferri E, Kreisberg RA, Bar RS, eds. *Advances in endocrinology and metabolism*, vol. 2. Chicago: Mosby Year Book, 1991:59–76.
4. Refetoff S, Weiss RE, Usala SJ. The syndromes of resistance to thyroid hormone. *Endocr Rev* 1993;14:348–399.
5. Gershengorn MC, Weintraub BD. Thyrotropin-induced hyperthyroidism caused by selective pituitary resistance to thyroid hormone. A new syndrome of inappropriate secretion of TSH. *J Clin Invest* 1975;56:633–643.
6. Kaplan MM, Swartz SL, Larsen PR. Partial peripheral resistance to thyroid hormone. *Am J Med* 1982;70:1115–1121.
7. Refetoff S, Weiss RE, Usala SJ, Hayashi Y. The syndromes of resistance to thyroid hormone: update 1994. In: Negro-Vilar A, Braverman LE, Refetoff S, eds. *Endocrine reviews monographs: 3. Clinical and molecular aspects of diseases of the thyroid*. Bethesda, MD: Endocrine Society Press, 1994;336–343.
8. Beck-Peccoz P, Chatterjee VKK. The variable clinical phenotype in thyroid hormone resistance syndrome. *Thyroid* 1994;4:225–232.
9. Usala SJ, Bale AE, Gesundheit N, et al. Tight linkage between the syndrome of generalized thyroid hormone resistance and the human c-erbAβ gene. *Mol Endocrinol* 1988;2:1217–1220.
10. Usala SJ, Menke JB, Watson TL, et al. A new point mutation in the T3-binding domain of the c-erbAβ thyroid hormone receptor is tightly linked to generalized thyroid hormone resistance. *J Clin Endocrinol Metabol* 1991;72:32–38.
11. Usala SJ, Menke JB, Watson TL, et al. A homozygous deletion in the c-erbAβ thyroid hormone receptor gene in a patient with generalized thyroid hormone resistance: isolation and characterization of the mutant receptor. *Mol Endocrinol* 1991;5:327–335.
12. Sakurai A, Bell GI, DeGroot LJ. Dinucleotide repeat polymorphism in the human thyroid hormone receptor β gene (THRB) on chromosome 3. *Nucleic Acids Res* 1990;19:6661–6662.
13. Fein HG, Burman KD, Djuh Y, et al. Tight linkage of the human c-erbA gene with the syndrome of generalized thyroid hormone resistance is present in multiple kindreds. *J Endocrinol Invest* 1991;14:219–223.
14. Ono S, Schwartz ID, Mueller OT, Root AW, Usala SJ, Bercu BB. Homozygosity for a dominant negative thyroid hormone receptor gene responsible for generalized thyroid hormone resistance. *J Clin Endocrinol Metab* 1991;73:990–994.
15. Takeda K, Sakurai A, DeGroot LJ, Refetoff S. Recessive inheritance of thyroid hormone resistance caused by complete deletion of the protein-coding region of the thyroid hormone receptor β gene. *J Clin Endocrinol Metab* 1992;74:49–55.
16. Behr M, Loos U. A point mutation Ala299 to Thr in the hinge domain of the c-erbAβ thyroid hormone receptor in a family with generalized thyroid hormone resistance. *Mol Endocrinol* 1992;61:1119–1126.
17. Parilla R, Mixson AJ, McPherson JA, McClaskey JH, Weintraub BD. Characterization of seven novel mutations of the c-erbAβ gene in unrelated kindreds with generalized thyroid hormone resistance. Evidence for two "hot spot" regions of the ligand binding domain. *J Clin Invest* 1991;88:2123–2130.
18. Weiss RE, Weinberg M, Refetoff S. Identical mutations in unrelated families with generalized resistance to thyroid hormone occur in cyto-

19. Geffner ME, Su F, Ross SN, et al. An arginine to histidine mutation in codon 311 of the c-erbAβ gene results in a mutant thyroid hormone receptor that does not mediate a dominant negative phenotype. *J Clin Invest* 1993;91:538–546.
20. Weiss RE, Stein MA, Duck SC, et al. Low intelligence but not attention deficit hyperactivity disorder is associated with resistance to thyroid hormone caused by mutation R316H in the thyroid hormone receptor β gene. *J Clin Endocrinol Metab* 1994;78:1525–1528.
21. Adams M, Matthews C, Collingwood TN, Tone Y, Beck-Peccoz P, Chatterjee VKK. Genetic analysis of 29 kindreds with generalized and pituitary resistance to thyroid hormone. *J Clin Invest* 1994;94:506–515.
22. Meier CA, Dickstein BM, Ashizawa K, et al. Variable transcriptional activity and ligand binding of mutant β1 Te receptors from four families with generalized resistance to thyroid hormone. *Mol Endocrinol* 1992;6:248–258.
23. Zavacki AM, Harney JW, Brent GA, Larsen PR. Dominant negative inhibition by mutant thyroid hormone receptors is thyroid hormone response element and receptor isoform specific. *Mol Endocrinol* 1993;7:1319–1330.
24. Brent GA, Moore DD, Larsen PR. Thyroid hormone regulation of gene expression. *Ann Rev Physiol* 1991;53:17–25.
25. Wondisford FE, Steinfelder HJ, Nations M, Radovick S. AP-1 antagonizes thyroid hormone receptor action on the thyrotropin-subunit gene. *J Biol Chem* 1993;268:19217–19223.
26. Baniahmad A, Tsai SY, O-Malley BW, Tsai MJ. Kindred S thyroid hormone receptor is an active and constitutive silencer and repressor for thyroid hormone retinoic acid responses. *Proc Natl Acad Sci USA* 1992;89:10633–10637.
27. Fondell JD, Roy AL, Roeder RG. Unliganded thyroid hormone receptor inhibits formation of a functional preinitiation complex: implications for active repression. *Genes Dev* 1993;7:1400–1410.
28. Nagaya T, Madison LD, Jameson JL. Thyroid hormone receptor mutant that causes resistance to thyroid hormone. *J Biol Chem* 1992;267:13014–13019.
29. Hughes MR, Malloy PJ, Kieback DG, et al. Point mutations in the human vitamin D receptor gene associated with hypocalcemic rickets. *Science* 1988;242:1702–1705.
30. Glass CK. Differential recognition of target genes by nuclear receptor monomers, dimers, and heterodimers. *Endocr Rev* 1994;15:391–407.
31. O'Donnell AL, Koenig RJ. Mutational analysis identifies a new functional domain of the thyroid hormone receptor. *Mol Endocrinol* 1990;4:715–720.
32. Hao E, Menke JB, Smith AM, et al. Divergent dimerization properties of mutant β1 thyroid hormone receptors associated with different dominant negative activities. *Mol Endocrinol* 1994;8:841–851.
33. Yen PM, Sugawara A, Refetoff S, Chin WW. New insights on the mechanisms of the dominant negative effect of mutant thyroid hormone receptor in generalized resistance to thyroid hormone (GRTH). *J Clin Invest* 1992;90:1825–1831.
34. Forman BM, Yang CR, Au M, Casanova J, Ghysdael J, Samuels HH. A domain containing leucine-zipper-like motifs mediate novel in vivo interactions between the thyroid hormone and retinoic acid receptors. *Mol Endocrinol* 1989;3:1610–1626.
35. Hayashi Y, Sunthornthepvarakul T, Refetoff S. Mutations of CpG dinucleotides located in the triiodothyronine T_3-binding domain of the thyroid hormone receptor (TR) β gene that appears to be devoid of natural mutations may not be detected because they are unlikely to produce the clinical phenotype of resistance to thyroid hormone *J Clin Invest* 1994;94:607–615.
36. Magner JA, Petrick P, Menezes-Ferreira M, Weintraub BD. Familial generalized resistance to thyroid hormones: report of three kindreds and correlation of patterns of affected tissues with the binding of [125I] triiodothyronine to fibroblast nuclei. *J Endocrinol Invest* 1986;9:459–469.
37. Cugini Jr CD, Leidy Jr JW, Chertow BS, et al. An arginine to histidine mutation codon 315 of the c-erbAβ thyroid hormone receptor in a kindred with generalized resistance to thyroid hormones results in a receptor with significant 3,5,3'-triiodothyronine binding activity. *J Clin Endocrinol Metab* 1992;74:1164–1170.
38. Mixson AJ, Hauser P, Tennyson G, Renault JC, Bodenner DL, Weintraub BD. Differential expression of mutant and normal beta-T3 receptor alleles in kindreds with generalized resistance to thyroid hormone. *J Clin Invest* 1993;91:2296–2300.
39. Hayashi Y, Janssen OE, Weiss RE, Murata Y, Seo H, Refetoff S. The relative expression of mutant and normal thyroid hormone receptor genes in patients with generalized resistance to thyroid hormones determined by estimation of their specific messenger RNA products. *J Clin Endocrinol Metab* 1993;76:64–69.
40. Klann RC, Torres B, Menke JB, Holbrook CT, Bercu BB, Usala SJ. Competitive PCR quantitation of c-erbAβ, c-erbAα1, and c-erbAα2 messenger RNA levels in normal heterozygous and homozygous fibroblasts of kindred S with thyroid hormone resistance. *J Clin Endocrinol Metab* 1993;77:969–975.
41. Weiss RE, Marocci C, Bruno-Bossio G, Refetoff S. Multiple genetic factors in the heterogeneity of thyroid hormone resistance. *J Clin Endocrinol Metab* 1993;76:257–259.
42. Dulgeroff AJ, Geffner ME, Koyal SN, et al. Bromocriptine and triac therapy for hyperthyroidism due to pituitary resistance to thyroid hormone. *J Clin Endocrinol Metab* 1992;75:1071–1075.
43. Kunitake JM, Hartman N, Henson LC, et al. 3,5,3'-triiodothyroacetic acid therapy for thyroid hormone resistance. *J Clin Endocrinol Metab* 1989;69:461–466.
44. Beck-Peccoz P, Mariotti S, Guillausseau PJ. Treatment of hyperthyroidism due to inappropriate secretion of thyrotropin with the somatostatin analog SMS 201–995. *J Clin Endocrinol Metab* 1989;68:208–213.
45. Hauser P, Zametkin AJ, Martinez P, et al. Attention deficit hyperactivity disorder in people with generalized resistance to thyroid hormone. *N Engl J Med* 1993;328:997–1001.
46. Weiss RE, Stein MA, Trommer B, Refetoff S. Attention deficit hyperactivity disorder and thyroid function. *J Pediatr* 1993;123:539–545.

CHAPTER 13

Oncogenes and Thyroid Cancer

Michael T. McDermott

Thyroid cancer accounts for approximately 1% of all diagnosed invasive malignancies. There are four major types of thyroid cancer: papillary, follicular, anaplastic, and medullary. Papillary and follicular carcinomas arise from thyroid follicular cells. Because they retain many characteristics of normal thyroid cells, they are referred to as differentiated thyroid carcinomas. Anaplastic carcinomas also arise from thyroid follicular cells, but they lose all normal features as they acquire highly invasive properties. Medullary carcinoma arises from the parafollicular C cells, which normally function to produce calcitonin.

Through the study of molecular biology, it has become apparent that thyroid cancer, like other malignancies, results from genetic aberrations within affected cells. Investigation of these abnormalities holds the key to our understanding of why cancers develop, why they grow and metastasize, and how they may be prevented, controlled, or cured. Some of the fruits of these endeavors are already available for clinical application, and there is great promise for much more to come. In this chapter, I will review the definitions, genetics, and molecular mechanisms by which these alterations are believed to cause malignant growth, with particular emphasis on those concepts most relevant to cancer of the thyroid gland.

ONCOGENES AND TUMOR SUPPRESSOR GENES

The cells of the body have a life cycle that consists of three major transitional stages: cell division, cell differentiation, and cell death (Fig. 1). Developing tissues initially undergo prolific cell division, resulting in a rapid increase in immature tissue mass. At some defined point, cells begin differentiating into mature forms, which carry out the functions characteristic of their particular tissue type. As they later become senescent, cells undergo programmed cell death, or apoptosis. A diverse group of proteins serve as the signals and the effectors that instruct cells when to divide, when to differentiate, and when to die. Neoplasia, or tumor growth, occurs when cell division is augmented and/or there is a failure of cells to undergo differentiation or senile apoptosis.

Genes that encode proteins that promote normal cell division are termed proto-oncogenes. Proto-oncogenes may develop mutations, some of which result in the production of proteins that are qualitatively overactive or quantitatively increased, promoting excessive cell division (1–6). These mutated proto-oncogenes are referred to as oncogenes. Other genes, known as tumor suppressor genes, encode proteins that normally restrain cell division or promote differentiation or apoptosis. Mutations that inactivate tumor suppressor genes may also predispose to tumor growth (6–9). Cells undergoing unregulated cell division because of the presence of an oncogene or an inactive tumor suppressor gene are said to be transformed.

Mutations of genetic material are frequent in nature. There are approximately 3 billion nucleotide base pairs in each cell and all must be duplicated faithfully with every cell division. Spontaneous mutations occur at a rate of about two per million base pairs, or 6000 per cell division. Additional mutations develop in response to exposure to environmental mutagens such as radiation, chemicals, and viruses. Over 99% of these mutations are promptly corrected by a set of proteins comprising the DNA repair system (see Fig. 1), but a small fraction persist and may cause disease.

Germline mutations are those that are present in a parent or occur during gametogenesis and are inherited through the sex cells. Such mutations may be present in every cell in the offspring's body. Somatic mutations, on

---

M. T. McDermott: Department of Endocrinology, University of Colorado Health Sciences Center, Denver, Colorado 80262.

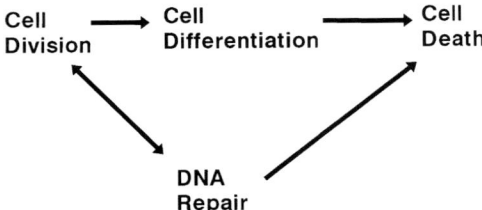

FIG. 1. The three transitional stages in the life of a cell. Immature cells initially undergo rapid cell division. Once a critical mass is reached, they differentiate into functional cells and perform their intended activities. Eventually they become senescent and undergo programmed cell death or apoptosis. When damaged DNA is detected during DNA replication, cell division ceases and repair proteins attempt to repair the DNA. The cell then either resumes division or proceeds to apoptosis.

the other hand, appear after fertilization. If they occur early in the developing embryo they may affect multiple tissues, whereas those arising later in embryogenesis or after birth may involve only one tissue or even one cell.

Genetic mutations that convert proto-oncogenes into oncogenes are called activating or gain-of-function mutations, whereas those that disable tumor suppressor genes are referred to as inactivating or loss-of-function mutations (10,11). Oncogenes tend to be dominantly expressed, so disease often develops in individuals who are heterozygous for the mutation. Tumor suppressor gene inactivation, on the other hand, is recessively expressed, and disease appears only in homozygotic individuals who have lost both of their homologous loci. In many hereditary cancer syndromes, patients are born as whole body heterozygotes as a result of a germline mutation in one tumor suppressor gene locus. Then, if a somatic mutation inactivates the other normal locus later in life, the individual develops cancer.

Thus, tumors may arise because of the heterozygous development of an oncogene or the homozygous loss of a tumor suppressor gene. Such mutations presumably confer upon a cell a growth or survival advantage that permits monoclonal expansion of its progeny. Moreover, when cell division is excessive and unregulated, new mutations occur more frequently. Hence, with time, rapidly growing tumor cells tend to acquire additional mutations that give them further selective survival advantages. As a result, it is not surprising that in highly malignant and metastatic tumors, multiple activated oncogenes and/or inactivated tumor suppressor genes may be detected.

NORMAL TRANSDUCTION OF CELLULAR GROWTH SIGNALS

The mechanisms by which oncogenes and inactivated tumor suppressor genes predispose to tumor formation are best understood in the context of a simple model of growth signal transduction (Fig. 2). Accordingly, an extracellular molecular signal is generated and binds to a specific signal receptor on a cell membrane. The binding of the signal to the receptor results in activation of intracellular messengers, which relay the message to the nucleus by activating nuclear transcription factors. These DNA-binding proteins attach to the promotor regions of specific genes and modulate their transcription of messenger RNA (mRNA). The mRNA is then translated into regulatory proteins, which direct the cell to undergo further division, differentiation or apoptosis.

SIGNAL TRANSDUCTION IN THYROID CELLS

The major known signal for thyroid cell growth and function is thyrotropin (TSH), a glycoprotein hormone that binds to specific TSH receptors (TSH-R) on the cell membrane (Fig. 3). The TSH-R is a protein that has a large extracellular domain, a middle segment that traverses the cell membrane seven times, and a short intracellular portion. When TSH binds to the extracellular domain, it stimulates the transmembrane and intracellular regions to activate an intracellular messenger cascade. The first step in the cascade is the dissociation of the adjacent guanine nucleotide stimulatory protein (GsP) into its three subunits: alpha, beta, and gamma. The alpha subunit has two important properties: it is activated by binding to guanosine triphosphate (GTP) and it possesses intrinsic GTP degrading (GTPase) activity. The free alpha subunit binds to a GTP molecule, forming an active

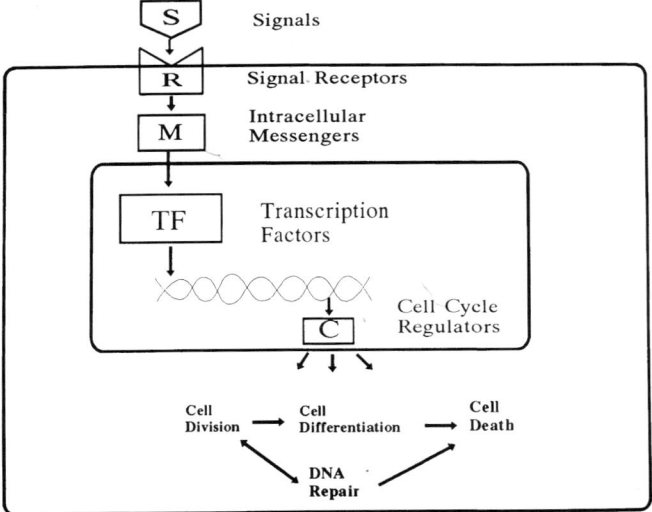

FIG. 2. A growth signal transduction model. An extracellular signal binds to a membrane receptor, resulting in the generation of active intracellular messengers that transmit the message to the nucleus by activating nuclear transcription factors. These activated proteins then bind to specific DNA sequences to govern the transcription rate of messenger RNA, which will be translated into the regulatory proteins that direct the cell to continue dividing, to differentiate, or to die.

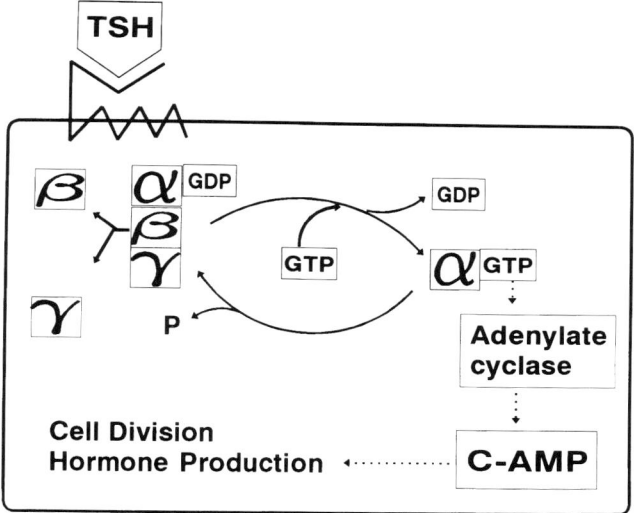

FIG. 3. TSH signal transduction in thyroid cells. TSH binds to the large extracellular domain of the TSH receptor (TSH-R), resulting in dissociation of the guanine nucleotide stimulatory protein (GsP) into its three subunits: alpha, beta, and gamma. Alpha releases a bound guanosine diphosphate (GDP) and attaches to a guanosine triphosphate (GTP) molecule, forming an active dimer that stimulates cyclic adenosine monophosphate (cAMP) production. By its intrinsic GTPase, alpha then converts GTP back to GDP, inactivating the dimer. This pathway promotes both cell division and hormone synthesis.

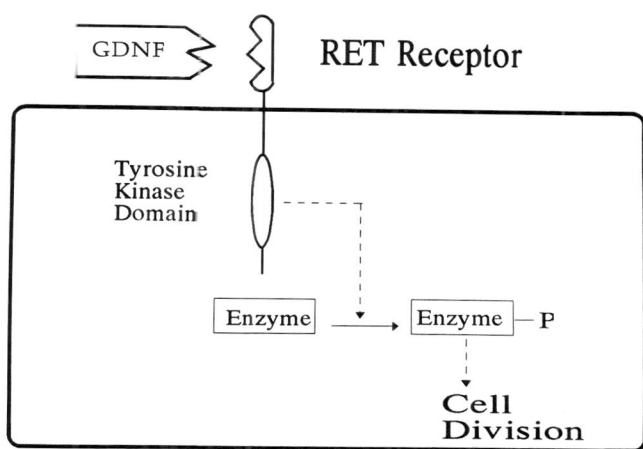

FIG. 4. The Ret receptor. GDNF binds to the Ret receptor extracellular domain. This greatly enhances the intrinsic tyrosine kinase activity of the intracellular domain, which then stimulates, by phosphorylation, downstream enzymes that participate in a pathway involved in cell division.

dimeric complex that stimulates the adenylate cyclase pathway, generating cyclic adenosine monophosphate (cAMP). Soon thereafter, the alpha subunit utilizes its intrinsic GTPase activity to convert the bound GTP to guanosine diphosphate (GDP), thereby terminating the activity of the alpha–GTP complex.

The increased cAMP stimulates additional proteins to enter the nucleus and phosphorylate transcription factors, such as Myc, Jun, and Fos. Thus activated, these transcription factors bind to specific DNA sequences in the regulatory regions of TSH responsive genes. There they modulate the transcription of mRNA, which is translated into the specific regulatory proteins that commit the thyroid cell to continued cell division, to differentiation, or to apoptosis.

There are numerous other signal transduction pathways in thyroid cells, but their physiologic roles are less well defined. The Ret receptor belongs to a family of single transmembrane receptors possessing intrinsic tyrosine kinase activity (Fig. 4). Tyrosine kinases are enzymes that stimulate other functional proteins by phosphorylating their tyrosine residues. The receptor has an extracellular domain, a single transmembrane segment, and an intracellular portion. The ligand or signal that binds to the Ret receptor is the glial cell line derived neurotrophic factor (GDNF) (11a). When it binds, the receptor's intracellular portion acquires enhanced tyrosine kinase activity, enabling it to phospho-

rylate proteins that are components of a signal transduction pathway that promotes primarily cell division.

Ras proteins are intracellular messengers that participate in another signalling pathway (Fig. 5). The Ras proteins are like the GsP alpha subunits in that they bind GTP and possess intrinsic GTPase activity. In the basal state, Ras proteins are tethered to the cell membrane, bound in an inactive complex to GDP. When an extracellular growth sig-

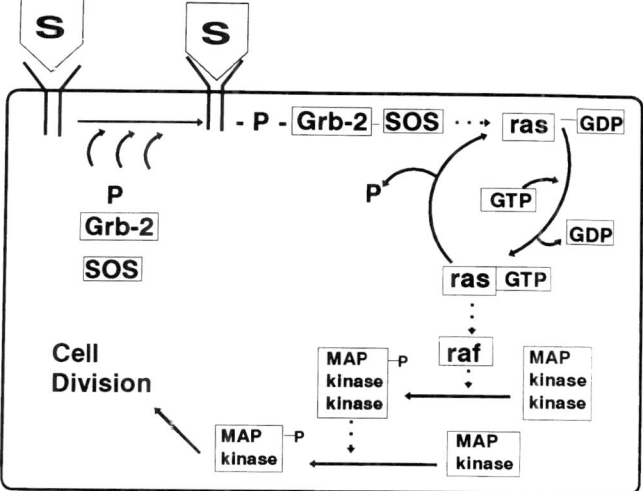

FIG. 5. The Ras signalling system. A ligand binds to a Ras-associated receptor, resulting in the sequential engagement of a protein complex that releases an inactive Ras–GDP dimer from the inner side of the cell membrane. Ras immediately dissociates from GDP and binds to GTP, forming a highly active dimer that stimulates the map kinase cascade. By its intrinsic GTPase, Ras then converts GTP back to GDP, inactivating the dimer. This pathway promotes primarily cell division.

nal binds to a membrane receptor, the receptor's intracellular domain becomes phosphorylated. This activated receptor then sequentially engages two proteins, Grb and Sos, which in turn release the Ras–GDP complex into the cytoplasm. Ras quickly dissociates from GDP and binds a new GTP molecule, forming an active Ras–GTP dimer that turns on a cascade involving map (mitogen-activated protein) kinase, eventually resulting in the stimulation of cell division. Subsequently, the Ras protein utilizes its intrinsic GTPase activity to disable itself by converting the bound GTP to GDP.

THYROID ONCOGENES

According to our model (see Fig. 2) and the current concepts about growth signal transduction in thyroid cells (see Figs. 3–5), thyroid oncogenes may be classified as genes that encode abnormal signal, receptor, messenger, transcription factor, or regulatory proteins that promote excessive unregulated thyroid cell division. Similarly, inactivated tumor suppressor genes may be classified as genes that are unable to produce functional signal, receptor, messenger, transcription factor, or regulatory proteins to restrain thyroid cell division, or to promote normal differentiation or apoptosis (12–16).

SIGNAL PROTEINS

Graves' disease is an autoimmune disorder in which altered B-cell genes encode autoantibodies, termed thyroid stimulating immunoglobulins (TSI), that bind to and activate the membrane TSH-R of the thyroid gland (Fig. 6). Typically, this results in thyroid cell hyperplasia and hyperfunction. However, there is also evidence that patients with Graves' disease, presumably caused by excessive TSH-R stimulation by TSI, have an increased risk of developing differentiated thyroid carcinoma, and further, that these tumors may be more aggressive than other well-differentiated thyroid neoplasms (17–20). Convincing data in this arena are scanty at present but active investigation is currently ongoing.

SIGNAL RECEPTOR PROTEINS

Autonomously functioning thyroid nodules are benign tumors that produce thyroid hormone of their own accord, without the need for TSH stimulation. Numerous patients with these nodules have been discovered to have activating mutations in the gene regions that code for the transmembrane segments of the TSH-R (21–27). These mutations result in the production of a TSH-R that is constitutively or basally overactive, without the requirement for TSH binding (26,27). Constitutively active TSH-Rs stimulate both cell division and hormone production in the affected cell line, resulting in expansion of a hormone-producing clone of thyroid cells (Fig. 7).

Medullary carcinoma of the thyroid (MCT), a malignancy of the parafollicular C cells, accounts for approximately 4% to 10% of all thyroid cancers. It is a sporadic tumor in the majority of cases but appears in a familial pattern in about 10%. Familial MCT is an autosomal dominant disorder that occurs in three forms: isolated familial MCT, MCT associated with the multiple endocrine

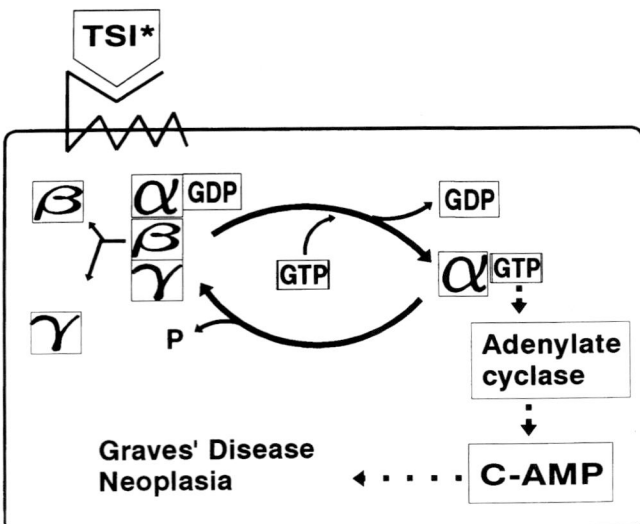

FIG. 6. Thyroid stimulating immunoglobulins. In Graves' disease, abnormal B-cell genes encode autoantibodies that bind to the TSH-R and hyperstimulate the TSH signal pathway in all thyroid cells, leading to diffuse toxic goiter and, in some cases, neoplasia.

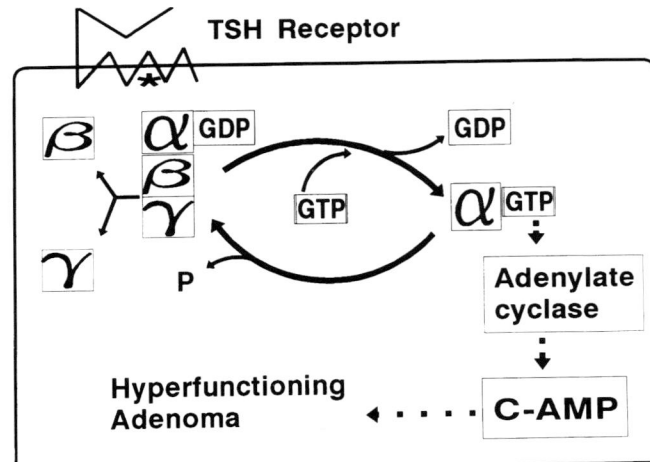

FIG. 7. Constitutively active TSH-R. Point mutations in the *TSH-R* gene regions that code for the transmembrane segments of the TSH-R produce a receptor that is activated in the basal state, without the need for TSH binding. This causes continuous overstimulation of the TSH signal pathway in the proband cell and its progeny, resulting in the development of an autonomously functioning thyroid nodule.

neoplasia (MEN) IIA syndrome, and MCT associated with the MEN IIB syndrome. Nearly all cases of familial MCT have been shown to result from point mutations in the regions of the proto-oncogene encoding the transmembrane and intracellular domains of the Ret receptor (28,29). The resultant Ret receptors are constitutively active, functioning without a need for ligand binding (Fig. 8). This produces continuously high levels of intracellular tyrosine kinase activity, which sets in motion downstream pathways that eventually lead to C-cell neoplasia. The *Ret/MCT* oncogene has also been detected in some sporadic MCTs (30,31). This suggests that sporadic MCT, generally a unifocal tumor, sometimes develops from a somatic *Ret* mutation in a single cell; familial MCT, in contrast, is a multifocal disorder that usually results from a germline *Ret* mutation affecting all cells. Consistent with this is the coexistence of pheochromocytomas, also containing the *Ret* oncogene, in patients with MEN IIA and MEN IIB syndromes (32,33).

A different type of mutation in the *Ret* proto-oncogene has been detected (34–36) in approximately 11% to 25% of papillary thyroid carcinomas (PTCs). The mutation involves a gene rearrangement that deletes the extracellular domain of the Ret receptor and interposes an activating segment in the intracellular domain (Fig. 9). The result is a constitutively active intracellular receptor segment that generates a continuous excess of tyrosine kinase activity. The reason the *Ret/PTC* oncogene causes thyroid follicular cell neoplasia, whereas the *Ret/MCT* oncogene selectively transforms parafollicular C cells, is unknown at present.

Met and TRK are other membrane receptors possessing intrinsic tyrosine kinase activity that is normally stimulated by cognate ligand binding. Constitutively activating mutations of the genes encoding these receptors may also be involved in the pathogenesis of some PTCs. Further investigation in this field is ongoing and should be illuminating.

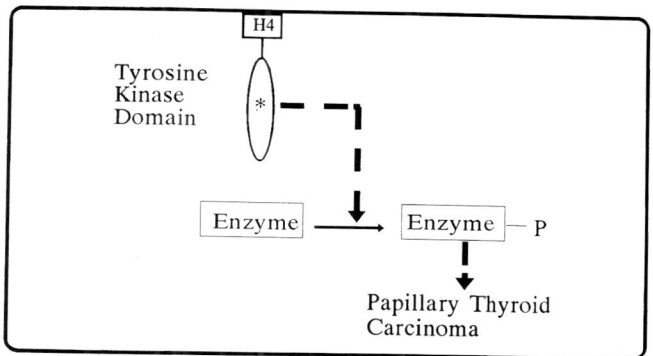

FIG. 9. Constitutively active Ret receptor in papillary thyroid carcinoma. Deletion/rearrangement mutations in the *Ret* gene result in basal hyperactivity of the intracellular tyrosine kinase domain. These mutations are often found in papillary thyroid carcinoma.

INTRACELLULAR MESSENGER PROTEINS

Approximately 25% of benign functioning thyroid adenomas have been found to harbor mutations in the proto-oncogene coding for the alpha subunit of GsP (37–39). These mutations result in the production of an alpha subunit that retains the ability to bind GTP but lacks intrinsic GTPase activity (Fig. 10). The abnormal alpha proteins thus form active complexes with GTP and generate excessive cAMP because they have no GTPase activity for self-deactivation. The overproduction of cAMP then leads to functioning tumors characterized by increased cell division and function.

In contrast, about 30% of nonfunctioning thyroid tumors, both adenomas and carcinomas, contain *Ras* mutations (39–45). Analogous to the situation with GsF, mutations of the *Ras* proto-oncogene have been found to result in the production of a Ras protein which lacks intrinsic GTPase activity. Thus, it can bind GTP to form an active complex, but, lacking GTPase activity, it cannot turn the signal off (Fig. 11). This results in overstimulation of the map kinase pathway, which promotes cell growth but not hormone production.

TRANSCRIPTION FACTORS

The proto-oncogenes that encode the transcription factors, Myc, Jun, and Fos, sometimes develop gain-of-function mutations that cause markedly increased synthesis of these nuclear factors. This may result in the overproduction of regulatory proteins that favor cell division, leading

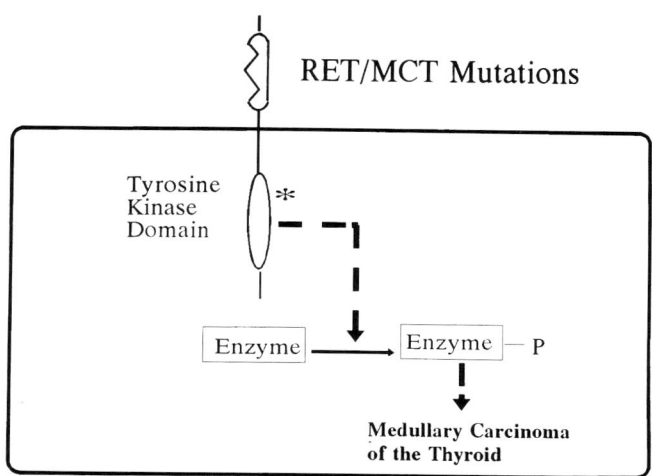

FIG. 8. Constitutively active Ret receptor in familial medullary carcinoma of the thyroid. Point mutations in the gene regions that encode the Ret receptor's intracellular tyrosine kinase domain result in increased basal enzyme activity. These mutations predispose to diffuse hyperplasia and multifocal neoplasia of thyroid parafollicular C cells.

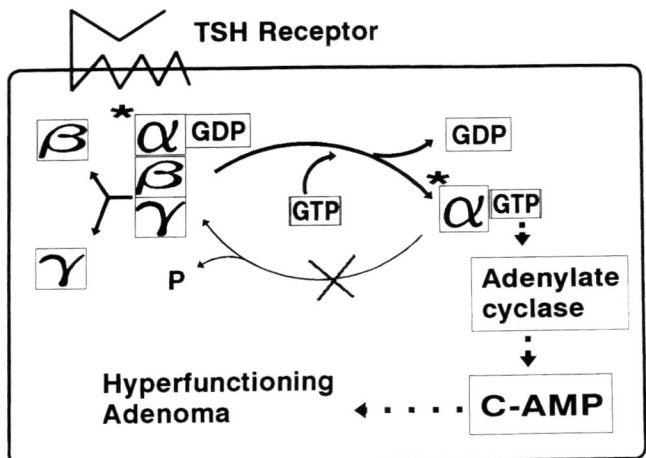

FIG. 10. Constitutively active GsP alpha subunit. Point mutations in the gene that codes for the alpha subunit of GsP produce an alpha protein which has retained its GTP binding properties but lost its GTPase activity, rendering it unable to deactivate the alpha–GTP dimer. This leads to hyperactivity of the TSH signal pathway and the development of hyperfunctioning follicular adenomas.

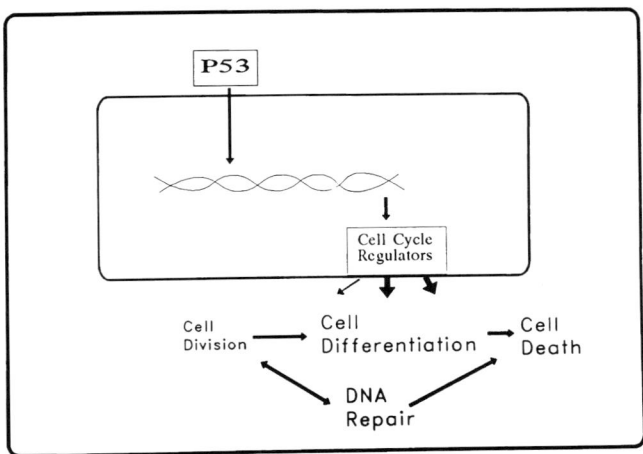

FIG. 12. Normal p53 function. The p53 protein enters the nucleus, where it binds to specific DNA sequences in the promoter regions of target genes to control the production rate of regulatory proteins that inhibit cell division and promote DNA repair, cell differentiation, or apoptosis.

to neoplasia. Oncogenes overexpressing Myc and Fos have been detected in some thyroid carcinomas (46,47), but their overall frequency is, at present, unknown.

Another transcription factor, p53, stimulates the production of regulatory proteins that inhibit cell division and promote cell differentiation, DNA repair, and apoptosis (48–51). Thus, the gene for p53 is a tumor suppressor gene. The p53 protein forms multimers (particularly tetramers) in the cytoplasm and enters the nucleus, where it binds to DNA and stimulates the production of these regulatory proteins (Fig. 12). p53 is then degraded into inactive peptides.

A *p53* gene mutation may result in the production of a p53 protein that cannot enter the nucleus, thereby being unable to properly control regulatory protein production (Fig. 13). Meanwhile, the abnormal p53 protein accumulates in the cell; cellular p53 levels may, therefore, actually be increased.

Mutations of the *p53* gene are the most common known genetic abnormalities in all of human cancer, be-

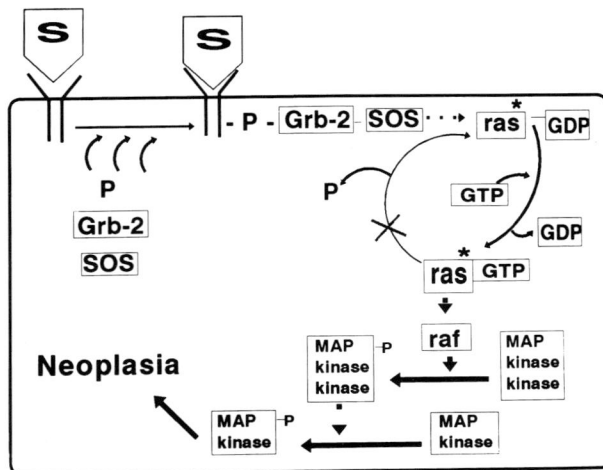

FIG. 11. Constitutively active Ras proteins. Point mutations in a *Ras* gene produce a Ras protein that can bind GTP but lacks GTPase activity and thus cannot deactivate the Ras–GTP dimer. The result is continuous overstimulation of the map kinase cascade. These mutations have been detected in nonfunctioning thyroid adenomas and carcinomas.

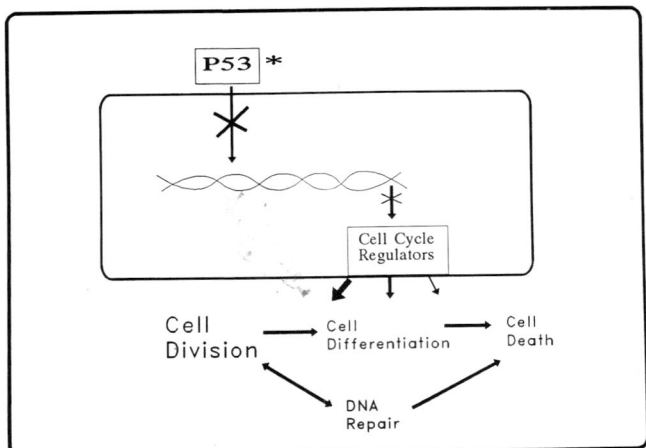

FIG. 13. Loss of p53 function. Mutations of the *p53* gene produce a p53 protein that is unable to bind to DNA and modulate the production of regulatory proteins. The result is continued cell division and failure of DNA repair, of cell differentiation, and of senile apoptosis. These mutations are found in undifferentiated or anaplastic thyroid carcinomas.

ing present in up to 50% of all malignant tumors (51). They are not usually detected in differentiated thyroid carcinomas but have been found in up to 20% of anaplastic thyroid carcinomas (52–56). This suggests that *p53* gene mutations are more likely to occur in cells already transformed by another oncogene. It further suggests that they herald the development of a more aggressive phenotype and a poorer prognosis.

REGULATORY PROTEINS

The last step in this signal transduction model is the production of the regulatory proteins that commit a cell to continued division, to differentiation, or to apoptosis. Mutations of the proto-oncogenes encoding these regulatory proteins would predispose to malignant transformation if they altered cellular activity in favor of cell division. No such oncogenes have been described in thyroid cancer but mutations of the gene encoding cyclin D have been detected in some human neoplasias, and the field remains a fertile ground for research.

DNA REPAIR PROTEINS

As discussed above, approximately 6000 mutations occur each time a cell divides. However, most mutations are detected and corrected by another set of proteins that comprise the DNA repair system (see Figs. 1,2). If the tumor suppressor genes that encode one or more of these repair proteins become mutated, the number of mutations persisting in a cell's genome may increase dramatically. Again, no inactivated tumor suppressor genes of this type are known to be involved in thyroid cancer, but a prototypical example of this mechanism of disease is xeroderma pigmentosum, where congenitally defective DNA repair results in a dramatic increase in skin cancers.

MULTIPLE HITS IN THYROID CANCER

A number of different oncogenes and at least one inactivated tumor suppressor gene have been found in various types of thyroid neoplasia (Table 1). Some are primarily associated with benign functioning nodules (GsP, TSH-R) and others with nonfunctioning nodules, both benign and malignant (Ras). Some are found in all carcinoma types (Myc, Fos), but others are seen primarily in papillary carcinomas (Ret/PTC, Met, TRK); one has been detected only in anaplastic thyroid carcinoma (p53). Because it is believed that once a cell has been transformed by any mutation, its progeny become increasingly likely to develop additional mutations, it is probable that many thyroid cancers develop as a result of more than one genetic abnormality (19,20). A proposed scheme is shown (Fig. 14).

TABLE 1. *Genetic aberrations in thyroid neoplasms*

Gene product category	Gene product	Thyroid phenotype
Signals	TSI	Graves' disease
		Neoplasia
Signal receptors	TSH-R	HFA
	Ret/PTC	PTC
	Met	PTC
	TRK	PTC
	Ret/MCT	MCT
Intracellular messengers	GsP	HFA
	Ras	NFA, FC, PTC
Transcription factors	Myc	FC, PTC, AC
	Fos	FC, PTC, AC
	p53	AC

TSI, thyroid stimulating immunoglobulins; TSH-R, TSH receptor; HFA, hyperfunctioning follicular adenoma; PTC, papillary thyroid carcinoma; MCT, medullary carcinoma of the thyroid; NFA, nonfunctioning follicular adenoma; FC, follicular carcinoma; AC, anaplastic carcinoma.

Accordingly, when a thyroid cell develops a genetic mutation that gives it a reproductive or survival advantage, there is clonal expansion of its progeny. Because TSH-R and GsP stimulate a pathway that is involved in both cell growth and function, activating mutations of their genes tend to promote the development of benign hyperfunctioning adenomas. Ras, on the other hand, participates primarily in a growth pathway, so that *Ras* gene mutations lead to the development of transformed cells

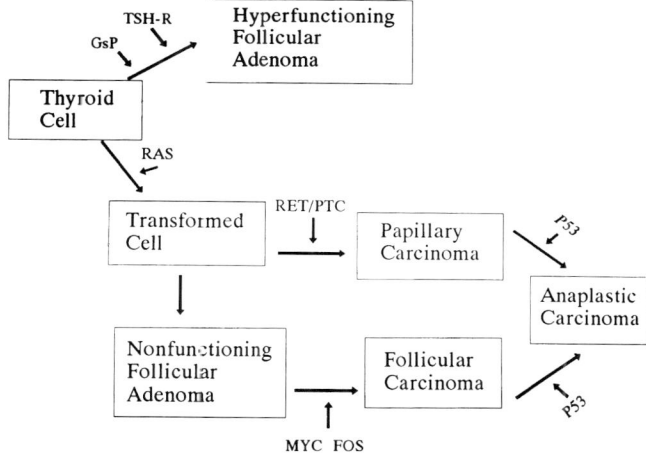

FIG. 14. Oncogenes and thyroid neoplasia. Genetic mutations such as TSH-R and GsP stimulate both cell division and function, predisposing to the development of hyperfunctioning follicular adenomas. *Ras* mutations, in contrast, promote primarily cell division, resulting in transformed follicular cells that are prone to develop further oncogenic mutations. Additional *Ret/PTC* mutations then lead to the low grade malignant characteristics of papillary thyroid carcinoma, whereas *p53* mutations cause progression to highly malignant anaplastic carcinoma.

characterized by rapid division, loss of normal function, and predisposition to other genetic mutations. In this setting, the emergence of a new *Ret/PTC* mutation may produce the disordered growth and low grade invasiveness characteristic of PTC. Should this cell line develop an additional mutation resulting in the loss of function of the *p53* gene, the cells may lose all growth restraints and become a highly invasive anaplastic carcinoma.

CLINICAL IMPLICATIONS

The study of oncogenes and tumor suppressor genes has provided scientists with extremely valuable insights into normal cell physiology and the pathobiology of cancer development. Although some aspects remain within the realm of basic research, many of the discoveries have, or should soon have, important clinical utility in the areas of diagnosis, prognosis, and treatment.

Diagnosis

Some oncogenes and inactivated tumor suppressor genes are characteristic of certain tumor types (see Table 1). In the foreseeable future, pathologic material obtained at surgery, by fine-needle aspiration (FNA), or from archived samples could be screened with an oncogene panel to facilitate the determination of a specific diagnosis.

Oncogene panels might also be helpful in the preoperative evaluation of follicular neoplasms. The differentiation of follicular adenomas from follicular carcinomas by FNA is difficult, because the cytologic differences are usually quite subtle. However, if oncogenes encoding excess proteins, such as Myc and Fos, turn out to be specific for carcinoma, testing for these mutations may greatly enhance our ability to make this important distinction preoperatively.

Testing for familial MCT is another area in which oncogene screening has great promise. This autosomal dominant disorder is transmitted, on average, to 50% of an affected individual's offspring. Once a patient is diagnosed with MCT, family members must also be screened for the disease. Screening has traditionally involved measuring serum calcitonin levels after the intravenous administration of pentagastrin, calcium, or both. However, these tests have unsatisfactory accuracy. Furthermore, they do not become positive until either C-cell hyperplasia or frank malignancy is present. At present, it is recommended that the tests be repeated annually in all members of affected kindreds until age 35. Ret/MCT genetic screening of peripheral blood mononuclear cells, on the other hand, has a sensitivity of over 99%, can make the diagnosis at birth, and needs to be done only once in each family member. Although not yet widely available, testing for the *Ret/MCT* oncogene will likely obviate the need for most prospective calcitonin screening for the familial MCT syndromes in the future.

Prognosis

Reasonably accurate prediction of the probable future course of a disease is important to both the physician and the patient. This is particularly true in the management of thyroid cancer. The majority of thyroid malignancies are indolent and do not affect the patient's life expectancy, but a significant minority recur locally or metastasize and are associated with morbidity and premature mortality. Prognosis is currently estimated on the basis of clinical features such as patient age, tumor size, histologic grade, and the presence or absence of local invasion and distant metastases. Oncogene screening of tumor tissue from primary or recurrent lesions may in the future allow more accurate prognostication based on the types and numbers of genetic mutations detected.

Treatment

Thyroid cancers are currently treated by surgery, radioactive iodine, and levothyroxine administration. However, controversy remains over issues such as the optimal extent of surgery, the use and dosage of radioactive iodine, and the degree of levothyroxine suppression. Oncogene screening could offer several potential therapeutic advantages in the future. It may allow us to decide with prescience whether a patient should receive a more aggressive or less aggressive course of treatment. It may also be that certain mutations predispose a tumor to respond more favorably to a specific therapeutic approach. Finally, understanding the molecular genetics and signalling aberrations present in a tumor may allow us to tailor specific immunologic or chemotherapeutic agents to destroy tumor cells or to promote their differentiation into more mature, less aggressive cell types.

REFERENCES

1. Cline MJ, Slamom DJ, Lipsick JS. Oncogenes: implications for the diagnosis and treatment of cancer. *Ann Intern Med* 1984;101:223–233.
2. Gordon H. Oncogenes. *Mayo Clin Proc* 1985;60:697–713.
3. Druker BJ, Mamon HJ, Roberts TM. Oncogenes, growth factors, and signal transduction. *N Engl J Med* 1989;321:1383–1391.
4. Krontiris TG. Molecular medicine: oncogenes. *N Engl J Med* 1995;333:303–306.
5. Latchman DS. Transcription-factor mutations and disease. *N Engl J Med* 1995;334:28–33.
6. Friend SH, Dryja TP, Weinberg RA. Oncogenes and tumor-suppressing genes. *N Engl J Med* 1988;318:618–622.
7. Weinberger RA. Tumor suppressor genes. *Science* 1991;254:1138–1145.
8. Marshall CF. Tumor suppressor genes. *Cell* 1991;64:313–326.
9. Knudson AG. Antioncogenes and human cancer. *Proc Natl Acad Sci USA* 1993;90:10914–10921.
10. Samara G, Hurwitz M, Sawicki M, Passaro E. Molecular mechanisms of tumor formation. *Am J Surg* 1992;164:389–396.
11. Hurwitz M, Sawicki M, Samara G, Passaro E. Diagnostic and prognostic molecular markers in cancer. *Am J Surg* 1992;164:299–306.

11a. Durbec P, Marcos-Gutierrez CV, Kilkenny C, et al. GDNF signalling through the Ret receptor tyrosine kinase. *Nature* 1996;381:789–793.
12. Melmed S. Oncogenes and the thyroid. *Thyroid Today* 1988;11(1):1–7.
13. Fagin JA. Genetic basis of endocrine disease. 3: Molecular defects in thyroid gland neoplasia. *J Clin Endocrinol Metab* 1992;75:1398–1400.
14. Fagin JA. Molecular pathogenesis of human thyroid neoplasms. *Thyroid Today* 1994;17(3):1–6.
15. Clark OH, Elmhed J. Thyroid surgery-past, present and future. *Thyroid Today* 1995;18(1):1–9.
16. Williams ED. Mechanisms and pathogenesis of thyroid cancer in animals and man. *Mutat Res* 1995;333(1-2):123–129.
17. Farbota LM, Calandra DB, Lawrence AM, Paloyan E. Thyroid carcinoma in Graves' disease. *Surgery* 1985;98:1148–1152.
18. Filetti S, Belfiore A, Amir SM, Daniels GH, Ippolito O, Vigneri R, Ingbar SH. The role of thyroid-stimulating antibodies of Graves' disease in differentiated thyroid cancer. *N Engl J Med* 1988;318:753–759.
19. Belfiore A, Garofalo MR, Giuffrida D, Runello F, et al. Increased aggressiveness of thyroid cancer in patients with Graves' disease. *J Clin Endocrinol Metab* 1990;70:830–835.
20. Hales IB, McElduff A, Crummer P, Clifton-Bligh P, Delbridge L, et al. Does Graves' disease of thyrotoxicosis affect the prognosis of thyroid cancer. *J Clin Endocrinol Metab* 1992;75:886–889.
21. Paschke R, Tonacchera M, Van Sande J, Parma J, Vassart G. Identification and functional characterization of two new somatic mutations causing constitutive activation of the thyrotropin receptor in hyperfunctioning autonomous adenomas of the thyroid. *J Clin Endocrinol Metab* 1994;79:1785–1789.
22. Porcellini A, Ciullo I, Laviola L, Amabile G, Fenzi G, Avvedimento VE. Novel mutations of thyrotropin receptor gene in thyroid hyperfunctioning adenomas. Rapid identification by fine needle aspiration biopsy. *J Clin Endocrinol Metab* 1994;79:657–661.
23. Russo D, Arturi F, Wicker R, Chazenbalk GD, et al. Genetic alterations in thyroid hyperfunctioning adenomas. *J Clin Endocrinol Metab* 1995;80:1347–1351.
24. Ohno M, Endo T, Ohta K, Gunji K, Onaya T. Point mutations in the thyrotropin receptor in human thyroid tumors. *Thyroid* 1995;5:97–100.
25. Takeshita A, Nagayama Y, Yokoyama N, Ishikawa N, et al. Rarity of oncogenic mutations in the thyrotropin receptor of autonomously functioning thyroid nodules in Japan. *J Clin Endocrinol Metab* 1995;80:2607–2611.
26. Parma J, Duprez L, Van Sande J, Paschke R, et al. Constitutively active receptors as a disease-causing mechanism. *Mol Cell Endocrinol* 1994;100:159–162.
27. Van Sande J, Parma J, Tonacchera M, Swillens S, Dumont J, Vassart G. Somatic and germline mutations of the TSH receptor gene in thyroid diseases. *J Clin Endocrinol Metab* 1995;80:2577–2585.
28. Quadro L, Panariello L, Salvatore D, Carlomagno F, et al. Frequent RET proto-oncogene mutations in multiple endocrine neoplasia type 2A. *J Clin Endocrinol Metab* 1994;79:590–594.
29. Lips CJM, Landsvater RM, Hoppener JWM, Geerdink RA, Blijham G, et al. Clinical screening as compared with DNA analysis in families with multiple endocrine neoplasia type 2A. *N Engl J Med* 1994;331:828–835.
30. Hofstra RMW, Landsvater RM, Ceccherini I, Stulp RP, Stelwagen T, et al. A mutation in the RET proto-oncogene associated with multiple endocrine neoplasia type 2B and sporadic medullary thyroid carcinoma. *Nature* 1994;367:375–376.
31. Zedenius J, Larsson C, Bergholm U, Bovee J, Svensson A, Hallengren B, Grimelius L, Backdahl M, Weber G, Wallin G. Mutations of codon 918 in the RET proto-oncogene correlate to poor prognosis in sporadic medullary thyroid carcinomas. *J Clin Endocrinol Metab* 1995;80:3088–3090.
32. Smith DP, Eng C, Ponder BAJ. Mutations of the RET proto-oncogene in the multiple endocrine neoplasia type 2 syndromes and Hirschsprung disease. *J Cell Science* 1994;(suppl 18):43–49.
33. Mulligan LM, Ponder BAJ. Genetic basis of endocrine disease: multiple endocrine neoplasia type 2. *J Clin Endocrinol Metab* 1995;80:1989–1995.
34. Grieco M, Santoro M, Berlingieri MT, Melillo RM, Donghi R, Bongarzone I, Pierotti MA, Della-Porta G, Fusco A, Vecchio G. PTC is a novel rearranged form of the ret proto-oncogene and is frequently detected in vivo in human thyroid papillary carcinomas. *Cell* 1990;60(4):557–563.
35. Santoro M, Carlomagno F, Hay ID, Herrmann MA, Grieco M, et al. Ret oncogene activation in human thyroid neoplasms is restricted to the papillary cancer subtype. *J Clin Invest* 1992;89:1517–1522.
36. Jhiang SM, Mazzaferri EL. The ret/PTC oncogene in papillary thyroid carcinoma. *J Lab Clin Med* 1994;123:331–337.
37. Lyons J, Landis CA, Harsh G, Vallar L, Grunewald K, et al. Two G protein oncogenes in human endocrine tumors. *Science* 1990;249:655–658.
38. Dumont JE. Thyroid adenoma, Gsα expression and the cyclic adenosine monophosphate mitogenic cascade: a complex relationship [editorial] *J Clin Endocrinol Metab* 1995;80:1518–1520.
39. Goretzki PE, Lyons J, Stac-Phipps S, Rosenau W, et al. Mutational activation of RAS and GSP oncogenes in differentiated thyroid cancer and their biological implications. *World J Surg* 1992;16:576–582.
40. Schark C, Fulton N, Jacoby RF, Westbrook CA, Straus FH, Kaplan EL. N-ras 61 oncogene mutations in Hurthle cell tumors. *Surgery* 1990;108:994–1000.
41. Namba H, Gutman RA, Matsuo K, Alvarez A, Fagin JA. H-Ras protooncogene mutations in human thyroid neoplasms. *J Clin Endocrinol Metab* 1990;71:223–229.
42. Namba H, Rubin SA, Fagin JA. Point mutations of ras oncogenes are an early event in thyroid tumorigenesis. *Mol Endocrinol* 1990;4:1474–1479.
43. Karga H, Lee J-K, Vickery AL, Thor A, Gaz RD, Jameson JL. Ras oncogene mutations in benign and malignant thyroid neoplasms. *J Clin Endocrinol Metab* 1991;73:832–836.
44. Schark C, Fulton N, Tashiro T, Stanislav G, Jacoby R, et al. The value of measurement of RAS oncogenes and nuclear DNA analysis in the diagnosis of Hürthle cell tumors of the thyroid. *World J Surg* 1992;16:745–752.
45. Basolo F, Pinchera A, Fugazzola L, Fontanini G, Elisei R, Romei C, Pacini F. Expression of p21 ras protein as a prognostic factor in papillary thyroid cancer. *Eur J Cancer* 1994;30A(2):171–174.
46. Auguste LJ, Masood S, Westerband A, Belluco C, Valderamma E, Attie J. Oncogene expression in follicular neoplasms of the thyroid. *Am J Surg* 1992;164(6):592–593.
47. Romano ME, Gratone M, Karner MP, Moiguer S, Tetelbaum F, Romaro LA, Illescas E, Padin R, Cueva F, Burdman JA. Relationship between the level of c-myc mRNA and histologic aggressiveness in thyroid tumors. *Horm Res* 1993;39(3-4):161–165.
48. Frebourg T. Cancer risks from germline p53 mutations. *J Clin Invest* 1992;90:1637–1641.
49. Lane DP. p53, guardian of the genome. *Nature* 1992;358:15–16.
50. Marx J. How p53 suppresses cell growth. *Science* 1993;262:1644–1645.
51. Harris CC. Medical progress: clinical implications of the p53 tumor suppressor gene. *N Engl J Med* 1993;329:1318–1327.
52. Nakamura T, Yana I, Kobayashi T, Shin E, Karakawa K, Fujita S, Miya A, Mori T, Nishisho I, Takai S. p53 gene mutations associated with anaplastic transformation of human thyroid carcinimas. *Jpn J Cancer Res* 1992;83(12):1293–1298.
53. Fagin JA, Matsuo K, Karmakar A, Chen DL, Tang S-H, Koeffler HP. High prevalence of mutations of the p53 gene in poorly differentiated human thyroid carcinomas. *J Clin Invest* 1993;91:179–184.
54. Donghi R, Longoni A, Pilotti S, Michieli P, Porta GD, Pierotti MA. Gene p53 mutations are restricted to poorly differentiated and undifferentiated carcinomas of the thyroid gland. *J Clin Invest* 1993;91:1753–1760.
55. Zou M, Shi Y, Farid NR. p53 mutations in all stages of thyroid carcinomas. *J Clin Endocrinol Metab* 1993;77:1045–1048.
56. Donashi Y, Sugimura H, Sakamoto A, Mernyei M, Mori M, Oyama T, Machinami R. Stepwise participation of p53 gene mutation during dedifferentiation of human thyroid carcinomas. *Diagn Mol Pathol* 1994;3(1):9–14.

CHAPTER 14

Hyperthyroidism: Systemic Effects and Differential Diagnosis

Amy L. O'Donnell and Stephen W. Spaulding

SYSTEMIC EFFECTS OF HYPERTHYROIDISM

High circulating levels of thyroid hormones can affect almost all organ systems (Table 1). In the case of hyperthyroid due to Graves' disease, however, some of the signs and symptoms reflect extrathyroidal immunological processes rather than the excessive levels of thyroid hormone.

General Features

Typically, hyperthyroid patients are gaunt and restless, talk rapidly, and display emotional lability. Other classic signs and symptoms include sweating, heat intolerance, palpitations, insomnia, and warm, fine skin. Prominent eyes or a stare may be produced by increased thyroid hormone levels, but infiltrative eye signs signal the presence of Graves' disease. It is important to note that thyrotoxicosis may also present in an atypical fashion. Older patients in particular tend to show fewer findings and may present with only weight loss, cardiac symptoms, or a change in mental function. Elderly patients may also be taking medications or have coexisting diseases that can interfere with the diagnosis of hyperthyroidism. Furthermore, older patients are more likely to have a toxic thyroid nodule as the cause of their hyperthyroidism, and these patients tend to have fewer signs and symptoms than patients with Graves' disease. Some patients have "apathetic" hyperthyroidism and lack almost all of the usual clinical manifestations of thyrotoxicosis. Their behavior may lead one to consider, erroneously, a psychiatric diagnosis. Although apathetic hyperthyroidism is most commonly seen in elderly patients, it has also been reported in childhood and middle age (1–3).

Intermediary Metabolism

One of the most prominent symptoms in the hyperthyroid patient is heat intolerance. This symptom reflects an increase in the basal metabolism of many substrates and heat production by the cells in the body from an increased consumption of adenosine triphosphate (ATP) and oxygen. Patients tend to eat more, and some actually gain weight, but weight loss is the usual finding, and it becomes more pronounced with age. In addition to losing fat stores, hyperthyroid patients often lose muscle mass as well, making weakness a common complaint. In view of the fact that beta-adrenergic blocking agents are often used in the treatment of thyrotoxicosis, it is important to note that although propranolol did abolish the exaggerated calorigenic response to epinephrine, it did not affect the rate of protein breakdown in T_3-induced thyrotoxicosis in one experimental study (4).

Both glucose absorption and glucose production are increased in hyperthyroidism. Hyperthyroid patients often display impaired glucose tolerance, which reflects the combined effects of the increased caloric intake, the enhanced absorption of glucose, and the inappropriate persistence of hepatic glucose production in the presence of high glucose and insulin levels (5). These metabolic changes can also unmask a patient's underlying tendency toward developing type II diabetes. The effectiveness of insulin on peripheral tissue is essentially unaltered by hyperthyroidism (6).

A. L. O'Donnell: Department of Veterans' Affairs Western New York Healthcare System; and Department of Medicine, State University of New York at Buffalo, Buffalo, New York 14215.

S. W. Spaulding: Research and Development Service, Department of Veterans' Affairs Western New York Healthcare System; and Department of Medicine, State University of New York at Buffalo, Buffalo, New York 14215.

TABLE 1. *Overview: systemic effects of hyperthyroidism*

Organ system	Effects
General	Weight loss; heat intolerance; insomnia; fatigue; increased sweating; restlessness; glucose intolerance
Skin, hair, and nails	Skin warm, moist, and smooth; alopecia; pruritus; vitiligo; hyperpigmentation; pretibial myxedema; onycholysis
Bone and calcium	Elevated serum calcium, alkaline phosphatase, and markers of bone turnover; osteoporosis; acropachy
Neuromuscular	Muscle weakness (especially proximal); fatigue; tremor; myopathy; hypokalemic periodic paralysis; neuropathy
Mental	Hyperactivity; emotional lability; nervousness; anxiety; depression; distractibility; disorientation; delirium
Gastrointestinal	Frequent bowel movements or diarrhea; increased appetite; elevated liver enzymes
Respiratory	Dyspnea
Hematologic/immune	Anemia; hyperplasia of spleen, lymph nodes, and thymus
Cardiovascular	Tachycardia; palpitations; increased cardiac output; increased pulse pressure; dilated cardiomyopathy; atrial fibrillation; angina pectoris
Renal	Polyuria; polydipsia
Eyes	Lid retraction; lid lag; exophthalmos; conjunctivitis; diplopia; visual loss from optic nerve involvement
Endocrine/reproductive	Irregular menses; gynecomastia; impotence; decreased fertility

Both the synthesis and the clearance of cholesterol and triglycerides are increased, but the latter effect predominates, so that the serum levels of both are generally low in hyperthyroidism.

Skin, Hair, and Nails

The skin of the typical hyperthyroid patient is moist and warm, reflecting a homeostatic mechanism for dissipating the heat being generated in the body. The patient may complain of cutaneous flushing, perspiration at rest, and sweaty palms. The skin tends to have a smooth velvety texture and the hair is characteristically fine; in some instances, the hair may fall out in patches, or total alopecia may occur. Some hyperthyroid patients have developed generalized pruritus for unknown reasons, but it may be related to thyrotoxicosis-induced hepatic dysfunction (7). For unknown reasons, pigmentation may be increased, particularly in such areas as the knuckles and skin creases, whereas patches of vitiligo apparently reflect the autoimmune processes at work in Graves' disease.

Localized nonpitting edema on the shins can be as important as ophthalmopathy in establishing the diagnosis of Graves' disease. This "pretibial myxedema" can also occur elsewhere, generally on extensor surfaces. The lesion reflects the deposition of glycosaminoglycans in the subcutaneous connective tissue (8,9). The lesion is elevated above the surrounding tissue—often finely dimpled and hyperpigmented, or pruritic and red. Most patients with pretibial myxedema and Graves' disease also have ophthalmopathy (9,10). Another cutaneous change in Graves' disease causes the fingernail edge to separate from the nail bed (onycholysis), resulting in a dirty appearance to the nails.

Bone and Calcium Metabolism

Many aspects of bone and calcium metabolism can be affected by hyperthyroidism. Elevated blood levels of calcium, alkaline phosphatase, and osteocalcin (GLA protein, containing gamma-carboxyglutamic acid, which is produced by active osteoblasts and reflects bone formation) may be observed (11,12). Bone resorption is increased to a greater extent than new bone formation, so the urinary excretion of calcium and hydroxyproline is increased. Urinary pyridinoline cross-link excretion, which reflects bone resorption, is often elevated in patients with hyperthyroidism, and this may be a more sensitive marker of altered bone metabolism than osteocalcin or bone-specific alkaline phosphatase (11). Parathyroid hormone (PTH) and 1,25-dihydroxyvitamin D_3 levels tend to be low, a result of the increased release of calcium from bone. Consequently, the gut absorbs less calcium and phosphate. Note that increased bone turnover occurs despite the suppressed levels of PTH and of 1,25-dihydroxyvitamin D_3.

Longstanding endogenous hyperthyroidism may produce radiographic signs of osteoporosis, including transparency of vertebral bodies, widely spaced trabeculae, or actual compression fractures of the vertebral bodies. Hyperthyroidism also appears to be a risk factor for hip fractures (13). Dual energy x-ray absorptiometry shows a decrease in bone mineral density in patients with Graves' disease (14) or with toxic thyroid nodules (15), and treatment of hyperthyroidism often improves the bone density (14,16), although they do not always return to the values for age-matched controls. Postmenopausal women with a history of thyrotoxicosis, even if adequately treated in the past, appear to have a lower bone mineral density than age-matched controls (17).

Thyroid acropachy is soft-tissue swelling and subperiosteal formation of new bone, particularly in the distal phalanges, that resembles clubbing. It may occur in patients with Graves' disease, even in a single digit, but the etiology and pathogenesis is not yet clear (9).

Neuromuscular System

Muscle weakness and fatigue are common complaints in hyperthyroidism. Rarely, severe muscle wasting is the predominant symptom. Skeletal muscle is a target for thyroid hormone action, and high hormone levels increase mitochondrial enzyme activity, particularly in the slow muscle fibers. On physical examination, the deep tendon reflexes are hyperactive, with both contraction and relaxation phases being accelerated. The explanation for the rapid low-amplitude tremor noted when the tongue or hands are extended has not been clearly established; however, the symptoms often decrease after administration of beta-adrenergic blocking agents. Overtreatment with thyroid hormone reportedly increases the density of beta-adrenergic receptors in human skeletal muscle fibers (18). Beta-blockers have also been shown to improve the muscle weakness of Graves' disease (19). If the myopathy involves the oropharyngeal muscles, the resultant bulbar dysfunction might be confused with myasthenia gravis, which also can occur in association with Graves' disease. Another myopathy sometimes observed in association with hyperthyroidism is hypokalemic periodic paralysis. This disorder affects mostly Asian men, but it has also been reported to occur in Hispanics, American Indians, and Caucasians, as well as African Americans (20,21). Episodes may be precipitated by carbohydrate ingestion.

The hyperactivity, emotional lability, distractibility, nervousness, insomnia, and anxiety observed in hyperthyroidism reflect changes in the nervous system, although the mechanisms involved remain obscure. In children, these symptoms may be interpreted as hyperactivity or an attention deficit disorder. Neurotic anxiety, simple depression, or even disorientation or delirium can occasionally occur as a monosymptomatic presentation of hyperthyroidism, particularly in the elderly, and the true etiology can be easily missed. Parkinsonian-like or choreoathetoid symptoms can also occur in hyperthyroidism.

Gastrointestinal System

Hyperthyroid patients commonly complain of weight loss despite increased appetite. A prominent physiologic response to thyrotoxicosis in the GI tract is increased intestinal motility and malabsorption owing to the rapid transit time. These changes, along with the increased food intake, can result in frequent bowel movements, or even steatorrhea or diarrhea. In the elderly, however, constipation is as common as increased stool frequency, and anorexia rather than hyperphagia may be observed. Hepatic function may also be affected by hyperthyroidism. The etiology of the increased serum alkaline phosphatase, bilirubin, and transaminase levels has not been established, but in some instances they may reflect passive congestion of the liver secondary to heart failure. One study of five patients with hyperthyroidism found intrahepatic cholestasis, lobular inflammatory infiltrate with some eosinophils, and Kupffer cell hyperplasia on liver biopsies (22). Because of the alterations in hepatic function, the metabolism of various drugs may also be affected.

Respiratory System

The hyperthyroid patient's complaint of dyspnea probably reflects not only an increase in the basal consumption of oxygen and production of CO_2, but also an increased sensitivity to hypoxemia and hypercapnia, producing an inappropriate increase in respiratory drive (23,24). Weakness of respiratory muscles may also play a role in the dyspnea of hyperthyroidism (25). Occasionally, a large gland may produce wheezing caused by tracheal compression. There is no apparent effect of hyperthyroidism on airway responsiveness in patients with asthma (26,27).

Hematologic and Immune Systems

The hypermetabolism of hyperthyroidism can increase red blood cell production and red blood cell mass, presumably reflecting the increased need for oxygen. An even greater increase in plasma volume, however, may dilute the blood, causing a pseudoanemia. A real anemia may result from low folate or vitamin B_{12} levels; pernicious anemia has an increased incidence in Graves' disease, and there is a substantially increased incidence of anti-gastric parietal cell antibodies in this disorder. Certain human leukocyte antigen (HLA) types predominate in Graves' disease, although they vary among racial groups. A variety of autoimmune disorders occur with increased frequency in patients with Graves' disease and their families, including diabetes, adrenal insufficiency, premature gonadal failure, Sjögren's syndrome, idiopathic thrombocytopenic purpura, and myasthenia gravis, in addition to pernicious anemia. Hyperplasia of spleen, lymph nodes, and thymus may occur (Fig. 1), and there is also a slightly increased incidence of acute leukemia reported in Graves' disease.

Cardiovascular System

The cardiac output is increased in hyperthyroidism, as would be expected because of the increased demand for oxygen in peripheral tissues, and the increased blood flow to the skin, muscle, brain, thyroid, and kidneys. Clinically, the patient manifests a tachycardia and a bounding pulse; the widened pulse pressure reflects both increased cardiac output and decreased peripheral vascu-

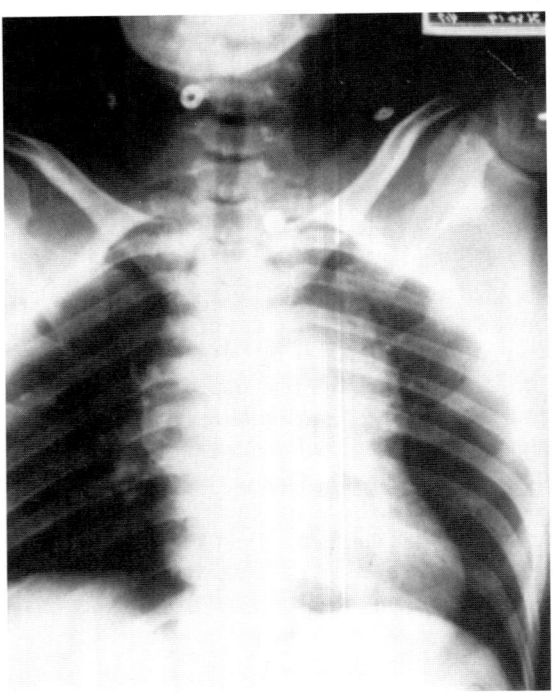 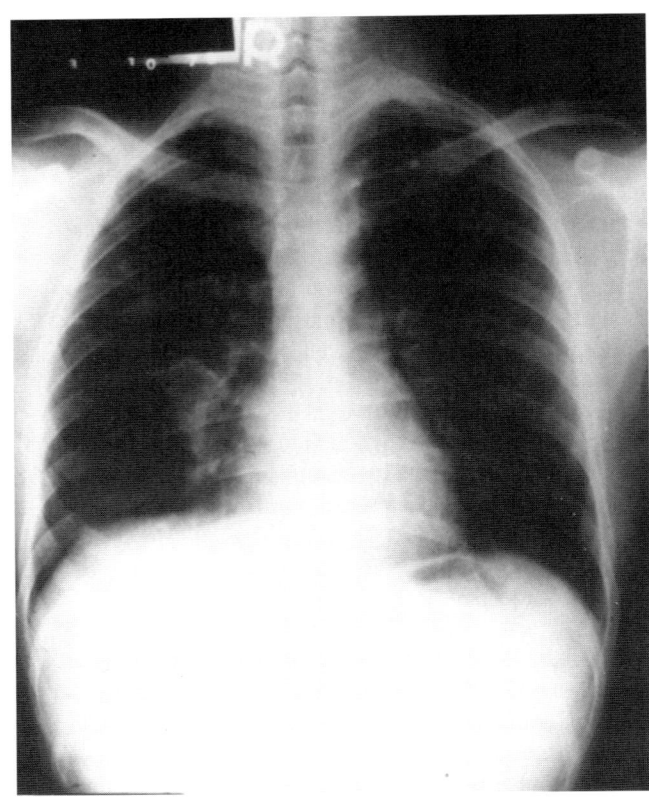

FIG. 1. A 20-year-old woman with Graves' disease was found to have a retrosternal mass (A). Hematologic evaluation was unremarkable at that time, and after 14 months of treatment with propylthiouracil, the thymic enlargement resolved (B).

lar resistance. The complaint of palpitations usually indicates a resting tachycardia.

Despite several clinical signs that might suggest hyperactivity of the sympathetic nervous system, the circulating levels of catecholamines are normal or even low in hyperthyroidism (28). However, an increase in cardiac beta-adrenergic receptors has been observed in experimental hyperthyroidism (29). Adrenergic receptors in several other tissues have been shown to be altered as well, and processes that mediate target organ responses to catecholamines intracellularly are probably also affected. Some of the hemodynamic responses to catecholamines in experimental human hyperthyroidism may remain normal (29), but the sensitivity of the heart rate and left ventricular shortening velocity appears to be increased (30). In patients with thyrotoxicosis, the intrinsic activity of the sinus node is increased, but this is not mediated by the autonomic nervous system (31). In addition to alterations in adrenergic receptor sensitivity, decreased parasympathetic tone may affect the basal heart rate in hyperthyroidism. Other common clinical findings reflecting the high cardiac output include a systolic ejection murmur and a gallop rhythm. Systolic and diastolic left ventricular function at rest is not necessarily depressed by hyperthyroidism (32). During exercise, the left ventricular ejection fraction may actually fall (33), but despite this apparently pathological response, frank congestive heart failure is not common in hyperthyroidism, unless the patient has underlying cardiac disease or atrial fibrillation has occurred. In one study of patients with both atrial fibrillation and thyrotoxicosis, half had a dilated cardiomyopathy with clinical congestive heart failure without evidence of other organic heart disease (mean age of those patients was 36) (34). There have been several other case reports of thyrotoxicosis causing a dilated cardiomyopathy, which is usually reversible with treatment of the hyperthyroidism. Mitral valve prolapse also appears to occur more commonly in patients with thyrotoxicosis (35). Hyperthyroidism can also exacerbate preexisting cardiac disease by precipitating atrial fibrillation, or by worsening angina pectoris or congestive heart failure (36,37). In elderly patients, cardiac symptoms may be the presenting feature of thyrotoxicosis. Simply the presence of a low serum thyrotropin level in clinically euthyroid patients 60 years of age or older was associated with a threefold higher risk of developing atrial fibrillation in one study (38). There is no clear evidence, however, that screening all clinically euthyroid patients with atrial fibrillation for occult hyperthyroidism will detect subclinical disease with any greater frequency than control subjects (39,40). Rarely, angina pectoris and myocardial infarction may occur in hyperthyroidism in the absence of coronary artery disease (41,42).

Experimental studies indicate that hyperthyroid heart muscle contracts more rapidly than normal. High levels of thyroid hormone alter the types and the amounts of myosin adenosine triphosphatase (ATPase) expressed in heart muscle, and an increase in beta myosin increases the contractility of cardiac muscle in the resting state. There is evidence that thyroid hormone has a hypertrophic effect on isolated myocytes, but cardiac hypertrophy may also result from the increased work load. Atrial natriuretic factor (ANF) is a peptide released from the heart in response to atrial distention. ANF causes natriuresis, relaxes vascular smooth muscle, and inhibits aldosterone secretion. Hyperthyroidism increases expression of ANF, which is an additional factor in considering fluid balance and vascular tone in this disease.

Renal System

Patients with hyperthyroidism often complain of increased thirst and urinary frequency. Renal blood flow is increased, as are glomerular filtration, tubular resorption, and electrolyte secretion, but blood electrolytes are maintained in the normal range. Patients who complain of polyuria and polydipsia may have a somewhat low osmolarity, and some data indicate that stimulation of thirst can be increased directly at a central nervous system level in hyperthyroidism (43).

Eye

Noninfiltrative disease of the eye muscles can occur in any type of hyperthyroidism, but it can also occur in euthyroid patients. Two common signs are lid retraction (which leaves a white rim of sclera above the limbus, making the patient appear to be staring in fright), and lid lag on downward gaze (which occurs when unbalanced muscular tension delays the downward motion of the lid). These findings may occur in any form of hyperthyroidism and in many other disease states.

On the other hand, infiltrative ophthalmopathy strongly indicates that the etiology of a case of hyperthyroidism is Graves' disease. Orbital computerized tomography (CT) can provide precise documentation of the anatomic changes. Perhaps the most common eye complaint in Graves' disease is a "gritty" feeling, often accompanied by other signs of conjunctivitis. Inflammation, fibroblast activation, and deposition of glycosaminoglycans produce swelling in the retro-orbital muscles and connective tissue, causing diplopia and proptosis (8,9,44). If the eyelid cannot be properly closed, corneal trauma can result. Vision can also be threatened if the muscles surrounding the optic nerve swell and entrap it because of the limited volume in the orbital space. Graves' ophthalmopathy is more commonly seen in women than in men, but the eye signs and symptoms tend to be more severe in men, and in patients over 50 to 60 years of age (45,46). Cigarette smoking increases the risk of developing ophthalmopathy, perhaps through the stimulation of orbital fibroblasts by tissue hypoxia. Because Graves' ophthalmopathy results from the extrathyroidal autoimmune process rather than from the excess levels of thyroid hormone, it can run a separate course from that of the thyroid.

Endocrine System

Hyperthyroidism increases the metabolism of a number of hormones. The half-life of cortisol is shortened, so both the number of bursts of adrenocorticotropic hormone (ACTH) and the resulting bursts of cortisol secretion are increased in order to maintain serum cortisol levels. Basal prolactin levels may be low, and the prolactin response to thyrotropin-releasing hormone (TRH) may be decreased.

Sex hormone–binding globulin is increased in hyperthyroidism, and thus total levels of serum estradiol and estrone are commonly high in hyperthyroid women. The free levels of these hormones, however, are generally maintained in the low normal range. Luteinizing hormone (LH) and follicle-stimulating hormone (FSH) levels tend to be slightly increased, perhaps reflecting the lower free estrogen levels. Midcycle surges of LH and FSH may be subnormal, but serum progesterone levels do increase at ovulation. Some hyperthyroid women develop menstrual abnormalities, and those with higher thyroid hormone levels or those who smoke may be at higher risk (47). Interestingly, if a patient with Graves' disease does become pregnant, her disease usually becomes easier to control, whereas postpartum exacerbations are common, probably reflecting alterations in immune processes during pregnancy.

Gynecomastia and a decrease in libido and potency are not uncommon in hyperthyroid men, yet total testosterone levels are elevated because of an increase in sex hormone–binding globulin levels. Free testosterone levels tend to be normal, but the extragonadal conversion of androgens to estrogens is increased, and total and free estradiol levels tend to be higher than normal. Thyrotoxicosis can also be a cause of male infertility (48).

Thyroid Gland

In Graves' disease, the thyroid is usually diffusely enlarged, although a retrosternal gland may be clinically inapparent. Superior vena cava syndrome has been reported to occur from enlargement of an intrathoracic goiter due to Graves' disease (49). Bruits caused by the marked increase in the blood flow to the Graves' disease gland through dilated capillary and venous beds are common, and they are relatively specific for Graves' disease as the cause of the hyperthyroidism. An overactive gland shows increased cellularity, the cells are tall and columnar rather than cuboidal, and they surround small amounts of colloid. Collections of lymphocytes often occur in Graves' disease.

Goiter may be less prominent in elderly patients, particularly if hyperthyroidism is a result of a single toxic adenoma. An asymmetrical thyroid gland is expected in the toxic adenoma or multinodular goiter, but such a gland can also occur in Graves' disease, particularly when the gland has previously suffered from some process that has affected it in a patchy fashion, such as Hashimoto's thyroiditis.

DIFFERENTIAL DIAGNOSIS OF HYPERTHYROIDISM

An Overview

Etiologies

Hyperproduction of thyroid hormone is most commonly a result of excessive stimulation of the gland by abnormal autoantibodies (Graves' disease), although the thyroid itself can be intrinsically responsible for overproduction (e.g., toxic adenoma). The disease can also arise from the ingestion of too much thyroid hormone. Occasionally, inflammatory processes that destroy thyroid tissue (thyroiditis) will cause transient hyperthyroidism as a result of the release of the thyroid hormones from the thyroglobulin stores in the gland. Rarely, hyperproduction of hormone is produced by high levels of thyroid stimulating hormone (TSH) or chorionic gonadotropin, or by oversupply of iodine to a gland that has defective regulatory mechanisms (Jod-Basedow).

History and Physical Examination

The history and physical examination can be of central importance in establishing the cause of a patient's hyperthyroidism. Important features include the duration of symptoms, the presence of a diffuse or focal enlargement of the thyroid, the presence of neck pain or a bruit in the gland, and particularly the presence of extrathyroidal manifestations of Graves' disease (see later) (Table 2).

Laboratory Tests

If a modern, very sensitive ("third generation") TSH assay is available, evidence that the serum TSH level is suppressed can be useful in establishing the diagnosis of primary thyroidal or exogenous hyperthyroidism, although if the level of TSH is not completely suppressed, other diagnoses need to be considered. If a sensitive TSH assay is not available, the TSH response to an intravenous injection of TRH can be used in its place to determine if pituitary thyrotrophs are suppressed. A low TSH in the presence of a normal free T_4 (thyroxine) level may sug-

TABLE 2. *Causes of hyperthyroidism: relative frequency and special clinical characteristics*

Etiology	Relative frequency[a]	Special characteristics
Graves' disease[b]	70%–85%	Ophthalmopathy, pretibial myxedema, thyroid bruit, TSH receptor antibodies
Thyroiditis	5%–25%	Low RAI uptake
Subacute granulomatous		Pain, tenderness in neck
Painless ("silent")		More common in postpartum women
Postradiation		After RAI therapy
Exogenous	Uncommon	Low RAI uptake
Iatrogenic		No goiter, patient taking thyroxine
Factitious		No goiter, low serum thyroglobulin
Iodine-induced		Usually underlying nodular goiter, exposure to iodide-containing contrast agents or drugs
Toxic multinodular goiter	5%–15%	Older patients, multiple nodules palpable or seen on scan
Toxic adenoma	3%–30%	Single nodule palpable or seen on scan, rest of gland suppressed
Thyroid carcinoma	Rare	Usually metastatic and clinically apparent
Ectopic hyperthyroidism	Very rare	Low RAI uptake, no goiter
Excessive TSH	Rare	TSH not suppressed
Pituitary tumor		May have compressive symptoms of tumor, excessive alpha subunit levels
Pituitary insensitivity to thyroxine		Alpha subunit level proportionate to TSH
Trophoblastic tumors	Rare	High hCG levels

[a]Overall frequency; in certain populations (e.g., the elderly, regions of endemic goiter), relative frequency may be altered.
[b]Including so-called Hashitoxicosis.
TSH, thyroid stimulating hormone, thyrotropin; RAI, radioactive iodine; hCG, human chorionic gonadotropin.

gest subclinical hyperthyroidism, which has a prevalence of about 1%, and is more common in older age groups and patients with nodular thyroid glands. In such patients, measurement of T_3 (triiodothyronine) by RIA (radioimmunoassay) (T_3RIA), measurement of free T_3, and/or a thyroid uptake test may be useful in determining whether the patient is truly hyperthyroid (50,51). A low TSH is not uncommon in elderly patients and thus by itself may not be a useful screening test (52–54). Furthermore, certain drugs (e.g., glucocorticoids, dopamine) can suppress the TSH level. Very rarely, excessive pituitary production of TSH can cause hyperthyroidism; in such cases, TSH is not suppressed by the high circulating levels of thyroid hormone.

In addition to the serum TSH level, both the serum level of thyroxine and a measure of thyroid hormone–binding proteins [e.g., a T_3 resin uptake (T_3RU)] should be determined in all patients whose symptoms suggest hyperthyroidism (see Chapter 4). This assessment of the circulating thyroxine level provides the confirmatory laboratory data needed for establishing the diagnosis of hyperthyroidism in the vast majority of cases. It is impossible to simply use a thyroxine determination by itself to estimate thyroid activity because of the variability in hormone-binding proteins, particularly thyroxine-binding globulin. If there is evidence for altered levels of thyroid hormone–binding proteins (i.e., the T_4 and the T_3 resin uptakes are not increased to the same extent), then a free T_4 determination (generally by dialysis) can be made to get a better idea of the metabolically important level of hormone.

Even when changes in the level of the binding proteins have been taken into account, the level of thyroid hormone in a hyperthyroid patient does not always correlate with the severity of the patient's symptoms. Occasionally, this may reflect a marked difference between the serum T_4 and T_3 levels. The majority of the circulating T_3 is produced by the thyroid gland in hyperthyroidism. Rarely, only the serum T_3 levels are above the normal range, resulting in so-called T_3 toxicosis. Serum T_3 levels are determined by radioimmunoassay, and it is important not to confuse the T_3RIA with the T_3RU, which measures unsaturated hormone binding sites, not T_3 levels. T_3 toxicosis appears to occur more frequently in toxic adenoma or in recurrent Graves' disease, particularly in regions where there is a relative deficiency of iodine in the diet. The reverse (high levels of T_4 with normal levels of serum T_3) occasionally can occur in hyperthyroid patients who have another serious illness, such as pneumonia or myocardial infarct, or who have received drugs that inhibit the peripheral conversion of T_4 to T_3, such as iodinated radiographic contrast agents. When these intercurrent illnesses or drug treatments end, the serum T_3 concentration rises into the hyperthyroid range.

The amount of radioactive iodine (RAI) taken up by the thyroid gland (the "RAI uptake") can provide confirmation of the diagnosis of hyperthyroidism, or point to its etiology, but it cannot be used as the sole measure of thyroid function (see Chapter 8). The distribution of isotope within the gland (the "RAI scan") can establish the presence of a solitary hot nodule, multinodularity, or the patchy pattern seen in Hashimoto's thyroiditis. In the latter case, determination of the serum antithyroglobulin and antimicrosomal (peroxidase) antibody levels in the blood can be useful, although high titers are not always diagnostic for Hashimoto's thyroiditis. Determinations of thyroid-stimulating immunoglobulins (TSI, or TSH receptor antibodies) are rarely useful in routine diagnosis. (Note that TSIs should not be confused with either thyroxine-binding globulin or thyroglobulin.)

Occasionally, the determination of serum thyroglobulin levels may be helpful in establishing factitious hyperthyroidism, in which case the high levels of thyroid hormone are accompanied by suppression of the thyroglobulin level (55).

Characteristic Features of the Different Causes of Hyperthyroidism

The relative frequencies of the causes of hyperthyroidism, and some of their special clinical characteristics discussed in this section, are shown in Table 2.

Graves' Disease

Graves' disease is the most common cause of hyperthyroidism and occurs most frequently in young women. It is an autoimmune disorder that can affect many systems in addition to the thyroid, including the eyes, the skin, and occasionally other organ systems as well. Classically, the thyroid is diffusely enlarged and all the usual symptoms of hyperthyroidism occur, but it is the extrathyroidal manifestations of Graves' disease that are the most useful in establishing the etiology of a patient's hyperthyroidism. (The absence of extrathyroidal manifestations does not eliminate Graves' disease as the cause of hyperthyroidism.) Thyroid-stimulating autoantibodies (TSH receptor antibodies) have been implicated both in the increase in thyroid function and in the hyperplasia of the thyroid gland observed in Graves' disease. Such autoantibodies have been detected using a variety of experimental procedures: those involving stimulation of biologic responses of intact thyroid tissue (i.e., cyclic adenosine monophosphate) appear to be the more specific, whereas those depending on inhibition of TSH binding to thyroid membranes may be more sensitive and easily performed but seem to be less specific. These antibodies interact with the TSH receptor, activating adenylate cyclase and other pathways as well; some gamma G immunoglobulins (IgGs) may stimulate thyroid growth without stimulating thyroid adenylate cyclase. It is not clear why a patient's lymphocytes should begin to produce thyroid-stimulating antibodies; possibly something associated with Graves' disease activates a normally suppressed population of B lymphocytes. It is even less clear what causes the extrathyroidal manifestations of Graves' disease, but they may develop before or after the hyperthyroidism develops; rarely, they may occur without hyperthyroidism ever appearing. Neither the titers nor even the detectability of TSH receptor antibodies correlates closely with severity of symptoms in individual cases. In some instances, anti-idiotypic antibodies against the thyroid-stimulating antibodies have also been demonstrated, and they could be involved in altering the potency of circulating thyroid-stimulating antibodies.

Graves' disease can undergo spontaneous remission, often accompanied by the disappearance of detectable thyroid-stimulating antibodies. Sometimes "blocking antibodies" may have developed, but more frequently, autoimmune destruction of the thyroid has occurred. (The concurrent development of Hashimoto's disease and Graves' disease is sometimes termed Hashitoxicosis.) Even when Graves' patients are in clinical remission, evidence of suppression of the pituitary–thyroid axis may persist, suggesting the continued production of less potent thyroid-stimulating antibodies that no longer cause clinical hyperthyroidism, but that stimulate enough hormone output from the thyroid to suppress the pituitary's production of TSH.

There are some well-recognized genetic risk factors for Graves' disease. There is an increased association with certain HLA haplotypes, which seems to vary from one ethnic group to another. Some families show a disposition toward the development of a spectrum of thyroid conditions in addition to Graves' disease, including idiopathic hypothyroidism, Hashimoto's thyroiditis, or high titers of antithyroid antibodies.

Histologic examination of the thyroid in Graves' disease reveals increased vascularity and microvascularity, and focal collections of lymphocytes that occasionally show lymphoid germinal centers.

Hyperthyroidism Caused by Thyroiditis

Subacute Thyroiditis

Subacute thyroiditis sometimes follows a viral infection. Symptoms of local pain, pain radiating to the ears, and signs of tenderness and hard areas in the thyroid usually make the diagnosis obvious. Clinical features that may help in distinguishing it from acute thyroiditis (see later) include the absence of adenopathy and the absence of involvement of surrounding structures. Transient clinical manifestations of hyperthyroidism are common, and hyperthyroid blood tests are nearly always observed. The RAI uptake, in contrast, is suppressed as a result of damage to the function of the gland. The hyperthyroid phase generally subsides over a period of weeks, and it is often followed by a hypothyroid period, with low serum thyroxine and T_3RU levels but an elevated RAI uptake, caused by both the recovery of thyroid function and the action of high TSH levels resulting from the low circulating levels of thyroid hormone. The acute phase may be confused with hemorrhage into a thyroid nodule, suppurative thyroiditis, or a rapidly growing tumor. Histologically, subacute thyroiditis is characterized by the presence of foreign-body giant cells as well as by leukocytes invading follicles. Despite this damage, the great majority of patients eventually recover normal thyroid function with only symptomatic therapy. Beta-adrenergic blocking agents may ameliorate the transient symptoms of thyrotoxicosis (see Chapter 15), and aspirin or corticosteroids can control the associated pain.

Acute suppurative thyroiditis is a rare condition. Severe pain in the thyroid may radiate to the ears, reflecting the underlying pyogenic infection in the gland. A fever and other toxic symptoms arise from an acute infection of the gland, generally caused by extension of bacterial infection into surrounding structures, and are not thought to reflect thyroid hormone release. The presence of tender adenopathy is often helpful in establishing the diagnosis.

Painless Thyroiditis

Painless thyroiditis, seen commonly in postpartum women, resembles subacute thyroiditis in its clinical course; it is generally self-limited, of 3 to 6 months' duration. Its histologic picture, on the other hand, often resembles chronic autoimmune thyroiditis, but the lymphocytic infiltration does not usually proceed to destroy the follicular cells. As in subacute thyroiditis, after the initial thyrotoxic phase, these patients frequently undergo a period of hypothyroidism. One clinical feature that should provoke suspicion of the diagnosis is the existence of thyrotoxicosis in a patient with a small, nontender goiter. The radioiodine uptake is low, indicating that thyroid function is impaired, thus serving to warn the clinician not to employ thyroid ablative therapy with radioiodine in this form of hyperthyroidism.

Radiation Thyroiditis

The release of preformed stores of thyroid hormone after radiation damage to a gland [e.g., after treatment with iodine-131 (^{131}I)] occasionally can produce thyrotoxic symptoms a week or so after therapy. This consequence is more common if the patient's initial hyperthyroidism was not first brought under control with medications. Pain or tenderness of the neck may not always develop along with the symptoms of hyperthyroidism.

Exogenous Hyperthyroidism

Iatrogenic Hyperthyroidism

If patients are given 300 µg of levothyroxine or 75 µg of liothyronine a day, most will suppress their secretion of TSH, and if the dose is given long enough, they will develop clinical signs of hyperthyroidism. Some individuals, however, will develop symptoms of clinical hyperthyroidism if given only a replacement dose of thyroid hormone (i.e., ≤150 µg levothyroxine); generally, they have underlying thyroid autonomy. This situation is encountered clinically when a physician attempts to suppress a multinodular goiter with thyroid hormone (see Chapter 27). Iatrogenic hyperthyroidism occurs because an autonomous region in the goiter adds enough hormone to the circulation that, when combined with the additional exogenous dose, thyrotoxicosis is produced.

Another way that physicians occasionally may be misled is by thinking that a patient's low serum T_4 represents hypothyroidism, when it actually represents low serum thyroid-binding protein. Treatment will then inadvertently precipitate hyperthyroidism. In these instances of iatrogenic disease, the thyroidal radioiodine uptake will be suppressed, and the serum TSH and thyroglobulin levels will be low, also indicating suppression of the thyroid.

Factitious Hyperthyroidism

Patients may overdose themselves with thyroid hormone for a variety of reasons, most commonly in an ill-conceived attempt to regulate their weight. Patients with psychiatric disturbances may induce hyperthyroid symptoms with thyroid hormone. Such patients may adamantly deny self-overdosage, but demonstrating suppression of the radioiodine uptake and/or the serum thyroglobulin concentration will provide evidence to support the diagnosis of hyperthyroidism resulting from exogenous hormone (55). Some patients have inadvertently taken an excess of thyroid hormone in the form of health-food-store nutritional supplements containing desiccated thyroid (56), or in hamburger that contained thyroid tissue (57). Again, such intake of thyroid hormone may be diagnosed through the measurement of thyroglobulin, which will be inappropriately low compared to the levels observed in patients with genuine thyrotoxicosis, or by fecal thyroxine levels (58), although this test is not widely available.

Iodide-Induced Hyperthyroidism

In regions where dietary intake of iodine is low, the initial introduction of supplemental iodine to the diet is known to increase the incidence of hyperthyroidism in the population up to fivefold for several years. Presumably, such patients had overactive thyroids, but they were unable to obtain enough iodine to permit overproduction of hormone until the diet was supplemented.

Patients on normal iodine diets also can develop hyperthyroidism after receiving pharmacologic doses of iodide, usually from iodide-containing radiographic contrast agents (59) or drugs, particularly amiodarone (60). This seems to happen most often in patients who have a multinodular goiter or thyroid adenoma. The thyroids in such patients do not down-regulate their iodine uptake properly and so the unprotected gland uses the additional iodide to produce excessive amounts of thyroid hormone.

Drug-Induced Hyperthyroidism

Drugs, such as lithium and amiodarone, have been associated with the development of both thyrotoxicosis and hypothyroidism. Lithium carbonate can decrease the secretion of thyroid hormones from the thyroid gland, and this commonly causes a goiter. It has even been used in the treatment of thyrotoxicosis. Lithium does not affect iodide uptake, however, and appears to be connected to an increased risk for the development of hyperthyroidism (61). It has been postulated that lithium may predispose patients to the development of autoimmune thyroid disease (61). Amiodarone is an iodinated compound, and it releases large amounts of iodide into the circulation. The pathogenesis of amiodarone-induced thyrotoxicosis is not completely established, but this condition is felt to have at least two different etiologies. In patients with underlying thyroid disease, thyrotoxicosis may result from the iodide load, as discussed. There is also some evidence for a direct toxic effect of the amiodarone on thyroid cells, with subsequent release of thyroid hormones (60,62). Like lithium, amiodarone has also been used in the treatment of hyperthyroidism.

Toxic Multinodular Goiter

Although the basic causes of the multinodular goiter remain poorly understood, repeated division of autonomous cells gradually forms areas of hyperplasia that grow until they become clinically apparent, autonomously functioning nodules (63). Although such regions are autonomous, they are usually either insufficiently active—or they receive insufficient iodide—to produce an excess of thyroid hormone. Such so-called warm nodules ordinarily do not cause problems because their oversecretion of hormone is compensated for by decreased production from the remainder of the gland. Generally, the development of hyperthyroidism from such a region of autonomy occurs very slowly, because autonomous tissue is usually less efficient in producing thyroid hormone than normal. Administration of large amounts of iodide (as in x-ray contrast agents or amiodarone) to individuals with autonomous nodules, however, may provide enough substrate to precipitate frank hyperthyroidism.

Clinical features of toxic multinodular goiter that are useful in making the diagnosis include the fact that the disease occurs in an older population than that of Graves' disease, and, perhaps as a consequence, cardiac symptoms tend to be more common. The goiter may be obvious, and palpation of the neck usually reveals the thyroid to be multinodular, but it can be retrosternal, and hyperextension of the neck may be necessary before palpation reveals the enlarged thyroid. A thyroid scan generally provides clear evidence of multiple nodular regions, many with little uptake, but with at least one hot area. Demonstrating that the serum TSH is suppressed provides confirmation that the thyroid is autonomous.

Toxic Adenoma

As with the toxic multinodular goiter, the solitary toxic adenoma occurs more frequently in elderly patients. A solitary toxic nodule is considered a tumor, albeit benign, unlike the hyperfunctioning nodules observed in multinodular goiter. Somatic mutations in the TSH receptor gene (64) or in a G-protein gene (65,66) have been demonstrated to cause constitutive activation of adenylyl cyclase and result in the formation of hyperfunctioning thyroid adenomas in some, but not all, cases. What appears to be a solitary nodule clinically, however, often turns out to be simply a very active nodule in a multinodular goiter when a thyroid scan is performed.

Physical examination generally reveals a single palpable nodule, usually greater than 3 cm in diameter. There is little palpable evidence of the remainder of the gland, because the excessive production of hormone by the nodule shuts off pituitary production of TSH, and the remainder of the gland becomes atrophic. A thyroid scan is useful for confirming these physical findings. If clinical signs of hyperthyroidism are present, but the serum T_4 level is not elevated, a serum T_3 determination is in order, because T_3 toxicosis occurs more commonly in these patients. Formerly, diagnostic attempts were made to suppress the nodule's uptake of radioiodine by administration of exogenous T_3, but, as mentioned, this can exacerbate thyrotoxic symptoms, and it has largely been supplanted by simply determining whether the serum TSH level is suppressed (see Chapters 22 and 27.)

Thyroid Carcinoma

Even though it may be well differentiated histologically, thyroid carcinoma is very inefficient at hormonogenesis. Nonetheless, occasional patients with longstanding follicular carcinoma have developed hyperthyroidism, which has been postulated to result either from the tumor's production of thyroid hormone (67) or from the presence of TSIs, possibly from the tumor's stimulating the autoimmune process (67,68). Obviously, thyroid carcinoma can coexist along with thyrotoxicosis from other causes, but there is no evidence for a direct causal relationship with TSIs, and the incidence of carcinoma is probably similar to that in euthyroid individuals.

Ectopic Hyperthyroidism

Ectopic rests of thyroid tissue can occur in the ovary (struma ovarii) or in dermoid tumors or teratomas. They may show laboratory evidence of increased thyroid function, but evidence that such ectopic tissue is the sole cause of hyperthyroidism has been difficult to obtain (69).

Excessive Thyroid Stimulating Hormone

Pituitary Adenomas

Excessive secretion of TSH from the pituitary is a very rare cause of hyperthyroidism. Thyrotroph adenomas are the least common of the functional pituitary adenomas, and they represent less than 1% of this group (70). A pituitary adenoma, in addition to oversecreting TSH, may also oversecrete growth hormone or prolactin. Such pituitary tumors characteristically also secrete a disproportionately high level of the alpha subunit shared by pituitary glycoprotein hormones, and they may even secrete excess amounts of FSH. Neither the secretion of intact TSH nor of the alpha subunit is consistently responsive to TRH. Pituitary surgery is usually effective therapy.

Nonneoplastic Pituitary Secretion of TSH

Patients with nonneoplastic pituitary secretion of TSH represent an unusual subgroup of the syndrome of thyroid hormone resistance—namely, selective pituitary resistance to thyroid hormone. In this subgroup, most peripheral tissues do respond to the high levels of thyroid hormone produced by the thyroid, resulting in the symptoms of thyrotoxicosis, whereas the pituitary gland is relatively resistant and only shuts off TSH secretion when T_4 is at a hyperthyroid level (71). Unlike the pituitary adenoma that oversecretes TSH, the amount of pituitary alpha subunit secreted in these patients is proportionate to the secretion of TSH. TSH secretion from the pituitary in these cases tends to respond to TRH. There is some overlap with the syndrome of generalized resistance to thyroid hormone, especially in patients with few signs or symptoms of thyrotoxicosis, and these forms of thyroid hormone resistance may belong to the same spectrum of thyroid hormone resistance with variable expression.

Trophoblastic Tumors

Hydatidiform mole, choriocarcinoma, and embryonal carcinoma of the testis can cause hyperthyroidism, due to massive overproduction of human chorionic gonadotropin (hCG) (72). Although hCG has only a small amount of intrinsic thyroid-stimulating activity, if it is present in very high levels, it is sometimes capable of producing hyperthyroidism. Symptoms of hyperthyroidism are usually more subtle than the serum levels of thyroid hormone would suggest, possibly because of the short duration of the disease or the primary manifestations of the tumor.

Pregnancy

Pregnant women with hyperemesis gravidarum have an increased incidence of transient thyrotoxicosis, which appears to be related to higher hCG levels, or to hCG with higher thyroid-stimulating activity, than those pregnant patients without hyperemesis (73,74).

ACKNOWLEDGMENTS

These studies were supported in part by a Buswell Fellowship from the State University of New York at Buffalo (A.L.O.), and by the Office of Research and Development, Department of Veterans Affairs (A.L.O. and S.W.S.)

REFERENCES

1. Palacios A, Cohen MA, Cobbs R. Apathetic hyperthyroidism in middle age. *Int J Psychiatry Med* 1991;21:393–400.
2. Grewal RP. Apathetic hyperthyroidism in an adolescent. *J Psychiatry Neurosci* 1993;18:276.
3. Teelucksingh S, Pendek R, Padfield PL. Apathetic thyrotoxicosis in adolescence. *J Intern Med* 1991;229:543–544.
4. Gelfand RA, Hutchinson-Williams KA, Bonde AA, Castellino P, Sherwin RS. Catabolic effects of thyroid hormone excess: the contribution of adrenergic activity to hypermetabolism and protein breakdown. *Metabolism* 1987;36:562–569.
5. Karlander S-G, Khan A, Wajngot A, Torring O, Vranic M, Efendic S. Glucose turnover in hyperthyroid patients with normal glucose tolerance. *J Clin Endocrinol Metab* 1989;68:780–786.
6. Ahren B. Hyperthyroidism and glucose intolerance. *Acta Med Scand* 1986;220:5–14.
7. Tormey WP, Chambers JPM. Pruritis as the presenting symptom in hyperthyroidism [letter]. *Br J Clin Pract* 1994;48:224.
8. Smith TJ, Bahn RS, Gorman C. Connective tissue, glycosaminoglycans, and diseases of the thyroid. *Endocr Rev* 1989;10:366–391.
9. Weetman AP. Extrathyroidal complications of Graves' disease. *Q J Med* 1993;86:473–477.
10. Fatourechi V, Pajouhi M, Fransway AF. Dermopathy of Graves' disease (pretibial myxedema). Review of 150 cases. *Medicine* 1994;73:1–7.
11. Garnero P, Vassy V, Bertholin A, Riou JP, Delmas PD. Markers of bone turnover in hyperthyroidism and the effects of treatment. *J Clin Endocrinol Metab* 1994;78:955–959.
12. De Menis E, Da Rin G, Roiter I, Legovini P, Foscolo G, Conte N. Bone turnover in overt and subclinical hyperthyroidism due to autonomous thyroid adenoma. *Horm Res* 1992;37:217–220.
13. Wejda B, Hintze G, Katschinski B, Olbricht T, Benker G. Hip fractures and the thyroid: a case-control study. *J Intern Med* 1995;237:241–247.
14. Wakasugi M, Wakao R, Tawata M, et al. Change in bone mineral density in patients with hyperthyroidism after attainment of euthyroidism by dual X-ray absorptiometry. *Thyroid* 1994;4:179–182.
15. Foldes J, Tarjan G, Szathmari M, Varga F, Krasznai I, Horvath C. Bone mineral density in patients with endogenous subclinical hyperthyroidism: is this thyroid status a risk factor for osteoporosis? *Clin Endocrinol* 1993;39:521–527.
16. Rosen CJ, Adler RA. Longitudinal changes in lumbar bone density among thyrotoxic patients after attainment of euthyroidism. *J Clin Endocrinol Metab* 1992;75:1531–1534.
17. Franklyn J, Betteridge J, Holder R, Daykin J, Lilley J, Sheppard M. Bone mineral density in thyroxine treated females with or without a previous history of thyrotoxicosis. *Clin Endocrinol* 1994;41:425–432.
18. Martin WH 3rd, Korte E, Tolley TK, Saffitz JE. Skeletal muscle beta-adrenoceptor distribution and responses to isoproterenol in hyperthyroidism. *Am J Physiol* 1992;262:E504–E510.
19. Olson BR, Klein I, Benner R, Burdett R, Trzepacz P, Levey GS. Hyperthyroid myopathy and the response to treatment. *Thyroid* 1991;1:137–141.
20. Ober KP. Thyrotoxic periodic paralysis in the United States. Report of 7 cases and review of the literature. *Medicine* 1992;71:109–120.
21. Kilpatrick RE, Seiler-Smith S, Levine SN. Thyrotoxic hypokalemic periodic paralysis: report of four cases in black American males. *Thyroid* 1994;4:441–445.
22. Sola J, Pardo-Mindan FJ, Zozaya J, Quiroga J, Sangro B, Prieto J. Liver changes in patients with hyperthyroidism. *Liver* 1991;11:193–197.
23. Massey DG, Becklake MR, McKenzie JM, Bates DV. Circulatory and ventilatory response to exercise in thyrotoxicosis. *N Engl J Med* 1967;276:1104–1112.
24. Small D, Gibbons W, Levy RD, de Lucas P, Gregory W, Cosio MG. Exertional dyspnea and ventilation in hyperthyroidism. *Chest* 1992;101:1263–1273.
25. Siafakas NM, Milona I, Salesiotou V, Filadataki V, Tzanakis N, Bouros D. Respiratory muscle strength in hyperthyroidism before and after treatment. *Am Rev Respir Dis* 1992;146:1025–1029.
26. Hollingsworth HM, Pratter MR, Dubois JM, Braverman LE, Irwin RS. Effect of triiodothyronine-induced thyrotoxicosis on airway hyperresponsiveness. *J Appl Physiol* 1991;71:438–444.
27. Nakazawa T, Kobayashi S. Influence of antithyroidal therapy on asthma symptoms in the patients with both bronchial asthma and hyperthyroidism. *J Asthma* 1991;28:109–116.
28. Klein I, Levey GS. New perspectives on thyroid hormone, catecholamines, and the heart. *Am J Med* 1984;76:167–172.
29. Liggett SB, Shah SD, Cryer PE. Increased fat and skeletal muscle beta-adrenergic receptors but unaltered metabolic and hemodynamic sensitivity to epinephrine in vivo in experimental human thyrotoxicosis. *J Clin Invest* 1989;83:803–809.
30. Martin WH 3d, Spina RJ, Korte E. Effect of hyperthyroidism of short duration on cardiac sensitivity to beta-adrenergic stimulation. *J Am Coll Cardiol* 1992;19:1185–1191.
31. Valcavi R, Menozzi C, Roti E, et al. Sinus node function in hyperthyroid patients. *J Clin Endocrinol Metab* 1992;75:239–242.
32. Mintz G, Pizzarello R, Klein I. Enhanced left ventricular diastolic function in hyperthyroidism: noninvasive assessment and response to treatment. *J Clin Endocrinol Metab* 1991;73:146–150.
33. Forfar JC, Muir AL, Sawers SA, Toft AD. Abnormal left ventricular function in hyperthyroidism: evidence for a possible reversible cardiomyopathy. *N Engl J Med* 1982;307:1165–1170.
34. Wilson BE, Newmark SR. Thyrotoxicosis-induced congestive heart failure in an urban hospital. *Am J Med Sci* 1994;308:344–348.
35. Channick BJ, Adlin EV, Marks AD, et al. Hyperthyroidism and mitral valve prolapse. *N Engl J Med* 1981;305:497–500.
36. Aronow WS. The heart and thyroid disease. *Clin Geriatr Med* 1995;11:219–229.
37. Woeber KA. Thyrotoxicosis and the heart. *N Engl J Med* 1992;327:94–98.
38. Sawin CT, Geller A, Wolf PA, et al. Low serum thyrotropin concentrations as a risk factor for atrial fibrillation in older persons. *N Engl J Med* 1994;331:1249–1252.
39. Giladi M, Aderka D, Zeligman-Melatzki L, Finkelstein A, Ayalon D, Levo Y. Is idiopathic atrial fibrillation caused by occult thyrotoxicosis? A study of one hundred consecutive patients with atrial fibrillation. *Int J Cardiol* 1991;30:309–313.
40. Siebers MJ, Drinka PJ, Vergauwen C. Hyperthyroidism as a cause of atrial fibrillation in long-term care. *Arch Intern Med* 1992;152:2053–2064.
41. Glikson M, Freimark D, Leor R, Shechter M, Kaplinsky E, Rabinowitz B. Unstable anginal syndrome and pulmonary oedema due to thyrotoxicosis. *Postgrad Med J* 1991;67:81–83.

42. Phull PS, Collins CE, Norell MS, Thomas DJ. Variant angina in thyrotoxicosis. *Br J Clin Pract* 1993;47:17–18.
43. Evered DC, Hayter CJ, Surveyor I. Primary polydipsia in thyrotoxicosis. *Metabolism* 1972;21:393–404.
44. Bahn RS, Heufelder AE. Pathogenesis of Graves' ophthalmopathy. *N Engl J Med* 1993;329:1468–1475.
45. Kendler DL, Lippa J, Rootman J. The initial clinical characteristics of Graves' orbitopathy vary with age and sex. *Arch Ophthalmol* 1993;111: 197–201.
46. Perros P, Crombie AL, Matthews JN, Kendall-Taylor P. Age and gender influence the severity of thyroid-associated ophthalmopathy: a study of 101 patients attending a combined thyroid-eye clinic. *Clin Endocrinol* 1993;38:367–372.
47. Krassas GE, Pontikides N, Kaltsas T, Papadopoulou P, Batrinos M. Menstrual disturbances in thyrotoxicosis. *Clin Endocrinol* 1994;40: 641–644.
48. O'Brien IA, Lewin IG, O'Hare JP, Corrall RJ. Reversible male subfertility due to hyperthyroidism. *Br Med J Clin Res Ed* 1982;285:691.
49. Ishihara T, Kurahachi H, Hattori N, et al. Superior vena cava syndrome due to Graves' disease. *Intern Med* 1993;32:80–83.
50. Figge J, Leinung M, Goodman AD, et al. The clinical evaluation of patients with subclinical hyperthyroidism and free triiodothyronine (free T_3) toxicosis. *Am J Med* 1994;96:229–234.
51. Jackson RS, Jewkes R, Carter GD, Alaghband-Zadeh J. Are patients with low serum thyroid stimulating hormone and normal total thyroxine hyperthyroid? Usefulness of 99mTc pertechnetate uptake. *Ann Clin Biochem* 1991;28(4):331–334.
52. Sawin CT, Geller A, Kaplan MM, Bacharach P, Wilson PWF, Hershman JM. Low serum thyrotropin (thyroid-stimulating hormone) in older persons without hyperthyroidism. *Arch Intern Med* 1991;151:165–168.
53. Drinka PJ, Siebers M, Voeks SK. Poor positive predictive value of low sensitive thyrotropin assay levels for hyperthyroidism in nursing home residents. *South Med J* 1993;86:1004–1007.
54. Sundbeck G, Jagenburg R, Johansson PM, Eden S, Lindstedt G. Clinical significance of low serum thyrotropin concentration by chemiluminometric assay in 85-year-old women and men. *Arch Intern Med* 1991;151:549–556.
55. Mariotti S, Martino E, Cupini C, et al. Low serum thyroglobulin as a clue to the diagnosis of thyrotoxicosis factitia. *N Engl J Med* 1982;307: 410–412.
56. Eliason BC, Doenier JA, Nuhlicek DN. Desiccated thyroid in a nutritional supplement. *J Fam Pract* 1994;38:287–288.
57. Hedberg CW, Fishbein DB, Janssen RS, et al. An outbreak of thyrotoxicosis caused by the consumption of bovine thyroid gland in ground beef. *N Engl J Med* 1987;316:993–998.
58. Bouillon R, Verresen L, Staels F, Bex M, De Vos P, De Roo M. The measurement of fecal thyroxine in the diagnosis of thyrotoxicosis factitia. *Thyroid* 1993;3:101–103.
59. Martin FI, Tress BW, Colman PG, Deam DR. Iodine-induced hyperthyroidism due to nonionic contrast radiography in the elderly. *Am J Med* 1993;95:78–82.
60. Unger J, Lambert M, Jonckheer MH, Denayer P. Amiodarone and the thyroid: pharmacological, toxic, and therapeutic effects. *J Intern Med* 1993;233:435–443.
61. Barclay ML, Brownlie BE, Turner JG, Wells JE. Lithium associated thyrotoxicosis: a report of 14 cases, with statistical analysis of incidence. *Clin Endocrinol* 1994;40:759–764.
62. Bartalena L, Grasso L, Brogioni S, Aghini-Lombardi F, Braverman LE, Martin E. Serum interleukin-6 in amiodarone-induced thyrotoxicosis. *J Clin Endocrinol Metab* 1994;78:423–427.
63. Peter HJ, Gerber H, Studer H, Smeds S. Pathogenesis of heterogeneity in human multinodular goiter. *J Clin Invest* 1985;76:1992–2002.
64. Parma J, Duprez L, Van Sande J, et al. Somatic mutations in the thyrotropin receptor gene cause hyperfunctioning thyroid adenomas. *Nature* 1993;365:603–604.
65. Lyons J, Landis CA, Harsh G, et al. Two G protein oncogenes in human endocrine tumors. *Science* 1990;249:655–659.
66. Weinstein LS, Shenker A, Gejman PV, Merino MJ, Friedman E, Spiegel AM. Activating mutations of the stimulatory G protein in the McCune-Albright syndrome. *N Engl J Med* 1991;325:1688–1695.
67. Kasagi K, Takeuchi R, Miyamoto S, et al. Metastatic thyroid cancer presenting as thyrotoxicosis: report of three cases. *Clin Endocrinol* 1994;40:429–434.
68. Steffensen FH, Aunsholt NA. Hyperthyroidism associated with metastatic thyroid carcinoma. *Clin Endocrinol* 1994;41:685–687.
69. Kempers RD, Dockerty MB, Hoffman DL, Bartholomew LG. Struma ovarii-ascitic, hyperthyroid and asymptomatic syndromes. *Ann Intern Med* 1970;72:883–893.
70. Beckers A, Abs R, Mahler C, et al. Thyrotropin-secreting pituitary adenomas: report of seven cases. *J Clin Endocrinol Metab* 1991;72: 477–483.
71. Beck-Peccoz P, Forloni F, Cortelazzi D, et al. Pituitary resistance to thyroid hormone [review]. *Horm Res* 1992;38:66–72.
72. Giralt SA, Dexeus F, Amato R, Sella A, Logothetis C. Hyperthyroidism in men with germ cell tumors and high levels of beta-human chorionic gonadotropin. *Cancer* 1992;69:1286–1290.
73. Goodwin TM, Montoro M, Mestman JH, Pekary AE, Hershman JM. The role of chorionic gonadotropin in transient hyperthyroidism of hyperemesis gravidarum. *J Clin Endocrinol Metab* 1992;75:1333–1337.
74. Kimura M, Amino N, Tamaki H, et al. Gestational thyrotoxicosis and hyperemesis gravidarum: possible role of hCG with higher stimulating activity. *Clin Endocrinol* 1993;38:345–350.

CHAPTER 15

Medical Management of Hyperthyroidism: Theoretical and Practical Aspects

Jeffrey I. Mechanick and Terry F. Davies

There are many strategies to treat the diverse clinical scenarios of hyperthyroidism, and a wide array of medical protocols in the clinician's armamentarium. The common thread in medical management should always be the specific treatment of the underlying pathophysiology. National and international therapeutic variability stems from physicians' subtle preferences, as well as impressions concerning patient needs. These include future childbearing, surgical risk, compliance, appearance, allergies, diet, and other medical problems and associated drugs. This point is particularly borne out in the 1984 (1) and 1987 (2) surveys of the American Thyroid Association and the 1986 survey of the European Thyroid Association (3), in which there are geographic, temporal, and physician-to-physician differences in the approach to treating hyperthyroid Graves' disease (Fig. 1). Fortunately, hyperthyroidism is easily treatable and nearly always curable.

In this chapter, we will discuss only medical modalities for the treatment of hyperthyroidism. In the first section, various drugs with antithyroid activity will be discussed. Then, diverse hyperthyroid conditions and special considerations will be presented. Tables 1 and 2 are lists of the drugs used in various hyperthyroid conditions. Multiple approaches to each hyperthyroid condition will be described to provide the flexibility needed to treat each patient individually.

Since the first edition of this textbook, significant advances in the medical treatment of hyperthyroidism have occurred. These include controlled, prospective trials involving the block-replace method (see later) of using thionamides and thyroxine in the treatment of Graves' disease, and early intervention in the treatment of sub-clinical hyperthyroidism that predisposes the elderly to atrial tachyarrhythmias. In addition, granulocyte-colony stimulating factor has been used as a remedy for thionamide-induced bone marrow aplasia, and ultrasonography has been introduced to guide percutaneous intranodular ethanol injection for the treatment of nodular hyperthyroidism.

DRUG PROFILES

The Thionamides

Structure

Thionamides commonly refer to a class of structures capable of inhibiting thyroid hormone synthesis. They have in common a thiocarbamide backbone incorporated in a six-membered heterocyclic ring termed a thioureylene (Fig. 2). The two principal drugs used in the United States are propylthiouracil (6-n-propyl-2-thiouracil, PTU) and methimazole (1-methyl-2-mercaptoimidazole, MMI). Methimazole is also the active metabolite of carbimazole, a thionamide used in Europe. After Mackenzie et al. (4,5), Richter and Clisby (6,7), and Kennedy (8) described thiourea derivatives as being goitrogenic, Astwood tested hundreds of related agents in rats (9) and in humans (10) and found thiourea and thiouracil to be the most promising. In 1945, Gabrilove et al. (11) studied the effects of thiouracil at Mount Sinai Hospital on 51 patients with hyperthyroidism. Thirty-three patients responded to therapy, but in 11 patients severe toxic reactions developed (six with agranulocytosis), necessitating discontinuation of thiourea. The high frequency of agranulocytosis (12) prompted development and acceptance of PTU, which had a better side-effect profile and improved potency (13). In

---

J. I. Mechanick and T. F. Davies: Department of Medicine, Division of Endocrinology, The Mount Sinai School of Medicine, New York, New York 10029.

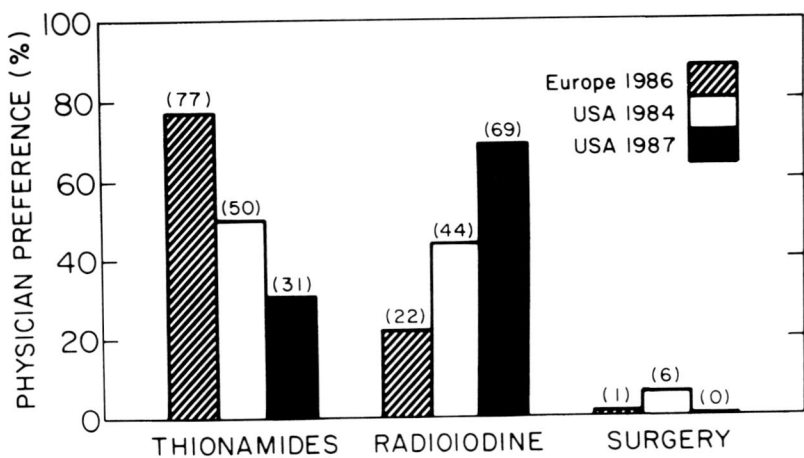

FIG. 1. Physician preferences for primary therapy of hyperthyroidism. (Data from refs. 1, 2, 3.)

an attempt to elucidate the relationship between drug structure and antithyroid activity, Jambut-Absil et al. (14) found that among various drugs containing nitrogen-carbon-sulfur groups, the Kc (electron-donating ability to form a charge-transfer complex with iodine) correlated with antithyroid activity.

Action

Intrathyroidal

Thionamides affect the thyroid epithelial cell organification process, coupling reaction, thyroglobulin immunoreactivity, local immunoregulatory mechanisms, and thyroidal cell growth (Fig. 3); there are no demonstrable effects on iodide uptake or hormonal release.

TABLE 1. *Some therapeutic agents used in hyperthyroidism*

Drug	Usual starting dose
Propylthiouracil (PTU)	200 mg po tid
Methimazole (MMI)	20 mg po bid
Propranolol	10–40 mg po qid
Saturated solution of potassium iodide (SSKI)	1–2 gtts po qd-tid
Compound solution of iodine (Lugol's solution)	2–5 gtts po qd-tid
Dexamethasone	2 mg po qid
Prednisone	40–60 mg po qd
Ipodate	1 g po qd
Lithium	300–450 mg po tid
Perchlorate	1 g po qd
Cholestyramine	2–4 g po bid–qid
Colestipol	5 g po 1–5 times a day
Octreotide	50–100 µg sq bid–tid
Diltiazem	120 mg po tid

po, by mouth; sq, subcutaneously; gtts, drops; bid, twice a day; tid, three times a day; qid, four times a day; qd, every day.

The thionamides inhibit iodination of tyrosine residues on the thyroglobulin molecule by interacting with the enzyme thyroid peroxidase (TPO). Specifically, the drugs inhibit initial TPO-mediated iodine oxidation and subsequent thyroglobulin iodination. MMI has been found to act as a potent free-radical scavenger (hydroxyl and iodine) (15). TPO inactivation may be reversible or irreversible, depending on the ratio of intrathyroidal drug to iodine concentrations (16–18). Irreversible TPO inactivation principally occurs in iodide-deficient states. On the other hand, when iodine levels are sufficient, a TPO intermediate is generated that iodinates and oxidizes the thionamide, although eventually TPO and iodide are regenerated (18). In this case, iodide is diverted from normal thyroglobulin iodination, yielding reduced synthesis of thyroid hormone. For a review of this mechanism, see Taurog et al. (19).

It is of interest that one *in vitro* study found that MMI irreversibly inhibits TPO, whereas PTU has a reversible effect (20). In addition, elevated intrathyroidal concentrations of thionamides inhibit their own metabolism or turnover (16). The duality of drug turnover and peroxidase inactivation pathways has been supported by the studies of Doerge (21).

Propylthiouracil exerts its inhibitory effects on organification within 4 hr and is dose dependent (22). Following a 100-mg dose of PTU, there is 72% inhibition of organification within 7 hr in euthyroid patients, and within 8 hr in hyperthyroid patients (23). Furthermore, serum PTU levels of 3 µg/mL or greater 4 hr after ingestion are associated with at least a 50% perchlorate-dischargeable iodine-123 (^{123}I) level (22). Although just 0.5 mg of MMI can inhibit organification, 10 to 25 mg is required to extend this effect for 24 hr (24). Following a 10 mg dose of MMI, there is 90% inhibition of organification within 12 hr in euthyroid patients, and within 8 hr in 8 of 11 hyperthyroid patients (23).

Thionamides may also inhibit the TPO-mediated coupling reaction and directly alter thyroglobulin structure

TABLE 2. *Matrix of hyperthyroid conditions and medical interventions discussed in this chapter*

Condition	Thionamides	β-Blockers	Stable iodine	Steroids	Ipodate	Lithium	Perchlorate	Bile-acid sequestrant
Graves' disease	+	+	+	+	+	+	−	+
Toxic nodular goiter	+	+	−	+	−	+	−	+
T_3 toxicosis	+	+	−	+	−	+	−	+
Trophoblastic disease	+	+	+	+	+	+	−	+
Thyroiditis[a]	−	+	−	+	−	−	−	+
Inappropriate TSH[b]	−	+	−	−	−	−	−	+
Postpartum thyroiditis	−	+	−	−	−	−	−	+
Thyrocardiac disease[c]	+	+	+	+	+	+	−	+
Accelerated hyperthyroidism	+	+	+	+	+	+	−	+
Iodine-induced hyperthyroidism	+	+	−	+	−	−	+	+
Factitious	−	+	−	−	−	−	−	+
Rare causes	+	+	−	+	−	−	−	+
Adjuvant therapy with RAI or surgery	+	+	+	+	+	+	−	+

[a] May also use salicylates or nonsteroidal anti-inflammatory drugs.
[b] May also use bromocriptine, pergolide, octreotide, T_3, TRIAC, or D-thyroxine.
[c] May also use calcium channel antagonists, digoxin, diuretics, and/or anticoagulants.
TSH, thyroid stimulating hormone; RAI, radioactive iodine.

(25–27). According to the model of Courtin et al. (28), there are four forms of TPO, depending on oxidation state and distribution of oxidizing equivalents: native, compound I, compound II, and compound III. Theoretically, compound I (two oxidized equivalents more than native peroxidase) catalyzes iodine oxidation and thyroglobulin iodination, and compound II (also with two oxidized equivalents but with a different distribution not requiring iodine binding) catalyzes the coupling reaction and production of thyroxine (28). Compound III is produced in conditions of hydrogen peroxide excess and is inactive; its formation is thought to be inhibited by iodine (28). This model is supported by the studies of Engler et al. (25), in which thionamides exhibit independent inhibition of the coupling reaction and the iodination reaction. Furthermore, because the coupling reaction appears to be more sensitive to thionamides, it is concluded that compound II is more sensitive to these drugs than compound I (25).

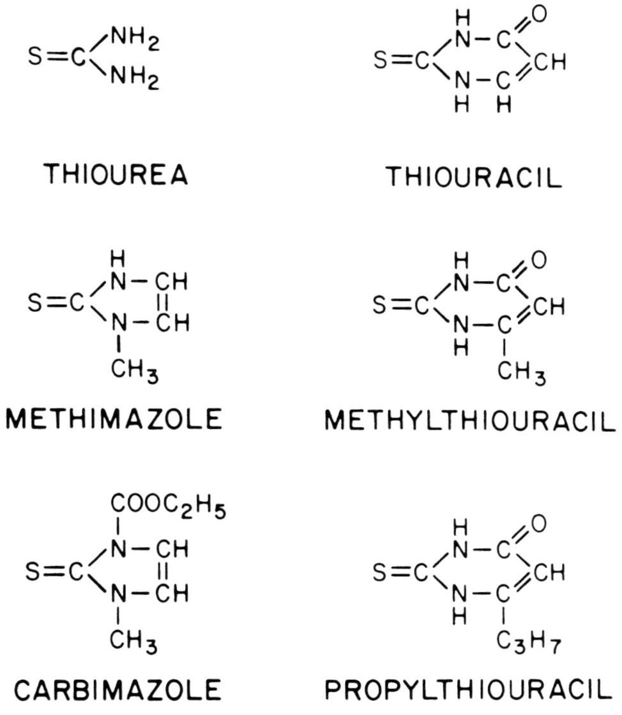

The third locus of intrathyroidal thionamide action is a direct alteration of the structure of thyroglobulin. Papapetrou et al. (26) demonstrated covalent binding of PTU to thyroglobulin; this effect was inhibited by iodine. The effects of thionamides were further described by Monaco et al. (27) as possibly impairing amino acid incorporation into the polypeptide backbone and attachment of necessary oligosaccharide chains. Alternatively, thionamides may alter the immunogenicity of the thyroglobulin molecule via inhibition of iodide organification (29). For a detailed and comprehensive review of thyroid hormone formation, see Nunez and Pommier (30).

The fourth locus of thionamide action is alteration of intrathyroidal immunoregulatory mechanisms that are central to the etiology of autoimmune thyroid disease. Because the relapse rate in hyperthyroid Graves' disease after thionamide therapy alone (30% to 60%) (31–35) is less than the relapse rate observed during treatment with beta-blockers alone (70%) (36), it is likely that thionamides affect the underlying pathophysiology in Graves' disease. The influence of thionamides on the immune system was first suspected in 1967 when Michie et al.

FIG. 2. Thionamide drug structures.

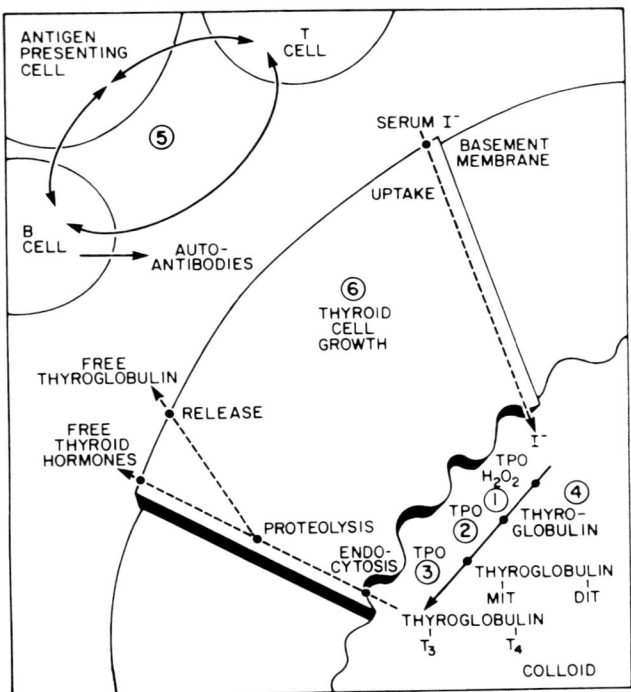

FIG. 3. Spectrum of action of thionamides. Key: (1) iodine oxidation; (2) thyroglobulin iodination; (3) coupling reaction; (4) thyroglobulin immunoreactivity; (5) local immunoregulation; and (6) thyroidal cell growth. TPO, thyroid peroxidase; MIT, monoiodotyrosine; DIT, diiodotyrosine.

(37) described reduction in thymic size following thionamide therapy. Since then, many studies have demonstrated a variety of effects of PTU and MMI on the immune system (Table 3).

We will examine the effects of thionamides on the immune system in terms of *in vitro* data, animal model data, and human data. *In vitro*, thionamides have been reported to decrease or impair thyroidal autoantibody secretion (38), [^{3}H]thymidine incorporation into lymphocytes (39), mitogenic activation of lymphocyte immunoglobulin production (40), antigen handling by primed accessory cells (41), antibody-dependent cell-mediated cytotoxicity (42), and elaboration of markers of T-cell activation [human leukocyte antigen (HLA-DR), gamma-interferon, and interleukin-2 receptors] (43). Thionamides have also been reported to increase T-suppressor-cell activity (44).

In the murine thyroiditis model (A/J mice immunized with heterologous human thyroglobulin), Davies et al. (45) observed decreased mononuclear thyroidal infiltration, follicular destruction, and splenic immune responses with MMI, although the circulating and intrathyroidally deposited antihuman thyroglobulin antibody was unchanged. Rennie et al. (46) also found that MMI reduced the degree of experimental autoimmune thyroiditis and circulating autoantibodies in the rat. However, addition of thyroxine abolished this effect. Because the *in vitro* studies mentioned used MMI at concentrations of approximately 10^{-4} M, unlikely to be maintained peripherally in tissues that do not concentrate thionamides, the effects of MMI *in vivo* are restricted to intrathyroidal immunosuppression rather than generalized immunosuppression. In clinical practice, it is likely that these intrathyroidal concentrations are achieved, because peak serum levels with standard doses are on the order of 10^{-6} M and thyroid to serum (T:S) concentration ratios range from 1.2 to 20 (4 to 8 hr after a 10-mg MMI dose or a 100-mg PTU dose in hyperthyroid patients) (47). This generates an average total intrathyroidal concentration in the 10^{-5} M range. Because there is heterogeneity of thyroid cell activity, higher intrathyroidal thionamide concentrations would occur.

Clinically, patients undergoing thionamide therapy may experience declines in thyroid autoantibodies. This effect was first described by Pinchera et al. (48) and later confirmed by others (38,49). Markers of infiltrating T-cell activation, such as HLA-DR antigen, gamma-interferon, and interleukin-2 receptors, are also reduced with thionamide therapy (50,51). In contrast to the *in vitro* findings mentioned, no effect on circulating T suppressor cells was noted after a 3- to 6-month course of carbimazole therapy (52). Generally, the thyroid-stimulating immunoglobulin response to thionamides is variable, may in part be idiosyncratic, and may also predict the eventual response to therapy (53).

Three theories have surfaced to explain these findings. The first asserts that there is a direct action of thion-

TABLE 3. *Reported effects of the thionamides on the immune system*

In vitro effects
Decreased [^{3}H]thymidine incorporation into lymphocytes
Decreased total immunoglobulin and antithyroid antibody secretion
Inhibition of mitogen-induced antithyroid antibody production
Impaired handling of antigens by primed accessory cells
Decreased antibody-dependent, cell-mediated cytotoxicity
Decreased markers of lymphocyte activation (HLA-DR, gamma-interferon, and interleukin-2 receptors)
In vivo effects
Antigen-induced murine thyroiditis
Decreased mononuclear thyroidal infiltration
Decreased follicular destruction
Decreased splenic immune response
Antigen-induced rat thyroiditis
Decreased thyroiditis
Decreased autoantibody
Human data
Induction of remission of autoimmune disease
Decreased antithyroid antibodies
Reduced lymphocytic infiltration
Decreased markers of lymphocyte activation
Transient rise in T-helper cells

amides on antibody-dependent cellular cytotoxicity. This is based on observations that killer (K) and natural killer (NK) lymphocyte populations decrease with thionamide treatment (42,54). However, a direct causal association is unlikely, because PTU and MMI are concentrated by peroxidase-containing cells and K and NK cells do not have peroxidase (55–57), and because Weetman et al. (58) found no in vitro effect of MMI on NK or K function.

The second theory (38,41,59–64) asserts that thionamides interfere with antigen handling by antigen-presenting cells (APC), macrophages, and monocytes. APCs are responsible for presenting antigen to local (intrathyroidal) T lymphocytes stimulating T and B cell differentiation and antithyroid antibody production. Moreover, APCs are peroxidase-positive, and it is postulated that interference with H_2O_2 generation (a scavenger effect) disrupts the requisite respiratory burst responsible for monokine generation.

A third possible mechanism is that suppression of the immune system caused by thionamides is the result of a primary modulation of thyroidal cell activity (65,66). According to this model, thionamides decrease (normalize) thyroidal production of thyroid hormone and thyroidal antigens as described. This interrupts the following sequence of events found in Graves' disease: (a) unregulated stimulation of thyroidal activity by anti-thyroid-stimulating-hormone-receptor antibody (TSHR-Ab), (b) enhanced production of thyroidal antigens and thyroid hormone, (c) thyroid hormone suppression of suppressor T cells, (d) enhanced T helper cell activity because of previous step [(c)] and because of stimulation by increased thyroidal antigens, (e) stimulation of B lymphocytes to produce more TSHR-Ab, and (f) increased gamma-interferon production by T helper cells (which increases HLA-DR expression, further stimulating T helper cells). In this model, there is no major immunosuppressive effect of thionamides on APCs or lymphocytes themselves.

This theory is supported by the findings of Romaldini et al. (67), in which disappearance of anti-TPO antibodies and TSHR-Abs paralleled attainment of the euthyroid state and not thionamide drug administration. However, this theory is not supported by the observation that both PTU and MMI inhibited lectin-induced major histocompatibility complex (MHC) class II (HLA-DR) antigen expression in crude human thyroid monolayer preparations (including lymphocytes) but had no effect on direct gamma-interferon induction of class II antigens in similar cell preparations (68). Lectin must have been acting via the lymphocytes themselves, which were inhibited by thionamides.

Thionamides may indirectly affect total thyroidal hormone production by influencing thyroidal cell growth. In the cloned normal rat thyroid cell line (FRTL-5), MMI inhibited insulin-like growth factor–induced cell growth that is not dependent on cyclic adenosine 3′,5′-cyclic monophosphate (cAMP) generation (69). In contrast, MMI did not inhibit TSH-induced, cAMP-dependent thyroid cell growth in this in vitro system (69).

Extrathyroidal

Because 70% to 90% of the daily production rate of the active thyroid hormone, triiodothyronine (T_3), originates from peripheral deiodination of serum thyroxine (T_4), interference with this mechanism would be desirable when treating hyperthyroid conditions. PTU, but not MMI, exerts noncompetitive inhibition of the type I 5′-monodeiodination enzyme found in liver, kidney, brain, and pituitary gland, but it does not affect the type II deiodinase found in brown adipose tissue, brain, and pituitary gland (70–73). Hypothyroid patients on replacement thyroxine therapy demonstrate a 25% to 30% reduction in serum T_3 with high doses of PTU, 750 to 1000 mg/day (71,72). In rat liver homogenates, PTU concentrations of 900 ng/mL (5.3×10^{-6} M) produced a 50% reduction in deiodinase activity (73). However, in euthyroid volunteers, therapeutic doses of PTU do not have a statistically significant effect on serum T_3 levels. On the other hand, after a single oral dose of PTU, a serum T_3 reduction occurs in hyperthyroid patients that is not dose dependent (Table 4) (22). After 5 days of therapy in hyperthyroid patients with PTU (750–900 mg/day) or MMI (60–90 mg/day), with or without iodide, there was a greater decrease in serum T_3 in the PTU groups compared to the MMI groups (74). This extrathyroical action of PTU is shared by various thyroid hormone analogs, of which reverse T_3 (rT_3) is the most potent (about 100 times more than PTU) (73). Theoretically, the inhibition of peripheral deiodinase activity by PTU should render hyperthyroid patients euthyroid earlier than that by MMI. However, in most instances this does not appear to be an important advantage, because it applies to large doses of the drug. PTU does not affect thyroid hormone membrane transport, binding to thyroxine-binding globulin or transthyretin (thyroxine-binding prealbumin), or nuclear or mitochondrial binding.

Clinical Pharmacokinetics

Propylthiouracil

Propylthiouracil is rapidly absorbed from the digestive system and appears in the blood within 20 to 30 min (24). Like other thioureas, PTU has a bioavailability of 80% to

TABLE 4. Effects of different doses of propylthiouracil (PTU) on 5′-monodeiodinase activity in hyperthyroid patients

PTU dose (mg)	Serum PTU level (µg/mL)	Serum T_3 reduction (%)
50	1.04	24
200	4.50	39
300	7.10	28

From ref. 22.

95% (75). Following a 300-mg dose, radioimmunoassayable PTU levels peak at 4.0 μg/mL in euthyroid patients and 7.1 μg/mL in hyperthyroid patients (Fig. 4) (22). The volume of distribution is 30 liters and it is 80% protein-bound in the serum. Because of its very low lipid solubility, there is low placental transfer and excretion into milk (Fig. 5). The serum half-life is 1 to 2 hr in young and old euthyroid and hyperthyroid patients (75,76) but 8.5 hr in patients with renal failure (77). This is because the majority of PTU, like MMI, is excreted in the urine, with only 3% excreted in the stool (78). By 24 hr, 83% of PTU is excreted in the urine as five sulfur-containing compounds: 61% as glucuronic acid, 0.5% to 5.7% as unchanged PTU, 8.1% to 8.9% as inorganic sulfur, and 7.7% to 10.9% as two minor metabolites (23). A double-antibody radioimmunoassay is available to monitor therapy (22).

Methimazole

Following a 30-mg dose of MMI, peak serum levels are 0.65 and 0.78 μg/mL in euthyroid and hyperthyroid patients, respectively (see Fig. 4), and approximately 1.31 μg/mL in patients with hepatic cirrhosis (78). MMI is lipid soluble with a volume of distribution of 40 liters and greater placental transfer and excretion into milk compared with PTU (see Fig. 5) (76). In fact, 8 hr after a 40-mg dose of MMI, there is a serum to milk ratio of 1.03 and a total of 70 μg of MMI in the milk (78). The half-life of MMI in euthyroid and hyperthyroid patients is 3 to 6 hr, but in hepatic cirrhosis it is 21.2 hr (75,78). By 48 hr, 63% to 72% of MMI is excreted into the urine as four sulfur-containing urinary compounds: 7.1% as unchanged MMI, 47% as an unknown major polar metabolite, 6.3% as inorganic sulfur, and 1.5% as a minor unknown metabolite (23). A double-antibody radioimmunoassay is also available to monitor MMI therapy (78).

General Remarks

Pharmacokinetic studies of thionamides support the concept of a two-compartment model with a rapid distribution phase and a slow elimination phase (23). Several factors influence the accumulation and oxidation of thionamides in the thyroid gland. A low dose of iodide increases accumulation and oxidation of MMI, whereas an iodine-deficient diet decreases it (23). The effects of iodide may be explained by its inhibition of organification (the Wolff-Chaikoff effect), decreased thyroid hormone secretion, and resultant increased TSH secretion (79). In fact, TSH and thyroid-stimulating autoantibodies enhance MMI and PTU accumulation but not oxidation (23). Doses of perchlorate and iodide that inhibit trapping decrease PTU accumulation by 30% (23). Thyroxine decreases MMI and PTU accumulation (and oxidation of MMI but not PTU) by inhibiting TSH secretion (23).

Thionamides gain entry into the thyroid gland via two mechanisms. At low concentrations, they are primarily transported by an active, saturable, TSH-regulated system (47). At higher concentrations, this system is saturated and the drugs passively diffuse into the thyroid cell (47). Accumulation of these drugs is dose dependent, with a plateau of unmetabolized intrathyroidal MMI concentrations occurring after three to four doses at 8-hr intervals (23). Intrathyroidal concentrations in hyperthyroid patients 8 hr after a 10-mg MMI dose or a 100-mg PTU dose are 0.74 μg/g tissue and 12.5 μg/g tissue, respectively (47).

Although there have been conflicting reports concerning changes in the half-life with and without hyperthy-

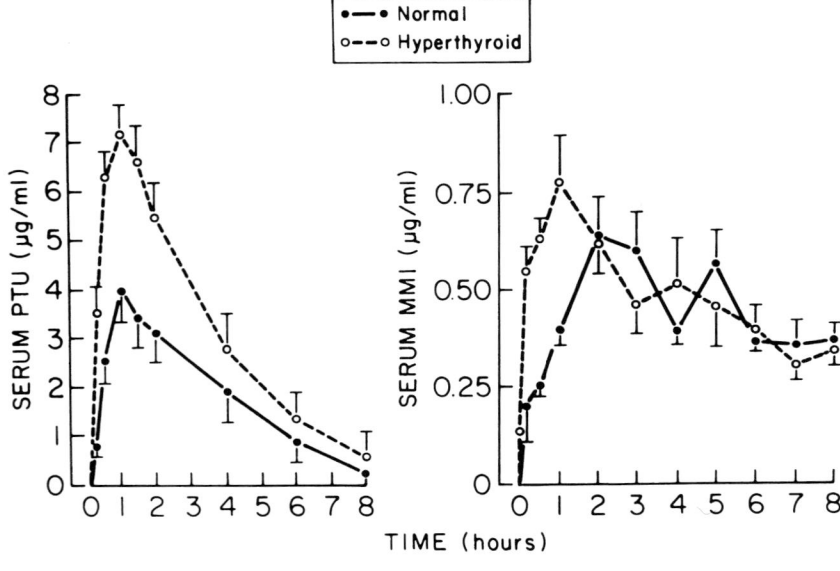

FIG. 4. Serum levels of PTU and MMI in normal and hyperthyroid patients after a 300-mg oral dose of PTU or a 30-mg oral dose of MMI. (From refs. 22, 78.)

TABLE 6. *Some comparisons between propylthiouracil and methimazole*

Parameter	Propylthiouracil	Methimazole
Average starting dose	200 mg po tid	20 mg po bid
Average maintenance dose	100–200 mg po tid	10–20 mg qd
Once-a-day dosing	Possible	Yes
Absorption/bioavailability	Rapid	Rapid
Serum half-life (hr)	1–2	3–6
Peak serum levels (μg/mL)	1–4	0.5–1.5
Thyroid/serum concentrations after 8 hr (dosage)	18.2 (100 mg po)	3.4 (10 mg po)
Intrathyroid levels (μg/g whole tissue) after 8 hr (dosage)	12.5 (100 mg po)	0.7 (10 mg po)
Placental tissue and milk excretion	Minimal	Significant
Organification inhibition after 8 hr (dosage)	60% (100 mg po)	90% (10 mg po)
Inhibition of deiodinase	Yes	No
Evidence for immunosuppression	Yes	Yes
Excretory route	Urine	Urine
Radioimmunoassay available	Yes	Yes
Toxicity		
Overall (%)	5	5
Granulocytopenia (%)	0.5	0.5
Dose-related	No	Yes

Adrenergic Antagonists

Actions

Antiadrenergic

Although reserpine (105) and guanethidine (106) have been used to treat hyperthyroidism, the principal adrenergic antagonist presently used is propranolol. This drug is generally prescribed for symptomatic relief of thyrotoxic symptoms (e.g., palpitations and tremor) despite a lack of significant action on thyroid function (107). Accordingly, propranolol does not replace primary therapy for thyrotoxicosis, such as thionamides, radioiodine, or surgery (108–110).

The utility of propranolol is historically based on the demonstration of enhanced sensitivity to catecholamines in the hyperthyroid state, which is lessened by adrenergic blocking agents (111–115). Specifically, propranolol, through blocking sympathetic action at the receptor level, would be expected to normalize the hyperadrenergic signs and symptoms associated with the thyrotoxic state. Even though there is increased beta-adrenergic receptor density in rat myocardium during experimental hyperthyroidism (116) and ostensible improvements in various cardiovascular parameters (heart rate, oxygen consumption, and myocardial contractility and efficiency) with propranolol therapy (117,118), other reports have failed to show any enhanced adrenergic sensitivity, adrenomedullary activity, or serum catecholamine levels with thyrotoxicosis (119–123). Forfar et al. (124) found similar nyctohemeral variations in heart rate, hemodynamic responses to exercise, and hemodynamic responses to propranolol in hyperthyroid and euthyroid patients. This supports the contention that there is no adrenergic cardiovascular hypersensitivity in hyperthyroidism and that it is the direct effects of thyroid hormone on the heart (inotropic and chronotropic) (125) that resets myocardial function at a higher level. Propranolol acts by inhibiting native sympathetic tone on the heart and peripheral tissues, eventually unmasking pure thyroid hormone effects. The possibility exists, nevertheless, that excessive thyroid hormone somehow modulates adrenergic action. Nonspecific findings, thought to result from adrenergic hyperactivity, such as tremor, palpitations, amenorrhea, stare, lid lag, and anxiety, may also improve with beta-blockade (126).

Effect on Thyroid Hormone Metabolism

Another possible action of propranolol is the inhibition of peripheral T_4 conversion to the active hormone T_3 (127,128). This activity would contribute to amelioration of hyperthyroid signs and symptoms beyond direct sympathetic blockade. Beta-adrenergic blockers inhibit hepatic microsomal 5'-deiodinase (propranolol, alprenolol, and the β_1-selective blockers atenolol and metoprolol) (129,130) and 5-deiodinase (only the β_1-selective blockers) (129). Variations in beta-blocker activity can be accounted for by fluctuations in serum levels of short-acting preparations (131) compared to longer-acting preparations (132) in patients with thyrotoxicosis. Nadolol, a long-acting, nonselective beta-blocker, has been reported to lower free T_4 and free T_3 levels (133).

Miscellaneous Actions

Additional effects of beta-blockers in hyperthyroidism include improvement in nitrogen balance (134), correction of associated hypercalcemia (135), reversal of associated bulbar dysfunction and proximal myopathy (136, 137), and relief of periodic paralysis (138).

Dosing and Special Precautions

When doses of 40 to 120 mg are given every 8 hr, a response to propranolol frequently occurs within 48 hr (108). The usual starting dose in mild hyperthyroidism is 20 mg qid and in moderate to severe hyperthyroidism, 40 mg qid. The dose is titrated to achieve a heart rate in the range of 70 to 80 beats per min.

Using beta-blockers becomes a problem when relative contraindications exist, such as congestive heart failure, bronchospastic disease, and diabetes mellitus. In congestive heart failure with thyrotoxicosis, a short-acting beta-blocker, such as esmolol, can be used with appropriate monitoring (telemetry or intensive care unit) depending on the severity and nature of the heart disease. Care should be given to withdraw the beta-blocker gradually when ischemic heart disease is present (128,139). When the history or physical examination is suggestive of bronchospastic disease, a β_1-cardioselective agent is preferable. Beta-blockers should not be withheld because of coexisting diabetes mellitus (insulin or noninsulin requiring); rather, careful observations must be made to monitor for and avoid symptomatically masked hypoglycemia.

Summary

Beta-blockers are ideal agents for early-phase therapy along with thionamides to initiate control of thyrotoxic symptoms prior to maintenance with thionamides, radioactive iodine therapy, or surgery. The various structures, side effect profiles, and pharmacology of the many antiadrenergic agents are beyond the scope of this section.

Iodides (Stable Iodine ^{127}I) Actions

The role of iodine as specific treatment for thyroid disease was introduced by Coindet in 1820 (140). In 1821, Coindet discovered that iodine could also precipitate thyrotoxicosis (141). Iodine-induced hyperthyroidism in patients with preexistent endemic goiter with autonomous nodular elements was first termed "Jod-Basedow" by Kocher in 1910 (142). Modern therapy with iodine was inspired by the report by Plummer in 1923 that preoperative treatment with iodine prevented thyrotoxic crises in patients with Graves' disease (143). Subsequently, large doses of iodine (10 drops/day of Lugol's solution) (144) were used to manage hyperthyroidism. In 1925, Kimball (144) studied 2659 patients with hyperthyroidism and found that prescribed iodine was the precipitating factor in 12%. Consequently, Kimball recommended a maximal iodine dosage for goiter in adults of 10 mg/day for less than a month. In 1930, Thompson et al. (145–147) demonstrated a dose-dependent reduction in maximal basal metabolic rate following iodine. They found the minimum adequate dose for reduction to be one drop (6 mg iodine) per day. The onset of action was 1 to 4 days. For details of the quantitative kinetics of the exchangeable thyroidal pool of organic iodine, and trapping and binding functions of the thyroid gland, see the early works of Quimby et al. (148) and Berson and Yalow (149,150).

By the 1940s, iodide was known to exert a number of effects on thyroidal activity. Specifically, in glands hyperplastic because of endemic iodine deficiency, physiologic amounts of iodide increased total thyroidal iodine content and normalized thyroid hormone secretion (151). In normal glands, prolonged pharmacologic amounts of iodide ingestion mimicked thionamides and gave rise to a hypothyroid state (151). In patients with hyperthyroid Graves' disease, iodides decreased thyroid function, but in patients with nodular goiter, iodides often induced hyperthyroidism (Jod-Basedow phenomenon) (151).

In 1944, Morton et al. (152) demonstrated the inhibitory effects of iodide on thyroid biosynthesis *in vitro*. Subsequently, the classic studies of Wolff and Chaikoff in 1948 (153,154) showed that large doses of iodide reversibly inhibited organification in the rat independent of the trapping apparatus. They hypothesized that this homeostatic mechanism prevents wasteful hormone production when the body is suddenly flooded with iodine. This finding was soon confirmed by Stanley (155) in humans. The Wolff-Chaikoff effect is thought to depend on high intrathyroidal free iodide concentrations (156,157), which create a thyroperoxidase–iodide complex incapable of organification and coupling.

Adequate short-term iodide prevents hormonogenesis, yet chronic administration may either produce hypothyroidism or fail to control thyrotoxicosis. By 1949, Wolff et al. (151) found that when iodides are given at inhibitory concentrations for a prolonged period of time, hormonogenesis resumes despite the high serum iodide levels. This "escape" from the Wolff-Chaikoff effect was later shown to be caused by an intrinsic, qualitative change in thyroidal function resulting in diminished iodide trapping, and it may be mediated by an iodinated organic inhibitor of iodine transport (158–160). Iodide autoregulation involves adenylate cyclase–cyclic AMP dependent and independent systems that control intrathyroidal glucose, amino acid, and phosphate transport (161). Decreased trapping would theoretically decrease intrathyroidal free iodide concentrations and disinhibit organification. Other conditions harboring organification defects, potentially enhanced by iodides, include radioiodine therapy (162–165), Hashimoto's thyroiditis (166), and Graves' disease (151). In the radioiodinated, Hashimoto's, and Graves' disease glands, escape may not occur at all, producing a hypothyroid state.

Besides affecting organification steps, iodides influence other aspects of thyroidal function (Table 7). In pa-

TABLE 7. *Spectrum of action of iodides*

Trapping
   Inhibition with prolonged exposure
Organification
   Inhibition (Wolff-Chaikoff effect)
   Escape from inhibition with prolonged exposure
Release
   Inhibition of TSH action on adenyl cyclase
   Inhibition of TSH-mediated thyroglobulin endocytosis
   Escape from inhibition of release with prolonged exposure
Growth
   Inhibition of proliferation
   Inhibition of gamma-IFN-induced MHC class II expression
   Direct cytotoxicity

tients with Graves' disease whose thyrotoxicosis responds to iodides, the effect is faster than that observed with thionamides alone. Iodides have been found to have a rapid inhibitory action on the release of thyroid hormones, possibly mediated through adenyl cyclase or interference with TSH-controlled proteolytic breakdown of thyroglobulin to its active form and subsequent endocytosis (167–169). This early effect is considerable in hyperthyroid patients but may be much more subtle in normal individuals.

The effect of iodides on synthesis and release of thyroid hormones is clinically significant in the thyrotoxic patient, with overt improvement within days. For example, by 4 days, the serum T_4 reduces by 50% on 90 mg/day (169), and by 4 to 11 days, the serum T_3 reduces by 47% on 150 mg/day (170). Escape from the inhibitory effect on release in 3 to 4 weeks is reflected by relapse in patients despite continued therapy (171). This may occur as intrathyroidal iodine accumulation promotes enhanced total thyroid hormone secretion despite continued reduction in the fractional secretion rate.

Other actions of iodides include a concentration-dependent inhibition on cellular growth and cyclic AMP production stimulated by TSH (172). Iodide has also been found to inhibit gamma-interferon induction of MHC class II antigen expression in proliferating rat cells (68). Last, and perhaps most important, iodide may initiate induction of autoimmune thyroiditis in genetically susceptible individuals by conferring immunogenicity to thyroglobulin, and/or via direct cytotoxicity resulting in an inflammatory response (173,173a).

Pharmacokinetics and Dosing

Following ingestion, iodine is reduced to iodide and then rapidly absorbed and trapped by the thyroid gland (174). Iodide is concentrated, to a lesser degree, in certain specialized tissues, such as uterine cervix, gastric parietal cells, breast, ova, and salivary glands. These lesser pools turn over more quickly than the thyroid gland and are partly in equilibrium with serum levels (83). Iodide is also rapidly excreted by the kidneys, and minimally in feces, sweat, and milk. The serum half-life of plasma iodide is 8 hr (83).

The daily iodine requirement is only 75 to 200 μg and is slightly increased with pregnancy to 250 μg (174). Iodine may be administered therapeutically in liquid form as saturated solution of potassium iodide (SSKI) or Lugol's solution (compound solution of iodine). The dose is diluted in 50 to 100 mL of water just prior to ingestion. One mL of SSKI contains 760 mg of iodine and 1 mL of Lugol's solution contains 125 mg of iodine. Moreover, 1 drop of SSKI equals 6 drops of Lugol's solution or the equivalent of 38 mg of iodine (the total body content is 20 to 50 mg) (174). Alternatively, iodide may be administered in solid form as sodium iodide (crystals, granules, or powder) or potassium iodide (300-mg tablets), or as an intravenous infusion of sodium iodide (100 mg/mL in 10-mL vials or 200 mg/mL in 20-mL vials). The advantages of the liquid form are that appropriately small doses in the range of 10 mg/day may be given easily, and SSKI and Lugol's solution are readily available in most pharmacies. However, oral liquid iodine has a poor taste, even when diluted with juice instead of water; for this reason, tablets are preferable. Unfortunately, low-dose tablet preparations are not widely available.

Side Effects

Toxicity of iodine may be either dependent or independent of thyroidal function. Thyroid-dependent iodide toxicity is indicated by iodide-induced hyperthyroidism, increased relapse rate in Graves' disease treated with thionamides (175,176), and precipitation of hypothyroidism in susceptible patients.

Reactions independent of thyroid metabolism include acute hypersensitivity reactions (angioedema, hemorrhagic skin lesions, and serum sickness) and chronic reactions (iodism) that are dose dependent and reversible with discontinuation of the iodide [brassy taste, burning mouth with parotid and salivary gland swelling and increased salivation, rhinitis, conjunctivitis, headache, cough, gastritis, bloody diarrhea, anorexia, depression, mild acneiform skin lesions, and, rarely, severely bizarre eruptions (iododerma)]. If chronic reactions are severe, renal iodide excretion may by increased by measures that promote chloride excretion, such as salt-loading or administration of loop or osmotic diuretics.

Summary

Iodides may be used in the following circumstances to control thyroid hormone excess: (a) preparation for thyroidectomy, (b) in combination with thionamides in early-phase medical treatment for severe thyrotoxicosis (174), (c) after radioactive iodine therapy, and (d) in patients allergic to thionamides.

Corticosteroids

Action

Corticosteroids have a wide spectrum of immunosuppressive actions and beneficial effects on hyperthyroidism (178–180). In patients with Graves' hyperthyroidism, administration of dexamethasone produces a rapid fall in serum T_3 and a rise in serum rT_3 (Fig. 6) (181–184). This suggests an inhibition of peripheral monodeiodination. Because dexamethasone also produces a fall in serum T_4, there may be decreased thyroidal hormone synthesis as well (182). In addition, agents with mineralocorticoid activity are capable of expanding the plasma volume sufficiently to reduce serum thyroid hormone concentrations. In light of the fact that corticosteroids can depress antibody production, it is reasonable to conclude that TSHR-Ab production in Graves' disease is affected. Five Graves' patients treated only with prednisone all experienced remissions, becoming clinically and chemically euthyroid (185). In addition to diminution in thyroidal size, these patients exhibited an interesting change in serum thyroxine binding distribution. Their thyroxine-binding globulin (TBG)-bound T_4 decreased, whereas transthyretin (thyroxine-binding prealbumin)-bound T_4 increased, compared to controls. The mechanism of this binding alteration is unknown. The indication for corticosteroid use in hyperthyroidism is limited to situations where rapid control is required.

Side Effects

The untoward reactions associated with corticosteroid use are manifold and will be discussed briefly here with regard to short-term therapy (less than a week or two). Patients treated with dexamethasone or prednisone for early-phase management of hyperthyroidism may develop dyspepsia or mild-to-severe behavioral disturbances. Antacids or H_2-receptor blockers may be given to patients complaining of epigastric discomfort. If acute behavioral changes occur, the drug should be stopped. Prednisone may rarely induce a hypokalemic alkalosis and edema. If this occurs, supplemental potassium should be prescribed. Hyperthyroid patients with severe congestive heart failure should not be treated with high doses of prednisone. Last, a noninsulin-dependent diabetic state may be unmasked with corticosteroid use. This side effect is not a contraindication to continue the steroid and, if refractory to dietary control, subcutaneous insulin should be used.

Summary

Corticosteroids are a useful adjunct in early-phase therapy to control severe accelerated hyperthyroidism. Their use is limited to a brief course, usually not exceeding 1 or 2 weeks. Corticosteroids are also useful in the management of painful subacute thyroiditis. The structure and pharmacokinetics of steroids are beyond the scope of this section.

Oral Cholecystographic Agents

Structure

The first report, in 1976, of gallbladder dyes (iopanoic acid, Telepaque) reducing serum T_3 levels introduced these agents as potential drugs for treating thyrotoxicosis (185). Iopanoic acid is a benzene ring substituted with an amino group, an isovaleric acid side chain, and three iodine atoms, and it superficially resembles thyroxine (Fig. 7). Ipodate and tyropanoate are related iodinated contrast agents shown to have antithyroid activity. Ipodate is the more potent; 63% of ipodate by weight is iodine.

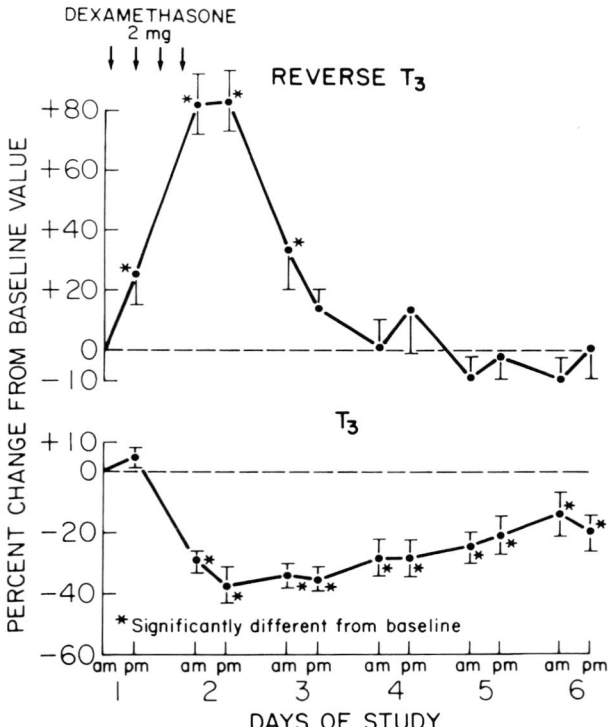

FIG. 6. Effects of dexamethasone on triiodothyronine (T_3) and reverse T_3 (rT_3) in hyperthyroid Graves' disease. Data are expressed as percent change from the baseline. Twice daily samples were obtained at 9 AM and 5 PM. Baseline T_3 = 94.4 ng/dL, and baseline rT_3 = 622 ng/dL. (From ref. 182.)

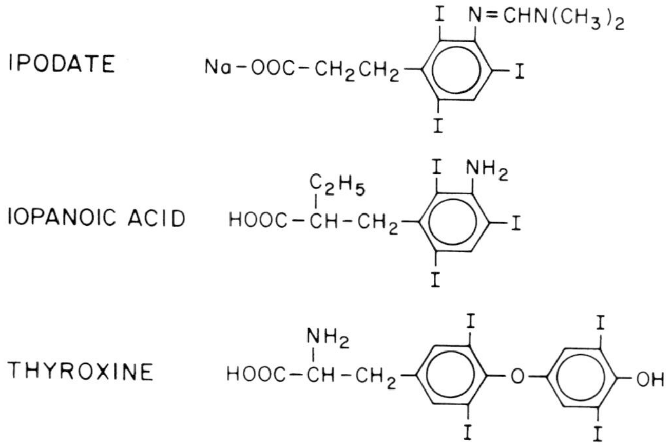

IPODATE   Na-OOC-CH₂CH₂—⟨phenyl with I, I, N=CHN(CH₃)₂⟩

IOPANOIC ACID   HOOC-CH(C₂H₅)-CH₂—⟨phenyl with I, I, NH₂⟩

THYROXINE   HOOC-CH(NH₂)-CH₂—⟨phenyl with I, I⟩-O-⟨phenyl with I, I, OH⟩

FIG. 7. Structure of thyroxine and two iodinated cholecystographic dyes used to treat hyperthyroidism.

Action and Pharmacokinetics

Since 1976, several studies have confirmed that ipodate produces decreased serum T_3 and increased rT_3 (186). The effects on T_4, however, depend on thyroid function: T_4 levels are increased in patients on supplemental thyroid hormone therapy and in euthyroid patients, and they are decreased in hyperthyroid patients (187). From these early studies, it was reasoned that ipodate acts to inhibit peripheral monodeiodinase activity and to block thyroid hormone release. The latter action is due to iodine liberated from metabolized ipodate. In addition, ipodate may affect cellular T_3 transport and nuclear binding (188).

The time course of ipodate action is impressive when compared to the effects of corticosteroids or stable iodine on serum T_3 and T_4. Whether it is administered as a single dose of 0.5, 1, or 3 g, or as 3-g doses given every 3 days, the serum T_3 is reduced by 50% to 62% in 24 hr (187,189–191). Following a 3-g dose, a 30% reduction in T_3 is seen in only 6 hr (184). This is comparable to the 65% reduction in 24 hr in serum T_3 with large and repeated doses of SSKI, PTU, and dexamethasone (192). In Graves' disease, the serum T_4 level is reduced 20% in 24 hr and is normal at 10 weeks with ipodate, 500 mg/day (191). Clinically, the Graves' disease patients studied displayed increases in body weight and reductions in heart rate and blood pressure with ipodate (189).

When regimens of PTU and propranolol with and without ipodate are compared, the ipodate regimen produces greater reductions in serum T_3 levels (193). Moreover, when ipodate alone is compared with PTU alone, reductions in heart rate and blood pressure are seen earlier with ipodate (190). A direct comparison between ipodate and stable iodine therapy was made by Roti et al. (Fig. 8) (194). Although ipodate clearly reduced serum T_3 earlier and to a greater degree (75% by day 5 for ipodate, compared to 64% by day 9 for iodine), a marked rebound effect in serum T_4 (23%) and T_3 (50%) was noted with ipodate but not iodine (194). This same rebound phenomenon was also observed for thyroxine levels using tyropanoate (195). The radioactive iodine uptake may normalize 7 days after discontinuation of ipodate therapy (500 mg/day) (191).

There are certain advantages to using ipodate and thionamides together. First, their effects on peripheral deiodination are thought to be additive, as PTU is a noncompetitive inhibitor and ipodate is a competitive inhibitor of 5'-monodeiodinase (196,197). Second, the effects of thionamides on thyroid hormone synthesis and immunomodulation in Graves' disease would complement the effects of ipodate. Even though thionamide therapy might prevent the rebound effect after ipodate use, the probability of eventual recurrence of Graves' disease, after thionamide and ipodate therapy, may be increased. This is because ipodate is associated with increased adipose iodine stores up to 1 year after use (198), and a high iodine intake has been linked to recurrence of Graves' disease after thionamide treatment. Therefore, although ipodate may be considered for short-term therapy to treat acute thyrotoxicosis, it is not indicated for use in long-term management of hyperthyroidism. Relapse of Graves' disease is frequent with long-term sodium ipodate therapy (199). A case of hyperthyroid Graves' disease has been reported to be resistant to thionamides after a 9-week course of ipodate (200). This observation

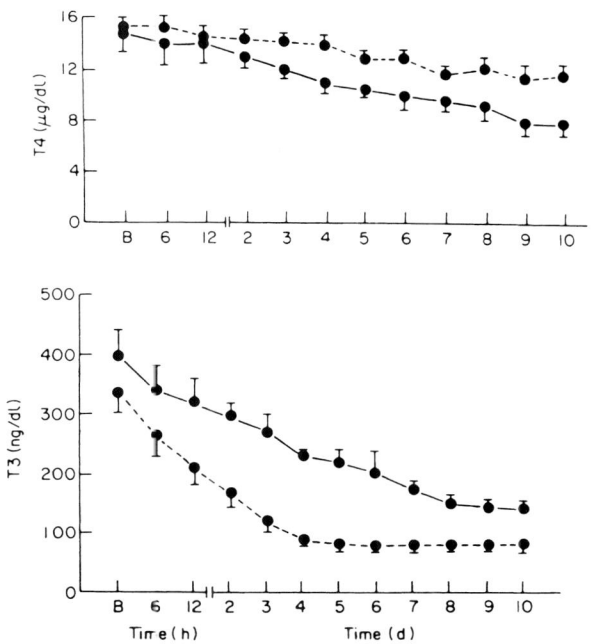

FIG. 8. Comparison of the effects of ipodate (• – – – •) and iodide (• ----- •) on serum T_3 and T_4 levels in patients with hyperthyroid Graves' disease. (From ref. 194.)

may be related to the aforementioned rebound effect or a subclinical Jod-Basedow phenomenon.

Side Effects

Ipodate is a safe therapeutic agent; no serious toxicity has been reported thus far. Side effects may include nausea, vomiting, and transient diarrhea (201). Theoretically, relinquished iodine from metabolized ipodate might precipitate a Jod-Basedow phenomenon.

Summary

In short, ipodate may be a suitable agent for early-phase treatment of thyrotoxicosis and as preparation for subtotal thyroidectomy, because of its rapid onset of action. Although it is effective as adjunctive therapy with thionamides and before treatment with radioiodine, judicious use should be exercised in light of adverse effects caused by serum T_3 rebound, potential thionamide resistance, and prolonged iodine storage in adipose tissue.

Lithium

Action

Although lithium has been employed as treatment for bipolar disorders since 1949 (202), it was not recognized as specific therapy for thyrotoxicosis until 1968 when Schou et al. (203) reported goiters in patients treated with lithium for 5 months to 2 years. The use of lithium has found a small niche in the armamentarium to combat hyperthyroidism, as an alternative to iodide therapy. It has a rapid action and, unlike iodides, does not preclude early radioiodine therapy once patients are rendered euthyroid. The chief action of lithium is inhibition of T_4 release (204–206).

The site of lithium action, like iodide action, appears to be suppression of TSH-stimulated cyclic AMP production and at a step beyond cAMP production (207). Lithium, like iodide, affects colloidal droplet formation and thyroglobulin hydrolysis in response to TSH and cyclic AMP (205). When serum lithium levels are maintained at 0.5 to 1.0 mEq/L (with a usual dose of 900 to 1500 mg/day), there is a 30% to 85% reduction in thyroidal iodide secretion by 12 hr (204); this compares to a 73% reduction after iodine administration (169). In a study of patients with Graves' disease treated with a 6-month course of lithium, euthyroidism was achieved in 8 of 11 patients by 2 weeks and was associated with a 35% reduction in the serum T_4 and T_3 (208). Even though no escape was noted in this study by 6 months, 7 of the 8 responders relapsed 1 to 4 weeks after discontinuation of treatment. Escape from lithium may occur in a similar manner to that of iodides, whereby intrathyroidal iodide accumulation overcomes the block and increases the total thyroid hormone secretory rate. Thionamides prevent eventual escape from lithium by preventing new thyroid hormone synthesis. The effect on thyroid hormone release by lithium is synergistic to iodide and not dependent on intrathyroidal iodine accumulation (209,210).

Pharmacokinetics and Dosing

Lithium is rapidly absorbed from the digestive tract and reaches peak levels by 4 hr with a serum half-life of 24 to 36 hr (83). Because lithium toxicity is dose dependent, a three-times-a-day regimen is preferred, despite its long half-life, to produce a relatively even serum plateau without toxic peaks (83). In the kidney, lithium undergoes about 80% resorption, mainly in the proximal tubule. Once lithium therapy is initiated (300–450 mg tid), levels must be meticulously monitored and maintained in a therapeutic range of 0.5 to 1.5 mEq/L, and lower (0.1 to 0.5 mEq/L) in persons over 60 years old.

Side Effects

Perhaps the best explanation for the relatively infrequent use of lithium as a major therapeutic modality in the treatment of hyperthyroidism is its side-effect profile (Table 8). Toxicity is clearly related to serum concentration and may occur with prerenal conditions that enhance proximal-tubular sodium resorption. Common side effects at therapeutic levels include malaise, nausea with rare vomiting, anorexia, and diarrhea in about a third to a half of patients (208). Other side effects are abdominal pain, weakness, fatigue, tremor, thirst, polyuria, leukocytosis, and flattened T waves on the electrocardiogram (EKG) (204). Rarely, toxicity is manifested at therapeutic levels by rash, alopecia, psychosis, seizure, nephrogenic diabetes insipidus, edema, and leg ulcers (204). Additional toxicity associated with levels above 2.0 mEq/L include stupor or coma, hypertonia and ataxia, dysarthria, focal neurologic deficits, proteinuria, and azotemia (204). Cardiac manifestations of lithium toxicity are ventricular arrhythmias and atrioventricular conduction delays. In addition, lithium therapy has been associated with progression of orbitopathy requiring surgical decompression, and lithium withdrawal induced a dramatic improvement of the exophthalmos (211). Hyperthyroidism itself has also been associated with lithium use and may result from the appearance of TSHR-Ab in susceptible individuals (212,213).

Lithium intoxication may be treated with an osmotic diuresis and intravenous sodium bicarbonate infusion, providing renal function is adequate. If toxicity is severe,

TABLE 8. *Side effects of lithium*

Side effects at therapeutic levels
Common
Nausea
Diarrhea
Anorexia
Malaise
Occasional
Polyuria
Abdominal pain
Fatigue
Thirst
Leukocytosis
Weakness
Tremor
Flattened T waves on EKG
Rare
Vomiting
Seizure
Rash
Psychosis
Leg ulcers
Alopecia
Arrhythmia
Nephrogenic diabetes insipidus
Hypercalcemia
Edema
Orbitopathy
Hypothyroidism
Hyperthyroidism
Side effects at toxic levels (>2.0 mEq/L)
Stupor
Hypertonia
Dysarthria
Proteinuria
Coma
Ataxia
Focal neurologic deficits
Azotemia

dialysis must be considered, although recovery will still be slow after reduction of serum lithium levels because of delayed reduction in intracellular ion concentration. Amiloride or thiazide diuretics may correct the nephrogenic diabetes insipidus.

Summary

Lithium may be employed as an adjunct to thionamides and steroids for rapid control of thyrotoxicosis (such as before surgery or in the presence of associated cardiac disease) when the patient has a history of untoward iodine reactions or when early radioiodine therapy is desired. There is no change in the 24-hr radioiodine uptake after a week of lithium therapy, 400 mg/day, and the retention of a standard dose of iodine-131 (^{131}I) is increased (214). Other advantages of lithium over iodine are the absence of Jod-Basedow phenomenon with nodular goiter and possibly a delayed escape. These advantages must be carefully weighed against the risks of toxicity.

Perchlorate

A discussion of perchlorate is included for historical interest only, because it is rarely recommended today as specific treatment for hyperthyroidism, with the possible exception of amiodarone-induced hyperthyroidism. The perchlorate discharge test is occasionally employed to assess organification defects, which may result from either inborn enzymatic defects or acquired disorders, such as autoimmune disease or treatment with thionamides, stable iodine, or radioactive iodine.

From the mid 1930s to the mid 1950s, various anionic substances were investigated for antithyroid activity (215–218). Perchlorate was found to be the most potent agent studied, preventing thyroidal iodide uptake, prompting rapid release of trapped iodide, and decreasing intrathyroidal iodide (218,219). Its effects in patients with Graves' disease were encouraging, resulting in normalization of the basal metabolic rate and protein-bound iodine within 2 to 8 weeks (220). Although perchlorate was effective, inexpensive, and initially thought to be safe, many reports of toxicity surfaced. At first, gastric irritation and hypersensitivity reactions consisting of rash, fever, sore throat, and lymphadenopathy were found (221). However, in the early 1960s, several reports of fatal aplastic anemia appeared, and larger studies, revealing an overall frequency of toxicity in the range of 2% to 18%, with 3% fatalities, dissuaded routine use of perchlorate as specific treatment for hyperthyroidism (222–225).

Other Drugs

Salicylates and nonsteroidal anti-inflammatory drugs are useful in treating thyroiditis. Dopamine receptor agonists (pergolide and bromocriptine), octreotide, and 3,5,3′-triiodothyroacetic acid (TRIAC) are used as treatment for TSH-dependent hyperthyroidism. Calcium channel blockers, digoxin, diuretics, and anticoagulants may be employed to manage thyrotoxic heart disease. Bile acid sequestrants, such as cholestyramine or colestipol, bind thyroxine in the gastrointestinal tract and are useful in the management of factitious and iatrogenic hyperthyroidism (Fig. 9) (226). Furthermore, in 15 patients with thyrotoxicosis (14 with Graves' and one with toxic nodule), a more rapid decline in thyroid hormone levels was seen with 2 weeks of treatment with cholestyramine, 4 g po qid, with individualized MMI dosing and propranolol 50 mg qid compared to the same regimen but without cholestyramine (227). Bile salt sequestrants are safe and may be added to any regimen to manage hyperthyroidism, provided the patient can tolerate medicine by mouth or via an enteric tube.

Summary of Drug Actions

The overactive thyroid cell can be inhibited at a variety of steps beginning with iodine uptake, subsequently in-

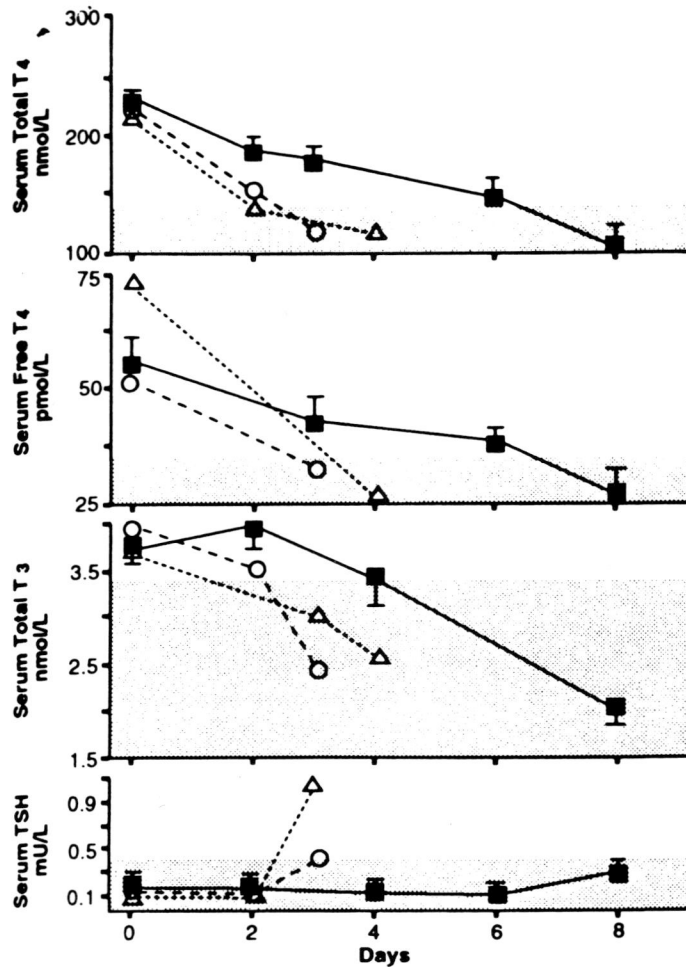

FIG. 9. Changes in thyroid function tests with cholestyramine, 4 gm qid, in two patients with iatrogenic hyperthyroidism (○——○; △——△) and three control patients (■——■). (From ref. 226.)

volving iodine activation, iodination, coupling, and thyroglobulin release, and culminating with the metabolism and action of thyroid hormones on peripheral tissue (Fig. 10). In the next two sections, regimens that exploit these vulnerable stages are constructed to treat the many distinct hyperthyroid diseases.

WHOM TO TREAT AND WHEN

Hyperthyroid Graves' Disease

Selection of Treatment Modality

There are three principal modalities for managing the thyrotoxic state. The options are medical therapy (most commonly with the thionamides) and destructive therapy, with either radioactive iodine (RAI) or subtotal thyroidectomy. Each of these choices has advantages and disadvantages. Ultimately, the decision is based on the particular patient and the medical support services available. Factors that impact on this decision are availability of an experienced thyroid surgeon, potential patient compliance and accessibility, risk–benefit analysis, particular medical/immunologic/nutritional conditions, socioeconomics and cost, dietary iodine, patient preferences, and physician experience and bias. Each modality is relatively safe and effective, so management of Graves' disease will continue to vary from physician to physician (see Fig.1).

Medical therapy for Graves' disease may be considered as (a) early-phase therapy for short-term control prior to definitive treatment with surgery or RAI, (b) primary therapy with only thionamides for 6 to 24 months, or (c) maintenance therapy with thionamides for long-term control.

Early-phase medical therapy is recommended in all cases of hyperthyroidism. Thionamides should be the mainstay of this approach unless previous toxicity has been demonstrated, in which case adjunctive therapy with iodine, steroids, propranolol, and/or ipodate may be used. Initial medical treatment is continued until the patient is rendered euthyroid (usually 1 to 6 weeks depending on severity and agents used). This approach affords the most rapid response and permits adequate time to fully discuss plans for definitive therapy with the patient.

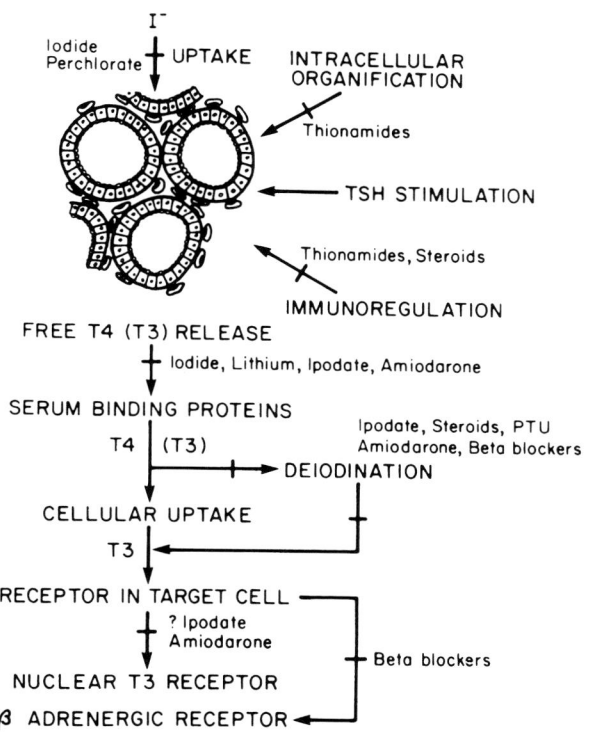

FIG. 10. Sites of action of various antithyroid drugs.

Advantages of thionamide use for primary therapy over RAI and surgery include lack of thyroidal destruction, a high response rate during treatment, and low cost. The principal disadvantages are the high relapse rate (30% to 60%) (31–35), variable degrees of compliance, and adverse reactions. The high relapse rate with thionamides must be weighed against the frequency of hypothyroidism following RAI therapy (90% or more) and surgery (20% to 50%) (34,228,229), as well as the uncommon anesthesia and surgical risks.

A theoretical disadvantage of destructive therapy using surgery or RAI is the reported increased risk of posttreatment orbitopathy or worsening of existing orbitopathy. This is a subject of great debate and several recent reports have supported this association. Tallstedt et al. (230) found that orbitopathy developed or worsened in 10% of patients treated medically, 16% treated surgically, and 33% treated with RAI. These results are supported by additional reports that RAI is causally associated with orbitopathy and dermopathy (231,232). Furthermore, thyroid carcinoma has been linked to radioactive iodine therapy for Graves' disease, although this association is outside most physicians' experience. This relationship remains to be clarified and is quite rare (0.17%) (233,234). The aggressive nature of these cancers is controversial.

Three significant surveys of thyroidologists have been conducted to examine trends and preferences in treating young Graves' disease patients (see Fig. 1) (1–3). The basic cases were a 29-year-old woman with a 70-g goiter, and a 43-year-old mother of two with a 40-g goiter with "moderate" hyperthyroidism (1–3). In these basic cases, Europeans clearly favor thionamides over RAI as primary therapy. Interestingly, American thyroidologists are divided, although there is a distinct preference for RAI over thionamides in the 1987 survey. There was a general international consensus that surgery had only a limited role in the primary treatment of Graves' disease unless the goiter was very large.

The decision to continue long-term treatment with thionamides depends on the absence of significant risk factors. Indicators associated with a high relapse rate on thionamides include large goiter; severe or long duration of symptoms; ophthalmopathy; high T_3 to T_4 ratio [greater than 20 (235,236)]; elevated and/or unaffected serum thyroglobulin level (237,238); early-phase (20 min or 4 hr) T_3-suppressed RAI uptake greater than 8% or 12%, respectively (239–243), or a 24-hr T_3-suppressed RAI uptake greater than 20% (244–246); suppressed supersensitive TSH levels (247); increased CD4 to CD8 ratios [greater than 2.5 (248,249)]; peripheral lymphocyte count less than 3000/mm^3; and demonstrable autoantibodies to the TSH receptor (53,250–255). In fact, Kawai et al. (256) showed that remission rates among patients with Graves' disease and (a) undetectable TSHR-Ab throughout MMI therapy, (b) TSHR-Ab levels that become detectable with MMI therapy, and (c) TSHR-Ab levels that were detectable pre-therapy and remained detectable throughout MMI therapy, were 77.4%, 36.4%, and 36.5%, respectively. The demonstration by bioassay of blocking, rather than stimulating, TSHR-Ab may portend eventual hypothyroidism after treatment for Graves' disease (250).

We do not consider all these parameters relevant to the decision to continue thionamide treatment. However, we do recommend obtaining a TSHR-Ab level at the time of diagnosis and, if previously positive, at the conclusion of the thionamide trial. Laboratory testing for stimulating antibodies is unnecessary in the setting of ostensible hyperthyroidism, because the patient serves as the bioassay. Therefore, we do not recommend the use of this test except in pregnant patients who have had destructive therapy for Graves' disease, in order to predict neonatal thyroid function.

Overall, we recommend a 6- to 24-month trial of thionamides in Graves' disease in all children and adults, particularly those with eye signs, except in cases of disfiguring goiter, suspicious thyroid lesions, advanced age, or the presence of severe medical illness such as cardiac, renal, or hepatic disease. Our rationale is based on a priority given to safety and a bias that thionamides theoretically have a salutary effect on the immune system and possibly offer control over the autoimmune response. We emphasize that the risks and benefits of the three treatment options ought to be thoroughly discussed with the patient and family to assess any special preferences or needs that may have impact on the decision.

Selection of Medical Agents and Dosing Strategies

There is no standard treatment protocol for thionamides. The physician first decides whether the thionamide used will be PTU or MMI; second, whether or not to use adjunctive therapy with beta-blockers, steroids, iodine, or ipodate; third, what dose should be initially implemented and how to adjust dosage thereafter; and finally, how long to treat.

The advantages and disadvantages of PTU and MMI have been discussed. PTU may be more suitable for cases of severe hyperthyroidism because of its inhibition of 5'-monodeiodinase activity. Theoretically, MMI is preferred in cases where compliance is a potential problem because of its longer half-life and greater potency. Both agents have been investigated with regard to once-a-day dosing and long versus short duration of treatment, and MMI appears to be more effective in this regard.

To critically review the extant literature on dosage and duration of therapy, it is necessary to emphasize the variability in experimental designs among the various studies. Even in the best controlled protocols, it is virtually impossible to assess the effects of the natural history of Graves' disease on treated subjects. That is, untreated or propranolol-treated Graves' disease patients exhibit spontaneous exacerbations and remissions that cannot always be predicted (109). Remission rates generally refer to attainment of the euthyroid state with ongoing treatment. Cure refers to persisting remission after discontinuation of the drug within the particular study follow-up period. Relapse refers to recurrence of the hyperthyroid state after remission and discontinuation of the drug; early relapse (within 3 to 6 months) is a "true" relapse, whereas late relapse (after 6 months) may reflect a natural exacerbation (239). Even though parameters of disease activity are available (e.g., TSHR-Ab titers), their measurements are often lacking in the early literature.

There are two issues to be considered for thionamide doses: high versus low dose, and single versus multiple daily doses. Because high, rather than low, doses of PTU (900–1200 mg/day compared to 300–600 mg/day) or MMI (40–80 mg/day compared to 10 mg/day) purportedly reach levels necessary for immunosuppression (22,81,257,258), clinical trials were undertaken to determine if relapse rates would be affected. Several trials have demonstrated greater effectiveness in controlling hyperthyroidism with higher doses compared to conventional doses (259–261).

When a decision is made to treat with sustained high-dose thionamides, supplemental T_4 or T_3 must be given to prevent iatrogenic hypothyroidism ("block-replace" therapy). Several single-arm prospective studies demonstrate comparable relapse rates with block-replace therapy compared to historical controls (53,242,262–266). Other controlled, prospective clinical studies have investigated the specific effect of combined T_4 and thionamides with mixed results. In 1983, Romaldini et al. (259) found that higher doses of thionamide with T_3 resulted in lower relapse rates (24.6%) than in patients treated with thionamides alone (58.4%; $p<0.001$). Hashizume et al. (266) and Kuo et al. (267) reported lower TSHR-Ab following MMI plus T_4 compared to MMI alone. This result was confirmed by Weetman et al. (268) after 6- and 12-month treatment intervals. In another single-arm study using daily MMI (20 mg) plus T_4 (75 µg), 19 of 28 patients (67.8%) treated were still in remission after 2 years, with lower TSHR-Ab levels and smaller thyroid glands than those not in remission (269).

Edmonds and Tellez (270) studied patients for 24 months and failed to demonstrate any difference in relapse rates. A 40-mg, compared with a 10-mg, daily MMI dosing schedule rendered more hyperthyroid patients euthyroid within the first 6 weeks of treatment but was associated with an increased rate of adverse effects without higher remission rates at 1 year (271). Similar findings were observed by Iriarte et al. (272), who found that combined therapy was associated with a lower recurrence rate at 1 year but no difference at 3 years. The only prognostic factor in this study was the size of the initial goiter: 100% of the patients who had had large thyroid glands had recurrences. Furthermore, Tamai et al. (273) studied randomly selected patients with Graves' disease treated with MMI plus T_4, versus MMI alone, and found no significant difference in TSHR-Ab titers after 2 years or recurrence after 3 years. In a study by McIver et al. (273a), recurrence of hyperthyroidism was not delayed or prevented, nor were TSHR-Ab levels significantly reduced, in patients treated with carbimazole and T_4 titrated to an undetectable TSH level, compared with patients treated with carbimazole alone titrated to a normal TSH level.

Taken together, these results indicate that high-dose thionamide therapy with simultaneous T_4 replacement may decrease TSHR-Ab more than thionamides alone, but by 1 to 2 years, TSHR-Ab and relapse rates are comparable to conventional treatment protocols with thionamides alone (relapse approximately 30% to 60% at 5 years) (31–35) (Table 9). That is, there does not appear to be a clear advantage of block-replace therapy on long-term prognosis.

Overall response rates depend on a variety of factors. Benker et al. and the European Multicenter Study Group (274) found the therapeutic response depended on MMI dose (high versus low), pretreatment T_3 level, goiter size, urinary iodide excretion (reflecting dietary iodine intake), and TSHR-Ab levels.

We presently recommend initiating thionamide therapy with MMI 20 mg bid or PTU 200 mg tid until the patient is euthyroid. In most cases, titrating the patient to normal T_4 levels with reducing doses of thionamides, regardless of the eventual dose, is adequate therapy. Alternatively, the

TABLE 9. Summary of prospective clinical trials of combined thyroxine with thionamides for Graves' disease[a]

Ref. #	Authors (yr)	Group A[c]	Group B	Design[d]	Study size	Duration (mo) Treatment[e]	Duration (mo) Follow-up[f]	Advantage to Group A[b] ↓TSHR-Ab	Advantage to Group A[b] ↓Relapse
262	Alexander et al. (73)	↑Carb+T₃	—	SA	105	13	40–70	—	No (49%)
53	Davies et al. (77)	↑Carb+T₃/T₄	—	SA	30	6	6	—	No (53%)
241	Wilkin et al. (81)	↑Carb+T₃	—	SA	35	18	6	—	No (57%)
259	Romaldini et al. (83)	↑MMI/PTU+T₄	↓MMI/PTU	C	113	10–30	17–81	Yes	Yes
263	Gossage et al. (83)	↑Carb+T₃	—	SA	27	12	12	—	No (41%)
264	Laurberg et al. (86)	↑MMI+T₄	—	SA	99	21–58	11–141	—	No (37%–82%)[g]
265	Young et al. (88)	↑Carb+T₄	—	SA	72	6–9	8–72	Yes	No (49%)
266	Hashizume et al. (91)	↓MMI+T₄	↓MMI	C	109	12	36	Yes	Yes
269	Perozim et al. (93)	↑MMI+T₄	—	SA	28	18–24	24	Yes	No (32%)
271	Reinwein et al. (93)	↓MMI+T₄	↑MMI+T₄	C	309	12	12	No	No
268	Weetman et al. (94)	↑Carb+T₄	↑Carb+T₄	C	100	6 vs. 12	12	—	No (41% vs. 35%)
270	Edmonds and Tellez (94)	↑Carb+T₄	↓Carb	C	70	12	24	—	No
272	Iriarte et al. (95)	↑Carb+T₄	↓Carb	C	66	24	36	—	No[h]
273	Tamai et al. (95)	↓MMI+T₄	↓MMI	C	195	12	12	—	No
273a	McIver et al. (96)	↑Carb+T₄[i]	↑/↓Carb[i]	C	53	18	3–18	No	No

[a] Randomized studies with a follow-up period after discontinuation of the thionamide to assess effects on TSHR-Ab status and relapse.
[b] Presence and absence of an advantage of combined thionamides + thyroxine therapy versus thionamides alone; TSHR-Ab during follow-up period; relapse rates in percentages for single-arm studies may be compared to historical controls with thionamides alone: 30%–60% (see text).
[c] Carb, carbimazole; MMI, methimazole; PTU, propylthiouracil; low dose, <20 mg/day Carb/MMI or <200 mg/day PTU; high dose, ≥ 20 mg/day Carb/MMI or ≥ 200 mg/day PTU.
[d] SA, single-arm study; C, controlled study.
[e] Time on thionamide and thyroid hormone.
[f] Time off thionamide.
[g] 82.5%, no goiter; 71.5%, small goiter; 37.0%, medium/large goiter; compared with 15.5% with multinodular goiter.
[h] Decreased relapse rate with block-replace regimen at 12 months but not at 36 months follow-up.
[i] Group A, titrated to undetectable TSH levels; Group B, titrated to normal TSH levels.

thionamide dose may be reduced and then maintained at 10 to 20 mg/day for MMI, or 200 to 400 mg/day for PTU, with supplemental thyroid hormone in patients who demonstrate a very narrow therapeutic window on thionamides alone. In those with severe orbitopathy, ongoing high-dose thionamides with T_4 replacement may have a salutary role on retro-orbital immunosuppression (Fig. 11) (275). There do not appear to be sufficient data at the present time to recommend the routine use of block-replace dosing in order to maximize the theoretical immunosuppressive effect of thionamides on intrathyroidal autoimmunity (276).

Single-dose therapy with MMI traditionally finds little resistance by physicians, but single-dose PTU therapy required controlled studies to demonstrate its efficacy. Several reports have shown that PTU may indeed be prescribed at a once-a-day frequency independent of dose amount without significant reduction in remission rates (277–282). Although more patients will experience remission with once-a-day dosing of MMI compared to PTU (36% for PTU compared to 77% for MMI) (Fig. 12) (280), once-a-day PTU yields euthyroidism sooner (8 weeks for PTU compared to 16 weeks for MMI) (283). Nevertheless, we do not use PTU on a once-a-day regimen. Besides, MMI is less expensive than PTU. MMI, 10 mg tid, has also been found to induce euthyroidism sooner than PTU 100 mg tid (284). Both MMI and PTU in solution have been administered rectally and found to be absorbed adequately to manage patients with hyperthyroidism (Fig. 13) (285,286).

Currently, there is no consensus on how long to continue thionamide therapy before withdrawing and monitoring for relapse. The general trend is to continue treatment for 6 to 24 months. Some physicians, including ourselves, favor a short course of 6 months (277,287), whereas others favor a longer course in selected patients (18 to 24 months) (228,288,289). In a prospective study of 114 patients with Graves' disease, 58% of patients treated with MMI for 6 months (30–60 mg daily at outset, 10–20 mg daily at end) relapsed, compared to only 38% treated similarly for 18 months (290). A longer period of time to gain euthyroidism may be expected in patients with large glands, because they have higher intrathyroidal free iodide stores that the thionamides must overcome. It has been postulated that these patients have an intrinsically enhanced trapping mechanism (291). Note, however, that increased relapse rates following thionamides are observed from 5 to 10 years after withdrawal of treatment (228).

Finally, the use of adjunctive medical therapy is recommended when the patient has moderate to severe hyperthyroidism, or when there is an urgency to attain the euthyroid state. We recommend using propranolol 20 to 40 mg qid initially to manage the hyperadrenergic symptoms attending the hyperthyroid state. This drug should be stopped when euthyroidism occurs and used with cau-

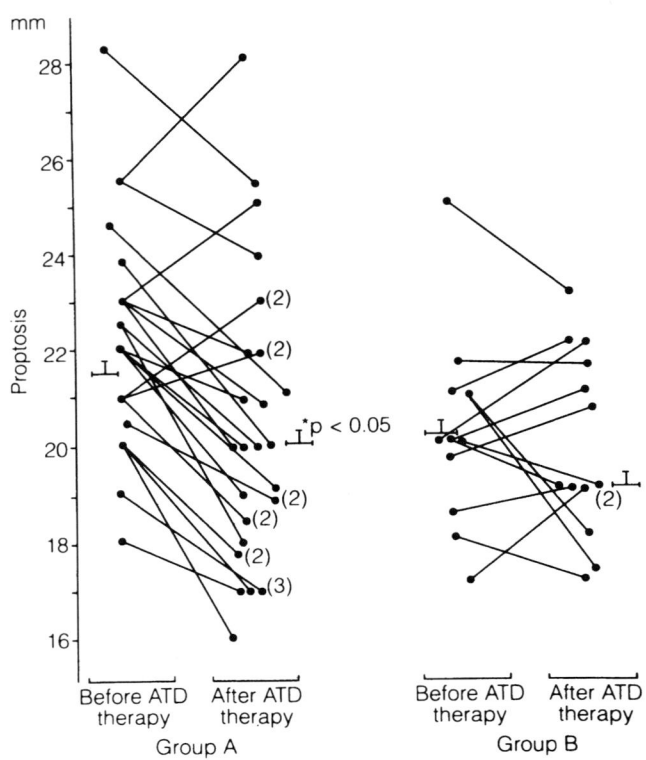

FIG. 11. Change in proptosis of more prominent eye with Hertel exophthalmometer in Graves' disease before and after block-replace regimen (Group A: high-dose MMI or PTU with T_3) or low-dose MMI or PTU and no T_3 (Group B). *Parentheses* indicate number of patients. *Bars* represent mean ± SEM. Reduction of mean proptosis was significant in Group A but not in Group B. (From ref. 275.)

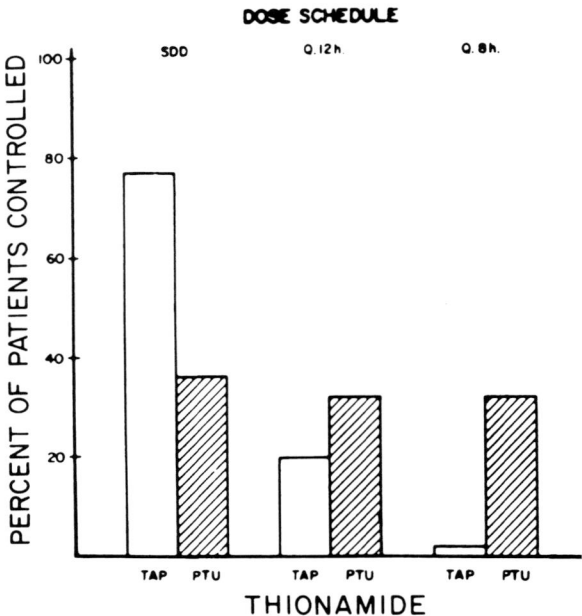

FIG. 12. Percent of patients controlled by different dose schedules of methimazole (TAP) and propylthiouracil (PTU). In the methimazole group, 77% of patients could be controlled with a single daily dose (SDD), although 21% required a twice-daily dose (q12h), and 2% a thrice-daily dose (q8h). In contrast, only 36% of patients in the PTU group could be controlled with SDD, with the remaining patients requiring q12h and q8h dosing. (From ref. 280.)

tion if there are any relative contraindications such as congestive heart failure, bronchospasm, or diabetes mellitus. Propranolol may be continued during primary treatment with thionamides when adrenergic symptoms are not yet fully controlled.

When hyperthyroidism is accelerated and rapid reduction in the serum T_3 level is desired, we recommend corticosteroids and iodine in addition to thionamides. If iodine is given (a minimum of 1 drop/day of SSKI or 2 drops/day of Lugol's solution), it should be administered at least 2 hr after the thionamide; if given earlier it may attenuate the thionamide effect. The administration of iodides has been associated with a high relapse rate caused by attenuation of intrathyroidal thionamide action (175, 176). Prednisone (60 mg/day) or dexamethasone (2 mg every 6 hr) is recommended when additional control is needed or if the patient has an allergy to iodine.

Monitoring Medical Therapy

Once thionamide therapy is initiated, the patient must understand that frequent follow-up visits are necessary. Depending on the initial severity of hyperthyroidism and

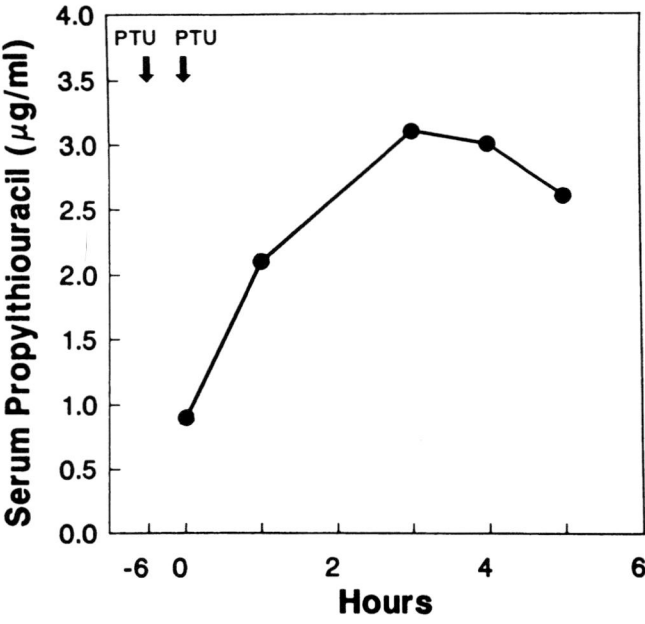

FIG. 13. Plasma propylthiouracil (PTU) levels in a Graves' disease patient with thyroid storm following the rectal administration of 400 mg of PTU in 60 mL Fleet mineral oil *(first arrow)* and in 60 mL Fleet phosphosoda *(second arrow)*. (From ref. 286.)

whether adjuvant therapy was instituted, frequency of visits should range from every 2 weeks to every 3 months. In the latter case, visits are oriented toward monitoring physical signs of hyperthyroidism so that adjuvant therapy may be stopped once the patient is euthyroid. Thereafter, or in the case of mild hyperthyroidism, bi- or trimonthly visits are maintained to follow the clinical exam (e.g., for thyroid size and heart rate), and chemical indices of thyroid function (specifically, a free thyroxine index and/or supersensitive TSH assay) are obtained. Thionamide doses are usually titrated to a chemically euthyroid state unless block-replace therapy is utilized.

The physician should also periodically follow serologic markers of disease activity such as TSHR-Ab, antithyroid peroxidase (microsomal) antibodies, and antithyroglobulin antibodies. Once the thionamide treatment schedule is completed, a 1-year observation period is started, to monitor for early (true) relapse. During this time, the serum T_3 rises before the serum T_4, producing an increased T_3 to T_4 ratio. Therefore, monitoring T_3 levels is very important during this period.

With appropriate testing, the physician is better equipped to advise the patient of the chances for permanent remission so that, if needed, an eventual recommendation for RAI treatment or surgery may not present a sudden shift in strategy. Patients with persistently suppressed supersensitive TSH levels and positive TSHR-Ab should be followed more closely than those without evidence of Graves' disease activity because of their increased risk for relapse (Fig. 14). On the other hand, the practical utility of measuring TSHR-Ab levels in individual patients to predict relapse or remission can be helpful (292). This is particularly true where TSHR-Ab titers remain very positive. Unfortunately, this applies to only a minority of patients. In addition, anti-TPO antibodies are a better predictor of intrathyroidal lymphocytic infiltration than TSHR-Ab (293) and may be measured to gauge the extent of residual autoimmune thyroiditis after thionamide discontinuation. Otherwise, patients should be seen every 3 months after discontinuation of thionamides to monitor chemical and clinical thyroidal status for hypothyroidism or recurrent hyperthyroidism.

If hyperthyroidism recurs, the likelihood of cure after another course of thionamides is reduced. These patients should be referred for RAI or surgery unless they prefer to take another course of medication. A guide to treating Graves' disease is given in Figure 15.

Toxic Multinodular Goiter and Toxic Adenoma (Plummer's Disease)

Overview

Development of nodular goiters is insidious and often presents late in life. Nodular goiters may present as a clinically euthyroid condition with TSH suppression and an absent response to thyrotropin-releasing hormone (TRH), signaling mild overproduction of thyroid hormone or overt clinical hyperthyroidism. When the patient is chemically or clinically hyperthyroid, treatment should be initiated.

In contrast to Graves' disease, where many follicles are overstimulated, there is distinct geographic variability within the gland in a toxic nodular goiter. Fewer hy-

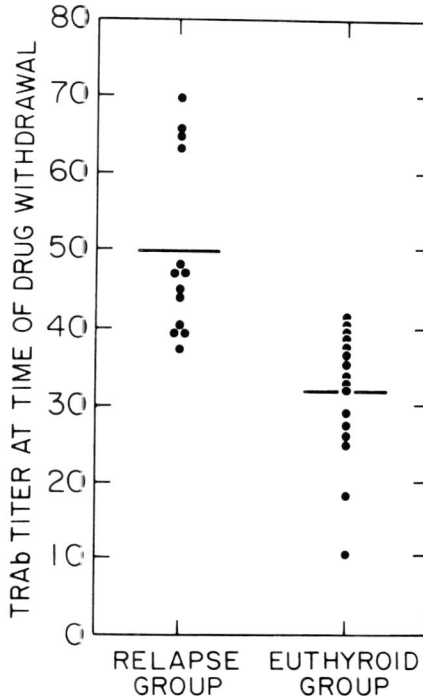

FIG. 14. TSHR-Ab titers at the time of withdrawal of thionamide therapy in patients found to be euthyroid or in relapse 2 months later. *Horizontal lines* indicate the mean TSHR-Ab titer. (From ref. 53.)

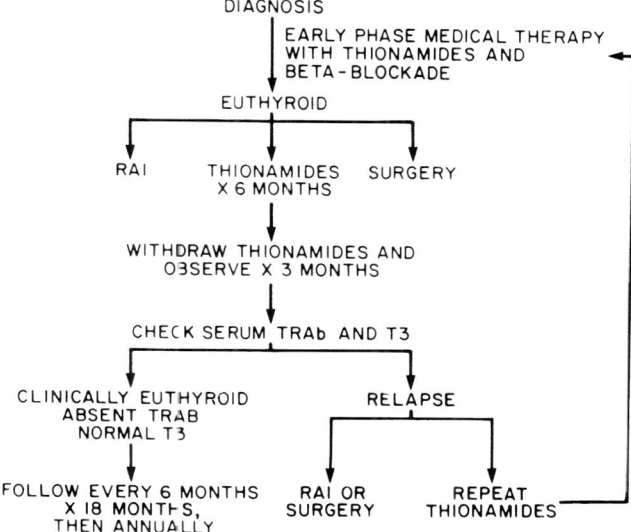

FIG. 15. A strategy for medical therapy of Graves' disease.

pothyroid complications to treatment develop compared to the Graves' disease gland. This is because (a) RAI preferentially accumulates in the active follicles, (b) normal glandular tissue does not undergo a high rate of mitosis that is susceptible to radiation damage, and (c) when surgery is performed, resection may be more confined than with the diffuse goiter of Graves' disease. In theory, a decreased frequency of iatrogenic hypothyroidism mitigates the advantage thionamides enjoy over RAI therapy and surgery with regard to safety. In light of the need for lifelong compliance when treating exclusively with thionamides and a relative urgency for euthyroidism in the usual setting of cardiac disease in the aged, the role of thionamides is relegated to early-phase, preparative, and adjunctive therapy rather than long-term treatment.

The etiology of nodular goiter may be related to intrathyroidal production of TSHR-Abs, which also act as growth-stimulating immunoglobulins (294,295). Therefore, the presence of thyrotoxicosis and TSHR-Abs in the setting of nodular goiter is simply a variant of Graves' disease. Kraiem et al. (296) demonstrated just such an autoimmune variant of toxic multinodular goiter, characterized by a diffuse but uneven technetium thyroidal uptake, younger age, presence of TSHR-Ab and ophthalmopathy, and concurrent development of goiter and hyperthyroidism. Therefore, these patients may be treated with thionamides for primary therapy.

Conventional Treatment

Thionamides may be used as combined primary therapy with RAI, affording an even lower incidence of iatrogenic hypothyroidism and an earlier remission compared to RAI alone (297). In addition, thionamides may be used for early-phase therapy for moderate to severe hyperthyroidism, with or without beta-blockers, prior to surgery. Thionamides are not recommended for definitive therapy: the 2-year relapse rate in patients with toxic multinodular goiter treated with thionamides alone was 95.1% compared to 34.1% in patients with Graves' disease (298). Iodine is generally not used in the management of nodular goiter because of the risk of iodine-induced hyperthyroidism. This is particularly true in regions of low iodine intake, which are associated with a greater incidence of toxic nodular goiter (299).

The approach to the patient with a toxic adenoma (toxic uninodular goiter) is essentially the same as with multinodular goiter. These adenomas should be managed with surgery or RAI therapy, and any medical treatment would be given early, as pretreatment, to rapidly control moderate to severe hyperthyroidism.

Unconventional Treatment

Recently, an alternative nonsurgical but invasive technique has been investigated for potential management of toxic, autonomously functioning thyroid nodules. This method involves percutaneous, sonographically guided ethanol intralesional injection (300–303). The procedure requires multiple injections for successful ablation and is frequently associated with local pain. Patients may also experience transient dysphonia resulting from injury to the recurrent laryngeal nerve. Intralesional injections are not the treatment of choice when rapid control is required, such as in elderly patients or those with thyrocardiac disease. However, when surgery is not possible and the nodule is small and not suppressing the surrounding thyroid tissue, intralesional injection is a relatively safe alternative.

Papini et al. (300) treated 20 women with toxic nodules with 2 to 4 mL sterile ethanol three to eight times, followed them for 12 months, and found that (a) all nodules demonstrated significant shrinkage, (b) TSH responded to TRH in 17 of 20 patients, and (c) scintigraphy normalized in 17 of 20 patients. Recurrence of hyperthyroidism following ethanol injection may be associated with excess iodine exposure (304).

T_3 Toxicosis

When T_3 toxicosis occurs, it is usually associated with toxic multinodular goiter or endemic iodine deficiency. Patients with unequivocal Graves' disease, who experience continued goitrous growth after a 6- to 24-month course of thionamide treatment, display persistent TSHR-Ab and hyperthyroidism with an increased serum T_3 to T_4 ratio (305). Low intrathyroidal iodide concentrations caused by thionamides, endemic iodine deficiency, or a trapping defect induce a shift in production of thyroid hormones from T_4 to T_3. Although this condition occurs in a wide range of situations, treatment is uniformly directed at managing the underlying thyroidal condition (i.e., with surgery or RAI).

Medical management is oriented toward early-phase control of the hyperthyroid state. This is best accomplished with thionamides and adjunctive agents, depending on the severity of symptoms. When the hyperthyroid state is mild, patients may be treated with beta-blockers alone prior to RAI therapy or surgery. However, in a study by Jones et al. (306), six of eight patients with T_3 toxicosis treated with propranolol alone, 160 mg/day, failed to become euthyroid by 6 months. This argues against propranolol as a sole therapy when thyroid symptoms are clinically significant. With severe T_3 toxicosis or when cardiac disease is present, we recommend adjunctive therapy with corticosteroids. In the United States, T_3 toxicosis often occurs with nodular disease, so we do not recommend the routine use of iodine or ipodate because of the risk of a Jod-Basedow phenomenon.

Trophoblastic Disease

Two types of gestational trophoblastic neoplasias (GTN) are associated with the hyperthyroid state: hydatidiform mole and choriocarcinoma. Partial molar pregnancy has also been associated with thyrotoxicosis (307). Primary treatment for hydatidiform mole is prompt surgical removal. Choriocarcinomas are treated with prompt institution of chemotherapy, with or without surgical resection. The associated hyperthyroidism results from elevated levels of human chorionic gonadotropin (β-hCG) (308) which stimulates the thyroidal TSH receptor via "specificity-crossover" (309). Generally, serum concentrations of β-hCG are proportional to tumor mass (310). Interestingly, hyperemesis gravidarum with transient hyperthyroidism may be due to β-hCG itself, as it also stimulates estradiol production through hCG receptor activation (Fig. 16) (311). This raises the possibility of a therapeutic role for thionamides in this situation.

The natural history of GTN is characterized by initial clinical euthyroidism and chemical hyperthyroidism, which may proceed to thyrotoxicosis, heart failure with pulmonary edema, and death (312,313). This dissociation of clinical and chemical thyroid status is partially explained by the lower T_3 to T_4 (314) and higher rT_3 to T_3 (312) ratios (indicative more of 5-monodeiodination than 5'-monodeiodination) in GTN compared to Graves' disease. These effects on monodeiodination activity are unclear.

Depending on severity, treatment consists of PTU or MMI 2 hr prior to iodide administration, preoperative oral or IV iodine (1 g over 8 to 12 hr preoperatively) to shorten postoperative hyperthyroidism, beta-blockers (preferably propranolol) 10 to 40 mg every 6 hr, sedation, and careful fluid and electrolyte replacement (312, 315–317). After surgery or aggressive chemotherapy, there will be a rapid fall in serum T_3, T_4, rT_3, and β-hCG levels (312). Beta-blockers should be continued postoperatively for 3 or 4 days, but the thionamides can be discontinued once the β-hCG, T_4, and T_3 are normalized and the patient is clinically euthyroid. Prognosis is usually favorable, although there have been reports of several patients experiencing thyrotoxic death despite adequate prophylaxis (312).

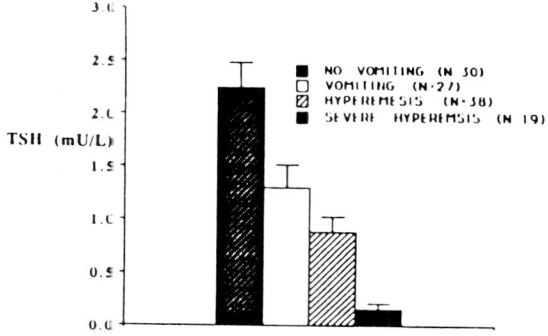
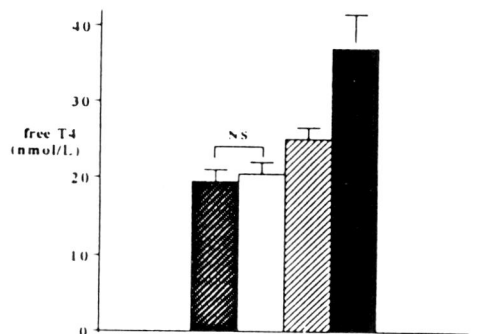
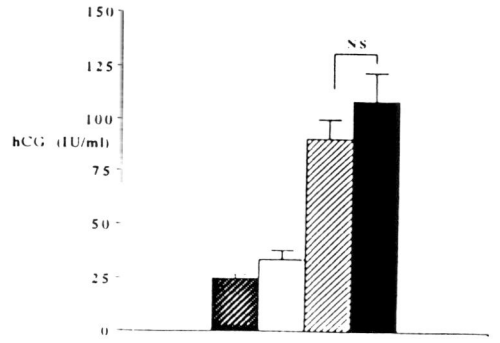

FIG. 16. Relationship between severity of vomiting during pregnancy and serum TSH, free T_4, and hCG levels (mean ± SEM). Hormone levels differed significantly ($p<0.05$) except where indicated otherwise. NS, not significant. (From ref. 311.)

Thyrotoxicosis and Thyroiditis

Patients with clinical and chemical thyrotoxicosis may be erroneously diagnosed as having Graves' disease or toxic nodular goiter, and they may be needlessly treated with thionamides, radioactive iodine, or surgery. Patients with thyroiditis typically have a depressed RAI uptake and spontaneously remit or become hypothyroid within several months. Subacute thyroiditis is typically short lived with spontaneous resolution, and it may be characterized on a pathologic basis as lymphocytic thyroiditis (LT) or granulomatous thyroiditis (GT). These conditions present as painless (silent) or, more commonly, painful thyroiditis, respectively. The association of hyperthyroidism with these states has been referred to as "spontaneous resolving hyperthyroidism" (SRH) (318). A thyrotoxic phase is produced by rapid leaking of thyroid hormones by the damaged and inflamed follicles. Although the natural course of these disorders is spontaneous resolution in the majority of patients, in LT-SRH, persistent hypothyroidism may be quite common, and recurrent hyperthyroidism is also seen (319). On the other hand, in GT-SRH, hypothyroidism and/or true recurrences are rare (320).

Patients with thyroiditis should not be treated initially with thionamides, RAI, or surgery. For those who are only mildly hyperthyroid, observation and treatment with salicylates, other nonsteroidal anti-inflammatory drugs, and propranolol may be appropriate, with monitoring of the erythrocyte sedimentation rate (321). If the patient develops severe pain and tenderness as well as severe hyperthyroidism, a brief (1-month) course of prednisone may be added (321). Initial doses should be 30 to 60 mg/day with a taper of 10 to 15 mg a week. Prednisone is associated with a rapid reduction in the pain and serum T_4 levels, resulting in normal T_3 and T_4 levels by 10 days and relief of symptoms as early as 24 hr. Corticosteroids, however, have no impact on the recurrence rate (321). Sodium ipodate, 0.5 g/day for 15 to 60 days, results in prompt normalization of serum T_3 with amelioration of clinical symptoms and should be considered a safe and effective therapy (322). The effect of additional thyroid hormone suppression therapy on long-term prognosis is still unclear, although it is effective in shrinking goiter size (321).

Surgery is reserved for patients with a protracted thyrotoxic course or recurrent disease, especially in the setting of other compromising medical problems such as cardiac disease. Patients should be followed for at least 3 years after presentation for hypothyroidism or recurrence. In LT-SRH, patients should be advised that the thyrotoxic course may run 2 to 5 months (318). If the hypothyroidism becomes clinically significant, replacement therapy should be started, and then the patient is weaned as euthyroidism appears. If hypothyroidism continues for more than 6 months, it will probably be permanent.

TSH-Dependent Hyperthyroidism

Hyperthyroidism associated with inappropriately elevated TSH levels results from pituitary or ectopic tumoral TSH production, abnormal hypothalamic control of thyrotroph activity, or selective pituitary thyroid hormone resistance (PThHR) (323,324). The management of tumoral secondary hyperthyroidism is primarily with surgery or irradiation. When a medical approach is desired in patients with TSH-secretion pituitary tumors, octreotide can control the hyperthyroidism (84%), decrease serum TSH (in 30 of 33 patients, with a mean decline of 74%), normalize thyroid hormones (73%), and reduce tumor volume (40%) (325).

Abnormal hypothalamic stimulatory regulation (via TRH, norepinephrine, and estrogens) or inhibitory regulation (via dopamine, somatostatin, serotonin, and corticosteroids) of TSH secretion can essentially produce a deranged integrated set-point to thyroid hormone feedback. This nontumoral state may be approached, for all practical purposes, as PThHR in which there are intact hypothalamic regulatory mechanisms but an intrinsically increased pituitary set-point or threshold (decreased sensitivity) to the negative feedback of thyroid hormones. This yields increased TSH levels, increased thyroid hormone levels, and a hypermetabolic state. TSH-dependent hyperthyroidism is an extraordinarily rare event. Even rarer is the clinical description of a patient presenting with encephalopathic symptoms (transient ischemic attack and seizure) and thyroid storm in the setting of Graves' disease and nonsuppressed TSH due to PThHR (326).

The ideal management of nontumoral inappropriate TSH secretion with hyperthyroidism would be to normalize the set-point to thyroid hormone feedback. In lieu of this approach, studies have concentrated on substances that have native inhibitory activity on thyrotroph function. Dopamine receptor agonists (bromocriptine and pergolide) are reported to have inconsistent effects on TSH suppression and are therefore not an optimal choice (327, 328). The long-acting somatostatin analog, octreotide, in doses of 50 to 100 µg bid to tid subcutaneously, decreases serum TSH, alpha subunit, and thyroid hormone levels (329–331). Management of nontumoral inappropriate TSH secretion with octreotide is less effective than that observed with TSH-producing tumors (332). Although dexamethasone, 2 mg po every 6 hr, has been consistently demonstrated to lower TSH and thyroid hormone levels, inevitable Cushing's syndrome and hypothalamic–pituitary–adrenal axis suppression militates against its long-term use (333). T_4 therapy may not adequately suppress TSH in PThHR, but once-a-day T_3, 25 to 50 µg, has been reported to produce clinical regression of hyperthyroidism (334). This remission occurs over a 2- to 3-month period.

The thyromimetic agent TRIAC (3,5,3′-triiodothyroacetic acid), at a dosage of 3 mg/day, produces near-normalization of TSH, T_4, and basal metabolic rate (331). TRIAC is a thyroid hormone analog that effectively inhibits TSH secretion but has poor peripheral thyroid hormone activity. There has been a report of cutaneous rash occurring with TRIAC therapy (335). Other thyromimetic agents, such as DIMIT (3,5-dimethyl-3-isopropyl-L-thyronine) deserve further investigation (331,336). Thionamides and RAI are discouraged because they may induce pituitary hyperplasia and adenoma formation. Beta-blockers are useful to assist in controlling the adrenergic signs and symptoms of hyperthyroidism. Overall, if faced with this rare situation, we recommend treatment with TRIAC or octreotide, beta-blockers as needed, and periodic monitoring of serum alpha subunit levels as an early indicator of recurrence. If the hyperthyroidism remains clinically significant despite all of the above medical therapies, thyroidectomy and L-thyroxine replacement titrated to slightly elevated serum free T_4 levels should be considered.

SPECIAL CONSIDERATIONS

Variation of Treatment with Age

Childhood and Adolescent Graves' Disease

The natural history of childhood Graves' disease, as with adults, is characterized by spontaneous remissions and exacerbations. However, in contrast to adults, remissions may be less frequent and recurrences more frequent (337). About one fifth of cases are diagnosed by age 10, with a peak activity by adolescence (338).

There is much debate in the literature concerning appropriate initial therapy: thionamides, subtotal thyroidectomy, or RAI treatment. The proponents of surgery argue that it affords rapid cure in virtually all patients and causes hypothyroidism in less than 50% and infrequent hypoparathyroidism (338,339). More recent studies do not observe damage to the recurrent laryngeal nerve, but close follow-up is indicated because of the incidence of frank or subclinical hypothyroidism (59% to 62%, compared to 2% with medical therapy) and recurrent hyperthyroidism (7% to 9%, compared to 22% with medical therapy) (340–342).

Radioactive iodine treatment has been traditionally discouraged because of the theoretical (unproven) risk of resultant thyroid cancer or leukemia and the frequent consequence of hypothyroidism, which might be deleterious to growth and development. Recent data on the use of radioactive iodine in children, however, are more positive. Hamburger (343) studied 239 patients ages 3 to 13, of whom 191 (80%) received RAI therapy (85% cured with one dose) without any increased incidence of congenital abnormalities in first-generation descendants. On the other hand, an association between the Chernobyl nuclear accident and a significantly increased number of thyroid cancers in children in Belarus, Ukraine, and Russia has been documented epidemiologically (344,344a).

Thionamides generally induce persistent remission in 40% to 75% of children studied (338,345,346), although side effects may be more common at an early age (347). We recommend medical therapy as first-line therapy in childhood Graves' disease because of its ease of use with minimal interruption in schooling and avoidance of destructive therapy. Thionamides may not be easy to employ if the child is uncooperative or has ineffective parental support, because compliance is of utmost importance. Adolescent patients are liable to avoid taking medications that do not have an immediate or noticeable effect and may require frequent counseling concerning the importance of compliance with therapy. Daily dosing of MMI makes this the thionamide of choice. Issues concerning monitoring, high or low doses, short- or long-term therapy, and adjunctive therapy are similar to those in adults, as described. Long-term treatment until after adolescence is recommended where possible. Subtotal thyroidectomy performed by an experienced pediatric thyroid surgeon should be considered for children and adolescents with large goiters that fail to regress with medical therapy. Radioiodine may be useful in children and adolescents with small glands who relapse after medical therapy.

Hyperthyroidism in the Elderly

The yearly incidence of hyperthyroidism in patients over the age of 60 years is 7 times that in younger patients (348). Furthermore, the spectrum of presenting symptomatology ranges from classical hyperkinetic findings to an apathetic picture. Apathetic hyperthyroidism may result from an age-related attenuation of thyroid hormone amplification of adrenergic tone. In Graves' disease, there may be an absence of ophthalmopathy and minimal thyroidal enlargement. Toxic multinodular goiter, however, is the most common cause of hyperthyroidism over age 60 (349). Hyperthyroidism in the elderly may be manifested by congestive heart failure, gastrointestinal distress, depression, anorexia and weight loss, hypercalcemia, accelerated osteoporosis with pathological fractures, or myopathy. True subclinical hyperthyroidism in the elderly is associated with atrial fibrillation and is discussed later.

Once a diagnosis is made, specific treatment may be instituted as in a young adult, with the following provisos. First, a special effort should be made to render the patient euthyroid as quickly as possible, as the hyperthyroid state is poorly tolerated by the aged. This may be accomplished with thionamides, but since they require time to be effective, adjunctive therapy with beta-blockers is recommended. Second, beta-blockers should be used cautiously, because cardiac decompensation is a significant risk. Once the patient is euthyroid, plans can be made for RAI ablation or surgery as appropriate.

Thyroid Disease: Pregnancy and the Neonate

Pregnancy and Graves' Disease

A diagnosis of hyperthyroid Graves' disease with pregnancy needs to be differentiated from the normal hyperthyroxinemia of pregnancy, in which there are increased total T_4 and T_3 levels (as a result of an estrogen-induced increase in thyroxine-binding globulin), but free T_4 and free T_3 levels remain normal. In contrast, Graves' hyperthyroidism is accompanied by elevated free thyroid hormone levels, suppressed TSH, and the presence of TSHR-Ab. Once diagnosed, this condition requires treatment because of the risk of spontaneous abortion and the deleterious effects of hyperthyroidism on the fetus. The fetus may become affected by TSHR-Ab crossing the placental barrier. Of 74 hyperthyroid neonates studied, 35% had hyperthyroidism for over 3 months, 27% developed psychomotor abnormalities, and 42% developed growth retardation (350).

Radioactive iodine is never used in pregnancy because of its effects on the fetal thyroid gland, which is able to concentrate iodine after the 12th developmental week. Surgery used to be the first-line treatment (351–353). Talbert et al. (353) reported a 92% live term birth rate with surgery, compared to 77% with thionamides. They argued that thionamides were hazardous because they could cross the placenta and cause small (nonobstructive) goiter formation (351,354,355), and the potential growth and intellectual impairment resulting from fetal hypothyroidism would be difficult to avoid. The subsequent use and acceptance of thionamides was primarily a result of the lack of fetal abnormalities and improved methods of monitoring dosing. In fact, thionamides may reduce the incidence of fetal malformation from maternal hyperthyroidism (356). The use of thionamides is justified by their ability to block the pathological action of TSHR-Ab on the fetal, as well as the maternal, thyroid gland.

Fetal goiter may develop in response to enhanced fetal TSH secretion resulting from excessive transplacental thionamide. Congenital goiter also occurs with adjunctive iodide treatment (obstructive goiter with dystocia) (357), inadequate hyperthyroid control, or a family history of goiter (355). Significantly, no intellectual or physical developmental abnormalities were found with thionamides (358,359), although MMI has been associated with aplasia cutis of the fetal scalp (356). Based on the data, we recommend medical treatment of pregnant Graves' disease patients and reserve surgery for those patients who are uncooperative, unreliable, unresponsive, or allergic to thionamides. In addition, those patients with very large goiters and severe local symptoms, as with nonpregnant patients, are candidates for surgery, preferably after the first trimester.

Because MMI has greater placental transfer than PTU, MMI has the advantage, in severe Graves' disease with very high TSHR-Ab titers, of protecting the fetal thyroid gland from the effects of maternal TSHR-Ab. However, when the activity of maternal Graves' disease is not severe, considerations of complications of thionamide use become predominant. Therefore, on theoretical grounds, in the majority of pregnant patients with Graves' disease, PTU is the preferred agent because of its minimal transplacental transfer and low excretion into milk. It should be noted, however, that when the records of 185 hyperthyroid pregnant patients were reviewed, of which 99 were treated with PTU and 36 with MMI, the outcomes were comparable with respect to (a) percent still hyperthyroid at delivery (32% versus 33%), (b) time to euthyroidism (7 versus 8 weeks), and (c) incidence of major congenital anomalies (3.0% versus 2.7%, respectively) (Fig. 17) (360). Furthermore, a block-replace treatment regimen has also been found to decrease TSHR-Ab and the postpartum recurrence rate in pregnant patients with Graves' hyperthyroidism (361) but is not to be recommended because the rate of T_4 transplacental transfer may not equal the rate of PTU transfer.

We recommend initiating treatment with a low thionamide dose (PTU, 50 mg qid; or MMI, 10 mg bid) to avoid fetal or maternal hypothyroidism. Theoretically, congenital goiter should not occur with thionamides as long as there is sufficient maternal placental T_4 transfer or fetal T_4 to suppress fetal TSH. As soon as a reduction in maternal free T_4 is detected (7 days to 4 weeks, depending on pretreatment thyroidal preformed hormone stores), the thionamide dose is rapidly decreased (PTU, 50 to 100 mg/day; or MMI, 5 to 10 mg/day). The endpoint is a free T_4 in the low toxic range, because chemically euthyroid mothers may still have reduced cord T_4 levels and neonates may have augmented cold-induced TSH rises on the first day of life (362,363). In addition, the fetal heart rate should be maintained between 120 and 160 beats per min on thionamides (364). By the third trimester, when activity of Graves' disease decreases even

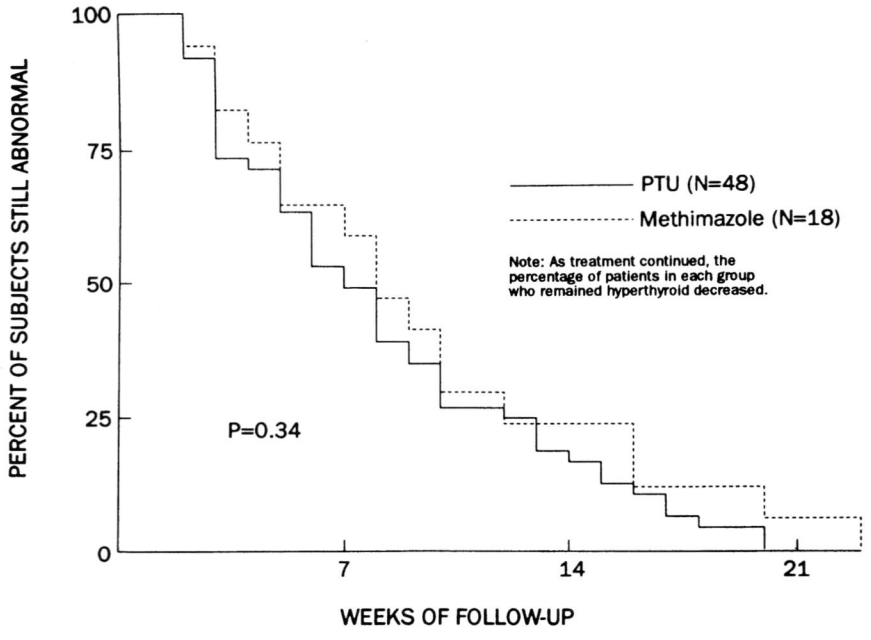

FIG. 17. Normalization of thyroid function in pregnant hyperthyroid patients treated with thionamides. PTU, propylthiouracil. (From ref. 360.)

without intervention as a result of the immunosuppressive effect of pregnancy, the thionamide dose should be no greater than 50 mg/day for PTU or 5 mg/day for MMI. Thionamides can often be discontinued during the third trimester as the immunosuppressive effects of pregnancy ensue. Therapy should be monitored by periodic intrauterine growth measurement, fetal heart rate assessment, and chemical/serologic indices (T_4, TBG, or T_3 resin uptake to determine a free T_4 index, and supersensitive TSH and TSHR-Ab levels) every 4 to 6 weeks. There do not appear to be any long-term deleterious effects of carefully monitored antithyroid therapy in pregnant women on the somatic growth, intellectual development, or thyroid function of their offspring (365).

Mothers previously treated for Graves' disease with surgery or RAI and on replacement T_4 therapy may still have stimulating TSHR-Ab present in their serum. Once a radioreceptor assay demonstrates the presence of TSHR-Ab, a thyroid cell bioassay should be performed to determine TSHR-Ab blocking and/or stimulating activity. If a stimulating TSHR-Ab is present, thionamides may be administered as above. In this case of maternal euthyroidism with demonstrable stimulating TSHR-Ab, a small dose of MMI might protect the fetus from hyperthyroidism. Such therapy, however, is difficult to monitor. If the bioassay reveals a blocking antibody to the TSH receptor, thionamides are withheld and careful monitoring must be undertaken to avoid fetal or neonatal hypothyroidism. Parenthetically, if hyperthyroidism due to nodular hyperthyroidism complicates pregnancy, thionamide dosing should be titrated to mild hyperthyroidism. This decreases the risk of fetal hypothyroidism in a situation in which thyroid-stimulating antibodies are not present but the fetal thyroid gland is still exposed to small amounts of thionamide.

Demonstration of an increased free T_4 index early in pregnancy has been found to be predictive of transient or persistent stimulation-induced postpartum hyperthyroidism (366). In addition, quantitation of stimulating TSHR-Ab may predict the development of neonatal hyperthyroidism. Munro et al. (367) found that of 13 mothers with long-acting thyroid stimulator (LATS)-protector (detected indirectly by mouse bioassay) greater than 20 units/mL, 12 delivered unequivocally thyrotoxic babies. Intra-amniotic TSH monitoring for fetal hypothyroidism is theoretically appropriate for cases of euthyroid mothers placed on thionamides because of the presence of TSHR-Ab (368). In addition, pelvic sonography may be utilized to monitor for neonatal goiter.

Four drugs may be considered as adjunctive therapy with pregnancy: supplemental thyroid hormone, iodine, dexamethasone, and propranolol. Although adding thyroid hormone to thionamides to cushion against maternal hypothyroidism was promulgated by various investigators from the early 1950s through the 1970s, most thyroidologists today use thionamides alone (369–371). This is because thyroid hormones do not cross the placental barrier well and can actually create a state of maternal euthyroidism, or even hyperthyroidism, and fetal hypothyroidism as a result of placental transfer of thionamides (353,372,373).

Because of the well-described and invariable risk of obstructive goiter with prolonged iodide use, the use of iodide is justified only with profound life-threatening thyrotoxicosis requiring prompt reduction of thyroid hormone release. Similarly, the use of dexamethasone should be limited to severe thyrotoxicosis and discontinued as soon as possible.

The debate over propranolol for thyrotoxicosis during pregnancy is founded upon the demonstration of its efficacy in controlling the adrenergic signs and symptoms of hyperthyroidism and the controversial association with placental insufficiency, intrauterine growth retardation, excessive uterine irritability, and fetal bradycardia, hypoglycemia, hyperbilirubinemia, and polycythemia (374–381). Propranolol may also be used preoperatively during pregnancy, but it should be used sparingly and stopped at least 24 to 48 hr prior to delivery.

Another circumstance in which iodides (IV), dexamethasone (2 mg every 6 hr for 24 hr), and propranolol are used is with uncontrolled thyrotoxicosis at the onset of labor. This condition may trigger accelerated thyrotoxicosis.

The Postpartum Thyroid Syndromes

Autoimmune thyroid diseases, like other autoimmune diseases such as rheumatoid arthritis and systemic lupus erythematosis, undergo spontaneous remissions during the latter half of pregnancy because of the suppression of humoral and cell-mediated immunity. It is thought that relapses of these diseases in the postpartum period result from immunological rebound (381a). Approximately 95% of postpartum hyperthyroidism cases are accounted for by the early phase of postpartum thyroiditis (PPT) (70% to 80%) and the onset of recurrence of authentic postpartum Graves' disease (PGD) (10% to 15%) (382). The various patterns of postpartum thyroid syndromes are depicted in Figure 18.

Postpartum thyroiditis usually occurs 4 to 9 months after delivery (383) and is autoimmune in nature and mostly confined to patients with thyroid autoantibodies. It is similar to what many physicians call silent thyroiditis. Hyperthyroidism results from rapid release of thyroid hormone from destruction of thyroid follicles, presumably by cytotoxic T cells and antithyroid antibodies. In patients with a history of Graves' disease, a destructive thyrotoxicosis may also occur postpartum, especially in patients who were euthyroid before pregnancy or have elevated anti-thyroid peroxidase (anti-TPO) antibodies (366). Patients with established but mild Hashimoto's thyroiditis may also experience PPT (366). In fact, postpartum silent thyroiditis may occur and mask the development of postpartum Graves' disease (384).

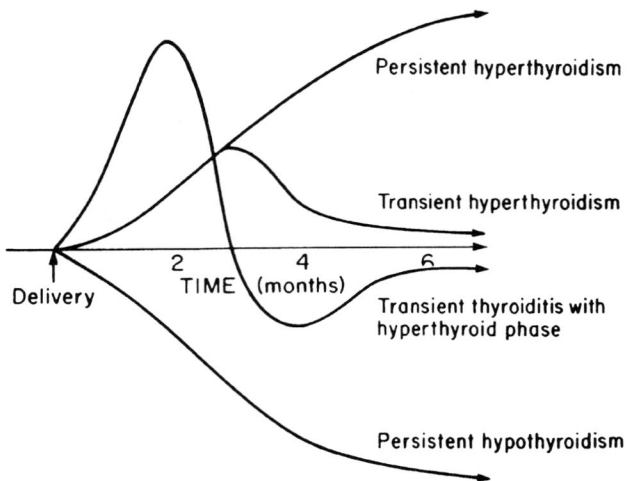

FIG. 18. Patterns of postpartum thyroid syndromes. (From ref. 383.)

Because the disease tends to be transient, the treatment of PPT is directed toward symptoms. If the patient is asymptomatic, no specific therapy is indicated and the patient is seen every 4 weeks because of the risk of subsequent hypothyroidism. If the patient is symptomatic, a brief course of propranolol (10 to 20 mg qid) may be used. Prophylaxis of mothers with elevated first trimester anti-TPO antibodies with steroids is contraindicated because of the low morbidity and excellent response of PPT to time and treatment. Thionamides are not recommended because resolution or progression to hypothyroidism occurs spontaneously and they would theoretically have little effect on a gland undergoing destruction and inactivation of organification mechanisms.

Postpartum Graves' disease is associated with recurrent TSHR-Ab. Symptoms occur 3 to 5 months after delivery, and the radioactive iodine uptake is elevated (366,383,385). PGD may be either transient or permanent (366). A thyroid scan (if the mother is not breast-feeding) or thyroid ultrasound should be performed to exclude toxic uni- or multinodular goiter. If the patient with PGD does not respond to thionamides, requires large doses of thionamides for control, or has recurrent disease, destructive therapy with RAI (if the mother is not breast-feeding) or surgery is recommended.

If thionamides are to be used while the mother is breast-feeding, low-dose PTU is preferred because of its poor concentration in milk compared to MMI, which has a serum to milk ratio of 1.03 (79,386). However, Lamberg et al. (387) described 12 infants who all remained euthyroid during 3 weeks of continued breast-feeding while their mothers received up to 10 mg/day of MMI. The mother should be made aware of the risks of neonatal hypothyroidism as well as other potential risks thionamides may have on her baby (although we are not aware of any reports of neonatal thionamide-induced fever, rash, or bone marrow suppression). In addition, the baby should have regular thyroid function testing. Based on these data, if the mother is allergic to PTU, MMI may be given at doses not exceeding 10 mg/day and the infant's thyroid function should be assessed at 2- to 4-week intervals (388). In any case, we believe mothers should not be actively dissuaded from breast-feeding simply because of low-dose thionamide therapy.

Neonatal Graves' Disease

Neonates born to mothers with Graves' disease are at a small but definite risk for hyperthyroidism dependent on the transplacental passage of TSHR-Ab. This risk may be gauged based on quantification of maternal stimulating TSHR-Ab during pregnancy, and cord blood thyroid function tests should be performed on all such newborns. Often, the neonate can be observed to have a goiter. There is a brief euthyroid period after birth, from hours to up to 10 days, resulting from the effects of prenatal thionamides on the fetal thyroid gland. The onset of neonatal hyperthyroidism, however, is rather dramatic, consisting of restlessness, sweating, fever, and tachycardia. This is followed by failure to thrive, cardiac failure, and death in 16% of patients (389). If the patient survives, there may still be developmental skeletal abnormalities (250). The hyperthyroid phase may last several months, reflecting the biologic half-life of the thyroid stimulator (390). It has also been suggested that the postnatal euthyroid period may be protracted by the presence of an immunoglobulin inhibitor of the thyroid stimulator (391). This syndrome should be distinguished from the rare form of dominantly inherited congenital hyperthyroidism associated with an activating mutation of the TSH receptor (391a).

Treatment for severe neonatal Graves' disease consists of thionamides [for example, PTU, 5 to 10 mg/kg per day in divided doses (317)]; iodine [1 drop Lugol's solution tid (317)]; sedation; digoxin for impending heart failure; propranolol [2 mg/kg per day in divided doses (392) to manage adrenergic signs]; fluids and electrolytes; steroids; and cooling blankets and oxygen as needed. In milder cases, neonates are successfully managed with propranolol alone. Neonates born to Graves' disease mothers should be carefully monitored, even if initially euthyroid.

Cardiac Disease and Thyroid Death

Medical therapy for thyrotoxicosis associated with cardiac manifestations should be limited to (a) early-phase treatment prior to destructive therapy and (b) the 12 weeks after RAI, before a therapeutic effect takes place. Thyrocardiac disease, first described by Levine and Sturgis in 1924 (393), embodies the spectrum of cardiomyopathies responsible for congestive heart failure, high-output heart failure, cardiomegaly, and atrial tachyarrhythmias in the setting of chemical hyperthyroidism. Thyroid death currently refers to mortality resulting from the combination of thyrotoxicosis and thyrocardiac disease.

An increased number of high-affinity adrenergic receptors have been identified in some tissues exposed to excessive thyroid hormones (116,394). In porcine myocardial cells, T_3 treatment increases the number of cell surface adrenergic receptors via genomic and nongenomic mechanisms (394a). T_3 treatment also potentiates beta-adrenergic receptor stimulation transduction via increasing cAMP production, calcium channel current, and calcium availability to contractile elements (394b). In humans, in vivo, T_3 treatment increases beta-adrenergic receptor sensitivity (394c). Summation of the adrenergic and thyroid hormonal effects on sensitive tissue will therefore be greater in thyrotoxicosis.

The high cardiac output state associated with thyrotoxicosis is caused by increased systemic oxygen consumption and demands, provoked by stimulation of mitochondrial oxidation–phosphorylation enzymes as well as the adenyl cyclase–cAMP system (102,395). However, most patients with cardiac failure in thyrotoxicosis have underlying organic heart disease. Cardiac output may be increased minimally at best, though not enough to meet the circulatory needs of the patient. The systemic vascular resistance is decreased because of peripheral vasodilation. This results from an accumulation of metabolites, increase in heat production, and enhanced beta-adrenergic receptor tone. Although arrhythmias are among the most frequent cardiac manifestations of hyperthyroidism, angina may also occur. Cardiac ischemia and pain can result from coronary artery vasospasm in hyperthyroidism rather than true atherosclerosis (396).

Accelerated Hyperthyroidism

Accelerated thyrotoxicosis is a potentially dangerous clinical condition with an overall mortality rate of 20% when crisis or storm exists (397). In a study of 33 patients suffering thyroid death, over 50% of the deaths occurred during the first 2 weeks of hospital admission, about half were in patients younger than 60 years of age, 15% were sudden and unexpected, 21% were within 3 weeks after RAI therapy, and 18% were due to major emboli (398). Myocardial infarction is rare with thyrocardiac disease (399). The cardinal symptoms of thyrocardiac disease are angina, exertional dyspnea and edema, and palpitations. It must be stressed that the elderly often present with apathetic hyperthyroidism manifested only by subtle cardiac signs and symptoms.

The underlying hyperthyroid state should be treated with thionamides to reduce thyroidal organification and production of hormones. Because their effect may take several weeks to impact clinically, additional agents are required to rapidly render the patient euthyroid. Iodine and/or dexamethasone, 2 mg every 6 hr, may be given to assist in rapid control. Ablative RAI therapy may be given as soon as the patient is euthyroid if iodine treatment has been avoided.

Congestive heart failure should be treated with digoxin, diuretics, and bed rest. Propranolol or diltiazem may be judiciously administered to control concomitant tachyarrhythmias unless the cardiac output is severely reduced. If there is significant hemodynamic compromise, intensive care monitoring is needed. When underlying organic heart disease is known or suspected, pulmonary arterial catheterization may provide useful information to monitor response to treatment.

Atrial fibrillation is present in 10% to 28% of thyrotoxic patients (400) and should be treated with both propranolol and digoxin. Because hyperthyroidism increases the renal clearance of digoxin, larger initial doses must be given to obtain therapeutic levels. Of 165 patients with thyrotoxic atrial fibrillation, 101 (61%) spontaneously converted following control of the thyrotoxic state (401). All spontaneous conversions occurred within 4 months after treatment (RAI and/or thionamides) or when the hyperthyroid state did not persist for more than 13 months. The remaining patients, still fibrillating, required DC cardioversion.

Because about a third of thyrotoxic patients with atrial fibrillation will eventually experience systemic embolization (400), and almost half of these after euthyroidism is attained (402), anticoagulation is recommended at the time of initial therapy unless specifically contraindicated. Thus the development of emboli, of which 10% are pulmonary (400), may be due to conversion of the aberrant rhythm to normal sinus rhythm. It should be noted that the hyperthyroid state potentiates the action of warfarin (403). When conditions preclude the use of beta-blockers, such as severe bronchospasm or diabetes, the calcium-channel blocker diltiazem (120 mg every 8 hr) may be tried to control the tachyarrhythmia (404). Because there are no prospective studies supporting the role of amiodarone, which blocks atrioventricular (AV) conduction (405), we can only suggest its use in extenuating circumstances in a carefully monitored setting (406). Angina pectoris may accompany the thyrotoxic state and is responsive to nitrates and calcium-channel blockers (407). Cardiac catheterization should not be performed until the patient is rendered euthyroid.

Rarely, cardiac arrhythmias and EKG changes can be associated with periodic paralysis (408). This condition is though to be related to catecholamine-mediated potassium uptake, which may be potentiated in certain patients. Thyroid hormone is known to directly stimulate Na^+-K^+-ATPase as well as the number and sensitivity of beta-adrenergic receptors. The treatment of thyrotoxic periodic paralysis consists of two parts. First, the hypokalemia is immediately corrected with parenteral potassium. However, great care must be exercised, because the hypokalemia is caused by intracellular shifts and not wasting, so hyperkalemia can result quickly. Second, the hyperthyroidism requires control. Initially, this is accomplished medically with propranolol (138) and thionamides, but definitive treatment is with radioiodine or subtotal thyroidectomy.

Subclinical Hyperthyroidism and Atrial Fibrillation in the Elderly

With the advent and availability of supersensitive TSH assays, suppressed TSH levels with normal T_4, free T_4 index (FTI), and T_3 levels have been noted. This condition is termed subclinical hyperthyroidism when overt signs of hyperthyroidism do not occur. The incidence of subclinical hyperthyroidism is about 1%, with lower female preponderance, more frequent association in the elderly, and an incidence of progression to frank hyperthyroidism in 5% (409). In a well-controlled prospective study over a 10-year period of 2007 patients 60 years old, Sawin et al. (410) found that the cumulative incidence of atrial fibrillation was 28% among those with low TSH values, compared to 11% with normal values. After correcting for other risk factors, this significant difference reflects a relative risk of 3.1. The etiology of hyperthyroidism in this setting is usually nodular thyroid disease, although Graves' disease can occur in older persons. From a practical standpoint, patients with subclinical hyperthyroidism over 60 years of age ought to be treated, preferably with radioiodine as described. In patients under 60 years old with subclinical hyperthyroidism, observation is a reasonable approach, reserving definitive therapy until frank hyperthyroidism develops.

Iodine-Induced Thyrotoxicosis Caused by Amiodarone, Contrast Dyes, and Other Iodinated Agents

The adverse effects of exogenous iodide on the thyroid gland are iodide-induced hypothyroid goiter, iodide-induced thyroiditis without hyperthyroidism (411,412), and iodide-induced thyrotoxicosis (IIT) (413). IIT is seen in patients with endemic (iodine-deficient) goiter, current or previous nonendemic goiter, normal (iodine-sufficient) gland and multinodular goiter, and Graves' disease (true Jod-Basedow phenomenon) (413). Traditionally, the mechanisms of IIT have been described as provision of substrate to an iodide-deficient gland (caused by inadequate dietary iodide or an impaired trapping mechanism) with autonomous components (414). However, demonstration of IIT in iodine-sufficient glands with (415) and without (416) goiter has raised the possibility that there must be underlying abnormal thyroid homeostasis. This defect might involve a reversible, abnormally high set-point (low sensitivity) to intrathyroidal iodide by autoregulatory mechanisms, such as the Wolff-Chaikoff effect (413). Such an abnormality might also result from an atypical thyroiditis (416) or chronic stimulation by TSH (413) or TSHR-Ab. An additional mechanism of IIT in normal glands may be release of organic iodide (thyroglobulin) and inorganic iodide from the cytotoxic effects of iodide (173). The released thyroglobulin may be structurally altered and highly immunogenic (26,27).

Amiodarone and Thyrotoxicosis

Amiodarone (2-n-butyl-3-[4'-diethylaminoethoxy-3', 5'-diiodobenzoyl]-benzofurane) is an antianginal, antiarrhythmic agent that is 37% iodine (Fig. 19) (417). The amiodarone metabolite, desethylamiodarone, noncompetitively inhibits T_3 binding to myocardial thyroid hormone receptor β_1 proteins and competitively binds to nuclear T_3 receptors, inducing tissue hypothyroidism (418). The parent compound, amiodarone, competitively binds to myocardial calcium channels but does not act as an antagonist to T_3 receptors (419,420). At doses of 400 to 600 mg/day, it inhibits transport of T_4, but not T_3, into the perfused liver as well as inhibiting 5'-monodeiodination of T_4 and rT_3; this leads to increased serum concentrations of these thyroid hormones (421,422). Consequently, serum T_3 levels are diminished. Within the first 3 months, basal and TRH-stimulated TSH levels are increased, but with continued therapy, TSH normalizes and is even suppressed, despite clinical euthyroidism (421,423). Amiodarone's resemblance to T_3 may cause the pituitary gland to respond as in a hyperthyroid state with TSH suppression (424).

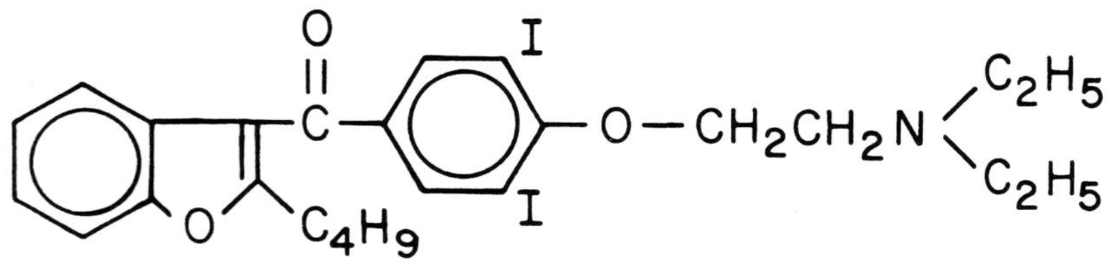

FIG. 19. Amiodarone structure.

Abnormal clinical thyroid status is found in 15% to 24% of patients treated with amiodarone (425). Hyperthyroidism is found in only 1% to 4% of patients treated with amiodarone (426). Because of its long half-life in muscle and fat stores, toxicity may be encountered long after the drug is stopped (416). Amiodarone–iodine-induced thyrotoxicosis (AIIT) can result from the effects of metabolized free iodide on the thyroid gland and can be detected by a raised T_3 or free T_3 level. Interestingly, Pinchera et al. (423) found 7 of 7 patients with AIIT and diffuse goiter to have TSHR-Ab. Here, amiodarone may also precipitate Graves' disease in susceptible individuals.

Alternatively, *in vitro* studies on rat FRTL-5 cells and primary cultures of human thyroid follicles have demonstrated the direct cytotoxicity of amiodarone, which is inhibited by perchlorate, dexamethasone, and to a lesser degree methimazole (427,428). This toxic effect may be potentiated by the excess iodide liberated by the drug.

The notion of thyrotoxicosis related to amiodarone exposure and an underlying inflammatory process has been popularized. Bartalena et al. (429) described two populations of amiodarone-treated patients with thyrotoxicosis. In the first group, with normal thyroid glands and no history of preexisting thyroid disease, serum interleukin-6 (IL-6) levels were very high and radioiodine uptake low, consistent with an amiodarone-induced thyroiditis. In the second group, with goiter and preexisting thyroid abnormalities, serum IL-6 levels were only slightly elevated and the radioiodine uptake normal or high, consistent with amiodarone-induced hyperthyroidism. Steroid, but not MMI, therapy normalized IL-6 and free T_3 levels despite persistently elevated urinary iodine excretion rates in patients with amiodarone-induced thyroiditis (Fig. 20) (429). On the other hand, patients with amiodarone-induced hyperthyroidism may respond better to conventional therapy with perchlorate and thionamides. The potential lethality of amiodarone-induced thyrotoxicosis is illustrated by a recent report of fatal hyperthyroidism in a cardiac transplant patient who had received amiodarone and total lymphoid irradiation with subsequent thyroid storm (430).

Patients treated with amiodarone should be monitored closely for concurrent or subsequent development of hyperthyroidism. Because the T_4 and free T_4 are expected to be high, serum T_3, free T_3, TSH, and thyroid antibodies should be followed. Moreover, neonates of mothers treated with amiodarone ought to be followed closely for thyroid dysfunction. Among 12 patients exposed to amiodarone during pregnancy, transient neonatal hypothyroidism and hyperthyroidism were each observed once (431).

Contrast Dyes and Other Iodinated Agents

There are many other iodinated agents, including topical agents and urographic and cholecystographic contrast dyes, that may cause IIT (Table 10). The amount of iodine in one dose of urographic and cholecystographic dyes is 10 g and 1 to 4 g, respectively, compared to 150 to 225 mg in amiodarone (412). In view of the millions of doses prescribed each year for these contrast agents, the extremely rare report of IIT is not surprising, because chronic administration is not undertaken. Such reports of IIT proba-

TABLE 10. *Iodinated agents used in clinical medicine*

Oral agents
Amiodarone
Beziodarone
Calcium iodide
Diiodohydroxyquin
Echothiphate iodide ophthalmic solution
Hydriodic acid syrup
Iodochlorhydroxyquin
Vitamins
Iodinated glycerol
Iodinated expectorants
Idoxuridine ophthalmic solution
Iodinated eye drops
Isopropamide iodide
Potassium iodide
Lugol's solution
Saturated solution potassium iodide
Parenteral preparations
Sodium iodide solution
Topical antiseptics
Diiodohydroxyquin cream
Iodine tincture
Iodoform gauze
Iodochlorhydroxyquin cream
Povidone iodine
Radiographic contrast agents
Diatrizoate meglumine and sodium
Iodinized oil
Iopanoic acid
Ipodate
Iothalamate
Metrizamide
Tyropanoate

Modified from ref. 432.

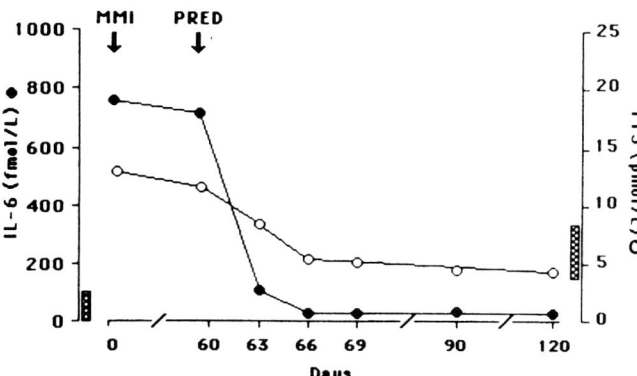

FIG. 20. Beneficial effect of steroids, but not MMI, on IL-6 and free T_3 levels in a patient with amiodarone-induced thyrotoxicosis. PRED, prednisone. (From ref. 429.)

bly reflect occult hyperthyroidism fortuitously uncovered by thyroid function testing. No prospective evaluations of routine use of cholecystographic agents, such as ipodate, have demonstrated an association with IIT (412).

Therapy

The therapies for IIT and AIIT are similar and fraught with the following predicaments: (a) intrathyroidal inorganic and organic iodine stores are large and impair the action of thionamides, (b) the use of therapeutic free iodide is precluded, and (c) there may be an exacerbation after discontinuation of the iodinated agent as thyroid hormone release is disinhibited. Treatment of AIIT is further complicated by the long half-life of amiodarone.

Conservative medical therapy is preferred, because the condition eventually resolves after discontinuation of the drug (in 3 to 6 months with a normal gland and 6 to 9 months with a goiter in AIIT) (432), and usually the hyperthyroidism is mild although the cardiac disease is life threatening. RAI therapy is contraindicated because of the low radioactive iodine uptake usually seen as the whole-body stable iodine pool is expanded. Surgery may be inappropriate in patients with ongoing thyrotoxicosis and/or cardiac disease.

For mild hyperthyroidism in IIT, the offending agent should be withdrawn. Although propranolol therapy may be helpful, beta-blockers synergize with amiodarone on atrioventricular conduction and should be used with caution. Prednisone (50 to 100 mg/day) (433) or prednisolone (1.5 mg/kg per day) (434) has been successful in producing a euthyroid state in approximately 20 days and is indicated when propranolol is ineffective or contraindicated. Despite its antithyroid secretory action, lithium is ineffective in IIT (435).

Thionamides are routinely used to block further organification, although their effect is not apparent for some weeks, depending on the amount of preformed hormone, and their use should be stopped once the patient is euthyroid. In severe hyperthyroidism, perchlorate and thionamides may be tried. Martino et al. (436) observed a remission by 16 to 36 days in seven of eight AIIT patients treated with potassium perchlorate, 1 g/day, and MMI, 40 mg/day, for up to 40 days. This is compared to six patients treated with MMI alone who remained thyrotoxic for 3 to 6 months. However, Newnham et al. (437) found that five patients with AIIT treated with PTU, 800 mg/day, and potassium perchlorate, 800 mg/day, did not become euthyroid until 7 to 19 weeks later. Perchlorate may have a role in treating severe IIT, but careful monitoring for development of leukopenia is mandatory. Of 60 consecutive patients without known thyroid disease undergoing coronary angiography, 33 demonstrated features of iodine excess on the thyroid gland 12 weeks later, and three patients developed latent hyperthyroidism (438). Twenty-six subsequent patients received prophylactic sodium perchlorate, 1 g, and MMI, 60 mg, 24 hours before and on the day of angiography, and none developed overt hyperthyroidism (one other patient had a second contrast dye procedure 2 weeks later without prophylaxis and did develop hyperthyroidism) (438).

If medical therapy is unsuccessful, surgical management is indicated (439). Surgery may be indicated when (a) thyrotoxicosis persists and the amiodarone must be continued to control cardiac disease, (b) the underlying gland is abnormal (presence of hot nodules or suspicious for neoplasm), or (c) medical therapy is ineffective. In 6 of 6 patients requiring near-total thyroidectomies at the Mayo Clinic, Brennan et al. (440) observed rapid correction of the thyrotoxicosis without any perioperative arrhythmias, and this has also been our own limited experience.

Factitious Hyperthyroidism

The treatment of surreptitious or inadvertent ingestion of thyroid hormones resulting in clinically significant hyperthyroidism consists of prompt discontinuation of the offending drug and control of symptoms with propranolol (441). Cholestyramine (2 to 4 g bid to qid) or colestipol (5 g 1 to 5 times a day), may be used to bind thyroxine in the gastrointestinal tract. Return to euthyroidism has been reported to occur in 3 to 4 days with cholestyramine therapy (442). A psychiatric referral should be considered in all cases of surreptitious use of thyroid hormones. Typically, there is an uncomplicated transition to the euthyroid state in 2 to 4 weeks without intervening hypothyroidism associated with the suppressed hypothalamic–pituitary–thyroidal axis.

Rare Causes of Hyperthyroidism

The hyperthyroidism associated with malignant infiltration of the thyroid gland (lymphoma, pancreatic carcinoma, breast cancer, malignant thymoma, and parathyroid carcinoma) (443–445) or infarction of an autonomous nodule (446) is caused by spillage of thyroid hormone from damaged follicles, and it is similar to the hyperthyroidism of thyroiditis. In the former condition, thyroid hormone spillage may be slow and protracted, requiring eventual surgical resection. In the latter case, hyperthyroidism is transient. In both, thyrotoxic signs and symptoms may be controlled with propranolol. Thyrotoxicosis has also been described with thyroid cancer, and with TSHR-Ab production (447,447a). Radiation thyroiditis may be seen after external beam radiotherapy and is extremely rare (448). Therapy consists of propranolol and steroids.

Struma ovarii (a very rare teratomatous ovarian tumor containing functioning thyroid tissue) and hyperfunctioning metastatic differentiated thyroid cancer are sources of ectopic thyroid hormone excess. Struma ovarii is best managed surgically, whereas thyroid metastasis should be treated with RAI or surgery. Again, medical management prior to surgery or RAI would consist of propranolol, thionamides, and/or steroids.

"Bovine" thyrotoxicosis has been reported to occur after ingestion of hamburger meat contaminated with thyroid tissue and is self-limited once the offending meat is taken away (449). In a related scenario, various vitamin supplements, which are largely unregulated by the U.S. Food and Drug Administration, contain desiccated bovine or porcine thyroid gland and can induce thyrotoxicosis even with the recommended dose (450). Graves' hyperthyroidism has also been described following long-term treatment with alpha-interferon therapy for chronic active hepatitis C (451).

Adjunctive Therapy with Radioactive Iodine

The purpose of adjunctive medical therapy with RAI treatment is to provide symptom control before and after administration of the radioisotope, potentially improving the effectiveness of RAI. We believe all patients are best rendered euthyroid prior to RAI treatment by using thionamides. This removes the danger of toxic radiation thyroiditis or accelerated hyperthyroidism (due to rapid release of T_4 and T_3 10 to 14 days after RAI) by decreased intrathyroidal iodine and preformed hormone concentrations. Because thionamides also reduce the 24-hr radioactive iodine uptake, they must be temporarily stopped at least 72 hr prior to RAI administration. During this time, there may even be a rebound increase in the uptake, although this is not usually seen in the presence of TSHR-Ab (452). Furthermore, because thionamides and iodine compete for iodination sites, thionamides should be restarted no sooner than 3 days after RAI. Propranolol (10 to 40 mg qid) may be administered alone (in mild cases) or with thionamides (in more severe cases), to manage thyrotoxic symptoms before and after RAI therapy.

Thionamides provide the advantage of an earlier restoration of euthyroidism after RAI treatment compared to treatment with propranolol alone (295,453). This is particularly important with coexistent cardiac disease, because the full effects of RAI may not be realized until 3 months after treatment, or even later. However, thionamides are associated with a higher relapse rate and frequency of permanent hypothyroidism (295,453,454). A higher failure rate has been associated with pretreatment with PTU, even if the PTU was discontinued 4 days before RAI and not restarted (455). However, a block-replace regimen with MMI effected an earlier response to RAI, without compromising the one-dose cure rate, compared with patients not receiving the thionamide (456). One cannot monitor the chemical effects of RAI on thyroid function while the patient is on thionamides (457). Therefore, 2 months after RAI treatment, the thionamides are stopped. A month later, the thyroid function tests are then checked.

Three other drugs have limited roles in adjunctive therapy with RAI treatment. Stable iodide initiated 7 days after RAI brings about the euthyroid state quicker than with RAI alone (457). Although there is a 60% transient hypothyroidism rate with iodide related to the frequent coexistent organification defect, the frequency of permanent hypothyroidism (58%) is the same as with RAI alone (457). The development of goiter was associated with transient hypothyroidism, whereas patients developing permanent hypothyroidism had normal or slightly enlarged glands (457).

Lithium carbonate, 400 mg/day, administered for 7 days prior to RAI and 7 days after RAI, increases retention of the radioactive iodine dose (211). This is most advantageous in treating patients with a small gland and rapid turnover, or young patients in whom a small RAI dose is preferred. At this dose, lithium has few side effects (211). When thyrotoxicosis is severe or when there are cardiac problems, propranolol and lithium may be added to the medical regimen. Steroids have been used in conjunction with RAI for control of accelerated hyperthyroidism. In addition, prednisone may also be administered at 0.4 to 0.5 mg/kg per day at the time of RAI treatment, continued at this dose for 1 month, and then weaned over a 3-month period as a prophylactic measure to decrease the risk of development or worsening of orbitopathy (458–460).

Perioperative Medical Management

Three drugs are primarily used in the management of thyrotoxic patients destined for surgical treatment. Historically, iodine was first introduced by Plummer (143) as an effective postoperative agent to prevent thyroid crisis. Prior to modern preoperative prophylaxis, the incidence of medical and surgical thyroid crisis was reported as high as 7% (461), with a mortality of 60% to 70% (462,463). Fear of postoperative storm engendered the routine use of iodine until it was noted clinically that some patients "escaped" the effect in as few as 10 days (167), whereas others experienced an exacerbation of their thyrotoxicosis (464). The potential of escape necessitates performing surgery within a 7- to 14-day period. It should be noted, however, that concentrations of free T_4 and free T_3 in venous thyroid effluent during emergency thyroidectomy for Graves' disease did not exceed peripheral levels, casting doubt on the need for routine preoperative medical therapy (465).

The advent of thionamides, however, provided an effective means to completely render the patient euthyroid prior to surgery, thereby decreasing the risk of thyroid crises. Following thionamide therapy for 1 to 3 months, the addition of iodine (SSKI or Lugol's solution, 2 to 5 drops bid to tid) within the last 7 to 14 days promotes involution of the gland, in part because of reduced thyroidal blood flow (466). Using thionamides affords greater flexibility in timing or arranging hospitalization for surgery. In patients intolerant to thionamides, lithium carbonate, 600 to 900 mg/day, may be considered preoperatively (Fig. 21) (467,468).

Propranolol has been used as single therapy in the preparation of mildly thyrotoxic patients for surgery. Because an effect on the heart rate is achieved by 24 hr, with a maximal effect attained by 3 to 4 days in most thyrotoxic patients, surgery may be scheduled as early as 3 to 4 days after propranolol is started (469). Metoprolol (100 mg bid) has been found to be an effective preoperative therapy in patients with asthma when propranolol cannot be used (470). Although it is debated whether propranolol alone can provide acceptable prophylaxis against postoperative thyroid crisis (471), Toft et al. (472) did not observe any episodes of crisis in 100 patients treated only with propranolol. They caution, however, that this is because a high standard of supervision was maintained, ensuring all doses were taken (titrating to a heart rate below 90 beats per min, not omitting the last presurgical dose, and continuing through surgery and for 7 postoperative days). Eighty percent of patients were euthyroid by 1 year, with 20% experiencing transient hypothyroidism between 3 and 6 months. In the minority of patients that do not respond to large doses of beta-adrenergic blockade (160 mg every 6 hr) (473), usually with a large goiter, addition of iodide can induce the euthyroid state (474). Propranolol with iodide has also been noted to bring about a firmer, less friable, more mobilizable gland that is less likely to bleed and contribute to surgical complications, than thionamides with iodide (475). Finally, the addition of iodide to propranolol may relax the standards necessary for propranolol-alone therapy.

An alternative to traditional preoperative therapy with thionamides, iodine, and propranolol for 4 to 6 weeks consists of steroids (dexamethasone 0.5 mg po q6h), ipodate (500 mg po q6h), and propranolol (40 mg po q8h) for 5 days. Of 14 patients so treated, all were clinically euthyroid by surgery on day 6, with a mean reduction in the serum T_3 of 65% and no adverse side effects (476). This approach is safe, effective, and of low cost, and it is particularly useful in patients unable to comply with the longer regimen.

In conclusion, for severe thyrotoxicosis requiring surgery, we recommend the combination of thionamides, propranolol, and iodide (477). In mild hyperthyroid cases, thionamides have been successfully omitted prior to surgery. Following surgery, thyroid function tests should be obtained every 4 to 8 weeks in case transient or permanent hypothyroidism occurs. If chemical hypothyroidism develops, indicated by a prolonged increase in the postoperative TSH level, supplemental T_4 should be added to the regimen.

REFERENCES

1. Dunn JT. Choice of therapy in young adults with hyperthyroidism of Graves' disease. *Ann Intern Med* 1984;100:891–893.
2. Solomon B, Glinoer D, Lagrasses R, Wartofsky L. *Management of hyperthyroidism due to Graves' disease: results of a survey of members of the ATA.* 63rd annual meeting of the American Thyroid Association, Montreal, September-October, 1988.
3. Glinoer D, Hesch D, Lagasse R, Laurberg P. *The management of hyperthyroidism due to Graves' disease in Europe in 1986. Results of an international survey.* 15th annual meeting of the European Thyroid Association, Stockholm, June-July, 1986.
4. Mackenzie JB, Mackenzie CG, McMollum EV. Effect of sulfanilylguanidine on the thyroid of the rat. *Science* 1941;94:518–519.
5. Mackenzie CG, Mackenzie JB. Effect of sulfonamides and thioureas on the thyroid gland and basal metabolism. *Endocrinology* 1943;32:185–209.
6. Richter CP, Clisby KH. Graying of hair produced by ingestion of phenylthiocarbamide. *Proc Soc Exp Biol Med* 1942;48:684–687.
7. Richter CP, Clisby KH. Toxic effect of bitter tasting phenylthiocarbamide. *Arch Pathol* 1942;33:46–57.
8. Kennedy TH. Thioureas as goitrogenic substances. *Nature* 1942;150:223–234.
9. Astwood EB, Sullivan J, Bissell A, Tyslowitz R. Action of certain sulfonamides and of thioureas upon the function of the thyroid gland of the rat. *Endocrinology* 1943;32:210–225.
10. Astwood EB. Treatment of hyperthyroidism with thiourea and thiouracil. *JAMA* 1943;122:78–81.
11. Gabrilove JL, Kert MJ, Soffer LJ. The use of thiouracil in the treatment of patients with hyperthyroidism. *Ann Intern Med* 1945;23:537–558.
12. Van Winkle W, Hardy SM, Hazel GR, et al. The clinical toxicity of thiouracil. *JAMA* 1946;130:343–347.
13. Astwood EB, Vanderlaan WP. Thiouracil derivatives of greater activity for the treatment of hyperthyroidism. *J Clin Endocrinol Metab* 1945;5:424–430.
14. Jambut-Absil AC, Buxeraud J, Claude J, Raby C. Drugs derived from thiazole and imidazole or with nitrogen-carbon-sulphur or tertiary amino groups: prediction of secondary antithyroid activity by UV/visible spectroscopy. *Arzneimittelforschung* 1987;37:772–777.
15. Taylor JJ, Willson RL, Kendall-Taylor P. Evidence for direct interactions between methimazole and free radicals. *FEBS Lett* 1984;176:337–340.
16. Taurog A. The mechanism of action of the thioureylene antithyroid drugs. *Endocrinology* 1976;98:1031–1046.
17. Davidson B, Soodak M, Neary JT, et al. The irreversible inactivation of thyroid peroxidase by methylmercaptoimidazole, thiouracil, and

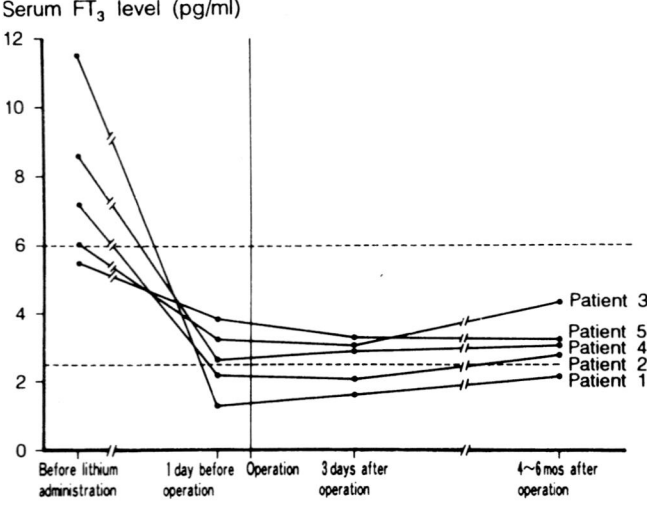

FIG. 21. Changes in serum free T_3 levels in five patients treated with lithium preoperatively. (From ref. 467.)

propylthiouracil in vitro and its relationship to in vivo findings. *Endocrinology* 1978;103:871–882.
18. Engler H, Taurog A, Luthy C, Dorris ML. Reversible and irreversible inhibition of thyroid peroxidase-catalyzed iodination by thioureylene drugs. *Endocrinology* 1983;112:86–95.
19. Taurog A, Dorris ML, Guziec FS. Metabolism of ^{35}S- and ^{14}C-labelled 1-methyl-2-mercaptoimidazole in vitro and in vivo. *Endocrinology* 1989:124:30–39.
20. Nagasaki A, Hikada H. Effect of antithyroid agents 6-propyl-2-thiouracil and 1-methyl-2-mercaptoimidazole on human thyroid iodide peroxidase. *J Clin Endocrinol Metab* 1976;43:152–158.
21. Doerge DR. Mechanism-based inhibition of lactoperoxidase by thiocarbamide goitrogens. *Biochemistry* 1988;27:3697–3700.
22. Cooper DS, Saxe VC, Meskell M, Maloof F, Ridgway EC. Acute effects of propylthiouracil (PTU) on thyroidal organification and peripheral iodothyronine deiodination: correlation with serum PTU levels measured by radioimmunoassay. *J Clin Endocrinol Metab* 1982; 54:101–107.
23. Marchant U, Lees JFH, Alexander WD. Antithyroid drugs. *Pharmacol Ther B* 1978;3:305–348.
24. Haynes RC, Murad F. Thyroid and antithyroid drugs. In: Gilman AG, Goodman LS, Gilman A, eds. *The pharmacologic basis of therapeutics*, 6th ed. New York: MacMillan, 1980;1397–1419.
25. Engler H, Taurog A, Dorris ML. Preferential inhibition of thyroxine and 3,5,3′-triiodothyronine formation by propylthiouracil and methylmercaptoimidazole in thyroid peroxidase-catalyzed iodination or thyroglobulin. *Endocrinology* 1982;110:190–197.
26. Papapetrou PD, Mothon S, Alexander WD. Binding of the ^{35}S or ^{35}S-propylthiouracil by follicular thyroglobulin in vivo and in vitro. *Acta Endocrinol (Copenh)* 1975;79:248–258.
27. Monaco F, Santolamazza C, De Ros I, Andreoli A. Effects of propylthiouracil and methylmercaptoimidazole on thyroglobulin synthesis. *Acta Endocrinol (Copenh)* 1980;93:32–36.
28. Courtin F, Deme D, Virion A, Michot JL, Pommier J, Nunez J. The role of lactoperoxidase-H$_2$O$_2$ compounds in the catalysis of thyroglobulin iodination and thyroid hormone synthesis. *Eur J Biochem* 1982;124:603–609.
29. Feldman A, Schwartz AE, Friedman EW, Davies TF. Inhibition of thyroglobulin secretion by antithyroid drugs: another mechanism for immunosuppression by thionamides. In: Medeiros-Neto G, Gaitan E, eds. *Frontiers in thyroidology*. New York: Plenum Press, 1985; 1535–1538.
30. Nunez J, Pommier J. Formation of thyroid hormones. *Vitam Horm* 1982;39:175–229.
31. Solomon DH, Beck JC, Vanderlaan WP, Astwood EB. Prognosis of hyperthyroidism treated by antithyroid drugs *JAMA* 1953;152: 201–205.
32. Hershman JM, Givens JR, Cassidy CE, Astwood EB. Long-term outcome of hyperthyroidism treated with antithyroid drugs. *J Clin Endocrinol Metab* 1966;26:803–807.
33. Leclere J. Antithyroid drugs a rational treatment for Graves' disease? *Horm Res* 1987;26:125–130.
34. Sugrue D, McEvoy M, Feely J, Drury MI. Hyperthyroidism in the land of Graves': results of treatment by surgery, radioiodine and carbimazole in 837 cases. *Q J Med* 1980;49:51–61.
35. Hedley AJ, Young RE, Jones SJ, Alexander WD, Bewsher PD, and Scottish Automated Follow-up Register Group. Antithyroid drugs in the treatment of hyperthyroidism of Graves' disease: long-term followup of 434 patients. *Clin Endocrinol (Oxf)* 1989;31:209.
36. Weetman AP. McGregor AM, Hall R. Evidence for an effect of antithyroid drugs on the natural history of Graves' disease. *Clin Endocrinol (Oxf)* 1984;21:163–172.
37. Michie W, Beck JS, Mahaffy RG, Honein EF, Fowler GB. Quantitative radiological and histological studies of the thymus in thyroid disease. *Lancet* 1967;1:691–695.
38. McGregor AM, Petersen MM, McLachlan SM, Rooke P, Smith BR, Hall R. Carbimazole and the autoimmune response in Graves' disease. *N Engl J Med* 1980;303:302–307.
39. Wall JR, Manwar GL, Greenwood DM, Walters BA. The in vitro suppression of lectin induced ^{3}H-thymidine incorporation into DNA of peripheral blood lymphocytes after the addition of propylthiouracil. *J Clin Endocrinol Metab* 1976;43:1406–1409.
40. Weiss I, Davies TF. Inhibition of immunoglobulin-secreting cells by antithyroid drugs. *J Clin Endocrinol Metab* 1981;53:1223–1228.
41. Weetman AP, McGregor AM, Hall R. Methimazole inhibits thyroid autoantibody production by an action on accessory cells. *Clin Immunol Immunopathol* 1983;28:39–45.
42. Pozzilli P, Sensi M, Andreani D. Inhibition of killer cell cytotoxicity induced by carbimazole in vitro. *J Endocrinol Invest* 1982;5:149–152.
43. Goldrath N, Eisenstein Z, Bank H, Shoham J. Anti-thyroid drugs and lymphocyte function. *Clin Exp Immunol* 1982;50:55–69.
44. Aoki R, Pinnamaneni M, DeGroot LJ. Studies on suppressor cell function in thyroid diseases. *J Clin Endocrinol Metab* 1979;48:803–810.
45. Davies TF, Weiss I, Gerber MA. Influence of methimazole on murine thyroiditis. *J Clin Invest* 1984;73:397–404.
46. Rennie DP, McGregor AM, Keast D, et al. The influence of methimazole on thyroglobulin-induced autoimmune thyroiditis in the rat. *Endocrinology* 1983;112:326–330.
47. Lazarus JH, Marchant B, Alexander WD, Clark DH. ^{35}S-antithyroid drug concentration and organic binding of iodine in the human thyroid. *Clin Endocrinol (Oxf)* 1975;4:609–615.
48. Pinchera A, Liberti P, Martino E, et al. Effects of antithyroid therapy on the long-acting thyroid stimulator and the antithyroglobulin antibodies. *J Clin Endocrinol Metab* 1969;29:231–238.
49. Bech K, Madsen SN. Influence of treatment with radioiodine and propylthiouracil on thyroid stimulating immunoglobulins in Graves' disease. *Clin Endocrinol (Oxf)* 1980;13:417–424.
50. Totterman THG, Anders Karksson F, Bengtsson M, Mendel-Hartvig I. Induction of circulating activated suppressor-like T cells by methimazole therapy for Graves' disease. *N Engl J Med* 1987;316:15–22.
51. Murakami M. Improvement of immunologic abnormalities associated with hyperthyroidism of Graves' disease during methimazole treatment. *Horm Metab Res* 1988;20:235–238.
52. Charreire J, Karsenty G, Bouchard P, Schaison G. Effect of carbimazole treatment on specific and nonspecific immunological parameters in patients with Graves' disease. *Clin Exp Immunol* 1984;57:633–638.
53. Davies TF, Evered DC, Smith RR, Yeo PPB, Clark F, Hall R. Value of thyroid-stimulating-antibody determinations in predicting short-term thyrotoxic relapse in Graves' disease. *Lancet* 1977;1:1181–1182.
54. Ferguson MM, Alexander WD, Conn IG, McDonald FG, Mairs RJ, Sweeney D. Are antithyroid drugs immunosuppressive? *Br Med J [Clin Res]* 1984;288:1004–1005.
55. Connell JMC, McCrudden DC, Small M, Ferguson MM, Alexander WD. Accumulation of thioureylene drugs in mouse salivary gland. *J Endocrinol* 1983;96:91–96.
56. Timonen T. Characteristics of fresh and cultured natural killer cells. *Clin Immunol Allergy* 1983;3:465–477.
57. Horwitz UA, Fakke AC. An Fc-bearing, third population of human mononuclear cells with cytotoxic and regulatory function. *Immunol Today* 1984;5:148–153.
58. Weetman AP, Gunn C, Hall R, McGregor AM. The absence of any effect of methimazole on in vitro cell-mediated cytotoxicity. *Clin Endocrinol (Oxf)* 1985;22:57–64.
59. McGregor AM, Ibbertson HK, Smith BR, Hall R. Carbimazole and autoantibody synthesis in Hashimoto's thyroiditis. *Br Med J* 1980;281:968–969.
60. Weetman AP, Gunn C, Hall R, McGregor AM. The accumulation of [^{35}S]methimazole by monocytes and macrophages. *Acta Endocrinol (Copenh)* 1984;107:366–370.
61. Weetman AP, Holt ME, Campbell AK, Hall R, McGregor AM. Methimazole and generation of oxygen radicals by monocytes: potential role in immunosuppression. *Br Med J* 1984;288:518–520.
62. McLachlan SM, Pegg CA, Atherton MC, et al. The effect of carbimazole on thyroid autoantibody synthesis by thyroid lymphocytes. *J Clin Endocrinol Metab* 1985;60:1237–1242.
63. Weetman AP, Gunn C, Hall R, McGregor AM. The absence of any effect of methimazole on in vitro cell-mediated cytotoxicity. *Clin Endocrinol (Oxf)* 1985;22:57–64.
64. Ratanachaiyavong S, McGregor AM. Immunosuppressive effects of antithyroid drugs. *Baillieres Clin Endocrinol Metab* 1985;14:449–467.
65. Volpe R, Karlsson A, Jansson R, Dahlberg PA. Evidence that antithyroid drugs induce remissions in Graves' disease by modulating thyroid cellular activity. *Clin Endocrinol (Oxf)* 1986;25:453–462.
66. Volpe R, Karlsson A, Jansson R, Dahlberg PA. Thyrostatic drugs act through modulation of thyroid cell activity to induce remissions in Graves' disease. *Acta Endocrinol Suppl (Copenh)* 1987;281:305–311.
67. Romaldini JH, Werner MC, Rodrigues HF, Teixeira VL, Werner RS, Farah CS, Bromberg N. Graves' disease and Hashimoto's thyroiditis; effects of high doses of antithyroid drugs on thyroid autoantibody levels. *J Endocrinol Invest* 1986;9:233–238.

68. Davies TF, Yang C, Platzer M. The influence of antithyroid drugs and iodine on thyroid cell MHC class II antigen expression. *Clin Endocrinol (Oxf)* 1989;31:125–135.
69. Taniguchi S, Yoshida A, Mashiba H. Direct effect of methimazole on rat thyroidal cell growth induced by thyrotropin and insulin-like growth factor I. *Endocrinology* 1989;124:2046–2051.
70. Morreale de Escobar C, Escobar del Rey F. Influence of thiourea, potassium perchlorate and thiocyanate and of graded doses of propylthiouracil on thyroid hormone metabolism in thyroidectomized rats, isotopically equilibrated with varying doses of exogenous hormone. *Endocrinology* 1962;71:906–913.
71. Saberi M, Sterling FH, Utiger RD. Reduction in extrathyroidal triiodothyronine production by propylthiouracil in man *J Clin Invest* 1975;55:218–223.
72. Geffner DL, Azukizawa M, Hershman JM. Propylthiouracil blocks extrathyroidal conversion of thyroxine to triiodothyronine and augments thyrotropin secretion in man. *J Clin Invest* 1975;55:224–229.
73. Chopra IJ. A study of extrathyroidal conversion of thyroxine (T_4) to 3,3′,5-triiodothyronine (T_3) in vitro. *Endocrinology* 1977;101:453–463.
74. Abuid J, Larsen PR. Triiodothyronine and thyroxine in hyperthyroidism. *J Clin Invest* 1974;54:201–208.
75. Kampmann JP, Hansen JM. Clinical pharmacokinetics of antithyroid drugs. *Clin Pharmacokinet* 1981;6:401–428.
76. McMurray JF, Gilliland PF, Ratliff CR. Bourland PD. Pharmacodynamics of propylthiouracil in normal and hyperthyroid subjects after a single oral dose. *J Clin Endocrinol Metab* 1975;41:362–364.
77. Alexander WD, Evans V, Macauleay A, Gallagher TF, Londono J. Metabolism of ^{35}S-labelled antithyroid drugs in man. *Br Med J* 1969;2:290–291.
78. Cooper DS, Bode HH, Nath B, Saxe V, Maloof F, Ridgway EC. Methimazole pharmacology in man: studies using a newly developed radioimmunoassay for methimazole. *J Clin Endocrinol Metab* 1984;58:473–479.
79. Aungst BJ, Vesell E, Shapiro JR. Unusual characteristics of the dose-dependent uptake of propylthiouracil by thyroid gland in vivo. *Biochem Pharmacol* 1979;28:1479–1484.
80. Williams RH, Kay GA. Further studies of the absorption, distribution, and elimination of thiouracil. *J Clin Endocrinol* 1944;4:385–393.
81. Jansson R, Dahlberg PA, Johansson H, Lindstrom B. Intrathyroidal concentrations of methimazole in patients with Graves' disease. *Baillieres Clin Endocrinol Metab* 1983;57:129–132.
82. Okuno A, Yano K, Inyaku F, et al. Pharmacokinetics of methimazole in children and adolescents with Graves' disease. *Acta Endocrinol (Copenh)* 1987;115:112–118.
83. Solomon DH. Treatment of Graves' hyperthyroidism. In: Ingbar SH, Braverman LE, eds. *Werner's The thyroid,* 5th ed. New York: JB Lippincott, 1986;987–1014.
84. Larsen PR, Ingbar SH. The thyroid gland. In: Wilson JD, Foster DW, eds. *Williams' Textbook of Endocrinology*, 8th ed. Philadelphia: WB Saunders, 1992;357–487.
85. Amrhein JA, Kenny FM, Ross D. Granulocytopenia, lupus-like syndrome, and other complications of propylthiouracil therapy. *J Pediatr* 1970;76:54–63.
86. Wiberg JJ, Nuttall FQ. Methimazole toxicity from high doses. *Ann Intern Med* 1972;77:414–416.
87. Cooper DS, Goldminz D, Levin AA, Ladensen PW, Daniels GH, Molitch ME, Ridgway EC. Agranulocytosis associated with antithyroid drugs: effects of patient age and drug dose. *Ann Intern Med* 1983;98:26–29.
88. Wall JR, Fang SL, Kuroki T, Ingbar SH, Braverman LE. In vitro immunoreactivity to propylthiouracil, methimazole, and carbimamole in patients with Graves' disease: a possible cause of antithyroid drug-induced agranulocytosis. *J Clin Endocrinol Metab* 1984;58:868–872.
89. Martelo OJ, Katims RB, Yunis AA. Bone marrow aplasia following propylthiouracil therapy. Report of a case with complete recovery. *Arch Intern Med* 1967;120:587–590.
90. Tamai H, Mukuta T, Matsubayashi S, Fukata S, Komaki G, Kuma K, Kumagai LF, Nagataki S. Treatment of methimazole-induced agranulocytosis using recombinant human granulocyte colony-stimulating factor (rhG-CSF). *J Clin Endocrinol Metab* 1993;77:1356–1360.
91. Magner JA, Snyder DK. Methimazole-induced agranulocytosis treated with recombinant human granulocyte colony-stimulating factor (G-CSF). *Thyroid* 1994;4:295–296.
92. Balkin MS, Buchholtz M, Ortiz J, Green AJ. Propylthiouracil (PTU)-induced agranulocytosis treated with recombinant human granulocyte colony-stimulating factor (G-CSF). *Thyroid* 1993;4:305–309.
93. Shabatai R, Shapiro MS, Orenstein D, Taragan R, Shenkman L. *Arthritis Rheum* 1984;27:227–229.
94. Takuwa N, Kojima I, Ogata E. Lupus-like syndrome: a rare complication in thionamide therapy for Graves' disease. *Endocrinol Jpn* 1981;28:663–667.
95. Hung W, August GP. A "collagen-like" syndrome associated with antithyroid therapy. *J Pediatr* 1973;82:852–854.
96. Shergy WJ, Caldwell DS. Polymyositis after propylthiouracil treatment for hyperthyroidism. *Ann Rheum Dis* 1988;47:340–343.
97. Griswold WR, Mendoza SA, Johnston W, Nichols LS. Vasculitis associated with propylthiouracil: evidence for immune complex pathogenesis and response to therapy. *West J Med* 1978;128:543–546.
98. Fedotin MS, Lefer LG. Liver disease caused by propylthiouracil. *Arch Intern Med* 1975;135:319–321.
99. Huang MJ, Li KL, Wei JS, Wu SS, Fan KD, Liaw YF. Sequential liver and bone biochemical changes in hyperthyroidism: prospective controlled follow-up study. *Am J Gastroenterol* 1994;89:1071–1076.
100. Liaw YF, Huang MJ, Fan KD, Li KL, Wu SS, Chen TJ. Hepatic injury during propylthiouracil therapy in patients with hyperthyroidism. *Ann Intern Med* 1993;118:424–428.
101. Singh A, Thakur R. Scintigraphic study of propylthiouracil induced submassive hepatic necrosis. *Clin Nucl Med* 1995;20:132–135.
102. Hirata Y, Tominga M, Ito IJ, Noguchi A. Spontaneous hypoglycemia with insulin autoimmunity in Graves' disease. *Ann Intern Med* 1974;81:214–218.
103. Lu CC, Lee JK, Lam HC, Yang CY, Han TM. Insulin autoimmune syndrome in a patient with methimazole and carbimazole-treated Graves' disease: a case report. *Chung Hua I Hseuh Tsa Chih (Taipei)* 1994;54:353–358.
104. Sammon TJ, Peden VH, Witzleben C, King JP. Disseminated intravascular coagulation complicating PTU therapy. *Clin Pediatr (Phila)* 1971;10:739–742.
105. Canary Jl, Schaaf M, Duffy BI, Kyle LH. Effects of oral and intramuscular administration of reserpine in thyrotoxicosis. *N Engl J Med* 1957;257:436–442.
106. Lee WY, Bronsky D, Waldstein SS. Studies of thyroid and sympathetic nervous system interrelationships. II. Effects of guanethidine on manifestations of hyperthyroidism. *J Clin Endocrinol Metab* 1962;22:879–885.
107. Wartofsky L, Dimond RC, Noel GL, Frantz AG, Earll JM. Failure of propranolol to alter thyroid iodine release, thyroxine turnover, or the TSH and PRL responses to thyrotropin-releasing hormone in patients with thyrotoxicosis. *J Clin Endocrinol Metab* 1975;41:485–490.
108. Vinik AI, Pimstone BL, Hoffenherg R. Sympathetic nervous system blocking in hyperthyroidism. *J Clin Endocrinol Metab* 1968;28:725–727.
109. McLarty DG, Brownlie BEW, Alexander WD, Papepetrou PD, Horton P. Remission of thyrotoxicosis during treatment with propranolol. *Br Med J* 1973;2:332–334.
110. Mazzaferri EL, Reynolds JC, Youny RL, Thomas CN, Parisi AF. Propranolol as primary therapy for thyrotoxicosis. *Arch Intern Med* 1976;136:50–56.
111. Lyon DM. The influence of the thyroid gland on the response to adrenaline. *Br Med J* 1923;1:966–967.
112. Schneckloth RE, Kurland GS, Freedberg AS. Effects of variation in thyroid function on the pressor response to norepinephrine in man. *Metabolism* 1953;2:546–555.
113. Gaffney TE, Braunwald E, Kahler RL. Effects of guanethidine on triiodothyronine induced hyperthyroidism in man. *N Engl J Med* 1961;265:16–20.
114. Goldstein S, Killip T. Catecholamine depletion in thyrotoxicosis. *Circulation* 1965;31:219–227.
115. Prichard BNC, McDevitt DG, Shanks RG. Uses of beta-adrenoceptor blocking drugs. *J R Coll Physicians Lond* 1976;11:35–57.
116. Williams LT, Lefkowitz RJ, Watanabe AM, Hathaway DR, Besch HR. Thyroid hormone regulation of β-adrenergic receptor number. *J Biol Chem* 1977;252:2787–2789.
117. Wiener L, Stout BD, Cox JW. Influence of beta sympathetic blockade (propranolol) on the hemodynamics of hyperthyroidism. *Am J Med* 1969;46:227–233.
118. Saunders J, Hall SE, Crowther A, Sonksen PH. The effect of propranolol on thyroid hormones and oxygen consumption in thyrotoxicosis. *Clin Endocrinol (Oxf)* 1978;9:67–72.

119. Amidi M, Leon DF, De Groot WJ, Kroetz FW, Leonard JJ. Effect of the thyroid state on myocardial contractility and ventricular ejection in man. *Circulation* 1968;38:229–239.
120. Howitt G, Rowlands DJ, Leung DYT, Logan WFWE. Myocardial contractility and the effects of beta-adrenergic blockade in hypothyroidism and hyperthyroidism. *Clin Sci* 1968;34:485–495.
121. Grossman W, Robin NI, Johnson LW, Brooks HL, Selenkow HA, Dexter L. The enhanced myocardial contractility of thyrotoxicosis: role of the beta-adrenergic receptor. *Ann Intern Med* 1971;74:869–874.
122. Wiswell JG, Hurwitz GE, Corohono V, Bing OHL, Child DL. Urinary catecholamines and their metabolites in hyperthyroidism and hypothyroidism. *J Clin Endocrinol Metab* 1963;23:1102–1106.
123. Christensen NJ. Plasma noradrenaline and adrenaline in patients with thyrotoxicosis and myxoedema. *Clin Sci Mol Med* 1973;45:163–171.
124. Forfar JC, Stewart J, Sawers A, Toft AD. Cardiovascular responses in hyperthyroidism before and during β-adrenoceptor blockade: evidence against adrenergic hypersensitivity. *Clin Endocrinol (Oxf)* 1982;16:441–452.
125. Symons C. Thyroid heart disease. *Br Heart J* 1979;41:257–262.
126. Grossman W, Robin NI, Johnson LW, Brooks H, Selenkow HA, Dexter L. Effects of beta blockade on the peripheral manifestations of thyrotoxicosis. *Ann Intern Med* 1971;74:875–879.
127. Verhoeven RP, Visser TJ, Docter R, Hennemann G, Schalekamp MADH. Plasma thyroxine, 3,3′,5-triiodothyronine and 3,3′,5′-triiodothyronine during β-adrenergic blockade in hyperthyroidism. *J Clin Endocrinol Metab* 1977;44:1002–1005.
128. Harrower ADB, Fyffe JA, Horn DB, Strong JA. Thyroxine and triiodothyronine levels in hyperthyroid patients during treatment with propranolol. *Clin Endocrinol (Oxf)* 1977;7:41–44.
129. Perrild H, Hansen JM, Skovsted L, Christensen LK. Different effects of propranolol, alprenolol, sotalol, atenolol and metoprolol on serum T_3 and serum rT_3 in hyperthyroidism. *Clin Endocrinol (Oxf)* 1983;18:139–142.
130. Lumholtz IB, Siersbaek-Nielsen K, Faber J, Kirkegard C, Friis TH. Effect of propranolol on extrathyroidal metabolism of thyroxine and 3,3′,5-triiodothyronine evaluated by noncompartmental kinetics. *J Clin Endocrinol Metab* 1978;47:587–589.
131. Rubenfeld S, Silverman VE, Welch KMA, Mallette LE, Kohler PO. Variable plasma propranolol levels in thyrotoxicosis. *N Engl J Med* 1979;300:353–354.
132. McAinsh J, Baber NS, Smith R, Young J. Pharmacokinetic and pharmacodynamic studies with long-acting propranolol. *Br J Clin Pharmacol* 1978;6:115–121.
133. Kashiwai T, Tada H, Tamaki H, Hidaka Y, Ito E, Iwatani Y, Amino N. Reducing effect of nadolol on serum levels of free thyroid hormones in hyperthyroidism. *Endocr J* 1994;41:717–723.
134. Georges LP, Santangelo RP, Mackin JF, Canary JJ. Metabolic effects of propranolol in thyrotoxicosis. 1. Nitrogen, calcium, and hydroxyproline. *Metabolism* 1975;24:11–21.
135. Rude RK, Oldham SB, Singer FR, Nicoloff JT. Treatment of thyrotoxic hypercalcemia with propranolol. *N Engl J Med* 1976;294:431–433.
136. Weinstein R, Schwartzman R, Levey GS. Propranolol reversal of bulbar dysfunction and proximal myopathy in hyperthyroidism. *Ann Intern Med* 1975;82:540–541.
137. Pimstone N, Marine N, Pimstone B. Beta-adrenergic blockade in thyrotoxic myopathy. *Lancet* 1968;2:1219–1220.
138. Conway MJ, Seibel JA, Eaton RP. Thyrotoxicosis and periodic paralysis: improvement with beta blockade. *Ann Intern Med* 1974;81:332–336.
139. Miller RR, Olsen HG, Amsterdam EA, Mason DT. Propranolol-withdrawal rebound phenomenon. *N Engl J Med* 1975;293:416–418.
140. Coindet JC. Decouverte d'un nouveau remede contre le goitre (iodine). *Ann de Chim et de Phys* 1820;15:49–59. As cited in: Friend DG. Iodide therapy and the importance of quantitating the dose. *N Engl J Med* 1960;263:1358–1360.
141. Coindet JF. *Ann de Chim et de Phys* 1821;16:252. As cited in: Lividas DP, Koutras DA, Souvatzoglou A, Beckers C. The toxic effects of small iodine supplements in patients with autonomous thyroid nodules. *Clin Endocrinol (Oxf)* 1977;7:121–127.
142. Kocher T. Uber Jod Basedow. *Archivfür Klinische Chirurgie* 1910;92:1166–1193. As cited in: Lividas DP, Koutras DA, Souvatzoglou A, Beckers C. The toxic effects of small iodine supplements in patients with autonomous thyroid nodules. *Clin Endocrinol (Oxf)* 1977;7:121–127.
143. Plummer HS. Results of administering iodine to patients having exophthalmic goiter. *JAMA* 1923;80:1955.
144. Kimball OP. Induced hyperthyroidism. *JAMA* 1925;85:1709–1710.
145. Thompson WO, Brailey AG, Thompson PK, Thorp EG. The range of effective iodine dosage in exophthalmic goiter. *Arch Intern Med* 1930;45:261–281.
146. Thompson WO, Thorp EG, Thompson PK, Cohen AC. The range of effective iodine dosage in exophthalmic goiter. *Arch Intern Med* 1930;45:420–429.
147. Thompson WO, Cohen AC, Thompson PK, Thorp EG, Brailey AG. The range of effective iodine dosage in exophthalmic goiter. *Arch Intern Med* 1930;45:430–455.
148. Quimby EH, Feitelberg S, Silver S. *Radioactive isotopes in clinical practice.* Philadelphia: Lea & Febiger, 1958.
149. Berson SA, Yalow RS. Quantitative aspects of iodine metabolism. The exchangeable organic iodine pool, and the rates of thyroidal secretion, peripheral degradation and fecal excretion of endogenously synthesized organically bound iodine. *J Clin Invest* 1954;33:1533–1552.
150. Berson SA, Yalow RS. The iodide trapping and binding functions of the thyroid. *J Clin Invest* 1955;34:186–204.
151. Wolff J, Chaikoff IL, Goldberg RC, Meier JR. The temporary nature of the inhibitory action of excess iodide on organic iodine synthesis in the normal thyroid. *Endocrinology* 1949;45:504–513.
152. Morton ME, Chaikoff IL, Rosenfeld S. Inhibiting effect of inorganic iodide on the formation in vitro of thyroxine and diiodotyrosine by surviving thyroid tissue. *J Biol Chem* 1944;154:381–387.
153. Wolff J, Chaikoff IL. Plasma inorganic iodide as a homeostatic regulator of thyroid function. *J Biol Chem* 1948;174:555–564.
154. Wolff J, Chaikoff IL. The inhibitory action of excessive iodide upon the synthesis of diiodotyrosine and of thyroxine in the normal rat. *Endocrinology* 1948;43:174–179.
155. Stanley MM. The direct estimation of the rate of thyroid hormone formation in man. The effect of the iodide ion on thyroid iodine utilization. *J Clin Endocrinol Metab* 1949;9:941–954.
156. Raben MS. The paradoxical effects of thiocyanate and of thyrotropin on the organic binding of iodine by the thyroid in the presence of large amounts of iodide. *Endocrinology* 1949;45:296–304.
157. Wildberger E, Von Gruenigen C, Kohler J, Kohler H, Studer H. Regulation of enzymatic iodothyronine synthesis in thyroglobulin by low concentrations of iodide. *Eur J Biochem* 1983;130:485–490.
158. Braverman LE, Ingbar SH. Changes in thyroidal function during adaptation to large doses of iodide. *J Clin Invest* 1963;42:1216–1231.
159. Childs DS, Keating FR, Rall JE, Williams MMD, Power MH. The effect of varying quantities of inorganic iodide (carrier) on the urinary excretion and thyroidal accumulation of radioiodine in exophthalmic goiter. *J Clin Invest* 1950;29:726–738.
160. Halmi NS. Thyroidal iodine transport. *Vitam Horm* 1961;19:133–163.
161. Tseng F-Y, Rani CSS, Field JB. Effect of iodide on glucose oxidation and ^{32}P incorporation into phospholipids stimulated by different agents in dog thyroid slices. *Endocrinology* 1989;124:1450–1455.
162. Kirkland RH. Impaired organic binding of radioiodine by the thyroid following radioiodine treatment of hyperthyroidism. *J Clin Endocrinol Metab* 1954;14:565–571.
163. Kieffer J, Medeiros-Neto GA, Rueda R, Pieron PR, Neto AC, Campusano L, Cintra ABU. Perchlorate test in hyperthyroid patients treated with radioactive iodine. *N Engl J Med* 1965;273:1326–1327.
164. Hagen GA, Ouellette RP, Chapman EM. Comparison of high and low dosage levels of ^{131}I in the treatment of thyrotoxicosis. *N Engl J Med* 1967;277:559–562.
165. Braverman LE, Woeber KA, Ingbar SH. Induction of myxedema by iodine in patients euthyroid after radioiodine or surgical treatment of diffuse toxic goiter. *N Engl J Med* 1969;281:816–821.
166. Paris J, McConahey WM, Tauxe WN, Woolner LB, Bahn RC. The effect of iodides on Hashimoto's thyroiditis. *J Clin Endocrinol Metab* 1961;21:1037–1043.
167. DeRobertis E. Cytological and cytochemical bases of thyroid function. *Ann NY Acad Sci* 1949;50:317–335.
168. Goldsmith RE, Eisele ML. The effect of iodide on the release of thyroid hormone in hyperthyroidism. *J Clin Endocrinol Metab* 1956;16:130–137.
169. Wartofsky L, Ransil BJ, Ingbar SH. Inhibition by iodine of the release of thyroxine from the thyroid glands of patients with thyrotoxicosis. *J Clin Invest* 1970;49:78–86.
170. Emerson CH, Anderson AJ, Howard WH, Utiger RD. Serum thyrox-

ine and triiodothyronine concentrations during iodide treatment of hyperthyroidism. *J Clin Endocrinol Metab* 1975;40:33–36.
171. Harden RM, Koutras DA, Alexander WD, Wayne EJ. Quantitative studies of iodine metabolism in iodide treated thyrotoxicosis. *Clin Sci* 1964;27:399–405.
172. Saji M, Isozaki O, Tsushima T, Arai M, Miyakawa M, Ohba Y, Tsuchiya Y, Sano T, Shizume K. The inhibitory effect of iodide on growth of rat thyroid (FRTL-5) cells. *Acta Endocrinol (Copenh)* 1988;119:145–151.
173. Bagchi N, Brown TR, Sundick RS. Thyroid cell injury is an initial event in the induction of autoimmune thyroiditis by iodine in obese strain chickens. *Endocrinology* 1995;136:5054–5060.
173a. Brown TR, Bagchi N. The role of iodine in the development of autoimmune thyroiditis. *Int Rev Immunol* 1992;9:167–182.
174. Friend DG. Iodide therapy and the importance of quantitating the dose. *N Engl J Med* 1960;263:1358–1360.
175. Thalassinos NC, Fraser TR. Effect of potassium iodide on relapse rate of thyrotoxicosis treated with antithyroid drugs. *Lancet* 1971;2:183–184.
176. Alexander WD, Harden RM, Koutras DA, Wayne E. Influence of iodine intake after treatment with antithyroid drugs. *Lancet* 1965;2:865–868.
177. Kasai K, Suzuki H, Shimoda SI. Effects of propylthiouracil and relatively small doses of iodide on early phase treatment of hyperthyroidism. *Acta Endocrinol (Copenh)* 1980;93:315–321.
178. Shapiro S. Further observations on feeding interrenal gland in cases of Graves' disease. *Endocrinology* 1924;8:666–676.
179. Hill SR, Reiss RS, Forsham PH, Thorn GW. The effect of adrenocorticotropin and cortisone on thyroid function: thyroid adrenocortical interrelationships. *J Clin Endocrinol Metab* 1950;10:1375–1400.
180. Wikholm G, Einhorn J. Effect of prednisolone and triiodothyronine on thyroid function in hyperthyroidism. *J Clin Endocrinol Metab* 1963;23:76–80.
181. Williams DE, Chopra IJ, Orgiazzi J, Solomon DH. Acute effects of corticosteroid on thyroid activity in Graves' disease. *J Clin Endocrinol Metab* 1975;41:354–361.
182. Chopra IJ, Williams DE, Orgiazzi J, Solomon DH. Opposite effects of dexamethasone on serum concentrations of 3,3′,5′-triiodothyronine (reverse T_3) and 3,3′,5-triiodothyronine (T_3). *J Clin Endocrinol Metab* 1975;41:911–920.
183. Burr WA, Ramsden DB, Griffiths RS, Black EG, Hoffenberg R. Effect of a single dose of dexamethasone on the concentration of thyroid hormones. *Lancet* 1976;2:58–61.
184. Duick DS, Warren DW, Nicoloff JT, Otis CL, Croxson MS. Effect of single dose dexamethasone on the concentration of serum triiodothyronine in man. *J Clin Endocrinol Metab* 1974;39:1151–1155.
185. Werner SC, Platman SR. Remission of hyperthyroidism (Graves' disease) and altered pattern of serum thyroxine binding induced by prednisone. *Lancet* 1965;2:751–755.
186. Burgi H, Wimpheimer C, Burger A, Zaunbauer W, Rosler H, Lemarchand-Beraud T. Changes of circulating thyroxine, triiodothyronine and reverse triiodothyronine after radiographic contrast agents. *J Clin Endocrinol Metab* 1976;43:1203–1210.
187. Wu SY, Chopra IJ, Solomon DH, Bennett LR. Changes in circulating iodothyronines in euthyroid and hyperthyroid subjects given ipodate (Oragraffin), an agent for oral cholecystography. *J Clin Endocrinol Metab* 1978;46:691–697.
188. Felicetta JV, Green WL, Nelp WB. Inhibition of hepatic binding of thyroxine by cholecystographic agents. *J Clin Invest* 1980;65:1032–1040.
189. Wu SY, Chopra IJ, Solomon DH, Johnson DF. The effect of repeated administration of ipodate (Oragraffin) in hyperthyroidism. *J Clin Endocrinol Metab* 1978;47:1358–1362.
190. Wu SY, Shyh TP, Chopra IJ, Solomon DH, Huang HW, Chu PC. Comparison of sodium ipodate (Oragraffin) and propylthiouracil in early treatment of hyperthyroidism. *J Clin Endocrinol Metab* 1982;54:630–634.
191. Shen DC, Wu SY, Chopra IJ, Huang HW, Shian LR, Bian TX, Jeng CY, Solomon DH. Long-term treatment of Graves' hyperthyroidism with sodium ipodate. *J Clin Endocrinol Metab* 1985;61:723–727.
192. Croxson MS, Hall TD, Nicoloff JT. Combination drug therapy for treatment of hyperthyroid Graves' disease. *J Clin Endocrinol Metab* 1977;45:623–631.
193. Sharp B, Reed AW, Tamagna I, Geffner DL, Hershman JM. Treatment of hyperthyroidism with sodium ipodate (Oragraffin) in addition to propylthiouracil and propranolol. *J Clin Endocrinol Metab* 1981;53:622–625.

194. Roti E, Robuschi G, Manfredi A, D'Amato L, Gardini E, Salvi M, Montermini M, Barlli AL, Gnudi A, Braverman LE. Comparative effects of sodium ipodate and iodine on serum thyroid hormone concentrations in patients with Graves' disease. *Clin Endocrinol (Oxf)* 1985;22:489–496.
195. Noguchi K, Suzuki H. A reevaluation of long-term treatment of hyperthyroidism with tyropanoate (TP), an oral cholecystographic agent: a comparison of the effects of TP with those of combined TP and methimazole. In: Medeiros-Neto G, Gaitan E, eds. *Frontiers in thyroidology*. New York: Plenum Press, 1985;1143–1146.
196. Chopra IJ. Inhibition of outer ring monodeiodination of T_4 reverse T_3 (rT_3) by some radiocontrast agents. *Clin Res* 1978;26:303A.
197. Chopra IJ. A study of extrathyroidal conversion of thyroxine (T_4) to 3,3′,5′-triiodothyronine (T_3) in vitro. *Endocrinology* 1977;101:453–458.
198. Costa A. The use of X-ray contrast media in the treatment of hyperthyroidism. *J Endocrinol Invest* 1979;2:461–462.
199. Roti E, Gardini E, Minelli R, Bianconi L, Braverman LE. Sodium ipodate and methimazole in the long-term treatment of hyperthyroid Graves' disease. *Metabolism* 1993;42:403–408.
200. Caldwell G, Errington M, Toft AD. Resistant hyperthyroidism induced by sodium ipodate used as treatment for Graves' disease. *Acta Endocrinol (Copenh)* 1989;120:215–216.
201. Ermans A-M, Bourdoux P. Long-term administration of iopanoic acid in a case of severe thyrotoxicosis factitia. In: Medeiros-Neto G, Gaitan E, eds. *Frontiers in thyroidology*. New York: Plenum Press, 1985;1137–1142.
202. Cade JFJ. Lithium salts in the treatment of psychotic excitement. *Med J Aust* 1949;2;349–355.
203. Schou MA, Amdisen A, Jensen SE, Olsen T. Occurrence of goitre during lithium treatment. *Br Med J* 1968;3:710–713.
204. Temple R, Berman M, Carlson HE, Robbins J, Wolff J. The use of lithium in Graves' disease. *Mayo Clin Proc* 1972;47:872–878.
205. Temple R, Berman M, Robbins J, Wolff J. The use of lithium in the treatment of thyrotoxicosis. *J Clin Invest* 1972;51:2746–2756.
206. Berens SC, Bernstein RS, Robbins J, Wolff J. Antithyroid effects of lithium. *J Clin Invest* 1970;49:1357–1367.
207. Mori M, Tajima K, Oda Y, Matsui I, Mashita K, Tarui S. Inhibitory effect of lithium on the release of thyroid hormones from thyrotropin-stimulated mouse thyroids in a perfusion system. *Endocrinology* 1989;124:1365–1369.
208. Lazarus JH, Richards AR, Addison GM, Owen GM. Treatment of thyrotoxicosis with lithium carbonate. *Lancet* 1974;2:1160–1162.
209. Boehm TM, Burman KD, Barnes S, Wartofsky L. Lithium and iodine combination therapy for thyrotoxicosis. *Acta Endocrinol (Copenh)* 1980;94:174–183.
210. Radvila A, Roost R, Burgi H, Kohler H, Studer H. Inhibition of thyroglobulin biosynthesis and degradation by excess iodide. Synergism with lithium. *Acta Endocrinol (Copenh)* 1976;81:495–506.
211. Byrne AP, Delaney WJ. Regression of thyrotoxic ophthalmopathy following lithium withdrawal. *Can J Psychiatry* 1993;38:635–637.
212. Persad E, Forbath N, Merskey H. Hyperthyroidism after treatment with lithium. *Can J Psychiatry* 1993;38:599–602.
213. Barclay ML, Brownlie BEW, Turner JG, Wells JE. Lithium associated thyrotoxicosis: a report of 14 cases, with statistical analysis of incidence. *Clin Endocrinol* 1994;40:759–764.
214. Turner JG, Brownlie BEW, Rogers TGH. Lithium as an adjunct to radioiodine therapy for thyrotoxicosis. *Lancet* 1976;1:614–615.
215. Barker MN. The blood cyanates in the treatment of hypertension. *JAMA* 1936;106:762–767.
216. Vanderlaan JE, Vanderlaan WP. The iodide concentrating mechanism of the rat thyroid and its inhibition by thiocyanate. *Endocrinology* 1947;40:403–416.
217. Wyngaarden JB, Wright BM, Ways B. The effect of certain anions upon the accumulation and retention of iodine by the thyroid gland. *Endocrinology* 1953;50:537–549.
218. Wyngaarden JB, Stanbury JB, Rapp B. The effects of iodide, perchlorate, thiocyanate, and nitrate administration upon the iodide concentrating mechanism of the rat thyroid. *Endocrinology* 1953;52:568–574.
219. Stanbury JB, Wyngaarden JB. Effect of perchlorate on the human thyroid gland. *Metabolism* 1952;1:533–539.
220. Godley AF, Stanbury JB. Preliminary experience in the treatment of hyperthyroidism with potassium perchlorate. *J Clin Endocrinol Metab* 1954;14:70–78.

221. Morgans ME, Trotter WR. Potassium perchlorate in thyrotoxicosis. *Br Med J* 1960;2:1086–1087.
222. Hobson QJG. Aplastic anaemia due to treatment with potassium perchlorate. *Br Med J* 1961;1:1368–1369.
223. Johnson RS, Moore WG. Fatal aplastic anaemia after treatment of thyrotoxicosis with potassium perchlorate. *Br Med J* 1961;1:1369–1371.
224. Krevans JR, Asper SP, Reinhoff WF. Fatal aplastic anemia following use of potassium perchlorate in thyrotoxicosis. *JAMA* 1962;181:162–164.
225. Barzilai D, Sheinfeld M. Fatal complications following use of potassium perchlorate in thyrotoxicosis. *Isr J Med Sci* 1966;2:453–456.
226. Shakir KMM, Michaels RD, Hays JH, Potter BB. The use of bile acid sequestrants to lower serum thyroid hormones in iatrogenic hyperthyroidism. *Ann Intern Med* 1993;118:112–113.
227. Solomon BL, Wartofsky L, Burman KD. Adjunctive cholestyramine therapy for thyrotoxicosis. *Clin Endocrinol (Oxf)* 1993;38:39–43.
228. Hoffman DA. Late effects of I-131 therapy in the United States. In: Boice JD, Fraumeni JF, eds. *Carcinogenesis*. New York: Raven Press, 1984;273–280.
229. Linquette M, Fossati P, Proye C. Une experience de traitement chirurgical de la maladie de Basedow. *Ann Endocrinol (Paris)* 1980;41:611–613.
230. Tallstedt L, Lundell G, Torring O, Wallin G, Ljunggren J-G, Blomgren H, Taube A, and The Thyroid Study Group. The occurrence of opthalmopathy after treatment for Graves' hyperthyroidism. *N Engl J Med* 1992;326:1733–1738.
231. Bartalena L, Marcocci C, Bogazzi F, Panicucci M, Lepri A, Pinchera A. Use of corticosteroids to prevent progression of Graves' ophthalmopathy after radioiodine therapy for hyperthyroidism. *N Engl J Med* 1989;321:1349.
232. Harvey RD, Metcalfe RA, Morteo C, Furmaniak W, Weetman AP, Bevan JS. Acute pre-tibial myxoedema following radioiodine therapy for thyrotoxic Graves' disease. *Clin Endocrinol* 1995;42:657–660.
233. Ozaki O, Ito K, Mimura T, Sugino K, Kitamura Y, Iwabuchi H, Kawano M. Thyroid carcinoma after radioactive iodine therapy for Graves' disease. *World J Surg* 1994;18:518–521.
234. Tezelman S, Grossman RF, Siperstein AE, Clark OH. Radioiodine-associated thyroid cancers. *World J Surg* 1994;18:522–528.
235. Takamatsu J, Kuma K, Mozai T. Serum triiodothyronine to thyroxine ratio: a newly recognized predictor of the outcome of hyperthyroidism due to Graves' disease. *J Clin Endocrinol Metab* 1986;62:980–983.
236. Yamada T, Takasu N, Sato A, Aizawa T, Koizumi Y. Pituitary thyroid feedback regulation in patients with Graves' disease during antithyroid drug therapy. *J Clin Endocrinol Metab* 1982;54:83–88.
237. Uller RP, Van Herle AJ. Effect of therapy on serum thyroglobulin levels in patients with Graves' disease. *J Clin Endocrinol Metab* 1978;46:747–755.
238. Kawamura S, Kishino B, Tajima K, Mashita K, Tarui S. Serum thyroglobulin changes in patients with Graves' disease treated with long-term antithyroid drug therapy. *J Clin Endocrinol Metab* 1983;156:507–512.
239. Leclère J, Ueda M, Hartemann P, et al. Traitement de l'hyperthyroidie par les antithyroidiens de synthese. *Ann Endocrinol (Paris)* 1980;41:95–105.
240. Alexander WD, Harden RM, Shimmins L, McLarty D, McGill P. Treatment of thyrotoxicosis based on thyroidal suppressibility. *Lancet* 1967;2:681–685.
241. Yamamoto M, Koizumi Y, Sato A, et al. Outcome of patients with Graves' disease after long-term medical treatment guided by triiodothyronine (T_3) suppression test. *Clin Endocrinol (Oxf)* 1983;19:467–476.
242. Wilkin TJ, Isles TE, Crooks J, Gunn A, Beck JS. Patterns of change in the early (20-minute) radioiodine uptake during carbimazole treatment for Graves' disease and their relationship to outcome. *J Clin Endocrinol Metab* 1981;52:1067–1072.
243. Yamada T, Totsuka Y, Kojma I, et al. Reappraisal of the 3,5,3′-triiodothyronine suppression test in the prediction of long-term outcome of antithyroid drug therapy in patients with hyperthyroid Graves' disease. *J Clin Endocrinol Metab* 1984;58:676–680.
244. Gardner DF, Utiger RD. The natural history of hyperthyroidism due to Graves' disease in remission: sequential studies of pituitary-thyroid regulation and various serum parameters. *J Clin Endocrinol Metab* 1979;49:417–421.
245. Slingerland DW, Sullivan JJ, Dell EE, Burrows BA. Thyroid suppression tests during treatment of hyperthyroidism. *Clin Endocrinol (Oxf)* 1976;5:415–418.
246. Werner SC. Response to triiodothyronine as index of persistence of disease in the thyroid remnant of patients in remission from hyperthyroidism. *J Clin Invest* 1956;35:57–61.
247. Bayer MF, Kriss JP, McDougall IR. Clinical experience with sensitive thyrotropin measurements: diagnostic and therapeutic implications. *J Nucl Med* 1985;25:1248–1256.
248. Edan G. A prospective longitudinal study in Graves' disease. OKT4/OKT8 ratio indicates treatment choice and thyrostimulating antibodies (TSAb) indicate treatment duration. Presented at the Ninth International Thyroid Congress, Sao Paulo, 1985;164.
249. Ludgate ME, McGregor AM, Weetman AP, et al. Analysis of T cell subsets in Graves' disease: alterations associated with carbimazole. *Br Med J* 1984;288:526–530.
250. Kasigi K, Iida Y, Konishi J, Misaki T, Arai K, Endo K, Torizuka K, Kuma K. Paired determination of thyroid-stimulating and TSH-binding inhibitory activities in patients with Graves' disease during antithyroid drug treatment. *Acta Endocrinol (Copenh)* 1986;111:474–480.
251. Arem R. When to choose radioactive iodine, drugs, or surgery. *Consultant* 1989;Jan:21–35.
252. Hardisty CA, Fowles A, Munro US. The effect of radioiodine and antithyroid drugs on serum long-acting thyroid stimulator protector (LATS-P). A three-year prospective study. *Clin Endocrinol (Oxf)* 1984;20:547–605.
253. Duprey J, Izembart M, Vallee G, Benazet-Louis M-F. Long-term prognostic value of the anti-TSH receptor autoantibodies (ATRAA) in Graves' disease treated with carbimazole. In: Medeiros-Neto G, Gaitan E, eds. *Frontiers in thyroidology*. New York: Plenum Press, 1985;1117–1119.
254. Teng CS, Yeung RTT. Changes in thyroid-stimulating antibody activity in Graves' disease treated with antithyroid drug and its relationship to relapse; a prospective study. *J Clin Endocrinol Metab* 1980;50:144–147.
255. Hegedus L, Hansen JM, Bech K, Kampmann JP, Jensen K, Andersen E, Hansen P, Karstrup S, Bliddal H. Thyroid stimulating immunoglobulins in Graves' disease with goiter growth, low thyroxine and increasing triiodothyronine during PTU treatment. *Acta Endocrinol (Copenh)* 1984;107:482–488.
256. Kawai K, Tamai H, Matsubayashi S, Mukuta T, Morita T, Kubo C, Kuma K. A study of untreated Graves' patients with undetectable TSH binding inhibitor immunoglobulins and the effect of anti-thyroid drugs. *Clin Endocrinol* 1995;43:551–556.
257. Cooper DS. Antithyroid drugs. *N Engl J Med* 1984;311:1353–1362.
258. Sitar DS, Hunninghake DB. Pharmacokinetics of propylthiouracil in man after single oral dose. *J Clin Endocrinol Metab* 1975;40:26–29.
259. Romaldini JH, Bromberg N, Werner RS, Tanaka LM, Rodrigues HF, Werner MC, Farah CS, Reis LC. Comparison of effects of high and low dosage regimens of antithyroid drugs in the management of Graves' hyperthyroidism. *J Clin Endocrinol Metab* 1983;57:563–570.
260. Benker G, Reinwein D, Creutzig, H, Hirche H, Alexander WD, McCruden D, Galvan G, Kahaly G, Beyer J, Lazarus JH, Schatz H, Schleusener H, Schneider HG, Ziegler R, Tegler L, Nilson OR. Effects of high and low doses of methimazole in patients with Graves' thyrotoxicosis. *Acta Endocrinol Suppl (Copenh)* 1987;281:312–317.
261. O'Malley BP, Rosenthal FD, Northover BJ, Jennings PE, Woods KL. Higher than conventional doses of carbimazole in the treatment of thyrotoxicosis. *Clin Endocrinol (Oxf)* 1988;29:281–288.
262. Alexander WD, McLarty DG, Horton P, Pharmakiotis AD. Sequential assessment during drug treatment of thyrotoxicosis. *Clin Endocrinol* 1973;2:43–50.
263. Gossage AAR, Crawley JCW, Copping S, Hinge D, Himsworth RL. Thyroid function and immunological activity during and after medical treatment of Graves' disease. *Clin Endocrinol* 1983;19:87–96.
264. Laurberg P, Hansen PEB, Iversen E, Jensen SE, Weeke J. Goitre size and outcome of medical treatment of Graves' disease. *Acta Endocrinol* 1986;111:39–43.
265. Young ET, Steel NR, Taylor JJ, Stephenson AM, Stratton A, Holcombe M, Kendall-Taylor P. Prediction of remission after antithyroid drug treatment in Graves' disease. *Q J Med* 1988;66:175–189.
266. Hashizume K, Ichikawa K, Sakurai A, Suzuki S, Takeda T, Kobayashi M, Miyamoto T, Arai M, Nagasawa T. Administration of thyroxine in treated Graves' disease: effects on the level of antibodies to thyroid-stimulating hormone receptors and on the risk of recurrence of hyperthyroidism. *N Engl J Med* 1991;324:947–953.

267. Kuo SW, Huang WS, Hu CA, Liao WK, Fung TC, Wu SY. Effect of thyroxine administration on serum thyrotropin receptor antibody and thyroglobulin levels in patients with Graves' hyperthyroidism during antithyroid drug therapy. *Eur J Endocrinol* 1994;131:125–130.
268. Weetman AP, Pickerill AP, Watson P, Chatterjee VK, Edwards OM. Tretament of Graves' disease with the block-replace regimen of antithyroid drugs: the effect of treatment duration and immunogenetic susceptibility on relapse. *Q J Med* 1994;87:337–341.
269. Perozim LM, Lima N, Knobel M, Cavaliere H, Medeiros-Neto G. Treatment of Graves' disease: effects of the administration of L-thyroxine associated with methimazole as a single daily dose. *Eur J Med* 1993;2:70–74.
270. Edmonds CJ, Tellez M. Treatment of Graves' disease by carbimazole: high dose with thyroxine compared to titration dose. *Eur J Endocrinol* 1994;131:120–124.
271. Reinwein D, Benker G, Lazarus JH, Alexander WD, and The European Multicenter Study Group on Antithyroid Drug Treatment. A prospective randomized trial of antithyroid drug dose in Graves' disease therapy. *J Clin Endocrinol Metab* 1993;76:1516–1521.
272. Iriarte GMJ, Lenas LF, Beroiz AI, Apinaniz EA, Erdozain RR, Torre EM. Recurrence of Graves-Basedow disease: the influence of treatment schedule. *Med Clin (Barc)* 1995;104:11–14.
273. Tamai H, Hayaki I, Kawai K, Komaki G, Matsubayashi S, Kuma K, Kumagai LF, Nagataki S. Lack of effect of thyroxine administration on elevated thyroid stimulating hormone receptor antibody levels in treated Graves' disease patients. *J Clin Endocrinol Metab* 1995;80:1479–1480.
273a.McIver B, Rae P, Beckett G, Wilkinson E, Gold A, Toft A. Lack of effect of thyroxine in patients with Graves' hyperthyroidism who are treated with an antithyroid drug. *N Engl J Med* 1996;334:220–224.
274. Benker G, Vitti P, Kahaly G, Raue F, Tegler L, Hirche H, Reinwein D, and the European Multicenter Study Group. Response to methimazole in Graves' disease. *Clin Endocrinol* 1995;43:257–263.
275. Bromberg N, Romaldini JH, Werner RS, Sgarbi JA, Werner MC. The evolution of Graves' ophthalmopathy during treatment with antithyroid drug alone and combined with triiodothyronine. *J Endocrinol Invest* 1992;15:191–195.
276. Paschke R, Vogg M, Kristoferitsch R, Aktuna D, Wawschinek O, Eber O, Usadel KH. Methimazole has no dose-related effect on the intensity of the intrathyroidal autoimmune process in relapsing Graves' disease. *J Clin Endocrinol Metab* 1995;80:2470–2474.
277. Greer MA, Meihoff WC, Studer H. Treatment of hyperthyroidism with a single dose of propylthiouracil. *N Engl J Med* 1956;272:888–891.
278. Kammer H, Srinivasan K. The use of antithyroid drugs in a single daily dose. *JAMA* 1969;209:1325–1327.
279. Greer MA, Kammer H, Bouma DJ. Short-term antithyroid drug therapy for the thyrotoxicosis of Graves' disease. *N Engl J Med* 1977;297:173–176.
280. Gwinup G. Prospective randomized comparison of propylthiouracil. *JAMA* 1978;239:2457–2459.
281. Mashio Y, Beniko M, Ikota A, Mizumoto H, Kunita H. Treatment of hyperthyroidism with a small single daily dose of methimazole. *Acta Endocrinol (Copenh)* 1988;119:139–144.
282. Barnes HV, Bledsoe T. A simple test for selecting the thioamide schedule in thyrotoxicosis. *J Clin Endocrinol Metab* 1972;35:250–255.
283. Bouma DJ, Kammer H. Single daily dose methimazole treatment of hyperthyroidism. *West J Med* 1980;132:13–15.
284. Okamura K, Ikenoue H, Shiroozu A, Sato K, Yoshinara M, Fujishima M. Reevaluation of the effects of methylmercaptoimidazole and propylthiouracil in patients with Graves' hyperthyroidism. *J Clin Endocrinol Metab* 1987;65:719–723.
285. Nabil N, Miner DJ, Amatruda JM. Methimazole: an alternative route of administration. *J Clin Endocrinol Metab* 1982;54:180–181.
286. Walter RM, Bartle WR. Rectal administration of propylthiouracil in the treatment of Graves' disease. *Am J Med* 1990;88:69–70.
287. Bouma DJ, Kammer H, Greer M. Follow-up comparison of short-term versus 1-year antithyroid drug therapy for the thyrotoxicosis of Graves' disease. *J Clin Endocrinol Metab* 1982;55:1138–1142.
288. Allannic H. Strategy for antithyroid drug therapy in Graves' disease. *Horm Res* 1987;26:146–153.
289. Slingerland DW, Burrows BA. Long-term antithyroid treatment in hyperthyroidism. *JAMA* 1979;242:2408–2410.
290. Allannic H, Fauchet R, Orgiazzi J, Madec AM, Genete B, Lorcy Y, Le Guerrier AM, Delambre C, Derennes V. Antithyroid drugs and Graves' disease: a prospective randomized evaluation of the efficacy of treatment duration. *J Clin Endocrinol Metab* 1990;70:675–679.
291. Arntzenius AB, Elte JWF, Frolich M, Haak A. The significance of the initial FT_4-index for the management of single daily dose methimazole treatment of hyperthyroidism. *Clin Endocrinol (Oxf)* 1988;29:239–247.
292. Feldt-Rasmussen U, Schleusener H, Carayon P. Meta-analysis evaluation of the impact of thyrotropin receptor antibodies on long-term remission after medical therapy of Graves' disease. *J Clin Endocrinol Metab* 1994;78:98–102.
293. Paschke R, Vogg M, Swillens S, Usadel KH. Correlation of microsomal antibodies with the intensity of the intrathyroidal autoimmune process in Graves' disease. *J Clin Endocrinol Metab* 1993;77:939–943.
294. Studer H, Peter HJ, Gerber H. Toxic nodular goiter. *Baillieres Clin Endocrinol Metab* 1985;14:351–372.
295. Schatz H, Ludwig I, Wiss F, Goretzki PE. Pathological and clinical implications of thyroid growth-stimulating immunoglobulins: evidence for their intrathyroidal production. *Acta Endocrinol Suppl (Copenh)* 1987;281:334–341.
296. Kraiem Z, Glaser B, Yigla M, Pauker J, Sadeh O, Scheinfeld M. Toxic multinodular goiter: a variant of autoimmune hyperthyroidism. *J Clin Endocrinol Metab* 1987;65:659–664.
297. Bliddal H, Hansen JM, Rogowski P, Johansen K, Friis T, Siersbæk-Nielsen K. ^{131}I treatment of diffuse and nodular toxic goitre with or without antithyroid agents. *Acta Endocrinol (Copenh)* 1982;99:517–521.
298. van Soestbergen MJ, van der Vijver AC, Graafland AD. Recurrence of hyperthyroidism in multinodular goiter after long-term drug therapy: a comparison with Graves' disease. *J Endocrinol Invest* 1992;15:797–800.
299. Kristensen HL, Vadstrup S, Knudsen N, Siersbaek-Nielsen K. Development of hyperthyroidism in nodular goiter and thyroid malignancies in an area of relatively low iodine intake. *J Endocrinol Invest* 1995;18:41–43.
300. Papini E, Panunzi C, Pacella CM, Bizzarri G, Fabbrini R, Petrucci L, Pisicchio G, Nardi F. Percutaneous ultrasound-guided ethanol injection: a new treatment of toxic autonomously functioning thyroid nodules? *J Clin Endocrinol Metab* 1993;76:411–416.
301. Livraghi T, Paracchi A, Ferrari C, Bergonzi M, Garavaglia G, Raineri P, Vettori C. Treatment of autonomous thyroid nodules with percutaneous ethanol injection: preliminary results. *Radiology* 1990;175:827–829.
302. Monzani F, Goletti O, Caraccio N, del Guerra P, Ferdeghini M, Pucci E, Baschieri L. Percutaneous ethanol injection treatment of autonomous thyroid adenoma: hormonal and clinical evaluation. *Clin Endocrinol (Oxf)* 1992;36:491–497.
303. Paracchi A, Ferrari C, Livraghi T, Reschini E, Macchi RM, Bergonzi M, Raineri P. Percutaneous intranodular ethanol injecction: a new treatment for autonomous thyroid adenoma. *J Endocrinol Invest* 1992;15:353–362.
304. Sandrock D, Olbricht T, Enrich D, Benker G, Reinwein D. Long-term follow-up in patients with autonomous thyroid adenoma. *Acta Endocrinol* 1993;128:51–55.
305. Wenzel KW, Lente JR. Syndrome of persisting thyroid stimulating immunoglobulins and growth promotion of goiter combined with low thyroxine and high triiodothyronine serum levels in drug treated Graves' disease. *J Endocrinol Invest* 1983;6:389–394.
306. Jones MK, Owens DR, Jones GR, Birtwell J. The effect of propranolol on thyroid hormones in T_3 toxicosis. *Clin Endocrinol (Oxf)* 1981;14:621–623.
307. Brittain PC, Bayliss P. Partial hydatidiform molar pregnancy presenting with severe preeclampsia prior to twenty weeks gestation: a case report and review of the literature. *Mil Med* 1995;160:42–44.
308. Davies TF, Taliadouros GS, Catt KJ, Nisula BC. Assessment of urinary thyrotropin-competing activity in choriocarcinoma and thyroid disease: further evidence for human chorionic gonadotropin interacting at the thyroid cell membrane. *J Clin Endocrinol Metab* 1979;49:353–357.
309. Davies TF, Platzer M. hCG-induced TSH receptor activation and growth acceleration in FRTL-5 thyroid cells, *Endocrinology* 1986;118:2149–2151.
310. Bagshawe KD. Immunological methods in the diagnosis and monitoring of tumours. In: Bageshawe KD, ed. *Medical oncology: medical aspects of malignant disease*. Oxford: Blackwell Scientific, 1976;245–267.
311. Goodwin TM, Montoro M, Mestman JH, Pekary AE, Hershman JM. The role of chorionic gonadotropin in transient hyperthyroidism of hyperemesis gravidarum. *J Clin Endocrinol Metab* 1992;75:1333–1337.
312. Norman RJ, Green-Thompson RW, Jialal I, Soutter WP, Pillay NL,

Joubert SM. Hyperthyroidism in gestational trophoblastic neoplasia. *Clin Endocrinol (Oxf)* 1981;15:395–401.
313. Hershman JM. Hyperthyroidism induced by trophoblastic thyrotropin. *Mayo Clin Proc* 1972;47:913–918.
314. Nagataki S, Mizuno M, Sakamoto S, Irie M, Shizume K, Nahao K, Galton VA, Arky RA, Ingbar SH. Thyroid function in molar pregnancy. *J Clin Endocrinol Metab* 1977;44:254–263.
315. Higgins HP, Hershman JM. The hyperthyroidism due to trophoblastic hormone. *Baillieres Clin Endocrinol Metab* 1978;7:167–175.
316. Hoffenberg R. Thyroid emergencies. *Baillieres Clin Endocrinol Metab* 1980;9:503–507.
317. Soutter WP, Norman R, Green-Thompson RW. The management of choriocarcinoma causing severe thyrotoxicosis. *Br J Obstet Gynaecol* 1981;88:938–943.
318. Nikolai TF, Brosseau J, Kettrick A, Roberts R, Beltaos E. Lymphocytic thyroiditis with spontaneously resolving hyperthyroidism (silent thyroiditis). *Arch Intern Med* 1980;140:478–482.
319. Nikolai TF, Coombs GJ, McKenzie AK. Lymphocytic thyroiditis with spontaneously resolving hyperthyroidism and subacute thyroiditis. Long-term followup. *Arch Intern Med* 1981;141:1455–1458.
320. Greene JN. Subacute thyroiditis. *Am J Med* 1971;51:97–108.
321. Nikolai TF, Coombs GJ, McKenzie AK, Miller RW, Weir J. Treatment of lymphocytic thyroiditis with spontaneously resolving hyperthyroidism (silent thyroiditis). *Arch Intern Med* 1982;142:2281–2283.
322. Chopra IJ, van Herle AJ, Korenman SG, Viosca S, Younai S. Use of sodium ipodate in management of hyperthyroidism in subacute thyroiditis. *J Clin Endocrinol Metab* 1995;80:2178–2180.
323. Gershengorn MC, Weintraub BD. Thyrotropin-induced hyperthyroidism caused by selective pituitary resistance to thyroid hormone. *J Clin Invest* 1975;56:633–642.
324. Weintraub BD, Gershengorn MC, Kourides IA, Fein H. Inappropriate secretion of thyroid-stimulating hormone. *Ann Intern Med* 1981;95:339–351.
325. Chanson P, Weintraub BD, Harris AG. Octreotide therapy for thyroid stimulating hormone-secreting pituitary adenomas. *Ann Intern Med* 1993;119:236–240.
326. Modignani RL, Venegoni M, Beretta F, Fassina S. Thyroid storm with encephalopathic syndrome due to Graves' disease and inappropriate secretion of thyrotropin. *Ann Ital Med Int* 1992;7:250–254.
327. Sriwatanakul K, McCormick K, Wolff P. Thyrotropin (TSH) induced hyperthyroidism: response of TSH to dopamine and its agonists. *J Clin Endocrinol Metab* 1984;58:255–261.
328. Connell JMC, McCruden DC, Davies DL, Alexander WD. Bromocriptine for inappropriate thyrotropin secretion. *Ann Intern Med* 1982;96:251–252.
329. Williams G, Kraenzlin M, Sandler L, Burrin J, Law A, Bloom S, Joplin GF. Hyperthyroidism due to non-tumoral inappropriate TSH secretion. Effect of a long-acting somatostatin analogue (SMS 201–995). *Acta Endocrinol (Copenh)* 1986;113:42–46.
330. Faglia G, Beck-Peccoz P, Piscitelli G, Medri G. Inappropriate secretion of thyrotropin by the pituitary. *Horm Res* 1987;26:7999.
331. Beck-Peccoz P, Piscitelli G, Cattaneo MG, Faglia G. Successful treatment of hyperthyroidism due to non-neoplastic pituitary TSH hypersecretion with 3,5,3'-triiodothyroacetic acid (TRIAC). *J Endocrinol Invest* 1983;6:217–223.
332. Beck-Peccoz P, Mariotti S, Guillausseau PJ, Medri G. Piscitelli G, Bertoli A, Barbarino A, Rondena M, Chanson P, Pinchera A, Faglia G. Treatment of hyperthyroidism due to inappropriate secretion of thyrotropin with the somatostatin analog SMS 201–995. *J Clin Endocrinol Metab* 1989;68:208–214.
333. Spanheimer RG, Bar RS, Hayford JC. Hyperthyroidism caused by inappropriate thyrotropin hypersecretion. *Arch Intern Med* 1982;142:1283–1286.
334. Rosler A, Litvin Y, Hage C, Gross J, Cerasi E. Familial hyperthyroidism due to inappropriate thyrotropin secretion successfilly treated with triiodothyronine. *J Clin Endocrinol Metab* 1982;54:76–82.
335. Chiarini V, Graziano E, Cremonin N, Leandri P, Tarroni A, Marinelli M. *Iperliroidismo da inappropriata secrezione di TSH: primi risultati della terapia con TRIAC*. Atti delle Terze Gionate Italiane della Tiroide, Tonno, 1985;18. As cited in: Fag lia (331).
336. Hamon P, Bovier-Lapierre M, Robert M, Peynaud D, Pugeat M, Orgiazzi J. Hyperthyroidism due to selective pituitary resistance to thyroid hormones in a 15 month old boy: efficacy of D-thyroxine therapy. *J Clin Endocrinol Metab* 1988;67:1089–1093.
337. Arnold MB, Talbot NB, Cope OC. Concerning the choice of therapy for childhood hyperthyroidism. *Pediatrics* 1958;21:47–53.
338. Hayles AB. Problems of childhood Graves' disease. *Mayo Clin Proc* 1972;47:850–853.
339. Hayles AB, Kennedy RLJ, Beahrs OH, Woolner LB. Exophthalmic goiter in children. *J Clin Endocrinol* 1959;19:138–151.
340. Andrassy RJ, Buckingham BA, Weitzman J. Thyroidectomy for hyperthyroidism in children. *J Pediatr Surg* 1980;15:501–504.
341. Buckingham BA Costin G, Roe TF, Weitzman JJ, Kogut MD. Hyperthyroidism in children. A re-evaluation of treatment. *Am J Dis Child* 1981;135:112–117.
342. Csaky G, Balazs G, Bako G, Ilyes I, Kalman K, Szabo J. Late results of thyroid surgery for hyperthyroidism performed in childhood. *Prog Pediatr Surg* 1991;126:31–40.
343. Hamburger JI. Management of hyperthyroidism in children and adolescents. *J Clin Endocrinol Metab* 1985;60:1019–1024.
344. Kreisel W. International program on the health effects of the Chernobyl accident. *Stem Cells* 1995;13(suppl 1):33–39.
344a. Abelin T, Averkin JI, Egger M, Egloff B, Furmanchuk AW, Gurtner F, Karotkovich JR, et al. Thyroid cancer in Belarus post-Chernobyl: improved detection or increased incidence. *Soz Praventivmed* 1994;39:189–197.
345. Lippe BM, Lardaw EM, Kaplan SA. Hyperthyroidism in children treated with long-term medical therapy: twenty five percent remission every two years. *J Clin Endocrinol Metab* 1987;64:1241–1245.
346. Vaidya V, Bongiovanni AM, Parks JS, Tenore A, Kirkland RT. Twenty-two years' experience in the medical management of juvenile thyrotoxicosis. *Pediatrics* 1974;54:565–570.
347. Hayles AB, Zimmerman D. Graves' disease in childhood. In: Ingbar SH, Braverman LE, eds. *Werner's The thyroid*, 5th ed. New York: JB Lippincott, 1986;1412–1426.
348. Ronnov-Jessen V, Kirkegaard C. Hyperthyroidism: a disease of old age? *Br Med J* 1973;1:41–43.
349. Hurley JR. Thyroid disease in the elderly. *Med Clin North Am* 1983;67:497–516.
350. Hollingsworth DR, Mabry CC, Reid MC. New observations in congenital Graves disease. In: *Thyroid research, proceedings of the 8th International Thyroid Congress, Sydney*. Oxford: Pergamon Press, 1980;587–592
351. Werner SC. Hyperthyroidism in the pregnant woman and neonate. *J Clin Endocrinol Metab* 1967;27:1637–1653.
352. Bell GO, Hall J. Hyperthyroidism and pregnancy. *Med Clin North Am* 1960;44:363–367.
353. Talbert LM, Thomas CG, Holt WA, Rankin P. Hyperthyroidism during pregnancy. *Obstet Gynecol* 1970;36:779–785.
354. Frisk AR, Josefsson E. Thiouracil derivatives and pregnancy. *Acta Med Scand Suppl* 1947;196:85–91.
355. Burrow GN. Neonatal goiter after maternal propylthiouracil therapy. *J Clin Endocrinol* 1965;25:403–408.
356. Momotani N, Ito K, Hamada N, Ban Y, Nishikawa Y, Mimura T. Maternal hyperthyroidism and congenital malformation in the offspring. *Clin Endocrinol (Oxf)* 1984;20:695–700.
357. Galina MP, Avnet NL, Einhorn A. Iodide during pregnancy. An apparent cause of neonatal death. *N Engl J Med* 1962;267:1124–1127.
358. McCarroll AM, Hutchinson M, McAuley R, Montgomery DAD. Long-term assessment of children exposed in utero to carbimazole. *Arch Dis Child* 1976;51:532–536.
359. Burrow GN, Bartsocas C, Klatskin EH, Grunt JA. Children exposed in utero to propylthiouracil. *Am J Dis Child* 1968;116:161–165.
360. Wing DA, Millar LK, Koonings PP, Montoro MN, Mestman JH. A comparsion of propylthiouracil versus methimazole in the treatment of hyperthyroidism in pregnancy. *Am J Obstet Gynecol* 1994;170:90–95.
361. Hashizume K, Ichikawa K, Nishii Y, Kobayashi M, Sakurai A, Miyamoto T Suzuki S, Takeda T. Effect of administration of thyroxine on the risk of postpartum recurrence of hyperthyroid Graves' disease. *J Clin Endocrinol Metab* 1992;75:6–10.
362. Cheron RG Kaplan MM, Larsen PR, Selenkow HA, Crigler JF. Neonatal thyroid function after propylthiouracil therapy for maternal Graves' disease. *N Engl J Med* 1981;304:525–528.
363. Momotani N, Noh J, Oyanagi H, Ishikawa N, Ito K. Antithyroid drug therapy for Graves' disease during pregnancy. *N Engl J Med* 1986;315:24–28.
364. Robinson PL, O'Mullane NM, Alderman B. Prenatal treatment of fetal thyrotoxicosis. *Br Med J* 1979;1:383–384.

365. Messer PM, Hauffa BP, Olbricht T, Benker G, Kotulla P, Reinwein D. Antithyroid drug treatment of Graves' disease in pregnancy: long-term effects on somatic growth, intellectual development and thyroid function of the offspring. *Acta Endocrinol* 1990;123:311–316.
366. Amino N, Tanizawa O, Mori H, Iwatani Y, Yomada T, Kurachi K, Kumahara Y, Mirai K. Aggravation of thyrotoxicosis in early pregnancy and after delivery in Graves' disease. *J Clin Endocrinol Metab* 1982;55:108–112.
367. Munro DS, Dirmikis SM, Humphries H, Smith T, Broadhead GD. The role of thyroid-stimulating immunoglobulins of Graves' disease in neonatal thyrotoxicosis. *Br J Obstet Gynaecol* 1978;85:837–843.
368. Kourides IA, Heath CV, Ginsberg-Fellner F. Measurement of thyroid-stimulating hormone in human amniotic fluid. *J Clin Endocrinol Metab* 1982;54:635–637.
369. Fraser TR, Wilkerson M. Simplified method of drug treatment for thyrotoxicosis using a uniform dosage of methyluracil and added thyroxine. *Br Med J* 1953;1:481–484.
370. Herbst AL, Selenkow HA. Combined antithyroid-thyroid therapy of hyperthyroidism in pregnancy. *Obstet Gynecol* 1963;21:543–550.
371. Herbst AL, Selenkow HA. Hyperthyroidism during pregnancy. *N Engl J Med* 1965;273:627–633.
372. Hamburger JI. Management of the pregnant hyperthyroid. The argument against combined antithyroid–thyroid therapy. *Obstet Gynecol* 1972;40:114–117.
373. Fisher DA. Thyroid function in the fetus. In: Fisher DA, Burrow GN, eds. *Perinatal thyroid physiology and disease.* New York: Raven Press, 1975;21–32.
374. Langer A, Hung CT, McA'Nulty JA, Harrigan JT, Washington E. Adrenergic blockade. A new approach to hyperthyroidism during pregnancy. *Obstet Gynecol* 1974;44:181–186.
375. Bullock JL, Harris RE. Young R. Treatment of thyrotoxicosis during pregnancy with propranolol. *Am J Obstet Gynecol* 1975;121:242–245.
376. Gladstone GR, Hordof A, Gersony WM. Propranolol administration during pregnancy: effects on the fetus. *J Pediatr* 1975;86:962–964.
377. Levy CA, Waite JH, Dickey R. Thyrotoxicosis and pregnancy. Use of preoperative propranolol for thyroidectomy. *Am J Surg* 1977;133:319–321.
378. Habib A, McCarthy JS. Effects on the neonate of propranolol administered during pregnancy. *J Pediatr* 1977;91:808–811.
379. Lieberman BA, Stirrat GM, Cohen SL, Beard RW, Pinker GD, Belsey E. The possible adverse effect of propranolol on the fetus in pregnancies complicated by severe hypertension. *Br J Obstet Gynaecol* 1978;85:678–683.
380. Pruyn SC, Phelan JP, Buchanan GC. Long-term propranolol therapy in pregnancy: maternal and fetal outcome. *Am J Obstet Gynecol* 1979;135:485–489.
381. Rubin PC. Beta-blockers in pregnancy. *N Engl J Med* 1981;305:1325–1328.
381a. Stagnaro-Green A. Postpartum thyroiditis: prevalence, etiology, and clinical implications. *Thyroid Today* 1993;16:1–11.
382. Walfish PG, Chan JYC. Post-partum hyperthyroidism. *Baillieres Clin Endocrinol Metab* 1985;14:417–447.
383. Amino N, Miyai K. Postpartum autoimmune endocrine syndromes. In: Davies TF, ed. *Autoimmune endocrine disease.* New York: Wiley, 1983;247–272.
384. Momotani N, Noh J, Ishikawa N, Ito K. Relationship between silent thyroiditis and recurrent Graves' disease in the postpartum period. *J Clin Endocrinol Metab* 1994;79:285–289.
385. Yabu Y, Amino N, Mori H, Miyai K, Tanizawa O, Takai SI, Kumahara Y, Matsuzuka F, Kuma K. Postpartum recurrence of hyperthyroidism and changes of thyroid-stimulating immunoglobulins in Graves' disease. *J Clin Endocrinol Metab* 1980;51:1454–1458.
386. Johansen K, Andersen AN, Kampmann JP, Hansen JM, Mortensen HB. Excretion of methimazole in human milk. *Eur J Pharmacol* 1982;23:339–341.
387. Lamberg BA, Ikonen E, Osterlund K, Teramo K, Pekonen F, Peltola J, Valimaki M. Antithyroid treatment of maternal hyperthyroidism during lactation. *Clin Endocrinol (Oxf)* 1984;21:81–87.
388. Cooper DS. Antithyroid drugs: to breast-feed or not to breast-feed. *Am J Obstet Gynecol* 1987;157:234–235.
389. Hollingsworth DR, Mabry CC. Congenital Graves' disease: four familial cases with long-term followup and perspective. *Am J Dis Child* 1976;130:148–155.
390. Wilkin TJ, Kenyon E, Isles TE. The behaviour of thyroid hormones in an infant with untreated neonatal thyrotoxicosis. *Clin Endocrinol (Oxf)* 1977;7:227–231.
391. Zakarija M, McKenzie JM, Hoffman WH. Prediction and therapy of intrauterine and late-onset neonatal hyperthyroidism. *J Clin Endocrinol Metab* 1986;62:368–371.
391a. Duprez L, Parma J, Van Sande J, Allgeier A, Leclere J, Schvartz C, Delisle M-J, Decoulx M, Orgiazzi J, Dumont J, Vassart G. Germline mutations in the thyrotropin receptor gene cause non-autoimmune autosomal dominant hyperthyroidism. *Nat Genet* 1994;7:396–401.
392. Smith CS, Howard NJ. Propranolol in treatment of neonatal thyrotoxicosis. *J Pediatr* 1973;83:1046–1048.
393. Levine SA, Sturgis CC. Hyperthyroidism masked as heart disease. *Boston Med Surg J* 1924;190:233–237.
394. Bilezikian JP, Loeb JN. The influence of hyperthyroidism and hypothyroidism on α- and β-adrenergic receptor systems and adrenergic responsiveness. *Endocr Rev* 1983;4:378–388.
394a. Yin Y, Vassy R, Nicolas P, Perret GY, Laurent S. Antagonism between T_3 and amiodarone on the contractility and the density of beta-adrenoceptors of chicken cardiac myocytes. *Eur J Pharmacol* 1994;261:97–104.
394b. Walker JD, Crawford FA Jr, Mukherjee R, Spinale FG. The direct effects of 3,5,3'-triiodo-L-thyronine (T_3) on myocyte contractile processes. Insights into mechanisms of action. *J Thorac Cardiovasc Surg* 1995;110:1369–1379.
394c. Martin WH. Triiodothyronine, beta-adrenergic receptors, agonist responses and exercise capacity. *Ann Thorac Surg* 1993;56(suppl 1):S24–34.
395. DeGroot LJ. Thyroid and the heart. *Mayo Clin Proc* 1972;47:864–871.
396. Moliterno D, DeBold CR, Robertson RM. Case report: coronary vasospasm—relation to the hyperthyroid state. *Am J Med Sci* 1992;304:38–42.
397. Lamberg BA. The medical thyroid crisis. *Acta Med Scand* 1959;164:479–496.
398. Parker JLW. Death from thyrotoxicosis. *Lancet* 1973;2:894–895.
399. Cheah JS, Lee GS, Chew LS. Myocardial infarction in thyrotoxicosis. *Med J Aust* 19711:393–395.
400. Yuen RWM, Gutteridge DH, Thompson PL, Robinson JS. Embolism in thyrotoxic atrial fibrillation. *Med J Aust* 1979;1:630–631.
401. Nakazawa HK, Sakurai K, Hamada N, Monotani N, Ito K. Management of atrial fibrillation in the post-thyrotoxic state. *Am J Med* 1982;72:903–906.
402. Staffurth JS, Gibberd MC, Fui ST. Arterial embolism in thyrotoxicosis with atrial fibrillation. *Br Med J [Clin Res]* 1977;2:688–690.
403. McIntosh TJ, Brunk SF, Kolln I. Increased sensitivity to warfarin in thyrotoxicosis. *J Clin Invest* 1970;49:63a.
404. Roti E, Montermini M, Roti S, Gardini E, Robuschi G, Minelli R, Salvi M, Bentivoglio M, Guiducci V, Braverman LE. The effect of diltiazem, a calcium channel-blocker drug, on cardiac rate and rhythm in hyperthyroid patients. *Arch Intern Med* 1988;148:1919–1921.
405. Oates JA, Wood AJJ. Drug therapy: amiodarone. *N Engl J Med* 1987;316:455–466.
406. Cauchie P, Decaux G, Unger J. Treatment of atrial fibrillation associated with hyperthyroidism by amiodarone and methimazole. *Int J Card Imaging* 1988;19:123–124.
407. Forfar JC, Caldwell GC. Hyperthyroid heart disease. *Baillieres Clin Endocrinol Metab* 1985;14:491–508.
408. Kilpatrick RE, Seiler-Smith S, Levine SN. Thyrotoxic hypokalemic periodic paralysis: report of four cases in black American males. *Thyroid* 1994;4:441–445.
409. Wiersinga WM. Subclinical hypothyroidism and hyperthyroidism. I. Prevalence and clinical relevance. *Neth J Med* 1995;46:197–204.
410. Sawin CT, Geller A, Wolf PA, Belanger AJ, Baker E, Bacharach P, Wilson PWF, Benjamin EJ, D'Agostino RB. Low serum thyrotropin concentrations as a risk factor for atrial fibrillation in older persons. *N Engl J Med* 1994;331:1249–1252.
411. Edmunds HT. Acute thyroiditis from potassium iodide. *Br Med J* 1955;1:354.
412. Marine D. Iodine in the treatment of diseases of the thyroid gland. *Medicine (Baltimore)* 1927;6:127–141.
413. Fradkin JE, Wolff J. Iodide-induced thyrotoxicosis. *Medicine (Baltimore)* 1983;62:1–20.
414. Ermans AM, Camus M. Modifications of thyroid function induced by chronic administration of iodide in the presence of "autonomous" thyroid tissue. *Acta Endocrinol (Copenh)* 1972;70:463–475.
415. Vagenakis AG, Wang C-A, Burger A, Maloof F, Braverman LE, Ing-

bar SH. Iodide-induced thyrotoxicosis in Boston. *N Engl J Med* 1972; 287:523–527.
416. Savoie JC, Massin JP, Thomopoulos P, Leger F. Iodine-induced thyrotoxicosis in apparently normal thyroid glands. *J Clin Endocrinol Metab* 1975;41:685–691.
417. Amico JA, Richardson V, Alpert B, Klein I. Clinical and chemical assessment of thyroid function during therapy with amiodarone. *Arch Intern Med* 1984;144:487–490.
418. Bakker O, van Beeren HC, Wiersinga WM. Desethylamiodarone is a noncompetitive inhibitor of the binding of thyroid hormone to the thyroid hormone β_1-receptor protein. *Endocrinology* 1994;134:1665–1670.
419. Gotzsche LBH. β-Adrenergic receptors, voltage-operated Ca^{2+}-channels, nuclear triiodothyronine receptors and triiodothyronine concentration in pig myocardium after long-term low-dose amiodarone treatment. *Acta Endocrinol* 1993;129:337–347.
420. Barlow JW, Curtis AJ, Raggatt LE, Loidl NM, Topliss DJ, Stockigt JR. Drug competition for intracellular triiodothyronine-binding sites. *Eur J Endocrinol* 1994;130:417–421.
421. Burger A, Dinichert D, Nirod P, Jenny M, Lemarchand-Beraud T, Valloton MB. Effect of amiodarone on serum triiodothyronine, reverse triiodothyronine, thyroxine and thyrotropin: a drug influencing peripheral metabolism on thyroid hormones. *J Clin Invest* 1976;58:255–265.
422. De Jong M, Docter R, van der Hoek H, Krenning E, van der Heide D, Quero C, Plaisier P, Vos R, Hennemann G. Different effects of amiodarone on transport of T_4 and T_3 into the perfused rat liver. *Am J Physiol Endocrinol Metab* 1994;266:E44–E49.
423. Pinchera A, Martino E, Aghini-Lombardi F, Pacchiarotti A, Lenziardi M, Braverman L. Amiodarone and the thyroid. In: Medeiros-Neto G, Gaitan E, eds. *Frontiers in thyroidology.* New York: Plenum Press, 1985;161–168.
424. Norman MF, Lavin TN. Antagonism of thyroid hormone action by amiodarone in rat pituitary tumor cells. *J Clin Invest* 1989;83:306–313.
425. Martino E, Safran M, Aghini-Lombardi F, Rajatanavin R, Lenziardi M, Fay M, Pacchiarotti A, Aonin N, Macchia E, Haffajee C, Odeguardi L, Love J, Bigalli A, Baschieri L, Pinchera A, Braverman L. Environmental iodine intake and thyroid dysfunction during chronic amiodarone therapy. *Ann Intern Med* 1984;101:28–34.
426. Borowski GD, Garofano CE, Rose LI. Effect of long-term amiodarone therapy on thyroid hormone levels and thyroid function. *Am J Med* 1985;78:443.
427. Chiovata L, Martino E, Tonacchera M, Santini F, Lapi P, Mammoli C, Braverman LE, Pinchera A. Studies on the in vitro cytotoxic effect of amiodarone. *Endocrinology* 1994;134:2277–2282.
428. Brennan MD, Erickson DZ, Carney JA, Bahn RS. Nongoitrous (type I) amiodarone-associated thyrotoxicosis: evidence of follicular disruption *in vitro* and *in vivo*. *Thyroid* 1995;5:177–183.
429. Bartalena L, Grasso L, Brogioni S, Aghini-Lombardi F, Braverman LE, Martino E. Serum interleukin-6 in amiodarone-induced thyrotoxicosis *J Clin Endocrinol Metab* 1994;78:423–427.
430. Hauptman PJ, Mechanick JI, Lansman S, Gass A. Fatal hyperthyroidism after amiodarone treatment and total lymphoid irradiation in a heart transplant recipient. *J Heart Lung Transplant* 1993;12:513–516.
431. Magee LA, Downar E, Sermer M, Boulton BC, Allen LC, Koren G. Pregnancy outcome after gestational exposure to amiodarone in Canada. *Am J Obstet Gynecol* 1995;172:1307–1311.
432. Martino E, Aghini-Lombardi F, Mariotti S, Bartalena L, Braverman L, Pinchera A. Amiodarone: a common source of iodine-induced thyrotoxicosis. *Horm Res* 1987;26:158–171.
433. Wimpfheimer C, Staubli M, Schadelin J, Studer H. Prednisone in amiodarone-induced thyrotoxicosis. *Br Med J [Clin Res]* 1982;284:1835–1836.
434. Manciet G, David JP, Tabarin A, Guillaume D, Villaret E, Roger P. In: Medeiros-Neto G, Gaitan E, eds. *Frontiers in thyroidology.* New York: Plenum Press, 1985;1173–1175.
435. Leger AF, Baulieu J, Malinsky M, Chomette G, Savoie J-C. Therapeutic aspects of iodine-induced thyrotoxicosis. *Ann Endocrinol (Paris)* 1977;38:86A.
436. Martino E, Aghini-Lombardi F, Mariotti S, et al. Treatment of amiodarone associated thyrotoxicosis by simultaneous administration of potassium perchlorate and methimazole. *J Endocrinol Invest* 1986;9:201–207.
437. Newnham HH, Topliss DJ, Le Grand BA, Chosich N, Harper RW, Stockigt JR. Amiodarone-induced hyperthyroidism: assessment of the predictive value of biochemical testing and response to combined therapy using propylthiouracil and potassium perchlorate. *Aust N Z J Med* 1988;18:37–44.
438. Fritsche H, Benzer W, Furlan W, Hammerle D, Langsteger W, Weiss P. Prevention of iodine-induced hyperthyroidism after coronary angiography. *Acta Med Austriaca* 1993;20:13–17.
439. Mulligan DC, McHenry CR, Kinney W, Esselstyn CB. Amiodarone-induced thyrotoxicosis: clinical presentation and expanded indications for thyroidectomy. *Surgery* 1993;114:1114–1119.
440. Brennan MD, Heerden JAV, Carney JA. Amiodarone-associated thyrotoxicosis (AAT): experience with surgical management. *Surgery* 1987;102:1062–1067.
441. Thyrotoxicosis Outbreak Study Group. An epidemic of thyrotoxicosis due to inclusion of bovine thyroid gland in ground beef. *Clin Res* 1986;34:713A.
442. Loughney MH, Burman KD. Unusual forms of thyrotoxicosis. *Adv Endocrinol Metab* 1994;5:349–392.
443. Shimaoka K, Van Herle AJ, Dindogau A. Thyrotoxicosis secondary to involvement of the thyroid gland with malignant lymphoma. *J Clin Endocrinol Metab* 1976;43:64–68.
444. Rosen IB, Strawbridge HG, Walfish PG, Brain J. Malignant pseudothyroiditis a new clinical entity. *Am J Surg* 1978;136:445–449.
445. Edmonds CJ, Thompson BD. Hyperthyroidism induced by secondary carcinoma in the thyroid. *Clin Endocrinol (Oxf)* 1978;8:411–415.
446. Hamburger JI, Taylor CI. Transient thyrotoxicosis associated with acute haemorrhagic infarction of autonomously functioning thyroid nodules. *Ann Intern Med* 1979;91:406–409.
447. Steffensen FH, Aunsholt NA. Hyperthyroidism associated with metastatic thyroid carcinoma. *Clin Endocrinol (Oxf)* 1994;41:685–687.
447a. Snow MH, Davies T, Rees Smith B, Ross WM, Evans RGB, Teng CS, Hall R. Thyroid stimulating antibodies and metastatic thyroid carcinoma. *Clin Endocrinol* 1979;10:413–418.
448. Fachnie JD, Rao SI. Painless thyroiditis with hyperthyroidism following external irradiation to the neck. *Henry Ford Hosp Med J* 1980;28:149–151.
449. Hedberg CW, Fishbein DB, Janssen RS, et al. Outbreak of thyrotoxicosis caused by the consumption of bovine thyroid gland in ground beef. *N Engl J Med* 1990;70:396–402.
450. Eliason BC, Doerier JA, Nuhlicek DN. Desiccated thyroid in a nutritional supplement. *J Fam Pract* 1994;38:287–288.
451. Koizumi S, Mashio Y, Mizuo H, Matsuda A, Matsuya K, Mizumoto H, Ikota A, Benito M, Iriuda Y. Graves' hyperthyroidism following transient thyrotoxicosis during interferon therapy for chronic hepatitis type C. *Intern Med* 1995;34:58–60.
452. Cavalieri RR. Quantitative *in vivo* tests. In: Ingbar SH, Braverman LE, eds. *Werner's The thyroid,* 5th ed. New York: JB Lippincott, 1986;445–458.
453. Aro A, Huttunen JK, Lamberg B-A, Pelkonen R, Ikkala E, Kuusisto A, Rissanen V, Salmi J, Tervonen S. Comparison of propranolol and carbimazole as adjuncts to iodine-131 therapy for hyperthyroidism. *Acta Endocrinol (Copenh)* 1981;96:321–327.
454. Velkeniers B, Vanhaelst L, Cytryn R, Jonckheer MH. Treatment of hyperthyroidism with radioiodine: adjunctive therapy with antithyroid drugs reconsidered. *Lancet* 1988;1:1127–1129.
455. Tuttle RM, Patience T, Budd S. Treatment with propylthiouracil before radioactive iodine therapy is associated with a higher treatment failure rate than therapy with radioactive iodine alone in Graves' disease. *Thyroid* 1995;5:243–247.
456. Kung AWC, Yau CC, Cheng ACK. The action of methimazole and L-thyroxine in radioiodine therapy: a prospective study on the incidence of hypothyroidism. *Thyroid* 1995;5:7–12.
457. Ross DS, Daniels GH, Stefano PD, Maloof F, Ridgway EC. Use of adjunctive potassium iodide after radioactive iodine (^{131}I) treatment of Graves' hyperthyroidism. *J Clin Endocrinol Metab* 1983;57:250–253.
458. Marcocci C, Bartalena L, Bogazzi F, Bruno-Bossio G, Pinchera A. Relationship between Graves' ophthalmopathy and type of treatment of Graves' hyperthyroidism. *Thyroid* 1992;2:171–178.
459. Bartalena L, Marcocci C, Bogazzi F, Panicucci M, Lepri A, Pinchera A. Use of corticosteroids to prevent progression of Graves' ophthalmopathy after radioiodine therapy for hyperthyroidism. *N Engl J Med* 1989;321:1349–1362.
460. Bartalena L, Marcocci F, Bogazzi F, Bruno-Bossio ML, Tanda G, Vanni E, Dell'Unto E, Martino E, Pinchera A. *Further studies on the course of Graves' ophthalmopathy (GO) following radioactive iodine*

(RAI) administration. 11th International Thyroid Congress, Toronto, 1995, #139.
461. Waldstein SS, Slodki SJ, Kaganiec I, Bronsky D. A clinical study of thyroid storm. *Ann Intern Med* 1960;52:626–642.
462. Bayley RH. Thyroid crisis. *Surg Gynecol Obstet* 1934;59:41–47.
463. Foss HL, Hunt HF, McMillan RM. Pathogenesis of crisis and death in hyperthyroidism. *JAMA* 1939;113:1090–1094.
464. Thompson WO, Thompson PK, Brailey AG, Cohen AC. Prolonged treatment of exophthalmic goiter by iodine alone. *Arch Intern Med* 1930;45:481–502.
465. Hermann M, Richter B, Roka R, Freissmuth M. Thyroid surgery in untreated severe hyperthyroidism: perioperative kinetics of free thyroid hormones in the glandular venous effluent and peripheral blood. *Surgery* 1994;115:240–245.
466. Marigold JH, Morgan AK, Earle DJ, Young AE, Croft DN. Lugol's iodine: its effect on thyroid blood flow in patients with thyrotoxicosis. *Br J Surg* 1985;72:45–47.
467. Takami H. Lithium in the preoperative preparation of Graves' disease. *Int Surg* 1994;79:89–90.
468. Mochinaga N, Eto T, Maekawa Y, Tsunoda T, Kanematsu T, Izumi M. Successful preoperative preparation for thyroidectomy in Graves' disease using lithium alone: report of two cases. *Surg Today* 1994;24:464–467.
469. Toft AD, Irvine WJ, Campbell RWF. Assessment by continuous cardiac monitoring of minimum duration of preoperative propranolol treatment in thyrotoxic patients. *Clin Endocrinol (Oxf)* 1976;5:195–198.
470. Dial P, Hastings PR. The use of a selective beta-adrenergic receptor blocker for the preoperative preparation of thyrotoxic patients. *Ann Surg* 1982;196:633–635.
471. Eriksson M, Rubenfeld S, Garber AJ, Kohler PO. Propranolol does not prevent thyroid storm. *N Engl J Med* 1977;296:263–264.
472. Toft AD, Irvine WJ, Sinclair I, et al. Thyroid function after surgical treatment of thyrotoxicosis. *N Engl J Med* 1978;298:643–647.
473. McDevitt DG. The assessment of β-adrenoceptor blocking drugs in man. *Br J Clin Pharmacol* 1977;4:413–425.
474. Feek CM, Sawers J, Irvine WJ, et al. Combination of potassium iodide and propranolol in preparation of patients with Graves' disease for thyroid surgery. *N Engl J Med* 1980;302:883–885.
475. Bewsher PD, Pegg CAS, Stewart DJ, Lister DA, Michie W. Propranolol in the surgical management of thyrotoxicosis. *Ann Surg* 1974;180:787–790.
476. Baeza A, Aguayo J, Barria M, Pineda G. Rapid preoperative preparation in hyperthyroidism. *Clin Endocrinol* 1991;35:439–442.
477. Mieny CJ, Franz RC, Med M, Venter ID. The management of severe hyperthyroidism. *World J Surg* 1982;6:689–695.
478. Kampmann JP, Johansen K, Hansen JEM, Helweg J. Propylthiouracil in human milk: revision of dogma. *Lancet* 1980;1:736–738.

CHAPTER 16

Iodine-131 Treatment of Hyperthyroidism

Sidney H. Sobel and Roland Bramlet

Hyperthyroidism may be managed by surgery, antithyroid drugs, radioactive iodine-131 (^{131}I) or, in certain circumstances, by a "watch-policy" (i.e., observation alone). Drug and surgical approaches are considered in detail elsewhere in this text (see Chapters 15 and 17).

The extraction of iodine as iodide by the thyrocytes (the hormone-producing cells of the thyroid gland) presents the unique potential for delivering beta and gamma radiation largely restricted to the thyroid gland by using the isotope ^{131}I. This isotope is concentrated and bound in the thyrocytes, where its ionizing radiations damage the nuclear reproductive mechanism of the cells. The damaged cells eventually disintegrate, resulting in the loss of production of thyroid hormone (1).

For practical purposes, hyperthyroidism may be divided into two major categories for which ^{131}I treatment may be indicated: (a) the nonautoimmune toxic nodule, including the autonomous functioning solitary nodule and the toxic multinodular goiter; and (b) the autoimmune causes, notably Graves' disease. Insofar as we know, ^{131}I does not affect the underlying causes of hyperthyroidism, which in fact are poorly understood, but only addresses the effects of the diseases, which cause an unregulated production of thyroid hormone.

Studies comparing practice patterns between Europe and the United States suggest that radioiodine treatment is prescribed for the majority of hyperthyroid indications in the United States for patients over the age of 45 and increasingly for younger patients, even into the early twenties and late teens (2). With increasing experience over decades of use, the concerns appear to be unfounded that ^{131}I treatment for hyperthyroidism may result in an increased incidence of leukemia, cancer, infertility, and genetic defects in treated patients and their offspring (3–5).

For the nonimmune causes of hyperthyroidism, including toxic multinodular goiter and autonomous solitary nodule, ^{131}I treatment is quite direct and, in concept, not too different from the surgeon's knife. The isotope is taken up selectively by the toxic nodules, which are then functionally destroyed. Because thyroid stimulating hormone (TSH) is suppressed at the time of ^{131}I treatment, the normal thyroid tissue will be relatively unstimulated; it will not take up any significant amount of the therapeutic isotope, and it is therefore largely spared the damaging effects of the isotope. Because of this built-in protection of the normal portion of the gland, the patient with the toxic nodular gland is likely to return to a euthyroid state after ^{131}I treatment (6).

Indeed, isotope treatment of these nonautoimmune types of hyperthyroidism would appear to be nearly ideal. It must be noted, however, that, except for the patient who is a poor surgical risk, surgery is still favored by many thyroidologists, who cite as their reasons expedience, rapid resolution of hyperthyroidism, a lower incidence of early hypothyroidism, slower progression to permanent hypothyroidism, resolution of any concerns that may exist regarding pathology, and, in the case of a large goiter causing compression and substernal extension, providing direct surgical correction of the compression (7). One must balance these reasons against the potential complications of surgery and the observations that ^{131}I treatment has caused significant reduction in volume of both toxic and nontoxic nodular goiter (8–10). The relatively poor uptake in the nontoxic portion of the gland of the patient with toxic adenoma and toxic multinodular goiter contrasts with the diffuse and relatively uniform uptake of ^{131}I throughout the thyroid gland of the Graves' disease patient, in whom there is a relatively global effect on the gland as a whole, and ultimate progression to hypothyroidism.

Three basic approaches have evolved for prescribing ^{131}I treatment of Graves' disease: The multiple low-dose

---

S. H. Sobel: Department of Radiation Oncology, University of Rochester School of Medicine and Dentistry, Rochester, New York 14642; and Finger Lakes Community Cancer Center, Clifton Springs Hospital and Clinic, Clifton Springs, New York 14432.
R. Bramlet: Rochester, New York 14610-3363.

method, the single high-dose method, and the calculated dose method. (The dosimetry of these methods is treated in detail later in this chapter.) It must be noted that for the Graves' disease patient, who has a uniform uptake of the isotope, hypothyroidism is inevitable regardless of the dosimetric method employed. Patients who receive the lower dose are more likely to require retreatment (i.e., more than one dose of ^{131}I). Although the low-dose patient may have a lower incidence of early hypothyroidism, that patient will progress to hypothyroidism at a rate of 3% per year. This relentless progression to hypothyroidism is likely the result of a combination of direct cellular damage by ^{131}I, as well as the natural history of this autoimmune disease (11).

In the single high-dose method, a dose of ^{131}I is selected that is highly likely to ablate thyroid function and render the patient hypothyroid in a few months. The maximum ambulatory dose is often chosen for this purpose. This method of dosing is frequently used in the elderly or cardiac patient in whom hyperthyroidism is complicating overall management. For the Graves' disease patient for whom there are no such overriding concerns, some clinicians still opt for the high-dose method because it brings the patient to the inevitable state of hypothyroidism more quickly and with less likelihood of treatment failure. This method has also been chosen in the case of failure following an initial ^{131}I treatment, regardless of dose, again in an effort to avoid further retreatment (12).

Of late there is a great deal of interest in finding a method that will define a dose for the individual that will minimize the need for retreatment, and that will not deliberately ablate the thyroid. By basing the dosage calculations on thyroid volume and uptake of iodine, we should be able to reduce the incidence of early hypothyroidism. Combining the newest ultrasonic methodology for determination of thyroid volume with a methodology that more accurately predicts the dose that will be effectively taken up and retained by the gland, one may expect a better outcome, with prompt (within 3 to 6 months) control of hyperthyroidism and prolongation of the interval before the development of hypothyroidism. Later in our discussion, we will review the work of Berg et al., which we believe provides a means for approaching that ideal more closely.

The Graves' disease patient may expect to become euthyroid or even hypothyroid within 3 to 6 months after ^{131}I treatment. If hyperthyroidism persists beyond 3 months, as evidenced by thyroid function studies, one should temporize for another 3 months, using as necessary antithyroid drugs in doses sufficient to maintain a euthyroid condition and beta-blockers to protect from the effects of release of T$_4$ from the damaged gland.

Persistence of goiter along with hyperthyroidism at 3 months after treatment usually means treatment failure. However, it is still recommended to wait the additional 3 months under protection of a beta-blocker and an antithyroid drug. Transient hypothyroidism may occur after several months. It is wise to delay T$_4$ replacement therapy until an additional 2 to 3 months have elapsed, allowing for the possibility that a rising TSH may raise the T$_4$ and T$_3$ to normal levels. On the other hand, an enlarging goiter in a patient who is euthyroid or hypothyroid at 3 months after ^{131}I may require T$_4$ replacement that will shrink the goiter and relieve the hypothyroidism (13).

One should also heed the warning of Beierwaltes (whose chapter in the previous edition of this text is highly recommended) not to be fooled by the patient who has an elevated T$_4$ with an elevated TSH several months after ^{131}I treatment. This patient may have been noncompliant in taking replacement T$_4$ and may have taken a higher "catch-up pulse dose" on the day of follow-up blood testing, resulting in misleading and confusing results (14).

CONSIDERATIONS FOR ANTITHYROID DRUGS

Although radioactive ^{131}I may be the preferred definitive treatment for most cases of Graves' disease in the United States (15–17), most patients when first seen in our clinic for this diagnosis are already on treatment with antithyroid drugs [propylthiouracil (PTU), methimazole (MMI)], which prevent the oxidation and binding of iodide in the thyroid gland. Furthermore, most patients will be continued on these drugs after ^{131}I treatment. Whereas the beta-blockers that are routinely prescribed in thyrotoxicosis have no such adverse effect on ^{131}I treatment and therefore may be continued throughout, the antithyroid drugs must be withdrawn for radioiodine to be effective. The length of time that the antithyroid drugs are withdrawn prior to ^{131}I treatment varies among clinics. Pharmacologically, PTU should be cleared from the system within 24 to 48 hours. In general, one would then wait approximately 7 days before iodine treatment, so that a clinically efficient uptake is reestablished. Then the determination of the critically important radioiodine uptake is done, which, together with the estimated or measured (by ultrasound) thyroid volume, guides the clinician in the timing and calculation of the dose of ^{131}I (17). If antithyroid drugs are to be reinstituted, this should not occur sooner than 8 days after the administration of ^{131}I,

---

*Iodine-131, like any other iodine absorbed into the bloodstream, circulates as the iodide. The amount of iodide extracted from the blood and concentrated in the thyroid gland is a function of a dynamic balance between the rate of entry into the gland and binding to protein on the one hand, and the passive diffusion back out into the bloodstream. Whereas the normal thyroid can concentrate iodide to 50 times that in plasma, the gland in Graves' disease can concentrate to several hundred times that in the plasma. In repeated passes of the blood through the hyperactive gland, additional amounts of the ^{131}I will be extracted and bound, contributing to the therapeutic effect on the gland (19). Antithyroid drugs, such as MMI and PTU, prevent the binding of iodide and thus lessen the potential effect, or effective dose, of the administered ^{131}I on the gland. At some point, the diminishing radioactivity, determined by the half-life of the isotope, will outweigh any additional benefit of the binding of the isotope. At that point, antithyroid drugs may be reinstituted. In practice, one would want to take advantage of the fact that ^{131}I has a physical half-life of 8 days. If antithyroid drugs are to be resumed, we recommend a delay of 8 to 12 days before doing so. This will assure a near-maximal effect of the dose administered.

and preferably 12 days after (18), so that the patient may benefit from the effects of recirculation of the isotope.*

Some clinicians have pretreated the patient with Graves' hyperthyroidism with antithyroid drugs (PTU and MMI) to potentiate the uptake of ^{131}I and to reduce the risk of exacerbation of toxic symptoms that may follow ^{131}I treatment. The rationale for this use of the antithyroid drugs derives from the observations that (a) PTU and MMI will cause depletion of T_4 as a result of blockage of the binding of iodide (20), (b) will cause a decrease in the size of the gland, and (c) within several days after their withdrawal, there may be an increase in the 24-hour uptake of ^{131}I, compared to the uptake prior to taking the antithyroid drug, possibly allowing a lower prescribed dose (21). One cannot overemphasize the importance of calculating a dose by determining the radioactive iodine uptake (RAIU) at the time of treatment, and also the gland volume. As will be discussed later, we prefer that RAIU be determined at several intervals. Clearly, the clinician must tailor the treatment and the management thereafter to the special circumstances that may apply in any particular case.

COMPLICATIONS

Complications of ^{131}I treatment are extremely uncommon. Thyroid storm, vascular and airway compromise, and acute thyroiditis present the greatest concerns. Headache, bone and joint pain, and stiffness have also been reported (22). Ophthalmopathy has been described as a complication of ^{131}I treatment of Graves' disease; this remains a subject of considerable controversy (23) and will not be reviewed here (see Chapter 17). It is not uncommon for a mild increase in thyrotoxicosis to occur within a few weeks of ^{131}I treatment. Where this may be of concern, as in the case of a high-risk cardiac patient, pretreatment with an antithyroid drug, preferably PTU, may be prescribed to reduce stored hormone; the antithyroid drug may be resumed posttreatment to inhibit peripheral conversion of T_4 to T_3 (15,16). A beta-blocker is usually prescribed as well.

Thyroid storm is a severe exacerbation of thyrotoxicosis. It is a result of the release of excessive amounts of thyroid hormone into the bloodstream from the injured gland. It is most often causally related to an acute severe infection in a thyrotoxic patient. Less often, it may occur postoperatively in a thyrotoxic patient who has not had sufficient preoperative preparation for thyroidectomy. It has only rarely occurred as a result of ^{131}I treatment. Because it may be life threatening, however, the symptoms and signs should be familiar to the treating physician and should be described to the patient receiving ^{131}I, especially a cardiac patient, so that no time is lost in the event that symptoms and signs do occur. The signs and symptoms of ^{131}I-induced thyroid storm appear at approximately 3 to 4 weeks after the dose of ^{131}I. High fever, even to 105°F, may occur, associated with delirium, aberrant behavior (even psychotic behavior), tachycardia, nausea, vomiting, diarrhea, dehydration, abdominal pain, cardiac arrhythmia, congestive heart failure, and shock-like collapse. (For the management of thyroid storm, the reader is referred to Chapter 40.)

Thyroiditis caused by ^{131}I is usually experienced within 1 week of treatment and presents with pain, tenderness, and swelling in the neck, sore throat, and dysphagia. These symptoms generally resolve spontaneously within a week and are treated symptomatically with anti-inflammatory and analgesic agents. It would be very unusual for thyroiditis to occur within the dose limitations for ambulatory patients set by state and national agencies. As in thyroid storm, if infection is suspected as a contributing factor, antibiotics should be prescribed. Damage to the laryngeal and tracheal cartilage and to the parathyroids has been reported but only with excessively high doses of radioiodine.

When an enlarged thyroid lies within the tight closed space of the thoracic inlet, acute radiation-induced thyroiditis might result in edema of the thyroid, which may in turn cause vascular and airway compromise. Thyroid imaging, which is a standard part of the workup of such patients, will disclose the size, shape, and extent of such a large toxic goiter, and it would allow the clinician to anticipate this uncommon complication. Pretreatment with antithyroid drugs should be considered in such extreme circumstances, to decrease the volume of the gland and the risk of this complication. Recent studies suggest that significant swelling of the thyroid does not occur secondary to ^{131}I treatment, and that, in fact, volume reduction occurs (9,21). Nonetheless, surgery may be preferable for the medically operable patient who presents with vascular or airway compromise, or in whom such risk is anticipated from imaging.

When ^{131}I treatment results in hypothyroidism, the commonly observed symptoms and signs of a slowed metabolism may be accompanied by headache and generalized muscle and joint discomfort. The headache is considered to be a result of pituitary swelling. Both of these symptoms clear promptly with thyroid hormone replacement.

CONTRAINDICATIONS TO ^{131}I TREATMENT

There are few absolute contraindications to ^{131}I treatment. These include: (a) pregnancy (24), (b) lactation in a nursing mother, and (c) insufficient uptake of ^{131}I. A relative contraindication is patient/family apprehension regarding radiation exposure. Questionable contraindications are age and "active exophthalmos." With respect to ophthalmopathy, the data are not sufficient to indict ^{131}I treatment as a cause, direct or indirect, of initial ophthalmopathy, or of worsening preexisting ophthalmopathy. Most clinicians both in the United States and abroad advise ^{131}I treatment of the patient with ophthalmopathy, some favoring doses of ^{131}I that will completely ablate the thyroid (and not just render the patient euthyroid or hypothyroid), others recommending concomitant administration of steroids (glucocorticoids) that will, in their experience, prevent the worsening of preexisting ophthalmopathy (25) and still others the subsequent administration of T_4 to reduce the occurrence of ophthalmopathy (26).

With respect to age, emotionalism interferes with an objective evaluation of risk, no matter how carefully the data are reviewed and presented. As far as current analysis can reveal, there should be no restriction in the prescribing of ^{131}I for patients in any age group; however, from a practical point of view, most clinicians are unlikely to prescribe ^{131}I for a patient under 15 years of age.

In discussing the effects and risks of ^{131}I treatment, many authors compare and merge data derived from external beam x-ray treatment with data derived from systemic ^{131}I. There are substantial radiobiologic differences between these sources and techniques of radiation. It can be misleading to extrapolate the data from one to the other, or to summate the effects of one with the other.

In the ^{131}I treatment of hyperthyroidism, it is most important to have an understanding of the nature of the therapy and to seek an optimal method for selecting the dose of radioiodine. The technology now exists for relatively simple and expeditious determinations of the factors necessary to calculate an effective dose. These techniques, including pertinent background information and methodology, are presented in the next section.

PHYSICAL PROPERTIES OF ^{131}I

Before ^{131}I can be effectively and safely used in the treatment of thyroid conditions, certain properties of this radionuclide and its radiations must be considered. Iodine occurs in nature in a stable state with 53 protons and 74 neutrons in the nucleus of each atom (iodine-127). Any variation in the number of neutrons creates an unstable state that results in a radioactive isotope of iodine. The form of radioiodine most suitable for therapy is ^{131}I, in which each atomic nucleus has an atomic number of 53 (53 protons) and an atomic mass of 131 (53 protons and 78 neutrons). ^{131}I is produced by neutron irradiation of tellurium dioxide in a nuclear reactor. This produces tellurium-131 which, by radioactive decay, spontaneously turns to ^{131}I. ^{131}I is also produced as a fission product during the fissioning of uranium in nuclear reactors. ^{131}I spontaneously turns to a stable state through a process whereby a neutron in a given atom throws out an electron (called a beta particle) at high velocity and in so doing turns into a proton. This means that the atomic number has moved up by one (from 53 to 54) and the atom is now xenon, atomic number 54, with a mass of 131. This form of xenon has a neutron-to-proton ratio that provides a stable condition, and the radioactive decay of this atom is now complete. It is this process of electron ejection that produces the beta radiation that is responsible for the major portion of the therapeutic effect of ^{131}I (Fig. 1).

The rate at which radioactive decay takes place is proportional to the number of atoms present. In mathematical terms, the decay rate, which is best expressed as a series of half-lives, is an exponential process. For example, if you start with a sample of ^{131}I in an amount designated as 100% at time zero, in 8.05 days after time zero there will be 50%, or one half, left. In 8.05 more days (16.1 days from time 0), you will have 25% of the original 100% left, or half of the first half. In 8.05 additional days (24.15 days from time 0), the amount will again fall by half to 12.5%, and the radioactive decay will continue in

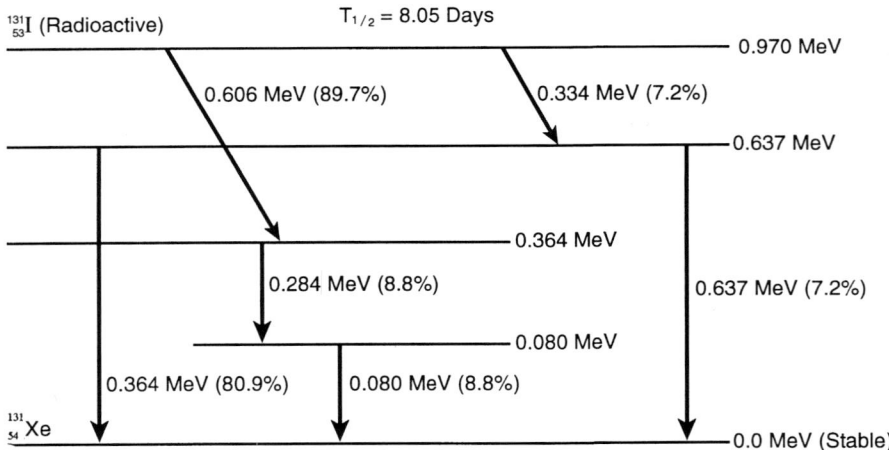

FIG. 1. Decay scheme showing the two major routes of radioactive decay for ^{131}I. *Horizontal lines* represent energy levels. *Lines sloping downward* to the right indicate beta particle emission. *Vertical lines* indicate gamma ray emission. The numbers for energy levels have been rounded off and may vary by ±0.001. This decay scheme accounts for 96.9% of the radiation from ^{131}I.

this fashion. (See Figs. 3,4 for graphs and the formula of amount of radioactivity versus time.) The radioactive decay rate varies greatly from radionuclide to radionuclide, with half-lives ranging from a fraction of a second to thousands of years. The rate at which radioiodine ($^{131}_{53}$I) changes to stable xenon ($^{131}_{54}$Xe) is such that the half-life is 8.05 days. There is no known way to change the rate of this reaction. In considering the decay of ^{131}I in the body, it should be noted that xenon is a nonreactive inert gas that escapes by way of the lungs.

The beta particles or electrons that are thrown out of decaying neutrons within the radioactive nucleus of ^{131}I have various energies. These energies are designated and measured in a unit called the electron volt. An electron volt is the amount of energy gained by an electron in falling through a potential difference of 1 volt. (This is a unit of energy and is not to be confused with the volt as an electrical potential difference term that applies to batteries or the electrical outlet in your home.) Because the electron volt is a very small unit, and because most beta particles have energies on the order of a million electron volts, the practical unit is a million electron volts, or a megavolt (MeV). The two major beta energies for ^{131}I are 0.606 MeV and 0.334 MeV. Although beta particles are ejected from ^{131}I atoms with considerable energy, they do not travel far through tissue (on the order of a couple of millimeters). Virtually no beta particles escape from the thyroid where iodine collects. This is the major reason that large doses of ^{131}I may be given without damage to the parathyroid glands. This is also the reason that dosage within the thyroid gland is not uniform. Areas that take up more iodine become radiation hot spots; areas of low uptake become cold spots. After the emission of a beta particle, the ^{131}I atom undergoes a further adjustment with the emission of electromagnetic energy in the form of gamma rays. By definition, the radiations that come from the nucleus, rather than from the outer part of the atom (the orbital electron rings), are designated as gamma and beta radiations. For ^{131}I, the major gamma radiation is at 0.364 MeV and at 0.637 MeV. These beta and gamma radiations account for 90% of the radiation from ^{131}I. The remaining 10% includes three additional beta modes and five additional gamma modes. Although gamma radiation contributes only 10% of the total radiation dosage, it still must be accounted for. When gamma rays are emitted within an organ, it is rare that complete energy absorption takes place within the organ. The gamma ray component of radiation dosage is much more uniform throughout the thyroid than is the beta ray component. Much of the gamma ray energy leaves through the surface of the patient, which makes it possible for a radiation detector in the vicinity of the patient to quantitatively determine the amount of radioactivity within.

Radioactive materials are measured, not in pounds or grams, but in disintegrations per second (dps). The standard in the c.g.s. (centimeter-gram-second) system is the number of disintegrations per second taking place in 1 gram of radium in equilibrium with its decay products. This very large number (3.7×10^{10} dps) is designated a curie (Ci). More practical subunits are the millicurie (mCi, or 3.7×10^7 dps) and the microcurie (μCi, or 3.7×10^4 dps). In the new standard international system of units, the basic unit is 1 dps, which is designated as the becquerel (Bq) (27). Because the becquerel is very small, the practical unit is the megabequerel (MBq, or 10^6 dps). The gigabequerel (GBq, or 10^9 dps) is a unit that is also often useful. The conversion factor from curies to bequerels is

$$1 \text{ Ci} = 3.7 \times 10^{10} \text{ Bq}.$$

In more practical units, it is

$$1 \text{ mCi} = 37 \text{ MBq}.$$

A table of commonly used conversions follows:

mCi	MBq	mCi	MBq	mCi	MBq
0.1	3.7	2.5	92.5	10	370
0.2	7.4	3.0	111	12	444
0.25	9.25	4.0	148	15	555
0.3	11.1	5.0	185	20	740
0.4	14.8	6.0	222	25	925
0.5	18.5	7.0	259	30	1110
1.0	37	8.0	296	40	1480
2.0	74	9.0	333	50	1850

Because the number and type of particles vary greatly with different radioactive materials, the amount of energy deposited in a given quantity of material exposed to radiation also varies. To get around this, a c.g.s. system unit of absorbed radiation dose called the rad (radiation absorbed dose) has been formulated. In the International System, the unit of absorbed dose is called the gray (Gy). One rad is equal to the absorption of 100 ergs of energy per gram of material. The gray is equal to the absorption of one joule of energy per kilogram of material. Thus absorption of one gray of energy by an object is equal to the absorption of 100 rads (1 Gy = 100 rad). The radiation dosage for thyroid treatment is usually specified in rads or grays, and the amount of radioiodine necessary to achieve this dosage is dispensed in terms of millicuries (mCi) or megabequerels (MBq).

RADIATION DOSIMETRY

Ionizing radiation disrupts chemical bonds throughout the cell and is particularly damaging to DNA, with the result that cellular dysfunction and death take place. The radiation dose delivered by an internally administered radionuclide depends on a number of factors:

1. The physical half-life of the radionuclide

2. The rate of biologic elimination of the radionuclide, or the biologic half-life
3. The energy and type of radiation emitted by the radioactive material during decay
4. The volume of tissue in which the radionuclide are distributed
5. The degree of homogeneity with which the radionuclide and its ionizing radiation are distributed

Items (1) and (3) are accurately known and the information is available from tables. For item (4), it is important to know the volume of the thyroid; the radiation dose given to a volume is inversely proportional to the volume in which the radioactive material is distributed. Clinical examination, x-ray studies, and nuclear scans have all been used to evaluate thyroid volume; however, the use of ultrasound imaging has greatly increased the accuracy of thyroid volume determination (28–31). In 1948, Marinelli et al. (32) postulated that the physical half-life of radioiodine, item (1), could be combined with the biological half-life of iodine in the thyroid, item (2), to give an effective half-life which would follow monoexponential decay (often simply referred to as exponential). At this point it may be well to review and clarify the half-life concept. Radioiodine disappears from any location, including the thyroid, by way of physical decay at a rate which is best described by the half-life. The decay rate is faster when much iodine is present but slows down as the amount decreases, and in such a fashion that no matter what amount we have at the time we begin measuring, we will, through physical decay, have only half of that amount left in eight days. By analogy we might say that we have a bucket with a magic hole in the bottom which lets water leak out at a faster or slower rate depending on the amount of water in the bucket. If I put in a lot of water the hole gets bigger and the water leaks out faster. If I put in a little water, the hole gets smaller and the water leaks more slowly; however, always half the water leaks out in a given time, e.g., 8 days. In mathematical terms we have a bucket with a hole that varies in size in a monoexponential manner according to the amount of water in the bucket. Half-life gives us a clue as to the size of the hole at any moment.

Frequently, physiologic elimination of a substance from the body proceeds in a monoexponential manner with a characteristic half-life. That half-life is referred to as the biologic half-life. Physiologic elimination of iodine from the thyroid follows a monoexponential pattern; however, its biologic half-life varies from patient to patient. (Now we have a bucket with two holes and we don't know how the size of the second hole varies.) The mathematical rules are such that if we have two monoexponential processes going on, we may combine them and determine an effective half-life reflecting the combined action. Fortunately, this effective half-life ($T_{1/2}$) is also monoexponential (see Figs. 3,4), and we have the equation

$$1/T_{1/2}\ \text{effective} = 1/T_{1/2}\ \text{physical} + 1/T_{1/2}\ \text{biologic}$$

Effective half-life for radioiodine in the thyroid can be determined by measuring radioiodine uptake at several different periods of time following iodine administration. In a particular case, Marinelli et al. (32) determined the effective half-life to be 6.5 days. In this case, the radiation dosage was 19% less when the dosage was calculated with the effective half-life rather than the physical half-life of the radioiodine. Since that time, the effective half-life has been widely used in ^{131}I dosage calculations for the thyroid, despite the fact that it has some serious limitations. Time zero, or the start of exponential decay, is taken at the moment of peak activity in the thyroid. Time zero, or the instant of peak activity, is usually estimated to be 24 hours after administration of the radioiodine dose. This may, or may not, be true in a particular case. Radiation dose to the thyroid during the period between the time the radioiodine dose is given and the time peak activity is reached is not included in dosage calculation. Effective half-life is seldom measured and is usually accepted as 5 or 6 days. Schmidt and Nadelhaft (33) have found effective half-life to vary from 3 to 8 days. Berg et al. (34) report a range of 1.6 to 7.5 days.

A change in effective half-life produces a significant change in the amount of radioiodine required to achieve a specific radiation dose to the thyroid. The accuracy of the estimate of effective half-life can be increased by measuring the radioactivity within the thyroid over a period of time following the administration of a dose of ^{131}I (31,34). Item (5) in the list, the degree of uniformity of dose, remains the most elusive factor. Uniform distribution is usually assumed but not necessarily achieved. Some have applied correction factors to thyroid volume determinations to account for nonuniformity (35).

A very simple approach to dosimetry is to give the patient 2 mCi (74 mBq) to 3 mCi (111 mBq) every 6 months until the patient becomes euthyroid without antithyroid medication. This method has been used for years in at least one well-known institution (30). This procedure has the advantage of minimizing the individual radiation dose and also the incidence of early hypothyroidism. Uptake studies are unnecessary. The major disadvantage is that multiple dosages may be required and it may be many months or years before thyrotoxicosis is controlled. Another dosage scheme is to give the largest statutory dose possible for an outpatient, now in excess of 30 mCi (1110 mBq or 1.11 GBq) in the United States. This method has the advantage of controlling the hyperthyroid state as quickly as possible. The need for retreatment is minimized. Once again, no uptake studies or scans are needed to determine dosage. The disadvantage is that most patients quickly become hypothyroid and require replacement therapy for the rest of their lives. The radiation exposure to the patients and those around them may be higher than necessary (36).

In the treatment of hyperthyroidism, the goal should be to minimize radiation exposure of the patient and to the environment, while eliminating the hyperthyroid state.

Therefore, the best methods should be used to optimize the radioiodine dose for the unique character of each patient's thyrotoxicosis. This is the thrust of much of the literature from the European and Scandinavian countries. It cannot be better said than in this 1994 quotation from Margaret Flower et al. (30):

> Many centers now prescribe a large initial dose of radioiodine with a view to rendering patients euthyroid quickly and accepting a high probability of hypothyroidism. This philosophy has never found favor at the Royal Marsden Hospital as we believe it to be suboptimal to replace one disease by another iatrogenic disease which is irreversible. Just because it is difficult to achieve euthyroidism, this should not become the excuse for not attempting optimal therapy.

The delivered absorbed dose method may be used to optimize dosage. In this method, a calculation is made relating the desired dose in grays to the amount of radioiodine to be given in megabequerels. The basic equation (34,37,38) is as follows:

$$\text{Amount of radioiodine to be given (MBq)} = \frac{23.4 \times \text{mass (g)} \times \text{absorbed dose (Gy)}}{\text{24-hr uptake (\%)} \times \text{5-day half-life}} \quad [1]$$

A typical absorbed dose for toxic adenoma is 150 Gy, and for diffuse uptake or Graves' disease, 100 Gy. The value of 23.4 is a constant, characteristic of the energy and type of radiation emitted by ^{131}I that gives rise to the tissue absorbed dose in MBq/Gy.

The mass of the thyroid is accepted as being equal to the volume. The volume of the thyroid may be determined by ultrasound scanning in three cross sections in sagittal, frontal, and transverse planes. Sagittal and transverse scans are done in the supine position with the neck hyperextended so that the sagittal and transverse planes are aligned with the actual orientation of the gland. Frontal scans are done in the left and right decubitus positions as described by Szebeni and Beleznay (28). Sections showing the maximal dimensions are used to calculate the volume of each lobe (28,31) according to the formula

$$\text{Volume equals } \pi/6 \times (a \times b \times c),$$

where a, b, and c are the height and the length of the cross-sectional axis (Fig. 2). If the volume of the isthmus cannot be measured, it may be estimated as 5% of the total volume of the two lobes.

$$V_{\text{isthmus}} = 0.05 \, (V_{\text{right lobe}} + V_{\text{left lobe}})$$

$$\text{Total thyroid } V = V_{\text{right lobe}} + V_{\text{left lobe}} + V_{\text{isthmus}}$$

The above calculation is based upon the concept that the lobes of the thyroid are ellipsoidal (28,30,31). If the thyroid is irregular in shape, cross-sectional slices may be taken at intervals along the length of the gland. The area and height of each slice may be used to determine slice volume. The slice volumes may then be summed to determine lobe volume. Computer programs are available to perform this type of numerical integration.

A major pitfall in volume determination by thyroid imaging is magnification. Measurements made on the image should have a one-to-one ratio with the gland dimensions; otherwise, magnification corrections are needed. When possible, a magnification marker should be used. For radionuclide scans, a capillary tube filled with a radioactive solution may be used to determine magnification. The length of the thyroid is sometimes best determined by radionuclide scan. This may be combined with ultrasound cross-sectional measurements. Magnetic resonance imaging provides ideal images for volume determination; however, the cost is not justified, except in large multinodular goiters where intrathoracic extension or tracheal compression is also to be evaluated (39). Positron emission tomography (PET) with radioiodine-124 (^{124}I) provides three-dimensional pictures of the functional volume of the thyroid rather than the anatomic volume demonstrated by ultrasound. Unfortunately, access to a cyclotron is required to produce ^{124}I. This requirement tends to limit PET scanning to research programs at large centers.

Turning attention to the denominator of equation (1), we find two factors, the 24-hour uptake and the 5-day half-life. It is assumed that the 24-hour uptake is a reasonably correct estimate of the maximum uptake. In most cases, uptake will have reached a peak in 20 to 24 hours; however, this is not always true. There is enough discrepancy to require consideration. Vemulakonda et al. (40) found that 17% of their patients had a 4-hour uptake higher than their 24-hour uptake, which indicates that the maximum uptake had been reached well before 24 hours. The time of peak activity and the amplitude of peak activity, as measured by the radioiodine uptake, are functions of the rate of iodine turnover in the gland. The rate of iodine turnover in the gland is measured by the effective half-life. The maximum uptake and the time of its appearance are functions of effective half-life. Maximum uptake does not always occur at 24 hours. It is assumed, not always correctly, that the accumulated radioiodine will leave the patient's thyroid in a monoexponential way (Figs. 3,4). This gives rise to a biologic half-life that exhibits the same behavior as that associated with radioactive elements. The amount of iodine in the thyroid, before its removal from the system (essentially by way of the kidneys), is 100%. After one half-life, 50% is left; after two half-lives, 25% is left, and so on. The effective half-life results from a combination of the physical half-life for the radioiodine and the biologic half-life for the elimination of the radioiodine from the thyroid. Whereas the half-life of ^{131}I is constant at 8.05 days, the biologic half-life varies greatly depending on thyroid function. As previously discussed, the effective

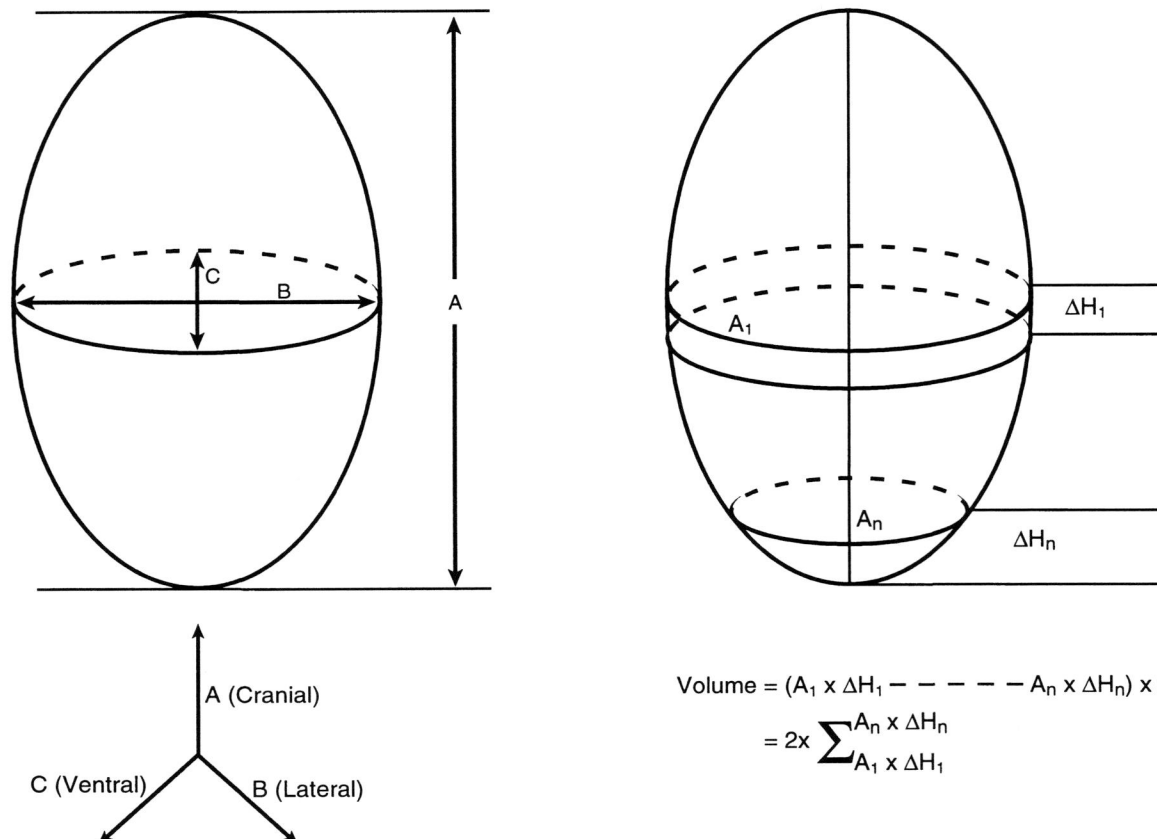

FIG. 2. Method for calculation of the volume of a thyroid lobe that is nonellipsoidal in shape. An ellipsoid is shown to demonstrate the method. Slices are cut through the figure. The volume of each slice is determined by multiplying the area of each slice by the thickness. The volumes so determined are added together to give the total volume. If the lobe is symmetrical, as shown here, the volume of half of it may be calculated, with the result being multiplied by 2 to obtain total volume.

half-life (e) is related to the physical (p) and biologic (b) half-lives by the following equations:

$$1/T^{1}/_{2}(e) = 1/T^{1}/_{2}(p) + 1/T^{1}/_{2}(b)$$

$$T^{1}/_{2}(e) = \frac{T^{1}/_{2}(p) \cdot T^{1}/_{2}(b)}{T^{1}/_{2}(p) + T^{1}/_{2}(b)}$$

$$T^{1}/_{2}(b) = \frac{T^{1}/_{2}(p) \cdot T^{1}/_{2}(e)}{T^{1}/_{2}(p) - T^{1}/_{2}(e)}$$

In practice, we determine the effective half-life by the RAIU procedure. Repeated direct measurement of thyroid radioiodine levels are made at frequent intervals over a period of time following radioiodine administration (see later section on Methods). The physical half-life for ^{131}I is a known value, available to us from tables containing the characteristics of various radionuclides. With the physical $T^{1}/_{2}$ for ^{131}I taken as 8.05 days, and the effective $T^{1}/_{2}$ measured, the relationship between effective half-life and biologic half-life is as follows for various values of effective half-life:

$T^{1}/_{2}$ effective	$T^{1}/_{2}$ biologic
1.60 days	2 days
2.67 days	4 days
4.01 days	8 days
5.36 days	16 days
6.43 days	32 days
7.11 days	64 days
7.57 days	128 days

In the average patient, the effective half-life is often considered to be 5 days, which corresponds to a biologic half-life of 13.2 days. Radiation dose depends not only on uptake but also on effective half-life. For a given uptake, the longer the effective half-life, the less radioactive iodine is required to achieve a given radiation dose.

Seed and Jaffe (41) and Freedberg et al. (42) have shown that the determination of uptake and effective half-life with a tracer dose of ^{131}I is a satisfactory predictor of the behavior of the therapeutic dose. In view of

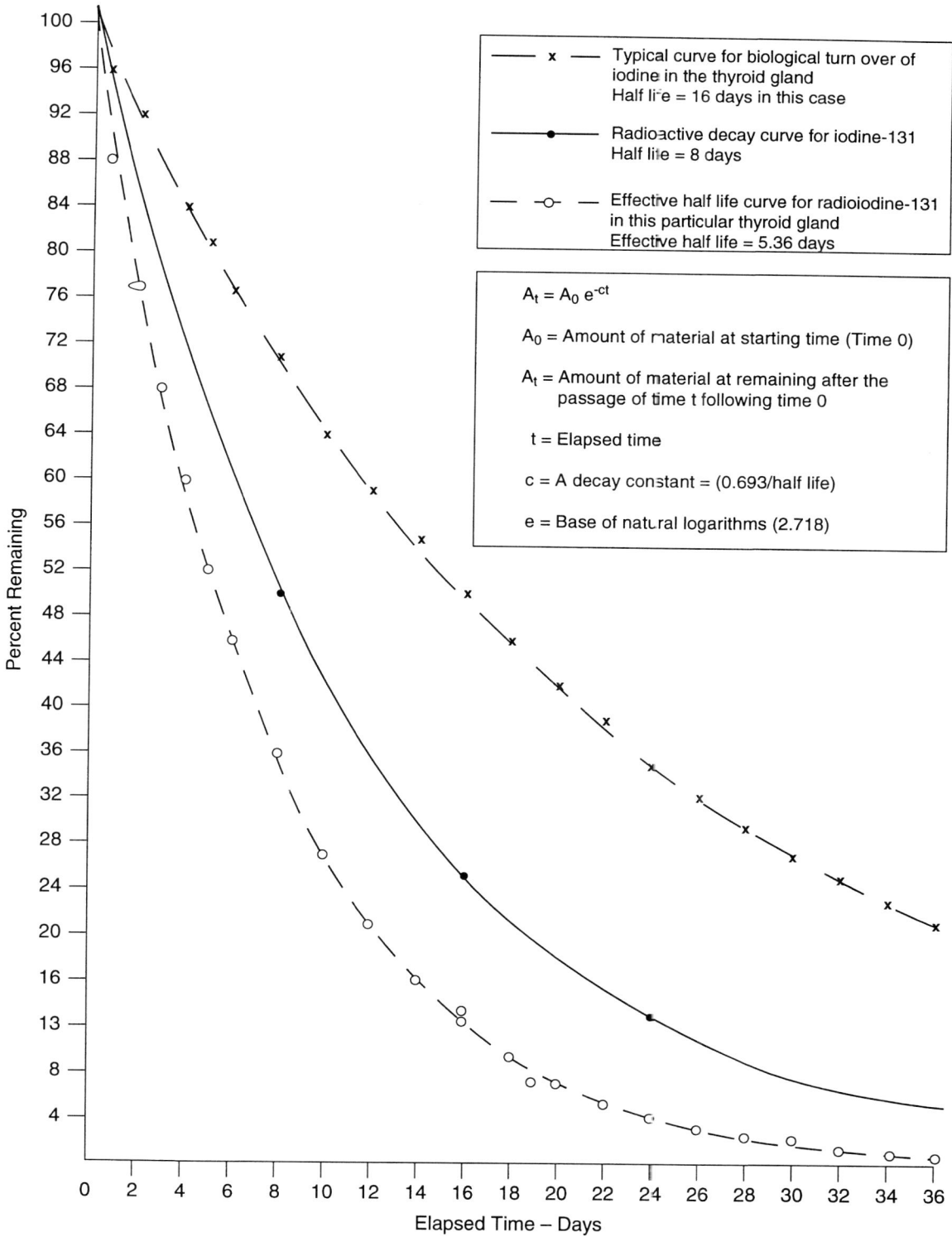

FIG. 3. The combination of biologic elimination and physical decay of ^{131}I gives rise to a combined process with an effective half-life shorter than either the biologic or physical half-life. Typical decay curves for all three are presented on rectangular coordinate paper.

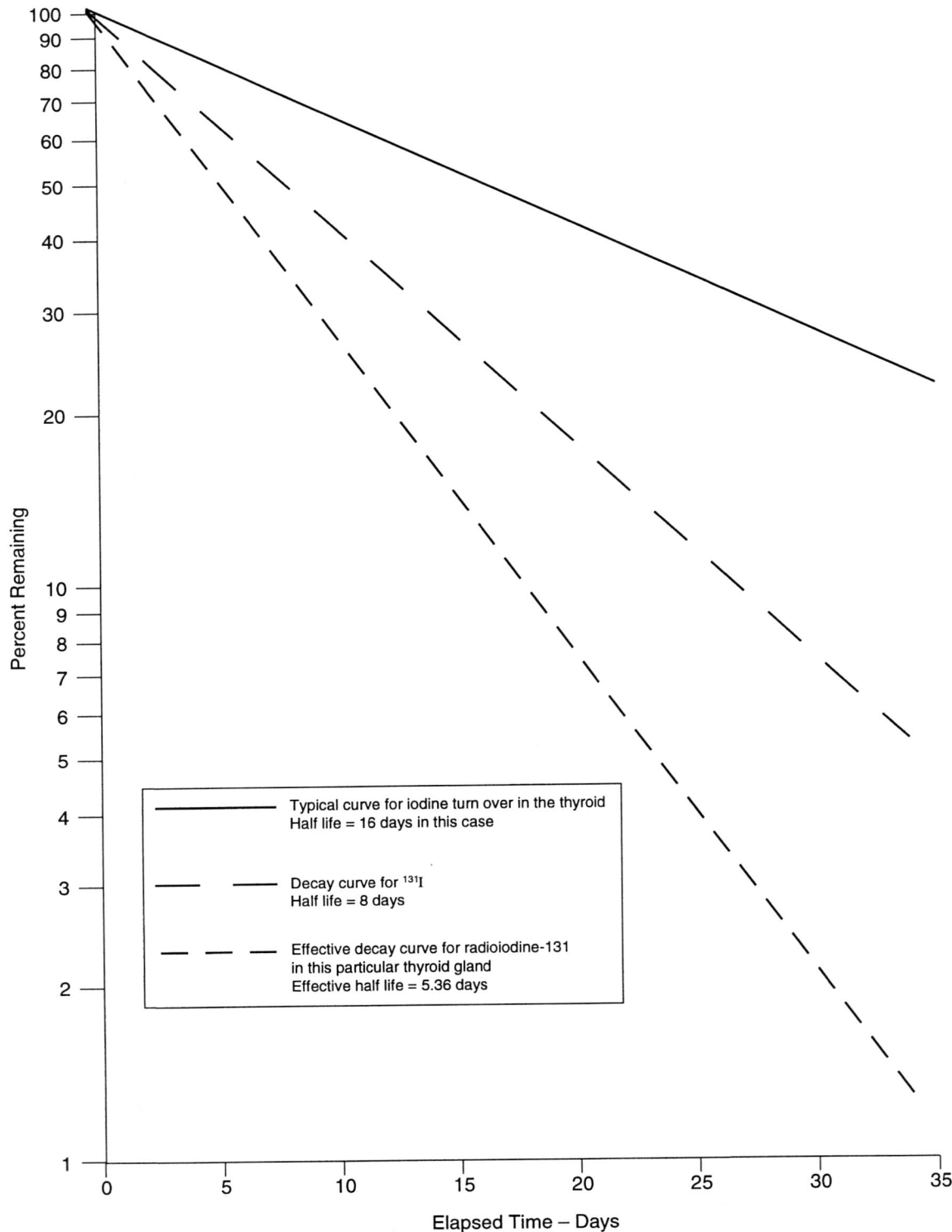

FIG. 4. The same curves that appear in Figure 3 are presented here on two-cycle semilogarithmic paper. Because the curves are now straight lines, the determination of any two points is sufficient to plot the curves over any range needed.

this, it is suggested that a kinetic study of the tracer dose be used to provide a better estimate of the effective half-life and also a better estimate of maximum uptake. For many years, the single 24-hour radioiodine uptake has been used as the basis for dosage calculations, based on the assumption that a 24-hour uptake is a reasonable estimate of maximum uptake. In a significant number of cases, this is not true. It has been proposed that uptake studies be done at other times for various reasons. Bockisch et al. (31) have measured uptake at 8, 24, 32, 48, 76, 96, and 192 hours for a rather complete study of iodine kinetics. They devised a system based upon one uptake performed at 96 hours, in which an empirically derived constant is used to compute therapeutic dosage. They point out that, at 96 hours, there is no rapid change in the declining activity curve, and hence little error is introduced if measurement is an hour or two early or late. With a 24-hour uptake, an error of 2 hours in measurement timing can be significant. At the other extreme, Vemulakonda et al. (40) reported the use of a 4-hour uptake test in Graves' disease patients. An algorithm, based on patient experience, is used to convert the 4-hour uptake to a 24-hour value, from which therapeutic calculations are made. They admit that, in the 15% of patients with rapid iodine turnover, this method may result in ineffective therapy. In favor of the 4-hour uptake, they cite reduced cost and increased patient convenience.

In reviewing iodine kinetics, we consider the relationship of effective half-life to radioiodine uptake. In the past, effective half-life has often been taken as a constant, with a value of 5 days, or perhaps 6 days, depending on opinion. Schmidt and Nadelhaft (33) examined effective half-life in 100 patients and found a range of 3 to 8 days. Eighty-two percent fell between 5 and 7 days, with an average of 6 days. Berg et al. (34) reported effective half-life as ranging from 1.6 days to 7.5 days in a review of 555 patients. They found iodine turnover rate to be more rapid (i.e., a shorter effective half-life) in Graves' disease than for toxic nodular goiter. Patients in both categories treated with antithyroid drugs were found to exhibit a significantly shorter effective half-life, even if medication was discontinued a week before radioiodine studies.

Berg et al. (34) suggested an ingenious modification to equation (1) that gives a better estimate of both uptake and effective half-life and results in a more accurate dose calculation. The method requires three uptake measurements to be made at 24, 48, and 96 hours (1, 2, and 4 days). Justifying their method, they stated, "Although this procedure is not laborious for the physician, especially when using computerized calculation, it does require extra effort from the patient. We are sure, however, that any inconvenience will be readily accepted by the patient(s) once they know that the method results in more accurate treatment."

$$\frac{\text{Amount of radioactivity to be given (MBq)}}{} = \frac{23.4 \cdot \text{mass (g)} \cdot \text{absorbed dose (Gy)}}{\text{estimated uptake} \cdot \text{effective } T_{1/2} \text{ (days)}} \quad [2]$$
(% at time 0) (calculated)

In equation (2), it is implicit that time zero is 24 hours. That is, the therapeutic effect is presumed to start in 24 hours. In equation (2), time zero has been shifted from 24 hours after administration of the dose of iodine to the time of administration of the dose. This provides an empirical link between the uptake level and the rate of iodine turnover in the thyroid. The shorter the effective half-life, the faster iodine turns over in the gland and the higher the estimated uptake at time zero. Because radiation dose to the thyroid occurs only while radioiodine is present in the thyroid, a larger amount of iodine is needed when there is fast turnover. If turnover is slow, the iodine remains in the gland for a long time and a smaller amount of radioiodine is needed to achieve a given radiation dose.

In the test procedure used by Berg et al. (34), the patient is given an oral dose of 0.5 MBq (13.5 µCi) of ^{131}I, and uptake measurements are made at 24 hours, 48 hours, and 96 hours (1, 2, and 4 days). We have taken the liberty of plotting the results on semilog paper to determine the estimated uptake at time zero and the effective half-life. Three examples are given, two from the data of Berg et al. (34), because they represent extreme cases.

Example 1. (Fig. 5)

Uptakes of 43%, 27%, and 18% were found at 24, 48, and 96 hours. On single-cycle semilog paper, the horizontal axis represents days. The vertical axis ranges from 100% at the top to 10% at the bottom. A straight line (line 1) is drawn through the 48-hour (27%) and 24-hour (43%) uptake points and extended through time zero (0). A second line (line 2) is drawn through the 96-hour uptake (18%) and through the 24-hour (43%) point and extended through time zero (0). The estimated uptake at time zero is taken half way between the zero time intercepts of lines 1 and 2 and is found to be 64%. Taking 32 (half of 64) and projecting to the right horizontally from the vertical axis, the effective half-life at the intercept with line 1 is 1.5 days. Line 1 represents the average turnover rate during the first 48 hours. The slope of this line reflects the effective half-life for this period. It should be remembered that 50% of the total radiation dosage will be delivered during the first half-life. The second line represents the average turnover rate during the first 96 hours. In the ideal situation, this line should be identical to, and an extension of, line 1. Experience has shown that the turnover rate tends to slow with time. This is very likely caused by recirculation and recapture of iodine released from the thyroid during or after the initial phase of iodine uptake. This tends to give a longer effective half-life, which is reflected in the slope of line 2. This longer half-life is compensated for by a reduction in estimated uptake at time zero. If line 2 is used for effec-

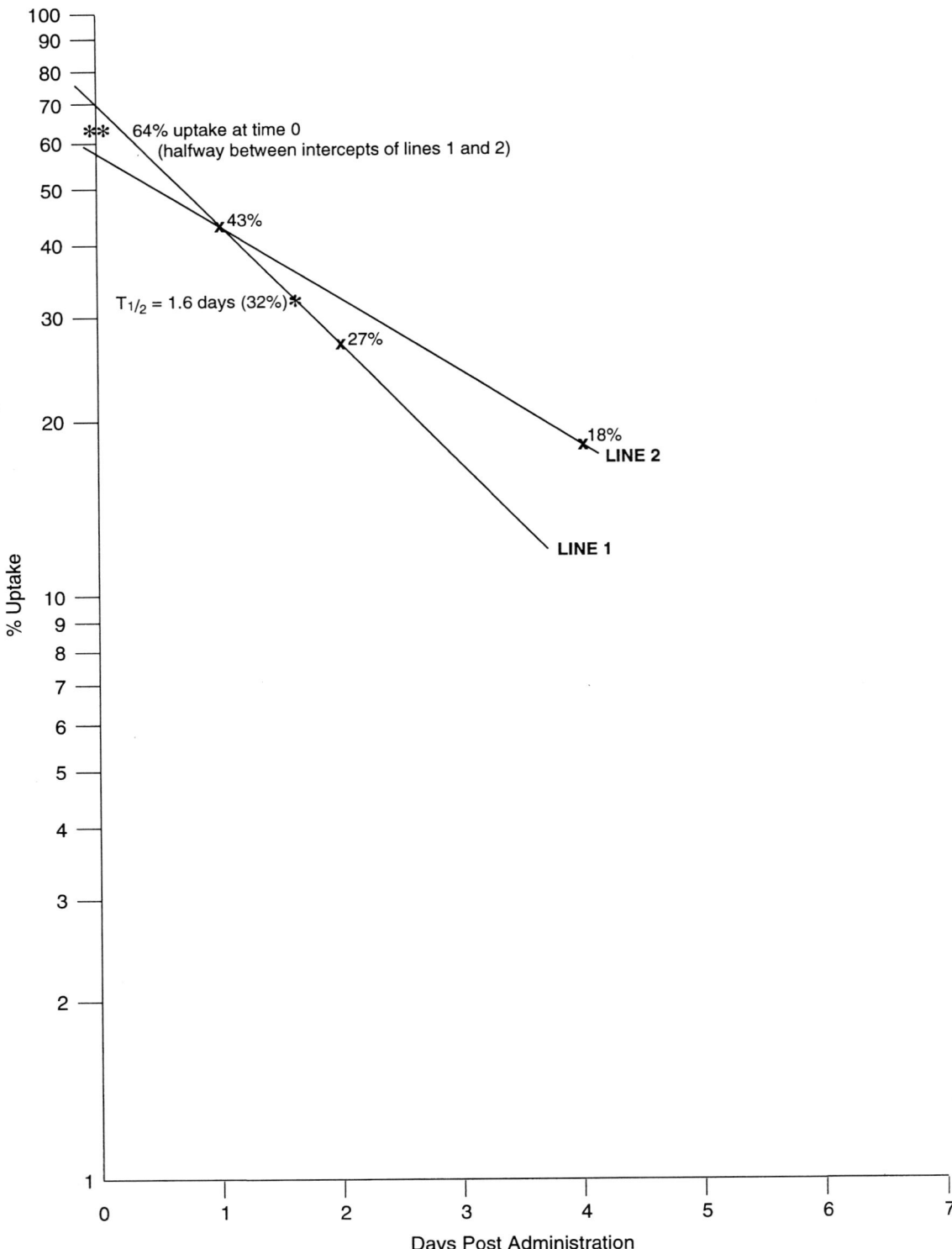

FIG. 5. Example of a patient with an average radioiodine uptake and an elevated rate of iodine turnover.

tive half-life calculation, effective half-life is extended to 2.4 days. Because 50% of the radiation dose is delivered during the first half-life, the effective half-life during the first 24- to 48-hour period is most relevant to calculations. The longer the radioiodine remains in the thyroid, the less will be needed to achieve a given radiation dosage. Whereas the 24-hour uptake is a measured value, the estimated uptake at time zero depends not only on the 24-hour uptake, but also on the effective half-life. A shorter effective half-life ($T_{1/2}$ effective) results in a higher uptake at time zero, a higher turnover rate of iodine, and a higher dose of radioiodine needed for a therapeutic effect. A longer effective half-life results in a lower estimated uptake at time zero, a lower iodine turnover rate, and a lower dose of iodine needed for a therapeutic effect. There is in this manner of calculation an element of inherent compensating adjustment.

Example 2. (Fig. 6)

Uptakes of 34%, 41%, and 40% were found at 24, 48, and 96 hours. Here, the uptake is rising beyond 24 hours. In this case, a line is drawn from the 96-hour point (40%) through the 48-hour point (41%) and extended through time zero (42%). The 24-hour value (34%) is ignored. In all cases where the uptake is still increasing at 48 hours, the effective half-life is taken as 7.5 days. In this rare situation, the thyroid is in effect trapping iodine but not releasing it, and loss of radioactivity in the thyroid is essentially a result of physical decay of the ^{131}I, which has a half-life of 8.05 days.

Example 3. (Fig. 7)

Uptakes of 64%, 55%, and 44% were found at 24, 48, and 96 hours. If these points are plotted on semilog paper and lines are drawn, as described in Example 1, the results are that the uptake at time zero is 73%, and the effective half-life is 4.7 days.

The results of these three examples can now be compared by computing the dosage arrived at by equation (1) versus equation (2) for each example. All calculations are made for a 35-gram gland that is to be given a radiation dose of 100 Gy.

Example no.	Equation (1) [24-hour uptake, 5-day $T_{1/2}(e)$]	Equation (2) [uptake at time 0, calculated $T_{1/2}(e)$]
1	381 MBq (10.3 mCi)	800 MBq (21.6 mCi)
2	482 MBq (13.0 mCi)	260 MBq (7.0 mCi)
3	256 MBq (6.9 mCi)	239 MBq (6.5 mCi)

In Example 1, which is typical of Graves' disease, the equation with the 5-day half-life resulted in an underdosing of the patient by a factor of 2, compared to the equation with the calculated half-life. In Example 2, which is typical of toxic nodular goiter, the equation with the 5-day half-life resulted in an overdosing of the patient by a factor of almost 2, compared to the equation with the calculated effective half-life. In Example 3, which is typical of toxic diffuse goiter or Graves' disease, the equation with the 5-day half-life gave a result close to the equation with the calculated effective half-life.

A major source of error in calculating ^{131}I dosage for the thyroid comes from the variation in effective half-life, which may range from less than 2 days to almost 8 days, a factor of 4. This may contribute greater error to dosage calculation than volume estimations, which contribute an error factor in the range of 1.5. By using the absorbed-dose calculation system described here, error can be minimized and dosage can be optimized for the individual patient to provide effective treatment with a minimum of radiation exposure.

A more sophisticated approach using Bayesian analysis in a computer program to provide estimates for iodine dosage in Graves' disease has been formulated by Merlé et al. (43). Bayesian analysis was first used by Sheiner et al. (44) to obtain an optimal dosage regimen for digoxin. Since then, Bayesian analysis has been applied to dosage calculations for a large number of drugs, particularly those with narrow therapeutic ranges (45). Bayesian estimation is most useful in situations where multiple doses of medication are given over a long period of time, and where it is desirable to limit the number of blood samples needed to monitor pharmacokinetics. Merlé et al. (43) have formulated Bayesian algorithms for calculation of dosage required in a situation where only one dose is given, as is the case for radioiodine.

The objective of Bayesian analysis is to increase the reliability of measurements made on a given variable over a period of time. If the reliability of the readings is increased, then the number of readings required to reach a certain level of accuracy may be decreased. Supplementary information is used to increase the reliability of determinations made on a given variable. Supplementary information may include covariates or variables statistically related to the variable in question, and retrospective data on the population to which the variable in question belongs. In the case of radioiodine dosage to the thyroid, the major variable is the iodine turnover rate, which is estimated by one or more uptake measurements performed at specified times.

Merlé and associates (43) have devised a Bayesian program for radioiodine kinetics that runs on a Macintosh II-SI (Apple Computer Inc.) with a mathematical co-processor. The program requires 2.5 megabytes (Mb) of available memory. The major variable used is the uptake study. Two external thyroid counts are performed at 2 hours and 168 hours after a test dose of radioiodine. Co-variables include the patient's body weight, height, age, and thyroid weight. There is no clear statistical relationship between any of the covariables and the thyroid uptake. Information is also obtained from a retrospective data file on 100 patients. This program appears to be re-

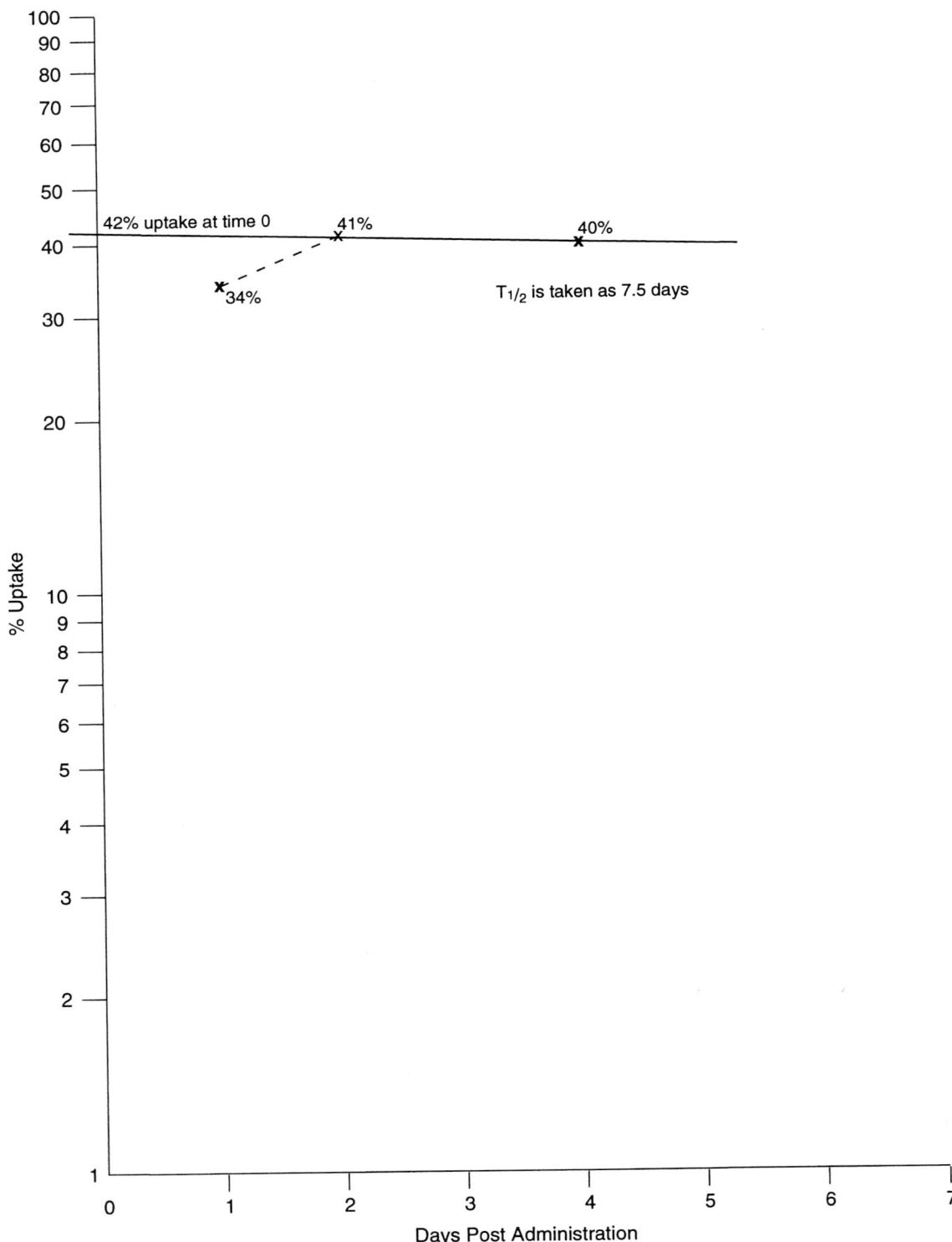

FIG. 6. Example of a patient with a low radioiodine uptake and a slow iodine turnover. In cases where the uptake level is still rising after 48 hours, the effective half-life is taken as 7.5 days.

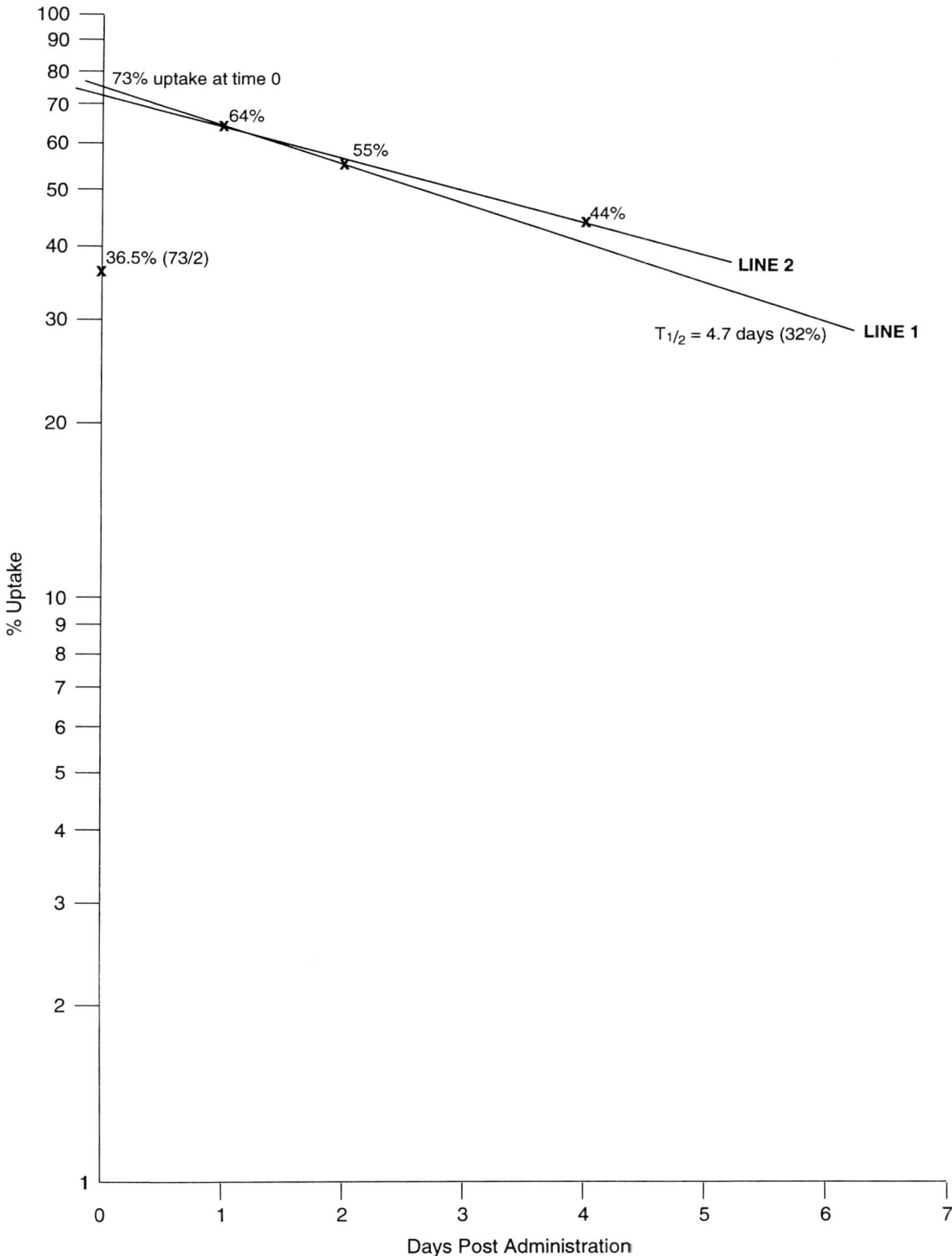

FIG. 7. Example of a patient with a high radioiodine uptake and a rapid iodine turnover. In rare instances, the uptake at time zero may extend above 100%. In this case, plot on the bottom half of two-cycle paper with 100% placed where the 10% line is shown in this graph. The next line up (now 20%) will become 200%. The lines extending downward will be 90%, 80%, and so on, to 10% at the bottom of the page. Divide the maximum uptake by 2 and find the effective half-life as usual.

stricted to patients with Graves' disease. If really relevant covariants can be found, this approach may become a desirable method.

METHODS

Every now and then someone reports that they have found the effective half-life for ^{131}I in a particular patient to be 10, 12, or more days. This signifies that some kind of mistake has been made in uptake measurement. The physical half-life of ^{131}I is 8.05 days. If iodine was collected in the thyroid and never released, the effective half-life would be identical to the physical half-life. Effective half-life can never be longer than the physical half-life. If a 24-hour uptake is used for a reference point as 100%, and the situation is such that maximum uptake peaks at some later time, then it may take longer than 8 days for the count rate to fall to half the 24-hour uptake. There are other pitfalls related to the instruments used for uptake measurement.

An uptake probe consists of a radiation detection crystal about 2 inches in diameter, in contact with an equivalent-sized photomultiplier tube. The sodium iodide detection crystal is transparent. When a photon of gamma radiation strikes the crystal, a flash of light is produced. The light strikes the photomultiplier tube, where the energy of the light flash is turned into an electrical impulse that is amplified and sent to a recording device. The light flash in the crystal is proportional in intensity to the energy of the gamma ray photon producing it, with the result that the amplified electrical impulse is proportional in amplitude to the energy of the gamma photon striking the crystal. The electronic system is usually equipped with a pulse height analyzer, which may be set for a specified photon energy (0.364 MeV for ^{131}I). Photons of other energies will be rejected and not counted. This reduces extraneous background count. It is best to set the pulse height analyzer before a study starts and then leave it alone. Any change in the pulse height analyzer setting will change the response of the system. If error is to be prevented, the response of the system must remain constant throughout the study. Before starting a study, put a weak sample of ^{131}I in front of the detector. Adjust the pulse height analyzer for maximal count rate and lock it. Uptake probes are equipped with flat field collimators that limit the probe's field of view to a region of interest such as the neck. A distance caliper is attached to the probe, so that a constant distance may be maintained between the source of radiation and the detecting crystal.

The thyroid uptake is performed with the aid of a neck phantom. In the United States, the most commonly used phantom is a lucite cylinder, 5 inches in diameter by 5 inches high, with an insert to hold a radioactive source to simulate the thyroid. The dimensions of this phantom are specified by the American National Standards Institute Standard N44.3. More anthropomorphic phantoms are provided by Radiology Support Devices of California and by Kyoto Kagaku Hyohon Company of Japan. Other standards for neck phantoms have been set forth by the International Council on Radiation Protection and by the Human Monitoring Laboratory in Canada. Kramer et al. (46) have compared these phantoms at short distances (12 cm or less) from neck to detector. There was considerable variation between phantoms at short distances. As neck-to-detector distance was increased, they found the difference between phantoms diminished to become insignificant at 30 cm.

The thyroid uptake is performed as follows. The radioiodine tracer dose (typically 0.2 MBq or 5.4 µCi of ^{131}I) as a capsule or liquid is placed in the neck phantom and counted for 1 or 2 minutes, at a distance of 20 to 30 cm between the surface of the phantom and the probe crystal. The count is recorded for reference, the tracer dose is removed from the phantom, and it is given to the patient. Twenty-four hours later, the uptake probe is placed over the patient's neck at the same distance as from the phantom and a count is made for the same period of time as for the phantom. A background count of 10 minutes is made in the room without any radioiodine present. (The background count is made to correct for cosmic rays from outer space or any traces of radioactive material in the environment.) The uptake is computed by the following formula:

$$^{131}\text{I uptake \%} = \frac{\left[\left(\frac{\text{patient neck count}}{\text{min}}\right) - \left(\frac{\text{background count}}{\text{min}}\right)\right] \cdot 100}{\left[\left(\frac{\text{phantom count}}{\text{min}}\right) \cdot 0.917\right] - \left(\frac{\text{background count}}{\text{min}}\right)}$$

The factor 0.917 corrects for 24 hours of physical decay of the ^{131}I. Another method is to set aside a sample of ^{131}I equivalent to the dose given to the patient. Twenty-four hours after administration, the patient and the reference sample are both counted. In this case, multiplication of the phantom count by the 0.917 decay factor is eliminated.

If the probe is placed close to the neck, particularly if a long-bore collimator is used, it may not cover the entire thyroid gland and a false low reading may be obtained. Also, any mistake in distance between the thyroid gland and the probe crystal will cause a significant error. Radiation intensity at the detector tends to vary inversely as the square of the distance between the detector and a small source. In theory, the inverse square law applies to a point source. In practice, a source is considered to approximate a point source when the distance between the source and the detector is at least 5 times the greatest dimension of the source. The inverse square equation works as follows:

$$I_2 = \frac{(D_1)^2}{(D_2)^2} \cdot I_1$$

I_1 is intensity at reference distance D_1. If the distance is changed to D_2, the intensity will be changed to I_2. For the purpose of demonstration, let us pick a very short distance of 10 cm (D_1) between source and detector. Let $I_1 = 100$. If the distance is now changed to 9 cm (D_2), we find I_2 to be $I_2 = (10)^2/(9)^2 \times 100 = 123.4$, a change of +23.4%. Now consider the situation where the change is from 10 to 11 cm: $I_2 = (10)^2/(11)^2 \times 100 = 82.6$, a change of −17.4%. If the reference distance is now changed to 30 cm, we find an increase to 31 cm causes a reduction in intensity of 6.3%. A decrease from 30 cm to 29 cm introduces an increase in intensity of +7%. Thus the error introduced by a change of 1 cm in distance is much less at a 30-cm source-to-detector distance than at a 10-cm source-to-detector distance.

Figure 8 is an example of good counting geometry. The region to be counted should not extend into the penumbra. The longer the collimator, the smaller the penumbra region will be. The smaller the penumbra, the better, because less background radiation will be included. In general, the longer the distance between the source and the detector, the less will be the error introduced by any discrepancy in the source-to-detector distance.

The scintillation detector is an event counter that counts nuclear disintegrations, one at a time, by responding to each one individually. A photon of radiation from a disin-

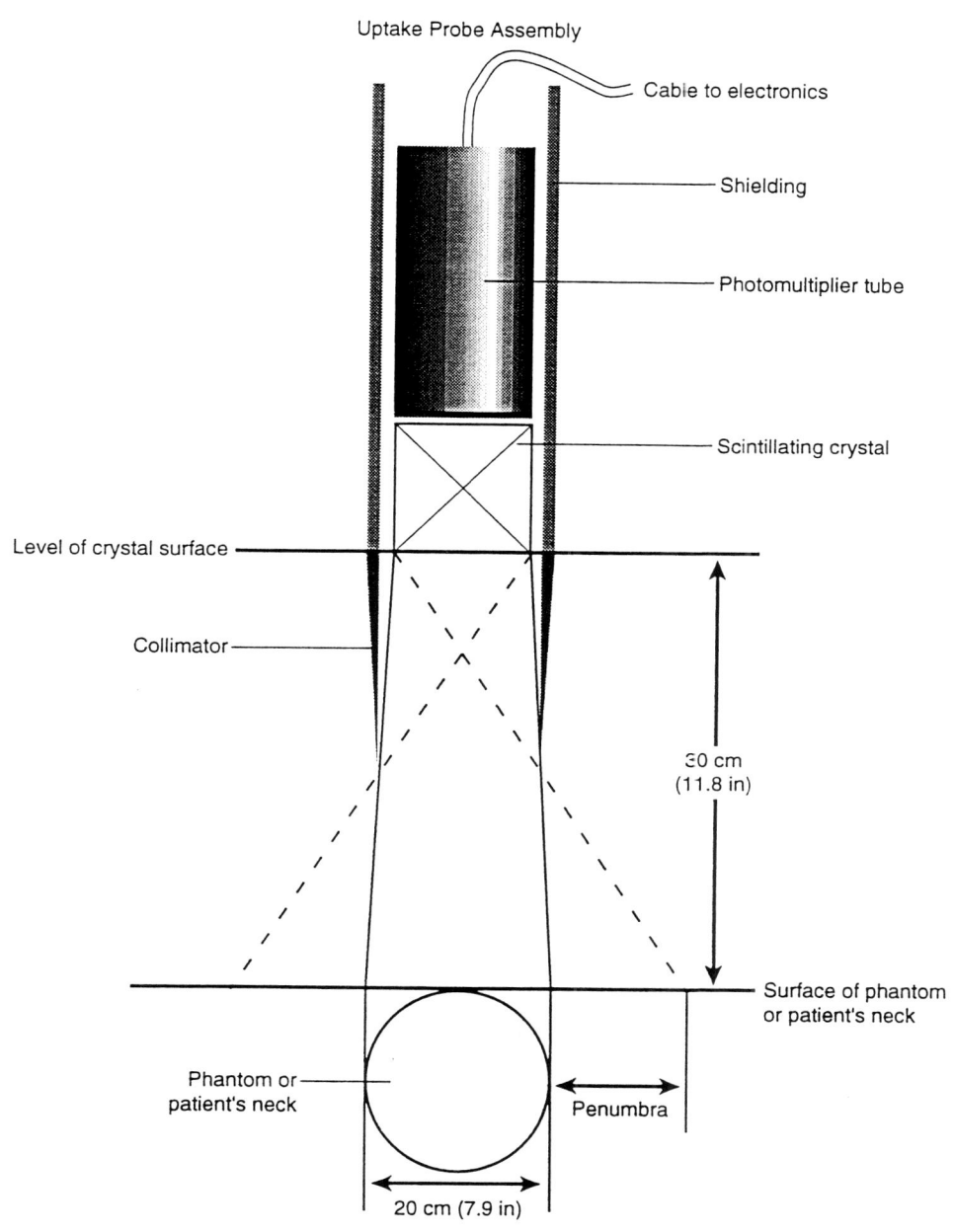

FIG. 8. Schematic diagram of a thyroid uptake probe (not to scale). Dimensions for good counting geometry are indicated. The region to be counted should not extend into the penumbra. The longer the collimator, the smaller the penumbra will be. The smaller the penumbra, the better, because less background radiation will be included.

tegrating atom strikes the detecting crystal, which starts a chain of events resulting in the number 1 being added to the reading on the recording device. During the time from when the photon strikes the crystal until the number is moved up on the recording device, the system cannot accept another event. This period is known as resolving time or, more descriptively, dead time (47). Any counts that occur during this period are missed and not recorded. Dead times may range from 1 μsec to 100 μsec. Dead-time losses may become significant for single-crystal detectors with long dead times and count rates as low as 1000 counts per second. A chart to correct for dead-time losses may be constructed by placing a small strong source at a long distance from the detector and then decreasing the distance. Readings are taken at points along the way as the source-to-detector distance is decreased. The starting point should be far enough away so that the count rate is not more than 500 counts per second. The true count rate at different distances may be calculated from the inverse square law (see preceding equation). Counts up to 500/sec may be taken as true counts, because dead-time loss at this counting rate should be negligible. The percent correction, C, needed may be calculated by

$$C = 100 \cdot \frac{(R_{true} - R_{observed})}{R_{observed}}$$

For example, for a true reading of +5000 counts/sec and an observed reading of 4500 counts/sec,

$$\frac{5000 - 4500}{4500} \cdot 100 = 11.1\%.$$

Correction factors higher than 20% should not be used. In cases where corrections larger than 20% are indicated, the amount of radioactivity in the test should be reduced to a range that the uptake counter can handle in a satisfactory manner.

Radioactive disintegration is a random process. The only prediction we can make about a given atom is that it will have a 50% chance of disintegrating during the next half-life. Even in a small amount of radioactive material, there are millions of atoms, and statistical predictions approach certainty when large numbers of events are involved. The precision in any measurement of radioactivity depends on the number of disintegrations counted. The relation between number of disintegrations counted and precision is given the by Poisson distribution: the standard deviation is proportional to the square root of the number of events observed. The standard deviation (s) is a measure of the error in the determination of a number of counts (N), and the relationship is $s = \sqrt{N}$. For example, if N is 900 counts, $s = \sqrt{900} = 30$. The value of N is then expressed as $N \pm s$. Nine hundred counts would be expressed as 900 ± 30, or $900 \pm 3\%$ to one standard deviation. This means that if this measurement were made many times, 68% of the time the result would fall within ±3.3%. Ninety-five percent of the time, the result would fall within two standard deviations, ±60 counts or ±6.6%, and 99.7% of the time, the result would be within ±90 counts or ±10%. Precision may be improved by increasing the number of counts, usually accomplished by counting for a longer period of time. To achieve a ±3% precision at a 99.7 confidence level requires 10,000 counts. A precision of ±6% will be obtained with 4444 counts. At the 99.7 confidence level, 370 out of 371 observations will be within limits. The number of counts needed to reach a certain precision at various confidence levels may be computed as follows, where N = number of counts and P = % variation.

1. Low precision: 2 out of 3 observations do not exceed P

$$N = \frac{10{,}000}{P^2}$$

2. Medium precision: 20 out of 21 observations do not exceed P at the 95% confidence level

$$N = \frac{40{,}000}{P^2}$$

3. High precision: 370 out of 371 observations do not exceed P at the 99.7% confidence level

$$N = \frac{90{,}000}{P^2}$$

Iodine-123 (^{123}I) has been used in some institutions for uptake studies to obtain better counting statistics with less radiation exposure to the patient (40,48). ^{123}I decays by electron capture, a process where a nuclear proton turns into a neutron by capturing an electron from an orbit outside of the nucleus. ^{123}I has a short half-life of 13.2 hours and emits no beta particles, so radiation dose to the patient is much reduced compared to ^{131}I, even though a larger amount of radioactivity is given in terms of disintegrations per second. Typically, 7.4 MBq (200 μCi) of ^{123}I is given for an uptake study.

Lee et al. (48) tested two commercial thyroid uptake probes (make and model not stated) and found a 10% dead-time loss at 1.85 MBq (50 μCi) and a 60% dead-time loss at 7.4 MBq (200 μCi) of ^{123}I when counted at a distance of 20 cm. They proposed doing uptake studies with a gamma camera to avoid dead-time error associated with probes. It should be noted that an uncorrected significant dead-time loss will result in an uptake value that is higher than the true reading, and the error may be quite large. Robeson and Margouleff (49) have tested a Nuclear Data model 62 probe and found it to demonstrate no significant dead-time loss when subjected to 4.44 MBq (120 μCi) of ^{123}I activity at a distance of 30 cm. The associated count rate was almost 5000 counts per second. It is reasonable to suspect that older probes may have longer dead times than newer models. In any case, probe linearity should be checked if a change is made from ^{131}I to ^{123}I for diagnostic studies.

Do not use effective half-life values determined with ^{123}I, for ^{131}I dosage calculation. If effective half-life is determined with ^{123}I, then dosage calculations for ^{131}I must be made as follows:

1. The biologic half-life must be determined from the measured effective half-life and the physical half-life of ^{123}I (13.2 hr).
2. Using the biologic half-life as shown and the physical half-life for ^{131}I, a new effective half-life is calculated for use with ^{131}I.

The use of ^{123}I studies to determine dosage for ^{131}I is subject to error and is not recommended.

RADIATION SAFETY

In general, the rules for safe transport, storage, and use of radioactive materials are provided as statutory regulations from the Nuclear Regulatory Commission or the state agency controlling the licensing of users. Additional rules may be set down by the facility's radiation safety officer. The general rule is to keep radiation exposure to all persons as low as is reasonably achievable. For external exposure, the safety factors are time, distance, and shielding. Exposure is directly proportional to the time an individual is around a radiation source: minimize time. In general, exposure varies inversely as the square of the distance from the source: maximize distance, handle sources with long-handled tools, and so on. The effectiveness of shielding is specific to the source: select shielding. ^{131}I and ^{123}I should be contained in lead pots of sufficient thickness, and suitable shielding should be provided as needed. The half-value thickness for ^{131}I in lead is 2.4 mm. That is, 2.4 mm of lead will reduce the intensity of the radiation passing through it by 50%. The half-value thickness for ^{123}I in lead is 0.5 mm. The radiologist's lead apron and gloves provide little protection against the 0.364-MeV gamma rays of ^{131}I; however, they are reasonably effective against the 0.027-MeV and 0.159-MeV gamma rays from ^{123}I. Time and distance work equally well for all radionuclides. However, shielding is dependent on the characteristics of the radiation from a given radionuclide.

Great care should be used to avoid contamination of the skin with radioactive material, and even greater care should be used to prevent internal contamination by swallowing, breathing, or absorbing (i.e., through the skin) radioactive material. The actual technique of dealing with radiation safety problems is best understood by describing the methods used in handling extreme emergency situations.

Situation 1.
A number of people are in the waiting room for various reasons, including a woman who is to receive a 20-MCi (740-MBq) capsule of ^{131}I. The woman is called and given the capsule. Twenty minutes later, it is discovered that, because of a similarity in names, the capsule has been given to the wrong patient who has a problem unrelated to the thyroid. The first step is an immediate gastric lavage with the gastric contents being collected and handled as radioactive material. A 5-gallon plastic pail is ideal for gastric lavage. About 100 mg of sodium hydroxide (household lye) is added to the pail to give an alkaline pH. About 1 mL of a saturated solution of potassium iodide should also be added to the pail to dilute the radioiodine, and 2 or 3 mL of toluene or mineral oil should also be added to prevent surface evaporation. All tubing, syringes, rubber gloves, towels, and any other materials used should be collected in plastic bags, labeled, dated, and sent to the radioactive storage area for disposal by decay. The area and all persons concerned should be monitored for radioactive contamination and should be treated accordingly. The patient should be given 1 mL of Lugol's solution, to be followed by 1-mL doses three times a day for the next 3 days.

Lugol's solution contains 5% iodine and 10% potassium iodide. One milliliter contains about 130,000 µg of iodine, and 1 mCi of ^{131}I contains 0.0081 µg of iodine. Normal daily intake of iodine by the thyroid is in the vicinity of 150 µg. If 1 mCi of radioiodine is diluted with 1 mL of Lugol's solution, then the probability that the thyroid will pick up a nonradioactive atom is 130,000 to 0.0081. Less than one atom in over a million picked up will be radioactive. This shows why Lugol's solution should be part of the first-aid kit in every place where radioiodine is used. A 24-hour measurement of radioiodine uptake should be made on the patient's thyroid to determine just how much iodine reached the thyroid.

Situation 2.
A nervous, hyperthyroid woman who is very fearful of radiation reluctantly comes in for a 20-MCi (740-MBq) capsule of ^{131}I. A few minutes after swallowing the capsule, she vomits, contaminating the floor and various linens. Paper towels should be immediately dropped into the spill to confine it. The patient should be removed to an adjacent room, where she can be checked with a radiation survey meter. Any contaminated clothing should be removed for storage. Clothing removal should be done with the patient standing on a disposable plastic sheet or while seated in a chair covered with disposable plastic. Skin contamination is dealt with as described later. The area of floor contamination should be roped off and radiation warning signs should be posted. Clean-up is a two-person job. One person should handle the survey meter and act as a guard to prevent intrusion. The person doing the cleaning should not handle the radiation survey meter. If the radiation survey meter is even slightly contaminated, it instantly becomes useless and it is very hard to decontaminate. It may be wise to put a plastic bag over the survey meter to protect it. Contaminated linen, instruments, and other materials should be collected, placed

in plastic bags, dated, and labeled. Surfaces should be scrubbed with a detergent containing a complexing agent, such as dishwashing detergent to which 1 mL of a saturated solution of potassium iodide is added. Mild abrasives may be used on certain surfaces. Use a sponge and avoid the use of a scrub brush, as the latter tends to splatter. Rubber gloves, plastic shoe covers, a face shield or disposable mask, along with a cap and gown should be used to prevent personal contamination. Using a sponge, start at the edge of the spill and work inwards toward the center. All washings should be collected and treated in the same fashion as the stomach washings mentioned previously. Decontamination may be considered satisfactory when readings on the survey meter are no more than twice background. All of the bagged linens and collected waste material may be sent to the radioactive storage area for disposal by decay or for disposal as directed by the radiation safety officer.

Contamination on the skin should be removed by repeated washing with soap and water at a designated sink. In persistent cases, a 4% solution of potassium permanganate may be used, although this is rather irritating to the skin. Contamination on the hands may sometimes be reduced by sweating it out in a rubber glove. Eye contamination should be washed out with commercial eye wash or 0.9% normal saline. Hair may be washed with regular shampoo, but if contamination is persistent, the hair may have to be cut.

For disposal by decay, the time needed depends on the physical half-life of the element involved. After the passage of seven half-lives, decay will have reduced the radioactivity present by a factor of 100. After ten half-lives, the activity present will be reduced by a factor of 1000. For ^{131}I, these time periods are 60 days and 90 days, respectively. After 90 days of decay, the collected items may be checked for activity. If it is no more than twice background level, linens may be sent to the laundry for return to regular service. Gloves, sponges, paper towels, and other materials may be thrown in ordinary trash. Liquids may be dumped down any toilet.

A decontamination kit should be assembled and kept available for quick use. It is suggested that the listed items be stored in 5-gallon plastic buckets with compression lids. The buckets may be used to collect liquid contamination. The buckets should contain the following:

1. A Geiger counter survey meter
2. Protective clothing
   A. Box of shoe covers
   B. Box of disposable plastic or rubber gloves
   C. Box of disposable surgical caps
   D. Box of disposable face masks
   E. Three disposable gowns
   F. One plastic face shield or disposable mask
3. Red and yellow rope for restricting contaminated areas
4. Radiation warning signs, adhesive and nonadhesive
5. Three plastic sheets, of sufficient size to cover examination table
6. Roll of paper towels and box of paper tissues
7. Box of 30-gallon plastic garbage bags, box of smaller plastic bags, box of labels for bags and marking pen
8. Sponges with and without abrasive backing
9. Decontaminating wash or detergent with complexing agent
10. Mild abrasive cleaner [such as sodium lauryl sulfate (e.g., Soft Scrub)]
11. Bottle of saturated solution of potassium iodide
12. Small long-handled forceps
13. Bottle of 4% solution of potassium permanganate or 5% acetic acid

REFERENCES

1. Berson SA, Yalow RS. The iodine trapping and binding functions of the thyroid. *J Clin Invest* 1955;34:186–204.
2. Solomon B, Glinder D, Lagasse R, Wartofsky L. Current trends in the management of Graves' disease, *J Clin Endocrinol Metab* 1990;70: 1518–1524.
3. Becker DV. Choice of therapy for Graves' hyperthyroidism. *N Engl J Med* 1984;311:464–466.
4. Saenger EL, Thoma GE, Tompkins EA. Incidence of leukemia following treatment of hyperthyroidism. Preliminary report of the cooperative thyrotoxicosis therapy follow-up study. *JAMA* 1968;205:855–862.
5. Freitas JE, Swanson DP, Gross, MD, Sisson JC. Optimal therapy for hyperthyroidism in children and adolescents? *J Nucl Med* 1979;20: 847–850.
6. Bertelsen J, Herskind AM, Sprogoe Jakobsen U, Hegedus L. Is standard 555 MBq 131-I therapy of hyperthyroidism ablative? *Thyroidology* 1992;4(3):103–106.
7. Huysmans DA, Hermus AR, Corstens FH, Barentsz JO, Kloppenborg PW. Large compressive goiters treated with radioiodine. *Ann Intern Med* 1994;121:757–762.
8. Hamburger JI, Hamburger SW. Diagnosis and management of large toxic multinodular goiters. *J Nucl Med* 1985;26:888–892.
9. Nygaard B, Faber J, Hegedus L. Acute changes in thyroid volume and function following 131-I therapy of multinodular goitre. *Clin Endocrinol* 1994;41:715–718.
10. Falk S. In: *Thyroid disease: endocrinology, surgery, nuclear medicine, radiotherapy.* Falk S, ed. New York: Raven Press, 1990:251.
11. Nygard B, Hegedus L, Gervil M, Hjalgrim H, Hansen BM, Soe-Jensen P, Hansen JM. Influence of compensated radioiodine therapy of thyroid volume and incidence of hypothyroidism in Graves' disease. *J Intern Med* 1995;238:491–497.
12. Farrar JJ, Toft AD. Iodine-131 treatment of hyperthyroidism: current issues. *Clin Endocrinol* 1991;35:207–212.
13. Beierwaltes WH. In: *Thyroid disease: endocrinology, surgery, nuclear medicine, radiotherapy.* Falk S, ed. New York: Raven Press, 1990:237.
14. Ibid. p. 239.
15. Bazzi MM, Bagchi N. Adjunctive treatment with propylthiouracil or iodine following radioiodine therapy for Graves' disease. *Thyroid* 1993;3:269–272.
16. Franklyn JA, Daykin J, Holder R, Sheppard MC. Radioiodine therapy compared in patients with toxic nodular or Graves' hyperthyroidism. *Q J Med* 1995;88:175–180.
17. Flower MA, Al-Saadi A, Harmer CL, McCready VR, Ott RJ. Dose-response study on thyrotoxic patients undergoing positron emission tomography and radioiodine therapy. *Eur J Nucl Med* 1994;21:531–536.
18. Velkeniers B, Vanhaelst L, Cytryn R, Jonckheer MH. Treatment of hyperthyroidism with radioiodine: adjunctive therapy with antithyroid drugs reconsidered. *Lancet* 1988;1127–1129.
19. Robertson JS. In: *Thyroid disease: endocrinology, surgery, nuclear medicine, radiotherapy.* Falk S, ed. New York: Raven Press, 1990:54.
20. DeGroot L, Larsen, PR, Hennemann G. *The thyroid and its diseases*, 6th ed. New York: Churchill Livingstone. 1996;428.

21. Kabadi U, Cech R. Therapeutic 131-I dose in hyperthyroidism; role of pretreatment with thionamide. *Thyroidology* 1994;6:87–92.
22. DeGroot L, Larsen PR, Hennemann G. *The thyroid and its diseases*, 6th ed. New York: Churchill Livingstone. 1996:430.
23. DeGroot LJ. Therapeutic controversies, radiation and Graves' ophthalmopathy. *J Clin Endocrinol Metab* 1995;80:339–340.
24. Spencer RP, Seevers RH Jr., Friedman AM. *Radionuclides in therapy*. Boca Raton: CRC Press, 1987;10.
25. Ursu HI, Dumitriul L, Grigorie D, Simescu M, Vaida E, Belgun M, Popovic D. Effects of radioiodine therapy in hyperthyroidism. *Romanian J Endocr* 1993;31:155–163.
26. Tallstedt L, Lundell G, Blomgren H, Bring J. Does early administration of thyroxine reduce the development of Graves' ophthalmopathy after radioiodine treatment? *Eur J Endocr* 1994;130:494–497.
27. Bjarngard B. Radiation therapy and SI units. *Int J Radiat Oncol Biol Phys* 1981;7:283–285.
28. Szebeni A, Beleznay E. New simple method for thyroid volume determination by ultrasonography. *J Clin Ultrasound* 1992;20:329–337.
29. Rasmussen SN, Hjorth L. Determination of thyroid volume by ultrasonic scanning. *J Clin Ultrasound* 1974;2:143–147.
30. Flower M, Al-Saadi A, Harmer V, McCready R, Ott R. Dose-response study on thyrotoxic patients undergoing positron emission tomography and radioiodine therapy. *Eur J Nucl Med* 1994;21:531–536.
31. Bockisch A, Jamitzky T, Derwanz R, Biersack J. Optimized dose planning of radioiodine therapy of benign thyroidal diseases. *J Nucl Med* 1993;34:1632–1641.
32. Marinelli LD, Quimby EH, Hine GJ. Dosage determination with radioactive isotopes. *Am J Roentgenol* 1948;59:260–268.
33. Schmidt CE, Nadelhaft J. Effective half life of radioactive iodine (I-131) in the hyperthyroid gland. *Lab Invest* 1953;2:133–139.
34. Berg GEB, Annika MMK, Holmberg ECV, Fink M. Iodine-131 treatment of hyperthyroidism: significance of effective half-life measurements. *J Nucl Med* 1996;37:228–232.
35. Emrich D, Erlenmaier U, Pohl M, Luig H. Determination of the autonomously functioning volume of the thyroid. *Eur J Nucl Med* 1993;20:410–414.
36. Shapiro B. Optimization of radioiodine therapy of thyrotoxicosis: What have we learned after 50 years? *J Nucl Med* 1993;34:1638–1641.
37. Reinhardt M, Emrich D, Krause T, Brautigam P, Nitsche E, Blattman H, Schumichen C, Moser E. Improved dose concept for radioiodine therapy of multifocal and disseminated functional thyroid autonomy. *Eur J Endocrinol* 1995;132:550–556.
38. Peters H, Fischer C, Bogner U, Reiners C, Schleusener H. Reduction in thyroid volume after radioiodine therapy of Graves' hyperthyroidism: results of a prospective randomized, multicentre Study. *Eur J Clin Invest* 1996;26:59–63.
39. Huysmans DAKC, De Haas MM, Van Den Broek WJM, Hermus ARMM. Magnetic resonance imaging for volume estimation of large multinodular goiters: a comparison with scintigraphy. *Br J Radiol* 1994;67:519–523.
40. Vemulakonda US, Atkins FB. Ziessman HA. Therapy dose calculation in Graves' disease using early I-123 uptake measurements. *Clin Nucl Med* 1996;21:102–105.
41. Seed L, Jaffe B. Comparison of the tracer dose and the therapeutic dose of I-131 as to thyroid uptake, effective half-life and roentgen dosage. *Radiology* 1954;65:551–561.
42. Freedberg AS, Kurland GS, Chamovitz DL, Ureles AL. A critical analysis of the quantitative I-131 therapy of thyrotoxicosis. *J Clin Endocrinol Metab* 1952;12:86–111.
43. Merlé Y, Mentré F, Mallet A, Aurengo A. Computer-assisted individual estimation of radioiodine thyroid uptake in Graves' disease. *Comput Methods Programs Biomed* 1993;40:33–41.
44. Sheiner LB, Rosenberg B, Melmon KL. Modelling of individual pharmacokinetics for computer-aided drug dosage. *Comput Biomed Res* 1972;5:441–459.
45. Thomson AH, Whiting B. Bayesian parameter estimation and population pharmacokinetics. *Clin Pharmacokinet* 1992;22:447–467.
46. Kramer GH, Olender G, Valahovich S, Hauck BM, Meyerhof DP. Comparison of the Ansi, RSD, KKH and BRMD thyroid neck phantoms for 125-I thyroid monitoring. *Health Phys* 1996;70:425–429.
47. Simpkin DJ. The effect of counting system deadtime on thyroid uptake measurements. *Med Phys* 1984;11:296–299.
48. Lee KH, Siegel ME, Fernandez OA. Discrepancies in thyroid uptake values use of commercial thyroid probe systems versus scintillation cameras. *Clin Nucl Med* 1995;20:199–202.
49. Robeson W, Margouleff D. Letter to the Editor Re: Dead Time Loss in Probes. *Clin Nucl Med* 1996;21:268–269.

CHAPTER 17

Surgical Treatment of Hyperthyroidism

Stephen A. Falk

Although most patients with hyperthyroidism are treated medically or with iodine-131 (^{131}I), surgery still has an important role. This chapter offers an in-depth look at practical and theoretical aspects of surgery for hyperthyroidism.

The chapter begins with a review of the pathogenesis and classification of hyperthyroidism, which puts into perspective the role of the surgeon in the treatment of hyperthyroidism. An important principle of this chapter is that the surgeon who understands the many aspects of hyperthyroidism in addition to having technical expertise during thyroidectomy will have maximal effectiveness in treating hyperthyroidism. These aspects are the pathogenesis of Graves' disease, toxic multinodular goiter, and toxic solitary nodule; the advantages and disadvantages of treatment options; the preoperative preparation of the patient; the extent of thyroid surgery (i.e., the size of the thyroid remnant); ways to reduce risks of thyroid surgery; and postoperative care and follow-up.

Since publication of the first edition of *Thyroid Disease* in 1990, several important advances have occurred, and these are included in the present text. New studies have clarified the incidence and prognosis of thyroid cancer in patients with Graves' disease. New and unusual indications for surgery for hyperthyroidism have been described, including thyroid storm unresponsive to medical therapy and amiodarone-induced thyrotoxicosis. A thorough review of the literature is presented as it relates to the question of whether surgery controls progression of thyroid-associated ophthalmopathy. New methods are reviewed to prepare the hyperthyroid patient for surgery; however, the older methods are still reliable and most often used.

S. A. Falk: Department of Surgery, University of Rochester School of Medicine and Dentistry, Rochester, New York 14610.

PATHOGENESIS AND CLASSIFICATION

Understanding the pathogenesis and classification of thyrotoxicosis will help clarify the role of surgery in treatment (1) (see also Chapter 14). Clinically, thyrotoxicosis is suspected in patients who present with one or more of its signs and symptoms, and it is confirmed by obtaining an elevated level of serum thyroxine (T_4) and/or triiodothyronine (T_3). As part of the evaluation, thyroid stimulating hormone (TSH) is also determined, and a thyroid scan and uptake, performed with one of the radioactive iodine preparations [most commonly, iodine-123 (^{123}I)], is obtained. The result of the thyroid uptake governs the differential diagnosis of thyrotoxicosis. Diseases can be classified into those characterized by increased radioactive iodine uptake by the thyroid gland and those characterized by decreased uptake.

Thyrotoxicosis with Hyperthyroidism (Increased Radioactive Iodine Uptake) Versus Thyrotoxicosis without Hyperthyroidism (Decreased Uptake)

Although the terms *hyperthyroidism* and *thyrotoxicosis* are often used synonymously, they are different. Diseases producing thyrotoxicosis (elevation of serum T_4 and/or T_3) fall into two groups—thyrotoxicosis with hyperthyroidism, and thyrotoxicosis without hyperthyroidism. Hyperthyroidism is defined as sustained thyroid hyperfunction, and diseases that produce hyperthyroidism are accompanied by an increased radioactive iodine uptake. Hyperthyroidism can be caused by the following:

A. Thyroid-stimulating immunoglobulins (TSI)
   1. Graves' disease
   2. Neonatal hyperthyroidism (occurs secondary to the transplacental passage of maternal TSI)
B. Autonomous (independent of TSH control) nodule or nodules in the thyroid gland (toxic solitary nodule,

toxic multinodular goiter). In A and B, the pituitary gland is normal and responds appropriately to elevated levels of T_4 and/or T_3 according to feedback inhibition. Serum TSH is absent or low.

C. Excessive secretion of pituitary thyrotropin, either with or without a pituitary tumor. Pituitary tumors secrete TSH in a manner not responsive to feedback inhibition. Despite elevated levels of T_4 and/or T_3, the tumor still secretes TSH, causing elevation of serum TSH levels. If there is no pituitary tumor, selective pituitary resistance to thyroid hormone may exist. The high level of serum TSH distinguishes C from A and B, where serum TSH level is low or absent.

D. Secretion of nonpituitary thyrotropin originating from:
  1. Trophoblastic tissues
    a. Choriocarcinoma, hydatidiform mole, embryonal carcinoma of testis. These rare tumors secrete large amounts of human chorionic gonadotrophin (HCG), which is structurally similar to TSH. HCG binds to TSH receptors on thyroid follicular cells, causing high iodine uptake and hyperthyroidism.
    b. Hyperthyroidism associated with hyperemesis gravidarum. HCG stimulates the TSH receptor.
  2. Ectopic locations (lung, gastrointestinal, prostatic, breast)

Some diseases producing thyrotoxicosis do not produce hyperthyroidism. These diseases are accompanied by a decreased radioactive iodine uptake by the thyroid gland. Thyrotoxicosis without hyperthyroidism can be caused by:

A. Excessive exogenous iodide (Jod-Basedow disease). Excess iodide from expectorants, amiodarone, radiographic contrast media, and topical antiseptics can cause thyrotoxicosis, especially in patients with multinodular goiter. The precise mechanism of thyrotoxicosis is unknown. Possibly, these patients have subclinical thyrotoxicosis and when given the substrate of iodine, their glands form excessive thyroid hormone. Since the body contains a large amount of iodine and the thyroid is saturated with iodine, a trace dose of radioactive iodine is taken up poorly by the gland, so uptake is low.

B. Ectopic secretion of thyroid hormone from:
  1. Functioning metastatic thyroid carcinoma. This is rare and may occur many years after thyroidectomy for the original carcinoma. It presents with the typical symptoms and signs of thyrotoxicosis, without the ophthalmopathy of Graves' disease. The pathology is usually follicular carcinoma. The carcinoma autonomously produces excessive levels of T_4 and/or T_3 independent of levels of serum TSH, T_4, and/or T_3. The pituitary gland is normal and responds appropriately to elevated levels of T_4 and/or T_3 according to feedback inhibition. Serum TSH is absent or low, and radioactive iodine uptake is low in the thyroid (if it is still present). Uptake may be high in the metastases. Because the carcinoma synthesizes thyroid hormone less efficiently than normal thyroid tissue, thyrotoxicosis occurs in patients with disseminated and large metastatic deposits.
  2. Struma ovarii. This is another extremely rare cause of thyrotoxicosis. A dermoid tumor or benign or malignant teratoma of the ovary contains ectopic, metabolically active thyroid tissue. Thyrotoxicosis occurs in only 5% to 10% of dermoids and teratomas that contain thyroid tissue. Struma ovarii presents with ascites, palpable ovarian mass, and, often, multinodular thyroid gland. Excessive T_4 and/or T_3 is produced by ovarian mass and often by the thyroid. If only ovarian mass produces excessive hormone, T_4 and/or T_3 suppresses TSH, resulting in low uptake of radioactive iodine by thyroid gland and high uptake by the mass. If both the ovarian mass and the thyroid gland produce excessive hormone, uptake is high in both locations.

C. Disruption of thyroid cell membranes with release of stored hormones.
  1. Subacute thyroiditis (de Quervain's, giant cell). This presents as acute, tender, and enlarged thyroid gland with fever, malaise, and other systemic signs. Viral infection disrupts follicular cells, releasing stores of thyroid hormone into the circulation, causing thyrotoxicosis. Inflammation prevents synthesis of T_4, so iodine uptake is low. Thyrotoxicosis occurs early in the disease and lasts as long as 9 weeks; it is followed by transient hypothyroidism (2 to 7 months), then by euthyroidism.
  2. Hashimoto's (lymphocytic) thyroiditis. This can present as an acutely enlarged, firm, and nonpainful gland with mild thyrotoxicosis (Hashitoxicosis). The thyrotoxicosis is self-limited and spontaneously resolves over weeks or months. Because of cell damage, iodine uptake is low and there are high titers of antithyroglobulin and antimicrosomal antibodies. Later in the course of Hashimoto's thyroiditis, thyroid status may become euthyroid or hypothyroid. Hypothyroidism causes elevated TSH, which produces goiter.

D. Exogenous thyroid hormone (factitious and medicamentosa). This can be distinguished from other etiologies that produce low iodine uptake by history and physical findings. If T_3 is overused, only serum T_3 will be elevated. If T_4 is overused, both serum T_4 and T_3 will be elevated. TSH is suppressed, causing a small thyroid with low radioactive iodine uptake. If the patient does not have underlying thyroid disease, serum thyroglobulin levels, which respond to TSH, will be normal or low. However, if the patient has any underlying thyroid disease or takes desiccated thyroid, thyroglobulin levels can be elevated. Therefore, a normal or low thyroglobulin level and thyrotoxicosis strongly point to an exogenous source; however, an elevated thyroglobulin level is not helpful in establishing this diagnosis.

By understanding the various diseases that produce thyrotoxicosis and hyperthyroidism, the surgeon can recognize unusual presentations of thyrotoxicosis that may be secondary to nonsurgical diseases. By understanding the pathophysiology of thyrotoxicosis and hyperthyroidism, the surgeon will better understand the results of thyroid scans and serum tests of thyroid function.

The role of the surgeon in the treatment of thyrotoxicosis and hyperthyroidism is to appreciate the differences among the multiple causes, and to know when surgery is warranted. Surgery of the thyroid gland for hyperthyroidism is indicated only in Graves' disease, toxic multinodular goiter, and toxic solitary nodule. Graves' disease accounts for 70% to 85% of all cases. The next most common cause is thyroiditis (5% to 25% of cases), in which ablative therapy with either surgery or radioactive iodine is contraindicated because the thyrotoxicosis is self-limited. Even thionamide drugs are not indicated in thyroiditis, because there is no excessive synthesis of thyroid hormone, just excessive release of hormone into the circulation. After Graves' disease and thyroiditis, in decreasing order of frequency, occur toxic solitary nodule (3% to 30%), toxic multinodular goiter (5% to 15%), and excessive exogenous iodide. All the other causes of thyrotoxicosis are rare. These diseases will be considered separately. The reader will refer to sources in neurosurgery (pituitary tumor), gynecology [trophoblastic tumors e.g., choriocarcinoma, hydatidiform mole, struma ovarii), and other disciplines (ectopic thyrotropin secreted by lung, gastrointestinal, prostatic, and breast malignancies) to complete a full review of surgery for thyrotoxicosis as seen in these rare diseases.

THE COMPLEMENTARY ROLE OF TREATMENT OPTIONS

Treatment of hyperthyroidism consists of medical therapy (thionamide drugs, iodine, and beta-blocking agents), ^{131}I, and surgery. All three treatments are safe and successful, and the clinician can consider their roles as complementary, and not conflicting, for patient benefit. Medical treatment is always used in conjunction with surgery for hyperthyroidism in order to prevent thyroid storm. Also, very often, medical treatment is used in conjunction with ^{131}I. One must consider the patient's age, gender, desire to have children, underlying medical diseases, and the personal philosophies of both the patient and physician to arrive at the most appropriate therapy (1).

When considering surgery as a treatment alternative for hyperthyroidism, the physician and patient should also consider the relative merits and disadvantages of ^{131}I treatment or prolonged administration of thionamides (also see Chapters 15 and 16). In addition to the three standard treatments, a novel approach was recently reported (2): successful treatment was accomplished in all 32 patients with Graves' disease by embolization of the thyroid gland through selective catheterization of thyroid arteries.

Before making a decision on treatment, the patient visits the internist or endocrinologist, the surgeon, and the nuclear medicine specialist. The patient hears the options together with the spoken and unspoken biases of the physicians. Because all three treatments are safe and successful, we have the luxury of choosing the best option based on patient needs. Although frequently performing thyroidectomy for hyperthyroidism, I also work closely in the management of patients who choose thionamides or ^{131}I treatment. I discuss in an objective manner the details of each treatment option. Patients are often pleasantly surprised and favorably impressed at this approach coming from the surgeon. I describe optimistically to my patients the alternatives available. Through this process, patients who choose surgery almost always are well informed and confident; their postoperative outcome is perceived as more satisfactory.

GRAVES' DISEASE

Benefits of Surgery

Surgery Is Rapid Treatment

Medical preparation for thyroidectomy (see later) can be accomplished within 6 weeks, in most cases, with thionamide therapy, and within 1 week with beta-blocking agents. When the surgery is followed by a 2- to 3-week period of recuperation (2 to 3 days of hospitalization), the patient has an excellent chance of completing the entire surgical experience within 3 to 9 weeks. Surgery offers permanent cure in the great majority of patients. With thionamide therapy, euthyroidism is also achieved rapidly, but this therapy must continue for at least 6 to 12 months, with frequent doctor visits and blood tests. Also, this treatment does not usually result in permanent correction of hyperthyroidism because of high relapse rate (see later). With ^{131}I, treatment is somewhat less rapid than that provided by surgery, because several months are needed before the hyperthyroidism is controlled.

Surgery Is Highly Safe

Probably the main hesitancy in recommending surgery is based on the risk of vocal cord paralysis and hypoparathyroidism (as discussed in Chapters 38 and 39, respectively). In numerous large series, these risks are small. Permanent vocal cord paralysis has been reported to occur in 0% (3), 0.4% (4), 0.5% (5), 0.6% (6), 1% (7),

2.1% (8), 2.2% (9), and 3.4% (10) of cases. Permanent hypoparathyroidism occurs in 0% (11–15), 0.4% (8), 0.6% (3,5), 0.8% (16), 1% (7,17), 1.3% (18), 1.5% (19), 1.9% (10), and 2.8% (20) of cases.

The major risks in prolonged thionamide therapy are also small (0.5% incidence of agranulocytosis per course of treatment). The risks of ^{131}I in terms of deleterious genetic, carcinogenic, teratogenic, and reproductive effects are only theoretical, and, after quite extensive study for over 40 years, they have not been demonstrated in adults or (especially) in children (21–23) (see Chapter 16). However, aggressive thyroid cancers have occurred after ^{131}I treatment, albeit rarely; a causal relationship has not been established (24,25).

Patients possess a healthy skepticism when presented with the good safety record of ^{131}I. Physicians are aware of the inherent difficulties in long-term follow-up studies of patients treated with ^{131}I. In addition, there is an established association between low-dose, low-energy external radiation to the thyroid and increased incidence of malignant and benign tumors of the thyroid and salivary glands (26): radiation was given to the thymus, tonsils, and adenoids and for acne, tinea, hemangioma, and cervical lymphadenitis. After a latent period of 20 to 30 years, thyroid tumors developed. The incidence of neoplasia increased linearly from a dose as low as 6.5 rads to 1500 rads. The incidence of thyroid carcinoma is 2% to 9% of all radiated persons, whereas the incidence of benign thyroid nodules is 9%. The difference between low-dose, low-energy external radiation therapy and ^{131}I (6000 to 10,000 rads) or high-dose, high-energy external radiation, used in the treatment of head and neck squamous cell cancer, is that high-energy external radiation ablates thyroid cells, whereas low-dose, low-energy external radiation may alter them to become neoplastic.

Although we present these explanations to patients, they often remain unconvinced of the completely benign role of ^{131}I. The length of follow-up information in ^{131}I-treated children is still short in comparison to their expected life span. Ideally, several generations should be studied for all adverse effects to be detected. Patients extrapolate from the disasters and attempted cover-ups at nuclear power plants at Three Mile Island and Chernobyl. Skepticism ensues from the reports of deteriorated and dangerous conditions at the Department of Energy nuclear power plants that manufactured plutonium for nuclear weapons despite previously repeated official statements that these plants are safe. It is little wonder that despite our reassurances regarding the known safety of ^{131}I, some patients will not accept this treatment.

The occurrence of hypothyroidism after treatment with ^{131}I and surgery is discussed at length in the literature (there are hundreds of articles addressing this topic). In clinical practice, I believe it is only a minor consideration in deciding on treatment, since hypothyroidism is easily diagnosed and treated. Nevertheless, there is the rare patient who insidiously slips into myxedema. Permanent hypothyroidism does not occur as a consequence of thionamide treatment. Hypothyroidism occurs frequently after both ^{131}I and surgery but more frequently after ^{131}I than after surgery. After ^{131}I, it occurs in 50% to 80% of cases [70% (27), 47.6% (28)]. After surgery, it occurs in 75% (29), 59.2% (15), 58% (30), 51% (31), 48.7%, 31% (8,9), 30% (32–34), 26.5% (10), 24% (14), 21% (3,35), 19% (36), 14% (37), 8.2% (19), and 5.8% (38) of cases.

Surgery Is Highly Successful

Surgery for Graves' disease reliably provides a cure with only a small chance of recurrent hyperthyroidism. Large series of thyroidectomy for Graves' disease show an incidence of recurrent hyperthyroidism in 9.8% (19), 7.7% (38), 7.5% (3), 6% (37), 4% (8), 3.2% (32,39), 2.6%, 1.2% (15), 1% (29), and 0.7% (9) of cases. Generally, a similar situation exists after treatment with ^{131}I, with the chance of recurrence depending on the dose of ^{131}I selected.

The small chance of recurrent hyperthyroidism after surgery is secondary to more than just the removal of the gland. Elevated preoperative levels of thyrotropin receptor antibody (also called thyroid-stimulating immunoglobulin, the mediator of thyroid stimulation in Graves' disease) became normal in 86% of Graves' disease patients after total thyroidectomy. Before surgery, thionamide therapy for at least 9 months failed to lower these levels. Therefore, the thyroid is an antigen that stimulates the production of thyrotropin receptor antibodies; thyroidectomy provided favorable immunosuppression for Graves' disease (13).

However, there is a high incidence of relapse after thionamides are withdrawn (see Chapter 15). For example, in one study (36), after 1 full year of treatment with carbimazole, the incidence of recurrent hyperthyroidism was 43% in the first year after completion of treatment. Subsequently, in years 2 through 5, 21%, 21%, 18%, and 13% of those remaining euthyroid at the start of each year relapsed. After 5 years, only 26% of patients remained euthyroid, with 74% relapsing. Other studies have confirmed a long-lasting remission in no more than 25% of unselected patients (40,41). Long-term remission ranges from 14% to 80% (42). Selection of patients has been attempted, to obtain a higher remission rate. The remission rate is 76% in patients with no goiter or a small goiter, but 37% in those with medium or large goiters (43). Relapse tends to occur in patients with high T_3 levels (44), high T_3/T_4 ratios (44), large goiter (43), greater clinical symptoms, certain human leukocyte antigen types (45), elevated levels of TSIs at the end of medical treatment (46–48), and elevated levels of antithyroid antibodies in children and young adults, but the predictive value of these characteristics is too inconsistent for clinical usefulness (40). Combined treatment for 1 year with T_4 and methimazole resulted in a significantly lower relapse rate and lower levels of TSIs than obtained with methimazole alone (49).

The success of ^{131}I and surgery in curing hyperthyroidism is a result of ablative therapy. Thionamides usually provide reversible treatment that can be looked upon as advantageous—there is the chance that a treatment for the underlying immunologic cause (TSIs) may be developed, and the patient could always undertake ^{131}I or surgery later. In the United States, the last 15 years has seen a change in the preference for treatment of Graves' disease from thionamides to ^{131}I. Surgery is chosen in a minority (less than 10%) of cases.

Surgery Provides Tissue for Diagnosis of Suspected Cancer

Knowledge of the incidence and prognosis of thyroid carcinoma occurring in Graves' disease patients would help to determine treatment (see also Chapter 28).

Incidence of Carcinoma in Graves' Disease

Two situations can arise: (a) patients with Graves' disease occasionally present with nodule(s) suspicious of carcinoma, and (b) carcinoma can be found after surgery for Graves' disease where a nodule was not clinically present.

Regarding the first situation, clinical experience and the scant literature on this topic generally support the concept that the chance that a solid and cold nodule is a well-differentiated adenocarcinoma is the same in Graves' disease and euthyroid patients—approximately 15% to 20% (50). However, Belfiore et al. (51) reported a 45.8% incidence of carcinoma in cold nodules in Graves' disease. The evaluation and use of needle biopsy in helping to select those patients with solid cold nodules for surgery are the same in Graves' disease and euthyroid cases. However, TSH suppression therapy cannot be used in Graves' disease cases because TSH is already suppressed, so the use of thyroidectomy to provide for final tissue diagnosis arises more frequently in Graves' disease cases.

Regarding the second situation, the carcinoma is an incidental finding. The incidence is small but variable, with reports of 0.5 to 1.5% (52–56), 2% (57,58), 2.3% (59), 2.9% (50,60), 4.3% (61), 5.1% (62), 6% (63), 8.7% (64), and 9.8% (51). The variable incidences can be caused by differences in extent of thyroidectomy, number of histologic sections examined, and prior exposure to neck radiation. The similarity of these incidences to the incidence of carcinoma in autopsy series in patients without a history of thyroid disease (see Chapter 28) supports the belief that carcinoma in Graves' disease cases without nodularity is an incidental finding of occult carcinoma (also called minimal or microcarcinoma), which exists frequently but will not progress to clinical cancer in the overwhelming majority of patients. Therefore, the possibility of finding occult carcinoma is not a justified reason for thyroidectomy for Graves' disease. However, some authors (57,65) interpret the literature as showing a higher incidence of carcinoma in Graves' disease than in euthyroid patients.

The incidence of carcinoma in toxic nodular goiter is less variable and reported as 3.1% (55), 3.9% (51), 4% (58), and 5% (60,63). When comparing the incidence of carcinoma in Graves' disease without clinical nodules versus toxic nodular goiter, incidence for Graves' disease shows a wider variation and a seemingly higher rate (0.5% to 9.9% in Graves' disease versus 3.1% to 5% in toxic nodular goiter). However, as shown in most studies that compare the two groups (52–55,58,60,62), the incidence of carcinoma is higher in toxic nodular goiter than in Graves' disease cases. This fact is expected, because patients with toxic nodular goiter have clinically enlarged nodules compared with the Graves' disease patients. One exception is the study by Belfiore et al. (51), which showed a higher incidence of carcinoma in Graves' disease (9.8%) than in toxic nodular goiter (3.9%).

Prognosis of Carcinoma in Graves' Disease

Studies comparing the prognosis of carcinoma in Graves' disease patients with carcinoma in patients with toxic nodular goiter and euthyroid patients show variable results. Some support a worse prognosis with markedly invasive growth and lymph node metastases (57,66). Belfiore et al. (51) found that in Graves' disease patients carcinomas were more often multifocal, larger, locally invasive, metastatic to lymph nodes or distant sites, and recurrent or persistent compared with carcinomas in euthyroid patients or in those with toxic nodules. TSI levels were present in the Graves' disease cases and absent in toxic nodule cases and were considered to play a role in the higher aggressiveness of carcinoma in Graves' disease patients. Reasoning for this role is as follows. Normal thyroid tissue and differentiated thyroid carcinoma have receptors for TSH. TSH stimulates growth and worsens prognosis of differentiated thyroid carcinoma. TSI mimics many of the effects of TSH on carcinoma and could worsen prognosis of carcinoma in Graves' disease (65,67). New understanding of the molecular biology of signal transduction in thyroid cells supports the role of TSI as a cause of Graves' disease and cancer. TSI, like TSH, activates an intracellular cascade (dissociation of guanine nucleotide–stimulatory protein and binding of its alpha subunit to guanine triphosphate, which stimulates adenylate cyclase to form cyclic AMP), which causes Graves' disease and cancer (see Chapters 11 and 13).

However, other studies report a similar prognosis of carcinoma in Graves' disease patients with carcinoma, in patients with toxic nodular goiter, and in euthyroid patients (59,61,68–70). The reported discrepancies may be secondary to patient selection with regard to age and gender (which are the most important factors in determining prognosis of thyroid carcinoma), stage and grade of carcinoma, cellular molecular genetic factors, local versus referral treatment center, geography of the study population, prior use of therapeutic head and neck radiation (in some of the older studies), criteria for surgery, and other unrecognized factors.

Surgery Is Useful for the Noncompliant Patient

The noncompliant patient who did not regularly take thionamide medication is often referred for surgery. Surgery provides more rapid control of hyperthyroidism compared with thionamides or ^{131}I; surgery more reliably provides permanent control compared with thionamides.

However, surgery for the noncompliant patient still presents many obstacles. Preparing such a patient for surgery to avoid thyroid storm requires frequent clinical evaluation and determinations of serum T_4 and T_3 right up to the time of surgery. Although it is true that once the patient lies down on the operating table, treatment is complete, the postoperative and long-term management of the patient is just beginning. The patient who was noncompliant before surgery almost always remains so during postoperative management, with the potential for significantly adverse consequences. After thyroidectomy for Graves' disease, some patients require calcium during the immediate postoperative period for temporary hypoparathyroidism and many ultimately require thyroid replacement therapy for hypothyroidism. Graves' disease is for life (until someone discovers how to modulate the immune response and control the stimulating immunoglobulin). Recurrent hyperthyroidism or hypothyroidism can occur at any time after any treatment.

Miscellaneous Indications for Surgery

Thyroid Storm Unresponsive to Medical Therapy

There is a widely held, yet erroneous, assumption that thyroid surgery for hyperthyroidism stimulates the intraoperative release of T_4 and T_3 into the circulation, increasing the risk of surgical storm. This belief is consistent with the known release of catecholamines and the development of hypertensive crisis from surgery for pheochromocytomas. However, Hermann et al. (71) studied patients undergoing thyroidectomy for hyperthyroidism who were prepared only with propanolol and not with antithyroid medications. Free T_4 and T_3 levels were at least 3 times normal. Intraoperative and postoperative levels of free T_4 and T_3 in the thyroid venous effluent (middle thyroid vein) did not exceed those in peripheral blood (cubital vein) in any patient. The long half-life of thyroid hormones (7 days for T_4, 1 day for T_3) accounts for the inability to detect differences in thyroid hormone levels in gland effluent versus peripheral blood; in contrast, catecholamines have short half-lives (minutes) so differences can be detected. Hermann et al. (71) concluded that thyroidectomy (and the associated manipulation of the gland) and the stress of surgery did not release thyroid hormones. Therefore, this mechanism cannot account for the development of intraoperative or postoperative storm. These findings suggest that immediate thyroidectomy should be considered for emergency treatment of thyroid storm. Thyroidectomy was used as treatment for storm after failure of medical management in five (72) and four (73) patients; all recovered completely. Thyroid storm unresponsive to medical therapy is a rare event for which thyroidectomy should be considered.

Amiodarone-Induced Thyrotoxicosis

Amiodarone, an antiarrhythmic and antianginal drug, is 37% iodine. Because of effects of metabolized free iodine, amiodarone can cause thyrotoxicosis. Treatment of the thyrotoxicosis is difficult because the drug has a prolonged half-life, cardiac decompensation due to underlying heart disease often occurs, discontinuation of amiodarone may not be possible, and standard treatment with thionamides and corticosteroids is often ineffective. Thyroidectomy was successfully used as treatment for amiodarone-induced thyrotoxicosis in one (74), six (75), and nine (76) patients. Thyroidectomy permits continued treatment with amiodarone. Thyroidectomy may be indicated for amiodarone-induced thyrotoxicosis when medical treatment is ineffective and amiodarone is necessary to treat cardiac disease.

Questionable Benefits of Surgery

Surgery Controls Progression of Thyroid Associated Ophthalmopathy

The effect of treatment of Graves' hyperthyroidism on the initiation and progression of infiltrative ophthalmopathy deserves attention. Infiltrative ophthalmopathy may precede, occur simultaneously with, or follow the hyperthyroidism. It may occur entirely independent of hyperthyroidism in the setting of euthyroidism (in which case it is called euthyroid Graves' disease) or it may occur associated with hypothyroidism. In these circumstances, the term *thyroid-associated ophthalmopathy* (TAO) is used to indicate ophthalmopathy associated with hyper-, hypo-, or euthyroid status. If one or more of the treatments of hyperthyroidism (thionamides, ^{131}I, surgery) favorably affected the incidence or severity of ophthalmopathy, this fact could become a decisive factor in choosing a treatment, because TAO is clinically evident in about 50% of patients with Graves' disease (77) and it is a serious problem leading to malignant exophthalmos in 8% (78).

Various groups from around the world have addressed this topic over many years. There are problems with this literature. Some studies draw conclusions based on a small patient sample. The period of observation is often too short to draw firm conclusions, because TAO is a chronic and variable disease. Many studies are not controlled, randomized, or prospective. Studies draw variable conclusions because they often do not control for known risk factors for TAO. These risk factors include (a) increased incidence in women, but increased severity in men and older (>60 years) patients, and (b) increased incidence in smokers (possibly through hypoxic stimulation on orbital connective tissue).

Some studies have shown that total thyroid ablation by surgery and/or ^{131}I, including the removal of all remnant thyroid tissue, decreases initiation and halts progression of TAO (78–82). These studies, which suggest that the presence of functioning thyroid tissue is necessary for TAO, include the following:

1. An uncontrolled study of 18 consecutive patients with progressive TAO who had functioning thyroid tissue showed marked improvement of TAO after ablation of thyroid remnants using high doses of ^{131}I (10–50 mCi) therapeutic for thyroid cancer (78).

2. A study of 88 consecutive patients showed overwhelming lack of initiation and cessation of progression of TAO after total thyroidectomy (79). All six patients with euthyroid Graves' disease showed improvement of TAO with complete regression of proptosis in two. None of 12 patients with thyrotoxic Graves' disease without TAO showed initiation of TAO after 9 years of follow-up. None of 70 patients with thyrotoxic Graves' disease with TAO showed progression of TAO, and 66 improved. All four patients not improving had remnant ectopic thyroid tissue. Although this study can be criticized because it was uncontrolled, the results are noteworthy for two reasons: surgery had an overwhelmingly beneficial effect on TAO, and the cases were probably not selected because the thyroidectomies were consecutive.

3. A retrospective, uncontrolled study showed that total thyroidectomy stabilized or improved TAO in 96% of Graves' disease cases with TAO (13).

4. A retrospective, controlled, nonrandomized study showed less progression of TAO in patients treated with thyroidectomy or ^{131}I compared with propylthiouracil (80).

5. An uncontrolled report of 503 patients with Graves' disease treated by total thyroidectomy or ^{131}I showed no initiation of TAO during a follow-up period of 8 to 32 years (mean, 12 years) (79,83).

6. An uncontrolled study of only four patients showed improvement of TAO after thyroidectomy (81).

7. A controlled, prospective, nonrandomized study with follow-up of only 1 year showed improvement of TAO after thyroidectomy but no change after ^{131}I (84).

8. An uncontrolled study of 27 children with Graves' disease with TAO treated by bilateral subtotal thyroidectomy showed remission in 18 (67%) and no progression in any during a mean 13.7-year follow-up (85).

9. Two studies have shown that total thyroidectomy caused more improvement of TAO compared with subtotal thyroidectomy (12,82); the amount of residual thyroid gland measured by 24-hour uptake of ^{131}I negatively correlated with improvement of TAO (82); thyrotropin receptor antibodies (mediators of thyroid stimulation in Graves' disease) became undetectable or normal in 88% of patients treated by total thyroidectomy, but in 41% treated by subtotal thyroidectomy (12). Winsa et al. (12) concluded that the thyroid is an antigen that stimulates the production of thyrotropin receptor antibodies, TAO is dependent on thyroid tissue, and total thyroidectomy may improve TAO.

10. Uncontrolled studies showed a beneficial effect of subtotal thyroidectomy on TAO in 50% (86) and 69% (87) of patients.

11. An uncontrolled, retrospective study with a 1- to 12-year follow-up, showed that of 50 patients with TAO, 54% improved and none worsened after bilateral subtotal thyroidectomy; of 31 patients without TAO, none developed TAO (15).

12. Corticosteroids and ^{131}I decreased the development of TAO in one study (88).

However, other studies have not supported the concept that total thyroid ablation by surgery and/or ^{131}I (including all remnant thyroid tissue) decreases initiation and halts progression of TAO; instead, they have shown that TAO is not affected by the treatment of hyperthyroidism (89–91). These studies, which are in keeping with the theory that the hyperthyroidism and TAO are separate phenomena, are as follows:

1. A controlled, retrospective, nonrandomized study of Graves' disease patients, comparing TAO after treatment with thionamides, thyroidectomy, or ^{131}I, showed no difference after 5 to 20 years of follow-up (91).

2. An uncontrolled study of only five patients with Graves' disease with severe TAO (four treated by total thyroidectomy, one by ^{131}I) found progression of TAO in all patients despite absence of thyroid remnant in 2 of the 4 surgical patients (89).

3. Although a prospective, randomized, and controlled study found no difference in TAO after thyroidectomy versus ^{131}I (92), this study can be interpreted to show that both methods are equally effective in controlling TAO.

4. Subtotal thyroidectomy did not have any significant effect on TAO (93).

5. ^{131}I treatment carried a higher risk (33%) for initiating or worsening TAO, compared with thionamide treat-

ment (10%) or thyroidectomy (16%) (94). Other studies also show a causal association of ^{131}I with TAO (95) and with pretibial myxedema (96). However, in another report, ^{131}I treatment caused no difference in TAO (97).

In summary, present evidence does not conclusively favor any one treatment for hyperthyroidism (thionamides, ^{131}I, surgery) over another to decrease the incidence or progression of TAO. However, a larger number of studies show an advantage of ablative therapy (thyroidectomy or ^{131}I) compared with medical therapy. Of the ablative treatments, surgery appears more effective than ^{131}I. Surveys of endocrinologists in the United States, Japan, and Europe show that surgery is used as primary treatment of Graves' disease in a small minority of patients (between 0% and 9%, depending on clinical circumstances). Total thyroidectomy appears to be an undervalued treatment for TAO of Graves' disease as long as surgical expertise can keep complications to a minimum. This is a controversial topic that will be elucidated as understanding of pathogenesis of TAO increases (see Chapter 18). Also, we need a large-scale, prospective, controlled, and randomized study to address the influence of treatment on the course of TAO. Because thyroidectomy is chosen as primary therapy in a minority of patients with Graves' disease, physicians are not willing to enter patients into such a study.

Disadvantages of Surgery

The cost for surgery (surgeon, anesthesia, operating room, hospitalization) is often assumed to be higher than the cost for ^{131}I or thionamide treatment. For ^{131}I this is true. After ^{131}I treatment, only several months of frequent doctor visits and tests of thyroid function are needed until hyperthyroidism is controlled. Also, ^{131}I is ablative, with little chance of recurrent hyperfunction. However, the cost for thionamide treatment is substantial and probably is equal to or greater than the cost of surgery. Thionamide treatment requires at least 6 to 12 months and sometimes 2 years of frequent doctor visits and laboratory tests of thyroid function. Also, the 50% of patients who relapse after thionamides go on to surgery or ^{131}I. Cost for treatment of these patients is clearly higher than if they had surgery or ^{131}I in the first place.

Only surgery requires hospitalization. Also, although surgery is safe (see preceding), it is the only therapy that can cause permanent vocal cord paralysis and permanent hypoparathyroidism, albeit infrequently. On rare occasions, ^{131}I can cause temporary vocal cord paralysis (98) and temporary hypoparathyroidism (99).

Preoperative Preparation

Preoperative preparation of the patient is crucial to avoid intraoperative or postoperative thyroid storm and to decrease the vascularity of the gland. A number of regimens have been used successfully.

Thionamides and Iodine, with or without Beta-Blockers

The safest regimen, and the one with which there is the greatest experience, is a combination of thionamide drugs and iodine, with or without beta-blocking agents. *Thionamide* is the proper pharmacologic term for antithyroid drugs. In the United States, propylthiouracil (PTU) (50-mg tablets) and methimazole (Tapazole) (5- and 10-mg tablets) are used. In Europe, methimazole and carbimazole are used. Thionamides inhibit the synthesis of T_4 and T_3.

Prior to starting thionamide drugs, the hyperthyroidism should be diagnosed and the exact etiology determined, because the thionamide drugs will affect the results of the thyroid scan as well as serum T_4, T_3, and TSH levels. The most common method of treatment is by the titration method, using a large dose initially and then lowering to the smallest dose that maintains euthyroidism. An initial dose of PTU 300 to 600 mg/day is usually used, but the dose can be lower for mild cases with small glands. Figure 1 graphically illustrates the important points in the preoperative preparation of the patient for thyroidectomy for Graves' disease. Once euthyroidism is reached, the dose is lowered to a maintenance dose, which is approximately one half of the initial dose. The patient should not be overtreated and rendered hypothyroid, a condition that predisposes to increase the size and vascularity of the gland under the influence of thyrotropin. (Low serum levels of T_4 and T_3 stimulate increased secretion of thyrotropin.) Thionamides are discontinued at the time of thyroidectomy, when the patient must be clinically and chemically euthyroid to avoid the possibility of intraoperative or postoperative thyroid storm. Propranolol may be started prior to the determination of the exact etiology of the hyperthyroidism, because this drug does not affect the results of thyroid scanning. However, propranolol inhibits the extrathyroidal conversion of T_4 to T_3, thereby causing a small decrease in serum T_3 concentrations (100). Propranolol may be used to control the symptoms and signs of hyperthyroidism. Propranolol is continued postoperatively and tapered over the first postoperative week.

In contrast to the titration method, another method, more frequently used in Europe than in the United States, continues the initial dosage once euthyroidism is achieved but adds exogenous thyroxine. This method, called high-dose or block-and-treat, secures nonfunction of the gland and provides for euthyroidism through exogenous thyroxine (4,101). Euthyroidism is maintained by titrating thyroxine and not PTU. This method was adopted based on histologic studies showing that thyroids obtained from patients prepared with thionamides and

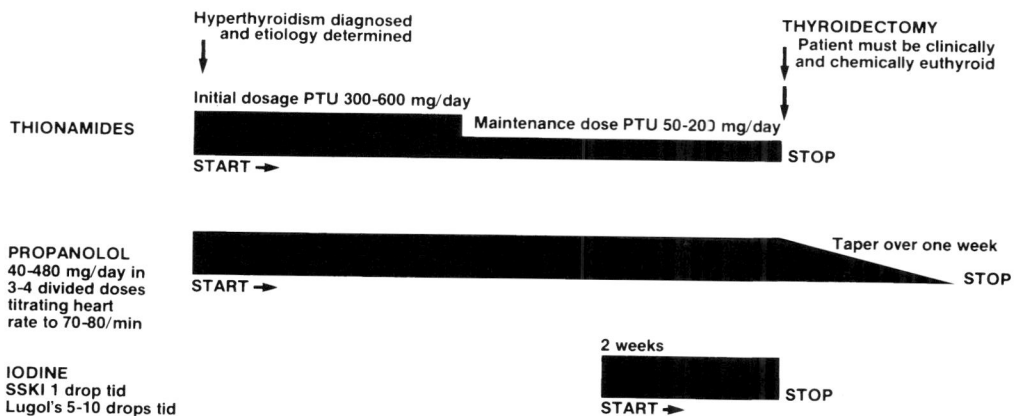

FIG. 1. The preoperative preparation for thyroidectomy of the patient with Graves' disease. PTU, propylthiouracil; SSKI, saturated solution of potassium iodide.

thyroxine contain the least amount of colloid when compared with thyroids from patients prepared with antithyroid drugs and iodine (101). Also, thyroids obtained from patients prepared with antithyroid drugs and thyroxine are most similar histologically to a normal gland (4). However, such observations do not translate into any real benefit, such as decreased blood loss during surgery or ease in performing surgery.

Also, the high-dose method is therapeutically illogical because the patient is intentionally overtreated with one drug and so requires another. It also increases the risks of toxic effects, especially agranulocytosis in patients treated with methimazole. Available data indicate that agranulocytosis is an idiosyncratic reaction—an autoimmune phenomenon not related to the dose of thionamide. This is true for any dose of PTU and for methimazole doses less than 40 mg/day. However, for doses of methimazole greater than 40 mg/day, the risk of agranulocytosis is dose related (102–104). Also, our understanding and knowledge of thionamide-induced agranulocytosis is still incomplete. Maintaining patients on unnecessarily high doses of thionamides so that they require exogenous thyroid (lest TSH rise and cause thyromegaly) gives certain extra risk with little or no benefit and appears not only ill advised but pharmacologically reckless in preparing the patient for surgery. However, when thionamides are used as primary therapy with the intention of inducing remission of Graves' disease, high-dose thionamides were initially reported to produce more remissions (by altering the immunogenicity of thyroid tissue) than low-dose thionamides (102). Here, the high-dose method may be worth the extra risk. However, more recent studies of high dose versus titration methods have failed to show any difference in remissions (105,106) (see Chapter 15).

With the proper use of thionamide drugs and iodine with or without beta-blocking agents, the risk of intraoperative or postoperative thyroid storm in reports totaling 2000 patients is zero (14,27,32,35,39,107).

Iodine

Before thionamides and ^{131}I became available in the 1940s, iodine was the main treatment for Graves' disease with or without surgery. Iodine has varying effects on the thyroid gland depending on its length of administration. Iodine inhibits release of T_4 and T_3 from the thyroid gland (108) and thus controls hyperthyroidism during its early administration (109). This action, which occurs within 24 hours and has a maximal effect after 2 weeks, is temporary, and the hyperthyroidism returns (110). In Graves' disease, large doses of iodine (radiographic contrast media) or prolonged use of iodine (expectorants) can worsen hyperthyroidism, as the iodine serves as a substrate for thyroid hormone synthesis (111). Also, in nodular goiter, iodine can worsen hyperthyroidism or induce hyperthyroidism (the Jod-Basedow phenomenon).

Preparing patients with thionamides alone results in a soft and friable gland at surgery, and these drawbacks are overcome by adding iodine (112), which decreases the vascularity of the gland and makes it firmer. This effect has been demonstrated histologically (113) and by using radioisotopic techniques that have shown decreased thyroid blood flow (114,115). The current use of iodine in thyroid surgery is to prepare the patient for surgery. Iodine is used for 2 weeks immediately prior to surgery, along with thionamide drugs and/or propranolol. Because iodine alone can worsen hyperthyroidism, the patient should be treated with thionamides and rendered euthyroid prior to giving the iodine. Iodine is discontinued on the day of surgery. Iodine is available as a saturated solution of potassium iodide (SSKI) (50 mg iodine per drop), of which 1 drop is administered three times daily, and as Lugol's solution (iodine plus potassium iodide, 6 mg iodine per drop), of which 5 to 10 drops is given three times daily. When SSKI causes side effects of parotitis or thyroiditis, iodinated glycerol (Organidin tincture, solution or tablets) has been successfully substituted. However,

Organidin is no longer available: it was recently discontinued because of its lack of effectiveness as a mucolytic, its original purpose.

Beta-Adrenergic Blockers

Many of the effects of hyperthyroidism are mediated through increased activity of the sympathetic nervous system. Beta-adrenergic receptor antagonists block many of the hyperadrenergic manifestations of hyperthyroidism. Propanolol also inhibits the peripheral conversion of T_4 into T_3 (116). Propranolol, alone (117–119a) or in combination with iodine (109), provides rapid control of the peripheral manifestations of hyperthyroidism and is useful for the preparation of the patient for surgery.

Because serum levels of propanolol are variable, especially in patients with hyperthyroidism, the dose needed to control hyperadrenergic signs and symptoms is variable (40 to 480 mg/day) (120). The optimal dose must be titrated for each patient. Propranolol has a short half-life of 3.2 hours (121) and an even shorter one in hyperthyroid patients (122), and it must be given three to four times daily and within 3 to 4 hours of surgery lest the chance of thyroid storm is increased (37). It must be restarted immediately after surgery either orally or, if this is not possible, intravenously. Because serum T_4 and T_3 become normal 3 to 4 days after thyroidectomy in patients prepared with propranolol only (123,124), beta-blocker treatment should be continued for at least 3 to 4 days after surgery and usually for 1 week.

Long- and short-acting beta-blockers have found roles in the preoperative preparation of the hyperthyroid patient. To avoid the frequent and impractical dosing of propranolol during the preoperative period, long-acting beta-adrenergic blocking agents [nadolol (Corgard) or atenolol (Tenormin)] have been used as the sole preoperative medication and found safe (125). They are usually given once daily and on the morning of surgery. The ultrashort-acting cardioselective beta-blocker esmolol, with only a 30-minute duration of action, is helpful in managing hyperthyroidism during the perioperative period (126–129).

Beta-adrenergic receptor blockers are classified into cardioselective (i.e., beta-1-selective) (atenolol, metoprolol, esmolol) and noncardioselective (propanolol, nadolol). Cardioselective blockers are preferred in patients with diseases that can be exacerbated by beta-blockade, including asthma and diabetes mellitus. A prospective randomized study comparing thyroidectomy groups prepared with metoprolol (a selective beta-1-blocker) versus thionamide and thyroxine showed similar thyroid consistency, vascularity, and operative blood loss (130). Other studies, although not as well controlled, reported similar findings (37,119,125). The selective beta-1-blocker metoprolol can be safely used without thyroid storm and offered shorter preoperative preparation time and shorter postoperative hospital stay in comparison to propanolol (131).

However, about 20% of patients treated solely with beta-blockers develop clinical signs of hyperthyroidism in the immediate postoperative period (119,122,124,130). Inadvertent omission of the beta-blocker 3 to 4 hours prior to surgery can result in this exacerbation of hyperthyroidism. Therefore, these patients need extremely close monitoring and often require intravenous treatment with propanolol or esmolol lest some develop thyroid storm. Although propranolol, alone (117–119a) or in combination with iodine (109), can be used for the preparation of the patient for surgery, such use of beta-blockers does carry risk of thyroid storm, which has occurred in these patients (119a,132–134). Thyroid storm carries a mortality rate of 28% to 100% (see Chapter 40).

In contrast, the incidence of thyroid storm is zero in numerous large series of patients, totaling 2000, prepared with standard thionamides (14,27,32,35,39,107). This difference in safety makes sense because thionamides render the patient clinically and chemically euthyroid as hormone synthesis is inhibited. Because propranolol only controls the peripheral adrenergic manifestations of hyperthyroidism and does not affect thyroid hormone synthesis, the patient is clinically euthyroid but still chemically hyperthyroid (109).

Advantages of beta-blockers over treatment with antithyroid drugs are faster relief of symptoms (within days), shorter preparation time (within a week), and more flexible timing of operation. I take advantage of the fast relief of symptoms and use beta-blockers initially and often throughout the preoperative period. I also use thionamides because of their extra margin of safety in preventing thyroid storm. I fail to see the shorter preparation time with beta-blockers as a practical advantage. In most busy practices, scheduling for surgery usually requires several weeks. Scheduling within a week of diagnosis usually indicates an urgent surgical problem, which Graves' disease is not. I prefer 8 weeks or so for the patient to become clinically and chemically euthyroid under thionamides and beta-blockers, during which time several visits with the surgeon provide the foundation for a successful surgical experience, as rapport is established, risks and alternative methods are explained, and all questions are answered. In my experience, the claimed advantage of more flexible timing of operation is more theoretical than real. Once the patient is euthyroid after thionamide preparation, surgery can be scheduled for any time, leaving, however, a 2-week period for iodine treatment just prior to surgery. Once iodine treatment begins, the patient is committed to the surgery, because if surgery is canceled, another course of iodine could theoretically worsen the hyperthyroidism. In a busy hospital where surgery is occasionally canceled because of lack of beds, patients with Graves' disease should be given priority.

The sole use of beta-blockers is reasonable in patients who have significant adverse reactions to thionamides, usually bone marrow suppression (agranulocytosis, thrombocytopenia, or aplastic anemia). Minor toxic effects, such as papular skin rashes, pruritus, fever, gastrointestinal upset, and arthralgias, usually resolve even with continued administration, or they can be taken care of by substituting another thionamide, because in only 20% of cases will these toxic effects be experienced with the other drug. However, if bone marrow suppression is encountered with one, the other thionamides will likely produce similar toxicity and so are contraindicated—in such cases preparation takes place with beta-blockers and iodine for 2 weeks before surgery. Beta-blockers also have an important role in controlling the signs and symptoms of thyrotoxicosis in patients requiring emergency surgery (when there is not time enough for the thionamides to work) and in patients with self-limited thyrotoxicosis secondary to subacute thyroiditis, Hashimoto's thyroiditis, and excessive exogenous thyroid hormone.

Lithium, Betamethasone, Iopanoic Acid, and Plasmapheresis

When thionamides produce adverse effects, a number of drugs (other than beta-blockers) either alone or in combinations can be used to prepare the hyperthyroid patient for thyroidectomy. Lithium carbonate (300 mg every 6 hours) has an effect similar to iodine and inhibits T_4 release from the thyroid gland. Lithium has been successfully used alone in the treatment of hyperthyroidism (136) and in preparation for surgery (137–139). Lithium has also been used with beta-blockers or glucocorticoids (139). However, a case of thyroid storm occurring after thyroidectomy was reported in a patient prepared with lithium and beta-blocker (140).

Radiographic contrast media that contain large amounts of iodine (iopanoic acid and iodate) are, like iodine, effective in decreasing thyroid hormone release from the gland (141). Iopanoic acid, betamethasone, and propanolol (142) and iopanoic acid and dexamethasone (143) are safe and effective.

Total and free thyroid hormone levels can be rapidly and safely lowered by plasmapheresis and peritoneal dialysis; these modalities are most useful in thyroid storm (144–148). The reader is referred to other chapters for insightful analysis—Chapter 15 for medical management of hyperthyroidism and Chapter 40 for thyrotoxic storm.

General Anesthesia in Thyroid Surgery

The reader is referred to Chapter 35 for a complete discussion of anesthetic considerations during thyroid surgery and in patients with hyper- and hypothyroidism. A rare occurrence was reported of an occult pheochromocytoma presenting as a hypertensive crisis and mimicking thyroid storm during thyroidectomy for hyperthyroidism (149).

The Extent of Surgery

An important consideration in surgery for Graves' disease is the extent of thyroidectomy. Three approaches can be taken: bilateral subtotal thyroidectomy (BST), total thyroidectomy (TT), or total lobectomy and contralateral subtotal lobectomy (TL plus SL). By each approach, the surgeon is determining the thyroid remnant—the amount of tissue of the posterior capsule intentionally left behind. BST yields bilateral remnants; TT yields no remnant; TL plus SL yields a unilateral remnant.

Thyroid Remnant

Determination of the Weight of the Thyroid Remnant

Studies concerned with the weight of the thyroid remnant have determined its weight in various ways. Ideally, to accurately measure the size of the remnant, a part of the resected gland, identical in size to the remnant, can be weighed.

Or, if a remnant of a specific weight is desired, a portion of the resected gland is trimmed under sterile conditions until it reaches the desired weight. This portion is used as a model and the remnant is trimmed to the same size (150). Within one surgical team, an accurate remnant size can be determined. It is unknown how often other teams obtain accurate weights and if we can with confidence compare weights across various studies. In addition, in most studies the thyroid remnant is not weighed but an estimate of weight is given (32,151). These estimates contain large inaccuracies and vary by at least 30% above or below the actual weight (152). Also, some studies express the weight of the remnant as a percentage of the weight of the gland (35), and because the weight varies depending on the size, these studies report patients with widely varying remnant weights.

Vascularity of Thyroid Remnant

The function of the thyroid remnant and parathyroid glands depends on an intact vascularity. Branches of the inferior thyroid artery supplying the remnant must be isolated and preserved. Unfortunately, the vascular integrity of the remnant is rarely mentioned in most studies. In fact, in some major centers reporting large series of thyroidectomies for Graves' disease (3,29,151,153), the main inferior thyroid arteries are routinely ligated. Such a technique is to be condemned because of the loss of blood supply to the remnant and parathyroid glands and the increased incidence of hypoparathyroidism.

What Is the Ideal Size of Thyroid Remnant?

Because of these varying factors in reporting remnant weight and its vascular integrity, it is not surprising that there are widely varying conclusions found in the literature regarding the thyroid remnant. The question of what is the ideal remnant size, if any (and, therefore, which operation to perform) was raised by Bartlett (154) in 1916 and since then has been debated in hundreds of articles; nevertheless, it is still controversial and will remain so. To understand why and to enable the reader to be comfortable with this controversy, I will relate the thyroid remnant to two issues—postoperative thyroid function and the risks of thyroid surgery.

Thyroid Remnant and Postoperative Thyroid Function

Thyroid Remnant and Hypothyroidism

The goal of surgery is to ensure permanent euthyroidism by leaving behind a certain thyroid remnant with no chance of hypothyroidism or recurrent hyperthyroidism. Unfortunately, this goal is often not realized because it is self-contradictory. The following studies show that leaving a certain thyroid remnant cannot reliably produce euthyroidism (with or without a chance of recurrent hyperthyroidism) and that hypothyroidism occurs regardless of remnant size.

1. Cusick et al. (3) left a 6- to 8-g remnant and produced a 21% incidence of clinical hypothyroidism at the 1-year follow-up and 30% at 5 years. They found a correlation between a smaller thyroid remnant and a greater chance of hypothyroidism.

2. Simms and Talbot (32) also left a 6-g remnant and produced a similar 30% incidence of hypothyroidism. Similarly, Kuma et al. (155) left a 6- to 7-g remnant that produced hypothyroidism in 33% of patients after a mean 9-year follow-up. In contrast, Noh et al. (156), leaving also a 6-g remnant, produced hypothyroidism in only 4% of patients, but recurrent hyperthyroidism occurred in 14%.

3. Reid (36), desiring to produce less hypothyroidism, left a larger remnant—10 g. Nevertheless, he still produced a 19% incidence of clinical hypothyroidism after 18 months follow-up.

4. Csaky et al. (85), despite leaving a large (6- to 10-g) remnant, obtained clinical hypothyroidism in 19.6% of cases and subclinical hypothyroidism in 50%.

5. Many authors report the type of operation and not remnant weight. Jortso et al. (33) performed BST and found a 30% incidence of clinical hypothyroidism. Contrary to the results of Cusick et al. (3), no difference in remnant size was found between the hypothyroid and euthyroid patients.

6. Sugrue et al. (35) also performed BST (described as a seven-eighth thyroidectomy) and produced hypothyroidism in 21% of patients after a long (30-year) follow-up.

7. Bradley et al. (150), leaving a large (10-g) remnant after BST, produced no hypothyroid patients after a 4-year follow-up, but, as expected, their rate of recurrent hyperthyroidism was unacceptably high at 6%.

8. Gough and Neill (157) also left a large (10-g) remnant and could not avoid a 9% rate of hypothyroidism.

Remnant size is the only factor under the direct control of the surgeon who attempts to leave a patient euthyroid. But, as these studies clearly show, manipulating the remnant does not produce euthyroidism in any predictable way but still leads to significant hypothyroidism. This is not surprising when we consider the changes that may occur in the remnant after surgery. It is known that lymphocytic infiltration of the thyroid gland tends to predispose to hypothyroidism. Graves' disease is often accompanied histologically by lymphocytic infiltration or may coexist with Hashimoto's thyroiditis (77). The lymphocytic infiltration or the thyroiditis reduces the functional capacity of the remnant thyroid tissue, predisposing to hypothyroidism. Also, the underlying disease process of Graves' disease can lead spontaneously to hypothyroidism, as related in the early descriptions of patients observed without treatment.

Thyroid Remnant and Recurrent Hyperthyroidism

Since we cannot predictably avoid hypothyroidism by manipulating the remnant, can we at least avoid recurrent hyperthyroidism? Almost always we can, by completely eliminating the remnant and performing TT. Even TT does not guarantee complete absence of recurrent hyperthyroidism because of thyroid tissue the surgeon may unintentionally leave behind. This tissue has been demonstrated by postoperative radioiodine scan in 71% of patients after total thyroidectomy (18). At any time after surgery, it can hypertrophy under the influence of TSIs and produce hyperthyroidism. Again, the thyroid remnant is the amount of tissue intentionally left behind at surgery. In BST, the surgeon intentionally leaves behind several grams of tissue of the posterior capsule on each side. TT represents only an attempt by the surgeon to remove all thyroid tissue, but this is often not accomplished. Thyroid tissue may be unintentionally left behind at surgery and predispose to persistent or recurrent hyperthyroidism. Locations of thyroid tissue that may be unintentionally left behind include the pyramidal lobe, the superior pole, posterior to Berry's ligament, the anterior tracheal wall, and adjacent to the parathyroid glands (at the superior pole or too much posterior capsule remnant left behind). Despite thyroid tissue that may unintentionally remain, the incidence of recurrent hyperthyroidism after total thyroidectomy is 0% (12,158).

Short of doing a TT, can we reduce the incidence of recurrent hyperthyroidism by preserving only a small remnant? Does remnant weight correlate with recurrence? Logic would say so, but the available data are conflicting.

Because of the difficulties in determining remnant weight, as discussed, comparing estimated remnant weight with recurrence across multiple studies is fraught with error. The following studies show that the incidence of recurrent hyperthyroidism cannot be predicted by remnant weight.

1. Bradley et al. (150) compared different studies and concluded that the incidence of recurrence is independent of remnant weight.
2. A 6-g remnant resulted in recurrent hyperthyroidism in 3.2% (32), 6% (155), 7.5% (3), and 14% (156) of cases by the 5-year follow-up.
3. A 3- to 5-g remnant resulted in recurrence in only 1.2% of cases (15).
4. Even a small remnant (2 to 4 g) results in a 7% recurrence rate (160).
5. Csaky et al. (85) produced recurrent hyperthyroidism in 11% of patients after BST.
6. Of great interest is the study of Winsa et al. (12), which showed that recurrent Graves' disease cases had a *smaller* remnant than present in euthyroid cases.

A more reliable judgment can be made where remnant weight was varied within one study. The following studies show that remnant size was correlated with recurrent hyperthyroidism.

1. Remnants greater than 21 g produced a 67% incidence of recurrence; between 11 and 20 g, 16%; less than 10 g, 7%. Therefore, leaving large remnants (>10 g) clearly correlates with recurrence (159).
2. Remnants greater than 6 g produced a 24% incidence of recurrence; between 4 and 6 g, 6%; less than 4 g, 0%.
3. Mitchie et al. (161,162) and Kasuga et al. (8) also found a difference depending on remnant size.

In contrast,

4. Tweedle et al. (163) found no difference in the incidence of recurrent hyperthyroidism with remnants of 6 to 12 g.
5. Cusick et al. (3) found no difference in the range of 5 to 10 g.

Clearly, the activity of Graves' disease in the thyroid remnant, and immunologic and other factors (see later), are stronger determinants of postoperative outcome than just the size of the remnant.

Also, recurrent hyperthyroidism continues to be a problem as patients are followed longer. Recurrent hyperthyroidism may occur at any time after surgery, with 57% of the cases occurring within the first 5 years and 43% after 5 years. In addition, 8% of the reported cases occur between 21 and 30 years after surgery, and 16% of the cases occur 30 years after thyroidectomy (BST) (35). Recurrent hyperthyroidism has been reported half a century after BST (164). These data emphasize the variable and life-long nature of Graves' disease.

Factors Besides Remnant Size Causing Recurrent Hyperthyroidism

Therefore, it is impossible to even approximate the chances of recurrence by leaving a certain remnant behind, and recurrence is an occasional and potentially life-long problem as long as any remnant exists. Patients with small remnants can develop recurrent hyperthyroidism because of multiple pathogenetic factors not related to remnant size. These factors include the following:

1. Age. Young patients, especially under 20 years (165,166), usually have a greater propensity for recurrence than older patients, but this is controversial (3).
2. Iodine intake. An increase in iodine intake may predispose to recurrence (167).
3. TSIs. Persistence of high titers of TSIs after surgery predisposes to recurrence (12,166,167a,168). Recurrence was found only in patients who had at the time of recurrence elevated titers of thyrotropin-binding-inhibitor immunoglobulin (which measures TSI and other thyrotropin receptor antibodies) (8). TSI may stimulate the thyroid remnant, leading to its hyperplasia and recurrence of hyperthyroidism. Disappearance of TSI after surgery is associated with a small chance of recurrent hyperthyroidism. Persistence of high titers of TSI after surgery is also associated with a high incidence of TAO (12).
4. Thyroid-associated ophthalmopathy (TAO). TAO, particularly at the time of thyroidectomy, is associated with an increased risk of recurrent hyperthyroidism (12). This association is mediated through elevated titers of TSI.
5. Autonomy of remnant. Autonomy (nonsuppressibility) of the thyroid remnant is also associated with recurrence of the hyperthyroidism. Autonomy is defined as the inability to decrease the thyroid remnant uptake of a ^{131}I trace dose by exogenous T_3 (a T_3 suppression test). When this happens, the remnant is autonomous (i.e., thyroid hormone production is not controlled by TSH), and the chance of recurrent hyperthyroidism increases. The thyroid in Graves' disease is, of course, autonomous. The gland or remnant, after treatment with thionamide drugs or surgery, respectively, often becomes nonautonomous (suppressible by the T_3 suppression test). These glands and remnants have the least chance of causing recurrent hyperthyroidism.
6. Natural history of Graves' disease. The underlying disease process of Graves' disease may enter a natural remission, decreasing the chance of recurrence of the hyperthyroidism.
7. Coexisting thyroid diseases. Graves' disease frequently coexists with Hashimoto's thyroiditis (77). The latter may reduce the functional capacity of the remnant thyroid tissue, decreasing the chance of recurrence.
8. Lymphocytic infiltration of the thyroid gland. Most studies show that less lymphocytic infiltration of the thyroid gland is associated with greater chance of recurrence

(33,156,165,166). However, a moderate or high grade of lymphocytic infiltration is associated with recurrence (8).

Therefore, to reduce the chance of recurrent hyperthyroidism, it is necessary to leave a progressively smaller remnant while performing BST, but even very small remnants will occasionally be associated with recurrence. TT (with no remnant) offers the least chance of recurrence.

Thyroid Remnant and Risks of Thyroid Surgery

A longstanding belief, and one that is properly becoming discredited, is that as less remnant is left behind and a TT or a near TT performed, there is necessarily an increased risk of vocal cord paralysis and hypoparathyroidism. Such an increased risk is real if the surgeon's primary purpose is to remove all thyroid parenchyma regardless of the consequences, as in cancer cases. (Even in cancer cases, I do not adhere to this philosophy, but rely on ^{131}I to eradicate small areas of residual thyroid tissue that I leave behind, if I feel their presence will aid the vascular integrity of parathyroid glands.) Rigid adherence to the goal of TT probably increases the incidence of hypoparathyroidism as compared with BST, as shown in some series (169). However, TT can be done safely by preservation of parathyroid glands and their blood supply. When this is accomplished, TT results in permanent hypoparathyroidism in 0% (11–13), 0.8% (16), 1% (17), 1.3% (18), and 2.8% (20) of cases. The parathyroids are found by following the inferior thyroid artery to the superior and inferior parathyroid arteries. The parathyroid glands are separated from the thyroid and allowed to fall away from the thyroid with intact vascularity. If this technique cannot be accomplished for at least two parathyroid glands, then a flexible response is warranted: TT is abandoned and a total lobectomy with contralateral subtotal lobectomy or a bilateral subtotal lobectomy (BST) is performed, because the remnant often contains parathyroid tissue and its blood supply.

The proper and modern technique of thyroidectomy requires identification and dissection of the recurrent laryngeal nerve from the thoracic inlet to the cricothyroid joint where it enters the larynx. Such a technique, done with proper instrumentation, lighting, and gentleness, is extremely safe and much safer than the old practice of not dissecting the nerve and assuming it is safely behind the thyroid remnant. The old practice invites nerve transection and/or contusion as the thyroid remnant is clamped, especially as the nerve courses under the ligament of Berry and then anteriorly as it enters the larynx. Mountain et al. (170) showed that the incidence of nerve paralysis is 3 to 4 times greater in cases where the nerve is not exposed than in cases where it is routinely exposed. Therefore, it is illogical to think that nerve paralysis is more common after TT than BST. In terms of nerve preservation, BST and TT are equally safe if the nerve is positively identified and traced throughout its course in the surgical field.

A Logical Approach to Extent of Surgery

Determining the extent of surgery for Graves' disease represents achieving a balance between the risks and benefits (of BST versus TT versus TL plus SL), as is true of most clinical decisions. There is no right or wrong answer. Each surgeon must decide on an approach individualized for each patient, arrived at during preoperative discussions with the patient, and depending on risks and benefits, modified by good surgical judgment of the findings at operation. Endocrinologists who dictate to surgeons the type of operation to be performed, and the surgeons who obey, are doing a disservice to their patients. This is also true for thyroid surgery for pathologies other than Graves' disease.

Preserve Parathyroid Tissue and Leave as Small a Remnant as Possible

My own approach is based on the following convictions. Permanent hypocalcemia is a very serious and life-long complication that is to be avoided if at all possible (even in cancer cases). Less serious, but still representing a colossal failure of surgery, is recurrent hyperthyroidism for which ^{131}I usually is necessary but not desirable, because it was avoided in the first place in favor of surgery. I do not consider hypothyroidism a complication of surgery, because it is an expected, natural sequela that is readily treatable.

Bearing in mind these convictions, I approach each case by attempting to perform TT, but only if I can dissect out and preserve at least two parathyroid glands and their intact arterial supply. TT can still be done with autotransplantation of vascular compromised parathyroids. However, the average success of fresh parathyroid autografts is 82% (171). Therefore, I prefer a subtotal lobectomy that will preserve parathyroid function in nearly all cases, rather than a total lobectomy and autotransplantation for parathyroids that do not readily dissect on a vascular pedicle. I do a subtotal lobectomy (SL) if I cannot identify at least one parathyroid on a side. With these principles in mind, I wind up with preferably a total lobectomy with contralateral subtotal lobectomy (TL plus SL), or a BST if I cannot do a TT. When performing BST or TL plus SL, I strive to leave as small a remnant as possible (especially in young patients who have a higher incidence of recurrent hyperthyroidism), but in so doing I strive never to compromise parathyroid tissue or its blood supply.

Possible Advantage of Total Lobectomy and Contralateral Subtotal Lobectomy

Total lobectomy plus SL is beneficial in that if hyperthyroidism recurs and ^{131}I treatment is not chosen, repeat thyroidectomy involves only one side, and the risks of recurrent laryngeal nerve injury and hypoparathyroidism decrease accordingly. In addition, TL plus SL may become the operation of choice if the unilateral remnant can be reliably preserved on a vascular pedicle (arterial blood coming from branches of the inferior thyroid artery, and venous return to the middle thyroid vein) and placed laterally in the neck far from parathyroid tissue and recurrent nerve. This is potentially a new operation, in the developmental stages, for Graves' disease that offers the advantage of allowing us to leave a larger remnant (less hypothyroidism) and the luxury of safe reoperation for recurrent hyperfunction of the remnant.

Postoperative Follow-Up

After TT and TL plus SL, hypothyroidism is an expected outcome. The patient is automatically placed on replacement therapy with thyroxine, with anticipation that such therapy will be life-long. The patient understands the need for therapy and the symptoms and signs of hypothyroidism and hyperthyroidism, whether medically induced or representing recurrent hyperfunction. After BST, the patient is followed clinically and chemically for hypothyroidism, taking into account the occurrence of temporary hypothyroidism owing to pituitary suppression, so that replacement therapy is not prematurely started (3,37) (see Chapter 39). Because hypothyroidism will eventually occur in many patients [21% (35), 30% (32), 31% (3)], vigilance in follow-up is needed for decades. This is an undesirable aspect of BST, because some patients are lost to follow-up and become severely hypothyroid before diagnosis. In contrast, patients who received TT or TL plus SL and are placed immediately on thyroxine probably have less chance of experiencing undiagnosed hypothyroidism, because they understand and accept, in preoperative counseling, the need for life-long replacement therapy.

TOXIC MULTINODULAR GOITER AND TOXIC SOLITARY NODULE

Definition of Terms

The literature regarding toxic nodules is often confusing, partly because some terms are variably defined. The following terms are defined:

Hot nodule. A nodule showing increased uptake of radioactive iodine on scan. A nodule that appears hot on technetium (Tc) scan must be rescanned with iodine, because only isotopes of iodine reveal the physiology of the nodule: Tc is only trapped by the thyroid, but iodine is trapped and organified into T_3 and T_4.
Autonomous nodule. A hot nodule that is independent of TSH control (i.e., it shows autonomy). All autonomous nodules are hot but only some hot nodules are autonomous.
Toxic nodule. An autonomous nodule that produces hyperthyroidism (clinical or subclinical). All toxic nodules are autonomous, but only some autonomous nodules are toxic.
Functioning nodule. This term is variably defined in the literature. Some authors mean autonomous, others mean toxic, and some mean both. Some authors even refer to a hot nodule as a functioning nodule. These varying definitions in the literature are also reflected in the hospital and clinic. If you ask your colleagues (whether in internal, nuclear, or family medicine, or in endocrinology or surgery) to define these terms as I have done, you will hear these definitions and even some others. It is no wonder that many physicians find management of these nodules confusing. Because of the varying definitions of the term *functioning*, I avoid using the term. If it is used, it must be clearly defined.

Toxic Multinodular Goiter

Pathogenesis

The pathogenesis of toxic multinodular goiter (TMG) involves a progression in its development from nontoxic multinodular goiter. In most cases, a nontoxic multinodular goiter without autonomy will occur first. This goiter is dependent on TSH control and is suppressible, which means there is a normal TSH response to thyrotropin-releasing hormone (TRH) and it is suppressible by the T_3 suppression test. Because of this, it can be treated by thyroid suppression. This goiter may lead to the formation of a nontoxic multinodular goiter with autonomy. This goiter is autonomous or independent of TSH control and nonsuppressible (subnormal or absent TSH response to TRH, not suppressible by T_3 suppression test). Thus, it cannot be treated with thyroid suppression. This goiter may lead to the formation of the toxic multinodular goiter, in which case there are high levels of T_4 and T_3, and thyroid scan shows hot nodules. The high levels of T_4 and T_3 result in a low level of TSH because the pituitary is normal and responds appropriately, according to the principle of feedback inhibition. However, the nodules are autonomous of TSH control and continue to produce excessive thyroid hormone despite low levels of TSH.

Recent studies demonstrate a high prevalence (75%) of subclinical hyperthyroidism (suppressed TSH, lowered TSH response to TRH, with normal T_4 and T_3) in patients with nontoxic multinodular goiters without and with autonomy. Levels of basal TSH and TSH after TRH stimulation were lower in patients with multinodular goiter with autonomy than in patients with multinodular goiter without autonomy. Similarly, levels were lower in patients with multinodular goiter without autonomy than in controls. The number of nodules, and not their total volume, predicted hyperthyroidism (172).

Hyperthyroidism can be precipitated in the nontoxic multinodular goiter both with autonomy (173) and without autonomy, and it can be exacerbated in the TMG by iodides (expectorants, radiographic contrast media) (174). This is referred to as the Jod-Basedow phenomenon.

Clinical Features

The clinical features of TMG are considerably different from those of Graves' disease. TMG usually occurs after the age of 50 in patients with a preexisting history of a nontoxic multinodular goiter for many years. The hyperthyroidism is insidious in onset, is mild to severe, and is unaccompanied by the infiltrative ophthalmopathy and the dermopathy of Graves' disease. Like its precursor, nontoxic multinodular goiter, the incidence is many times higher in women than in men. In older patients, the hyperthyroidism may be masked, and the patient may present with cardiac findings such as atrial fibrillation, tachycardia, congestive heart failure, unexplained or accelerated angina, unexplained weight loss, anxiety, or insomnia. The elderly patient with hyperthyroidism may present with muscle wasting, and 20% of the patients with TMG have no thyromegaly on clinical examination.

Toxic Solitary Nodule

Pathogenesis

Most toxic solitary nodules (TSNs) are follicular adenomas, but rarely are they carcinomas (see later). There is progression in the development of TSN as there is with TMG. First, there is a nontoxic solitary hot nodule without autonomy. Thyroid scan shows a hot nodule that is dependent on TSH control and thus is suppressible by the T_3 suppression test. Also, the response of TSH to TRH is normal. This nodule can be treated by thyroid hormone. It may grow slowly and progressively increase in function over many years, leading to a nontoxic, solitary hot nodule with autonomy. This new nodule is independent of TSH control and nonsuppressible by the T_3 suppression test, and the response of TSH to TRH is subnormal or absent. Hence, this nodule cannot be treated with thyroid hormone. As it grows, this nodule produces more thyroid hormone, and the remaining thyroid tissue becomes increasingly inactive, with the appearance on scan of function only in the hot nodule. Radioactive iodine uptake may be increased, but the serum T_3 and T_4 levels are normal at this stage, with the T_3 level often at the upper range of normal. This nodule may then lead to the TSN. Usually, hyperthyroidism does not occur until the nodule is 2.5 cm to 3.0 cm in diameter.

Clinical Features

The TSN ordinarily occurs in patients in their 30s, 40s, or 50s. There are high serum levels of T_4 and T_3. Occasionally, the serum T_3 level becomes elevated before T_4 (T_3 toxicosis) (175) and radioactive iodine uptake is normal to high. The high levels of T_4 and T_3 cause a low level of TSH, but the nodule is autonomous of TSH control and continues to make excessive thyroid hormone despite low TSH levels. The symptoms and signs of hyperthyroidism are milder than in Graves' disease and are unaccompanied by the infiltrative ophthalmopathy and dermopathy.

Treatment of Hot and Autonomous Nodules

Treatment of the solitary hot nodule (nontoxic and suppressible) consists of either thyroid suppression or continued observation. If enlargement or other findings suggestive of malignancy occur, thyroidectomy can be performed.

Treatment of the nontoxic autonomous solitary hot nodule is controversial. There is little concern that an autonomous nodule is carcinoma, as this is a rare event, less than 1% according to most studies (176–179). Most of the reports have been individual case reports because of its rarity (180,181). Eyre-Brook and Talbot (182) found one follicular carcinoma in 60 surgically removed autonomous toxic nodules, and Horst et al. (183) found none in 306 patients. Although more recent studies show a higher rate [9 cancers in 227 toxic nodules (4%) (51), 2 in 40 toxic nodules (5%) (60), 8% of toxic nodules (63), and 2 of 17 autonomous nodules (12%) (184)], the consensus in the literature is that there is a very low chance that an autonomous nodule (toxic or nontoxic) will harbor carcinoma.

Can we predict which autonomous nodules will become toxic and how often? After a 6-year follow-up, 20% of autonomous nodules larger than 3 cm became toxic (175). After a 5-year follow-up, 15% of autonomous nodules of all sizes became toxic (185). Smaller nodules have less chance of turning toxic. Therefore, some physicians recommend only close follow-up of these patients to detect early hyperthyroidism. However, some recommend unilateral thyroid lobectomy; after lobectomy, all patients remain euthyroid on follow-up after 10 years (182). However, at least 80% of these operations will be unnecessary (i.e., at least 80% of the patients do not become hyperthyroid) (175). Another study showed a mean incidence of developing toxicity of 4% per year, with the incidence increasing during follow-up (3% in the first 7 years, 10% in the following years). Age, gender, nodule size (in contrast to the previous study), and initial scintigraphic appearance did not predict toxicity. However, after iodine excess (by history or elevated urinary iodine levels), 31% became toxic (186). Therefore, a prudent surgical approach is thyroid lobectomy for autonomous nodules, especially those larger than 3 cm in good-risk patients with a likelihood of iodine exposure who prefer quick resolution of the problem rather than long-term follow-up. ^{131}I is another treatment alternative.

Preoperative Preparation

Considerations for the preoperative preparation of the patient with TMG or TSN to eliminate the risk of thyroid storm are the same as in Graves' disease cases (see previous section). Maximal safety is assured with thionamides (with or without beta-blockers) until chemical and clinical euthyroidism is achieved. Because TMG and glands with TSN are not diffusely vascular, iodine is generally not used, especially because iodine can worsen the hyperthyroidism.

Treatment of TMG

Reasons for surgery as the treatment of choice for TMG are stronger than for the treatment of Graves' disease. In Graves' disease, long-lasting spontaneous and thionamide-induced remissions occur in no more than 25% of patients (40). This figure is even lower in patients with TMG. A recent study compared the relapse rate in patients with Graves' disease and TMG. After euthyroidism was achieved, all patients received thionamides for at least 1 year and were followed for a minimum of 2 years. Relapse occurred in 95% of patients with TMG and in 34% with Graves' disease (187). Long-term thionamide therapy for TMG is not desirable and ablative therapy (surgery or ^{131}I) is preferable.

In patients with TMG, large and often multiple doses of ^{131}I (>50 mCi) are necessary to produce control of the hyperthyroidism because of the large size of the goiter and the lower uptake of ^{131}I in comparison with Graves' disease. Such large doses are not considered undesirable in the older patient with TMG, but they are undesirable in the younger patient, although as discussed in a previous section and in Chapter 16, no long-term carcinogenic or mutagenic effects of ^{131}I have been proven. Although ^{131}I will treat the hyperthyroidism, clinical experience and reports (188) show it will not substantially reduce goiter size, compressive symptoms, or substernal extension, because TMG contains nonfunctioning nodules and areas of fibrosis and calcification. However, a recent study using magnetic resonance imaging showed significant reduction in thyroid volume and tracheal deviation and an increase in cross-sectional area of the tracheal lumen after treatment of toxic and nontoxic multinodular goiter with 100 µCi ^{131}I per gram of thyroid tissue (189). Generally, surgery is preferred over ^{131}I in patients with large goiter size and compressive symptoms. However, ^{131}I is preferable in patients in poor general health and less able to tolerate anesthesia and surgery. The younger the patient, the better the general medical status, and the larger the goiter, especially with substernal extension and compressive symptoms, the more strongly thyroidectomy is recommended over ^{131}I for TMG.

Treatment of Toxic Solitary Nodule

In deciding among thionamide, ^{131}I, and surgery as treatment for TSN, we must compare their success in terms of avoiding hyperthyroidism (recurrent or persistent) and hypothyroidism, and in terms of achieving nodule regression.

Avoiding Recurrent and Persistent Hyperthyroidism

Thionamides

In Graves' disease, long-lasting remissions occur in no more than 25% of patients (40) after thionamide treatment. This figure is even lower in patients with TSN, making long-term thionamide therapy less desirable and ablative therapy (surgery or ^{131}I) the preferable choice.

^{131}I

In treating TSN, ^{131}I is effective, although generally doses must be larger (25 to 40 mCi) (182) than those required for Graves' disease, making this therapy less desirable than surgery, especially in the younger age group. However, Ross (190) cured 90% of his cases with a mean dose of 10 mCi ^{131}I. The successful use of such low doses of ^{131}I has not been confirmed by other researchers. Eyre-Brook and Talbot (182) found a relapse rate of 73% in patients treated with doses of 1.2 to 15 mCi. McCormack and Sheline (191) found a relapse rate of 47% with doses of 6 to 14 mCi, but no relapses with doses of 28 to 56 mCi. O'Brien et al. (192), using a median dose of 29 mCi, found a 4.4% incidence of persistent hyperthyroidism and 0% incidence of recurrence. As higher doses of ^{131}I are used, recurrent or persistent hyperthyroidism and the need for retreatment decreases. The dose needed to avoid recurrent or persistent hyperthyroidism increases as the size of the nodule increases (see Chapter 16).

Surgery

A unilateral thyroid lobectomy cures all patients and does not result in any cases of recurrent or persistent hyperthyroidism (182,192).

Avoiding Hypothyroidism

Thionamides

Overtreatment can cause temporary hypothyroidism. However, there is no risk of permanent hypothyroidism during thionamide treatment, because this treatment is reversible.

^{131}I

There is a low incidence of hypothyroidism after ^{131}I treatment with reported rates of 0% (190,193), 35% (192), and 36% (194). These rates are much lower than those occurring after ^{131}I treatment for Graves' disease. In the latter, the entire gland receives a large radiation dose because the entire gland is under the uniform influence of TSIs. With TSN, only the nodule is autonomous; thyroid tissue surrounding the nodule and in the opposite lobe is suppressed because it is normal thyroid tissue with little or no TSH stimulation. Because the suppressed thyroid tissue does not receive a substantial dose of ^{131}I, the incidence of hypothyroidism is low. As higher doses of ^{131}I are used, there is a greater risk of hypothyroidism. As doses are lowered, there is less hypothyroidism, but there is an increased need for retreatment for recurrent and persistent hyperthyroidism.

Surgery

After unilateral thyroid lobectomy for TSN, the incidence of hypothyroidism is also low, with reported rates of 14.3% (195) and 22% (192).

Achieving Nodule Regression

Although ^{131}I does not cause thyroid cancer and the chance of a toxic nodule being a cancer is extremely small, persistence of the nodule after any treatment is often worrisome for patient and doctor. If the nodule persists, careful follow-up is necessary. The ideal treatment would provide complete nodule regression. After thionamide treatment, there is little chance of nodule regression, because once the thionamides are stopped, the chance of recurrent hyperthyroidism is excellent. After ^{131}I treatment, complete nodule regression occurred in 56.3% (192), 36% (94), and 2.2% (190) of cases. As higher doses of ^{131}I are used, there is greater chance of complete nodule regression. Thyroid lobectomy, of course, provides absolute removal of the nodule and the added benefit of tissue in cases of suspected carcinoma.

Conclusion

In addition to thionamides, surgery, and ^{131}I, injection of sclerosing agents such as ethanol can be, but seldom are, used for toxic and autonomous, nontoxic nodules. For toxic nodules, ethanol failed to control hyperthyroidism in 9% of patients and nodules regressed by 60% in volume. Exacerbation of hyperthyroidism and temporary vocal cord paralysis can occur. Multiple injections (3 to 13) are needed (196,197).

Surgery provides absolute cure with no recurrent or persistent hyperthyroidism and total removal of the nodule. Hypothyroidism occurs similarly as after ^{131}I. Surgery also provides tissue in cases of suspected carcinoma. Therefore, surgery is the treatment of choice for most patients with TSN. The only objections are the need for an operation, increased costs compared with ^{131}I, and the risks specifically caused by surgery, but these risks are minimal. Because unilateral thyroid lobectomy is performed, the risk of vocal cord paralysis is minimal and the risk of hypoparathyroidism is zero (182).

Extent of Surgery

This topic has been discussed in detail in the preceding section on Graves' disease. Several large studies comparing the results of BST for Graves' disease and TMG show that recurrent hyperthyroidism remains a problem in Graves' disease patients (3.2% incidence) but not for those with TMG (0% incidence) (32,39). For this reason, total thyroidectomy or total lobectomy and contralateral subtotal lobectomy in Graves' disease cases is preferred when this can be done safely. Otherwise, BST can be done. In surgery for TMG, BST certainly seems adequate treatment to avoid recurrent hyperthyroidism, and it offers the benefit of leaving enough remnant to decrease the chance of hypothyroidism.

There are three choices in surgery for TSN: nodulectomy, subtotal lobectomy, and total lobectomy. The minimal thyroid operation is a subtotal or total lobectomy. For many reasons, this is the standard when malignancy is suspected. Enucleation or nodulectomy of solitary nodules is to be condemned, because pathologic evaluation to diagnose carcinoma requires analysis of the tumor–capsule–thyroid interface to identify capsular invasion (see Chapter 6). Also, a frozen section diagnosis of a nodule may prove benign, but a permanent section malignant. If only a nodulectomy was done, reoperation with its attendant higher risks would be required to complete the total lobectomy. However, if a lobectomy had been done in the first place, frequently no further surgery would be required, even for a malignant nodule. Although malignancy is usually not suspected in TSNs, these considerations still apply to their proper surgical removal. If the surgeon performs a nodulectomy, most probably the proper identification of the recurrent laryngeal nerve and parathyroid tissue will be dispensed with and thus complications will increase. Also, a TSN may represent the first manifestation of toxic multinodular goiter. Histologic and radioautographic studies (198) have shown autonomous micronodules in the extranodular thyroid tissue in 76% of patients with a large, solitary, autonomous toxic nodule, so removing just the nodule frequently leaves behind autonomous tissue that may produce future toxicity. Reoperation of these patients is associated with higher complications. Therefore, it does not seem logical to perform a nodulectomy—it is more dangerous and often fails to remove enough tissue to diagnose and treat the patient adequately. I favor total lobectomy over subtotal lobectomy for reasons discussed in the section titled, Thyroid Remnant and Risks of Thyroid Surgery. However, both are excellent treatments and can be used on the basis of the surgeon's judgment.

SPECIAL CONSIDERATIONS IN SURGERY FOR HYPERTHYROIDISM

Various rare congenital thyroid abnormalities and complications of hyperthyroidism can result in unusual presentations of hyperthyroidism. Of 102 patients with hemiaplasia of the thyroid gland, 32 were reported to be associated with hyperthyroidism. Of these 32, the cause of hyperthyroidism was Graves' disease in 22, TSN in 7, and TMG in 3 (199). In addition to congenital absence of a thyroid lobe, patients may have acquired absence of a lobe (because of prior unilateral thyroid lobectomy for benign or malignant disease) and may develop hyperthyroidism. Superior vena cava syndrome can rarely be caused by intrathoracic thyroid enlargement caused by TMG (200).

ACKNOWLEDGMENT

The author thanks Neal Goldman, M.D., for his many helpful suggestions during the preparation of this manuscript.

REFERENCES

1. Falk SA. Hyperthyroidism: a surgeon's perspective. In: English GM, ed. *Otolaryngology*. Philadelphia: Harper & Row, 1985;4–70.
2. Galkin EV, Grakov BS, Protopopov AV. First clinical experience of radio-endovascular functional thyroidectomy in the treatment of diffuse toxic goiter. *Vestn Rentgenol Radiol* 1994;3:29–35.
3. Cusick EL, Krukowski ZH, Matheson NA. Outcome of surgery for Graves' disease re-examined. *Br J Surg* 1987;74:780–783.
4. Heimann P, Martinson J. Surgical treatment of thyrotoxicosis: results of 272 operations with special reference to preoperative treatment with anti-thyroid drugs and L-thyroxine. *Br J Surg* 1975;62:683–688.
5. Khadra M, Delbridge L, Reeve TS, et al. Total thyroidectomy: its role in the management of thyroid disease. *Aust N Z J Surg* 1992;62:91–95.
6. Pimpl W, Rieger R, Waclawiczek HW, et al. The technique of recurrent laryngeal nerve exposure within the scope of interventions of the thyroid gland. *Wien Klin Wochenschr* 1992;104:439–442.
7. Melliere D, Scattolini G, Germain V, et al. The results of 300 operations for hyperthyroidism. *Nouv Presse Med* 1980;9:2121–2124.
8. Kasuga Y, Sugenoya A, Kobayashi S, et al. Clinical evaluation of the response to surgical treatment of Graves' disease. *Surg Gynecol Obstet* 1990;170:327–330.
9. Blondeau P, Wolfeler L, Rene L. Surgical treatment for Graves' disease. *Ann Chir* 1978;32:779–787.
10. Sugrue D, McEvoy M, Feeley J, et al. Hyperthyroidism in the land of Graves: results of treatment by surgery, radioiodine and carbimazole in 837 cases. *Q J Med* 1980;49:51–61.
11. Reeve TS, Delbridge L, Cohen A, Crummer P. Total thyroidectomy: the preferred option for multinodular goiter. *Ann Surg* 1987;206:782–786.
12. Winsa B, Rastad J, Akerstrom G, et al. Retrospective evaluation of subtotal and total thyroidectomy in Graves' disease with and without endocrine ophthalmopathy. *Eur J Endocrinol* 1995;132:406–412.
13. Winsa B, Rastad J, Larsson E, et al. Total thyroidectomy in therapy-resistant Graves' disease. *Surgery* 1994;116:1068–1075.
14. Ozoux JP, de Calan L, Portier G, Rivallain B, Favre JP, et al. Surgical treatment of Graves' disease. *Am J Surg* 1988;156:177–181.
15. Patwardhan NA, Moront M, Rao S, et al. Surgery still has a role in Graves' hyperthyroidism. *Surgery* 1993;114:1108–1113.
16. Perzik SL. The place of total thyroidectomy in the management of 909 patients with thyroid disease. *Am J Surg* 1976;132:480–483.
17. Clark OH. Total thyroidectomy: the treatment of choice for patients with differentiated thyroid cancer. *Ann Surg* 1982;196:361–370.
18. Attie JN, Khafif RA. Preservation of parathyroid glands during total thyroidectomy. *Am J Surg* 1975;130:399–404.
19. Palestini N, Valori MR, Carlin R, et al. Mortality, morbidity and long term results in surgically treated hyperthyroid patients. *Acta Chir Scand* 1985;151:509–513.
20. Jacobs JK, Aland JW, Ballinger JF. Total thyroidectomy. *Ann Surg* 1983;197:542–548.
21. Dobyns BM, Sheline GE, Workman, et al. Malignant and benign neoplasms of the thyroid in patients treated for hyperthyroidism: a report of the cooperative thyrotoxicosis therapy follow up study. *J Clin Endocrinol Metab* 1974;38:976–988.
22. Safa AM, Schumacher OP, Rodriguez-Antunez A. Long term follow up results in children and adolescents treated with radioactive iodine (^{131}I) for hyperthyroidism. *N Engl J Med* 1975;292:167–171.
23. Fujii H. A long-term follow-up study of late-onset hypothyroidism and prognosis of hyperthyroid patients treated with radioiodine. *Jpn J Nucl Med* 1991;28:1067–73.
24. Ozaki O, Ito K, Mimura T, et al. Thyroid carcinoma after radioiodine therapy for Graves' disease. *World J Surg* 1994;18:518–521.
25. Tezelman S, Grossman RF, Siperstein AE, et al. Radioiodine-associated thyroid cancers. *World J Surg* 1994;18:522–528.
26. Maxon HR, Thomas S, Saenger EL, Buncher CR, Kereikas JG. Ionizing radiation and the induction of clinically significant disease in the human thyroid gland. *Am J Med* 1977;63:967–978.
27. Nofal MM, Beierwaltes WH, Patno ME. Treatment of hyperthyroidism with sodium iodide: a 16 year experience. *JAMA* 1966;197:605–610.
28. Leese GP, Jung RT, Scott A, et al. Long term follow-up of treated hyperthyroid and hypothyroid patients. *Health Bull* 1993;51:177–183.
29. Farnell MB, Van Heerden JA, McConahey WM, et al. Hypothyroidism after thyroidectomy for Graves' disease. *Am J Surg* 1981;142:535–538.
30. Kasuga Y, Sugenoya A, Kobayashi S, et al. Significance of values of thyrotropin binding inhibitor immunoglobulins and appearance of intrathyroidal lymphocytes at subtotal thyroidectomy for Graves' disease. *J Am Coll Surg* 1994;178:589–594.
31. Sugino K, Mimura T, Toshima K, et al. Follow-up evaluation of patients with Graves' disease treated by subtotal thyroidectomy and risk factor analysis for post-operative thyroid dysfunction. *J Endocrinol Invest* 1993;16:195–199.
32. Simms JM, Talbot CH. Surgery for thyrotoxicosis. *Br J Surg* 1983;70:581–583.
33. Jortso E, Lennquist S, Lundstrom B, Norrby K, Smeds S. The influence of remnant size, antithyroid antibodies, thyroid morphology, and lymphocyte infiltration on thyroid function after subtotal resection for hyperthyroidism. *World J Surg* 1987;11:365–371.
34. Blondeau P. Surgical treatment of hyperthyroidism. *Bull Acad Natl Med* 1991;175:1065–1073.
35. Sugrue DD, Drury MI, McEvoy M, Heffernan SJ, O'Malley E. Long term follow up of hyperthyroid patients treated by subtotal thyroidectomy. *Br J Surg* 1983;70:408–411.
36. Reid DJ. Hyperthyroidism and hypothyroidism complicating the treatment of thyrotoxicosis. *Br J Surg* 1987;74:1060–1062.
37. Toft AD, Irvine WJ, Sinclair I, McIntosh D, et al. Thyroid function after surgical treatment of thyrotoxicosis: a report of 100 cases treated with propranolol before operation. *N Engl J Med* 1978;298:643–647.
38. Noguchi S, Murakami N, Noguchi A. Surgical treatment for Graves' disease: a long term follow-up of 325 patients. *Br J Surg* 1981;68:105–108.

39. Melliere D, Etienne G, Becquemin JP. Operations for hyperthyroidism. *Am J Surg* 1988;155:395–399.
40. Orgiazzi J. Management of Graves's hyperthyroidism. *Endocrinol Metab Clin North Am* 1987;16:365–389.
41. Bouma DJ, Kammer H, Greer MA. Follow up comparison of short term versus 1 year antithyroid drug therapy for the thyrotoxicosis of Graves' disease. *J Clin Endocrinol Metab* 1982;55:1138.
42. Klein I, Becker DV, Level GS. Treatment of hyperthyroid disease. *Ann Intern Med* 1994;121:281–288.
43. Laurberg P, Buchholtz-Hansen PE, Iverson E, et al. Goiter size and outcome of medical treatment of Graves' disease. *Acta Endocrinol (Copenh)* 1986;111:39.
44. Takamatsu J, Kuma K, Mozai T. Serum triiodothyronine to thyroxine ratio: a newly recognized predictor of the outcome of hyperthyroidism due to Graves' disease. *J Clin Endocrinol Metab* 1986;62:980.
45. Burman KD, Baker JR. Immune mechanisms in Graves' disease. *Endocr Rev* 1985;6:183.
46. Wilson R, McKippop JH, Hendersen N, et al. The ability of the serum thyrotrophin receptor antibody (TRAb) index and HLA status to predict long-term remission of thyrotoxicosis following medical therapy for Graves' disease. *Clin Endocrinol* 1986;25:151–156.
47. Schleusener H. Prospective multicentre study on the prediction of relapse after antithyroid drug treatment in patients with Graves' disaese. *Acta Endocrinol* 1989;120:689–701.
48. Gossage AAR, Crawly JCW, Copping S, et al. Thyroid function and immunological activity during and after medical treatment of Graves' disease. *Clin Endocrinol* 1983;19:87–96.
49. Hashizume K, Ichikawa K, Sakurai, et al. Administration of thyroxine in treated Graves' disease. Effects on the level of antibodies to thyroid-stimulating hormone receptors and on the risk of recurrence of hyperthyroidism. *N Engl J Med* 1991;324:947–953.
50. Pacini F, DiCoscio GC, Anelli S, et al. Thyroid carcinoma in thyrotoxicosis patients treated by surgery. *J Endocrinol Invest* 1988;11:107–112.
51. Belfiore A, Garofalo MR, Giuffrida D, et al. Increased aggressiveness of thyroid cancer in patients with Graves' disease. *J Clin Endocrinol Metab* 1990;70:830–835.
52. Hancock BW, Bing RF, Dirmikis SM, et al. Thyroid carcinoma and concurrent hyperthyroidism. *Cancer* 1977;39:298–302.
53. Wahl RA, Goreyzki P, Meybier H, et al. Coexistence of hyperthyroidism and thyroid cancer. *World J Surg* 1982;6:385–390.
54. Riger R, Pimpl W, Money S, et al. Hyperthyroidism and concurrent thyroid malignancies. *Surgery* 1989;106:6–10.
55. Chou F, Sheen-Chen S, Chen Y, et al. Hyperthyroidism and concurrent thyroid cancer. *Int Surg* 1993;78:343–346.
56. Sokal JE. Incidence of malignancy in toxic and nontoxic nodular goiter. *JAMA* 1954;154:1321–1325.
57. Ozaki O, Ito K, Kobayashi K, et al. Thyroid carcinoma in Graves' disease. *World J Surg* 1990;14:437–440.
58. Krause U, Olgricht T, Metz K, et al. Frequency of thyroid gland carcinoma in hyperthyroidism. *Deutsche Med Wochenschr* 1991;116:201–206.
59. Ahuja S, Ernst H. Hyperthyroidism and thyroid carcinoma. *Acta Endocrinol* 1991;124:146–151.
60. Zanella E. Surgical therapy of the autonomous thyroid nodule. *Minerva Endocrinol* 1993;18:165–167.
61. Kasuga Y, Sugenoya A, Kobayashi S, et al. The outcome of patients with thyroid carcinoma and Graves' disease. *Surg Today* 1993;23:9–12.
62. Farbota LM, Calandra DB, Lawrence AM, et al. Thyroid carcinoma in Graves' disease. *Surgery* 1985;98:1148–1153.
63. Terzioglu T, Tezelman S, Onaran Y, et al. Concurrent hyperthyroidism and thyroid carcinoma. *Br J Surg* 1993;80:1301–1302.
64. Shapiro SJ, Friedmann NB, Perzik SL, et al. Incidence of thyroid carcinoma in Graves' disease. *Cancer* 1970;26:1261–1270.
65. Mazzaferri EL. Thyroid cancer and Graves' disease. *J Clin Endocrinol Metab* 1990;70:826–829.
66. Behar R, Arganini M, Wu TC, et al. Graves' disease and thyroid cancer. *Surgery* 1986;100:1121–1127.
67. Filetti S, Belfiore A, Amir SM, et al. The role of thyroid-stimulating antibodies of Graves' disease in differentiated thyroid cancer. *N Engl J Med* 1988;318:753–759.
68. Nicolosi A, Addis E, Calo PG, et al. Hyperthyroidism and cancer of the thyroid. *Minerva Chir* 1994;49:491–495.
69. Hales IB, McElduff A, Crummer P, et al. Does Graves' disease or thyrotoxicosis affect the prognosis of thyroid cancer. *J Clin Endocrinol Metab* 1992;75:886–889.
70. Yeo PP, Wang KW, Sinniah R, et al. Thyrotoxicosis and thyroid cancer. *Aust N Z J Med* 1982;12:589–593.
71. Hermann M, Richter B, Roka R, et al. Thyroid surgery in untreated severe hyperthyroidism: perioperative kinetics of free thyroid hormones in the glandular venous effluent and peripheral blood. *Surgery* 1994;115:240–245.
72. Frilling A, Goretzki PE, Horster FA, et al. Subtotal thyroid gland resection as therapy for thyrotoxic crises. *Dtsch Med Wochenschr* 1990;115:735–739.
73. Schaaf L, Grescher M, Paschke R, et al. Thyrotoxic crisis in Graves' disease: indication for immediate surgery. *Klin Wochenschr* 1990;68:1037–1041.
74. Farwell AP, Abend SL, Huang SK, et al. Thyroidectomy for amiodarone-induced thyrotoxicosis. *JAMA* 1990;263:1526–1528.
75. Brennan MD, Heerden JAV, Carney JA. Amiodarone-associated thyrotoxicosis: experience with surgical management. *Surgery* 1987;102:1062–1067.
76. Meurisse M, Hamoir E, D'Silva M, et al. Amiodarone-induced thyrotoxicosis: is there a place for surgery? *World J Surg* 1993;17:622–626.
77. Falk SA, Birken EA, Ronquillo A. Graves' disease associated with histologic Hashimoto's thyroiditis. *Otolaryngol Head Neck Surg* 1985;93:86–91.
78. Bauer FK, Catz B. Radioactive iodine therapy for progressive malignant exophthalmos. *Acta Endocrinol (Copenh)* 1966;51:15–28.
79. Catz B, Perzik SL. Total thyroidectomy in thyrotoxic and euthyroid Graves' disease. *Am J Surg* 1969;118:434–439.
80. Gwinup G, Elias AN, Aseler MS. Effect on exophthalmos of various methods of treatment of Graves' disease. *JAMA* 1982;247:2135–2138.
81. Marushak D, Faurschon S, Blichert-Toft M. Regression of ophthalmopathy in Graves' disease following thyroidectomy. *Acta Ophthalmol (Copenh)* 1984;82:767–779.
82. Vana S, Rezek P, Lukas J, et al. Surgical treatment of endocrine orbital disease. *Vnitr Lek* 1992;38:897–902.
83. Catz B. Controversies in the management of Graves' ophthalmopathy. In: Falk SA, ed. *Thyroid disease: endocrinology, surgery, nuclear medicine and radiotherapy.* New York: Raven Press, 1990;275–277.
84. Sanchez J, Pradas J, Martinez O, et al. Graves' ophthalmopathy after subtotal thyroidectomy and radioiodine therapy. *Br J Surg* 1993;80:1134–1136.
85. Czaky G, Balazs G, Bako G, et al. Late results of thyroid surgery for hyperthyroidism in childhood. *Prog Pediatr Surg* 1991;26:31–40.
86. Huo BZ, Du RY, Huang CT, et al. The fate of exophthalmos after subtotal thyroidectomy in hyperthyroidism. *Chin Med J* 1988;101:137–140.
87. Frilling A, Goretzki PE, Grussendorf M, et al. The influence of surgery on endocrine ophthalmopathy. *World J Surg* 1990;14:442–445.
88. Bartalena L, Marcocci C, Bogazzi F, et al. Use of corticosteroids to prevent progression of Graves' ophthalmopathy after radioiodine therapy for hyperthyroidism. *N Engl J Med* 1989;321:1349–1352.
89. Werner SC, Feind CR, Aida M. Graves' disease and total thyroidectomy: progression of severe eye changes and decrease in serum long acting thyroid stimulator after operation. *N Engl J Med* 1967;276:132–138.
90. Peguegnat EP, Mayberry WE, McConahey WM, Hanson KC. Large doses of radioiodide in Graves' disease: effect on ophthalmopathy and long-acting thyroid stimulator. *Mayo Clin Proc* 1967;42:802.
91. Calissendorff BM, Soderstrom M, Alveryd A. Ophthalmopathy and hyperthyroidism—a comparison between patients receiving different antithyroid treatments. *Acta Ophthalmol (Copenh)* 1986;64:698–703.
92. Vazquez-Chavez C, Nishimura ME, Espinosa SL, et al. Effect of the treatment of hyperthyroidism on the course of exophthalmos. *Rev Invest Clin* 1992;44:241–247.
93. Levitt M, Edis A, Agnello R, et al. The effect of subtotal thyroidectomy on Graves' ophthalmopathy. *World J Surg* 1988;12:593–597.
94. Tallstedt L, Lundell G, Torring O, et al. Occurrence of ophthalmopathy after treatment for Graves' hyperthyroidism. *N Engl J Med* 1992;326:1733–1738.
95. Bartalena L, Marcocci C, Bogazzi F, et al. Use of corticosteroids to prevent progression of Graves' ophthalmopathy after radioiodine therapy for hyperthyroidism. *N Engl J Med* 1989;321:1349.
96. Harvey RD, Metcalfe RA, Morteo C, et al. Acute pre-tibial myxoedema following radioiodine therapy for thyrotoxic Graves' disease. *Clin Endocrinol* 1995;42:657–660.
97. Sridama V, Degroot LJ. Treatment of Graves' disease and the course of ophthalmopathy. *Am J Med* 1989;87:70–73.

98. Robson AM. Vocal cord paralysis after treatment of thyrotoxicosis with radioiodine. *Br J Radiol* 1981;54:632.
99. Burch WM, Pasillico JT. Hypoparathyroidism after ^{131}I therapy with subsequent return of parathyroid function. *J Clin Endocrinol Metab* 1983;57:398–401.
100. Wiersinga WM, Touber JS. The influence of β-adrenoreceptor blocking agents on plasma thyroxine and triiodothyronine. *J Clin Endocrinol Metab* 1977;45:293–298.
101. Bergfelt G. Preoperative treatment of thyrotoxicosis with antithyroid drugs and thyroxine. *J Clin Endocrinol* 1961;21:72–79.
102. Romaldini JH, Bromberg N, Werner RS, et al. Comparison of effects of high and low dosage regimens of antithyroid drugs in the management of Graves' hyperthyroidism. *J Clin Endocrinol Metab* 1983;57:563–570.
103. Cooper DS, Goldminz D, Levin AA, Ladenson PW, et al. Agranulocytosis associated with antithyroid drugs. *Ann Intern Med* 1983;98:26–29.
104. Cooper DS. Antithyroid drugs. *N Engl J Med* 1984;311:1353–1362.
105. Edmonds CJ, Tellez M. Treatment of Graves' disease by carbimazole: high dose with thyroxine compared to titration dose. *Eur J Endocrinol* 1994;131:120–124.
106. Reinwein D, Benker G, et al. and the European Multicenter Group on Antithyroid Drug Treatment. A prospective randomized trial of antithyroid drug dose in Graves' disease therapy. *J Clin Endocrinol Metab* 1993;76:1516–1521.
107. Califano G, Abate S, Ferulano GP, Danzi M. Surgery of toxic goiter: indications and long term results. *Ital J Surg Sci* 1985;15:233–237.
108. Wartofsky L, Rausil BJ, Ingbar SH. Inhibition by iodine of the release of thyroxine from the thyroid glands of patients with thyrotoxicosis. *J Clin Invest* 1970;49:78–86.
109. Feek CM, Sawers SA, Irvine WJ, et al. Combination of potassium iodide and propranolol in preparation of patients with Graves' disease for thyroid surgery. *N Engl J Med* 1980;302:883–885.
110. Emerson CH, Anderson AJ, Howard WH, Utiger RD. Serum thyroxine and triiodothyronine concentrations during iodide treatment of hyperthyroidism. *J Clin Endocrinol Metab* 1975;40:33–36.
111. Thompson WO, Thompson PK, Bailey G, Cohen AC. Prolonged treatment of exophthalmic goiter by iodine alone. *Arch Intern Med* 1930;45:481–502.
112. Bartels EC. Use of thiouracil in the preoperative preparation of patients with severe hyperthyroidism. *Ann Intern Med* 1945;22:365–372.
113. Reinhoff WF Jr. The histologic changes brought about in cases of exophthalmic goiter by the administration of iodine. *Bull Johns Hopkins Hosp* 1925;37:385–406.
114. Marigold JH, Morgan AK, Earle DJ, Young AE, Croft DN. Lugol's iodine: its effect on thyroid blood flow in patients with thyrotoxicosis. *Br J Surg* 1985;72:45–47.
115. Brownlie BEW, Turner JG, Ellwood MA, Rogers TGH, Armstrong DI. Thyroid vascularity-documentation of the iodide effect in thyrotoxicosis. *Acta Endocrinol (Copenh)* 1977;86:317–322.
116. Harrower ADB, Fyffe JA, Horn DB, et al. Thyroxine and triiodothyronine levels in hyperthyroid patients during treatment with propranolol. *Clin Endocrinol* 1977;7:41–44.
117. Zonszein J, Santangelo RP, Mackin JF, et al. Propranolol therapy in thyrotoxicosis: a review of 84 patients undergoing surgery. *Am J Med* 1979;66:411–416.
118. Lee TC, Coffey RJ, Curier BM, et al. Propranolol and thyroidectomy in the treatment of thyrotoxicosis. *Ann Surg* 1982;195:766–773.
119. Lennquist S, Jortso E, Anderberg B, Smeds S. Beta blockers compared with antithyroid drugs as preoperative treatment in hyperthyroidism: drug tolerance, complications, and postoperative thyroid function. *Surgery* 1985;98:1141–1146.
119a. Lee KS, Kim K, Hur KB, Kim CK. The role of propranolol in the preoperative preparation of patients with Graves' disease. *Surg Gynecol Obstet* 1986;162:365–369.
120. Rubenfeld S, Silverman VE, Welch KMA, et al. Variable plasma propranolol levels in thyrotoxicosis. *N Engl J Med* 1979;300:353–354.
121. Shand DG, Nuekolls EM, Oates JA. Plasma propranolol levels in adults. *Clin Pharmacol Ther* 1970;11:112.
122. Feely J, Hamilton WF, Forrest AL, et al. Beta-blocking drugs and thyroid function. *Br Med J [Clin Res]* 1977;2:1352.
123. Toft AD, Irvine WJ, McIntosh D, et al. Propranolol in the treatment of thyrotoxicosis by subtotal thyroidectomy. *J Clin Endocrinol Metab* 1976;43:1312–1316.
124. Anderberg B, Kagedal B, Nilsson OR, et al. Propranolol and thyroid resection for hyperthyroidism. *Acta Chir Scand* 1979;145:297–303.
125. Gerst PH, Fildes J, Baylor P, Zonszein J. Long acting beta-adrenergic antagonists as preparation for surgery for thyrotoxicosis. *Arch Surg* 1986;121:838–840.
126. Thorne AC, Bedford RF. Esmolol for peri-operative management of thyrotoxic goiter. *Anesthesiology* 1989;71:291–294.
127. Byrd RC, Sung RJ, Marks J. Safety and efficacy of esmolol for control of ventricular rate in supraventricular tachycardia. *J Am Coll Cardiol* 1984;3:394–399.
128. Brunette DD, Rothong C. Emergency department mangement of thyrotoxic crisis with esmolol. *Am J Emerg Med* 1991;9:232–234.
129. Isley WL, Dahl S, Gibbs H. Use of esmolol in managing a thyrotoxic patient needing emergency surgery. *Am J Med* 1990;89:122–123.
130. Adlerberth A, Stenstrom G, Hasselgren P. The selective beta 1-blocking agent metoprolol compared with antithyroid drug and thyroxine as preoperative treatment of patients with hyperthyroidism. *Ann Surg* 1987;205:182–188.
131. Vickers P, Garg KM, Arya R, et al. The role of selective beta 1-blocker in the preoperative preparation of thyrotoxicosis: a comparative study with propanolol. *Int Surg* 1990;75:179–183.
132. Eriksson M, Rubenfeld S, Garber AK, et al. Propranolol does not prevent thyroid storm. *N Engl J Med* 1977;296:263–264.
133. Jamison MH, Done JH. Postoperative thyrotoxic crisis in a patient prepared for thyroidectomy with propranolol. *Br J Clin Pract* 1979;33:82–83.
134. Jones DK, Solomon S. Thyrotoxic crisis masked by treatment with beta-blockers. *Br Med J* 1981;283:659–660.
135. Strube PJ. Thyroid storm during beta blockade. *Anaesthesia* 1984;39:343–346.
136. Lazarus JH, Addison GM, Richards AR, et al. Treatment of thyrotoxicosis with lithium carbonate. *Lancet* 1974;2:1160–1163.
137. Mochinaga N, Eto T, Maekawa Y, et al. Successful preoperative preparation for thyroidectomy in Graves' disease using lithium alone: report of two cases. *Surg Today* 1994;24:464–467.
138. Takami H. Lithium in the preoperative preparation of Graves' disease. *Int Surg* 1994;79:89–90.
139. Tsunoda T, Mochinaga N, Eto T, et al. Lithium carbonate in the preoperative preparation of Graves' disease. *Jpn J Surg* 1991;21:292–296.
140. Reed J, Bradley EL. Postoperative thyroid storm after lithium preparation. *Surgery* 1985;98:983–986.
141. Wu S-Y, Chopra IJ, Solomon DH, et al. The effect of repeated administration of ipodate (Oragrafin) in hyperthyroidism. *J Clin Endocrinol Metab* 1978;47:1358–1361.
142. Baeza A, Aguato J, Barria M, et al. Rapid preoperative preparation in hyperthyroidism. *Clin Endocrinol* 1991;35:439–442.
143. Perez JA, Silva R, Norambuena L, et al. Shortened preoperative preparation in diffuse hyperthyroid goiter: experience in 34 patients. *Rev Med Chile* 1991;119:1123–1127.
144. Neimark MI, Merkulov IV. The choice of a program of discrete plasmapheresis in the preoperative preparation of patients with diffuse toxic goiter. *Anesteziol Reanimatol* 1990;5:62–65.
145. Lukomskii GI, Alekseeva ME, Ivanova NA, et al. Plasmapheresis in preoperative care of patients with thyrotoxicosis. *Khirurgiia* 1991;4:102–105.
146. De Rosa G, Testa A, Menichella G, et al. Plasmapheresis in the therapy of hyperthyroidism associated with leukopenia. *Haematologica* 1991;76(suppl 1):72–74.
147. Ashkar FS, Katims RB, Smoak WM, et al. Thyroid storm treatment with blood exchange and plasmapheresis. *JAMA* 1970;214:1275–1279.
148. Tajiri J, Katsuya H, Kiyokaya T, et al. Successful treatment of thyrotoxic crisis with plasma exchange. *Crit Care Med* 1984;12:536–537.
149. Ambesh SP. Occult pheochromocytoma in association with hyperthyroidism presenting under general anesthesia. *Anesth Analg* 1993;77:1074–1076.
150. Bradley EL, DiGirolamo M, Tarcan Y. Modified subtotal thyroidectomy in the management of Graves' disease. *Surgery* 1980;87:623–629.
151. Hedley AJ, Bewsher PD, Jones SJ, et al. Late onset hypothyroidism after subtotal thyroidectomy for hyperthyroidism: implications for long term follow up. *Br J Surg* 1983;70:740–743.
152. Hedley AJ, Michie W, Duncan T, et al. The effect of remnant size in the outcome of subtotal thyroidectomy for thyrotoxicosis. *Br J Surg* 1972;59:559–563.
153. Ramus NI. Hypocalcemia after subtotal thyroidectomy for thyrotoxicosis. *Br J Surg* 1984;71:589–590.
154. Bartlett W. Subtotal thyroidectomy. *Trans South Surg Assoc* 1916;29:387–407.

155. Kuma K, Matsuzuka F, Kobayashi A, et al. Natural course of Graves' disease after subtotal thyroidectomy and management of patients with postoperative thyroid dysfunction. *Am J Med Sci* 1991;302:8–12.
156. Noh SH, Soh EY, Park CS, et al. Evaluation of thyroid function after bilateral subtotal thyroidectomy for Graves' disease—a long term follow-up of 100 patients. *Yonsei Med J* 1994;35:177–183.
157. Gough AL, Neill RW. Partial thyroidectomy for thyrotoxicosis. *Br J Surg* 1974;61:939–942.
158. Perzik SL. Total thyroidectomy in the management of Graves' disease: a review of 282 cases. *Am J Surg* 1976;131:284–287.
159. Makiuchi M, Miyakawa M, Sugenoya A, Furihata R. An evaluation of several prognostic factors in the surgical treatment for thyrotoxicosis. *Surg Gynecol Obstet* 1981;152:639–641.
160. Olsen WR, Nishiyama RH, Groeber LW. Thyroidectomy for hyperthyroidism. *Arch Surg* 1970;101:175.
161. Mitchie W, Pegg CAS, Bewsher PD. Prediction of hypothyroidism after partial thyroidectomy for thyrotoxicosis. *Br J Med* 1972;1:13–17.
162. Mitchie W. Whiter thyrotoxicosis. *Br J Surg* 1975;62:673–682.
163. Tweedle DEF, Collings A, Evered DC, Johnstone IDA. Thyroid remnant size and its relationships to hypothyroidism after partial thyroidectomy. *Br J Surg* 1976;63:150.
164. Thomson JA, Wilson R, McKillop JH. Relapse of Graves' disease half a century on. *Br J Surg* 1986;73:896.
165. Okamoto T, Fujimoto Y, Obara T, et al. Retrospective analysis of prognostic factors affecting the thyroid functional status after subtotal thyroidectomy for Graves' disease. *World J Surg* 1992;16:690–695.
166. Okamoto T, Fujimoto Y, Obara T, et al. Unfavorable characteristics in patients with early postoperative recurrence of Graves' disease after subtotal thyroidectomy. *J Jpn Surg Soc* 1993;94:1043–1046.
167. Alexander WD, Harden R, Koutras D, et al. Influence of iodine intake after treatment with antithyroid drugs. *Lancet* 1965;2:866.
167a. Mori Y, Matoba N, Miura S, et al. Clinical course and thyroid stimulating hormone (TSH) receptor antibodies during surgical treatment of Graves' disease. *World J Surg* 1992;16:647–653.
168. Hedley AJ, Ross IP, Beck JS, et al. Recurrent thyrotoxicosis after subtotal thyroidectomy. *Br J Med* 1981;4:258–261.
169. Chonkich GD, Petti GH, Goral W. Total thyroidectomy in the treatment of thyroid disease. *Laryngoscope* 1987;97:897–900.
170. Mountain JC, Stewart GR, Colcock BP. The recurrent laryngeal nerve in thyroid operation. *Surg Gynecol Obstet* 1971;133: 978–980.
171. Saxe AW, Spiegel AM, Marx SJ, Brennan MF. Deferred parathyroid autografts with cryopreserved tissue after reoperative parathyroid surgery. *Arch Surg* 1982;117:538–543.
172. Rieu M, Bekka S, Sambor B, et al. Prevalence of subclinical hyperthyroidism and relationship between thyroid hormonal status and thyroid ultrasonographic parameters in patients with non-toxic nodular goiter. *Clin Endocrinol* 1993;39:67–71.
173. Blum M, Kranjac T, Park CM, Engleman RM. Thyroid storm after cardiac angiography with iodinated contrast medium: occurrence in a patient with a previously euthyroid autonomous nodule of the thyroid. *JAMA* 1976;235:2324–2325.
174. Vagenakis AG, Wang C, Burger A, et al. Iodine induced thyrotoxicosis in Boston. *N Engl J Med* 1972;287:523.
175. Hamburger JE. Evolution of toxicity in solitary nontoxic autonomously functioning thyroid nodules. *J Clin Endocrinol Metab* 1980;50:1089–1093.
176. Becker FO, Economon PG, Schwartz TB. The occurrence of carcinoma in "hot" thyroid nodules: report of two cases. *Ann Intern Med* 1963;58:877.
177. Hamburger JE. Solitary autonomously functioning thyroid lesions: diagnosis, clinical features, and pathogenetic considerations. *Am J Med* 1975;58:740.
178. Hoving J, Piers DA, Vermey A, et al. Carcinoma in hyperfunctioning thyroid nodule in recurrent hyperthyroidism. *Eur J Nucl Med* 1981;6: 131.
179. Rosa GD, Testa A, Maurizio M, et al. Thyroid carcinoma mimicking a toxic adenoma. *Eur J Nucl Med* 1990;17:179–184.
180. Clement K, Levy L, Coutris G, et al. Thyroid cancer revealed by a suppressive hot nodule. *Presse Med* 1991;20:2191–2193.
181. Michigishi T, Mizukami Y, Shuke N, et al. An autonomously functioning thyroid carcinoma associated with euthyroid Graves' disease. *J Nucl Med* 1992;33:2024–2026.
182. Eyre-Brook IA, Talbot CH. The treatment of autonomous functioning thyroid nodules. *Br J Surg* 1982;69:577–579.
183. Horst W, Rosler H, Schneider C, et al. 306 cases of toxic adenoma: clinical aspects, findings in radioiodine diagnostics, radiochromatography and histology; results of ^{131}I and surgical treatment. *J Nucl Med* 1967;8:515–528.
184. Mizukami Y, Michigishi T, Nonomura A, et al. Autonomously functioning (hot) nodule of the thyroid gland. A clinical and histopathologic study of 17 cases. *Am J Clin Pathol* 1994;101:29–35.
185. Fumarola A, Sciacchitano S, Danese D, et al. The autonomous nodule. Clinical aspects. *Minerva Endocrinol* 1993;18:147–154.
186. Sandrock D, Olbricht T, Emrich D, et al. Long-term follow-up in patients with autonomous thyroid adenoma. *Acta Endocrinol* 1993;128: 51–55.
187. van Soestbergen MJ, van der Vijver JC, et al. Recurrence of hyperthyroidism in multinodular goiter after long-term drug therapy: a comparison with Graves' disease. *J Endocrinol Invest* 1992;15: 797–800.
188. Heimann P. Should hyperthyroidism be treated with surgery? *World J Surg* 1978;2:281–287.
189. Huysmans DA, Hermus AR, Corstens FH, et al. Large compressive goiters treated with radioiodine. *Ann Intern Med* 1994;121:757–762.
190. Ross DS, Ridgway EC, Daniels GH. Successful therapy of solitary toxic thyroid nodules: relatively low dose ^{131}I with low prevalence of hypothyroidism. *Ann Intern Med* 1984;101:488–490.
191. McCormack KR, Sheline GE. Long term studies of solitary autonomous thyroid nodules. *J Nucl Med* 1967;8:701.
192. O'Brien T, Gharib H, Suman VJ, et al. Treatment of toxic solitary thyroid nodules: surgery versus radioactive iodine. *Surgery* 1992;112: 1166–1170.
193. Blum M, Shenkman L, Hollander CS. The autonomous nodule of the thyroid: correlation of patient age, nodule size and functional status. *Am J Med Sci* 1975;269:43–50.
194. Goldstein R, Hart IR. Follow-up of solitary autonomous thyroid nodules treated with ^{131}I. *N Engl J Med* 1983;309:1473–1476.
195. Bransom CJ, Talbot CH, Henry L, et al. Solitary toxic adenoma of the thyroid gland. *Br J Surg* 1979;66:590–595.
196. Papini E, Panunzi C, Petrucci L, et al. Long-term results of echographically guided percutaneous ethanol injection in the treatment of the autonomous thyroid nodule. *Minerva Endocrinol* 1993;18: 173–179.
197. Livraghi T, Ferrari C, Paracchi A, et al. Percutaneous ethanol injections in the treatment of autonomous thyroid nodules. *Minerva Endocrinol* 1993;18:187–189.
198. Miller JM, Horn RC, Block MA. The autonomous functioning thyroid nodule in the evolution of nodular goiter. *J Clin Endocrinol Metab* 1967;27:1264.
199. Ozaki O, Ito K, Mimura T, et al. Hemiaplasia of the thyroid associated with Graves' disease: report of three cases and a review of the literature. *Surg Today* 1994;24:164–169.
200. Ishihara T, Kurahachi H, Hattori N, et al. Superior vena cava syndrome due to Graves' disease. *Int Med* 1993;32:80–83.

CHAPTER 18

Thyroid-Associated Ophthalmopathy: Etiology and Pathogenesis

Tomasz Bednarczuk, John S. Kennerdell, and Jack R. Wall

Despite the considerable effort made during the last two decades, the etiology and pathogenesis of the inflammatory eye disorder that frequently accompanies autoimmune thyroid disease, and its natural history, are still poorly understood. Often called Graves' ophthalmopathy, this disorder is more logically called thyroid-associated ophthalmopathy (TAO), which emphasizes that it is not unique to Graves' disease (GD). Although TAO is now accepted as an autoimmune-mediated inflammation of the extraocular muscle and periorbital connective tissue, the nature of the primary antigen(s) and the mechanisms for tissue damage and eye muscle (EM) dysfunction remain unclear.

Relationship to Autoimmune Thyroid Disease

Approximately 90% of patients with ophthalmopathy have associated Graves' hyperthyroidism (1–3). In about half of the remaining patients, the eye disorder is associated with Hashimoto's thyroiditis, and the rest have no overt thyroid disease. More detailed analysis of these latter patients has shown that probably all patients with ophthalmopathy have some form of chronic autoimmune thyroid disease, which becomes overt with prolonged follow-up. In one study, 22 euthyroid patients with ophthalmopathy not associated with goiter, antithyroid antibodies, or overt thyroid disease were tested for subclinical GD and Hashimoto's thyroiditis, using several immunologic markers and aspiration needle biopsies. Some evidence for thyroid autoimmunity was found in all patients (4).

Not only do almost all patients with ophthalmopathy have an associated autoimmune thyroid disorder, but also the great majority of patients with Graves' hyperthyroidism have eye signs or EM swelling on orbital imaging. The true prevalence of established ophthalmopathy in patients with Graves' hyperthyroidism is, however, unclear and depends mainly on the way in which the eye disorder is defined. Clinically apparent ophthalmopathy develops in 10% to 25% of patients with GD if lid signs are excluded, and in 30% to 50% if lid signs are included. Ophthalmopathy, defined as increased EM thickness, is present in 70% to 90% of patients with GD when sensitive imaging techniques such as orbital ultrasonography, computed tomography (CT) (Fig. 1), or magnetic resonance (MRI) are used (5–9). There is also a close temporal relation between the onset of the two disorders; in 80% of patients, hyperthyroidism and ophthalmopathy develop within 2 years of each other (10).

Predisposing Factors

The mechanism for the loss of tolerance to self antigens in TAO is unknown, although it is likely to involve both genetic and environmental factors. Race is an important predisposing factor: for example, ophthalmopathy is 6 times more frequent in Caucasians than in Asian Indians with GD living in the same region (11). Attempts to find a genetic-susceptibility locus have been mostly unsuccessful. Studies that compared human leukocyte antigen (HLA) alleles in patients with GD, with and without severe ophthalmopathy, have failed to reveal any consistent important differences between the two groups. The prevalences of HLA-DR4 and HLA-DRw6 were increased in African American patients with GD (12), whereas HLA-Bw46 and HLA-B35 alleles were more

---

T. Bednarczuk: Department of Endocrinology, Medical Research Center, Polish Academy of Science, 02-097 Warsaw, Poland.

J. S. Kennerdell and J. R. Wall: Department of Ophthalmology, Allegheny General Hospital and Medical College of Pennsylvania, and Hahnemann University, Pittsburgh, Pennsylvania 15212.

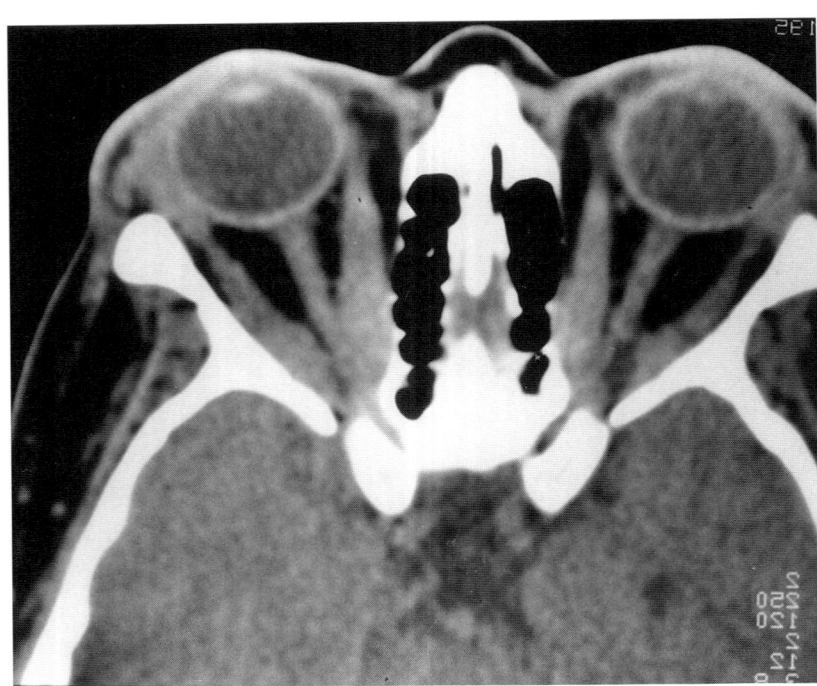

FIG. 1. Orbital CT scan in a patient with severe thyroid-associated ophthalmopathy showing extraocular eye muscle enlargement, particularly in its posterior one third, and resulting proptosis.

prevalent in Chinese and Japanese patients, respectively (13,14), although there was no significant difference between GD patients with and those without eye signs. The well-recognized association of HLA-DR3 with GD in Caucasians may be slightly stronger with eye disease in certain areas (e.g., Hungary), but not in others (15–17). Studies of other candidate susceptibility genes encoding immunoglobulin allotypes, and T-cell receptor polymorphism, have also been unrevealing (15,17).

The sex distribution is more nearly equal in patients with overt ophthalmopathy than in those with Graves' hyperthyroidism without eye signs; whereas the ratio of women to men in all patients with GD is approximately 10:1, it is only 2.5:1 in patients with severe ophthalmopathy (18,19). The peak incidences occur at 40 to 44 years and 60 to 64 years in women, and at 45 to 49 years and 65 to 69 years in men (18). The severity of TAO increases with advancing age, especially in men (19,20).

Smoking is an important risk factor for the development of ophthalmopathy in various ethnic groups (11,21). Furthermore, the duration of smoking and the amount smoked are both directly related to the prevalence and severity of the eye disorder (22,23). Despite this strong epidemiologic evidence, the mechanisms whereby smoking exerts its effects are unknown. Greater tobacco usage in male patients with GD may be a reason for the relatively increased proportion of men developing TAO. Another important predisposing factor is severe stress of many types, which almost always antedates the onset of GD (24).

The potential initiation or aggravation of ophthalmopathy as a result of treatment for hyperthyroidism is an issue of immense clinical relevance and will be discussed in more in detail in Chapter 15. Treatment of GD with antithyroid drugs or subtotal thyroidectomy appears to have little, if any, effect on the ophthalmopathy (25). Whether or not radioactive iodine treatment has any significant influence, either positively or negatively, on the development or progression of ophthalmopathy is controversial. Radioiodine may double the risk of eye signs developing or worsening, at least in the short term (25,26). In contrast, other studies found approximately equal incidences of clinically significant ophthalmopathy among patients treated with iodine-131 (^{131}I), surgery, or antithyroid drugs (27). Abnormal thyroid function may also be an important risk factor for developing TAO: in a retrospective study of 90 patients referred for evaluation of ophthalmopathy, euthyroidism was less frequent in those with severe eye signs (28), and posttreatment hypothyroidism seems to be associated with a higher incidence of progressive ophthalmopathy, although the mechanism remains unclear (26,29).

Clinical Features

The clinical signs and symptoms of TAO are the consequence of inflammation in the EM, the surrounding loose connective tissue, and possibly the lachrymal gland and eyelids, with secondary effects on the optic nerve and corneum (30,31). The soft-tissue inflammatory process is manifest as watering of the eyes, pain, discomfort, injection, and swelling of the lids and conjunctiva (Fig. 2). Muscle inflammation may lead to blurred vision, diplopia

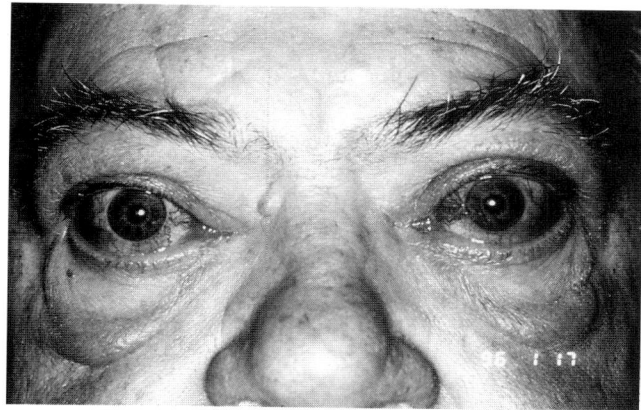
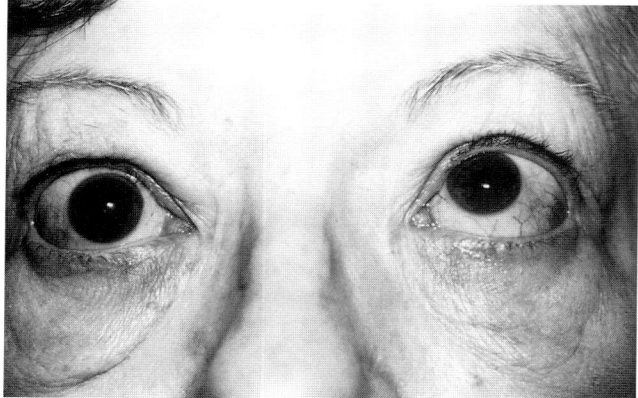

FIG. 2. A patient with thyroid-associated ophthalmopathy and severe eye muscle inflammation resulting in restricted movement of the eyes.

due to discoordinated function of the extraocular muscles, and, in a small proportion of patients, ophthalmoplegia. The increased volume of edematous EM and orbital fat within the unyielding orbital walls results in proptosis. Proptosis is bilateral in 80% to 90% of affected patients; in contrast to true unilateral ophthalmopathy, asymmetric eye involvement is quite common (30). Optic neuritis occurs in TAO as a result of apical compression due to enlargement of the EM. Optic nerve dysfunction is a rare manifestation of TAO that, if untreated, leads to an irreversible deficit in visual acuity and, occasionally, blindness. Once the disease progresses and the muscles become scarred and fixed, double vision may disappear (31). Compromised EM function, manifest as decreased movement of the eye in one or more directions (see Fig. 2), can be quantified. As the inflammation "burns out," previously watery eyes may become dry, which, along with exposure because of proptosis and lid retraction, may lead to corneal ulceration and scarring. Retraction of the upper eyelid is among the most common ocular findings in GD (32). Eyelid changes may result from enhanced sympathetic stimulation of Müller's muscle, autoimmune inflammation of this muscle, increased tone and overreaction of the levator superioris, or a combination of these.

The signs and symptoms of TAO are quite variable, and each may follow its own course in time and severity (1). Some patients have extreme proptosis with very little evidence of periorbital edema or EM dysfunction. Others have predominantly a massive soft-tissue swelling around the eyes, excessive tearing, eye pain, and sensitivity to light, whereas a small proportion of patients may be primarily bothered by double vision resulting from EM dysfunction, without significant proptosis, orbital pain, or other signs of soft-tissue inflammation. This latter variant of TAO is called ocular myopathy (33). Of all patients with ophthalmopathy, only a small minority have disease of sufficient severity to consider the use of anti-inflammatory or immunosuppressive drugs, and only 3% to 5% will require aggressive intervention such as surgical decompression. Most of the symptoms and signs of ophthalmopathy are likely to resolve or improve spontaneously without specific therapy over a 1- to 5-year period (34).

Orbital Pathology

There are two main schools of thought concerning the nature of the orbital inflammatory reaction in TAO, namely, the orbital connective tissue (OCT) school, which favors the orbital fibroblast as being the primary target in TAO, and the EM school, which believes that the EM is the more important site of autoimmune attack. It is now generally agreed, however, that the extraocular (eye) muscle and the loose, fatty OCT are *both* targets of autoantibodies and T lymphocytes in this disorder and that the characteristic exophthalmos and EM swelling are caused by inflammation in both compartments. It is, however, unclear whether the autoimmune reactions are restricted to the orbit or part of a more generalized inflammatory disorder, and whether EM inflammation precedes that in the OCT, as we have postulated (35), or is secondary to OCT inflammation, as others believe (36). Finally, it cannot be doubted that antibodies reactive with EM antigens, in particular a 64-kDa EM protein (see later) are early and reliable markers of ophthalmopathy, and that a cytotoxic effect of such antibodies would be a good explanation for the EM damage of TAO.

NORMAL ANATOMY AND HISTOLOGY OF THE ORBIT

Studies of the normal orbital anatomy and histology are important for an understanding of the pathophysiology of TAO. Orbital tissues are unique in structure and function (36), which may account in part for the targeting of the disease in the orbit. The bony orbit is cone shaped and opened only to the front. The volume of the orbital cavity is 29 mL, and 70% of the orbital content is occupied by retrobulbar and peribulbar structures, namely, EMs, extensive connective tissue, vessels, nerves, and fat (37–39).

The eye movements are finely controlled by six striated extraocular muscles. Two additional muscles, the levator palpebrae superioris, which is striated, and Müller's muscle, which is composed of smooth muscle fibers, control the movements of the upper eyelid. All of these muscles, with the exception of the inferior oblique, arise from Zinn's annulus, a tendinous ring in the orbital apex.

The extraocular muscle tissue comprises muscle fibers, connective tissue, nerve fibers, Schwann cells, and blood vessels. There are obvious morphologic differences between the EM and skeletal muscles (38,40). In the EM, there is a considerable amount of interstitial tissue between the muscle fibers, whereas in skeletal muscle the muscle cells are more tightly packed. Because of the fine control required by the EMs, the innervation rate is higher; the nerve to muscle ratio in EM is 1:5, compared to 1:50 in the semitendinous muscle. The EMs are highly vascularized, although lymphatics cannot be convincingly demonstrated. A few high endothelial venules, which permit the migration of lymphocytes from the circulation, are found in the normal orbital tissue. EM and orbital connective tissue contain significant numbers of HLA class II positive cells, predominantly macrophages, capillary endothelial cells, and T lymphocytes (38,40,41).

Apart from the extraocular muscles, an additional supportive system for the pear-shaped bony orbit is provided by the orbital connective tissue. The supporting connective tissue framework is divided into distinct anterior and posterior portions (38).

ALTERED ANATOMY AND HISTOLOGY IN TAO

Macroscopic Changes

To the surgeon and the pathologist, the orbital contents appear to be glistening and edematous. The individual muscles are enlarged; they have a firm, rubbery consistency (39,42,43) and are resistant to passive stretching. Not all the muscles appear to be affected by the disease to the same extent. The inferior rectus, medial rectus, and superior rectus are most often involved, whereas the inferior oblique and lateral rectus are involved to a far less extent. In some patients, the orbital connective tissue is also expanded, and in a few patients the lachrymal gland is markedly increased in size (44).

Histologic Changes

The major pathological changes occurring in the orbital tissues that are responsible for the gross appearance include the following:

1. Lymphocyte infiltrations
2. Increased fibroblast number
3. Increased mucopolysaccharide content
4. Interstitial edema
5. Increased collagen production and fibrosis
6. Degenerative changes in eye muscle fibers

These changes are seen predominantly within the interstitium of the EM, confirming that the extraocular muscles are the main site of the autoimmune process in TAO. The histologic findings are not consistent and vary in degree in different patients. Some discrepancies could be explained by the fact that only small amounts of orbital tissue are usually available from patients with TAO for study, and the tissue is typically obtained during a quiescent stage of chronic disease, often following treatment with corticosteroids or radiotherapy.

A mixed mononuclear cell infiltration, an important marker of the autoimmune reaction, is found mostly within the extraocular muscles and the surrounding connective tissue (Fig. 3). The infiltration can be observed throughout the muscle but is usually most extensive in their middle and posterior thirds (40,42,45). Many mononuclear cells appear to surround blood vessels in the endomysium and perimysium. The infiltrating mononuclear cells are predominantly T lymphocytes (45,46). Fat and connective tissue infiltration, which can be pronounced in ophthalmopathy, is not found in all cases (45–47). The meninges of the optic nerve and the tendons of EM are typically not inflamed.

The EM are enlarged, mainly because of an increased amount of endomysial connective tissue, large amounts of glycosaminoglycans (GAGs), and interstitial edema. Light microscopy and electron microscopy studies have revealed that, in addition to the inflammatory infiltration, the major alterations appear to be proliferation of fibroblasts, and active acid GAGs and collagen synthesis (40,42–44). Because GAGs consist mainly of hyaluronic acid, which has a profound water-binding capacity, there is increased osmotic pressure in the orbit and resulting interstitial edema (48). Early diffuse fibrosis within the muscle, in association with sites of GAG synthesis, has been reported (42). Dense orbital scarring is the end stage and is associated with severe muscle atrophy and loss of function (39). Although the muscles typically show degenerative changes and loss of striation (39), in many instances the myofibrillar structure is normal (43). However, subsarcolemmal deposits in the myofibers, which consist of collections of glycogen rosettes with intermixed lipid deposits, have been shown by electron microscopy (42).

Histologic changes found in the levator palpebrae superioris muscle and Müller's muscle are different from those in the oculorotary muscles (49–51). The connective tissue of the levator–superior oblique muscle complex shows only scant inflammation and fibrosis. Enlargement of individual levator muscle fibers is a primary cause of the levator muscle hypertrophy in TAO (49). On electron microscopy, Müller's muscle cells demonstrate contrac-

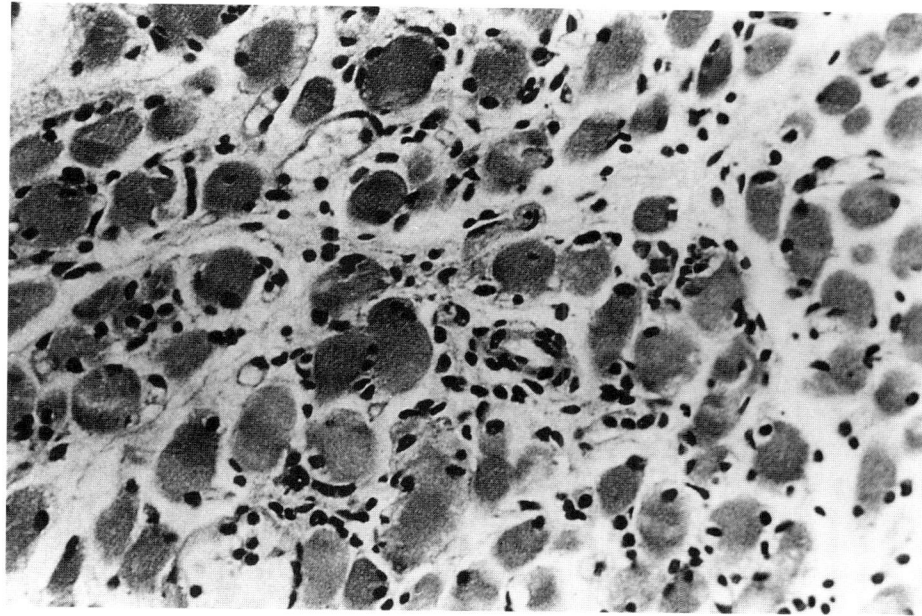

FIG. 3. Histologic examination of eye muscle tissue from a patient with thyroid-associated ophthalmopathy, showing increased numbers of lymphocytes around the individual muscle fibers.

tile degenerative changes (51). Swollen EM can cause a compressive optic neuropathy by impinging on the optic nerve at the Zinn's annulus (42). The posterior third of the muscle is most affected by the swelling. Within the optic nerve, loss of large axons has been demonstrated.

An inflammatory infiltration within the connective tissue is found in the lachrymal gland as well. Fibrosis occurs to a mild degree in this tissue and typically results in only a mild atrophy of the glandular elements (39).

IMMUNOHISTOCHEMISTRY

Several groups have carried out immunohistochemical studies of orbital tissue from patients with TAO, and they have demonstrated abnormal expression of heat shock proteins (HSP), intracellular adhesion molecules, and HLA-DR antigens, which are commonly detected on target cells in other autoimmune disorders.

The major histocompatibility gene complex (MHC) class II antigens, in particular HLA-DR, are important in the presentation of foreign or self antigens by antigen-presenting cells. Class II antigens are regularly presented on macrophages, B lymphocytes, and activated T cells. Aberrant HLA-DR expression seems to play an important role in the pathogenesis of thyroid autoimmunity (52). In normal EM, the interstitial cells (macrophages, fibroblasts) and endothelial cells may express HLA-DR (30,40,41). In biopsy specimens of orbital tissues from patients with severe TAO, marked HLA-DR immunoreactivity was detected in fibroblasts in the perimysial connective tissue (40,45,53,54) and in adipocytes in the retrobulbar adipose tissue (47). Recently, it has been shown that EM cells also express HLA-DR, especially in tissue from untreated patients with eye disease of short duration. In patients with stable ophthalmopathy following immunosuppressive therapy or irradiation therapy, those molecules were not expressed (41).

Heat shock proteins are highly conserved proteins that aid in the protection of cells under stressful stimuli and have immunomodulatory functions. Recently, HSP expression in autoimmune target cells, including thyroid cells, has been reported to play an important role in the development of autoimmune reactions, most likely at the level of antigen processing (55). HSP-70 expression by the EM cells was found in patients with TAO, especially in those with eye disease of short duration (41).

Adhesion molecules are immunomodulatory proteins that play an important role in lymphocyte activation, localization, and presentation of antigen to immunocompetent cells. In orbital tissue biopsies from patients with severe TAO, strong immunoreactivities for intercellular adhesion molecule-1 (ICAM-1) and lymphocyte function antigen-3 (LFA-3) were detected in endothelial cells of blood vessels, in perimysial fibroblasts surrounding muscle fibers (54), and in retrobulbar adipose tissue cells (47). Vascular endothelium also revealed strong immunoreactivity for endothelial leukocyte adhesion molecule-1 (ELAM-1) and vascular cell adhesion molecule-1 (VCAM-1) (54).

In conclusion, infiltration of the EM and surrounding connective tissue by mononuclear cells (in particular, T lymphocytes), enlargement of the fibroblasts, accumulation of hydrophilic GAGs, and interstitial edema, are characteristic histologic findings in TAO. Expression of immunomodulatory molecules (such as HLA-DR, HSP-70, and adhesion proteins) on fibroblasts, EM cells, and adipocytes is likely to play a crucial role in triggering and maintaining the autoimmune inflammation within the orbit.

In Vitro Studies

The orbital inflammation in TAO appears to result in an increased secretory activity of the fibroblasts. Experimental studies have shown that the lymphocyte and its products, including interferon gamma (IFN-γ), interleukin-1 alpha (IL-1α), transforming growth factor-beta (TGF-β), and leukoregulin, are responsible for the stimulation of GAG secretion by the retro-orbital fibroblasts. IFN-γ and, especially, leukoregulin are potent stimulators of GAG production in retro-ocular fibroblasts, but do not affect its synthesis in dermal fibroblasts (56,57). Additionally, hypoxia may cause a significant increase in GAG production (49). Similarly, orbital fibroblasts are stimulated to proliferate *in vitro* following treatment with certain cytokines, namely, IL-1α, IL-4, and TGF-β (59). Glucocorticoid treatment inhibited cytokine-stimulated proliferation and GAG production by orbital fibroblasts (57,59,60).

Cytokines have several effects of potential relevance to the development of orbital autoimmune inflammation, including the induction of HLA-DR, HSP, and adhesion molecules in retro-orbital tissue cells. Treatment with IFN-γ *in vitro* induced HLA-DR expression in cultured retro-orbital fibroblasts (61) and EM cells (62).

The adhesion of lymphocytes to retro-ocular fibroblasts from patients with severe TAO can be induced by interaction with LFA-1 and ICAM-1 (63). The surface expression of ICAM-1 has been demonstrated in orbital fibroblasts *in situ* following stimulation with Graves' disease immunoglobulin G (IgG), IFN-γ, IL-1α, and tissue necrosis factor-α (TNF-α) (63). The effect of Graves' disease IgG appeared to be specific for orbital fibroblasts from TAO patients. HSP-70 expression in orbital fibroblasts could be induced by inflammatory cytokines and various cellular stresses, and suppressed by prednisolone and antithyroid drugs (63–66). HSP-70 was detected on the surface of cultured orbital fibroblasts from patients with TAO, but not on those from normal subjects (65).

In conclusion, the orbital connective tissue cells, especially the fibroblasts surrounding the EM fibers, seem to be extremely sensitive to stimulation by cytokines and other soluble proteins released in the course of an immune reaction. Extraocular fibroblasts respond differently from dermal fibroblasts following cytokine stimulation, which may in part explain the anatomic localization of ophthalmopathy in the orbit.

Cell-Mediated Immunity in TAO

The initial event in the development of both cell-mediated immunity and the humoral reaction is antigen recognition by CD4+ helper T lymphocytes. Unfortunately, there is very little available information about T-cell function and status in TAO (67). For obvious reasons, earlier investigations have used circulating T cells in their studies of putative sensitization to orbital antigens. However, peripheral blood T cells may have little or no relationship to those within the orbital compartment and may comprise very few specifically sensitized cells. More recent studies have been performed on lymphocytes obtained from the retro-orbital tissues. These studies have to be judged cautiously, as a modification of T-cell function during tissue culture and cloning may occur.

Circulating T Cells

The analysis of circulating T-cell phenotypic specificity in TAO has revealed an increase in CD8+ (cytotoxic/suppressor) T cells in patients with severe disease. During successful corticosteroid therapy, the number of CD8+ T lymphocytes typically returns to the normal range (68). In contrast, a different pattern is seen in Graves' hyperthyroidism without ophthalmopathy. The function and specificity of these CD8+ lymphocytes remain to be established.

In earlier studies of the possible role of cell-mediated immunity in TAO, measurement of migration inhibition factor (MIF) was taken as a parameter of T-cell sensitization to putative orbital antigens by several groups (69). One study showed a positive MIF response in all patients with exophthalmos and hyperthyroidism, in two thirds of euthyroid patients with exophthalmos, and in 30% of patients with GD without overt ophthalmopathy (70). Further purification of the crude orbital fractions that had been used to demonstrate lymphocyte sensitization in the MIF assay led to identification of an EM membrane antigen that was claimed to be thyroglobulin (71). These results remain uncertain and could not be confirmed by other investigators (72).

Sensitization of peripheral T cells to EM antigens was also demonstrated using a lymphocyte proliferation assay. T cells from patients with TAO responded to a human EM membrane antigen preparation, although there was no correlation with the severity of the eye signs. Moreover, there was an identical response with skeletal muscle antigen (73). Further fractionation of EM membranes revealed a low grade and heterogeneous response to multiple antigens (74,75). Study of recombinant proteins, identified by screening an orbital cDNA library with sera from patients with TAO, have also failed to elucidate the nature of the putative EM antigen(s) (75).

Cell-mediated immunity to orbital antigens has also been studied using the leukocyte procoagulant activity assay (76). Preparations of pig EM membrane and human thyroid membrane fractions induced a significant response both in patients with TAO and in those with autoimmune thyroid disease without evident ophthalmopathy. EM cytosol, orbital connective tissue cytosol, and membrane fractions of both tissues did not evoke a significant response in either group. Natural killer (NK) cell cytotoxicity against EM cell targets does not seem to play a role in the pathogenesis of TAO (77).

Lachrymal gland antigens have not been studied in detail, although in one series of experiments, sensitization of peripheral T cells to membrane fractions of human lachrymal gland was demonstrated in the majority of patients with TAO (78).

Retrobulbar T Cells

The infiltrating orbital mononuclear cells comprise B lymphocytes and the more abundant T lymphocytes, antibody secreting plasma cells, macrophages, and, occasionally, mast cells. The T lymphocytes (mainly activated) and memory cells (CD45RO+) belong to both helper/inducer (CD4+) and suppressor/cytotoxic (CD8+) subsets (45,46). Cytokines, including IFN-γ, TNF-α, and IL-1α, have been detected in frozen tissue specimens of orbital connective tissue from patients with severe TAO; immunoreactivity was noted in the cytoplasm of infiltrating mononuclear cells and the adjacent connective tissue cells (46).

CD4+ and CD8+ T cells can be divided into three major subsets based on the lymphokines they produce (79). These are the Th1 cells which produce IFN-γ and IL-2, Th2 cells which secrete IL-4 and IL-5, and the Th0 cells which have no restriction in their lymphokine production. Lymphokines produced by each Th cell subset are inhibitory for the opposing subset, which drives CD4+ T lymphocytes towards either the Th1 or Th2 phenotype. In autoimmunity, the majority of T cells are of the Th1 subclass (79). Although there is much overlap, most T-cell clones obtained from sites of active inflammation are of the Th1 subclass, with the exception of largely antibody-mediated diseases such as Graves' hyperthyroidism (GH) (80) and myasthenia gravis (81), where the Th2 subclass predominates. There is also evidence that whereas Th1 cells may contribute to the pathogenesis of organ-specific autoimmune diseases, Th2 cells may prevent them (82).

Recent studies have attempted to determine the function and pattern of cytokines secreted by orbital infiltrating T cells. In one study, the cultured lymphocytes were mainly of CD8+/CD45RO cells and they secreted IL-4, IFN-γ and IL-10 upon activation (83), suggesting that the cells could be involved in both cell-mediated and humoral immune responses. Cultured T-cell lines proliferated in response to autologous orbital and skin fibroblasts in an MHC class I restricted manner, but not to a crude EM extract or a purified derivate of *Mycobacterium tuberculosis*. One T-cell line displayed cytotoxicity against fibroblasts (83). In another study, retro-orbital-derived T-cell clones comprised almost equal proportions of CD4+ and CD8+ cells (84). In this study, cultured lymphocytes displayed cytolytic activity and secreted mainly IL-2, IFN-γ, and TNF-α, consistent with TAO being a T-cell–driven type I helper (Th1) disorder (84).

A different cytokine profile was found when transcripts for cytokines expressed by infiltrating T cells were tested for using polymerase chain reaction (PCR) amplification of reverse transcribed mRNA. In this study, McLachlan et al. (85) showed that activated orbital T cells were mainly of the type 2 helper (Th2) cell phenotype, which secretes IL-4 and IL-5, known to play important roles in antibody production (both) and in suppressing cell-mediated immunity (IL-4). Contradictory data reported by groups who used expanded orbital lymphocytes (86) could be in part explained by a modification of T-cell function during tissue culture.

Molecular analysis of retro-orbital T-cell receptor genes in untreated patients with severe TAO of recent onset indicated a limited degree of variability of T-cell receptor variable region gene usage (87). In contrast, greater diversity of T-cell receptor gene usage was noted in patients with more chronic, inactive disease. This study supports the notion that orbital tissue–infiltrating T cells in patients with TAO are participating in a primary immune response, in which a limited number of T-cell clones are activated against specific antigens rather than in a nonspecific inflammatory response to multiple antigens.

In conclusion, T cells are likely to play a central role in the pathogenesis of TAO. Although there is evidence for T-cell sensitization to various orbital antigens (namely, EM membrane antigens, connective tissue cells, and lachrymal gland proteins), the nature of the principal autoantigen(s) is unknown. The studies have so far failed to determine whether T cells are primarily involved in a cell-mediated (Th-1) or a humoral (Th-2) immune response. Further phenotypic and functional analysis of infiltrating lymphocytes in orbital tissue from patients with early stages of TAO will hopefully elucidate their role in the pathogenesis of the eye disorder.

Humoral Immunity in TAO

Considerable effort has been made over the past several years to identify autoantigens involved in the humoral component of TAO. The possible significance of autoantibodies in the pathogenesis of TAO has been considered since the first reports of exophthalmos in neonates born to mothers with TAO (87–89); eye symptoms in neonates are usually transient and their clinical course consistent with the known half-life of IgG (90). The reported effectiveness of plasmapheresis treatment of active ophthalmopathy (91,92) further suggests that autoantibodies reactive with orbital antigens may play a role in the pathogenesis of TAO. However, investigations of the humoral response in TAO using different antigens and assays have given diverse and inconsistent results.

Autoantibodies Against Eye Muscle Antigens

Since the first report of circulating antibodies reactive with a soluble (cytosolic) EM antigen (93), considerable evidence has been obtained to support the EM as the primary target of autoantibodies in TAO (94,95). Serum EM-reactive antibodies have been detected using an enzyme-linked immunosorbent assay (ELISA) (96–99), *Staphylococcus* protein A binding (100,101), immunoblotting (102–104), antibody-dependent cell-mediated cytotoxicity (ADCC) assays (105), and immunofluorescence (106,107) (Fig. 4, top). The presence of immunoglobulins IgA and IgE in orbital muscles (108,109) has been shown in *in situ* studies.

Among the EM membrane proteins separated by SDS-polyacrylamide gel electrophoresis and detected in Western blotting, a 64-kDa membrane antigen seems to be the most specific and most closely related to ophthalmopathy in patients with thyroid autoimmunity (Fig. 4, bottom). This antigen is probably derived from a larger protein of approximately 200 kDa that is reduced by treatment with mercaptoethanol to proteins of 55, 64, and 95 kDa (110). Studies of the tissue specificity of the 64-kDa antigen showed it to be expressed in human thyroid and EM tissue, but probably not in other skeletal muscle (102,111). The corresponding autoantibodies were detected in sera from 75% of patients with severe active orbital inflammation of short duration (112), in the majority of patients with ocular myopathy (113) (a subgroup of TAO in which EM involvement is not accompanied by OCT inflammation), and in 50% of patients with lid lag but no other signs of progressive ophthalmopathy (104,114). These antibodies were often accompanied by reactivity to the 50-, 55-, 70-, and 95-kDa proteins. Titers of anti-64-kDa antibodies tend to be low (less than 1:100) in normals whose sera are reactive with that antigen, in GD patients without overt eye symptoms, and in patients with TAO of longer duration. On the other hand, high titers (1:200 to 1:6400) were found in the majority of patients with TAO and recent symptoms (104,115). In an earlier study, we found that all patients with GH who developed signs of ophthalmopathy had detectable anti-64-kDa-protein antibodies 2 to 4 months prior to the onset of the eye disease (104). Antibodies reactive with a native preparation of the 64-kDa protein were detected in sera from 67% patients with TAO, in 30% of those with GH without evident ophthalmopathy, but in only 11% of patients with Hashimoto's thyroiditis (HT) without eye disease, and in 9% of normals (116). The finding of positive reactivity many months *before* the onset of TAO makes

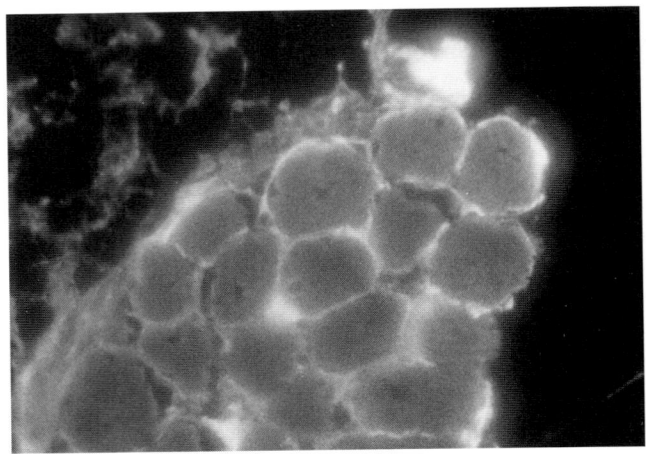

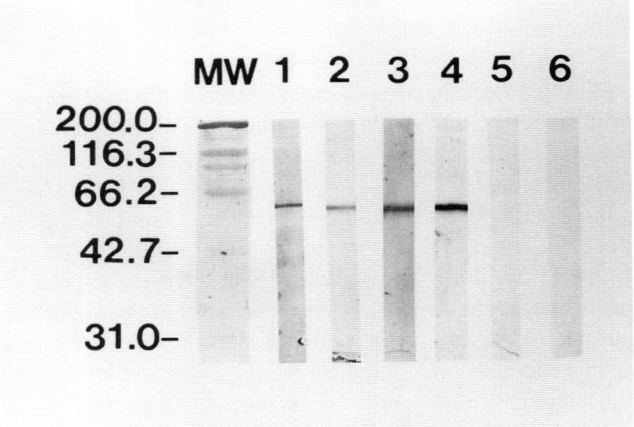

FIG. 4. Top: Immunofluorescence test for serum antibodies reactive with eye muscle antigens, showing staining of the eye muscle plasma membrane and endomysium. **Bottom:** Immunoblot test for eye muscle antibodies, showing reactivity of sera from patients with TAO (lanes 1–4), but not normals (lanes 5–7), with a protein of 64 kDa. MW, molecular weight standards.

improbable the notion that anti-64-kDa antibodies are secondary to the orbital inflammatory process. Antibody titers decreased after successful plasmapheresis treatment of patients with severe and active disease (117).

These findings of serum antibodies reactive with EM proteins, in particular a 64-kDa protein, in TAO, have been confirmed by several groups. Hiromatsu et al. (115) found a close relationship between levels of antibodies to a rat 64-kDa protein, measured as band density ratio by comparing to reactivity at 60 kDa, and ophthalmopathy, and low levels in normals. Dakovska and her colleagues essentially confirmed our findings of antibodies to EM membrane antigens of 55, 64, and 95 kDa in patients with TAO (118); these workers did not find such antibodies in sera from normal subjects (118). Boucher et al. (119) and Wengrowicz et al. (120) found antibodies against the 64-kDa protein in significant proportions of patients with active TAO. The latter workers also confirmed our finding of antibodies to a 55-kDa EM protein, which they found in over 50% of patients. Chang et al. (121) demonstrated antibodies reactive with the 55- and 64-kDa proteins in the majority of patients with TAO.

In contrast, some other investigators have found no evidence that EM membrane antibodies are present in a significant proportion of TAO patients (73,122–125). Kendler et al. (126) showed immunoreactivity against a 64-kDa protein was detected in equal proportions of patients with TAO, GD and no ophthalmopathy, and normal subjects. Decrease of serum antibody activity after absorption with thyroid fractions (123,124) and skeletal muscle (100,126), liver (122,126), and brain membranes (126) may reflect nonspecific affinity of autoantibodies to various tissues in these studies, or broad cross-reactivity. Polyreactive natural autoantibodies in normal sera have been shown to react with various conserved antigens, and their presence is known to be increased in several autoimmune disorders. Controversies concerning the prevalences of EM antibodies in normal subjects and the tissue specificity of the corresponding antigens may reflect differences in antigen preparation, subject selection, and the techniques used. Overall, the existence of serum EM antibodies in TAO has been well established and significant correlations between their levels and parameters of the eye disorder (2,35) suggest that they have a pathogenic role. Detection of serum EM autoantibodies also has prognostic value in patients with GH without overt ophthalmopathy.

Efforts to define EM antigens at the molecular level have not yet been successful (127,128). One group (129) reported the cloning and characterization of a 63- to 64-kDa protein obtained by screening a thyroid cDNA library with sera from patients with Hashimoto's thyroiditis. The initial fragment, called D1, seemed, in preliminary studies, to share an epitope with the 64-kDa protein (130). The full-length protein, called 1D, has been extensively studied (131). Recent experiments have revealed important differences between these two 64-kDa proteins. These findings include differences in their isoelectric points (6.2 for the 64-kDa protein and 9.2 for 1D) and glycosylation patterns (110,132), and reactivities with the corresponding antibodies in immunofluorescence and immunoblotting (133).

Autoantibodies Against Orbital Fibroblasts

The presence of serum autoantibodies reactive with OCT antigens in TAO has been also been demonstrated (134). Using an ELISA, it has been shown that IgG from TAO sera binds significantly better than IgG from normal serum, to retro-ocular TAO fibroblasts (135). A follow-up study, in which immunoblotting was used to detect autoantibodies, showed that more than half the sera from patients with GD recognized a 23-kDa protein found in fibroblasts (136). Other investigators were unable to reproduce these findings (125,135). The titer of these IgG antibodies did not correlate with the severity of eye symptoms and they were not disease or organ specific (133,136–138).

Organ Nonspecific Antibodies in Graves' Disease

A variety of organ nonspecific antibodies have been demonstrated in the sera from patients with GD. These include antinuclear antibodies (ANAs), which have been demonstrated by binding assay, in ELISA, and by indirect immunofluorescence (139–142). In a recent study using the latter technique, ANAs were detected in 31% of patients with ophthalmopathy but in no patient with GH without clinically evident eye involvement (131). In this study, 10% of patients with ophthalmopathy also had antibodies reactive with an uncharacterized connective tissue/perimysial antigen(s) (141). Smooth muscle and mitochondrial antibodies have been demonstrated in some studies (143,144) but not in others (145). Although the significance of the antibodies in GD and TAO is presently unclear, the findings confirm the widespread antigen reactivity in this disorder.

Biological Activity of Autoantibodies in TAO

Although the existence of serum antibodies reactive with EM in TAO has been well established, their role in the development of the EM damage that characterizes TAO remains unclear. Cytotoxic antibodies against human EM cells, measured in an ADCC assay, were demonstrated in about 60% of patients with TAO (62,77,105), and levels of cytotoxicity, expressed as percent specific lysis, correlated with the clinical status assessed as intraocular pressure and American Thyroid Association (ATA) class (105). The ADCC assay seems to be very specific for the eye disorder: the greatest prevalence of cytotoxic antibodies, 75%, is found in patients with "euthyroid ophthalmopathy" (ophthalmopathy associated with subclinical thyroiditis) from an iodine deficiency area (146). A recent ADCC study using a new nonradioactive assay for measuring cell lysis revealed that, although there is good evidence for cytotoxicity against cultured EM cells in TAO, only a few patients have positive reactivity against orbital fibroblast (147). As discussed above, there is good circumstantial evidence that such antibodies may play a role in the EM damage of TAO, although this has not yet been proven.

Limited data about other possible biologic actions of autoantibodies in TAO are available (94). Anti-EM antibodies are able to stimulate [^{3}H]thymidine incorporation into DNA of myocytes (148) and creatine kinase production (149) in cultured myocytes.

Immunoglobulin G preparations from hyperthyroid patients with TAO and monoclonal antibodies to the thyrotropin (TSH)-receptor-stimulated collagen biosynthesis in human fibroblasts as measured by [^{3}H]proline incorporation (150). Graves' IgG was able to induce a 72-kDa HSP in thyroid cells and Graves' retro-ocular fibroblasts, as well as ICAM-1 expression in orbital fibroblasts (63,64). Although autoantibodies can interact with an insulin-like growth factor receptor expressed on the orbital fibroblasts (151), they do not influence fibroblast metabolism and do not stimulate their proliferation. Attempts at identifying specific antibodies in TAO that stimulate GAG synthesis have been unsuccessful (151–153).

In conclusion, there is good evidence for humoral immunoreactivity against several EM antigens, although their pathogenic role is unclear. The antigen that seems to be most closely associated with the eye disorder is a 64-kDa protein. EM autoantibodies could serve as diagnostic or prognostic markers in TAO. OCT-specific antigens have been less convincingly identified. The biologic activity of autoantibodies in TAO suggest that they may be relevant in the pathogenesis of TAO, although this needs to be proven. Alternatively, autoantibodies against EM and OCT could arise secondarily as a result of local inflammation in the orbit. The precise role of such antibodies will be elucidated only when the target antigens have been cloned (154).

POSSIBLE PATHOGENIC MECHANISMS

Link Between the Eye and Thyroid
(See also Chapter 17)

The unique association of ophthalmopathy with thyroid autoimmunity, especially GH, may be best explained by immunological cross reactivity against thyroid and orbital tissue–shared antigen(s) (2,35). Circulating T cells and antibodies in patients with GD directed against an antigen on thyroid follicular cells may recognize antigenic epitopes that are shared by tissues contained in retro-orbital tissue. Those investigators and clinicians who believe that ophthalmopathy occurs because of cross reactivity against thyroid and orbital tissue-shared antigen(s) expect ophthalmopathy to improve after total removal or ablation of the thyroid gland, whereas those who believe that treatment with radioactive iodine is associated with release of the thyroid and orbital tissue antigen expect a flare-up of the eye disorder, or its development. There is support for both effects. Moreover, ocular manifestations similar to those of GD have occurred in patients after neck irradiation for nonthyroidal neoplasm (155), supporting the notion that the underlying mechanism is autoimmunity against orbital- and thyroid-shared antigen(s).

A logical starting point for thyroid- and orbital tissue–shared proteins is the antigens that have been characterized in autoimmune thyroid disease. Immunoreactive thyroglobulin (Tg)-like material found in EM pointed to one candidate (71), and interest was renewed recently with the discovery that Tg shares sequence homology with muscle acetylcholinesterase (ACHE), an enzyme that hydrolyzes the neurotransmitter acetylcholine. It has been demonstrated that a Tg-ACHE shared epitope was recognized by autoantibodies from patients with autoimmune thyroid disease (156,157). The reaction was more often found in patients with GD, two thirds of whom had antibodies to the epitope, sometimes in the absence of reactivity with the native Tg molecule. The significance of these findings remains to be established. The reason that recognition of the antigen is restricted to EM and occurs mostly in GD (Tg antibodies being more frequent in Hashimoto's thyroiditis) is unclear.

Another candidate for a shared antigen is the TSH receptor (TSH-R) (158). Using PCR amplification, the extracellular domain of the human TSH-R has been detected in cultured OCT, and in fibroblasts derived from abdominal skin and pretibial skin from patients with TAO and normal subjects. (159). The presence of TSH-R mRNA has been also reported in retro-orbital fat (160, 161) and other extrathyroidal tissues (162,163). The level of expression is low compared to thyroid, and some other studies have not been able to confirm its presence in retrobulbar tissues (164). However, immunoenzymatic and immunofluorescent studies confirmed the presence of TSH receptor, or an immunologically related protein, in cultured human retrobulbar fibroblasts obtained from patients with TAO (165). A genomic point mutation in an immunogenic region of the TSH-R is associated with autoimmune thyroid disease in women, especially those with GD with extrathyroidal manifestations (166). The effects of anti-TSH-R antibodies on retro-orbital tissue cells are unclear. Stimulation of collagen production by monoclonal anti-TSH-R antibodies was reported in one study (150), but these results have not been confirmed by others (167). TSH does not stimulate GAG synthesis *in vitro* (168), and clinically there is no close correlation between anti-TSH receptor antibody titers and the severity of eye disease (reviewed in ref. 35). High TSH-R antibody concentrations are associated with thyroid-associated dermopathy (169), which in turn almost invariably coexists with ophthalmopathy (1). Although the possible role of TSH-R as a major antigen in TAO is an interesting hypothesis, the presence of functionally active and/or immunogenic TSH receptor protein within the retro-orbital tissue remains to be established.

A thyroid- and EM-shared protein, with a calculated molecular weight of 63 to 64 kDa, called 1D, was cloned by M. Ludgate and coworkers from a thyroid cDNA expression library (129). This protein has been extensively studied in our laboratory and is shown to be the target of antibodies in the serum of about 40% of patients with thyroid autoimmunity with or without eye involvement (131). 1D, which shares 60% sequence homology with the muscle protein tropomodulin, is also expressed in many tissues apart from the orbit and thyroid (170) and is now known to be different from the 64-kDa protein identified in immunoblotting (35).

An extensively studied 64-kDa protein that is expressed in EM and thyroid is also a good candidate for a relevant target antigen in TAO (2,94,95). Cytotoxic antibody reactivity against a shared 64-kDa protein may explain the development of ophthalmopathy in patients with thyroid autoimmunity (171), although this is not universally accepted (3,36). We have postulated that TAO may be a two-stage disease (172). In a clinically silent stage of the eye disease, the 64-kDa protein is recognized by orbital CD4+ T cells and antibodies and initiates an inflammatory reaction. At this stage, the EMs are enlarged on orbital imaging. A second stage of the disease, in which cytotoxic mechanisms are postulated to play a more important role, occurs in about 25% of these patients. Subsequent connective tissue inflammation associated with nonspecific fibroblast stimulation, accumulation of GAGs, and fibrosis contributes to the EM damage (172).

One other possible mechanism for the link is a genetically determined loss of tolerance to both thyroid and striated muscle/connective tissue antigens, manifest as an autoimmune attack against the TSH-R (or thyroperoxidase in the case of Hashimoto's thyroiditis), and muscle autoantigens such as the 64-kDa protein, respectively. However, this is speculative.

Role of the Fibroblast as Autoimmune Target in TAO

It is now widely accepted that fibroblasts, in addition to synthesizing extracellular matrix and collagen, play an important role in various inflammatory and immune reactions. As discussed, there is evidence that fibroblasts may be the target cells in TAO; these cells express HSP-70, HLA-DR, and ICAM-1, proteins that are known to serve various immunomodulatory functions and assist in antigen processing and presentation and are recognized by both antibodies and T cells in TAO. Paracrine/autocrine interactions between orbital fibroblasts and infiltrating lymphocytes and macrophages may a play a central role in the evolution of TAO. Upon activation, T cells and macrophages populating the retro-orbital space are known to secrete a variety of cytokines into the surrounding tissue; IFN-γ, TNF-α, IL-1α, and other cytokines have been detected in orbital tissue from patients with TAO. Effects of potential relevance to the orbital disease include stimulation of GAG synthesis and induction of MHC class II molecules, HSPs, and adhesion molecules in retro-orbital fibroblasts (158). Variable sensitivity of fibroblasts from different anatomic regions to cytokine stimulation and hormonal regulation have been demonstrated (59,168, 173,174), which may be relevant to the localization of connective tissue inflammation in the orbit.

Possible Role of the Lachrymal Gland in TAO

Lachrymal gland swelling and inflammation have also been identified in patients with ophthalmopathy (1). There is also some evidence for immunoreactivity against lachrymal gland antigens in patients with ophthalmopathy associated with GD, although the nature of putative lachrymal antigens is unknown (78). Studies of the lachrymal fluid further indicate that an inflammatory process in the orbit associated with TAO may affect the lachrymal gland. Increased levels of IgA (175) and manganese superoxide dismutase activity (176) were found in tears from patients with active ophthalmopathy. The lachrymal gland may play a role in the pathogenesis of ophthalmopathy, either as a target of the autoimmune reactions of TAO or by directing lymphocyte trafficking to the orbit.

TAO as a Generalized Disorder of the Connective Tissue and Skeletal Muscle

A vexing problem that confronts those who study this complex disorder is to determine whether TAO is primarily a local (organ-specific) or a general (systemic) autoimmune disorder. Indeed, there is growing evidence to support the notion that GD is an autoimmune inflammatory disorder of the striated muscle (including eyelid and heart muscle), connective tissue (including that in the skin), orbit, and the ends of long bones and fingers, associated with inflammation of the thyroid gland and perhaps the lachrymal gland (141,177).

Although the true frequency of each is unknown, inflammation of the skin, skeletal muscle, and eyelid muscle can be demonstrated in significant proportions of patients with GD. Mild myopathy is probably much more common than generally believed (178), proximal muscle weakness often being admitted on direct questioning of patients with GH. In addition, lymphocytes are frequently found in muscle biopsies from patients with GD (179). Some of the cardiac abnormalities that frequently accompany Graves' hyperthyroidism may also be explained by a systemic immunological reaction against cardiac muscle. These muscle disorders may be either clinically mild, and therefore ignored by both patient and physician, or subclinical and unrecognized because of lack of specific diagnostic tests.

Pretibial myxedema is also much more common than suggested by current dogma; in a study by Salvi et al. (180) in which ultrasound was used to measure skin thickness, the skin disorder was identified in 30% of patients with GD, which was confirmed by biopsy in all cases where this was performed. As discussed, the lachrymal gland may also be a site of inflammation in TAO, and GD is associated with other organ specific and organ nonspecific autoimmune disorders in about 10% of cases.

Evidence for generalized inflammation of the muscle and connective tissue supports the notion that GD may be a collagen-like disorder, the orbital and thyroid inflammatory processes being the most prominent features of a systemic disease.

Mechanism for Localization in the Orbit

Although phenotypic and functional differences between cultured fibroblasts from various anatomic regions have been shown, antigenic differences have not been well defined; retro-orbital T-cell lines recognized both orbital and skin fibroblasts (181), and antibodies binding to retro-orbital fibroblasts often cross react with fibroblasts from other sites (125,182). Finally, specific retro-orbital fibroblast antigens could not be demonstrated by immunoblotting (137). Detection of RNA encoding the hTSH-R in fibroblasts from involved and uninvolved sites (see previous), and in both patients and healthy individuals, could provide further evidence for a generalized immunological involvement of fibroblasts in GD.

Similarly, the extraocular muscles have unique features compared to other striated muscles, including a greater number of spindles, a greater blood flow, and more abundant nerve fibers (183), although there is no evidence for a different antigenic pattern; for example, T cells from patients with autoimmune thyroid disease proliferated in response to striated muscle antigens of either extraocular or skeletal muscle origin (73). Not only is the skeletal muscle autoimmune reaction of GD mainly localized to the extraocular [and possibly eyelid (114)] muscles, but it is usually more severe in some of these muscles (inferior recti) than others [other recti, obliques (1)]. Anatomic and other features, such as the restrictive nature of the bony container, may be responsible for the clinical expression in the orbit. Other possibilities include (a) an unusual concentration of target antigen(s), (b) increased sensitivity of involved muscles to cytotoxic antibodies, and (c) variable effects of factors associated with the autoimmune reactions of GD (such as thyroid hormone, TSH, or inflammatory cytokines) on autoantigen gene expression.

In conclusion, the nature of primary autoantigen(s) and the exact pathogenic mechanism of orbital inflammation in TAO have not been established. Of various orbital tissues and organs, the EM and the orbital connective tissue are generally considered the most likely sites of the autoimmune reaction(s). There is also some evidence to support the notion that GD could be considered a multisystem autoimmune disorder, in which the damage is restricted to the thyroid, connective tissue of the skin and the orbit, extraocular and other skeletal muscle, and possibly the lachrymal gland. The primary event is postulated to be generalized loss of tolerance to thyroid antigens, resulting in production of autoreactive T cells and a variety of autoantigens. Activated T cells are recruited to infiltrate the orbit via certain adhesion molecules (ICAM-1, VCAM-1). Autoantibodies and lymphocytes may interact with the primary target cell (fibroblast or EM) exhibiting a shared antigen with the thyroid follicular cells. Activated T cells release cytokines into the surrounding tissue, which may stimulate cell proliferation, GAG and collagen synthesis by fibroblasts, and expression of immunomodulatory molecules on fibroblasts, muscle cells, and adipocytes. Expression of adhesion molecules, HSP, and HLA-DR by retro-orbital tissue cells may further direct T-cell migration and targeting. Fibroblast GAG and collagen production results in edema and characteristic swelling of the muscles and connective tissue, which causes clinical features. Impairment in venous drainage as a result of superior rectus muscle enlargement and/or increased orbital fat may lead to venous congestion (184). Progression of the ongoing inflammatory activities within the orbit may eventually lead to massive fibrosis of EM interstitial and retro-orbital connective tissue.

SUMMARY

The exact pathogenic mechanism of TAO remains unclear, and extensive studies of this disorder have often resulted in conflicting data. Well-known technical difficulties, including the limited access to orbital tissues from patients with active and early disease, lack of an animal model, and poor reproducibility of some of the immunological techniques used are in part responsible for this confusing situation. The self-limited course of the ophthalmology, as well as its variable temporal relation with the onset of Graves' hyperthyroidism, has further complicated the investigation of the disease and the interpretation of the results.

A number of important details about the disorder have, however, been worked out in recent years. TAO is almost certainly an autoimmune disorder of the orbit and is an almost constant accompaniment of GD. There is evidence for the existence of cellular and humoral autoimmune responses to orbital fibroblasts, extraocular muscles, and the lachrymal gland. Which of these mechanisms is of primary importance is as yet unclear. Many investigators support the notion that TAO may be part of a more generalized disorder of the connective tissue and striated muscle.

The primary antigen(s) recognized by immunocompetent cells and autoantibodies has not been definitely identified. Some good candidates, among them a TSH receptor protein and an EM membrane antigen of 64 kDa, have been partially characterized. Although it is uncertain which component of the autoimmune reaction (humoral or cell mediated) plays the more important role, it is likely that both are important for full clinical expression and propagation of the disease process within the orbit. The orbital fibroblasts are likely to play a major pathogenic role in ophthalmopathy. These cells seem to be extremely sensitive to stimulation by cytokines and other soluble proteins, and by immunoglobulins released in the course of an immune reaction. Fibroblasts secrete large amounts of GAGs and also participate in maintaining the autoimmune reaction. More knowledge about the pathogenesis of TAO is essential to better judge which therapies for the thyroid gland improve or worsen ophthalmopathy, and to develop preventive strategies and more effective and less troublesome therapies for the patients.

REFERENCES

1. Burch HB, Wartofsky L. Graves' ophthalmopathy: current concepts regarding pathogenesis and management. *Endocr Rev* 1993;14: 747–793.
2. Wall JR, Boucher BA, Salvi M, et al. Pathogenesis of thyroid associated ophthalmopathy: an autoimmune disorder of the eye muscle associated with Graves' hyperthyroidism and Hashimoto's thyroiditis. *Clin Immunol Immunopathol* 1993;68:1–8.
3. Weetman AP. Thyroid-associated eye disease: pathophysiology [editorial]. *Lancet* 1991;338:25–28.
4. Salvi M, Zhang ZG, Haegert D, et al. Patients with endocrine ophthalmopathy not associated with overt thyroid disease have multiple thyroid immunological abnormalities. *J Clin Endocrinol Metab* 1990; 70:89–94.
5. Forrester JV, Sutherland GR, McDougall IR. Dysthyroid ophthalmopathy: orbital evaluation with B-scan ultrasonography. *J Clin Endocrinol Metab* 1977;45:221–224.
6. Enzmann DR, Donaldson SS, Kriss JP. Appearance of GD on orbital computed tomography. *J Comput Assist Tomog* 1979;3:815–819.
7. Trokiel SL, Jakobiec FA. Correlation of CT scanning and pathologic features of ophthalmic GD. *Ophthalmology* 1981;88:553–564.
8. Forbes G, Gorman CA, Brennan MD, Gehring DC, Ilstrup DM, Earnest F. Ophthalmopathy of Graves' disease: computerized volume measurements of the orbital fat and muscle. *Am J Neuroradiol* 1986; 7:651–656.
9. Villadolid MC, Yokoyama N, Izumi M, et al. Untreated GD patients without clinical ophthalmopathy demonstrate a high frequency of extraocular muscle (EOM) enlargement by magnetic resonance. *J Clin Endocrinol Metab* 1995;80:2830–2833.
10. Gorman CA. Temporal relationship between onset of Graves' ophthalmopathy and diagnosis of thyrotoxicosis. *Mayo Clin Proc* 1983; 58:515–519.
11. Tellez M, Cooper J, Edmonds C. Graves' Ophthalmopathy in relation to cigarette smoking and ethnic origin. *Clin Endocrinol* 1992;36: 291–294.
12. Sridama V, Hara Y, Fauchet R, De Groot LJ. HLA immunogeneic heterogeneity in black American patients with GD. *Arch Intern Med* 1987;147:229–231.
13. Kawa A, Nakamura S, Nakasawa M, et al. HLA-B35 and B5 in Japanese patients with GD. *Acta Endocrinol* 1977;86:754–757.
14. Inoque D, Sato K, Maeda M, et al. Genetic differences shown by HLA typing among Japanese patients with euthyroid Graves' ophthalmopathy, GD and Hashimoto's thyroiditis: genetic characteristics of euthyroid Graves' ophthalmopathy. *Clin Endocrinol* 1991;34:57–62.
15. Kendall-Taylor P, Stephenson A, Stratton A, Papiha SS, Perros P, Roberts DF. Differentiation of autoimmune ophthalmopathy from Graves' hyperthyroidism by analysis of genetic markers. *Clin Endocrinol* 1988;28:601–610.
16. Weetman AP, Zhang L, Webb S, Shine B. Analysis of HLA-DQB and HLA DPB alleles in GD by oligonucleotide probing of enzymatically amplified DNA. *Clin Endocrinol* 1990;33:65–71.
17. Weetman AP, So AK, Warner CA, Foroni L, Fells P, Shine B. Immunogeneic markers in Graves' ophthalmopathy. *Clin Endocrinol* 1988;28:619–628.
18. Bartley GB, Fatourechi V, Kadrmas EF, et al. The incidence of Graves' ophthalmopathy in Olmsted County, Minnesota. *Am J Ophthalmol* 1995;120:511–517.
19. Perros P, Crombie AL, Matthews JNS, Kendall-Taylor P. Age and gender influence the severity of thyroid-associated ophthalmopathy: a study of 101 patients attending a combined thyroid eye-clinic. *Clin Endocrinol* 1993;38:367–372.
20. Kendler DL, Lippa J, Rootman J. The initial clinical characteristics of Graves' orbitopathy vary with age and sex. *Arch Ophthalmol* 1993;11: 197–201.
21. Shine B, Fells P, Edwards OM, Weetman AP. Association between Graves' ophthalmopathy and smoking. *Lancet* 1990;335:1261–1264.
22. Bartalena L, Martino E, Marcocci E, et al. More on smoking habits and Graves' ophthalmopathy. *J Endocrinol Invest* 1989;12:733–737.
23. Prummel MF, Wiersinga WM. Smoking and risk of GD. *JAMA* 1993; 269:479–482.
24. Sonino N, Girelli ME, Boscaro M, Fallo F, Busnardo B, Fava GA. Life events in the pathogenesis of GD. A controlled study. *Acta Endocrinol* 1993;128:293–296.
25. Tallstedt L, Luncell G, Torring O, et al. Occurrence of ophthalmopathy after treatment for Graves' hyperthyroidism. *N Engl J Med* 1992; 326:1733–1738.
26. Kung AW, Yau CC, Cheng A. The incidence of ophthalmopathy after radioiodine therapy for GD: prognostic factors and the role of methimazole. *J Clin Endocrinol Metab* 1994;79:542–546.
27. Sridama V, De Groot LJ. Treatment of GD and the cause of ophthalmopathy. *Am J Med* 1989;87:70–73.
28. Prummel MF, Wilmar MD, Wiersinga M, Kornneef L, Berghout A, van der Gaag R. Effects of abnormal thyroid function on the severity of Graves' ophthalmopathy. *Arch Intern Med* 1990;150:1098–1101.
29. Sjoberg HE, Saar M, Bostrom, L, Lundell G, Tallstedt L. Observations on progress periods in Graves' ophthalmopathy. *Acta Endocrinol* 1989; 121:179–181.
30. Wiersinga WM, Smit T, van der Gaag R, Mouritis M, Koorneef L. Clinical presentation of Graves' ophthalmopathy. *Ophthalmic Res* 1989;21:73–82.
31. Wall JR. Pathogenesis and management of thyroid associated ophthalmopathy: an update. *Thyroid Today* 1991;14:1–9.
32. Char DH. The ophthalmology of GD. *Med Clin North Am* 1991;75: 97–119.
33. Solovyeva TP. Endocrine ophthalmopathies. Problems of rational classification. *Orbit* 1989;8:193.
34. Perros P, Crombie AL, Kendall-Taylor P. Natural history of thyroid associated ophthalmopathy. *Clin Endocrinol* 1995;42:45–50.
35. Kiljanski J, Nebes V, Wall JR. The ocular muscle cell is a target of the immune system in endocrine ophthalmopathy. *Int Arch Allergy Immunol* 1995;106:204–212.
36. Bahn RS. The fibroblast is the target cell in the connective tissue manifestations of GD. *Int Arch Allergy Immunol* 1995;106:213–218.
37. Campbell RJ. Immunology of Graves' ophthalmopathy: retrobulbar histology, histochemistry. *Acta Endocrinol (Copenh)* 1989;121(suppl 2):9–16.
38. van der Gaag R, Schmidt ED, Koornneef L. Retrobulbar histology and immunohistochemistry in endocrine ophthalmopathy. In: Kahaly G, ed. Endocrine ophthalmopathy. Immunological and clinical aspects. *Dev Ophthalmol* 1993;25:1–10.
39. Campbell JR. Pathology of Graves' ophthalmopathy. In: Gorman CA, Waller A, Dyer S, eds. The eye and orbit in thyroid disease. New York: Raven Press, 1984.
40. Tallstedt L, Norberg R. Immunohistochemical staining of normal and Graves' extraocular muscle. *Invest Ophthalmol Vis Sci* 1988;29: 175–184.
41. Hiromatsu Y, Tanaka K, Ishisaka N, et al. Human histocompatibility leukocyte antigen-DR and heat shock protein-70 expression in eye muscle tissue in thyroid associated ophthalmopathy. *J Clin Endocrinol Metab* 1995;80:685–691.
42. Hufnagel TJ, Hickey WF, Cobbs NH, Jakobiec FA, Iwamo T, Eagle RC. Immunohistochemical and ultrastructural studies on the external orbital tissues of a patient with GD. *Ophthalmology* 1984;91:1411–1419.
43. Kroll AJ, Kuwabara T. Dysthyroid ocular myopathy. *Arch Ophthalmol* 1966;76:244–257.
44. Riley FC. Orbital pathology in GD. *Mayo Clin Proc* 1972;47:975–979.
45. Weetman AP, Cohen S, Gatter KC, Fells P, Shine B. Immunohistochemical analysis of the retrobulbar tissues in Graves' ophthalmopathy. *Clin Exp Immunol* 1989;75:222–227.
46. Heufelder AE, Bahn R. Detection and localization of cytokine immunoreactivity in retro-ocular connective tissue in Graves' ophthalmopathy. *Eur J Clin Invest* 1993;23:10–17.
47. Kahaly G, Hansen C, Felke B, Dienes HP. Immunohistochemical staining of retrobulbar adipose tissue in Graves' ophthalmopathy. *Clin Immunol Immunopathol* 1994;73:53–62.
48. Smith TJ, Bahn RS, Gorman CA. Connective tissue, glycosaminoglycans, and diseases of the thyroid. *Endocr Rev* 1989;10:366–391.

49. Small RG. Enlargement of levator palpebrae superioris muscle in Graves' ophthalmopathy. *Ophthalmology* 1989;96:424–430.
50. Kagoshima T, Hori S, Inoute Y. Qualitative and quantitative analyses of Mueller's muscle in dysthyroid ophthalmopathy. *Jpn J Ophthalmol* 1987;31:646–654.
51. Rootman J, Patel S, Berry K, Nugent R. Pathological and clinical study of Mueller's muscle in Graves' ophthalmopathy. *Can J Ophthalmol* 1987;22:32–36.
52. Bottazzo GF, Pujol-Borrell R, Hanafusa T, Feldmann M. Role of aberrant HLA-DR expression and antigen presentation in induction of endocrine autoimmunity. *Lancet* 1983;2:1115–1119.
53. Bahn RS, Heufelder AE. Orbital connective tissue in endocrine ophthalmopathy. In: Kahaly G, ed. Endocrine ophthalmopathy. Molecular, immunological and clinical aspects. *Dev Ophthalmol* 1993;25:46–57.
54. Heufelder AE, Bahn RS. Elevated expression in situ of selectin and immunoglobulin superfamily type adhesion molecules in retroocular connective tissues from patients with Graves' ophthalmopathy. *Clin Exp Immunol* 1993;91:381–389.
55. Heufelder AE, Goellner JR, Wenzel BE, Bahn RS. Immunohistochemical detection and localization of a 72-kilodalton heat shock protein in autoimmune thyroid disease. *J Clin Endocrinol Metab* 1992;74:724–731.
56. Smith TJ, Bahn RS, Gorman CA, Cheavens M. Stimulation of glycosaminoglycans by interferon gamma in cultured human retroocular fibroblasts. *J Clin Endocrinol Metab* 1991;72:1169–1171.
57. Smith TJ, Wang H-S, Evans CH. Leukoregulin is a potent inducer of hyaluronan synthesis in cultured human orbital fibroblasts. *Am J Physiol* 1995;268:C382–C388.
58. Metcalfe RA, Weetman AP. Stimulation of extraocular muscle fibroblasts by cytokines and hypoxia: possible role in thyroid-associated ophthalmopathy. *Clin Endocrinol* 1994;40:67–72.
59. Smith TJ, Bahn RS, Gorman CA. Hormonal regulation of hyaluronate synthesis in cultured human retroocular and dermal fibroblasts: evidence for differences between retroocular and dermal fibroblasts. *J Clin Endocrinol Metab* 1989;69:1019–1023.
60. Heufelder AE, Bahn RS. Modulation of Graves' orbital fibroblast proliferation by cytokines and glucocorticoid receptor agonists. *Invest Ophthalmol Vis Sci* 1994;35:120–127.
61. Heufelder AE, Smith TJ, Gorman CA, Bahn RS. Increased induction of HLA-DR by interferon gamma in cultured fibroblasts derived from patients with Graves' ophthalmopathy and pretibial dermapathy. *J Clin Endocrinol Metab* 1991;73:307–313.
62. Hiromatsu Y, Fukazawa H, How J, Wall JR. Antibody-dependent cell-mediated cytotoxicity against human eye muscle cells and orbital fibroblasts in Graves' ophthalmopathy—roles of class II MHC antigen expression and γ-interferon action on effector and target cells. *Clin Exp Immunol* 1987;70:593–603.
63. Heufelder AE, Bahn RS. Graves' immunoglobulins and cytokines stimulate the expression of intercellular adhesion molecule-1 (ICAM-1) in cultured orbital fibroblasts. *Eur J Clin Invest* 1992;22:529–537.
64. Heufelder AE, Wenzel BE, Bahn RS. Enhanced induction of a 72 kDa heat shock protein in cultured retroocular fibroblasts. *Invest Ophthalmol Vis Sci* 1992;33:466–470.
65. Heufelder AE, Wenzel BE, Bahn RS. Cell surface localization of a 72 kilodalton heat shock protein in retroocular fibroblasts from patients with Graves' ophthalmopathy. *J Clin Endocrinol Metab* 1992;74:732–736.
66. Heufelder AE, Wenzel BE, Bahn RS. Methimazole and propylthiouracil inhibit the oxygen free radical-induced expression of a 72 kilodalton heat shock protein in Graves' retroocular fibroblasts. *J Clin Endocrinol Metab* 1992;74:737–742.
67. Weetman AP. The role of T lymphocytes in thyroid-associated ophthalmopathy. *Autoimmunity* 1992;13:69–73.
68. Feldberg NT, Sergott RC, Savino PJ, Blizzard JJ, Schatz NJ, Amsel J. Lymphocyte subpopulations in Graves' ophthalmopathy. *Arch Ophthalmol* 1985;103:656–659.
69. Arnold K, Weetman AP. Cell-mediated immunity in thyroid-associated ophthalmopathy. *Orbit* 1996;15:159–164.
70. Munro RE, Lamki L, Row VV, Volpe R. Cell-mediated immunity in the exophthalmos of GD as demonstrated by the migration inhibition factor (MIF) test. *J Clin Endocrinol Metab* 1973;37:286–292.
71. Mullin BR, Levinson RE, Friedman A, Henson DE, Winand RJ, Kohn LD. Delayed hypersensitivity in GD and exophthalmos: identification of thyroglobulin in normal human orbital muscle. *Endocrinology* 1977;100:351–366.
72. Kuroki T, Ruf T, Whelan L, Miller A, Wall JR. Antithyroglobulin monoclonal and autoantibodies cross-reactivity on orbital connective tissue antigen. A possible mechanism for the association of ophthalmopathy with autoimmune thyroid disorders. *Clin Exp Immunol* 1985;69:931–936.
73. Weetman AP, Fells P, Shine B. T and B cell reactivity to extraocular and skeletal muscle in Graves' ophthalmopathy. *Clin Exp Immunol* 1989;73:323–327.
74. Arnold K, Tandon N, Macintosh RS, Ludgate M, Weetman AP. T cell responses to orbital antigens in thyroid-associated ophthalmopathy. *Clin Exp Immunol* 1994;96:329–334.
75. Kiljanski J, Stolarski C, Nebes V, Wall JR. Cell-mediated immunity against predicted epitopes of the 64 kDa protein 1D and eye muscle fractions in patients with thyroid-associated ophthalmopathy. *J Endo Invest* 1996;19:284–292.
76. Cohen M, Salvi M, Miller A, Bernard N, Wall JR. Cell-mediated immunity to orbital tissue antigens in thyroid associated ophthalmopathy determined using the leukocyte procoagulant activity assay. *Autoimmunity* 1992;11:225–231.
77. Wang PW, Hiromatsu Y, Laryea EA, How J, Wall JR. Immunologically mediated cytotoxicity against human eye muscle cells in Graves' ophthalmopathy. *J Clin Endocrinol Metab* 1986;63:316–320.
78. Wall JR, Trewin A, Fang SL, Ingbar SH, Braverman LE. Studies of immunoreactivity to human lacrimal gland fractions in patients with GD. *J Endocrinol* 1979;10:79–91.
79. Kelso A. Th1 and Th2 subsets: paradigms lost? *Immunol Today* 1995;16:374–379.
80. Rees Smith B, McLachlan SM, Furmaniak J. Autoantibodies to the thyrotropin receptor. *Endocr Rev* 1988;9:106–121.
81. Lindstrom J, Shelton D, Fuji Y. Myasthenia gravis (review). *Adv Immunol* 1988;42:233–284.
82. Liblau RS, Singer SM, McDevitt HO. Th1 and Th2 + T cells in the pathogenesis of organ-specific autoimmune diseases [Review]. *Immunol Today* 1995;16:34–38.
83. Grubeck-Loebenstein B, Trieb K, Sztankay A, Holter W, Anderi H, Wick G. Retrobulbar T cells from patients with Graves' ophthalmopathy are CD8+ and specifically recognize autologous fibroblasts. *J Clin Invest* 1994;93:2738–2743.
84. De Carli M, D'Elios MM, Mariotti S, et al. Cytolytic T cells with Th1-like cytokine profile predominate in retroorbital lymphocytic infiltrates of Graves' ophthalmopathy. *J Clin Endocrinol Metab* 1993;77:1120–1124.
85. McLachlan SM, Prummel MF, Rapoport B. Cell-mediated or humoral immunity in Graves' ophthalmopathy? Profiles of T-cell cytokines amplified by polymerase chain reaction from orbital tissue. *J Clin Endocrinol Metab* 1994;78:1070–1074.
86. De Carli M, D'Elios MM, Mariotti S, Pinchera A. Cytolytic T cells with Th1-like cytokine profile predominate in retroorbital lymphocytic infiltrates of Graves' ophthalmopathy. *J Clin Endocrinol Metab* 1993;77:1120–1124.
87. Heufelder AE, Herterich S, Ernst G, Bahn RS, Scriba PC. Analysis of retroorbital T-cell antigen receptor variable region gene usage in patients with Graves' ophthalmopathy. *Eur J Endocrinol* 1995;132:266–277.
88. McKenzie JM. Neonatal GD. *J Clin Endocrinol Metab* 1964;24:660–668.
89. Singer J. Neonatal thyrotoxicosis. *J Pediatr* 1977;91:749–751.
90. McKenzie JM, Zakarija M. Pathogenesis of neonatal GD. *J Endocrinol Invest* 1978;2:183–189.
91. Kelly W, Longson D, Smithard D, Fawcitt R, Wensley R. An evaluation of plasma exchange for Graves' ophthalmopathy. *Clin Endocrinol (Oxf)* 1983;18:485–493.
92. Glinoer D, Etienne-Decerf J, Schrooyen M, et al. Beneficial effects of intensive plasma exchange followed by immunosuppressive therapy in severe Graves' ophthalmopathy. *Acta Endocrinol (Copenh)* 1986;111:30–38.
93. Kodama K, Sikorska H, Bandy-Dafoe P, Bayly R, Wall JR. Demonstration of a circulating autoantibody against a soluble eye muscle antigen in Graves' ophthalmopathy. *Lancet* 1982;2:1353–1356.
94. Nauman JA. Biological activity of antibodies circulating in endocrine ophthalmopathy. In: Kahaly G, ed. Endocrine ophthalmopathy. Molecular, immunological and clinical aspects. *Dev Ophthalmol* 1993;25:29–37.
95. Wall JR. Nature and significance of eye muscle autoantigens in endocrine ophthalmopathy. In: Kahaly G, ed. Endocrine ophthalmopa-

thy. Molecular, immunological and clinical aspects. *Dev Ophthalmol* 1993;25:77–85.
96. Atkinson S, Holcombe M, Kendall-Taylor P. Ophthalmopathic immunoglobulin in patients with Graves' ophthalmopathy. *Lancet* 1984; 2:374–376.
97. Miller A, Sikorska H, Salvi M, Wall JR. Evaluation of an enzyme-linked immunosorbent assay for the measurement of autoantibodies against eye muscle membrane antigens in Graves' ophthalmopathy. *Acta Endocrinol (Copenh)* 1986;113:514–522.
98. Kahaly G, Moncayo R, Bemetz U, Krause U, Beyer J, Pfeiffer EF. Eye muscle antibodies in endocrine exophthalmos: clinical and serological observations. *Horm Metab Res* 1989;21:137–141.
99. Kapusta M, Salvi M, Triller H, Gardini E, Bernard N, Wall JR. Eye muscle membrane reactive antibodies are not detected in serum or immunoglobulin fraction of patients with thyroid-associated ophthalmopathy using ELISA and crude membranes. *Autoimmunity* 1990;7: 33–40.
100. Faryna M, Nauman J, Gardas A. Measurement of autoantibodies against human eye muscle membranes in Graves' ophthalmopathy. *Br Med J* 1985;59:104–116.
101. Kadlubowski M, Irvine WJ, Rowland AC. The lack of specificity of ophthalmic immunoglobulins in GD. *J Clin Endocrinol Metab* 1986; 63:990–995.
102. Salvi M, Miller A, Wall JR. Human orbital tissue and thyroid membranes express a 64 kDa protein which is recognized by autoantibodies in the serum of patients with thyroid-associated ophthalmopathy. *FEBS Lett* 1988;232:135–139.
103. Bernard NF, Chung F, Teboul N, Zhang Z-G, Salvi M, Wall JR. Isotype and immunoglobulin subclass distribution of eye muscle membrane reactive antibodies in the serum of patients with thyroid-associated ophthalmopathy as detected in Western blotting. *Autoimmunity* 1990;10:57–63.
104. Miller A, Arthurs B, Boucher A, et al. Significance of antibodies reactive with a 64 kDa eye muscle membrane antigen in patients with thyroid autoimmunity. *Thyroid* 1992;2:197–202.
105. Hiromatsu Y, Cadarso L, Salvi M, Wall JR. Significance of cytotoxic eye muscle antibodies in patients with thyroid-associated ophthalmopathy. *Autoimmunity* 1990;5:205–213.
106. Mengistu M, Laryea EA, Miller A, Wall JR. Clinical significance of a new autoantibody against a human eye muscle soluble antigen detected by immunofluorescence. *Clin Exp Immunol* 1986;65:19–27.
107. Kandror V, Birjukova M, Kryukova I, Mkrtumova N, Konnova E. Some immunological correlations between thyroid pathology and ophthalmopathy. *Exp Clin Endocrinol* 1991;97:212–216.
108. Rosen C, Raikow RB, Burde RM, Kennerdell JS, Mosseri M, Scalise D. Immunohistochemical evidence for IgA1 involvement in Graves' ophthalmopathy. *Ophthalmology* 1992;99:146.
109. Raikow RR, Dalbow MH, Kennerdell JS, et al. Immunohistochemical evidence for IgE involvement in Graves' orbitopathy. *Ophthalmology* 1990;97:629–635.
110. Boucher A, Bernard N, Miller A, Rodien P, Wall JR. Physicochemical characterization of 64 kDa antigens in thyroid-associated ophthalmopathy. Proc 65th annual meeting of the American Thyroid Association, Rochester, Minnesota, September 1992. *Thyroid* 1992(suppl) [abstr].
111. Zhang ZG, Salvi M, Miller A, Bernard N, Arthurs B, Wall JR. Restricted tissue reactivity of autoantibodies to 64 kDa eye muscle membrane antigen in thyroid-associated ophthalmopathy. *Clin Immunol Immunopathol* 1992;62:183–189.
112. Salvi M, Bernard N, Miller A, Zhang ZG, Gardini E, Wall JR. Prevalence of antibodies reactive with a 64 kDa eye muscle membrane antigen in thyroid-associated ophthalmopathy. *Thyroid* 1991;1:207–213.
113. Sato M, Scalise D, Tyutyunikov A, Genovese C, Wall JR. Antibodies reactive with eye muscle and thyroid membrane antigens in early and late thyroid associated ophthalmopathy. In: Nagataki S, Mori T, Torizuka K, eds. 80 years of Hashimoto disease. *Excerpta Medica* 1993; 649–652.
114. Salvi M, Arthurs B, Miller A, Bernard N, Wall JR. Patients with upper eyelid retraction and eye muscle autoantibodies may have subclinical thyroid autoimmunity. *Clin Immunol Immunopathol* 1995;74: 44–50.
115. Hiromatsu Y, Sato M, Tanaka K, et al. Significance of anti-eye muscle antibody in patients with thyroid-associated ophthalmopathy by quantitative Western blot. *Autoimmunity* 1993;14:1–8.
116. Wall JR, Hayes M, Scalise D, et al. Native gel electrophoresis and isoelectric focusing of the 64 kDa protein shows that is an important target for serum autoantibodies in patients with thyroid-associated ophthalmopathy and not expressed in other skeletal muscle. *J Clin Endocrinol Metab* 1995;80:1226–1232.
117. Atabay C, Schrooyen M, Zhang Z-G, Salvi M, Glinoer D, Wall JR. Use of eye muscle antibody measurements to monitor response to plasmapheresis in patients with thyroid-associated ophthalmopathy. *J Endocrinol Invest* 1993;16:1–6.
118. Dakovska L, Vulkova H, Kovatchena R, et al. Anti-eye muscle antibodies in patients with thyroid-associated ophthalmopathy (TAO) [abstr]. *Proc Ann Balkan Congress of Endocrinology*, Bursa, Turkey, 1995.
119. Boucher A, Emond G, Richard M, Griffiths N, Beauregard H, Comtois R. Effects of the treatment of hyperthyroidism on the levels of eye muscle autoantibodies in Graves' patients [abstr]. *Proc 11th International Thyroid Congress*, Toronto, Canada, September 11–15, 1995.
120. Wengrowicz S, Puig-Domingo M, Soldevila J, de Leiva A. Prevalences of antibodies reactive with pig eye muscle membrane antigens in patients with thyroid-associated ophthalmopathy [abstr]. *Proc 11th International Thyroid Congress*, Toronto, Canada, September 11–15, 1995.
121. Chang TC, Chang TJ, Huang YS, Hua KM, Su RJ, Kao SCS. Identification of autoantigen recognized by autoimmune ophthalmopathy sera with immunoblotting correlated with orbital computed tomography. *Clin Immunol Immunopathol* 1992;65:161–166.
122. Ahmann A, Baker JR, Weetman AP, Wartofsky L, Nutman TB, Burman KD. Antibodies to porcine eye muscle in patients with Graves' ophthalmopathy: identification of serum immunoglobulins directed against unique determinants by immunoblotting and enzyme linked immunosorbent assay. *J Clin Endocrinol Metab* 1987;64:454–460.
123. Schifferdecker E, Ketzler-Sasse U, Boehm BO, Ronsheimer HB, Scherbaum WA, Schoffling K. Re-evaluation of eye muscle autoantibody determination in Graves' ophthalmopathy: failure to detect a specific antigen by use of enzyme-linked immunosorbent assay, indirect immunofluorescence and immunoblotting techniques. *Acta Endocrinol* 1989;121:643–650.
124. Weightman D, Kendall-Taylor P. Cross reaction of eye muscle antibodies with thyroid tissue in thyroid associated ophthalmopathy. *J Endocrinol* 1989;122:201–206.
125. Tandon N, Yan SL, Arnold K, Metcalfe RA, Weetman AP. Immunoglobulin class and subclass distribution of eye muscle and fibroblast antibodies in patients with thyroid associated ophthalmopathy. *Clin Endocrinol* 1994;40:629–639.
126. Kendler DL, Rootman J, Huber GK, Davies TF. A 64 kDa membrane antigen is a recurrent epitope for natural autoantibodies in patients with Graves' thyroid and ophthalmic diseases. *Clin Endocrinol* 1991; 35:539–547.
127. Elisei R, Weightman D, Kendall-Taylor P, Vassart G, Ludgate M. Muscle autoantigens in thyroid associated ophthalmopathy: the limits of molecular genetics. *J Endocrinol Invest* 1993;16:533–540.
128. Ludgate M. Back to the drawing board for antigens in endocrine ophthalmopathy? In: Kahaly G, ed. Endocrine ophthalmopathy. Molecular, immunological and clinical aspects. *Dev Ophthalmol* 1993;25:86–92.
129. Dong Q, Ludgate M, Vassart G. Cloning and sequencing of a novel 64 kDa autoantigen recognized by patients with autoimmune thyroid disease. *J Clin Endocrinol Metab* 1991;72:1375–1381.
130. Zhang ZG, Dong Q, Rodien P, et al. Antibodies in the serum of patients with autoimmune thyroid disorders react with a recombinant-98 amino acid fragment of a full length 64 kDa eye muscle membrane protein which is also expressed in the thyroid. *Autoimmunity* 1992;13: 151–157.
131. Bernard NF, Salvi M, Tyutyunikov A, Genovese C, Ludgate M, Wall JR. Antibodies against 1D, a recombinant 64 kDa membrane protein, are associated with ophthalmopathy in patients with thyroid autoimmunity. *Clin Immunol Immunopathol* 1994;70:225–233.
132. Boucher A, Bernard N, Miller A, Rodien P, Salvi M, Wall JR. Two dimensional gel electrophoresis identifies minor differences in immunologically cross-reactive 64 kDa autoantigens in the thyroid and eye muscle. *J Endocrinol Invest* 1994;17:7–13.
133. Salvi M, Bingoye F, Chung F, Wall JR. Affinity purification of orbital membrane antigens for the study of the pathogenesis of Graves' ophthalmopathy. *J Clin Endocrinol Metab* 1988;66:939–945.
134. Bahn R, Smith TJ, Gorman CA. The central role of the fibroblast in the pathogenesis of extrathyroidal manifestations of GD. *Acta Endocrinol (Copenh)* 1989;121:75–81.
135. Bahn RS, Gorman CA, Woloschak GE, David CS, Johnson PM, Johnson CM. Human retroocular fibroblasts in vitro: a model for the

study of Graves' ophthalmopathy. *J Clin Endocrinol Metab* 1987;65: 665–670.
136. Bahn RS, Gorman CA, Johnson CM, Smith TJ. Presence of antibodies in the sera of patients with GD recognizing a 23 kilodalton fibroblast protein. *J Clin Endocrinol Metab* 1989;69:622–628.
137. Perros P, Kendall-Taylor P. Antibodies to orbital tissues in thyroid-associated ophthalmopathy. *Acta Endocrinol (Copenh)* 1992;126:137–142.
138. Weightman D, Perros P, Sherif I, Janet F, Kendall-Taylor P. Autoantibodies to eye muscle and orbital fibroblasts in the pathogenesis of thyroid-associated ophthalmopathy. *Exp Clin Endocrinol* 1991;97: 197–201.
139. McDermott MT, West SG, Emlen JW, Kidd GS. Antideoxyribonucleic acid antibodies in GD. *J Clin Endocrinol Metab* 1990;71:509–511.
140. Loviselli A, Velluzi F, Pala R, et al. Circulating antibodies to DNA-related antigens in patients with autoimmune thyroid disorders. *Autoimmunity* 1992;14:33–36.
141. Kiljanski J, Barsouk A, Peele K, et al. Antibodies against striated muscle, connective tissue and nuclear antigens in patients with thyroid-associated ophthalmopathy: Is GD a collagen disorder? *Horm Res* 1995; 27:528–532.
142. Neri S, Gambuzza C, Biondi L, Baschieri L. Parameters of organ-specific and non-specific autoimmunity in patients with Basedow's disease and Basedow's ophthalmopathy. Changes induced by IVIG treatment. *Clin Ter* 1992;141:49–54.
143. McCombe PA, Chalk JB, Pender MP. Familial occurrence of multiple sclerosis with thyroid disease and systemic lupus erythematosus. *J Neurol Sci* 1990;97:163–171.
144. Loviselli A, Velluzzi F, Pala R, et al. A family study of the antiphospholipid syndrome associated with other autoimmune diseases. *J Rheumatol* 1992;19:1393–1396.
145. Gordon T, Isenberg D. Organ specific and multisystem autoimmune disease: part of a spectrum which may coexist in the same patient. *Clin Rheumatol* 1990;9:401–403.
146. Medeiros-Neto G, Zhang ZG, Lima L, Iacona A, Liberman A, Salvi M, Wall JR. Immunologically mediated cytotoxicity against human eye muscle and thyroid cells in euthyroid and thyrotoxic Graves' ophthalmopathy. *Autoimmunity* 1991;9:293–300.
147. Barsouk A, Wengrowitz S, Scalise D, et al. New assays for the measurement of serum antibodies reactive with eye muscle membrane antigens confirm their importance in thyroid-associated ophthalmopathy. *Thyroid* 1995;5:195–200.
148. Perros P, Kendall-Taylor P. Biological activity of autoantibodies from patients with thyroid-associated ophthalmopathy: in vitro effect on porcine extraocular myoblasts. *Q J Med* 1992;84:691–706.
149. Otto E, Krimmer U, Stover C, Beyer J, Kahaly G. Eye muscle antibodies in endocrine ophthalmopathy. In: Kahaly G, ed. Endocrine ophthalmopathy. Molecular, immunological and clinical aspects. *Dev Ophthalmol* 1993;25:93–100.
150. Rotella CM, Zonefrati R, Toccafondi R, Valente WA, Kohn LD. Ability of monoclonal antibodies to the thyrotropin receptor to increase collagen synthesis in human fibroblasts: an assay which appears to measure exophthalmogenic immunoglobulins in Graves' sera. *J Clin Endocrinol Metab* 1986;62:357–367.
151. Stover C, Otto E, Beyer J, Kahaly G. Humoral immunity and retrobulbar fibroblasts in endocrine ophthalmopathy. *Acta Endocrinol (Copenh)* 1992;126:394–398.
152. Westermark K, Lilja K, Karlsson FA. Effects of sera and immunoglobulin preparations from patients with endocrine ophthalmopathy on the production of hyaluronate and the incorporation tritiated thymidine in fibroblasts. *Acta Endocrinol (Copenh)* 1989;121:85–89.
153. Metcalfe RA, Davies R, Weetman AP. Analysis of fibroblast stimulating activity in IgG from patients with Graves' dermopathy. *Thyroid* 1993;3:207–212.
154. Carlos Jaume J, Portolano S, Prummel MF, McLachlan S, Rapaport B. Molecular cloning and characterization of genes for antibodies generated by orbital tissue-infiltrating B-cells in Graves' ophthalmopathy. *J Clin Endocrinol Metab* 1994;78:348–352.
155. Hancock SL, McDougall IR, Constine LS. Thyroid abnormalities after therapeutic external radiation (review). *Int J Radiol Oncol Biol Phys* 1995;31:1165–1170.
156. Ludgate M, Dong Q, Soreq H, Mariotti S, Vassart G. The pathophysiological significance of a thyroglobulin-acetylcholinesterase-shared epitope in patients with Graves' ophthalmopathy. *Acta Endocrinol* 1989;121:38–45.
157. Mappouras GD, Philippou G, Haralambus S, et al. Antibodies to acetylcholinesterase cross-reacting with thyroglobulin in myasthenia gravis and GD. *Clin Exp Immunol* 1995;100:336–343.
158. Heufelder AE. Pathogenesis of Graves' ophthalmopathy: recent controversies and progress. *Eur J Endocrinol* 1995;132:532–541.
159. Heufelder AE, Dutton CM, Sarkar G, Donovan KA, Bahn RS. Detection of TSH receptor RNA in cultured fibroblasts from patients with Graves' ophthalmopathy and pretibial dermopathy. *Thyroid* 1993;3: 297–300.
160. Feliciello A, Porcellini A, Ciullo I, Bonavolonta G, Avvedimento EV, Fenzi G. Expression of thyrotropin-receptor mRNA in healthy and GD retro-orbital tissue. *Lancet* 1993;342:337–338.
161. Endo T, Ohta K, Haraguchi K, Onaya T. Cloning and functional expression of a thyrotropin receptor cDNA from fat cells. *J Biol Chem* 1995;270:10833–10837.
162. Roselli-Rehfuss L, Robbins LS, Cone RD. Thyrotropin receptor messenger ribonucleic acid is expressed in most brown and white adipose tissues in the guinea pig. *Endocrinology* 1992;130:1857–1861.
163. Francis T, Burch HB, Cai W, et al. Lymphocytes express thyrotropin receptor-specific mRNA as detected by the PCR technique. *Thyroid* 1991;1:223–228.
164. Paschke R, Elisei R, Vassart G, Ludgate M. Lack of evidence supporting the presence of mRNA for the thyrotropin receptor in extra-ocular muscle. *J Endocrinol Invest* 1993;16:329–332.
165. Burch HB, Selletti D, Barnes SG, Nagy EV, Bahn RS, Burman KD. Thyrotropin receptor antisera for the detection of immunoreactive protein species in retroocular fibroblasts obtained from patients with Graves' ophthalmopathy. *J Clin Endocrinol Metab* 1994;78: 1384–1391.
166. Cuddihy RM, Dutton CM, Bahn RS. A polymorphism in the extracellular domain of the thyrotropin receptor is highly associated with autoimmune thyroid disease in females. *Thyroid* 1995;5:89–95.
167. Tao TW, Leu SL, Kriss JP. Biological activity of autoantibodies associated with Graves' dermopathy. *J Clin Endocrinol Metab* 1989;69: 90–99.
168. Korducki JM, Loftus SJ, Bahn RS. Stimulation of glycosaminoglycan production in cultured human retroocular fibroblasts. *Invest Ophthalmol Vis Sci* 1992;33:2037–2042.
169. Harvey RD, Metcalfe RA, Morteo C, Furmaniak W, Weetman AP, Bevan JS. Acute pretibial myxedema following radioiodine therapy for thyrotoxic GD. *Clin Endocrinol* 1995;42:657–660.
170. Zhang ZG, Wall JR, Bernard NF. Tissue distribution and quantitation of a gene expressing a 64 kDa antigen associated with thyroid-associated orbitopathy. *Clin Immunol Immunopathol* 1996;80:236–244.
171. Hiromatsu Y, Fukazawa H, Guinard F, Salvi M, How J, Wall JR. A thyroid cytotoxic antibody that cross-reacts with an eye muscle cell surface antigen may be the cause of thyroid associated ophthalmopathy. *J Clin Endocrinol Metab* 1988;67:565–570.
172. Wall JR, Salvi M, Bernard N, Boucher A, Haegert D. Thyroid-associated ophthalmopathy—A model for the association of organ-specific autoimmune disorders. *Immunol Today* 1991;12:150–153.
173. Berenson CS, Smith TJ. Human orbital fibroblasts in culture express ganglioside profiles distinct from those in dermal fibroblasts. *J Clin Endocrinol Metab* 1995;80:2668–2674.
174. Smith TJ, Sempowski GD, Wang HS, Del Vecchio PJ, Lippe SD, Phipps RP. Evidence for cellular heterogeneity in primary cultures of human orbital fibroblasts. *J Clin Endocrinol Metab* 1995;80: 2620–2625.
175. Khalili HA, deKeizer RJ, Kijlstra A. Analysis of tear proteins in Graves' ophthalmopathy by high performance liquid chromatography. *Am J Ophthalmol* 1988;106:186–190.
176. Barsouk A, Fraiture, Peele KA, et al. Increased manganese superoxide dismutase activity in lacrimal secretions (tears) from patients with thyroid-associated ophthalmopathy; correlation with eye muscle dysfunction [abstr]. *Proc 11th International Thyroid Congress*, Toronto, Canada, 1995, September 11–15.
177. Wall JR. Extrathyroidal manifestations of GD [editorial]. *J Clin Endocrinol Metab* 1995;80:3427–3429.
178. Olson BR, Klein JI, Benner R, Burdett R, Trzepacz P, Levey GS. Hyperthyroid myopathy and the response to treatment. *Thyroid* 1991;1: 137–141.
179. Dudgeon LS, Urquhart AL. Lymphorrhages in the muscle in exophthalmic goitre. *Brain* 1975;49:182–186.
180. Salvi M, De Chiara F, Gardini E, et al. Echocardiographic diagnosis of pretibial myxedema in patients with autoimmune thyroid disease. *Acta Endocrinol (Copenh)* 1994;131:113–119.

181. Stover C, Otto, Beyer J, Kahaly G. Cellular immunity and retrobulbar fibroblasts in Graves' ophthalmopathy. *Thyroid* 1994;4:161–165.
182. Arnold K, Metcalfe R, Weetman AP. IgA class fibroblast antibodies in patients with GD and pretibial myxedema. *J Clin Endocrinol Metab* 1995;80:3430–3437.
183. Porter JD, Baker RS. Muscles of a different "color": the unusual properties of the extraocular muscles may predispose or protect them in neurogenic and myogenic disease. *Neurology* 1996;46:30–37.
184. Hudson HL, Levin L, Feldon SE. Graves' exophthalmos unrelated to extraocular muscle enlargement. Superior rectus muscle inflammation may induce venous obstruction. *Ophthalmology* 1991;98:1485–1499.

CHAPTER 19

Thyroid-Associated Ophthalmopathy: Treatment

Ronald R. Reed

Thyroid ophthalmopathy is the presentation of infiltrative or inflammatory orbital disease in conjunction with thyroid dysfunction. Although this occurs almost exclusively in Graves' disease patients, it may also be seen in euthyroid patients, in primary hypothyroidism, and in Hashimoto's thyroiditis. (The ophthalmologic manifestations are identical irrespective of the type of autoimmune thyroid disease.) Hashimoto's thyroiditis accounts for only 3% of cases of thyroid ophthalmopathy.

Euthyroid patients with ophthalmopathy present more of a diagnostic dilemma because their circulating levels of triiodothyronine (T_3) and thyroxine (T_4) are normal. The majority of these patients represent Graves' disease patients in whom the ophthalmopathy has preceded the eventual onset of the hyperthyroidism.

There is, however, a small group of thyroid ophthalmopathy patients who remain euthyroid, but in whom the thyroid gland functions autonomously of the hypothalamic–pituitary axis. These patients are believed to represent a subset of Graves' disease, as their ophthalmologic signs and symptoms and orbital pathology are identical to those of Graves' disease patients. They can be identified by the presence of thyroid stimulating hormone (TSH)-receptor antibodies.

Patients with autoimmune thyroiditis or Hashimoto's disease make antithyroid antibodies. Despite this, less than 3% of Hashimoto's thyroiditis patients develop thyroid ophthalmopathy.

Primary hypothyroidism is an autoimmune thyroid disease in which a TSH-blocking antibody is produced. This binds the TSH-receptors on the thyroid follicles and prevents stimulation by circulating TSH.

Thyroid ophthalmopathy may be seen, but only rarely, without hyperthyroidism.

In summary, while the eponym *Graves' disease* originally referred only to patients with diffuse toxic goiter and hyperthyroidism, it now refers to a family of autoimmune thyroid diseases that involve one or more of the following: hyperthyroidism, ophthalmopathy, and infiltrative dermopathy. Among patients with thyroid ophthalmopathy, 90% have Graves' hyperthyroidism, 1% have primary hypothyroidism, 3% have Hashimoto's disease, and 5% are euthyroid.

Thyroid ophthalmopathy is a self-limiting autoimmune disease. Its clinical course is protean and characterized by remissions and exacerbations. Most cases run a variable course lasting 1½ to 3 years. The incidence is 16 cases per 100,000 population per year in women, and 2.9 cases per 100,000 population in men. The high incidence of thyroid ophthalmopathy can be further appreciated by the fact that 47% of 1409 expanding orbital lesions proved to be thyroid ophthalmopathy [1]. It may be difficult to understand why a systemic autoimmune disease can frequently be unilateral. In most Graves' disease patients, involvement that appears to be unilateral proves to be bilateral (but asymmetric) when magnetic resonance imaging (MRI) is used. Furthermore, MRI can often be used to demonstrate orbital involvement in Graves' disease patients who appear not to have orbitopathy. Seventy-one percent of untreated Graves' disease patients with no clinical ophthalmopathy have been shown to have enlarged extraocular muscles by MRI [2].

Thyroid ophthalmopathy has a clear bimodal distribution, with the major peak incidence occurring at age 40 years and a second minor peak incidence occurring at age 60 years.

There is a strong female predilection in thyroid ophthalmopathy (as there is in many autoimmune diseases), with a female-to-male ratio of 6:1. Although thyroid ophthalmopathy is more common in younger women, it is more severe in men and in patients of both sexes over age 50.

R. R. Reed: Pittsford, New York 14534.

Thyroid ophthalmopathy also has a genetic predisposition. It has long been known that there is an increased incidence of Graves' disease in certain families. Evidence for an immunogenetic predisposition has been shown in the high prevalence of HLA-DR3 cell markers in patients with Graves' disease (3).

Environmental factors probably also play a role in the genesis of this disease, because the rate of concordance is maximally 50% in identical twins (3). Smoking is one of the environmental factors affecting thyroid ophthalmopathy. It has been clearly shown to increase the incidence and severity of thyroid ophthalmopathy in Graves' hyperthyroid patients.

Thyroid orbitopathy is clinically the most common orbital disease. Sixty-four percent of all orbital inflammatory disorders are diagnosed as Graves' disease.

The temporal relationship between the onset of Graves' hyperthyroidism and the development of thyroid ophthalmopathy is very variable. The thyroid gland and the orbital fibroblasts are both only the end organs of a common autoimmune process. Yet the clinical course of the thyroid gland disease and the clinical course of the orbitopathy progress independently. The orbitopathy may predate the onset of the thyroid gland dysfunction, occur concurrently, or have its onset after years of thyroid disease remission (Fig. 1). Treatment of thyroid gland dysfunction by propylthiouracil (PTU) or methimazole (Tapazole), radioactive iodine-131 (^{131}I) ablation, or surgical resection does not appear to alter the course of the thyroid ophthalmopathy. There is, in fact, some evidence that treatment with radioactive ^{131}I may exacerbate the orbital disease by causing glandular destruction with release of thyroid antigens, giving an augmented autoimmune response.

In fact, most patients with Graves' disease either present with concurrent onset of thyroid gland and orbital involvement, or the two occur within a narrow time span (Table 1). This makes the diagnosis of thyroid ophthalmopathy obvious. Yet it must be kept in mind that a long temporal delay can exist between the onset of the thyroid gland disease and the orbitopathy. The orbital disease may begin 10 to 20 years after the thyroid disease has been successfully treated. At the time of presentation of orbital disease, the thyroid disease may have been a distant memory and the patient euthyroid for many years.

Similarly, one must be alert for patients whose orbitopathy precedes the onset of their thyroid gland disease. This occurs in 35% of patients who eventually become clinically hyperthyroid.

There is no laboratory test specific for thyroid ophthalmopathy. Therefore, clinical diagnosis relies on the presence of several clinical findings, without universal agreement on inclusion or exclusion criteria, which produces varying incidence rates in different clinical studies. This creates a scenario very similar to the problem of diagnosing demyelinating disease when clinical symptoms were the only available diagnostic criteria. As another example, with the advent of MRI, monoclonal cerebrospinal fluid antibodies, and visual evoked response (VER), the incidence of multiple sclerosis (MS) was found to have been grossly understated.

In summary, most patients with Graves' hyperthyroidism are found to have thyroid ophthalmopathy if MRI imaging is performed. Seventy-one percent of untreated Graves' disease patients with no clinical ophthalmopathy show extraocular muscle enlargement by MRI (3). Therefore, clinical examination methods are insufficient to diagnose very early degrees of thyroid ophthalmopathy in patients with autoimmune thyroid disorders who do not initially present with clinical ophthalmopathy.

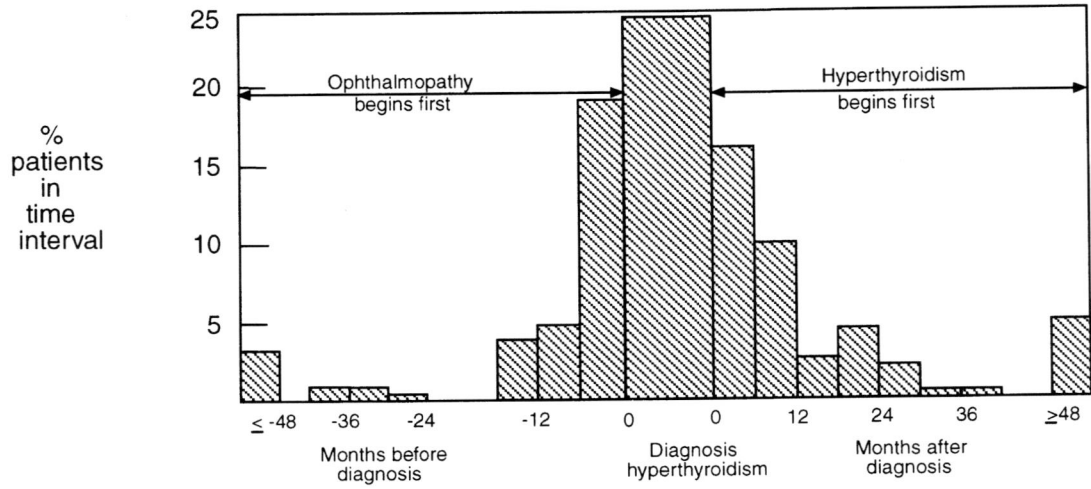

FIG. 1. Temporal relationship between the onset of Graves' ophthalmopathy and diagnosis of thyrotoxicosis. (From ref. 4.)

TABLE 1. *Temporal relationship between onset of thyroid ophthalmopathy and clinical hyperthyroidism*

Thyroid ophthalmopathy begins before hyperthyroidism	35%
Thyroid ophthalmopathy begins concurrently with hyperthyroidism	25%
Thyroid ophthalmopathy begins after hyperthyroidism	40%

PATHOPHYSIOLOGY

Thyroid ophthalmopathy is an autoimmune disease, involving both humoral and cell-mediated immunity of the crossfire type in which the thyroid and orbital tissues share common antigens. Crossfire-type reactions produce clinical disease manifestations because of shared antigenicity. There is no evidence that TSH, T_4, or other thyroid hormones have any role in thyroid ophthalmopathy.

Evidence for an immune basis for thyroid ophthalmopathy includes the following:

1. Ophthalmopathy involves lymphocytic infiltration of the orbit.
2. Ophthalmopathy is improved by plasmapheresis.
3. Thyroid ophthalmopathy has been transferred by bone marrow transplantation.
4. Thyroid ophthalmopathy may be partially suppressed by immunomodulation with corticosteroids and immunosuppressive agents.
5. Thyroid ophthalmopathy is seen in patients with other autoimmune diseases such as myasthenia gravis, celiac disease, and vitiligo.

The orbital antigenic site and the precise interplay between humoral and cell-mediated immunity is yet to be worked out. TSH-receptor antibodies are clearly the cause of the hyperthyroidism in Graves' disease, as they drive thyroid gland production. The demonstration of TSH receptors on extraocular muscles suggests a crossfire reaction. Yet the absence of any correlation between TSH-receptor antibody level and presence of thyroid ophthalmopathy fails to support this mechanism.

An autoimmune response to the 64-kDa antigen expressed on both thyroid and eye muscle membranes is an attractive theory. Unfortunately, IgG antibodies in many normal human sera can demonstrate binding to recurrent 64-kDa antigen. Therefore, the apparent specificity of the crossover represents only the natural autoantibodies reacting with recurrent autoepitopes, rather than a specific humoral antibody causing thyroid ophthalmopathy (5). So, although the clinical hyperthyroidism is a result of the production of TSH-receptor antibodies, there is no support for a humoral mechanism in thyroid ophthalmopathy. The evidence points to a cell-mediated mechanism.

Retrobulbar T cells in patients with thyroid ophthalmopathy have been shown to specifically recognize autologous retrobulbar fibroblasts. The retrobulbar fibroblasts are the major T-cell target in Graves' ophthalmopathy. Cytokine production may explain fibroblast proliferation, glycosaminoglycan secretion, and the secondary eye muscle enlargement (6).

Both retrobulbar and pretibial fibroblasts are likely the important effector cells in thyroid ophthalmopathy and pretibial dermopathy. Histologic similarities exist between the retrobulbar and the pretibial tissue in Graves' patients. In both there is lymphocytic infiltration and glycosaminoglycan production. Sensitized T cells release cytokines, including interferon-γ, which is capable of stimulating glycosaminoglycan production by fibroblasts. The accumulation of these hydrophilic mucopolysaccharides, with secondary edema, produces the clinical manifestations of thyroid ophthalmopathy and pretibial dermopathy. Only the fibroblasts from the retrobulbar and pretibial regions possess this unique immunological feature, which explains the site selectivity of Graves' disease (7).

Moreover, intrinsic differences in fibroblasts probably underlie the site-specific connective tissue manifestation seen with a specific autoimmune disease. Orbital and skin fibroblasts demonstrate different cytokine response domains. Prostaglandin E_2 (PGE_2) produces a rapid morphologic change in cultured orbital fibroblasts taken from Graves' patients. Skin fibroblasts fail to respond to PGE_2 (8).

In summary, the orbital fibroblast, rather than the extraocular muscle cell, is the autoimmune target in Graves' ophthalmopathy and pretibial dermopathy. Although the extraocular muscle bodies are grossly enlarged in thyroid ophthalmopathy, the muscle cells are histologically intact. The muscles are enlarged as a result of an accumulation of glycosaminoglycans between the muscle cells. These glycosaminoglycans are produced by fibroblasts that are stimulated by T-cell-secreted cytokines (9).

CLINICAL MANIFESTATIONS OF THYROID OPHTHALMOPATHY

The majority of Graves' disease patients have thyroid ophthalmopathy. Even in Graves' patients without clinically detectable ophthalmopathy, MRI demonstrates extraocular muscle involvement in 71%.

Periorbital Manifestations

Thyroid ophthalmopathy can produce swelling and chemosis of the lids and periorbital region due to edema. There is increased thickness to the periorbital fat pad (Fig. 2).

Lids

Upper eyelid retraction is historically one of the hallmark signs of thyroid ophthalmopathy, occurring in ap-

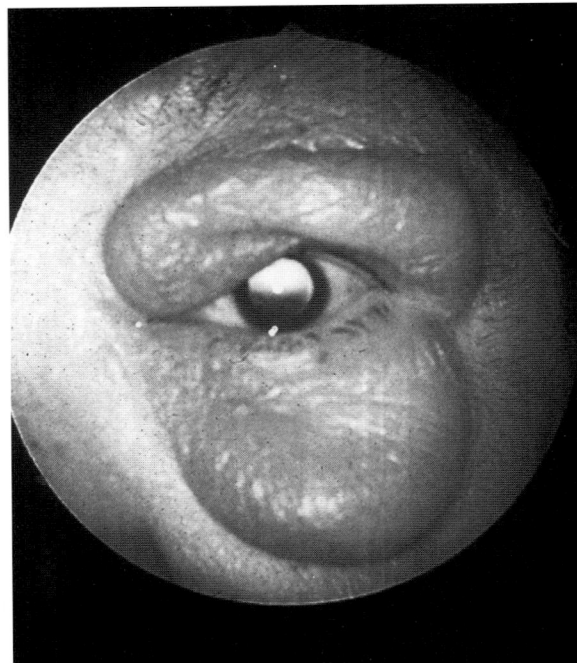

FIG. 2. Marked swelling and chemosis of the lids and periorbital region resulting from thyroid ophthalmopathy.

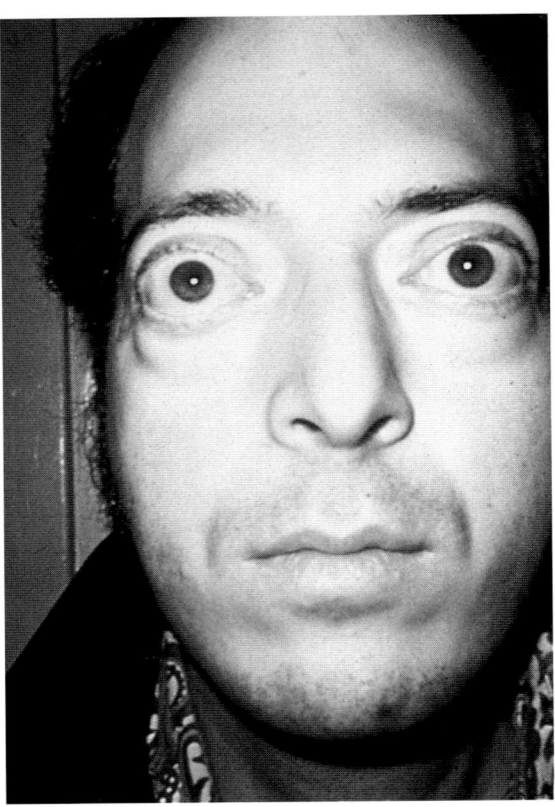

FIG. 3. Bilateral asymmetric lid retraction with exposed sclera above and below corneal limbus.

proximately 75% of patients at the time of diagnosis. In normal eyes, the upper lid covers 1.5 mm of superior cornea, and the top border of the lower lid is at the lower corneal edge. Lid retraction is present if either (a) the upper lid is at or above the superior corneal border or (b) more than 1 mm of exposed sclera is visible below the cornea (Fig. 3).

Lid retraction has three different mechanisms. First, it can result from increased Müller's muscle tone due to high levels of circulating catecholamines in patients who are endocrinologically hyperthyroid. Second, it may result initially from inflammation and later from fibrosis and retraction of the levator muscle. Third, lid retraction may occur indirectly from proptosis of the globe with secondary exposure. This mechanism is not unique to thyroid ophthalmopathy.

Fat prolapse into the upper and lower lids may occur as a result of increased orbital volume. This results from stimulation of orbital fibroblasts to produce glycosaminoglycans (GAG). The hydrophilic mucopolysaccharides secondarily imbibe water and swell the orbital contents. One eponymic sign that deserves mention in the context of thyroid ophthalmopathy is von Graefe's sign, which is upper eyelid lag on downgaze. The descent of the upper lid is momentarily delayed as the patient looks down. This is present either unilaterally or bilaterally in 50% of patients with thyroid ophthalmopathy at the time of initial diagnosis.

Globe

The globe may be involved by the presence of subconjunctival edema, which occurs on the same basis as periorbital edema. The conjunctival and scleral vessels may be grossly engorged from orbital congestion with secondary compromise of orbital venous drainage (Fig. 4). More often, the scleral injection is limited to the insertions of the rectus muscles.

Exophthalmos of one or both eyes affects approximately 60% of patients with thyroid ophthalmopathy. Proptosis, which may be either bilateral or unilateral, is a hallmark sign of thyroid ophthalmopathy (Fig. 5). Often visible grossly, it can be measured and followed by serial Hertzel exophthalmometer measurements. The Hertzel exophthalmometer is a device consisting of 45-degree mirrors that allow visualization of the corneal apex from a lateral view. A difference between both orbits of greater than 1.5 mm is considered abnormal. A reading for any orbit greater than 20 mm in a Caucasian patient is also abnormal. Higher readings exist in blacks because of shallow orbits.

The cause of the proptosis is swelling of the extraocular muscles and orbital fat as a result of GAG synthesis by orbital fibroblasts. A less common cause of proptosis

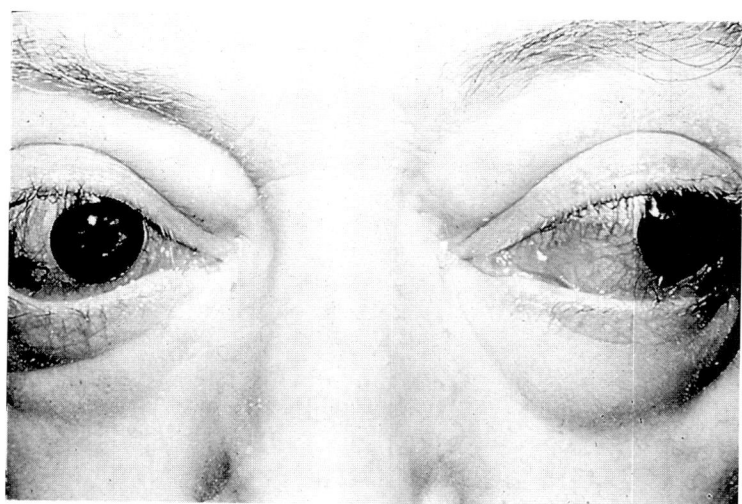

FIG. 4. Acute congestive thyroid ophthalmopathy with grossly engorged conjunctival and scleral vessels.

in thyroid ophthalmopathy is superior orbital vein compression by isolated enlargement of the superior rectus muscle. Hudson et al. (10) recently demonstrated on quantitative computed tomography (CT) scan that superior rectus muscle volume correlated with proptosis, whereas medial, lateral, and inferior rectus muscles did not correlate with proptosis. A prominent ophthalmic vein was seen to accompany isolated enlarged superior rectus muscle. This suggests that superior rectus muscle enlargement alone may produce reduced venous outflow from the orbit, and secondary venous congestion and orbital fat volume expansion.

Cornea

Corneal exposure caused by either severe proptosis or lid retraction may cause corneal desiccation. In its mild form, it will cause a superficial punctate keratitis, with the symptoms of irritation and foreign body sensation. In its severe form, frank corneal ulceration, pain, and potential visual loss may result.

Extraocular Muscles

Extraocular muscle involvement is common in thyroid ophthalmopathy. Forty percent of patients with the disease demonstrate restrictive myopathy, and 17% complain of diplopia. Extraocular muscle (EOM) enlargement on CT or MRI scan is the definitive diagnostic sign of orbital involvement in thyroid disease. Even in Graves' disease patients without clinically detectable ophthalmopathy, EOM involvement can be demonstrated on MRI in 71% of patients. MRI and CT scanning of the EOMs of patients with thyroid ophthalmopathy shows enlargement of the EOMs with a *normal* muscle tendon (Figs. 6,7). Other orbital inflammatory processes, such as primary orbital myositis or pseudotumor, do not demonstrate sparing of the muscle tendon.

Thyroid ophthalmopathy involves the inferior rectus muscle most frequently. Next most commonly involved is the medial rectus, followed by the superior rectus, and, last, the lateral rectus. For inexplicable reasons, the oblique muscles are rarely involved. Thyroid ophthalmopathy commonly causes a vertical muscle imbalance and in fact is the most common cause of vertical diplopia in the adult population. The inflammatory process initially causes inflammation, which is then followed by hypertrophy and eventually fibrosis of the extraocular muscles. This mechanically displaces the globe in the direction of the involved muscle. Inferior rectus involvement produces a hypotropia, or inferiorly displaced globe. Medial rectus muscle involvement causes an internal rotation of the globe. Fibrosis and foreshortening of the rectus muscles may tether the globe. Restriction of upgaze due to inferior rectus fibrosis is the most commonly observed motility disturbance seen in thyroid ophthalmopathy (Figs. 8,9).

In summary, thyroid ophthalmopathy is the most common cause of vertical diplopia in the adult population. Initially, this may be present in upgaze only, but with further fibrosis of the inferior rectus, it can produce vertical diplopia in primary gaze. Vertical diplopia, which may be permanent and not always curable with strabismus surgery, is the most common debilitating symptom of thyroid ophthalmopathy.

Optic Nerve

Thyroid ophthalmopathy may progress to rapid and sometimes irreversible visual loss if the patient develops optic neuropathy. Five percent of thyroid ophthalmopathy patients go on to develop optic neuropathy. The mechanism of thyroid optic neuropathy has traditionally been

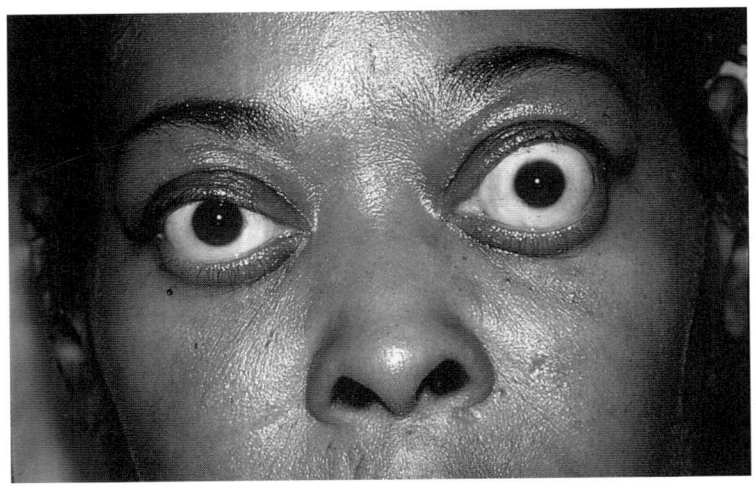
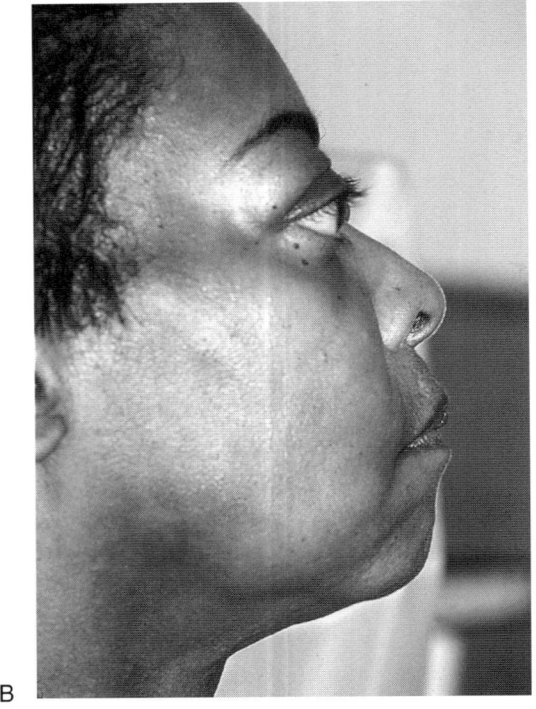
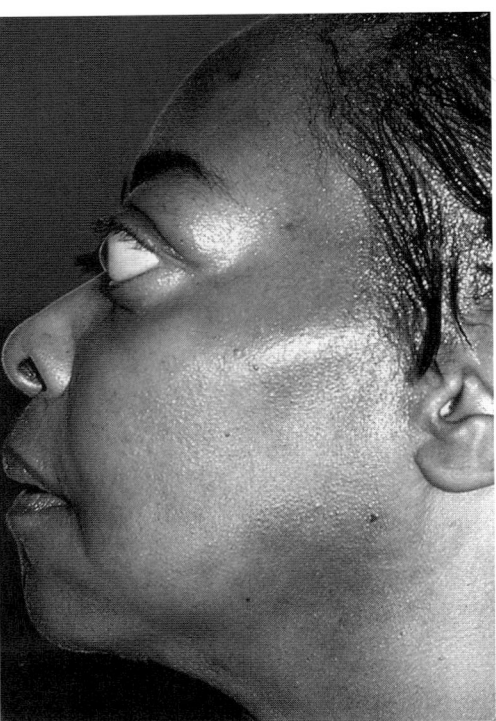

FIG. 5. A: Unilateral proptosis caused by thyroid ophthalmopathy. **B,C:** Lateral views of the same patient.

accepted as a compressive optic neuropathy. Grossly enlarged extraocular muscles produce a tight orbital apex and can compress the optic nerve as it exits through the muscle cone.

More recently, it has been shown that severe orbital venous stasis is an additional causative factor for thyroid optic neuropathy. Color Doppler imaging has been used to evaluate superior ophthalmic vein blood flow. In thyroid ophthalmopathy, orbits with demonstrated orbital apical crowding observed on MRI color Doppler showed reversal of direction of blood flow in the superior ophthalmic vein. Nakase et al. recently reported that reversal of flow in the superior ophthalmic vein (posteroanterior flow) was detected in 44% of thyroid ophthalmic orbits with optic neuropathy, as opposed to 7% of those without optic neuropathy (11). Reversed blood flow in the superior ophthalmic vein strongly supports the existence of severe stasis in those orbits.

A minority of patients may demonstrate evidence of *anterior* ischemic optic neuropathy. Evidence for an ischemic etiology comes from optic nerve changes seen in some patients with thyroid optic neuropathy. They may demonstrate peripupillary: flame-shaped hemorrhages, disc swelling, and bundle defects in the visual field. This

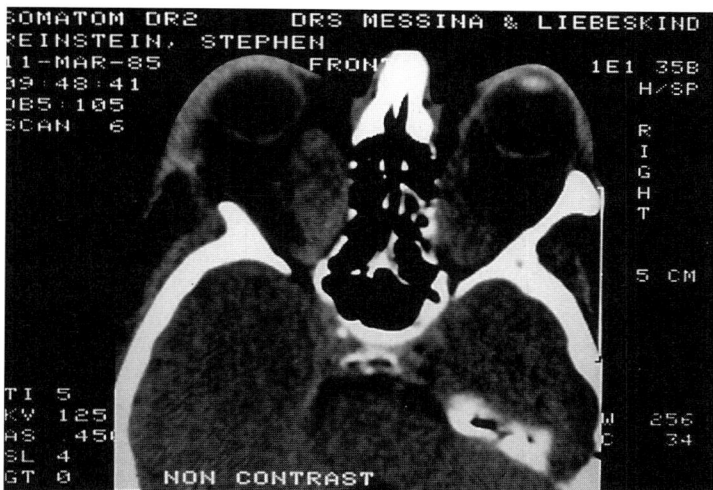

FIG. 6. Noncontrast MRI axial view demonstrates massive enlargement of both medial rectus muscles. Note normal muscle insertion.

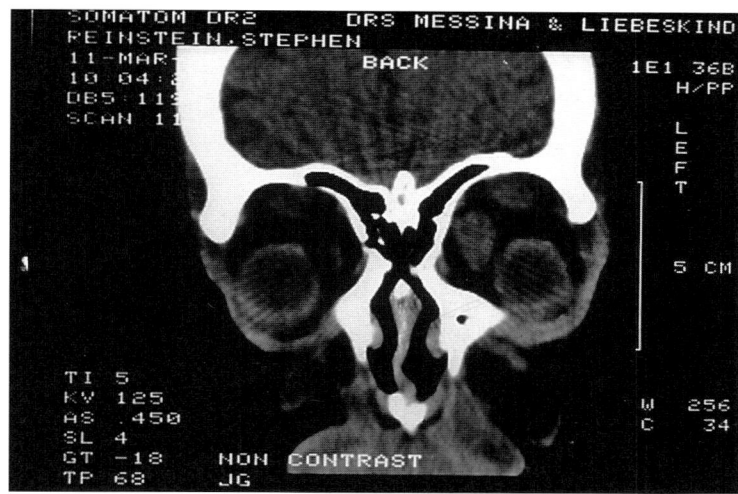

FIG. 7. Coronal view (MRI) of same patient shows enlargement of inferior, medial, and superior rectus muscles with normal-sized lateral rectus muscle.

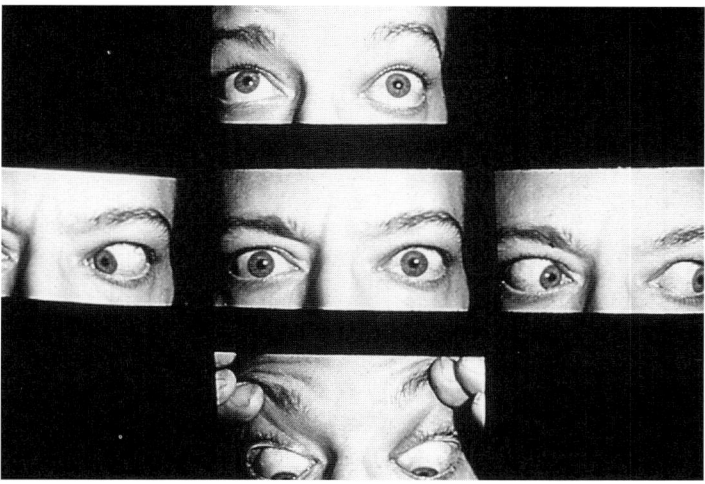

FIG. 8. Diplopia in upgaze caused by fibrosis of the left inferior rectus. Note also intense injection over horizontal rectus muscle tendon insertion.

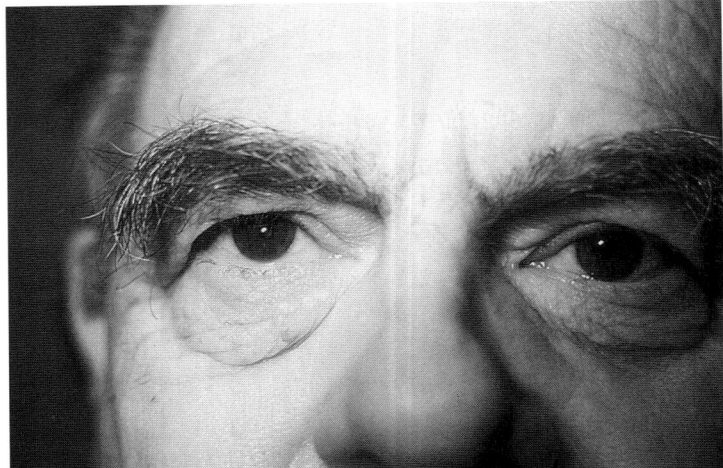

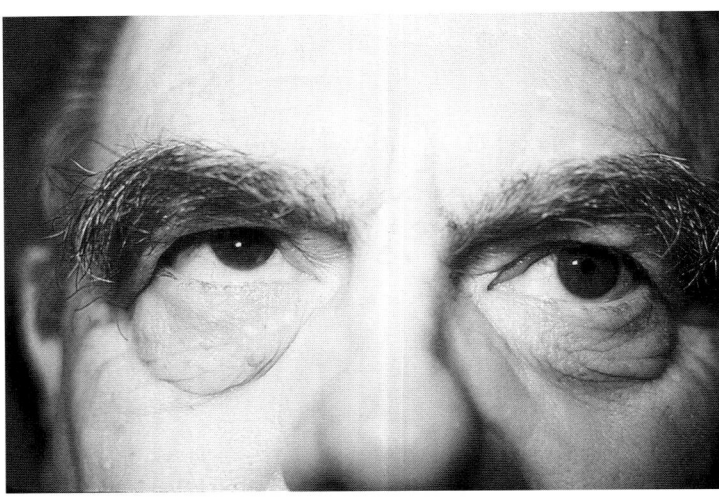

FIG. 9. A: Left hypodeviation caused by inferior rectus fibrosis, producing vertical diplopia in primary gaze. **B:** Tight inferior rectus tethers left globe and prevents elevation.

clinical pattern suggests that in some patients the optic neuropathy may be anterior and ischemic in nature (12) (Fig. 10).

In summary, the optic neuropathy seen in thyroid ophthalmopathy is probably primarily compressive in nature as a result of a tight orbital apex. Superior ophthalmic vein obstruction with severe venous stasis is probably a further aggravating etiologic cause and explains the anterior ischemic optic neuropathy signs that are sometimes seen in thyroid optic neuropathy.

Thyroid optic neuropathy often develops in eyes without marked proptosis. The course of thyroid ophthalmopathy optic neuropathy can be devastating. Trobe et al. (13) reported that in untreated eyes with thyroid optic neuropathy, 21% had a final visual acuity of 20/100 or worse, and 18% were legally blind.

Vision loss is a rare but devastating consequence of thyroid ophthalmopathy. Approximately 5% of patients with thyroid ophthalmopathy will develop optic neuropathy. Unfortunately, the optic neuropathy is often insidious. Many patients do not have marked proptosis. Because orbital apex compression is the most common mechanism, a posterior optic neuropathy develops. Therefore, the involved eye fails to show any observable disc changes. Visual field testing will most commonly reveal a central scotoma, although a significant percentage of patients will have nonspecific generalized field constriction. The minority of patients who demonstrate fundus changes consistent with anterior ischemic optic neuropathy often show an altitudinal defect on visual field exam. Visually evoked response testing will demonstrate both a decrease in amplitude and a delay in conduction. This pattern is seen with any compressive optic neuropathy and is not specific to thyroid disease. In only the minority of patients who demonstrate an ischemic neuropathy component do we see disc swelling and nerve-fiber-layer hemorrhages. Because optic neuropathy can develop in patients without marked proptosis, there is no way to identify those patients at risk.

In summary, because thyroid optic neuropathy is primarily a result of compression at the orbital apex, there are no observable signs. Fundus exam remains normal

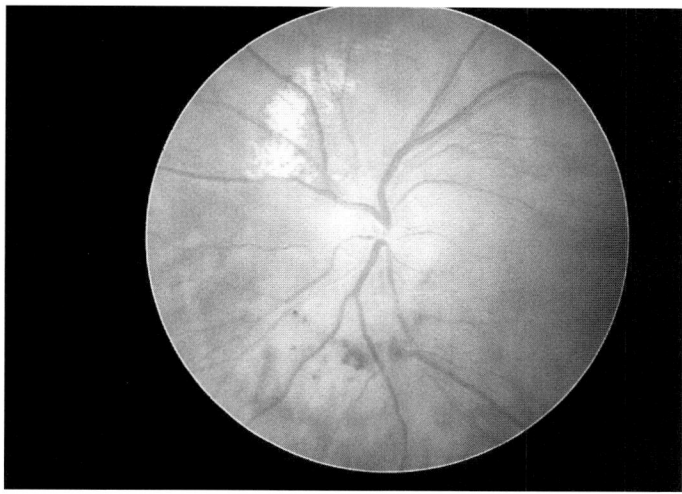

FIG. 10. Thyroid optic neuropathy presenting as anterior ischemic optic neuropathy with swollen disc and surrounding exudate with peripapillary exudative retinal detachment.

and does not alert one to the insidious process occurring at the orbital apex. Because the degree of proptosis does not correlate with the incidence of thyroid optic neuropathy, there is no satisfactory way to identify those patients at risk. Only periodic assessment of visual acuity and visual fields will detect thyroid optic neuropathy.

CLASSIFICATION

In 1969, Werner and the ad hoc committee of the American Thyroid Association proposed a classification of the orbital signs in Graves' disease. This system divided the eye changes in Graves' disease into seven classes that are widely known by the mnemonic NOSPECS (Table 2).

Although this classification system is often used in clinical practice, it has serious limitations. First, the classification system defines merely the severity of involvement but not the stages of progression of the disease. For instance, a patient may develop severe profound vision loss due to optic nerve involvement, yet have minimal or absent proptosis. Thyroid ophthalmopathy does not progress through a series of defined stages. More important, the classification system does not indicate disease activity or remission.

TABLE 2. *Abridged classification of ocular changes in Graves' disease*

Class	Ocular signs and symptoms
0	**N**o signs or symptoms
1	**O**nly signs, no symptoms (lid lag, lid retraction, stare, proptosis < 3 mm)
2	**S**oft tissue involvement (conjunctival edema or injection, lid chemosis)
3	**P**roptosis > 3 mm
4	**E**xtraocular muscle involvement
5	**C**orneal involvement (caused by exposure)
6	**S**ight loss (caused by optic nerve involvement)

The classification of thyroid ophthalmopathy really needs to be made on immunological profiles. As this is an immunological disease, these profiles serve as predictors of disease severity, disease activity, and incidence of ophthalmologic involvement, and as possible predictors for efficacy of therapy. To date no such immunoprofile classification system exists.

RELATIONSHIP OF THYROID OPHTHALMOPATHY TO THYROID STATUS

The thyroid gland and the orbital fibroblasts have in common that they are both end organs involved in a common immunological disease. Management of the thyroid involvement and its thyrotoxic state is much easier than treatment of thyroid ophthalmopathy. There are three good options for endocrinologic thyroid control: (a) surgical resection, (b) radioactive iodine ablation, and (c) antithyroid drugs.

Correction of the thyrotoxicosis by any of these three modalities has no beneficial effect on thyroid ophthalmopathy. After control of thyrotoxicosis, both lid retraction and stare may be lessened. This is a result of a reduction in the excess sympathetic stimulation of thyrotoxicosis, and not of altering the orbital disease. Although endocrine control of hyperthyroidism does not positively influence thyroid ophthalmopathy, controversy surrounds the question of an adverse effect from ^{131}I treatment.

Radioactive iodine for the treatment of Graves' hyperthyroidism may have an adverse effect on thyroid ophthalmopathy. ^{131}I treatment may increase the frequency of developing Graves' ophthalmopathy or aggravate preexisting ophthalmopathy. A study by Tallstedt and the thyroid study group in Sweden randomly assigned patients with Graves' disease to treatment with antithyroid drugs, subtotal thyroidectomy, or ^{131}I therapy. Whereas there was no significant difference in the frequency of the development or in the worsening of ophthalmopathy among the medically and surgically treated patients, thyroid ophthalmopathy prevalence and severity increased in the ^{131}I treated patients. Ophthalmopathy developed or worsened in 33% of the patients treated with ^{131}I, as compared with 10% of those treated medically and 16% of those treated surgically (14).

A possible explanation put forward to explain this finding is that antigenic leakage from the ^{131}I-damaged thyroid gland may lead to subsequent increased production of autoantibodies that crossreact with antigens shared by the thyroid and the orbit. Serum concentrations of thyrotropin-receptor antibodies decrease gradually during the first year after surgical or medical treatment. Following treatment with ^{131}I, serum thyrotropin-receptor antibodies actually increase during the first year.

A supporting prospective study by Pinchera and associates (15) revealed that while radioiodine administration had no effect on patients free from preexisting eye disease, exacerbation of ocular disease occurred in 53% of patients who had definite ophthalmopathy before radioiodine treatment.

Pinchera et al. also found that concomitant administration of corticosteroids prevented the radioiodine-associated exacerbation of eye disease. Oral glucocorticosteroids probably work by suppressing the anamnestic response to released thyroid antigens. They concluded that patients with thyrotoxicosis and ocular involvement should receive oral corticosteroids concomitant with radioiodine.

If antigenic overlap is the etiology of thyroid ophthalmopathy, thyroid ablation should not be expected to end the problem. If humoral immunity to TSH-receptor thyroid antigen starts the process, crossfire reaction with orbital antigen can continue the process, even if all of the thyroid antigens are removed.

Tallstedt et al. (14) suggested that the pretreatment serum T_3 concentration may be a predictive factor for the development or worsening of thyroid ophthalmopathy. A pretreatment T_3 less than 5 nmol/L carried a 10% risk of development or worsening of ophthalmopathy following I^{131}. This risk increased to 58% if the pretreatment T_3 concentration was greater than or equal to 5 nmol/L. This is not believed to be a direct effect of T_3. T_3 has no effect on glycosaminoglycan synthesis by orbital fibroblasts. It probably reflects the severity of the metabolic, and therefore also the inciting immunological, disease.

In summary, treatment of the Graves' thyrotoxicosis does not positively influence thyroid ophthalmopathy. Radioiodine therapy may aggravate thyroid orbital disease. Corticosteroids may attenuate the exacerbation of ophthalmopathy that would otherwise occur after radioiodine treatment.

TREATMENT

When discussing the treatment of thyroid ophthalmopathy, two clinical points must be remembered: (a) thyroid ophthalmopathy is self-limited in the majority of patients; and (b) the protean clinical course of thyroid ophthalmopathy, with marked variation between patients and propensity for spontaneous remissions and exacerbations, makes treatment claims suspect. Therefore, only a small percentage of patients with thyroid ophthalmopathy actually require treatment. Less than 10% of patients develop severe orbital involvement requiring treatment. Any proposed treatment must have a better outcome than the natural course of the untreated disease.

Evaluating the efficacy of any treatment is made even more difficult by the fact that thyroid ophthalmopathy has two clinical stages: the active inflammatory stage and the inactive fibrotic stage.

The autoimmune stage has an active inflammatory period lasting 3 to 36 months, followed by an inactive fibrotic stage. It is often difficult to determine the transition point from active inflammatory to fibrotic disease. Obviously, therapy directed at stage one inflammation (i.e., corticosteroids, immunosuppressive agents, orbital irradiation) would be totally ineffective in the burned-out fibrotic setting of stage two. Sergott and colleagues (16) attempted to separate these two stages by determining immune activity. Theoretically, this should determine which patients would benefit from corticosteroid or immunosuppressive therapy.

The symptoms of lid retraction, proptosis, and diplopia can be present in either stage of the disease. The major shortcoming of clinical treatment studies is that they have not specified the disease stage of the patients undergoing treatment. By combining patients with active inflammatory disease and those with inactive fibrotic disease, they obtained different clinical outcomes with the same therapy.

The only patients who are definitely stage one active inflammatory disease are those with recent onset (less than 3 months) of orbital disease, or those with recent onset of thyroid optic neuropathy.

In summary, 90% of patients with thyroid ophthalmopathy require no treatment at all. Their orbital disease will either eventually go into spontaneous remission or the signs and symptoms are not of sufficient severity to justify therapeutic intervention. If therapeutic intervention is required for the orbital disease, it may encompass one or more of the following: (a) medical therapy, (b) orbital irradiation, or (c) surgical intervention.

Control of Hyperthyroidism

Control of the patients' hyperthyroidism will decrease or eliminate only the lid retraction and its resultant stare. This occurs by decreasing the exaggerated alpha-adrenergic tone of the Müller's muscle secondary to the high levels of circulating catecholamines seen in the thyrotoxic state. Eyelid retraction is the most common ophthalmic feature of autoimmune thyroid disease, being present in

90% of patients at some point in their clinical course (15). No other factor of thyroid ophthalmopathy responds to endocrinologic control of hyperthyroidism. When lid retraction is reduced, the proptosis may appear to be reduced, but in actuality the degree of proptosis measured by Hertzel exophthalmometry and MRI scans is unchanged.

Alpha-Adrenergic Blocking Agents

Mild eyelid retraction can be managed by topical adrenergic blocking drugs, which rapidly inhibit the release of norepinephrine from sympathetic nerve endings that innervate Müller's muscle. This accounts for the almost immediate, but transient, production of ptosis (~1.5 mm) that is seen with topical guanethidine. With continued use, the tissue stores of norepinephrine become slowly depleted, eventually creating a chemical sympathectomy. Therefore, the topical guanethidine sulfate (5%), administered initially four times per day, can then be tapered (tid, bid, qd, qod, every 2 weeks), giving control of lid retraction with lower concentrations and/or less frequent instillation of guanethidine. An effect on lid retraction is usually seen by 72 hours. Topical guanethidine is not without local side effects that may limit its use. Pupillary constriction and dilation of conjunctival vessels occur in almost all patients. These side effects are usually tolerable, but intense conjunctival injection may limit its use in some patients. The major cause of guanethidine intolerance is the development of a superficial keratitis due to corneal toxicity. Fortunately, systemic side effects are not observed with topical guanethidine, which has a role in (a) mild lid retraction, (b) asymptomatic lid retraction, and (c) lid retraction that is present until the hyperthyroidism is controlled.

Botulinum-A

Botulinum-A toxin may also be used to control eyelid retraction in patients with thyroid ophthalmopathy. Injection of botulinum-A toxin into the levator muscle can produce a ptosis lasting 3 to 4 months (17). Serial injections can be used.

Corticosteroids

The use of corticosteroids in the treatment of thyroid ophthalmopathy has the appeal of logic. First, thyroid ophthalmopathy is an autoimmune disease and should respond to immunomodulation. Furthermore, corticosteroids suppress lymphocytic infiltration of tissue and in addition have been shown to decrease glycosaminoglycan production by orbital fibroblasts (16). Unfortunately, the clinical results of corticosteroid therapy for thyroid ophthalmopathy do not live up to their promise.

Corticosteroids would be expected to be of benefit only to patients in the active inflammatory stage of the disease. This is borne out by the fact that greatest steroid efficacy is seen in patients who present with acute onset of inflammatory orbital signs: periorbital edema, rapid onset of proptosis, and ophthalmoplegia.

The efficacy of corticosteroid therapy in thyroid ophthalmopathy depends on whether the orbital disease is in the acute inflammatory stage or the inactive fibrotic stage. Corticosteroids suppress orbital infiltration by lymphocytes which mediate orbital and periorbital edema and infiltration. Corticosteroids have also been shown to suppress the synthesis of GAG by orbital fibroblasts. Therefore, the most dramatic response to corticosteroids is seen in patients who present with abrupt onset of inflammatory orbital thyroid disease. These patients present with rapidly developing periorbital soft-tissue edema, proptosis, and ophthalmoplegia. Similarly, they may also show an abrupt clearing of all orbital signs within 72 hours.

The corticosteroids must be continued for the entire active inflammatory stage of the disease, or thyroid ophthalmopathy rapidly returns. This may be as short as 3 months or as long as 36 months.

High doses of steroids are required to produce a therapeutic response. The initial starting dosage is 40 to 100 mg of oral prednisone for 2 to 4 weeks, followed by a gradual tapering of 5 mg/day every week. Attempts to taper the required high dose of steroids at any time during the acute phase results in rapid return of ophthalmic symptoms. Most patients demonstrate a floor of 30 mg of prednisone daily, below which they cannot be tapered without breaking through and rebounding.

All components of thyroid ophthalmopathy do not respond equally to corticosteroid therapy. Periorbital soft-tissue edema gives the most predictable response. Diplopia responds minimally or not at all. Proptosis is unresponsive to corticosteroids. Thyroid optic neuropathy inconsistently responds to high dose corticosteroids, and even when it does respond, visual acuity usually declines when an attempt is made to lower the steroid dosage. Most patients with thyroid optic neuropathy are corticosteroid failures and require orbital irradiation or combined therapy of irradiation and orbital decompression.

The high doses of corticosteroids required, the inability to taper doses to safe levels, and the long duration of the active inflammatory phase limit their usefulness. Alternate-day steroid dosing, although less immunosuppressive to patient host defenses, is totally ineffective in thyroid ophthalmopathy. Long-term high dose corticosteroid therapy is not justifiable because of its risk-to-benefit ratio. Complications of high dose corticosteroids go far beyond the cushingoid habitus and include steroid myopathy, steroid-induced pseudotumor and optic nerve swelling, skeletal changes with compression fractures of the spine, emotional lability and insomnia, glucose control problems in diabetics and the production of clinical diabetes in nondiabetics, and the rare but potentially fatal hyperosmolar nonketotic coma.

Local injections of steroids, although they lack systemic side effects, have no demonstrable effect on thyroid ophthalmopathy. In addition, there is significant risk in injecting into tight orbits.

In summary, corticosteroids, either in the form of oral prednisone or intravenous methylprednisone, may dramatically reverse periorbital soft-tissue edema and chemosis. They have a minimal effect on diplopia and no effect on proptosis. Thyroid optic neuropathy inconsistently responds to high dose corticosteroids with the result that most patients require orbital irradiation with or without orbital decompression. The high failure rate and intolerable side effects limit the usefulness of corticosteroids in thyroid ophthalmopathy. Their major efficacy is (a) in those patients who present with a dramatic onset of inflammatory disease that comes on over several days, and (b) in patients with thyroid optic neuropathy who require rapid onset immunosuppression as a temporizing modality before orbital irradiation and/or orbital decompression.

Immunosuppressive Agents

The side effects of systemic steroids make their long-term use unacceptable for most patients. This led several investigators to try immunomodulation by other immunosuppressive agents. Cyclosporine, which is used after renal transplantation, has also been used for autoimmune posterior uveitis. Cyclosporine is an 11-amino-acid metabolite produced by a species of fungus. It inhibits immunocompetent T lymphocytes by blocking the production and release of interleukin-2 or T-cell growth factor.

In a randomized double-blind trial of prednisone (60 mg) versus cyclosporine for thyroid ophthalmopathy, prednisone was effective in 61% whereas cyclosporine was effective in only 22% of cases (18). Prednisone produced more drug-induced side effects. Cyclosporine is not without risk, as it may cause renal and liver toxicity. Although it does not produce the bone marrow suppression seen with other cytotoxic drugs, cyclosporine has been associated with development of lymphomas in renal transplant patients.

In summary, the role of cytotoxic drugs in thyroid ophthalmopathy is uncertain. The therapeutic response is less than prednisone. Although it may be argued that the incidence of side effects is lower with cyclosporine than with prednisone, the severity of side effects, including life-threatening carcinogenesis, is greater. The risk-to-benefit ratio does not support the use of cyclosporine for thyroid ophthalmopathy.

Orbital Radiation

The concept of orbital radiation resulted from the use of pituitary radiation to treat Graves' disease 50 years ago. The prevailing theory in the 1940s was that the pituitary produced hormonal factors that caused exophthalmos. The older radiation delivery systems were poorly collimated and sometimes led to inadvertent orbital irradiation. Only those patients with inadvertent orbital irradiation showed improvement of the thyroid ophthalmopathy.

Retrobulbar irradiation takes advantage of the differential radiosensitivity of the cell mix of orbital tissue in thyroid ophthalmopathy. Radiosensitivity of a cell population increases with (a) the ratio of nuclear chromatin to cell mass, (b) the mitotic potential of the cell, and (c) the degree of undifferentiation. Lymphocytes have a high index in all categories and therefore are the most exquisitely sensitive cell line. Lymphocyte reproductive death occurs with doses below 1 gray (Gy).

Orbital fibroblasts, possessing a low degree of differentiation and a high proliferative potential, are intermediate on the scale of sensitivity to ionizing radiation. At the other end of the spectrum, the most radioresistant cells are those that are highly differentiated and have lost the ability to divide, referred to as fixed postmitotic cells. Included in this class are both striated muscle and neural tissue.

Retrobulbar irradiation appears to be effective by killing orbital lymphocytes and fibroblasts. Sensitized T lymphocytes induce fibroblasts to synthesize GAG, which is very hydrophilic, imbibes water, and produces orbital edema. Orbital fibroblasts are sensitive to low dose radiation. Lymphocyte reproductive death occurs with doses below 1 Gy. Interphase death occurs with doses above 1 Gy. Therefore, retrobulbar radiation might suppress both the mediators (lymphocytes) and the effectors (fibroblasts) of the inflammatory reaction in the orbit (19).

Technique

The standard protocol for orbital irradiation in thyroid ophthalmopathy is to deliver a total dose of 20 Gy, fractioned into ten 2-Gy doses given over 2 weeks. The dosage is calculated at midline and delivered through posteriorly angled portals to avoid the lens of the contralateral eye. A fractionated dosage schedule is used to minimize irradiation injury to the optic nerve and extraocular muscles. The divided dose schedule takes advantage of the differentiated recovery rate of cells to sub-lethal radiation damage. The more radioresistant neural and striated muscle cells have the capacity to rapidly repair single-strand DNA breaks. Therefore, the 24-hour interval between irradiation treatments is sufficient to allow DNA repair. Lymphocyte and fibroblasts repair DNA breaks very slowly and never fully recover before the next dosage of irradiation. This cumulative sub-lethal damage results in cell death.

Results

As the mechanism of action of orbital irradiation is suppression of lymphocytes and possibly fibroblasts, it is effective only in the acute inflammatory stage of the disease. Therefore, the interval between the onset of orbitopathy and the start of treatment should be expected to greatly influence the success rate, because irradiation works by shortening the acute active phase.

Improvement in thyroid ophthalmopathy is seen beginning 1 to 2 weeks after irradiation and may continue for 18 weeks. Edema and chemosis of the conjunctiva, lids, and periorbital tissues show the most dramatic response. Extraocular muscle size is not influenced by orbital irradiation. Shine and associates concluded this on CT analysis of patients who received orbital irradiation during the acute active phase and then underwent repeat CT scan 5 years later (20). They also found a change in the CT picture of these muscles with time. They noted an increased definition of low-density areas within the muscles that may represent fatty replacement in the extraocular muscles in zones that were initially infiltrated with GAG.

Motility restriction and diplopia are also unaffected by orbital irradiation. The course of the proptosis in the irradiated patients was found to be no different from that in the control group. This would correlate with the static enlarged muscle size seen on serial CT scans.

The response to orbital irradiation appears to parallel that to oral prednisone. Therefore, a trial course of oral prednisone can be given to determine whether a specific patient will respond to orbital irradiation. The effects of orbital irradiation are less dramatic but more prolonged than those of prednisone. Whereas the side effects of oral prednisone are systemic, the side effects of orbital irradiation are local. The major risk is radiation-induced retinopathy, which begins after 18 to 36 months. The retinal capillary bed may show patchy obliteration with areas of nonperfusion and ischemia. There may be scattered retinal hemorrhages, exudate, and the development of retinal neovascularization. Radiation retinopathy closely resembles the retinal picture of diabetic retinopathy, but without the microaneurysms (Figs. 11,12). Therefore, orbital irradiation is contraindicated in patients with diabetic retinopathy because of increased risk of accelerated microangiopathy. Orbital irradiation is also contraindicated in patients receiving chemotherapy, because it potentiates the effect of irradiation, making orbital dosage calculation inaccurate. Finally, orbital irradiation causes the potential (albeit low) risk of development of orbital sarcomas.

In summary, the response of thyroid ophthalmopathy to orbital irradiation parallels that of corticosteroids. The effects of orbital irradiation are less dramatic in onset but more prolonged than those of prednisone. The soft-tissue changes, consisting of edema and chemosis of the conjunctiva, lids, and periorbital area, show the most marked improvement. Thyroid optic neuropathy can sometimes be controlled in the long term with orbital irradiation alone. Motility restriction and proptosis are unaffected by orbital irradiation.

Prednisone Versus Orbital Radiation

When offered two choices of lymphocytic suppression, does one therapy have the edge over the other, in terms of either efficacy or safety? Prummel and associates did a randomized double-blind trial of oral prednisone versus radiotherapy in Graves' disease. They concluded that radiotherapy and oral prednisone are *equally effective* as initial treatments in patients with moderately severe thyroid ophthalmopathy. A beneficial response was seen in 50% of the prednisone treatment group and in 40% of the radiation group. Side effects were more common and more severe in the prednisone group.

The last question to be answered in the comparison between orbital radiation and oral prednisone is, Although the therapies are equally effective, is either significantly effective?

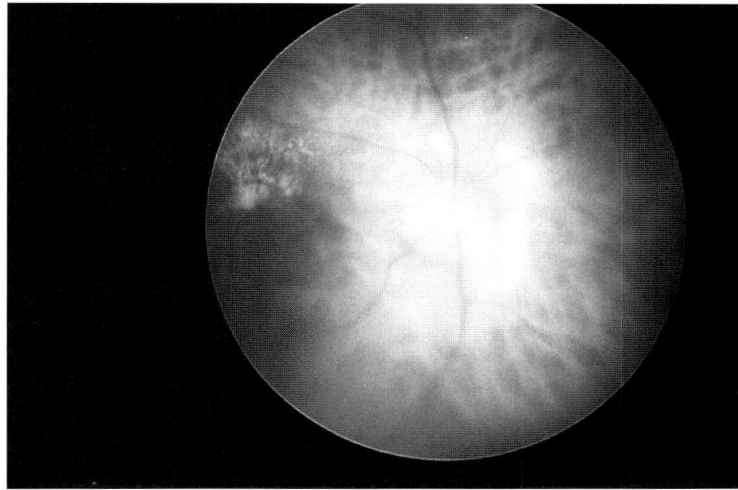

FIG. 11. Radiation-induced optic neuropathy, 18 months after orbital irradiation.

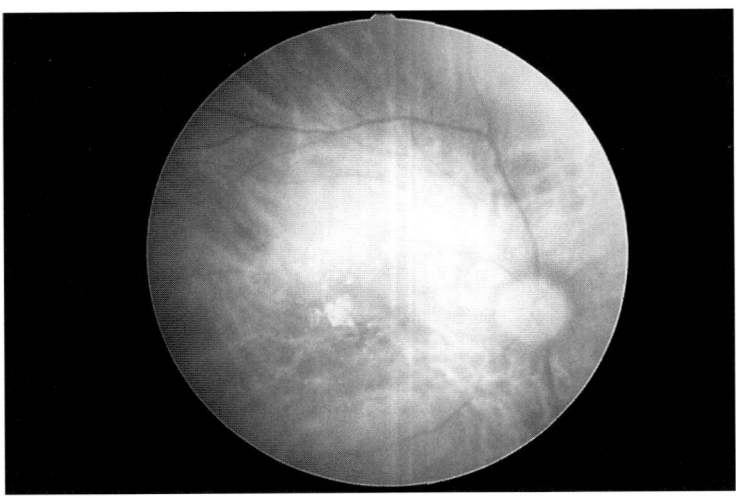

FIG. 12. Same patient as Figure 11, 8 months later. Patient has resolution of disc swelling and peripapillary retinal exudate. Ischemic maculopathy persists with hard exudate resolving. Vision has decreased from 20/30 to count fingers.

In Prummel's study, 75% of all patients, whether treated with irradiation or prednisone, eventually required rehabilitative surgery. So the efficacy of either treatment is modest at best. Neither cures the disease. Neither prevents progression to the fibrotic stage with lid retraction, gaze restriction, diplopia, or optic nerve compressive neuropathy. Does treatment of thyroid ophthalmopathy with corticosteroids or orbital irradiation in patients today positively influence where they will be 5 years hence? The vacuum created by the absence of facts is filled with a plethora of opinions.

Surgical Treatment of Thyroid Eye Disease

Neither oral prednisone nor orbital radiation reduces the incidence of the necessity for surgical treatment in thyroid ophthalmopathy. Bartley and associates (19) determined the frequency of surgical intervention in patients with Graves' ophthalmopathy over a period of 15 years. Twenty percent of their patients underwent one or more surgical procedures. The distribution of frequency of surgical procedures was eyelid surgery, 12%; strabismus surgery, 9%; and orbital decompression, 7%.

Their study further found that the relative risk of undergoing surgery was 2.6 times greater in patients over 50 years old. This is further confirmation of the clinical observation that, whereas the incidence of thyroid ophthalmopathy *decreases* with age, the severity of orbital involvement *increases* with age.

Eyelid Surgery

Eyelid surgery is the most commonly performed surgical procedure for Graves' patients. This is not surprising, because eyelid retraction is the most frequent sign of thyroid ophthalmopathy at the time of diagnosis. Eyelid retraction may result from (a) excessive sympathetic tone to the Müller's muscles in the thyrotoxic state, (b) inflammation of the eyelid retractors, (c) eventual fibrosis of the levator muscle, (d) pseudo-eyelid retraction as a result of proptosis, and (e) fixation duress. All of these have been previously discussed except fixation duress, which is upper eyelid retraction that occurs in patients with contracture of the inferior rectus muscle. These patients must maintain increased tone and overaction of the ipsilateral synergistic superior rectus and levator muscles to maintain the globe in primary position.

Indications

Surgical correction of eyelid retraction in thyroid ophthalmopathy is done for two purposes: (a) exposure keratitis and (b) cosmesis. The latter is the indication in the majority of cases.

Surgical Technique

The technique employed depends on the amount of lid retraction to be corrected. Two to 3 mm of upper eyelid retraction can be corrected by extirpation of Müller's muscle alone. The procedure has changed only minimally since originally described by Henderson in 1965 (18). Henderson's technique involves a posterior transconjunctival approach. Müller's muscle is detached from the tarsal plate and dissected free of the levator aponeurosis for 10 mm. Müller's muscle is then recessed by a graded amount.

One problem observed postoperatively with this procedure was the creation of a nasal ptosis. Putterman (21) corrected this by excising only the lateral two thirds of Müller's muscle and allowing it to retract. The nasal third was left untouched to prevent lateral/nasal lid height asymmetry.

Correction of more than 3 mm of upper eyelid retraction can be accomplished only if one also does a graded recession of the levator. Combining Müller's and levator recessions can correct up to 7 mm of lid retraction. Henderson (18) originally did a tenotomy of the levator aponeurosis at the upper tarsal border. Putterman (21) replaced this by a graded recession of the levator from a posterior approach. This was performed by incising the levator at the tarsal border and stripping it layer by layer until the desired lid height was obtained.

Harvey and Anderson (20) introduced an anterior approach to accomplish two things: (a) a complete excision of Müller's muscle from the upper tarsal border to 10 mm superiorly, and (b) recession of the levator aponeurosis by three double-armed absorbable gut sutures.

In 1994, Ceisler and associates (22) proposed a new technique for correcting moderate to severe upper eyelid retraction secondary to Graves' disease. Their technique consisted of (a) Müllerotomy just inferior to Whitnall's ligament, (b) recession of the levator aponeurosis, and (c) medial transposition of the lateral levator aponeurosis to reduce the temporal elevation of thyroid eyelid retraction.

The two unique components of their technique are (a) weakening of the lateral portion of the retractors by graded medial transposition with preservation of the medial horn of the levator aponeurosis to prevent nasal/lateral eyelid asymmetry, and (b) use of Müller's muscle as an autogenous spacer between the upper tarsal border and the levator aponeurosis.

Many surgeons have abandoned the use of eyebank sclera in the upper lid as a spacer material, sutured between the upper tarsal border and the levator aponeurosis. Problems with the use of allogeneic eyebank sclera include (a) host-versus-graft inflammatory reaction, (b) production of lid thickening, and (c) unpredictable percentage of graft shrinkage.

Preserved eye bank sclera is still the treatment of choice for lower eyelid retraction. The graft is sutured in place between the lower tarsal border and the retractors of the lower lid. Nasal or ear cartilage may also be used as spacer material (Fig. 13).

Orbital Decompression

Only 3% to 5% of patients with Graves' disease have ophthalmopathy severe enough to require any treatment. Yet a small percentage of thyroid ophthalmopathy patients develop marked orbital-content enlargement. This increase in volume of orbital contents with a fixed orbital volume, which creates several of the features seen in thyroid ophthalmopathy, is initially compensated for and partially relieved by proptosis. There is a limit to forward globe displacement, however, as it is tethered by the rectus muscles and optic nerve. Further increases in orbital content volume may compress and impede orbital venous drainage and cause the sudden onset of lid and conjunctival chemosis and congestion. An increase in extraocular muscle mass in the orbital apex may produce thyroid optic neuropathy.

All of these features that result in volume disparity can be addressed by attempting to shrink orbital contents (e.g., by corticosteroids, irradiation, or immunosuppression) or by expanding orbital volume by decompression. Failure to respond to medical therapy, imminently threatened vision secondary to corneal exposure, or compressive neuropathy are indications for immediate orbital decompression. Other indications are (a) severe congestive ophthalmopathy, (b) thyroid optic neuropathy, (c) exposure keratitis with a threatened cornea, and (d) cosmesis secondary to disfiguring proptosis.

In the Mayo Clinic series of 428 orbital decompressions by Garrity and associates (23), the indications were as follows: optic neuropathy, 51%; severe orbital inflammation, 27%; proptosis, 16%; exposure keratitis, 5%; and intolerance to steroids, 1%. Optic neuropathy was diagnosed if patients had one or more of the following: (a) afferent pupillary defect, (b) acquired dyschromatopsia, (c) visual field defect, or (d) optic disc edema. Severe congestive ophthalmopathy is defined as severe chemosis resulting in conjunctival prolapse, severe conjunctival congestion, and eyelid edema.

Transantral orbital decompression can be described as follows: the antrum is entered through a sublabial incision. The antral and ethmoid sinuses are exenterated; bone is removed from the medial orbital wall up to the ethmoid roof, and bone along the orbital floor is removed up to the infraorbital nerve.

Fatourechi et al. (24) reported that, of patients with reduced visual acuity preoperatively, 65% were better after decompression, 24% were the same, and 11% were worse. The disturbing fact was in that those patients whose vision was 20/20 before decompression, 15% were worse after decompression. Visual fields improved in 91% of patients after decompression, and 94% had partial or total resolution of disc edema. Severe orbital inflammation was reduced or improved in 90%. Exposure keratitis was improved or resolved in 92%. Proptosis was reduced by a mean of 4.7 mm (Table 3). This result is consistent with the anticipated proptosis reduction with a two-wall procedure.

Of those patients without diplopia preoperatively, 64% developed diplopia postoperatively. Seventy percent of all patients required strabismus surgery, but 16% still had

TABLE 3. *Anticipated proptosis reduction from decompression*

Decompression technique	Proptosis reduction
1-wall	0–4 mm
2-wall	3–6 mm
3-wall	6–10 mm
4-wall	10–17 mm

persistent double vision. Transantral orbital decompression has a higher incidence of induced diplopia than other techniques, because this technique allows a greater decompression of the posterior ethmoids, thereby allowing more soft tissue to prolapse.

Cerebrospinal fluid leaks were seen in 3.5% of patients. This is not unexpected, because part of the ethmoid sinus is the floor of the cranial fossa. Upper eyelid retraction is often made worse as the globe settles posteriorly and inferiorly while the lid remains fixed. On the other hand, lower eyelid retraction often improves. Lower eyelid entropion may also follow decompression, as the orbital contents, including eyelid retractors, drop inferiorly into the open antrum, pulling the attached lower lid as well. This entropion is most marked nasally as the orbital floor is decompressed only nasal to the infraorbital nerve.

Orbital decompression is clearly indicated for treatment of visual loss due to compressive optic neuropathy, exposure keratitis, or severe congestive orbitopathy. The morbidity of this procedure does not engender many surgeons to embrace it as a purely cosmetic procedure.

Recently, Lyons and Rootman (25) reported their results on a series of 34 patients who underwent orbital decompression solely for cosmetic correction of disfiguring exophthalmos. The entry criterion was exophthalmometry of greater than 22 mm in men or greater than 19 mm in women. A transcutaneous approach was used for both two- and three-wall decompressions because of a lower incidence of postoperative motility problems compared to transantral decompression. When diplopia arose *de novo* after decompression, it either resolved spontaneously or was cured by one strabismus surgery. The authors felt that the orbital decompression did not complicate the management of strabismus. They supported the position that cosmesis for the correction of disfiguring proptosis is a valid indication for decompression surgery in a disease that peaks in 39-year-old women (Fig. 14).

Strabismus Surgery

Thyroid ophthalmopathy is the most common cause of diplopia of acute onset in the adult population. Diplopia is the most common debilitating feature of thyroid ophthalmopathy. The inferior rectus is the most commonly involved muscle, followed by the medial rectus, less commonly the superior rectus, and rarely the lateral rectus. Inexplicably, the oblique muscles are seldom involved. Because the most common muscle involved is the inferior rectus, the most common presenting motility disturbance is limitation of upgaze. With further fibrosis and constriction of the inferior rectus, a downward displacement of the globe is seen. Patients with vertical muscle imbalances become symptomatic with diplopia very early, because there is normally very limited vertical fusion. The average vertical fusional amplitude is 2 to 4 diopters (1° to 2°), meaning that any deviation that exceeds this results in diplopia. Involvement of the medial rectus initially produces diplopia in lateral gaze, later followed by horizontal diplopia worse at a distance than near.

The motility disturbance often fluctuates widely during the acute inflammatory stage of the disease. For this reason, it is initially best treated with paste-on Fresnel prisms in an attempt to obtain single vision in primary gaze and downgaze. If this is not possible, occlusion of one eye may be necessary until the active stage of the disease is over. Steroids and orbital irradiation have little or no effect, even in the inflammatory stage, on thyroid motility disturbances. Some acute cases of motility disturbance clear completely when the acute phase is over. If the final residual muscle imbalance in the inactive fibrotic stage is less than or equal to 10 diopters, it is usually best managed by prisms. Deviations greater than this require surgical correction. No consideration for surgical correction should be given until the motility picture has been stable and unchanging for a minimum of 6 months.

In considering strabismus surgery for thyroid eye disease, the following points should be noted.

1. It is important that all thyroid motility patients have realistic and modest expectations of strabismus surgery. Success is defined as being free of diplopia in primary gaze and downgaze, with or without the use of supplemental prisms. Freedom from diplopia in all directions of gaze is not always possible.

2. Patients with severe proptosis (>25 mm) and restrictive myopathy pose a unique challenge. Strabismus surgery performed in eyes with severe proptosis may result in vision-threatening exposure keratitis. The mechanism for this is that the fibrotic extraocular muscles tether the globe and limit the proptosis. Recession of a fibrotic rectus muscle may allow for additional proptosis and corneal decompensation.

3. Orbital decompression may exacerbate the motility problem. Removal of an orbital wall allows the adjacent rectus muscle to herniate into the enlarged space. This further rotates the globe in the direction of the prolapsed rectus muscle. For example, orbital floor decompression can increase the hypotropia, and medial wall decompression can increase the esotropia. Therefore, all strabismus surgery should follow, not precede, any required orbital decompression.

4. Muscle recessions are the procedure of choice. Muscle resection should be avoided because the muscle to be resected is itself fibrotic to some degree and may limit rotation in the direction away from the resected muscle.

5. Always preserve some degree of downgaze, as this is critical for reading. This can be accomplished by (a) undercorrecting the hypotropia, or (b) limiting inferior rectus recession to 8 mm or less.

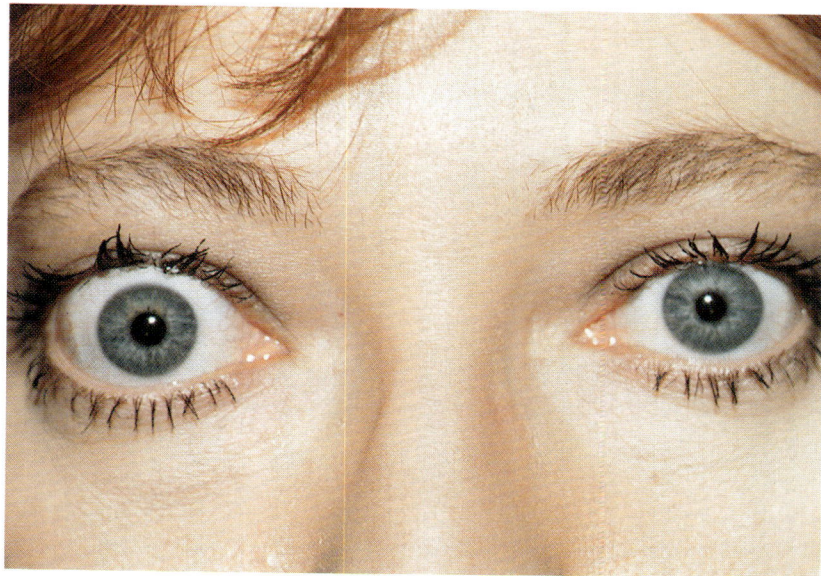

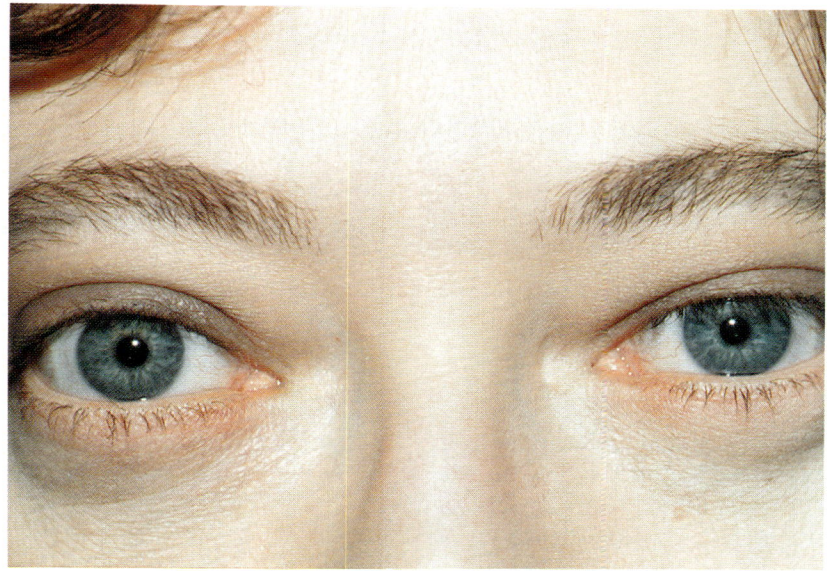

FIG. 13. Correction of upper and lower lid retraction by scleral graft lid lengthening (15) preoperative and (16) postoperative. (Courtesy of David H. Saunders, MD.)

6. Recession of a tight contracted inferior rectus muscle can reduce upper eyelid retraction by eliminating fixation duress. Inferior rectus recession of more than 4 mm can create lower eyelid retraction. Therefore, all strabismus surgery should precede any planned eyelid surgery.

7. No strabismus surgery should involve more than any two rectus muscles at a single procedure because of the risk of producing anterior segment ischemia. In strabismus surgery for thyroid ophthalmopathy, there have been isolated reports of anterior segment ischemia even when the surgery has been confined to only two muscles (25).

8. Limited elevation and adduction may be caused by a fibrotic inferior rectus muscle alone. This is because the inferior rectus plays a secondary role in adduction. Therefore, forced duction testing must be done at the time of surgery, after the inferior rectus has been recessed, to determine if the medial rectus requires surgery. Also, the adducting effect of the inferior rectus is magnified if medial wall orbital decompression has been done previously. This is because the inferior rectus muscle may move medially and change the vector of its pull.

9. Recession of both the inferior rectus and the medial rectus may create an A-pattern exotropia. The resulting exotropia in downgaze may produce diplopia when reading.

10. The clinical rule of 2.5 prism diopters of correction for each 1 mm of inferior rectus recession is not a hard-

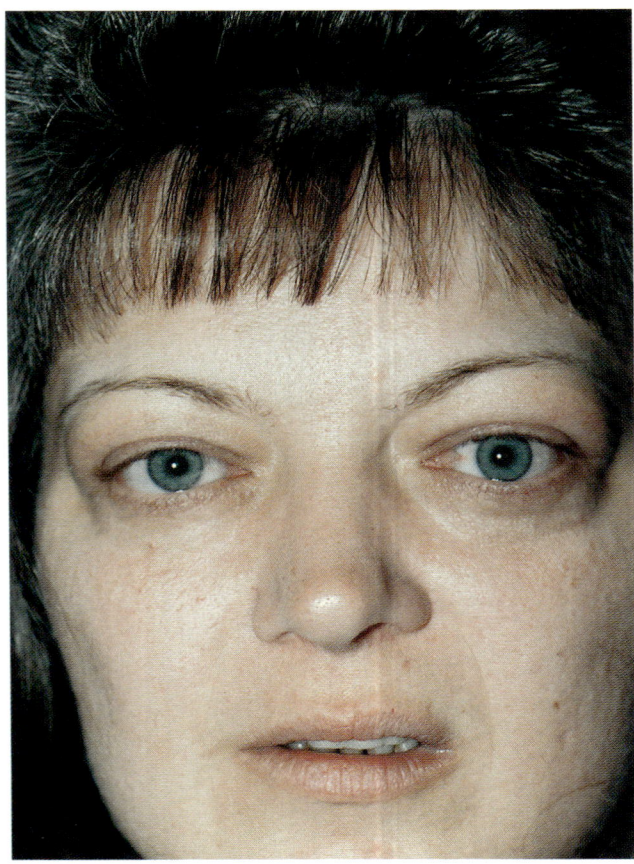 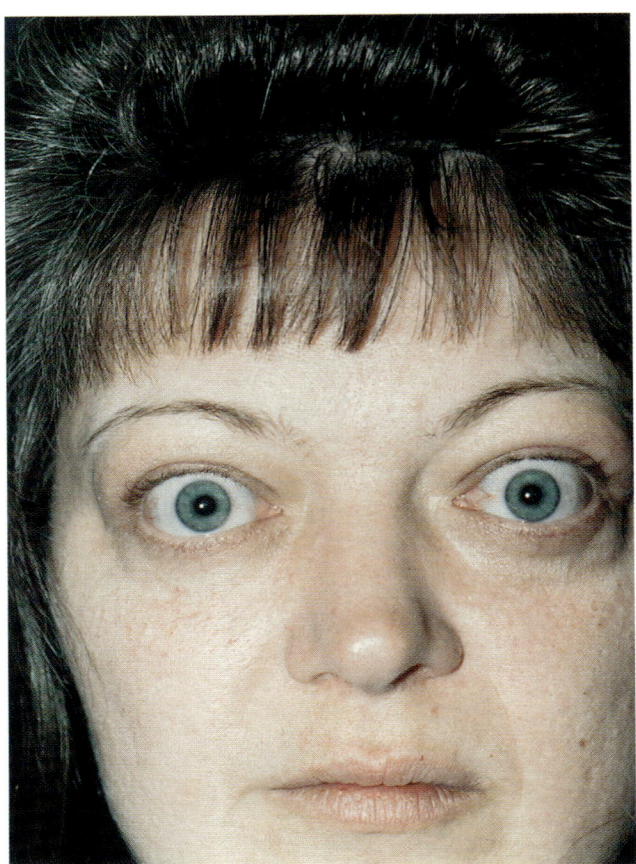

FIG. 14. Bilateral orbital decompression: floor and medial wall, preoperative and postoperative. (Courtesy of David H. Saunders, MD.)

and-fast rule. The standard nomograms to determine how far a muscle should be recessed are often highly inaccurate in thyroid orbits. This unpredictability of response results from several features seen in thyroid patients:

a. Fibrotic extraocular muscles in thyroid patients often have extensive adhesions that actually create a disparity between the anatomic insertion and the mechanically functional insertion.
b. Thyroid extraocular muscles with fatty replacement and fibrosis do not give the same response per millimeter of recession.
c. Reactivation of active inflammatory disease may cause further muscle contraction.
d. Fibrosis anterior to the point of muscle reattachment may cause forward creep of the mechanical insertion, acting as a muscle advancement.

This lack of predictability has led to the almost universal adoption of adjustable sutures in thyroid strabismus surgery to improve accuracy.

11. Last, presbyopic patients are usually poor bifocal candidates because of the incommitant nature of their strabismus. Therefore, they are often best served with separate distance and reading glasses.

When taking on the challenge of surgical rehabilitation of patients with severe thyroid ophthalmopathy who may require orbital decompression, strabismus surgery, and/or correction of lid retraction, it must be remembered that orbital decompression adversely affects both motility and lid retraction, and that motility surgery may affect lid retraction. Therefore, the inviolate rule for the order of surgical correction is: first, orbital decompression, if required; second, strabismus surgery; third, lid surgery.

SUMMARY

I will conclude with my opening thought that thyroid ophthalmopathy is a self-limiting autoimmune disease. Its clinical course varies widely between patients and is characterized by remissions and exacerbations in each patient. Thyroid ophthalmopathy has two stages of disease activity: an acute inflammatory phase and an inactive fibrotic stage. Attempts to shorten the active inflammatory phase include the use of corticosteroids, the use of immunosuppressive agents, and orbital irradiation. The results are modest at best.

Although the acute inflammatory phase is self-limited, unfortunately the debilitating symptoms caused by proptosis, motility restriction, lid retraction, and compressive optic neuropathy are permanent. Rehabilitative surgery can offer patients with severe thyroid ophthalmopathy relief from corneal pain, elimination of double vision, the opportunity to look "normal," and preservation of vision.

REFERENCES

1. Rootman J. *Diseases of the orbit.* Philadelphia: JB Lippincott, 1988.
2. Villadolid MC, Yokoyama N, et al. Untreated Graves' disease patients without clinical ophthalmopathy demonstrate a high frequency of extraocular muscle enlargement by magnetic resonance. *J Clin Endocrinol Metab* 1995;80(1):2830–2833.
3. Schleusener H, Bogner V, et al. The relevance of genetic susceptibility in Graves' disease and immune thyroiditis. *Exp Clin Encocrinol* 1991;97:127–132.
4. Gorman CA. *Mayo Clin Proc* 1983;58:517.
5. Kendler DL, Rootman J, et al. The 64kDa membrane antigen is a recurrent epitope for natural autoantibodies in patients with Graves' thyroid and ophthalmic disease. *Clin Endocrinol* 1991;35(6):539–547.
6. Grubeck-Loebenstein B, Trieb K, et al. Retrobulbar T cells from patients with Graves' ophthalmopathy are CD8+ and specifically recognize autologous fibroblasts. *J Clin Invest* 1994;93(6):2738–2743.
7. Bahn RS, Henfelder AE. Retrobulbar fibroblasts: important effector cells in Graves' ophthalmopathy. *Thyroid* 1992;2(1):89–94.
8. Smith TJ, Wang HS, et al. Prostaglandin E_2 elicits a morphological change in cultured orbital fibroblasts from patients with Graves' ophthalmopathy. *Proc Natl Acad Sci USA* 1994;91(11):5094–5098.
9. Bahn RS. The fibroblast is the target cell in connective tissue manifestions of Graves' disease. *Int Arch Allergy Immunol* 1995;106(3):213–218.
10. Hudson HL, Levin L, Feldon SE. Graves' exophthalmos unrelated to extraocular muscle enlargement, superior rectus muscle inflammation may induce venous obstruction. *Ophthalmopathy* 1991;98:1495–1499.
11. Nakase Y, Osanai T, et al. Color Doppler imaging of orbital venous flow in dysthyroid optic neuropathy. *Jpn J Ophthalmol* 1994;38(1):80–86.
12. Dosso A, Safran AB, et al. Anterior ischemic optic neuropathy in Graves' disease. *J Neurophthalmol* 1994;14(3):170–174.
13. Trobe JD, Glaser JS, Laflamme P. Dysthyroid optic neuropathy, clinical profile and rationale for management. *Arch Opthalmol* 1978;96:1199.
14. Tallstedt L, Lundell G, et al. Occurrence of ophthalmopathy after treatment for Graves' hyperthyroidism. *N Engl J Med* 1992;326:1733–1738.
15. Pinchera A, Bartalena L, Marcocci C. Therapeutic controversies: radiation and Graves' ophthalmopathy. *J Clin Endocrinol Metab* 1995;80(2):342–344.
16. Sergott RC, Felberg NT, Savino PJ, et al. Graves' ophthalmopathy—immunologic parameters related to corticosteroid therapy. *Invest Ophthalmol Vis Sci* 1981;20:173–182.
17. Biglan AW. Control of eyelid retraction associated with Graves' disease with botulinum-A toxin. *Ophthalmic Surg* 1994;25(3):186–188.
18. Henderson JW. Relief of eyelid retraction, a surgical procedure. *Arch Ophthalmol* 1965;74:205–216.
19. Bartley GB, Fatourechi V, et al. The treatment of Graves' ophthalmopathy in an incidence cohort. *Am J Ophthalmol* 1996;121:200–206.
20. Harvey JT, Anderson RL. The aponeurotic approach to eyelid retraction. *Ophthalmology* 1981;88:513–524.
21. Putterman AM. Surgical treatment of thyroid-related upper eyelid retraction. Graded Mueller's muscle excision and levator recession. *Ophthalmology* 1981;88:507–512.
22. Ceisler EJ, Shore JW, et al. Results of Muellerotomy and levator aponeurosis transposition for the correction of upper eyelid retraction in Graves' disease. *Ophthalmology* 1995;102:483–492.
23. Garrity JA, Valah F, et al. Results of transantral orbital decompression in 428 patients with severe Graves' ophthalmopathy. *Am J Ophthalmol* 1993;116:533–547.
24. Fatourechi V, Garrity JA, et al. Graves' ophthalmopathy: results of transantral orbital decompression performed primarily for cosmetic indications. *Ophthalmology* 1994;101:938–942.
25. Lyons CJ, Rootman J. Orbital decompresssion for disfiguring exophthalmos in thyroid orbitopathy. *Ophthalmology* 1994;101:223–230.

CHAPTER 20

Clinical Manifestations and Differential Diagnosis of Hypothyroidism

Alice C. Chiu and Steven I. Sherman

Hypothyroidism is the clinical state resulting from an insufficient amount of circulating thyroid hormone to support normal body functions. Although cretinism or congenital hypothyroidism has been known since antiquity, thyroid hormone deficiency was not postulated as the cause until 1871 by Fagge (1). Soon thereafter, Gull described the adult form of hypothyroidism, referring to it as "a cretinoid state supervening in adult life in women" (2). Within 10 years, the Clinical Society of London deemed the problem significant enough to create a committee to investigate the subject of "myxœdema," using the term coined by Ord (3). The committee's monograph, published in 1888, continues to provide a significant fund of information about the clinical and pathological aspects of hypothyroidism (4). Today, however, the term *hypothyroidism* should not be used interchangeably with *myxedema*, the latter denoting a more advanced state of thyroid hormone deficiency associated with deposition of glycosaminoglycans in interstitial tissues.

That hypothyroidism occurs more commonly in women escaped neither Gull (2) nor his colleagues. The female-to-male ratio in hypothyroidism ranges from 2:1 to 8:1 in various epidemiologic surveys. Similarly, the increasing prevalence of the disease with advancing age was recognized in the nineteenth century. The prevalence of unsuspected overt hypothyroidism, defined as the combination of clinical and biochemical findings of hypothyroidism, ranges from 1 to 18 cases per 1000 persons (5,6). Subclinical hypothyroidism, defined as a serum thyroid stimulating hormone (TSH) level between 5 and 20 mU/L in asymptomatic patients, occurs with a frequency of 2.5% to 10% (5,6). In contrast, the prevalence of hypothyroidism (defined as an elevation of serum TSH above the upper normal limit) in geriatric populations may be as high as 20% (7). Using the more stringent criterion for hypothyroidism (i.e., a TSH level >10 mU/L), the prevalence of hypothyroidism is 1% to 6% in women over 50 years of age, and 7.1% in women over 60 years of age. Laboratory diagnosis of hypothyroidism is discussed in Chapter 4.

CAUSES OF HYPOTHYROIDISM

The various causes of hypothyroidism are listed in Table 1. Primary hypothyroidism constitutes the great majority of the cases. In iodine-replete regions, autoimmune thyroid diseases and thyroablative therapy cause the majority of cases of hypothyroidism. However, worldwide, iodine deficiency is the leading cause of hypothyroidism. Although most patients with chronic hypothyroidism are treated with thyroid hormone replacement therapy, regardless of the etiology, every attempt should be made to determine the cause of hypothyroidism. This is especially true in cases of secondary or tertiary hypothyroidism, in which concomitant hormonal insufficiencies may require therapy. Reversible hypothyroidism may also occur as a result of transient thyroiditis, or drugs and food with antithyroid effects. A thorough history and physical examination supplemented with basic thyroid function tests will generally provide the necessary diagnostic information. Other laboratory tests or imaging procedures can be ordered as indicated on an individual basis.

Primary Hypothyroidism

Autoimmune Thyroid Disease

Although chronic autoimmune thyroiditis is most commonly diagnosed in middle-aged or older women, it can

---

A. C. Chiu and S. I. Sherman: Baylor College of Medicine, Houston, Texas 77030.

TABLE 1. *Causes of Hypothyroidism*

Primary hypothyroidism
    Autoimmune thyroid disease
        Hashimoto's thyroiditis
        Postpartum thyroiditis
        Silent thyroiditis
    Postablative hypothyroidism
        Surgery
        Radioiodide therapy
        External beam radiotherapy
    Biosynthetic defects
        Congenital enzymatic defects
        Antithyroid drugs
        Goitrogenic foods and medications
        Iodine deficiency
        Iodine excess (e.g., amiodarone, SSKI radiocontrast dye, iodine-containing antitussives, kelps)
    Subacute thyroiditis
    TSH-unresponsiveness syndrome
Central hypothyroidism
    Tumors
        Pituitary adenomas, craniopharyngiomas, meningiomas
    Infiltrative diseases
        Sarcoidosis, eosinophilic granulomas, metastatic tumors
    Sheehan's syndrome
    Postradiotherapy
    Trauma
    Autoimmune hypophysitis
    Defective TSH

SSKI, saturated solution of potassium iodide; TSH, thyroid stimulating hormone.

be found in men and women from childhood through senescence. The thyroid glands of these patients can be either goitrous or atrophic. The goitrous variant is commonly known as Hashimoto's thyroiditis, whereas the atrophic variant has been termed idiopathic hypothyroidism, Gull's disease, and primary myxedema. Histologically, these two disorders share the features of lymphocytic infiltration and fibrosis. Hashimoto's disease is also characterized by thyroid follicular hyperplasia, plasma cell infiltration, and germinal centers. Many patients with serologic or histologic evidence of autoimmune thyroiditis are clinically euthyroid and have normal circulating thyroid hormone levels. However, evidence of autoimmune thyroiditis increases the risk of subsequently developing clinical hypothyroidism (8–10).

Both humoral and cell-mediated immune mechanisms have been implicated in the pathogenesis of autoimmune thyroiditis. Circulating antibodies to thyroid peroxidase (TPO) and thyroglobulin are present in up to 95% and 70% (11), respectively, of patients with chronic autoimmune thyroiditis. Significant titers of these antibodies may identify euthyroid patients at risk of developing overt thyroid failure (9) or postpartum thyroiditis (12). Anti-TPO antibodies (previously termed antimicrosomal antibodies) have been shown *in vitro* to be able to fix complement and are cytotoxic to human thyroid follicular cells (13). Antibodies that interfere with binding of TSH to its receptor on the follicular cell can block physiologic thyroid stimulation (14) and contribute to both permanent and transient hypothyroidism in 10% to 40% of patients. Produced by intrathyroidal T cells in Hashimoto's thyroiditis, interferon-γ (IFN-γ) and tumor necrosis factor-α (TNF-α) may have inhibitory actions on thyroid growth and functions. They may also induce follicular cells to produce interleukin-6, leading to B-lymphocyte proliferation (15). IFN-γ can also induce thyrocytes to express major histocompatibility complex (MHC) class II molecules, which then turn thyrocytes into antigen-presenting cells, capable of stimulating autoreactive T cells by presentation of endogenous autoantigens. TNF may augment this effect of IFN-γ on thyrocytes (16). Although it is unlikely that the expression of MHC class II molecules by thyrocytes represents the initiating process of autoimmune thyroiditis, it may very well play an important role in the maintenance and amplification of the disease process through its interactions with T cells.

Transient hypothyroidism may occur as part of the course of silent thyroiditis (17) and of postpartum thyroiditis (18), both of which have autoimmune etiologies. These disorders are characterized by subacute development of thyroid inflammation, typically without death of follicular cells. The initial inflammatory phase may produce thyrotoxicosis as a result of the release of preformed thyroid hormone from disrupted follicles. Radioactive iodine uptake during the thyrotoxic stage is markedly decreased. In 50% to 75% of patients, a hypothyroid phase subsequently occurs, lasting up to several months. However, about 5% develop permanent hypothyroidism. Because the hyperthyroid phase is often clinically overlooked, patients frequently present during the hypothyroid phase. Goiter is variably present in both silent and postpartum thyroiditis. Thyroid autoantibodies are frequently positive in postpartum thyroiditis and can be used as a predictor for the development of thyroiditis when identified during pregnancy or the early postpartum period (12,19). Women who develop postpartum thyroiditis are at higher risk for chronic autoimmune thyroiditis in later years (20); this increased risk does not apply to patients with silent thyroiditis, however. Histologically, the transient thyroiditides are characterized by lymphocytic infiltration without germinal centers, plasma cells, or fibrosis. Because of the transient nature of the disease, patients often require only short-term symptomatic relief with thyroid replacement therapy. A syndrome similar to silent thyroiditis can be provoked in patients treated with the cytokines IFN-α and interleukin-2, drugs used for the treatment of various viral infections and malignancies (21,22).

Postablative Hypothyroidism

Transient hypothyroidism can occur in patients who undergo surgical resection of a single thyroid lobe for nodular disease. However, thyroid function usually recovers rapidly unless autoimmune thyroiditis is also present (23).

Thyroidectomy for Graves' disease may be followed by hypothyroidism, depending on the extent of surgery. In patients who have an aggressive thyroidectomy, TSH levels rise within 1 to 2 weeks of surgery and overt hypothyroidism occurs within 4 weeks (24). Spontaneous recovery from hypothyroidism can occur by stimulation of the remaining thyroid tissue, either by TSH or by thyroid stimulating immunoglobulins. However, the underlying autoimmune process may lead to progressive destruction of the thyroid remnants and eventually permanent hypothyroidism, which develops in about 1% of patients each year (25).

Patients treated with iodine-131 (^{131}I) for Graves' disease frequently develop hypothyroidism, at least 50% during the first year of treatment (26). The larger the administered dose of ^{131}I, the more likely the occurrence of early hypothyroidism. After radioiodine treatment, the underlying autoimmune inflammation and the radiation-induced vasculitis lead to eventual hypothyroidism in 90% of patients, regardless of the ^{131}I dose (27). In contrast, hypothyroidism is uncommon after ^{131}I treatment for toxic nodular disease. The lack of radioiodine uptake in the extranodular tissue allows recovery of euthyroidism after normalization of TSH.

External beam radiotherapy for lymphoma or head and neck carcinomas is usually given in doses of more than 20 Gy (2000 rad). Thyroidal exposure is sufficient to produce hypothyroidism, and the risk of eventual hypothyroidism increases with higher doses (28,29). As with other causes of postablative hypothyroidism, subclinical hypothyroidism may be present for many years before disease becomes symptomatic. Transient thyrotoxicosis resulting from radiation-induced thyroiditis may precede the development of both transient and permanent hypothyroidism (28).

Congenital Biosynthetic Defects

In addition to congenital absence of the thyroid, rare congenital enzymatic defects in the various steps of thyroid hormone synthesis can lead to hypothyroidism in newborns and infants. Because inheritance usually follows an autosomal recessive pattern, homozygotes are more severely affected and can be diagnosed early. Goiter is common, resulting from elevated TSH levels, but it may not be readily appreciated during the newborn period. Neonatal thyroid screening is thus essential for early detection and treatment of congenital hypothyroidism.

Congenital defects may involve any of the steps involved in thyroid hormone synthesis. Partial or complete flaws in iodide transport (30) into the follicular cell are associated with hypothyroidism, goiter, and low radioiodine uptake into both the thyroid and the salivary glands. Because of various quantitative and qualitative abnormalities in TPO function, impaired iodide oxidation and organification can occur in a heterogeneous group of syndromes (31). Organification defects lead to a condition in which there is increased iodine uptake but an inability to attach the iodine to tyrosine residues. Perchlorate discharge tests are therefore typically positive and diagnostic in these patients. The combination of goiter, congenital hypothyroidism resulting from impaired iodotyrosine coupling, and congenital sensorineural deafness is termed Pendred's syndrome (32,33). Abnormal primary structure and glycosylation of thyroglobulin can also lead to dysfunctional organification and coupling (34). Finally, the thyroid with insufficient iodotyrosine deiodinase is unable to recirculate and reuse iodotyrosines, thereby causing excessive iodine loss (35,36). Treatment of congenital biosynthetic defects generally consists of thyroid hormone replacement, but high dose iodine supplementation is appropriate for patients with deiodinase deficiency.

A rare cause of congenital hypothyroidism is the syndrome of TSH unresponsiveness. Mutations in the TSH receptor lead to decreased response to TSH stimulation (37). In general, patients appear to be well compensated with normal to low-normal levels of thyroid hormones and elevated TSH, but without goiter. In cases in which the mutation occurs in the postreceptor $G_s\alpha$, hypothyroidism can be a part of Albright's hereditary osteodystrophy syndrome.

Acquired Biosynthetic Defects

Thyroid hormone synthesis can be impaired by compounds both environmental and pharmacologic. Naturally occurring and industrial goitrogens (e.g., thiocyanate, resorcinol, and dinitrophenol) rarely cause hypothyroidism, except in patients with underlying thyroid disease. Excessive doses of thiouracil derivatives (propylthiouracil, carbimazole, and methimazole) used in the treatment of hyperthyroidism will cause reversible goitrous hypothyroidism.

Lithium carbonate, commonly used to treat psychiatric disease, decreases the release of thyroid hormones, affects intrathyroidal iodide regulation, and may alter extrathyroidal T^4 to T^3 conversion (38,39). Up to 15% of patients taking lithium may develop overt hypothyroidism; the frequency of subclinical disease is at least twice as high. Autoimmune thyroid disease may contribute to the risk of lithium-induced hypothyroidism. However, lithium itself may have immune-modulating effects and may trigger autoimmune thyroid disease in genetically susceptible persons (40,41). Because both the risk of developing hypothyroidism and the complications in this patient group are significant, patients taking lithium should have their thyroid function monitored before and during therapy.

Iodine deficiency ranks as the most common cause of thyroid biosynthetic failure worldwide. In severely iodine-deficient areas, cretinism is found in up to 15% of the population. With lesser degrees of iodine deficiency, euthyroid goiter is more typical. Certain goitrogen-containing foodstuffs, such as cassava and millet, can confound iodine deficiency and contribute to hypothyroidism in areas of borderline deficiency. Iodine supplementation of salt, drinking water, or prepared foods, or intermittent iodized oil injections, can prevent the devastating problem of cretinism in endemic areas (42).

On the other hand, iodine when taken in excess can inhibit both thyroid hormone release and synthesis. Although milligram quantities of iodine consumed daily can cause mild transient decreases in serum T_4 levels, clinical hypothyroidism rarely results unless there is coexistent thyroid disease such as autoimmune thyroiditis (43). Thyroids previously ablated with radioiodine are especially sensitive to the inhibitory effects of iodine excess (44). Even the normal thyroid can fail when exposed chronically to hundreds of milligrams daily of iodine, as has been described among populations with exceedingly high dietary intake from seaweed or water. Important sources of excess iodine include certain antitussives, topical antiseptics, and natural foodstuffs such as kelp and dulse. Radiographic contrast dye is another important iatrogenic source of excess iodine.

Amiodarone is an iodinated benzofuran widely used to treat cardiac arrhythmias. Because the drug is stored in adipose tissue, amiodarone has a prolonged half-life (25 to 100 days). The initial response to amiodarone is inhibition of T_4-to-T_3 conversion, with transient elevation of the TSH levels (45). Generally, TSH levels return to normal and most patients taking amiodarone have euthyroid hyperthyroxinemia (46). However, chronic hypothyroidism can result in as many as 22% of patients taking amiodarone, particularly in iodine-replete regions (47). As with other instances of iodine-induced hypothyroidism, patients with underlying thyroid diseases such as autoimmune thyroiditis are most susceptible to the thyroid inhibitory effects of amiodarone (48,49).

Thyroiditis

In addition to autoimmunity, inflammation of the thyroid gland can result from infection and inflammatory processes of uncertain etiology. Usually, the hypothyroidism is transient and requires only symptomatic therapy.

Subacute thyroiditis (de Quervain's, granulomatous, or nonsuppurative thyroiditis) usually presents with a painful goiter, malaise, myalgias, fatigue, and fever in a patient with a preceding viral upper respiratory illness (50). Because of the release of preexisting hormone from disrupted follicles, an initial thyrotoxic phase is common. Hypothyroidism is usually transient, lasting weeks to months. A characteristic laboratory feature in subacute thyroiditis is marked elevation of the erythrocyte sedimentation rate. Radioiodine uptake measured during the thyrotoxic stage is suppressed. In contrast to autoimmune causes of thyroiditis, antithyroid antibodies are generally absent or are only transiently present (51). Histologic evidence of subacute thyroiditis includes granulomatous inflammation, giant cell infiltration, and fibrosis. Treatment of this disorder includes salicylates or glucocorticoids to suppress the inflammatory response, and β-adrenergic-receptor blockers for symptoms of thyrotoxicosis. In the hypothyroid phase, thyroid hormone can be administered to symptomatic patients.

Riedel's thyroiditis (invasive fibrous thyroiditis) is a variant of a rare generalized fibrosing disorder (52,53). The gland may be totally or partially replaced by dense fibrous tissue, often extending beyond the gland capsule into extrathyroidal tissues. Associated conditions include retroperitoneal, orbital, pulmonary, and mediastinal fibrosis. Typical symptoms and signs include neck pressure, dysphagia, dyspnea, and rapid enlargement of a stony hard thyroid gland. Depending on the extent of thyroidal involvement, hypothyroidism may be seen in fewer than half of patients.

Miscellaneous Causes of Primary Hypothyroidism

Infections of the thyroid gland are a rare cause of thyroiditis and transient hypothyroidism (54). Infiltrative disorders such as progressive systemic sclerosis, sarcoidosis, amyloidosis, hemochromatosis, and cystinosis are associated with goiter, but hypothyroidism appears to be a rare complication.

Central Hypothyroidism

Due to the trophic and regulatory effects of TSH on the thyroid gland, disorders of TSH production or function can cause hypothyroidism. However, even in the absence of TSH, a basal level of thyroid hormone synthesis persists. Therefore, circulating T_4 and T_3 levels are typically not as low in central hypothyroidism as they are in primary thyroidal failure.

Pituitary Disorders

Pituitary disorders may directly affect TSH production. Defective TSH production can either be congenital or acquired, and it can occur either as an isolated deficiency or part of a plurihormonal deficiency. Congenital hypothyroidism resulting from absent or defective TSH production has been reported (55,56). Patients with this disorder are born with features of congenital nongoitrous hypothyroidism. Despite low levels of T_3 and T_4, TSH levels may be low or inappropriately normal. In isolated TSH deficiency, single nucleotide mutations in the β-subunit gene of TSH have been identified as the cause of the autosomal recessive disorder (57). In cases with combined anterior pituitary hormone deficiency, TSH deficiency often coexists with growth hormone (GH) and prolactin deficiencies (58). Absence of normal Pit-1, a pituitary transcription factor essential to normal pituitary development, leads to a hypoplastic pituitary gland and multiple hormone insufficiencies (59). The identification and treatment of newborn infants with TSH deficiency can prevent the complications of congenital hypothyroidism. However, screening programs that depend on newborn TSH levels can miss this rare diagnosis.

More common causes of central hypothyroidism are acquired destructive processes affecting the pituitary gland. These generally produce multiple pituitary hormone deficiencies, although any combination is possible. Infiltrative processes (such as sarcoidosis, giant cell granulomas, and lymphocytic hypophysitis) or infectious processes (such as syphilis, tuberculosis, and parasitic diseases) may all involve the pituitary gland. In particular, lymphocytic hypophysitis has been reported to cause acquired isolated TSH deficiency (60,61). Antipituicyte antibodies have been identified in this syndrome, and an autoimmune etiology is likely (62). Neoplastic diseases such as pituitary adenoma, craniopharyngioma, and metastatic disease to the pituitary (e.g., renal cell cancer, leukemia, and breast cancer) may cause acquired TSH deficiency. These mass lesions either destroy normal pituicytes or compress the pituitary stalk, thereby disrupting the portal supply of trophic factors from the hypothalamus. Patients with plurihormonal deficiency exhibit features of hypothyroidism, as well as those of gonadotrophin, adrenocorticotropic hormone (ACTH), and GH deficiencies.

Hypothalamic Disorders

Disorders of hypothalamic function can affect the pituitary production of TSH by altered synthesis or by release of trophic factors, particularly thyrotropin-releasing hormone (TRH). Neoplastic diseases such as germinomas, craniopharyngiomas, and meningiomas often cause defective TRH secretion. Infiltrative diseases such as sarcoidosis, histiocytosis X, and granulomatous disease, and infections such as tuberculosis, fungal infection, and syphilis can also affect the hypothalamus. Again, plurihormonal deficiency typically occurs. Diabetes insipidus is a frequent feature as a result of impairment of vasopressin production and release. Cranial or head and neck irradiation in cancer patients can also lead to hypothalamic hypothyroidism (63,64). Because dopamine transport to the pituitary is frequently affected, mild hyperprolactinemia is commonly seen in these patients.

CLINICAL MANIFESTATIONS OF HYPOTHYROIDISM

The clinical signs and symptoms of hypothyroidism occur as a result of deficient thyroid hormone actions.

Because chronic hypothyroidism usually develops over a span of years, the clinical features may develop insidiously and not be readily noticed. In contrast, severe hypothyroidism occurring after thyroiditis or ablation is usually associated with a rapid onset of symptoms. Complicating the recognition of hypothyroidism is the nonspecific nature of symptoms. Among patients in a general medical practice presenting with the most common symptoms of hypothyroidism (constipation, weight gain, menstrual irregularities, fatigue, depression, cold intolerance, and galactorrhea), only 4% are actually hypothyroid, and fewer than 2% have a TSH level at least 5 mU/L above normal (65). In contrast, more specific symptoms and signs include slow movements, coarse skin, decreased sweating, hoarseness, paresthesias, cold intolerance, periorbital edema, and delayed deep tendon reflex relaxation (66). Wide variability in clinical presentation can further confound clinical recognition of the disorder. Nonetheless, an appreciation of the clinical manifestations of hypothyroidism is necessary to provide the appropriate degree of clinical suspicion for the diagnosis.

Neuromuscular System

Muscular symptoms such as stiffness, cramps, aches, and weakness are frequent complaints in hypothyroid patients. On examination, a prolonged relaxation phase of deep tendon reflexes is common, perhaps secondary to delayed calcium ion recovery by the sarcoplasmic reticulum (67). Myoedema, also known as the mounding phenomenon, is rarely seen.

Other myopathies, such as polymyositis, polymyalgia rheumatica, and myasthenia gravis, may also be seen more commonly in hypothyroidism. The association of myasthenia gravis and hypothyroidism, although less frequent than that seen with hyperthyroidism, underlines the shared autoimmune basis of the diseases. Hereditary hypothyroid myotonia and muscular pseudohypertrophy (Kocker-Debré-Sémélaigne syndrome) in children and the Hoffman syndrome in adults are characterized by muscle enlargement, particularly of the gastrocnemius muscle. In contrast to the increased muscle bulk, muscle strength is reduced or normal (68,69). Aside from bradykinesia and proximal muscle weakness, the Hoffman syndrome is also characterized by painful spasms and stiffness.

On muscle biopsy, the most common abnormalities in hypothyroidism are types I and II fiber atrophy, elevated central nuclear counts, interstitial edema, loss of striation, and glycogen inclusions (70,71).

Increased serum levels of creatine kinase (CK) are frequently found in hypothyroidism, regardless of the presence of overt myopathy. Fractionation studies revealed a preponderance of the MM isotype. The elevated CK level is likely related both to a decrease in the enzyme clearance rate in hypothyroidism and to sarcoplasmic damage. Aldolase, aspartate transaminase, and lactate dehydrogenase levels are also elevated, but these are less sensitive or specific indicators of muscle dysfunction (69).

Neuropathic symptoms such as paresthesia, painful dysesthesia, focal muscle weakness, and deafness can all result from compression of peripheral nerves. Particular nerves more commonly affected in hypothyroidism include the median nerve and cranial nerves II, V, VII, and VIII. Peripheral nerve biopsy often shows nonspecific abnormalities such as mucinous infiltration of the perineurium and endoneurium, axonal degeneration, segmental demyelination and remyelination, and decreased number of large myelinated nerve fibers (67).

Central nervous system dysfunction in hypothyroidism can cause a wide variety of signs and symptoms. Typical findings in severe hypothyroidism include lethargy, depression, and impairment of memory without other evidence of intellectual deficits. Speech is often slowed. In occasional cases, reversible dementia can be caused by hypothyroidism. In contrast, "myxedema madness" is characterized by agitation, rapid speech, inappropriate wit, and delusional behavior. Cerebellar ataxia can occur, characterized by gait disturbance, dysarthric speech, intention tremors, dysmetria, and poor coordination. Thyroid hormone is crucial to normal brain development; severe mental retardation can be one of the most prominent findings in untreated congenital hypothyroidism.

Cardiovascular System

The multifaceted effects that thyroid hormones exert on the cardiovascular system occur both directly on the myocardium, and indirectly through effects on the sympathetic nervous system and basal metabolism (72). T_3 increases the activity of cardiac sarcoplasmic reticulum calcium-ATPase (affecting diastolic relaxation), and it may increase myocardial sensitivity to adrenergic stimulation (73). By altering the duration of depolarization and repolarization of myocardial cell membranes, thyroid hormones directly increase heart rate. Thyroid hormone–induced oxygen consumption in peripheral tissues leads to relative tissue hypoxia and arteriolar vasodilatation, reducing afterload and increasing cardiac output (74).

As a result of these and other physiologic effects, patients with thyroid hormone deficiency commonly present with bradycardia, reduced systolic contractility, prolonged ventricular diastolic relaxation, and increased systemic vascular resistance. Diastolic hypertension occurs secondary to the altered systemic resistance combined with increased blood volume. Heart sounds may be diminished, and cardiomegaly may be detected radiographically. Pericardial effusion may occur in up to 30% of patients and is best detected with the use of an echocardiogram (75). Because of the slow accumulation of the effusion, pulsus paradoxus and cardiac tamponade rarely occur. The effusate is characterized by a high protein content and the presence of mucopolysaccharides (76,77). Electrocardiographic changes commonly include sinus bradycardia, low QRS voltage, prolonged QT interval, and diffuse flattening or inversion of the T waves (76). Conduction abnormalities also occur more commonly in hypothyroidism.

Cardiac output is frequently decreased because of increased systemic vascular resistance and diminished stroke volume. In the setting of intrinsic cardiac disease, congestive heart failure is often exacerbated. Care must be exercised in the use of digitalis glycosides, as clearance is slowed and toxicity more likely. Reversible dilated cardiomyopathy can, rarely, be secondary to hypothyroidism (78,79).

Caution must be practiced in the treatment of hypothyroidism in patients with known coronary artery disease. Counterbalancing effects of thyroid hormone on myocardial oxygen consumption make it difficult to predict whether hypothyroid patients will experience worsened or improved cardiac ischemia with thyroid hormone therapy. When intervention is essential to treat coronary artery disease, coronary artery bypass surgery and percutaneous transluminal coronary angioplasty can both be performed, with minimal increased morbidity that can be managed expectantly (80,81).

Respiratory System

In uncomplicated hypothyroidism, measurements of lung volumes generally show normal values. However, coexisting obesity may lead to moderate reductions in inspiratory capacity, expiratory reserve volume, vital capacity, residual volume, and total lung capacity (82). In these cases, once weight loss occurs, lung volumes return to normal. Both hypoxic and hypercapnic ventilatory drives are impaired, leading to alveolar hypoventilation (83).

Pleural effusions are occasionally found in hypothyroidism, although usually in association with pericardial and peritoneal effusions (84,85). As a result of increased capillary permeability, hypothyroid pleural effusates have moderate protein elevation. The volume of effusion is generally small, and the patients are asymptomatic.

In some hypothyroid patients, obstructive sleep apnea can result from mucopolysaccharide infiltration of the tongue and upper airway (86). Hypotonic upper airway muscles may be unable to compensate for pharyngeal narrowing that occurs in the supine position. After initiation of thyroid hormone replacement, arrhythmias can complicate hypothyroid sleep apnea, as more rapid normalization of oxygen consumption leads to worsening hypoxemia (87). Thus, respiratory support with continuous positive airway pressure may be necessary despite hormone therapy.

Gastrointestinal System

Gastrointestinal dysfunction is common in thyroid disease. Indeed, constipation, obstipation, or even megacolon resulting from decreased gut motility may be the cardinal presenting feature of hypothyroidism (88–90). The gallbladder may be hypotonic or dilated, and impaired vascular permeability may lead to ascites (88).

Intestinal absorption is generally normal in hypothyroidism, although myxedematous infiltration of intestinal mucosa can rarely cause malabsorption. Patients with autoimmune thyroiditis are at increased risk for the development of pernicious anemia and achlorhydria resulting from atrophic gastritis. Calcium absorption is increased in hypothyroidism. Pancreatic function is usually normal (88).

In the absence of simultaneous liver disease, serum levels of alanine transaminase, γ-glutamyltransferase, bilirubin, and alkaline phosphatase are generally normal in hypothyroid patients. However, aspartate transaminase levels may be increased as a result of impaired metabolic clearance of the muscle-derived enzyme (91). The yellowish appearance that may be noted in the skin of hypothyroid patients, caused by hypercarotenemia, should not be confused with jaundice; scleral and mucous membranes are generally anicteric.

Integumentary System

The hypothyroid skin is generally pale with a tinge of yellowish discoloration, a result of the combined effects of elevated serum and tissue carotene levels (a consequence of the decrease in carotene metabolism), anemia, and decreased cutaneous blood flow. It is also accompanied by nonpitting edema, secondary to increased accumulation of mucopolysaccharides and fluids in the dermis. Typically, this swelling is most marked around the eyes and hands. The skin also feels dry and cool, related to the decrease in eccrine and apocrine secretion. Peripheral vasoconstriction contributes to the cool sensation of the skin (92).

Cutaneous appendages are commonly affected in hypothyroidism. Hair is often dry, brittle, and coarse in texture. Alopecia occurs commonly on the scalp and the lateral eyebrows (93). Thickening and slow growth of the nails are often noted. Hirsutism has been reported in children with hypothyroidism.

Skeletal System

Thyroid hormone is essential for normal skeletal growth and maturation. In neonatal and childhood hypothyroidism, delayed skeletal maturation and growth retardation are caused by deficient GH and insulin-like growth factor-1 (IGF-1; somatomedin-C) secretion (94, 95). Thyroid hormone itself may also play a significant role in skeletal maturation independent of its effect on GH and IGF-1. In adults, hypothyroidism is characterized by decreased bone turnover and a prolonged bone remodeling cycle. Elevated parathyroid hormone (PTH) levels may result from mild resistance, as evidenced by lower serum calcium increments following administration of exogenous PTH (96,97). In turn, increased PTH leads to increased 1,25-dihydroxyvitamin D, causing the relative increase in calcium absorption (98). Serum calcium and inorganic phosphate levels are usually normal, as is bone mineral density.

Hematopoietic System

Mild anemia is a common feature in hypothyroidism, occurring in about 25% of untreated patients (99,100). Although decreased plasma volume may mitigate the reduction in total red cell mass, normochromic normocytic anemia is a consequence of decreased erythropoietin synthesis (100). In general, red cell survival appears to be normal in hypothyroidism. Except for iron deficiency caused by hypothyroidism-induced menorrhagia, thyroid hormone deficiency rarely affects serum ferritin, iron, or total iron-binding capacity (99). Macrocytic anemia can result from malabsorption of either folate or vitamin B_{12}. As many as 10% of patients with hypothyroidism caused by autoimmune thyroiditis have pernicious anemia (100,101). Hypothyroid dyslipidemia can lead to increased membrane lipid content, also causing macrocytosis.

White blood cell and platelet counts are usually normal in hypothyroidism, unless there is coexistent pernicious anemia or folate deficiency causing low cell counts. Despite reports of decreased platelet adhesiveness, few hypothyroid patients have abnormal bleeding times (102). Similarly, decreased levels of factors VIII, IX, XI, and XII may be seen as the result of the general decrease in protein synthesis (102,103). Fibrinolytic activity is also decreased (103). However, clinically significant bleeding is infrequent.

Endocrine and Metabolic Systems

Pituitary Gland

Hyperprolactinemia is common in primary hypothyroidism, caused by stimulation of the lactotroph by TRH, and occasionally leading to galactorrhea. In severe cases of primary hypothyroidism, thyrotroph hyperplasia may occur, misidentified in sellar imaging as a mass lesion. In addition to decreased nocturnal secretion of GH, the response to insulin-induced hypoglycemia and GH-releasing hormone is blunted. Hypothyroidism also causes both reduced IGF-1 production and end-organ resistance to IGF-1.

Adrenal Glands

Despite delayed cortisol clearance in hypothyroidism, cortisol production rates and circadian rhythmicity remain essentially normal (104). Direct stimulation of adrenal glands with ACTH frequently yields normal cortisol responses (105). However, cortisol response to insulin-induced hypoglycemia and metyrapone may be subnormal, indicating slightly impaired hypothalamic–pituitary control over cortisol production (106).

Hypoadrenalism may coexist with hypothyroidism in patients with either autoimmune polyglandular failure or hypopituitarism. Because delayed cortisol clearance can preserve "normal" serum cortisol levels, adrenal insufficiency can be masked in patients with hypothyroidism. With reversal of thyroid hormone deficiency, symptomatic adrenal insufficiency can develop acutely if unsuspected. Therefore, patients at risk for simultaneous adrenal and thyroid insufficiency need to be evaluated for both conditions, and glucocorticoid therapy should be initiated along with thyroid hormone when appropriate. Occasional reversal of hypothyroidism has been reported after treatment of primary adrenal insufficiency with glucocorticoids (107).

Plasma norepinephrine levels are elevated in hypothyroid patients, regardless of the presence or absence of hypertension (108). However, epinephrine levels are generally unchanged. Impaired responsiveness to adrenergic stimulation may exist in hypothyroidism (109).

Gonadal Function

In hypothyroid children of both genders, sexual maturation is often delayed. Hypothyroidism is a common cause of primary amenorrhea that should be considered early in the diagnostic evaluation. Of note, when primary amenorrhea is a result of Turner's syndrome, thyroid function should also be evaluated, given the increased frequency of autoimmune thyroiditis. Premature thelarche, premature menarche, and central precocious puberty have also been reported (110). Macro-orchidism has been described in more than 75% of prepubertal hypothyroid boys (111). Testicular biopsy obtained before puberty shows a predominance of tubular component. If left untreated, testicular atrophy and involution may occur.

Amenorrhea, both primary and secondary, can be a result of hyperprolactinemia in primary hypothyroidism. In less severe hypothyroidism, menorrhagia and irregular anovulatory cycles are a common complaint. Infertility and galactorrhea may be seen in these cases, as well as hirsutism. Those who became pregnant without the benefit of thyroid hormone replacement therapy have a higher rate of pregnancy wastage, premature labor, and small-for-gestational-age infants (112).

In hypothyroid men, a hypergonadotrophic state has been described consistent with testicular resistance to gonadotropins (113). Testosterone and sex-hormone-binding globulin levels are generally low, with impotence and decrease in libido being reported in some. However, free testosterone levels may be normal. Semen analysis is usually normal, and hydrocele may be seen.

Lipoproteins

Fasting hyperlipidemia occurs in most hypothyroid patients. Multiple mechanisms account for the various combinations of lipid abnormalities that have been recognized for over 60 years (114,115). Primary defects include reduced activities of the hepatic low-density-lipoprotein (LDL) receptor, lipoprotein lipase, triglyceride lipase, microsomal β-hydroxy-β-methylglutaryl-coenzyme A reductase, and cholesterol 7α-reductase, and increased adipocyte lipolysis. Variations in the LDL-receptor gene may affect the magnitude of impaired LDL clearance induced by hypothyroidism (116). As a result of combinations of these abnormalities, patients may have elevated LDL-cholesterol, normal or elevated triglycerides, normal or elevated high-density-lipoprotein (HDL) cholesterol, and elevated nonesterified fatty acids. Of patients with primary hypothyroidism, normal lipid values are seen only in 8%, type IIa hyperlipidemia is seen in 56%, type IIb in 34%, and type IV in 2% (117). Patients with central hypothyroidism accompanied by adrenal insufficiency tend to have lesser degrees of hyperlipidemia, with a greater proportion of hypertriglyceridemic phenotypes. Although the exact etiology is uncertain, lipoprotein (a) levels may also be increased in hypothyroidism. Finally, the combined defects in lipoprotein lipase and hepatic triglyceride lipase may lead to an unusual pattern of postprandial lipemic changes, particularly among the subtypes of HDL cholesterol (118).

Hypothyroidism may be the cause of secondary hyperlipidemia in 4% of patients with hypercholesterolemia. The frequency of overt hypothyroidism appears to be twice that expected in the general population, justifying measurement of the serum TSH level in all hyperlipidemic patients (119).

Fluids and Electrolytes

Severely hypothyroid patients frequently complain of swelling and have nonpitting edema because of increased capillary permeability and interstitial hydrophilic mucopolysaccharides. Total body water and sodium content in these patients are frequently elevated; however, effective circulating volume is decreased. Plasma renin, aldosterone, creatinine, and atrial natriuretic factor levels are usually normal or low, and renal blood flow is decreased in proportion to the cardiac output and volume status of the patient.

Euvolemic hyponatremia is an important complication of severe hypothyroidism. Free water clearance is often decreased, which can be demonstrated by delayed water excretion following an acute water-loading test (120). Urine osmolality is inappropriately elevated for the degree of plasma hypo-osmolality. Although increased antidiuretic hormone secretion has been reported, vasopressin response to saline-loading test is generally normal (121). Postoperative hyponatremia occurs more commonly in unsuspected hypothyroid patients (80).

Metabolism

Hypothyroidism leads to decreased oxygen consumption and carbon dioxide production, yielding a decreased basal metabolic rate. Substrate catabolism is reduced, and appetite is frequently depressed. As a result, weight gain can be secondary to increased fat stores as well as fluid retention.

Although glucose metabolism is normal in patients without diabetes, hypothyroid diabetics may have greater difficulty controlling their blood sugars. Clearance of exogenous insulin is slowed, leading to higher risk for hypoglycemia (122).

Altered pharmacokinetics of many medications occurs in hypothyroidism. Of particular importance is delayed clearance of drugs with a narrow therapeutic range, such as digoxin, theophylline, and phenytoin. Because catabolism of vitamin K–dependent clotting factors is decreased, warfarin requirements may be increased in hypothyroidism, and doses may need to be reduced following thyroid hormone replacement therapy (123).

SPECIAL PRESENTATIONS OF HYPOTHYROIDISM

Subclinical Hypothyroidism

The term *subclinical hypothyroidism* was coined to describe patients who had biochemical indications of thyroid hormone deficiency, but who were otherwise asymptomatic with respect to their thyroid function. Although various criteria have been proposed to define it, subclinical hypothyroidism might best be described as applying to patients whose TSH level is elevated but whose free thyroid hormone levels remain within the population's normal range. In some, this represents an early stage of a progressive decline towards overt hypothyroidism; in others, thyroid function tests remain unchanged during follow-up, or they might actually normalize. Appropriate recognition of patients at risk for progression allows early intervention and prevention of symptomatic disease.

The most common etiology for subclinical hypothyroidism that can progress to clinical disease is autoimmune thyroiditis. Patients with a serum titer of antimicrosomal antibodies greater than 1:1600 and an elevated TSH have a 5% to 7% annual risk of developing overt hypothyroidism, and higher incidences have been reported in patients with higher ranges of TSH levels (8–10). The presence of thyroid antibodies or mildly elevated basal TSH alone is less predictive of subsequent clinical disease. Like autoimmune thyroiditis, subclinical hypothyroidism is particularly frequent in the older age groups, with a female preponderance. About 20% of healthy persons older than 60 years of age have TSH levels greater than normal on routine screening, and most of them have normal thyroid hormone levels (7). Other patients at risk for subclinical disease include those who have undergone previous thyroablative therapy (such as radioiodide or surgery for Graves' disease), those who have received external beam radiotherapy to the neck for treatment of nonthyroidal malignancies, and those treated with cytokines.

The role of thyroid hormone replacement therapy in asymptomatic patients with elevated TSH levels has been controversial. The cost of therapy and subsequent monitoring, and the risk of complications of overtreatment might temper enthusiasm for treatment. Nevertheless, potential benefit can be obtained in certain patients from therapy, and all patients diagnosed with subclinical hypothyroidism need consideration for therapy. Given the likelihood of progression of autoimmune thyroiditis in patients with elevated antimicrosomal antibodies and TSH levels, thyroid hormone therapy can certainly be justified on the basis of preventing clinical disease (124). A similar argument can be made for treatment of other patients at risk for progressive disease. More important perhaps, subclinically hypothyroid patients who are "asymptomatic" may report improvement in subjective indicators of thyroid hormone status, as demonstrated in a placebo-controlled randomized trial (125). Patients with mild cardiac dysfunction characterized by impaired systolic contractility, may also show detectable improvement after hormone therapy for subclinical hypothyroidism. In patients with concomitant increases in LDL cholesterol, thyroid hormone treatment may help to ameliorate the hyperlipidemia (125). Finally, goiter secondary to chronic TSH stimulation of thyroid growth may shrink following treatment of subclinical hypothyroidism.

Therefore, therapy for subclinical hypothyroidism can be recommended in patients at risk for progression to overt, symptomatic disease. In addition, a therapeutic trial of levothyroxine can be considered in patients with hypercholesterolemia, impaired cardiac contractility, goiter, or mild nonspecific symptoms that might be consistent with thyroid hormone deficiency. Doses of hormone should be kept to the minimum needed to reduce the TSH level to the lower half of the normal range; conservative dosing is particularly important in patients with Graves' disease, in whom the risk of iatrogenic thyrotoxicosis is significant. The treatment of hypothyroidism is also discussed in Chapter 27.

Myxedema Coma

Myxedema coma represents a systemic state of severely decompensated hypothyroidism, generally triggered by one of a variety of precipitating clinical events (Table 2). It occurs most commonly in elderly patients and carries a poor prognosis. Prompt clinical diagnosis is essential for institution of life-saving thyroid hormone therapy.

Two cardinal features of myxedema coma are altered state of consciousness and hypothermia. The degree of hypothermia may often be severe and underestimated by the use of clinical thermometers that cannot register less than 96°F. Many of the usual features of hypothyroidism are generally obvious, including facial and periorbital puffiness; coarse, dry hair; dry, sallow skin; bradycardia; and delayed reflex relaxation. In moribund patients, areflexia may be seen. Hypoventilation is invariably present, and the patient may require mechanical ventilatory support. The factors causing respiratory failure include impaired hypoxic and hypercapnic ventilatory drives (83, 127), respiratory muscle weakness (128), myxedematous swelling of the airway, and pleural effusion. The use of sedatives, narcotics, tranquilizers, or anesthetics may further contribute to the depression of the respiratory center. Cardiovascular complications of hypothyroidism can be exaggerated, particularly vasoconstriction. Active rewarming should therefore be avoided, as induced vasodilatation can lead to cardiovascular collapse (129,130).

Hyponatremia is common, generally responsive to fluid restriction (131,132). Hypoglycemia may be secondary to decreased gluconeogenesis and decreased insulin clearance (129,130). Impaired counterregulatory responses to hypoglycemia are also thought to occur. Adrenal insufficiency needs to be considered in all patients with myxedema coma, as the ability to mount an adrenocortical response to stress may be impaired. Further, initiation of thyroid hormone therapy may increase cortisol clearance. Therefore, high-dose glucocorticoid administration is prudent (133).

Once myxedema coma is suspected, therapy should be initiated promptly. Essential laboratory studies that should be done prior to treatment include thyroxine, TSH, cortisol, electrolytes, routine chemistries, and arterial blood gases. However, thyroid hormone therapy should be started without results of the thyroid function tests. Levothyroxine sodium and/or liothyronine should be given intravenously, as gastrointestinal motility and absorption are likely impaired (129). Liothyronine may have an important role in therapy, as deiodinase activity is often deficient (see Chapter 27).

Essential supportive therapy includes passive external warming, appropriate cultures and empiric antibiotics, and mechanical ventilation for patients with respiratory failure. Fluid restriction is often necessary for hyponatremia, but judicious use of hypertonic saline solution and diuretics is occasionally necessary. Vasopressors are generally not recommended and must be used with extreme caution (130).

Neonatal Hypothyroidism

Thyroid hormones are crucial to both the physical and neurologic development of the infant. Unfortunately, the clinical diagnosis of congenital hypothyroidism during the neonatal period may not always be evident. To facilitate rapid early diagnosis and correction, neonatal screening programs have been established, using thyroxine and/or TSH assays done from blood collected on filter papers. Abnormal results are then confirmed by serum assays. Thyroid screening is done in conjunction with other screening programs for inborn errors of metabolism (e.g., PKU and galactosemia). In the first 1 million North American infants screened for congenital hypothyroidism, the incidence of congenital hypothyroidism was 1 in 3700 live births (134). The incidence of primary hypothyroidism was estimated to be 1 in 4300 live births, and that of secondary or tertiary hypothyroidism was 1 in 68,000 births. Aplastic or hypoplastic thyroid glands accounted for the majority of cases of primary hypothyroidism. Identification of congenital hypothyroidism and early treatment is a cost-effective means of improving patient neurologic outcome (135,136).

REFERENCES

1. Fagge CH. On sporadic cretinism, occurring in England. *Medico-Chir Trans* 1871;54:155.
2. Gull WW. On a cretinoid state supervening in adult life in women. *Trans Clin Soc London* 1874;7:180–185.
3. Ord WM. On myxoedema, a term proposed to be applied to an essential condition in the "cretinoid" affection occasionally observed in middle-aged women. *Medico-Chir Trans* 1878;61:57.
4. London Clinical Society. *Report of a committee of the Clinical Society of London to investigate the subject of myxoedema*. London: author; 1888.
5. Tunbridge W, Evered D, Hall R, et al. The spectrum of thyroid disease in a community. *Clin Endocrinol* 1977;7:481–493.
6. Helfand M, Crapo L. Screening for thyroid disease. *Ann Intern Med* 1990;112:840–849.
7. Sawin C, Chopra D, Azizi F, Mannix J, Bacharach P. The aging thyroid: increased prevalence of elevated serum thyrotropin levels in the elderly. *JAMA* 1979;242(3):247–250.
8. Tunbridge W, Brewis M, French J, et al. Natural history of autoimmune thyroiditis. *Br Med J* 1981;282:258–259.
9. Rosenthal M, Hunt W, Garry P, Goodwin J. Thyroid failure in the el-

TABLE 2. *Common Precipitants of Myxedema Coma*

Infection
Trauma
Drugs (e.g., narcotics, sedatives, anesthetics, tranquilizers, diuretics)
Cerebrovascular accident
Congestive heart failure
Hypothermic exposure

derly. Microsomal antibodies as discriminant for therapy. *JAMA* 1987; 258(2):209–213.
10. Gordin A, Lamberg BA. Spontaneous hypothyroidism in symptomless autoimmune thyroiditis. A long-term follow-up study. *Clin Endocrinol* 1981;15:537–543.
11. Murakami Y, Takamatsu J, Sakane S, Kuma K. Serum levels of antibodies against thyroglobulin and microsomes in relation to thyroid function in patients with Hashimoto thyroiditis: analysis with various antibody measurements. In: Nagataki S, Mori T, Torizuka K, eds. *80 years of Hashimoto disease.* Amsterdam: Elsevier Science, 1993; 235–239.
12. Hayslip CC, Fein HG, O'Donnell VM, Friedman DS, Klein TA, Smallridge RC. The value of serum antimicrosomal antibody testing in screening for symptomatic postpartum thyroid dysfunction. *Am J Obstet Gynecol* 1988;159:203–209.
13. Bogner U, Schleusener H, Wall JR. Antibody-dependent cell mediated cytotoxicity against human thyroid cells in Hashimoto's thyroiditis but not Graves' disease. *J Clin Endocrinol Metab* 1984;59: 734–738.
14. Konishi J, Iida Y, Endo K, et al. Inhibition of thyrotropin-induced adenosine 3'5'-monophosphate increase by immunoglobulins from patients with primary myxedema. *J Clin Endocrinol Metab* 1983;57: 544–549.
15. Pinchera A, Mariotti S, Chiovato L. Current concepts of Hashimoto disease. In: Nagataki S, Mori T, Torizuka K, eds. *80 years of Hashimoto disease.* Amsterdam: Elsevier Science, 1993;533–538.
16. Weetman AP. Autoimmune thyroiditis: predisposition and pathogenesis. *Clin Endocrinol* 1992;36:307–323.
17. Nikolai TJ, Brosseau J, Kettrick MA. Lymphocytic thyroiditis with spontaneously resolving hyperthyroidism (silent thyroiditis). *Arch Intern Med* 1980;140:478–482.
18. Amino N, Mori H, Iwatani Y. High prevalence of transient postpartum thyrotoxicosis and hypothyroidism. *N Engl J Med* 1982;306:849–852.
19. Rasmussen NG, Hornnes PJ, Hoier-Madsen M, Feldt-Rasmussen U, Hegedus L. Thyroid size and function in healthy pregnant women with thyroid autoantibodies. Relation to development of postpartum thyroiditis. *Acta Endocrinol* 1990;123:395–401.
20. Othman S, Phillips DIW, Parkes AB, et al. A long-term follow-up of postpartum thyroiditis. *Clin Endocrinol* 1990;32:559–564.
21. Schwartzentruber DJ, White DE, Zweig MH, Weintraub BD, Rosenberg SA. Thyroid dysfunction associated with immunotherapy for patients with cancer. *Cancer* 1991;68:2384–2390.
22. Vassilopoulou-Sellin R, Sella A, Dexeus FH. Acute thyroid dysfunction (thyroiditis) after therapy with interleukin-2. *Horm Metab Res* 1992;24:434–438.
23. Geerdsen JP, Frolund L. Thyroid function after surgical treatment of nontoxic goiter. A randomized study of postoperative thyroxine administration. *Acta Med Scand* 1986;220:341–345.
24. Tamai H, Suemastu H, Kurokawa N, Esaki M. Alterations in circulating thyroid hormones and thyrotropin after complete thyroidectomy. *J Clin Endocrinol Metab* 1979;48:54–58.
25. Hedley AJ, Bewsher PD, Jones SJ, et al. Late onset hypothyroidism after subtotal thyroidectomy for hyperthyroidism: implications for long-term follow-up. *Br J Surg* 1983;70:740–743.
26. Cunnien AJ, Hay ID, Gorman CA, Offord KP, Scanlon PW. Radioiodine-induced hypothyroidism in Graves' disease: factors associated with the increasing incidence. *J Nucl Med* 1982;23:978–983.
27. Sridama V, McCormick M, Kaplan EL, Fauchet R, DeGroot LJ. Long-term follow-up study of compensated low-dose I-131 therapy for Graves' disease. *N Engl J Med* 1984;311:426–432.
28. Hancock SL, Cox RS, McDougall IR. Thyroid diseases after treatment of Hodgkin's disease. *N Engl J Med* 1991;325:599–605.
29. Grande C. Hypothyroidism following radiotherapy for head and neck cancer: multivariate analysis of risk factors. *Radiother Oncol* 1992; 25:31–36.
30. Wolff J. Congenital goiter with defective iodide transport. *Endocr Rev* 1983;4:240–254.
31. Medeiros-Nieto G, Stanbury JB. Defective organification of iodide. In: Medeiros-Nieto G, Stanbury JB, eds. *Inherited disorders of the thyroid system.* Boca Raton: CRC Press, 1994;53–80.
32. Medeiros-Nieto G, Stanbury JB. Pendred's syndrome: association of congenital deafness with sporadic goiter. In: Medeiros-Nieto G, Stanbury JB, eds. *Inherited disorders of the thyroid system.* Boca Raton: CRC Press, 1994;81–105.
33. Pendred V. Deaf mutism and goitre. *Lancet* 1896;2:532.
34. Kusakabe T. A goitrous subject with defective synthesis of diiodotyrosines due to thyroglobulin abnormalities. *J Clin Endocrinol Metab* 1973;37:317–325.
35. Kusakabe T, Miyake T. Defective deiodination of I-131-labelled L-diiodotyrosine in patients with simple goiter. *J Clin Endocrinol Metab* 1963;23:132–139.
36. Medeiros-Nieto G, Stanbury JB. The iodotyrosine deiodinase defect. In: Medeiros-Nieto G, Stanbury JB, eds. *Inherited disorders of the thyroid system.* Boca Raton: CRC Press, 1994;139–159.
37. Codaccioni JL, Carayon P, Michel-Bechet M, Foucault F, Lefort G, Pierron H. Congenital hypothyroidism associated with thyrotropin unresponsiveness and thyroid cell membrane alterations. *J Clin Endocrinol Metab* 1980;50:932–937.
38. Mannisto PT. Effect of lithium on deiodinating activity of various rat tissues in vitro. *Acta Endocrinol* 1974;76:260–272.
39. Salata R, Klein I. Effects of lithium on the endocrine system. *J Lab Clin Med* 1987;110:130–136.
40. Wilson R, McKillop JH, Crocket GT, et al. The effect of lithium therapy on parameters thought to be involved in the development of autoimmune thyroid disease. *Clin Endocrinol* 1991;34:357–361.
41. Calabrese JR, Gulledge AD, Hahn K, et al. Autoimmune thyroiditis in manic-depressive patients treated with lithium. *Am J Psychiatry* 1985; 142:1318–1321.
42. Stanbury J, Ermans A, Hetzel B, Pretell E, Querido A. Endemic goitre and cretinism: public health significance and prevention. *WHO Chronicle* 1974;28:220–228.
43. Paul T, Meyers B, Witorsch RJ, et al. The effect of small increases in dietary iodine on thyroid function in euthyroid subjects. *Metabolism* 1988;37:121–124.
44. Braverman LE, Woeber KA, Ingbar SH. Induction of myxedema by iodide in patients euthyroid after radioiodine or surgical treatment of diffuse toxic goiter. *N Engl J Med* 1969;281:816–821.
45. Hershman JM, Nademanee K, Sugawara M, et al. Thyroxine and triiodothyronine kinetics in cardiac patients taking amiodarone. *Acta Endocrinol* 1986;111:193–199.
46. Figge H, Figge J. The effects of amiodarone on thyroid hormone function: a review of the physiology and clinical manifestations. *J Clin Pharmacol* 1990;30:588–595.
47. Martino E, Safran M, Aghini-Lombardi F, et al. Environmental iodine intake and thyroid dysfunction during chronic amiodarone therapy. *Ann Intern Med* 1984;101:28–34.
48. Lombardi A, Martino E, Braverman L. Amiodarone and the thyroid. *Thyroid Today* 1990;13(2):1–7.
49. Martino E, Aghini-Lombardi F, Mariotti S, et al. Amiodarone iodine-induced hypothyroidism: risk factors and follow-up in 28 cases. *Clin Endocrinol* 1987;26:227–237.
50. Greene JN. Subacute thyroiditis. *Am J Med* 1971;51:97–108.
51. Nikolai TF, Coombs GJ, McKenzie AK. Lymphocytic thyroiditis with spontaneously resolving hyperthyroidism (silent thyroiditis) and subacute thyroiditis: long term follow-up. *Arch Intern Med* 1981; 141: 1455–1458.
52. Woolner L, McConahey W, Beahrs O. Invasive fibrous thyroiditis (Riedel's struma). *J Clin Endocrinol Metab* 1956;17:201–219.
53. Hay ID, McConahey WM, Carney JA, Woolner LB. Invasive fibrous thyroiditis (Riedel's struma) and associated extracervical fibrosclerosis: Bowlby's disease revisited. *Ann Endocrinol* 1982;42:29A.
54. Berger SA, Zonzein J, Villamena P, Mittman N. Infectious diseases of the thyroid gland. *Rev Infect Dis* 1983;5:108–122.
55. Miyai K, Azukizawa M, Kumahara Y. Familial isolated thyrotropin deficiency with cretinism. *N Engl J Med* 1971;285:1043–1048.
56. Labbe A, Dubray C, Gaillard G, Besse G, Assali P, Malpuech G. Familial growth retardation with isolated thyroid-stimulating hormone deficiency. *Clin Pediatr* 1984;23:675–678.
57. Hayashizaki Y, Hiraoka Y, Tatsumi K, et al. Deoxyribonucleic acid analyses of five families with familial inherited thyroid stimulating hormone deficiency. *J Clin Endocrinol Metab* 1990;71:792–793.
58. Tatsumi K, Kiyai K, Notomi T, Amino N, Mizuno Y, Kohno H. Cretinism with combined hormone deficiency caused by a mutation in the Pit 1 gene. *Nat Genet* 1992;1:56–58.
59. Parks JS, Kinoshita E, Pfafle RW. Pit-1 and hypopituitarism. *Trends Endocrinol Metab* 1993;4:81–85.
60. Cosman F, Post KD, Holub DA, Wardlaw SL. Lymphocytic hypophysitis: report of 3 new cases and review of literature. *Medicine* 1989;68:240–256.
61. Thodou E, Asa SL, Kontogeorgos G, Kovacs K, Horvath E, Ezzat S.

Lymphocytic hypophysitis: clinicopathological findings. *J Clin Endocrinol Metab* 1995;80:2302–2311.
62. Ozawa Y, Shishiba Y. Recovery from lymphocytic hypophysitis associated with painless thyroiditis: clinical implications of circulating antipituitary antibodies. *Acta Endocrinol* 1993;128:493–498.
63. Samaan NA, Schultz PN, Yang KP, Vassilopoulou-Sellin R. Endocrine complications after radiotherapy for tumors of the head and neck. *J Lab Clin Med* 1987;109:364–372.
64. Samaan NA, Bakdash MM, Caderao JB, Cangu A, Jesse RHJ, Ballantyne AJ. Hypopituitarism after external irradiation: evidence for both hypothalamic and pituitary origin. *Ann Intern Med* 1975;83:771–777.
65. Schectman JM, Kallenberg GA, Shumacher RJ, Hirsch RP. Yield of hypothyroidism in symptomatic primary care patients. *Arch Intern Med* 1989;149:861–864.
66. Billewicz WZ, Chapman RS, Crooks J, et al. Statistical methods applied to the diagnosis of hypothyroidism. *Q J Med* 1969;38:255–266.
67. Laycock M, Pascuzzi R. The neuromuscular effects of hypothyroidism. *Semin Neurol* 1991;11(3):288–289.
68. Mastaglia F, Ojeda V, Sarnat H, Kakulas B. Myopathies associated with hypothyroidism: a review based upon 13 cases. *Aust NZ J Med* 1988;18:799–806.
69. Klein I, Levey GS. Unusual manifestations of hypothyroidism. *Arch Intern Med* 1984;144:123–128.
70. McKeran R, Slavin G, Ward P, Paul E, Mair W. Hypothyroid myopathy: a clinical and pathological study. *J Pathol* 1980;132:35–54.
71. Evans RM, Watanabe I, Singer PA. Central changes in hypothyroid myopathy: a case report. *Muscle Nerve* 1990;13:952–956.
72. Polikar R, Burger A, Scherrer U, Nicod P. The thyroid and the heart. *Circulation* 1993;87(5):1435–1441.
73. Dillmann WH. Biochemical basis of thyroid hormone action in the heart. *Am J Med* 1990;88:626–630.
74. Klein I. Thyroid hormone and the cardiovascular system. *Am J Med* 1990;88:631–637.
75. Kerber R, Sherman B. Echocardiographic evaluation of pericardial effusion in myxedema. *Circulation* 1975;52:823–827.
76. Aber CP, Thompson GS. The heart in hypothyroidism. *Am Heart J* 1964;68(3):428–429.
77. Davis PJ, Jacobson S. Myxedema with cardiac tamponade and pericardial effusion of "gold paint" appearance. *Arch Intern Med* 1967;120:615–619.
78. MacKerrow SD, Osborn LA, Levy H, Eaton RP, Economou P. Myxedema-associated cardiogenic shock treated with intravenous triiodothyronine. *Ann Intern Med* 1992;117:1014–1015.
79. Ladenson PW, Sherman SI, Baughman KL, Ray PE, Feldman AM. Reversible alterations in myocardial gene expression in a young man with dilated cardiomyopathy and hypothyroidism [published erratum appears in *Proc Natl Acad Sci U S A* 1992;89(18):8856]. *Proc Natl Acad Sci U S A* 1992;89(12):5251–5255.
80. Ladenson PW, Levin AA, Ridgway EC, Daniels GH. Complications of surgery in hypothyroid patients. *Am J Med* 1984;77:261–266.
81. Sherman SI, Ladenson PW. Percutaneous transluminal coronary angioplasty in hypothyroidism. *Am J Med* 1991;90(3):367–370.
82. Wilson WR, Bedell GN. The pulmonary abnormalities in myxedema. *J Clin Invest* 1960;39:42–55.
83. Zwillich C, Pierson D, Hofeldt F, Lufkin E, Weil J. Ventilatory control in myxedema and hypothyroidism. *N Engl J Med* 1975;292:662–665.
84. Gottehrer A, Roa J, Stanford G, Chernow B, Sahn S. Hypothyroidism and pleural effusions. *Chest* 1990;98:1130–1132.
85. Sachdev Y, Hall R. Effusions into body cavities in hypothyroidism. *Lancet* 1975;1:564–565.
86. Rajagopal K, Abbrecht P, Derderian S, et al. Obstructive sleep apnea in hypothyroidism. *Ann Intern Med* 1984;101:491–494.
87. Grunstein R, Sullivan C. Sleep apnea and hypothyroidism: mechanisms and management. *Am J Med* 1988;85:775–779.
88. Miller L, Gorman C, Go V. Gut-thyroid interrelationships. *Gastroenterology* 1978;75:901–911.
89. Shafer R, Prentiss R, Bond J. Gastrointestinal transit in thyroid disease. *Gastroenterology* 1984;86:852–855.
90. Patel P, Hughes RWJ. An unusual case of myxedema megacolon with features of ischemic and pseudomembranous colitis. *Mayo Clin Proc* 1992;67:369–372.
91. Babb R. Associations between diseases of the thyroid and the liver. *Am J Gastroenterol* 1984;79(5):421–423.
92. Feingold K, Elias P. Endocrine-skin interactions: cutaneous manifestations of pituitary disease, thyroid disease, calcium disorders, and diabetes. *J Am Acad Dermatol* 1987;17(6):921–940.
93. Freinkel R, Freinkel N. Hair growth and alopecia in hypothyroidism. *Arch Dermatol* 1972;106:349–352.
94. Chernausek SD, Underwood LE, Utiger RD, Van Wyk JJ. Growth hormone secretion and plasma somatomedin-C in primary hypothyroidism. *Clin Endocrinol* 1983;19:337–344.
95. Chernausek SD, Turner R. Attenuation of spontaneous, nocturnal growth hormone secretion in children with hypothyroidism and its correlation with plasma insulin-like growth factor 1 concentrations. *J Pediatr* 1989;114(6):968–972.
96. Castro JH, Genuth SM, Klein L. Comparative response to parathyroid hormone in hyperthyroidism and hypothyroidism. *Metabolism* 1975;24(7):839–848.
97. Bouillon R, De Moor P. Parathyroid function in patients with hyper- or hypothyroidism. *J Clin Endocrinol Metab* 1974;38:999–1004.
98. Bouillon R, Muls E, De Moor P. Influence of thyroid function on the serum concentration of 1,25-dihydroxyvitamin D_3. *J Clin Endocrinol Metab* 1980;51(4):793–797.
99. Fein H, Rivlin R. Anemia in thyroid diseases. *Med Clin North Am* 1975;59:1133–1145.
100. Green S, Ng J. Hypothyroidism and anaemia. *Biomed Pharmacother* 1986;40:326–331.
101. Horton L, Coburn J, England J, Himsworth R. The haematology of hypothyroidism. *Q J Med* 1975;45:101–124.
102. Edson JR, Fecher DR, Doe RP. Low platelet adhesiveness and other hemostatic abnormalities in hypothyroidism. *Ann Intern Med* 1975;82:342–346.
103. Rennie J, Bewsher P, Murchison L, Ogston D. Coagulation and fibrinolysis in thyroid disease. *Acta Haematol* 1978;59:171–177.
104. Iranmanesh A, Lizarralde G, Johnson M, Veldhuis J. Dynamics of 24-hour endogenous cortisol secretion and clearance in primary hypothyroidism assessed before and after partial thyroid hormone replacement. *J Clin Endocrinol Metab* 1990;70(1):155–161.
105. Havard C, Saldanha V, Bird R, Gardner R. Adrenal function in hypothyroidism. *Br Med J* 1970;1:337–339.
106. Lessof M, Lyne C, Maisey M, Sturge R. Effect of thyroid failure on the pituitary-adrenal axis. *Lancet* 1969;1:642–643.
107. Gharib H, Hodgson S, Gastineau C, Scholz D, Smith L. Reversible hypothyroidism in Addison's disease. *Lancet* 1972;1:734–735.
108. Manhem P, Hallengren B, Hansson B. Plasma noradrenaline and blood pressure in hypothyroid patients: effect of gradual thyroxine treatment. *Clin Endocrinol* 1984;20:701–707.
109. Polikar R, Kennedy B, Ziegler M, Smith J, Nicod P. Decreased sensitivity to adrenergic stimulation in hypothyroid patients. *J Clin Endocrinol Metab* 1990;70(6):1761–1764.
110. Buchanan CR, Stanhope R, Adlard P, Jones J, Grant DB, Preece MA. Gonadotrophin, growth hormone and prolactin secretion in children with primary hypothyroidism. *Clin Endocrinol* 1988;29:427–436.
111. Jannini E, Ulisse S, D'Armiento M. Thyroid hormone and male gonadal function. *Endocr Rev* 1995;16(4):443–459.
112. Thomas R, Reid R. Thyroid disease and reproductive dysfunction. *Obstet Gynecol* 1987:789–798.
113. Wortsman J, Rosner W, Dufau M. Abnormal testicular function in men with primary hypothyroidism. *Am J Med* 1987;82:207–212.
114. Epstein AA, Lande H. Studies on blood lipoids: the relation of cholesterol and protein deficiency to basal metabolism. *Arch Intern Med* 1922;30:563–577.
115. Mason RL, Hunt HM, Hurxthal L. Blood cholesterol values in hyperthyroidism and hypothyroidism—their significance. *N Engl J Med* 1930;203:1273–1278.
116. Wiseman S, Powell J, Humphries S, Press M. The magnitude of the hypercholesterolemia of hypothyroidism is associated with variation in the low density lipoprotein receptor gene. *J Clin Endocrinol Metab* 1993;77:108–109.
117. O'Brien T, Dinneen S, O'Brien P, Palumbo P. Hyperlipidemia in patients with primary and secondary hypothyroidism. *Mayo Clin Proc* 1993;68:860–866.
118. Sherman SI, Scott L, Morrisett JD. Postprandial lipemia in severe hypothyroidism. *Program and abstracts; 10th International Congress of Endocrinology*, June 12–15. San Francisco, CA: Endocrine Society Press, 1996;639.
119. Oettgen P, Ginsburg G, Horowitz G, Pasternak R. Frequency of hypothyroidism in adults with serum total cholesterol levels >200 mg/dl. *Am J Cardiol* 1994;73:955–957.

120. Derubertis FR, Michelis M, Bloom ME, Mintz DH, Field JB, Davis BB. Impaired water excretion in myxedema. *Am J Med* 1971;51:41–53.
121. Hochberg Z, Benderly A. Normal osmotic threshold for vasopressin release in the hyponatremia of hypothyroidism. *Horm Res* 1983;17:128–133.
122. Elgee N, Williams R. Effects of thyroid function on insulin-I131 degradation. *Am J Physiol* 1955;180:13–15.
123. Van Oosterom A, Kerkhoven P, Veltkamp J. Metabolism of the coagulation factors of the prothrombin complex in hypothyroidism in man. *Thromb Haemost* 1979;41:273–285.
124. Tibaldi J, Barzel U. Thyroxine supplementation. Method for the prevention of clinical hypothyroidism. *Am J Med* 1985;79:241–243.
125. Cooper DS, Halpern R, Wood LC, Levin AA, Ridgway EC. L-thyroxine therapy in subclinical hypothyroidism. *Ann Intern Med* 1984;101:18–24.
126. Arem R, Patsch W. Lipoprotein and apolipoprotein levels in subclinical hypothyroidism. Effects of levothyroxine therapy. *Arch Intern Med* 1990;150:2097–2100.
127. Domm BM, Vassallo CL. Myxedema coma with respiratory failure. *Am Rev Respir Dis* 1975;107:842–845.
128. Laroche C, Cairns T, Moxham J, Green M. Hypothyroidism presenting with respiratory muscle weakness. *Am Rev Respir Dis* 1988;138:472–474.
129. Jordan R. Myxedema coma: pathophysiology, therapy, and factors affecting prognosis. *Med Clin North Am* 1995;79:185–194.
130. Nicoloff J, LoPresti J. Myxedema coma: a form of decompensated hypothyroidism. *Endocrinol Metab Clin North Am* 1993;22:279–290.
131. Royce P. Severely impaired consciousness in myxedema—a review. *Am J Med Sci* 1971;261(1):46–50.
132. Pettinger WA, Talner L, Ferris TF. Inappropriate secretion of antidiuretic hormone due to myxedema. *N Engl J Med* 1965;272:362–364.
133. Blum M. Myxedema coma. *Am J Med Sci* 1972;264:432–443.
134. Fisher DA, Dussault JH, Foley TP, et al. Screening for congenital hypothyroidism: results of screening one million North American infants. *J Pediatr* 1979;94:700–705.
135. Barnes N. Screening for congenital hypothyroidism: the first decade. *Arch Dis Child* 1985;60:587–592.
136. Illig R, Largo R, Qin Q, Torresani T, Rochiccioli P, Larsson A. Mental development in congenital hypothyroidism after neonatal screening. *Arch Dis Child* 1987;62:1050–1055.

CHAPTER 21

Thyroiditis

Paul D. Woolf

Thyroiditis has been conveniently classified into categories that reflect either the rapidity of onset or the duration of disease (1) (Table 1). In order of increasing chronicity, the categories are acute suppurative; subacute, which includes both granulomatous and lymphocytic or painless (silent) thyroiditis; and chronic, which encompasses chronic lymphocytic (Hashimoto's thyroiditis) and fibrous thyroiditis (Riedel's struma). Painless thyroiditis may be further divided into sporadic and postpartum forms. Both acute suppurative thyroiditis and Riedel's struma are extremely rare, whereas the others are relatively common causes of thyroid dysfunction.

ACUTE SUPPURATIVE THYROIDITIS

Acute suppurative thyroiditis is a very uncommon thyroid abnormality. It affects both sexes equally and children disproportionately. In a review of 153 cases, the average age was 30.6 years for men and 35.1 for women (2). In adults, preexisting thyroid disease is present in over two thirds of cases (2), but in children a left pyriform fistula is demonstrable in the vast majority (3,4). An antecedent infection is frequently present with either hematogenous or local spread to the thyroid. The occurrence of an upper respiratory infection in the presence of pyriform fistula is a particularly common predisposing feature (3). Pain, tenderness, fever, dysphagia, erythema, and localized warmth are present in the vast majority of patients (2,3). Fluctuance may appear later. The trachea can be deviated, and in one report patients presented with a neck mass in the absence of systemic symptoms (4). Although bilateral involvement may occur, the left lobe is preferentially involved, particularly in children, because of the pyriform fistula (5). In the presence of a fistula, recurrences are common and fistulectomy results in permanent cure (5). It is important to distinguish this potentially life-threatening illness from other conditions causing acute thyroidal pain, including subacute thyroiditis (see later), hemorrhage into a thyroid nodule, or a complication resulting from the administration of chemotherapy through a Hickman catheter (6).

Laboratory data reveal a white blood cell count that is usually elevated, but it may be normal when the infection is caused by anaerobic organisms. Thyroid function studies are generally normal (2,3) (Table 2), but occasionally triiodothyronine (T_3) or thyroxine (T_4) levels are low. The iodine-131 (^{131}I) uptake is low in 40% of patients and the thyroid scan is typically abnormal, demonstrating either focal or uniform abnormalities (2).

A number of different pathogens have been isolated, but in children they generally mirror the pharyngeal flora (3). *Staphylococcus* has been identified in one third of adult patients, and in two thirds of isolates in pure culture. There have been scattered case reports of a variety of gram-negative organisms, many of which are oral pathogens, including *Brucella melitensis* (7), *Capnocytophaga ochracea* (8), *Eikenella corrodens* (9), *Haemophilus influenzae* (10), *Moraxella nonliquefaciens* (11), *Salmonella paratyphi* (12), and *Serratia marcescens* (13). Mixed aerobic and anaerobic infections are infrequently present, whereas anaerobic infections of the thyroid may occur following spread from distant sites (2). An 8.6% mortality rate has been reported in one review, but the majority of the deaths occurred in patients not treated for their infection. Residua of the acute thyroiditis are uncommon. Transient hypothyroidism (which may require replacement therapy), vocal cord paralysis, disruption of regional sympathetics, and recurrences have all been reported (2).

Nonbacterial infections of the thyroid gland are distinctly uncommon. Thirty-one cases were compiled by Berger et al. (2) over an 80-year period. Twenty-six pa-

P. D. Woolf: Departments of Medicine, Pathology, and Laboratory Medicine, University of Rochester School of Medicine and Dentistry, Rochester, New York 14642.

TABLE 1. Classification of thyroiditis syndromes

Type of thyroiditis	Relative frequency	Histology	Outcome
Hashimoto's	Very common	Lymphocytic infiltration with germinal centers, fibrosis, and Hürthle cell change	Eventual hypothyroidism
Subacute granulomatous	About 1/40 as common as Hashimoto's	Giant cell infiltration with microabscesses and follicular disruption	Recovery >90%; <10% of patients have persistent goiter and hypothyroidism
Subacute painless lymphocytic			
Sporadic	Uncommon	Lymphocytic infiltration with follicular disruption	Recovery about 75%; persistent goiter and hypothyroidism are more often seen in postpartum form
Postpartum	Seen in 5.5% of postpartum women		
Acute suppurative	Rare	Abscess formation with bacteria or fungi	Recovery
Reidel's struma	Very rare	Dense fibrotic pattern	Progressive obstruction

Modified from ref. 1.

tients were infected by *Aspergillus* and were immunologically compromised. *Coccidioides immitis, Candida,* and *Allescheria boydii* have also been reported. Treatment with excision and amphotericin B may be successful, but the diagnosis is most frequently made at autopsy. The diagnosis of cryptococcal thyroiditis has been made by fine-needle thyroid aspiration, but the thyroidal involvement typically presents as part of systemic illness (14). Tubercular involvement of the thyroid is currently extremely rare, and when found, it may not have been suspected on clinical grounds (15).

Parasitic infections of the thyroid are rare. Both syphilis (2) and *Chlamydia psittaci* (16) have involved the thyroid. In the pre-AIDS (acquired immunodeficiency syndrome) era, echinococcosis was the most common parasitic infection of the thyroid (2). However, the advent of AIDS may alter the pathogenic spectrum, causing acute thyroiditis; several cases of *Pneumocystis carinii* infection of the thyroid, diagnosed by thyroidal aspiration, have been reported (17). The disease may present as part of a systemic illness or masquerade as subacute thyroiditis. Either hyperthyroid, or hypothyroid function along with suppressed thyroidal ^{131}I uptake is found. The thyroid may be unilaterally or diffusely enlarged, and tenderness is not universally present. Most of these patients were receiving pentamidine prophylaxis when thyroiditis developed. Treatment with intravenous pentamidine and oral sulfamethoxazole-trimethoprim may reduce thyroid size and clear the infection (17).

PAINLESS THYROIDITIS

Starting in the early 1970s, a new form of thyroid inflammatory disease began to receive increasing attention under a variety of names: painless thyroiditis, silent thyroiditis, painless subacute thyroiditis, subacute nonsuppurative thyroiditis, atypical ("silent") subacute thyroiditis, lymphocytic thyroiditis with spontaneously resolving hyperthyroidism, hyperthyroiditis, lymphocytic thyroiditis, autoimmune disease and thyroiditis, and postpartum painless thyroiditis.

It was characterized by the complete absence of pain, despite thyroidal destruction and temporary thyroid dysfunction, during which the typical patient passes through four phases—hyperthyroid, euthyroid, hypothyroid, and euthyroid—over a 1-year period (Fig. 1). In 1980, the data from 112 patients were reviewed (18). Since then, many more reports have appeared that have further clarified the clinical course and pathophysiology

TABLE 2. Laboratory findings in acute bacterial thyroiditis

	No. of cases (%) with indicated laboratory level[a]		
Laboratory findings	Elevated	Depressed	Normal
Leukocyte count	47/64 (73)	0/63	17/63
Thyroid function studies			
Triiodothyronine conc.[b]	4/19	0/19	16/20
Thyroxine conc.	3/24	0/24	22/25
Protein-bound iodine conc.	5/12	2/12	5/12
Thyroid-stimulating hormone conc.	0/13	1/13	12/13
Basal metabolic rate	11/12	1/12	0/12
^{131}I uptake/24 hr	3/27	11/26	12/26
Regional uptake on thyroid scan	0/29	27/30 (90)	3/29

[a]No. of patients exhibiting indicated change/no. for whom such information is recorded.
[b]Conc., serum concentration.
From ref. 2.

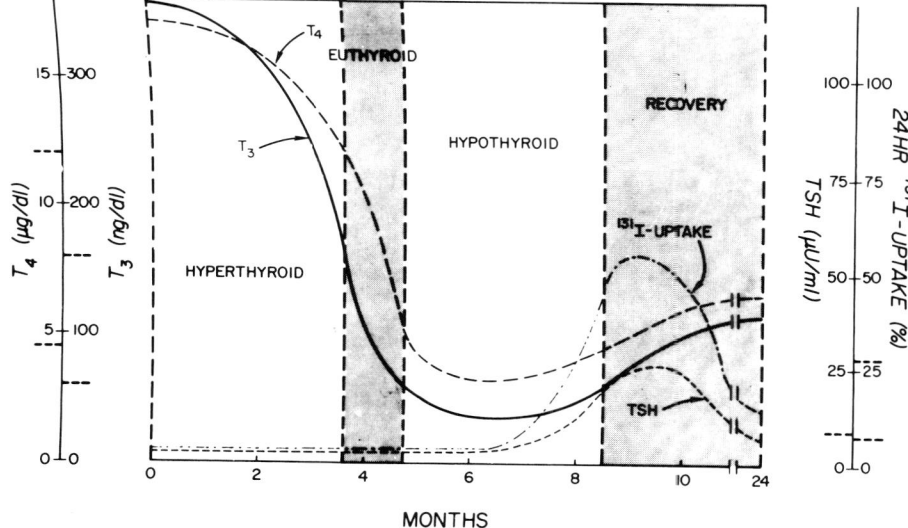

FIG. 1. Schematic representation of the course of 40% of the patients going through the four phases of thyroiditis. The remaining 60% never became hypothyroid and remained euthyroid after recovering from the hyperthyroidism. The *dashed lines* on the ordinate are the limits of the normal range. (From ref. 18, with permission.)

Incidence

Painless thyroiditis has been reported in all ages from 4.8 to 93 years, but the median is the middle of the fourth decade. As is true for most thyroid disorders, women are more likely to be affected than men, with a prevalence ratio of from 1.5 to 3, to 1. Reports have appeared from many sections of the United States, Canada, Europe (particularly Sweden), and Japan, but the frequency of both sporadic and postpartum forms varies widely. The former accounted for under 5% of all causes of hyperthyroidism in Philadelphia (19), Brooklyn (20), and coastal Virginia (21), but 15% in Texas (22) and 23% in Wisconsin (23). Nikolai et al. (23) reported a 255% increase over a 4-year interval. The incidence of postpartum thyroiditis shows similar diversity (24) (Table 3), ranging from none in Denmark (25) or Saudi Arabia (34) to 17% in Wales (31). However, these differences may be partly a result of earlier postpartum evaluation in the groups reporting the highest frequency. Postpartum thyroiditis has also been reported following abortions (18).

Clinical Presentation

The sporadic form of painless thyroiditis typically presents with signs and symptoms of hyperthyroidism (18). The onset is usually abrupt, unlike that in patients with Graves' disease, because it is caused by the sudden release of preformed thyroid hormone secondary to disruption of follicular integrity. The hyperthyroidism lasts an average of 3.6 (2.0, SD) months, but it may persist for up to 1 year. As expected, symptoms of nervousness, weight loss, palpitations, heat intolerance, and fatigue predominate. Although generally mild, there have been reports of patients who have required hospitalization for prominent cardiac symptoms. Patients do not have exophthalmos or pretibial myxedema, unless they have preexisting Graves' disease, but they may have eye signs, such as lid lag and stare, caused by increased sympathetic tone. The thyroid gland is usually firm and only modestly enlarged, but in one third of patients it may be 2 to 3 times normal size. The enlargement is almost always symmetrical. The complete absence of thyroidal pain or tenderness distinguishes these patients from those in the thyrotoxic phase of subacute granulomatous thyroiditis.

Treatment

Because of the transient and generally mild nature of the hyperthyroidism, most patients do not require treatment. When sympathetic symptoms are prominent, they will respond to adrenergic blockade. Propranolol in doses of 20 to 160 mg/day has been found to be effective. The use of prednisone, starting at 50 mg/day and tapering to 20 mg/day over 4 weeks, decreased the length of time for thyroid tests to return to normal by nearly 75% (35), but it is rarely required. Because the disease is self-limited, because the thyrotoxicosis is caused by release of preformed hormone and not by new hormone synthesis, and because the thyroid gland is incapable of trapping iodine (see later), it is inappropriate to treat these patients with either radioactive iodine or antithyroid drugs. Indeed, the latter may needlessly prolong subsequent hypothyroidism.

TABLE 3. Prevalence of thyroid dysfunction in the postpartum period as reported in nine epidemiologic studies from various parts of the world

Study area (ref.)	Number of women investigated	Time interval of blood sampling (mo after delivery)[a]	Number of women (%) with postpartum thyroid dysfunction	Number of women with permanent thyroid dysfunction	Number of hypothyroid women with thyroid microsomal autoantibodies (% of all hypothyroid women)
Japan (26)	507	3 (3–8)	28 (5.5)	1	14 (93)
Sweden (27)	460	2–5 (2–12)	30 (6.5)	1	21 (95)
New York (28)	212	1–2 (1–3)	4 (1.9)	?	—
Wisconsin (29)	238	0–3 (0–12)	16 (6.7)	3	6 (67)
Denmark (30)	591	3 (3–12)	23 (3.9)	3	13 (93)
Wales (31)	220[b]	0–12[b]	49 (16.7)[b]	1	23 (82)
Thailand (32)	570	3.5 (1.5–6)	9 (1.1)	1	7 (77)
Canada (33)	1376	1–12	82 (6.0)	2	?
Saudi Arabia (34)	277	1–2	0	0	0

[a]Within parentheses are given the time intervals of blood sampling in selected women.
[b]The study group was selected from an unselected group of 901 women. The percentage given is an estimation for the unselected group based on the composition of the study group.
Modified from ref. 24.

Laboratory Evaluation

During the thyrotoxic phase, thyroid hormone levels may be mildly to quite elevated, ranging from 86% to 352% of the upper limits of normal for T_4 and 100% to 444% for T_3 (18). Compared to patients with Graves' disease, patients with painless thyroiditis have lower free T_4, T_3, free T_3, and T_3 resin uptake values, but comparable concentrations of total T_4 (36). As a consequence, a $T_3:T_4$ ratio of 20 appears to completely differentiate between the two disorders. As expected, thyroid stimulating hormone (TSH) levels are depressed. The ability of the thyroid to trap iodine is markedly impaired; the radioactive iodine uptake is severely depressed or absent and the gland does not respond to exogenous TSH (18). Consequently, thyroidal iodine clearance is markedly diminished. Because of the thyroidal destruction, protein-bound iodine (PBI) levels are disproportionately elevated; thyroglobulin levels are very elevated and may remain so for up to 2 years (37). As a result of the sudden release of iodinated products, urinary iodide excretion is high (18,37) and significantly greater during both sporadic and postpartum forms of painless thyroiditis than during Graves' disease (38,39). The presence of antithyroid antibodies is variable (40). Antimicrosomal antibodies are present more frequently and in higher titer than antithyroglobulin antibodies (41) and are associated with transient hypothyroidism (42) or subclinical hypothyroidism following resolution of the acute process (40). Nonspecific indicators of inflammation—white blood count and erythrocyte sedimentation rate—are generally normal, in contrast to subacute thyroiditis (21). Therefore, it is the sudden onset of thyrotoxicosis in the absence of thyroidal pain and an ^{131}I uptake of below 5% that is the hallmark of painless thyroiditis.

With exhaustion of intrathyroidal hormone stores and the inability of the gland to synthesize more, 50% of patients will become clinically or biochemically hypothyroid for 1 to 8 months after a euthyroid interval of 1 to 6 weeks (18). The remainder stay euthyroid. During hypothyroidism, TSH levels become elevated. As the thyroid undergoes repair, its ability to trap iodine returns prior to organification. Thus, the 24-hour ^{131}I uptake becomes normal to supranormal and TSH responsiveness returns, but the response to perchlorate may be abnormal (21,37). A minority of those who become hypothyroid require replacement therapy, but such patients seldom need it for more than a few months. Prednisone treatment, although it shortens the thyrotoxic phase, does not prevent subsequent hypothyroidism (35). Complete resolution of thyroid dysfunction averages 6.4 months, but there is a wide dispersion about the mean (18). Measurement of thyroidal iodine-127 (^{127}I) reveals depressed iodine content for 2 or more years, along with persistence of elevated circulating thyroglobulin levels (37).

Prognosis

Although the vast majority of patients recover normal thyroid function, continuing thyroid disease has been reported with high frequency. In one series, two thirds of patients displayed abnormalities (43). In another, 23 of 54 patients had persistent goiters and 3 became hypothyroid (40). One of them had been treated with prednisone, but never recovered normal thyroid function, while the remaining two became hypothyroid 1 and 2 years after apparent recovery. Recurrences of painless thyroiditis are known to occur (18). In the series of 54 patients reported by Nikolai et al. (40), single recurrences were documented at 1- to 3-

year intervals in five patients and two and three recurrences in a sixth and seventh patient. Patients with multiple recurrences can be successfully treated with radioactive iodine ablation after resolution of the acute process (44). Patients with subacute thyroiditis, in contrast, seldom have persistent thyroid abnormalities or relapses (40).

Clusters of patients with laboratory data suggestive of painless thyroiditis are uncommon. Two large epidemics occurring 1 year apart centered in eastern Nebraska and western Minnesota were initially thought to be due to painful thyroiditis, but they were subsequently found to be caused by hamburger meat contaminated by beef thyroid glands (see later) (45,46). In a recent report, five employees of a nursery school presented within a 10-day interval with what appeared to be typical illnesses (47). Of interest is the report of a wife and husband who developed painless thyroiditis and subacute thyroiditis, respectively, within 3 weeks of each other (48).

Postpartum Thyroiditis

Postpartum thyroiditis shares many of the features of the sporadic form of painless thyroiditis and both have occurred in the same patient (49,50). A familial form of postpartum thyroiditis has been reported (51). However, the hyperthyroidism, if present at all, is usually quite mild. In fact, in an early series, 14 cases of hypothyroidism were found 3 to 5 months postpartum, and it was only after subsequent pregnancies in two patients that a hyperthyroid phase was detected 4 to 6 weeks after delivery (52). In a follow-up study, two thirds of women demonstrating postpartum thyroid disease were thyrotoxic 3 months after delivery (26). In the remainder, it is unclear whether the thyrotoxic phase failed to occur or if it was missed because of the overlap in symptomatology between the transient mild thyrotoxicosis and the changes in lifestyle brought on by a new baby (29). Although there has been speculation that postpartum psychosis may be precipitated by the hyperthyroidism of postpartum thyroiditis, this is an infrequent occurrence. In two series totaling 967 women, five women developed psychiatric symptoms requiring assistance or hospitalization (53). In another study, no differences in thyroid function were found between 30 women hospitalized for postpartum psychosis and 30 matched control subjects (54).

Complement-fixing microsomal antibodies are detected in a majority of women (55–57). Indeed, one of the striking features of postpartum thyroiditis is the association of antimicrosomal antibodies with the severity of the disorder; that is, the degree of hypothyroidism, determined by TSH levels, correlates with microsomal antibody titers obtained both early in pregnancy and 5 to 7 months postpartum (27). Fully 70% of women with an antibody titer above 6400 developed elevated TSH levels. A family history of thyroid disease and a history of smoking more than 20 cigarettes per day also may be predictive of the occurrence of postpartum thyroiditis, but antithyroglobulin antibodies, parity, and breast-feeding are not (24). Although administration of L-thyroxine prevents hypothyroid symptoms, it does not alter the course of the disease (58). It is curious that among women who have high antithyroid antibody titers, postpartum thyroid dysfunction is 3 times more likely to occur when the baby is a girl (59), but this finding has not been confirmed (24). There is an extraordinary recurrence rate of postpartum thyroiditis with subsequent pregnancies (29,60).

The acute course and management of postpartum thyroiditis are similar to the sporadic form of the disorder (41,52). Persistent thyroidal dysfunction can develop with striking frequency. Three-year follow-up of 25 women revealed that 12 had goiters, and 3 of these 12 became permanently hypothyroid (29). In this group, family history of thyroid disease in first-degree relatives was notably high. The Japanese have also reported the development of permanent hypothyroidism in 10 of 71 women followed for at least 5 years (61). Half of the ten remained persistently hypothyroid, whereas the other five had relapses more than 1 year after recovery. Similar data have been reported from Sweden (24). A 23% incidence of hypothyroidism was found in Wales 2 to 4 years postpartum (62). Associated factors included high antimicrosomal antibody titers at 16 weeks of gestation, severity of the hypothyroid phase, multiparity, and a history of spontaneous abortion. Subtle thyroid dysfunction can be detected even in euthyroid women (63). Of concern, however, is the report of decreased growth during the first 30 days in infants born of mothers affected by postpartum thyroiditis (64), despite normal maternal and baby thyroid hormone levels and gestational ages; Apgar scores and birth weight and length were comparable to those of babies born to unaffected women.

It is important to distinguish postpartum thyroiditis (destruction-induced thyrotoxicosis) from Graves' disease (persistent thyrotoxicosis), which commonly ameliorates during pregnancy (Fig. 2). Compounding the difficulty is a transient form of Graves' disease that appears to be reactivated by the termination of pregnancy. Differentiation between the two disorders, however, can be made readily by a 24-hour ^{131}I uptake test (65).

Etiology

The etiology of either form of painless thyroiditis remains speculative. Viral studies have been generally negative (23,41), although there is a case report following a rubella infection (66). Two cases were reported after radiotherapy for Hodgkin's disease (67), and several patients developed painless thyroiditis after surgery (68,69). It is quite clear that the immune system is involved, but it remains to be determined if the immunological dysfunction is directly causative. Painless thyroiditis has been

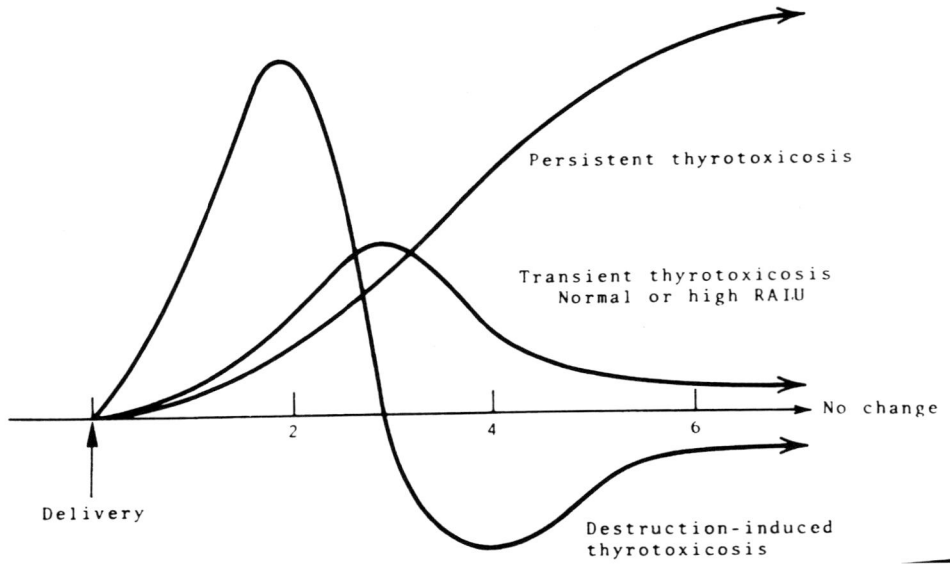

FIG. 2. Changes of free thyroxine index in various types of postpartum thyrotoxicosis. Numbers indicate months postpartum. RAIU, radioactive iodine uptake. (From ref. 61, with permission.)

found in patients with a wide variety of autoimmune diseases, including Graves' disease, Addison's disease, ovarian failure, lymphocytic hypophysitis, systemic lupus erythematosus, Sjögren's syndrome, systemic sclerosis, and rheumatoid arthritis. Nearly a quarter of patients with postpartum thyroiditis have first-degree relatives with autoimmune disease (70). The development of postpartum thyroiditis in 9 of 40 patients with type I diabetes mellitus is very intriguing, indicating the need for routine postpartum thyroid screening in this patient population (71). Anti-DNA antibodies have been reported during the thyrotoxic phases of both the sporadic (72) and the postpartum forms (73) of painless thyroiditis, as well as during postpartum exacerbations of Graves' disease. They are not, however, present during normal pregnancies or in the thyrotoxic phase of subacute thyroiditis (73). There are also clear associations between the major histocompatibility antigens and the incidence of painless thyroiditis, which are modified by ethnic background. In North America, human leukocyte antigen (HLA)-DR3 and HLA-DR5 are present in increased frequency in the postpartum forms of the disorder, and HLA-DR3 in the sporadic forms (74). This is in contrast to the association with HLA-DR4 among Swedish women who have elevated antimicrosomal antibody titers (75). Among Japanese women HLA-DR3, DR8, DR9, A26, Bw52, Bw62, and Cw7 are more prevalent (60). The same study reported that 6 of 9 women with antithyroglobulin titers above 12,000 and HLA-DRw9 and/or HLA-B51 became permanently hypothyroid.

The most cogent argument for an autoimmune etiology, however, is the thyroid pathology. In all cases studied of both sporadic and postpartum thyroiditis during the early phases of the disorder, the thyroid gland is prominently infiltrated with lymphocytes (18,76,77) (Fig. 3). The infiltration may be focal or diffuse, but even the two thirds of the samples that are focal demonstrate up to 50% replacement by lymphocytes (76). Lymphoid follicles are frequently present and giant cells are common in disrupted follicles, but granulomas are absent. Follicle destruction is striking, but it is of varying degree. Hürthle cells are not prominent and fibrosis is usually minimal, distinguishing painless thyroiditis from Hashimoto's thyroiditis. Specimens obtained later in the patient's course demonstrate minimal or mild lymphocytic infiltration and reconstitution of follicular architecture (76) (see Fig. 3). Immunohistochemical lymphocyte analysis reveals normal distributions of T and B cells *within* thyroidal lymph follicles (76), but T lymphocytes overwhelmingly predominate *between* thyroid follicles (76,78). In postpartum patients, a relative decrease in intrathyroidal suppressor/cytotoxic (OKT8+) T cells is present and the intrathyroidal helper to suppressor/cytotoxic (OKT4+/OKT8+) T cell ratio is increased (78). Although the preponderance of data suggests that there are no abnormalities in circulating lymphocyte function (79) or type (76,78), a recent study demonstrated that activated mature, activated helper/inducer, and activated suppressor/cytotoxic T cells are more numerous in both the hyperthyroid and recovery phases of painless thyroiditis than in healthy volunteers (80). Nevertheless, it remains unclear whether these observations are causative or are simply a reflection of the immunological response to an antecedent insult.

Data from the use of cytokines for the treatment of cancer or chronic hepatitis C suggest their possible role as mediators of the transient thyroidal destruction. Patients receiving interleukin-2 together with tumor necrosis factor α or α-interferon developed the classic biochemical

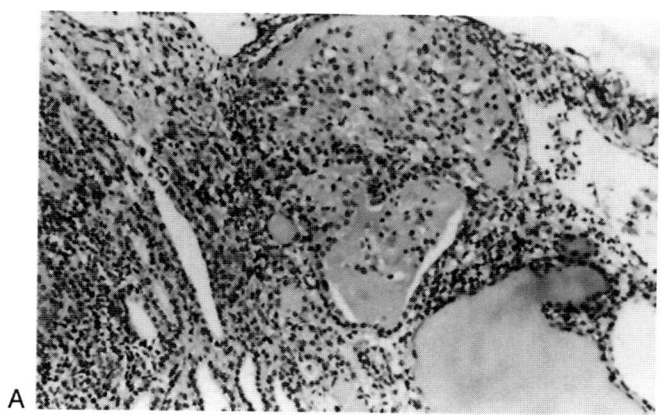 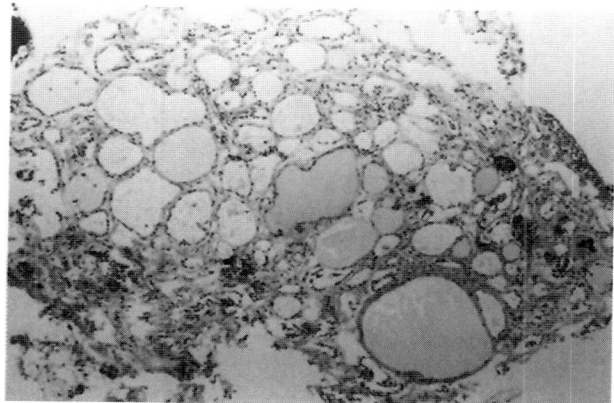

FIG. 3. The first biopsy during thyrotoxic phase (A) shows marked follicular destruction and diffuse lymphocytic infiltration, characteristic of silent thyroiditis. (×100.) The second biopsy during late recovery phase (B) shows that the degree of follicular destruction is markedly decreased and the thyroid is almost normal. (×40.) (From ref. 76, with permission.)

pattern of painless thyroiditis (81). Twenty-one percent of patients receiving interleukin-2 along with lymphokine-activated killer cells developed transient hypothyroidism (82). Four of eight patients receiving interleukin-2 with interferon α-2a for at least three cycles developed typical painless thyroiditis; all three aspirated patients had cytologic evidence of thyroiditis (83). Several patients developed a nontender thyroiditis in association with rising thyroidal antibody titers after α-interferon administration (84,85), whereas the two patients with preexisting thyroid antibodies (of the 25 treated) developed reversible thyroid dysfunction when treated with granulocyte-macrophage colony-stimulating factor (GM-CSF) (86).

Differential Diagnosis

Destruction-induced thyrotoxicosis (painless lymphocytic and subacute granulomatous thyroiditis) must be differentiated from several other conditions that closely mimic it (Table 4). The distinction between subacute granulomatous thyroiditis and painless thyroiditis is relatively straightforward. Clinically, the absence of pain will usually suffice, but there are occasional patients with subacute granulomatous thyroiditis in whom pain is not prominent. However, because their management and clinical courses are virtually identical, the distinction is not critical. Both struma ovarii and metastatic thyroid carcinoma can cause hyperthyroidism, but they are quite uncommon. Whole-body scanning will demonstrate the ectopic source of thyroid hormone synthesis. Iodide-induced hyperthyroidism must be strongly considered in all patients with a low ^{131}I uptake. Originally described during iodine supplementation in typical "goiter belts" (the Jod-Basedow phenomenon), it has been reported to occur in areas of iodine sufficiency (87,88). Excessive iodine exposure may precede the hyperthyroidism by 1 to 40 months, but in eight cases, the hyperthyroidism occurred during treatment. The ^{131}I uptake is below 3%, but, unlike painless and subacute thyroiditis, it responds to exogenous TSH. After passing through a short hypothyroid phase, most patients recover normal thyroid function after iodide removal. Occasional patients require definitive therapy for persistent hyperthyroidism. The sparse pathologic data available fail to show an inflammatory process (87,88).

Clearly factitious or iatrogenic hyperthyroidism must be included in the differential of thyrotoxicosis with a suppressed ^{131}I uptake. Although readily suspected, it may be difficult to document. Suppression of normally circulating thyroglobulin (89) may be helpful in this regard. Contamination of food products with animal-derived thyroid hormone presents a similar clinical picture (45,46,90). The occurrence of thyrotoxicosis in Cracow, Poland, in the early 1950s among slaughterhouse workers fed sausage made from thyroid glands was reported by Dymling and Becker as an anecdote (90).

Another outbreak involving 49 people occurred between January and March, 1984, in southeastern Nebraska (46). All ages were affected, with a median of 36 years. The highest attack rates were 5.7 and 5.5 cases per 1000 population among persons in the fourth and fifth decades of life. There was no apparent sex preference. Multiple members were involved in four families; the onset of their symptoms appeared up to 24 days apart. Typical symptoms of thyrotoxicosis were present; 15 were treated with beta-blockade, and five required hospitalization. None had thyroidal enlargement or pain. Thyroid hormone levels were elevated; thyroglobulin levels were not suppressed in the seven patients tested. A low ^{131}I uptake was found in all nine patients evaluated. Urinary iodide excretion was not elevated; there were no significant changes in mean antibody titers against all viruses tested. HLA-DR3 was significantly more prevalent in patients than in controls. Patients became euthyroid within 2 months. One patient relapsed within 3 months and two others became

TABLE 4. Laboratory data for various types of atypical thyrotoxicosis

	Subacute granulomatous thyroiditis	Painless lymphocytic thyroiditis	Hashitoxicosis	Iodine-induced thyrotoxicosis	Presumed hamburger induced[a]
T4 (µg/dL)	(N = 12) 16.3 ± 1.4	(N = 113) 17.0 ± 4.9	—	(N = 10) 12.9 ± 0.8	(N = 49) 19.8 ± 5.8
Free T4 (µ/dL)	(N = 6) 3.9 ± 0.9	(N = 3) 4.2 ± 0.9	—	(N = 4) 5.2 ± 0.9	(N = 17) 7.1 ± 1.8
T3 (µg/dL)	(N = 6) 173 ± 39	(N = 43) 346 ± 125	—	(N = 4) 280 ± 47.5	(N = 3) 330 ± 164
PBI (µg/dL)	(N = 6) 8.7 ± 1.9	(N = 11) 11.9 ± 2.8	(N = 13) 11.0 ± 1.0	(N = 10)[b] 27.8 ± 5.5	—
TSH (µU/mL)	(N = 5) <0.1	(N = 11) 2.0 ± 0.5	—	(N = 1) 0	(N = 5) <5
TRH (Δ) stimulation	(N = 5) <0.1	(N = 3) 0	—	(N = 1) 0	—
^{131}I uptake	(N = 11) 1.7 ± 0.6	(N = 48)[c] 1.2 ± 1.1	(N = 6) 48.3 ± 8.1	(N = 10) 2.0 ± 0.3	(N = 9) <6%
TSH stimulation	(N = 1) 7	(N = 8) 1.9 ± 1.8	—	(N = 8) 27.6 ± 8.8	—
Urinary I (µg/24 h)	—	(N = 15) 827 ± 532	—	(N = 9) 916 ± 162	(N = 12) 42.9 ± 30.1
Serum inorganic I (µ/dL)	—	(N = 2) 1.1	—	—	—
Antibodies (% increased) Thyroglobulin					
TRC	(N = 14) 21%	(N = 34) 10%	(N = 3)% 100	(N = 5) neg	(N = 16) 19%
RIA	—	(N = 7) 100%	—	—	—
Microsomal					
CF	(N = 8) 0%	(N = 16) 0%	(N = 5) 100%	—	(N = 16)
Fluorescent	—	57%	—	—	19%
ESR (% elevated)	(N = 12) 86%	(N = 29) 48%	—	(N = 8) 63%	(N = 8) 25%
HLA	B35	DR3[d]	—	—	DR3

[a]From ref. 26.
[b]Total serum iodine.
[c]Below 5% in 17 episodes, but actual values given in 48.
[d]DR5 is also associated with pregnancy-related cases.
TRC, tanned red cell antithyroglobulin; RIA, radioimmunoassayable antithyroglobulin; cF, complement fixation; PBI, protein-bound iodine; TSH, thyroid stimulating hormone; TRH, thyrotropin-releasing hormone; ESR, erythrocyte sedimentation rate; HLA, human lymphocyte antigen.
Modified from ref. 18.

transiently hypothyroid with elevated TSH levels. Thus, this outbreak of transient thyrotoxicosis appeared to have features typical of painless thyroiditis. However, follow-up investigation, after the appearance of another cluster of hyperthyroidism proven to be caused by hamburger contaminated by beef thyroid glands, demonstrated significant associations between this illness and the purchase of hamburger meat from the one supermarket that obtained its ground beef from a meat packer that practiced trimming gullets. In this procedure, part of the thyroid gland may be removed along with the neck muscle. The second outbreak of food-induced thyrotoxicosis occurred 15 months after the one in Nebraska and was centered in southwestern Minnesota and the adjacent areas of South Dakota and Iowa (45). Ultimately, 121 patients were involved. One of the keys to finding the offending agent was provided by the observation that the sole vegetarian of an extended family was the only unaffected individual (91). Further investigation found thyroid tissue in boxes of beef trimmings and in ground beef. Nine samples of implicated ground beef contained 43.7 µg/g of iodine, 11.4 µg/g T4, and 0.67 µg/g T3. Thus, the typical quarter-pound hamburger contained 1300 µg of T4 and 76 µg of T3, or 14 times the average replacement dose for a hypothyroid individual. Following these revelations, the United States Department of Agriculture prohibited the use of gullet trimming on August 29, 1985. Although the new regulation should prevent additional epidemics of this form of factitious hyperthyroidism, they may still take place on a sporadic basis. Indeed, some of the isolated cases in the past may have been caused by this practice.

SUBACUTE THYROIDITIS

Incidence

Although described as early as 1825, it was not until 1895 that 18 cases of subacute thyroiditis were reported as "thyroiditis acuta simplex," and in 1904 reports of the pathology were compiled from the literature by De Quervain (92). Subacute thyroiditis has been reported in all age groups from 3 to 76 years, but the fifth decade is most common. Only 9% of patients are under 30 years of age (43). Women predominate, with a proportion of from 3 to 6, to 1. Subacute thyroiditis accounted for 0.8% of referrals to one thyroid clinic (93) and 5% to 6% of all patients with thyroid disease (92).

Clinical Presentation

The illness is characterized by the abrupt onset of pain and tenderness over the thyroidal bed. The pain may radiate to the angles of the jaw or ears, masquerade as pharyngitis, or, rarely, present as chest pain. Although usually bilateral, it may first involve one side before migrating to the contralateral lobe in 30% of patients. Subacute thyroiditis has also been reported in a patient with thyroid hemiagenesis (94). In severe cases, the overlying skin may be erythematous and so tender that the mere thought of anything touching it evokes pain. Temperatures up to 102°F are common, and temperatures of up to 105°F have been reported. Malaise, fatigue, and weakness are frequently present. An antecedent viral prodrome is reported in approximately one third of cases. The white blood cell count is usually elevated and the erythrocyte sedimentation rate is invariably high. It is not surprising, therefore, that subacute thyroiditis may be confused with a suppurative process. Indeed, cases of positive gallium-67 citrate scans in subacute thyroiditis contribute to this confusion (95,96).

Thyrotoxic symptoms are prominent and it is not unusual for patients to be able to state their onset precisely. A 10- to 12-pound weight loss is common and associated with anorexia (92). Nervousness, tremor, palpitations, heat intolerance, and excessive sweating may all be present. Patients may have a stare, but proptosis is absent. Tachycardia and a widened pulse pressure have been reported. The thyroid gland is tender, often exquisitely so, and invariably enlarged. Although the goiter is usually modest and symmetrical, enlargement up to 10 times normal size has been described. About one third of patients have a localized firmness (92); cervical lymphadenopathy is rare. Although seldom reported, there have been several cases of complications, including liver dysfunction, splenomegaly, pancreatic inflammation, glucose intolerance, and mild anemia, all of which improved during recovery of the subacute thyroiditis (97). Unexplained fever and weight loss (98), myopathy (99), and vocal cord paralysis (100) have all been reported. Serum ferritin levels are significantly elevated and are higher than those present in patients with Graves' disease (101).

Patients typically undergo four phases of illness: hyperthyroid, euthyroid, hypothyroid, and recovery (102) (see Fig. 1). In this respect, subacute thyroiditis and painless thyroiditis, both sporadic and postpartum, are similar (21). The hyperthyroid phase, lasting 1 to 3 months, coincides with the period of thyroidal destruction. With disruption of follicular integrity, thyroid hormone and thyroglobulin flood the circulation (103); thyroglobulin levels follow the course of the disease (104). Because the thyroid is no longer capable of trapping iodine, the ^{131}I uptake is low, usually below 5%, and iodine stores are reduced in excess of 50% (37,105). However, the iodine retained in the thyroid is organified because abolition of the thyroid trap by perchlorate administration does not cause thyroidal iodine release (37). In patients with unilateral involvement, a thyroid scan may localize the abnormality to one side. However, with continued outpouring of T_3 and T_4, TSH levels are suppressed, causing uniform thyroidal suppression. There is no TSH response to thyrotropin-releasing hormone (TRH); administration of large amounts of TSH may increase the radioactive iodine uptake, but only in the uninvolved portions of the gland (106).

With exhaustion of hormonal stores and inability to synthesize new hormone, the patient passes through a euthyroid phase lasting 1 to 3 weeks. Hormone levels fall within the normal range. The ^{131}I uptake may become elevated, but this generally does not occur until later. The gland remains enlarged and firm, but it is no longer tender (92).

Severely affected patients (25% to 50% of the total) pass through a hypothyroid phase of 2 to 6 months, in which T_3 and T_4 levels are low and TSH concentrations high. Symptomatic individuals may require temporary thyroid replacement. Recovery of the ^{131}I uptake to often supranormal levels may precede TSH elevation (107). Recovery of normal thyroid function is the rule, and there have been very few reports of permanent thyroid dysfunction or goiter (40). Late recurrences are quite rare but can occur after more than 10 years (108). Nevertheless, abnormalities in thyroidal ^{127}I content (37), circulating thyroglobulin levels (37), or sensitivity to iodine-induced hypothyroidism (109) may persist for 2 or more years.

Pathology

Early in the course of subacute thyroiditis, the thyroid becomes infiltrated with neutrophils, large mononuclear monocytes, and lymphocytes. The thyroid follicles become hyperplastic with disruption of the epithelial lining. The characteristic multinuclear giant cells form from histiocytes. Immunohistochemical evaluation of the giant cells reveals that they generally contain lysozyme, vimentin, α1-antitrypsin, and thyroxine, but thyroglobulin is much less frequently present (110). The interstitium is edematous and infiltrated by lymphocytes and histiocytes. Carcinoembryonic antigen (CEA) is found in the center of granulomas in the acute stage, and carcinoma antigen 19-9 is present most strongly during the late stages of subacute thyroiditis (111). As the gland heals, follicles regenerate with minimal fibrosis (106). Caseation, hemorrhage, and calcification are generally not present.

Treatment

Treatment of subacute thyroiditis is directed toward pain relief and amelioration of the hyperthyroid symptoms. Glucocorticoids (prednisone 40 mg/day in divided doses) ameliorates pain within 24 hours (106) and leads to a return of thyroglobulin levels to normal within 4 weeks (112). The dosage should be tapered over the course of 1 month, but relapses may occur in 20% of patients (92,102). Less symptomatic individuals may be treated with salicylates or nonsteroidal anti-inflammatory agents. External irradiation between 200 and 2000 rads has been used in the past (92), but its use should be condemned. The thyrotoxic symptoms can be successfully managed with beta-blockade. Specific antithyroid therapy should be avoided, because it is not helpful in this transient disorder. Because the hyperthyroidism is caused by release of preformed thyroid hormone, antithyroid drugs are ineffective and are likely to prolong and worsen the hypothyroidism.

Differential Diagnosis

Subacute thyroiditis must be distinguished from several other entities. The presence of thyroidal tenderness and depressed ^{131}I uptake should readily distinguish it from Graves' disease. However, there have been several patients who have had both types of dysfunction spanning several years (113,114). Subacute thyroiditis needs to be differentiated from other causes of anterior neck pain, some of which are potentially life threatening (Table 5). Tenderness, fever, and elevated white blood cell count all suggest acute suppurative thyroiditis, an extremely rare condition (see preceding). The suppressed uptake in subacute thyroiditis, or signs of suppuration, should lead to the correct diagnosis, but the involvement of a single lobe with an abnormality on thyroid scan and a positive gallium scan may make the differentiation more difficult. Hemorrhage into a cyst or nodule may mimic subacute thyroiditis. A prior history of a thyroid nodule is helpful, but the failure of the process to migrate and involve the entire gland, the aspiration of blood, and the appropriate

TABLE 5. *Differential diagnosis of the painful anterior neck mass*

Subacute granulomatous thyroiditis*
Acute hemorrhage into thyroid cyst or adenomatoid nodule*
Acute hemorrhage into thyroid carcinoma
Acute suppurative thyroiditis
Rapidly enlarging thyroid carcinoma
Painful Hashimoto's thyroiditis
Infected thyroglossal duct cyst
Infected branchial-cleft cyst
Cellulitis of anterior neck

*Subacute granulomatous thyroiditis and hemorrhage into a cyst or adenoma probably account for more than 90% of all cases.
From ref. 115.

ultrasound picture should clarify the picture. Hashimoto's thyroiditis may occasionally present with pain (106). In these patients, the ^{131}I uptake may be low to slightly elevated, and antithyroid antibodies are generally of high titer. Trauma to the thyroid gland from martial arts (116) or seat belt use (117) may cause thyroidal pain and tenderness, but thyroid tests remain normal and the diagnosis should be self-evident.

Pathogenesis

The pathogenesis of subacute thyroiditis is unknown. Although an association between subacute thyroiditis and HLA-Bw35 has been found in Caucasians and in Chinese (118), it is generally felt that subacute thyroiditis is not an autoimmune disorder. However, there are changes in several immunological parameters that appear to be secondary to thyroidal destruction. Thyroid-binding inhibitory immunoglobulin titers are present in all patients with subacute thyroiditis and may disappear during recovery. However, changes in titer do not parallel the course of the illness (119). The same study also reported the appearance of thyroid-stimulating antibodies in low titer in some patients. Antibodies to thyroglobulin and microsomes may appear in relatively low titer in approximately half the patients, persisting for several months or becoming permanent (120). Autoantibodies to several novel thyroidal antigenic determinants have also been found that persist without change in levels for at least 39 months (121) and may be responsible for the persistence of subtle thyroidal defects. It is of interest that two patients have been reported who had recurrent episodes of typical subacute thyroiditis, but who had thyroidal amyloid deposition and not pathologic features of subacute thyroiditis (122).

Several viruses have been incriminated on the basis of changing viral antibody titers, including influenza, Coxsackie, adenovirus, echovirus, and mumps (120). In Italy, a high prevalence of subacute thyroiditis has been reported during the summer, coinciding with the seasonal distribution of enteroviruses (123). However, viral inclusion bodies have not been demonstrated in electron microscopic studies (106). The mumps virus has been grown from thyroidal biopsies of two patients during an outbreak of 11 cases of subacute thyroiditis occurring in a mumps epidemic (124), but other reports have not found this association. Additional evidence for environmental factors are the reports of the simultaneous occurrence of subacute thyroiditis in identical twins (125) and an outbreak of atypical subacute thyroiditis among 21 residents of the Dutch town of Winterswijk, including five affected members of two families (126).

HASHIMOTO'S THYROIDITIS

Incidence

Hashimoto's thyroiditis was initially described 80 years ago and is now recognized as an autoimmune destruction of the thyroid gland of unknown etiology. It is by far the most common of all thyroid disorders, affecting up to 2% of the population, 95% of whom are women (127). The incidence of 0.3 to 1.5 cases per 1000 population per year (128) is undoubtedly an underestimate, given the insidious nature of the disease. It affects all ages but is especially common in the 30- to 50-year age group. An incidence of 0.8% to 1.6% has been reported in adolescent girls, whereas it is present in 14% to 17% of routine postmortem specimens in the United Kingdom and Japan, respectively (128). Hashimoto's thyroiditis is particularly prevalent among patients with Down and Turner's syndromes (128).

Etiology and Pathogenesis

Thyroid disease in general, but particularly Hashimoto's thyroiditis, has a strong genetic component. Thyroid antibodies are found with high frequency among first-degree relatives and there is a high degree of concordance among twins and triplets (128). The prevalence of thyroid antibodies in the siblings of affected children is reported to be 71% if both parents have antibodies, and 54% or 29% if only one or neither parent is positive.

The etiology of Hashimoto's thyroiditis is unclear, but it is thought to be an interplay of genetic and environmental components. Although viruses have been incriminated, to date there is no compelling proof (129,130). Enhanced iodine intake is associated with an increase in thyroid autoantibodies, and thyroglobulin rich in iodine is more antigenic (129). Early studies demonstrated that Hashimoto's thyroiditis is closely associated with the HLA system. Patients are 3.4 times more likely to have the HLA-DR5 locus, whereas patients with primary myxedema (atrophic thyroiditis) have a relative risk of 5.7 for HLA-DR3 and HLA-B8. However, other HLA-DR specificities have been found in non-Caucasian populations (129).

The pathogenesis of the disorder is complex and has been recently reviewed (129). It is clearly an autoimmune disease with evidence of both cellular and humoral features. The interactions of genetic predisposition, antigenic presentation, T-cell responses, and thyrocytes form a cascade (131). The B-cell responses are more straightforward. Depending on the method used, antithyroglobulin antibodies are present in 55% to 90% of patients. Patients with negative thyroid serology may still be capable of producing thyroid antibodies within thyroid lymphoid tissue (132). Antibodies are generally IgG, but IgA and IgM antibodies to thyroglobulin have also been described. Thyroglobulin antibodies of the IgG4 class are overrepresented (129). Although they do not fix complement, they may participate in antibody-dependent cell-mediated cytotoxicity. Antibodies to thyroid microsomes (thyroperoxidase) are more universally present in high titer (128,133). They are polyclonal and distributed across all four IgG subclasses and both light chains. They recognize at least six different epitopes, including the site for catalytic peroxidation (129). Immune complexes have been found around the follicular basement membrane along with terminal complement complexes (129). In response, the thyrocyte may express adhesion molecules, which are important for cytotoxic T-cell recognition. However, even patients with negative antibody studies may still demonstrate cellular evidence of Hashimoto's thyroiditis using fine-needle aspiration (133). Growth-stimulating antibodies have also been demonstrated in most patients with Hashimoto's thyroiditis (134).

Clinical Presentation

The thyroid gland in Hashimoto's thyroiditis is generally symmetrically enlarged with fine nodularity. However, its size is variable, depending on the amount of fibrosis and lymphocytic infiltration and the degree of compensatory hyperplasia (127). The gland is very firm to rock hard. Distinct nodules are uncommon, and their presence, particularly if of recent onset or rapidly growing, should raise the suspicion of a thyroid lymphoma, which is present with greater frequency in patients with Hashimoto's thyroiditis than in the general population (135,136). Local symptoms are rarely present. Although only occasionally tender (137), a pathologically proven form has been reported with clinical features suggestive of subacute thyroiditis (138).

The natural history of Hashimoto's thyroiditis is variable. Hayashi et al. followed 43 patients for 10 to 20 years (139). Five of 13 patients failing to take thyroid replacement became hypothyroid and one developed thyrotoxicosis. Goiter size decreased in 57% of treated patients and in 23% of the untreated. In another series, 3 of 52 patients became hypothyroid over 14 years (140), and a 2% incidence of clinical hypothyroidism per year has been reported among patients with positive thyroid antibodies and elevated TSH levels (141). In a study of 46 children with autoimmune thyroiditis, 22 were either hypothyroid or subclinically hypothyroid (142). At the end of the follow-up period, which averaged 6.5 years, 17 individuals were hypothyroid, but there was extensive interchange among the three groups. Because of the progression to overt hypothyroidism, thyroid replacement should be administered to all patients with biochemical, as well as clinical, hypothyroidism. Specific therapy to prevent disease progression is generally of little help. Glucocorticoids may arrest the disease process, but their side effects outweigh their potential benefit. Surgery should be reserved for those very rare patients who manifest compressive symptoms.

At the time of presentation, thyroid hormone levels may be normal or low, depending on the degree of destruction. An elevated TSH in the presence of normal T_4 or T_3 levels may presage clinical hypothyroidism. The thyroid scan classically demonstrates a "salt and pepper" pattern. The 24-hour ^{131}I uptake may be low, normal, or elevated. An elevated uptake may be caused by a defect in organification demonstrable by perchlorate administration or by diminished intrathyroidal iodine content (127). Both conditions may lead to reduced thyroid hormone synthesis.

Pathology

The thyroid of the patient with Hashimoto's thyroiditis is infiltrated with lymphocytes and plasma cells forming lymphoid follicles with occasional germinal centers. Thyroid follicles are disrupted and some follicular epithelium demonstrates oxyphilic cytoplasmic changes characteristic of Hürthle or Askanazy cells. Fibrosis of varying degrees is present. Psammoma bodies have been reported in one patient without evidence of papillary carcinoma (143). Some authors make further pathologic distinctions (128). In the fibrous variation, the gland is very firm and replaced by dense fibrosis that does not extend beyond the capsule, distinguishing it from Riedel's struma (see later). In other glands, atrophic changes may predominate, leading to myxedema. Epithelial atrophy and fibrosis are prominent when there is less lymphocytic infiltration. Finally, the thyroiditis may be focal. This variation is quite common, being present in 25% of women at autopsy; the degree of abnormality correlates with the presence and titer of thyroid antibodies.

Cytologically, Hashimoto's thyroiditis can be diagnosed by the presence of lymphoid infiltration of follicles, follicular cells with oxyphilic (Hürthle cell) changes of varying degrees, polymorphous lymphocyte populations, and histiocytes. Multinuclear giant cells may be present on occasion. Tangles of chromatin are frequently present (144). The presence of abundant lymphocytes and polymorphous Hürthle cells distinguishes this lesion from a Hürthle cell neoplasm (145), whereas thyroidal non-Hodgkin's lymphomas have relatively uniform, large, malignant-appearing lymphocytes with prominent nucleoli (145). In a large series of patients, thyroid cytology correlated with thyroid function (146).

Association with Autoimmune Disease and Lymphoma

Autoimmune disorders are present in higher frequency in patients with Hashimoto's thyroiditis than in the general population. These include adrenal insufficiency, alopecia areata, biliary cirrhosis, diabetes mellitus, hypoparathyroidism, pernicious anemia, and the connective tissue diseases rheumatoid arthritis, lupus erythematosus, progressive systemic sclerosis, and Sjögren's syndrome. A 16% to 41% incidence of mitral valve prolapse has been reported in two large series (147,148).

Patients with Hashimoto's thyroiditis are also at increased risk for developing a B-cell lymphoma of the thyroid. In a study of 829 patients, four were found versus 0.06 expected (relative risk 66) (135). Similar observations have been reported from Japan (136) during 45,600 patient-years of observation. Hamburger and colleagues have reviewed their experience with thyroid lymphoma (149). Twenty-four of the 30 patients had evidence of Hashimoto's thyroiditis, 19 by serologic tests and the remainder by biopsy or surgery. Thirteen were under the age of 60, and seven of these were under 40 years. Eight of the patients were men and they tended to be younger. Discrete nodules were present in 19, and the remainder had multinodular or diffuse goiters. Local symptoms are common and include pain and tenderness, hoarseness, tracheal compression, and vocal cord paralysis. Monoclonal gammopathies may be present (150) and disappear following successful treatment (151), which consists of irradiation and/or chemotherapy. When the disease is confined to the thyroid, the 5-year survival is 75% to 85%, compared to 40% when it extends to surrounding neck structures and 5% when it is disseminated (149).

INVASIVE FIBROUS THYROIDITIS (RIEDEL'S STRUMA)

Incidence

Riedel's struma is an extremely uncommon thyroid disorder. It may occur alone or be associated with sclerosis of the mediastinum, retroperitoneum, orbit, and biliary tract (152–154). A 1988 review of 178 patients (154) revealed findings similar to Hay's update of an earlier series from the Mayo Clinic (155), in which 37 cases occurring between 1920 and 1984 were reported (153).

During this interval, 57,000 thyroidectomies were performed at the Mayo Clinic on 3.5 million registered patients. The operative incidence of 0.06% and the incidence among outpatients of 1.06 per 100,000 clearly overemphasizes its true prevalence (153). Women are 4 times more likely to be affected, and it generally occurs in the fourth and fifth decade of life (range, 23 to 67 years).

Clinical Presentation

Patients typically present with a thyroidal mass that has been present from 2 months to 5 years. Obstructive symptoms are uncommon and usually mild (156). The thyroid is fixed and rock hard. Within affected areas, the gland is replaced *in toto* by a fibrotic process that extends beyond the capsule to involve the surrounding structures, including the sternothyroid muscles and occasionally the internal jugular vein and carotid artery (156). Both the trachea and esophagus may be affected. Hypoparathyroidism develops because of involvement of the parathyroid glands by the fibrous process. In the series of Woolner et al., 6 of 20 patients had bilateral involvement and all were myxedematous (156). Thyroid hormone levels are normal two thirds of the time and low in all but 4% of the remainder (154), depending on the degree of replacement. A thyroid scan will demonstrate focal to uniform absence of isotopic accumulation. The white blood cell count and erythrocyte sedimentation rate are usually normal but can be elevated.

Pathology

Early pathologic lesions demonstrate intense infiltration of the thyroid parenchyma by lymphocytes, plasma cells, neutrophils, and eosinophils (154). Initially dense fibrous bands separate the thyroid into progressively smaller nodules, before the entire gland is replaced by fibrosis and collagen. Small and medium-sized veins are infiltrated by lymphocytes and plasma cells. The inflammatory changes, luminal obliteration, and ultimately sclerosis have also been seen in patients with multifocal fibrosis (154).

Association with Hashimoto's Thyroiditis

In the past, there has been controversy concerning the relationship between Riedel's struma and end-stage Hashimoto's thyroiditis. A 45% (153) to 64% (154) incidence of antithyroid antibodies has been found in the former, and there is a case report of a patient who had features of both processes, including extensive involvement of perithyroidal tissues by fibrosis, high titers of antimicrosomal and antithyroglobulin antibodies, and the presence of lymphoid follicles with germinal centers (157). However, the presence of a vasculitis, fibrous invasion beyond the capsule, effacement of thyroid architecture, and hyalinization of the connective tissue, and the absence of Hürthle cells, generally distinguishes the two entities (Table 6). Unlike the situation with Hashimoto's thyroiditis, association with autoimmune diseases is uncommon, although a patient with both Riedel's struma and pernicious anemia has been reported (158).

Treatment

Treatment of Riedel's struma is palliative surgery to remove obstructive symptoms. Subtotal resection should not be attempted because the surgical planes and landmarks have been obliterated. Treatment with glucocorticoids has been successful in a small number of patients (158,159). Untreated, the disease process is usually slowly progressive, although it may stabilize or regress (153). However, two of the patients in Woolner's series with unilateral involvement developed disease in the contralateral lobe within 2 years (155), and 12 of 37 developed extrathyroidal fibrosclerosis involving the orbit, mediastinum, or abdomen during an extended period of follow-up (153).

THYROIDITIS INTERRELATIONSHIPS

The interrelationships among the various causes of thyroiditis and their relationships to other causes of hyperthyroidism are of great interest. Both Riedel's struma and acute suppurative thyroiditis are separate entities, although the latter may be confused with granulomatous (subacute) thyroiditis. Currently, most authors believe that painless thyroiditis and granulomatous thyroiditis are distinct, despite their identical clinical courses over the near term, for the following reasons:

1. The pathologic changes in painless thyroiditis include infiltration of the gland by lymphocytes and some plasma cells. Hürthle cells, germinal centers, and fibrosis

TABLE 6. *Comparison of clinical and pathologic features of Riedel's and Hashimoto's thyroiditis*

Clinicopathologic feature	Riedel's thyroiditis	Hashimoto's thyroiditis
Sex	Women and men	Women
Age	Any age	Older than 45 years
Thyroid status	Euthyroid	Hypothyroid
Gross morphology	Localized	Diffuse
Connective tissue	Hyalinized	Delicate
Gland architecture	Effaced	Preserved
Capsule	Invasion	No invasion
Vascular changes	Vasculitis	Absent

From ref. 154.

may be present. In contrast, granulomatous thyroiditis is typified by the presence of neutrophils, large mononuclear cells, and giant cells.

2. Persistence of thyroid dysfunction, including goiter and permanent hypothyroidism, is common in painless thyroiditis, but it is very infrequent or absent in granulomatous thyroiditis. In the former, antithyroid antibodies are present in high titer in most patients, whereas they are seldom present in the latter. Even then they tend to be transient and in low titer.

3. The two disorders are associated with completely different HLA haplotypes (HLA-DR3 in sporadic, and HLA-DR3 and HLA-DR5 in postpartum thyroiditis, compared with HLA-B35 in the granulomatous form).

4. Elevated white blood cell counts and erythrocyte sedimentation rates are almost universally present in granulomatous thyroiditis and infrequently present in lymphocytic thyroiditis.

5. In reports of the last 15 years, thyroidal pain has been virtually absent in biopsy-proven patients with lymphocytic thyroiditis, whereas patients with pain have had the histologic picture of granulomatous thyroiditis (43). Current data suggest that painless thyroiditis is a form of Hashimoto's thyroiditis (Fig. 4).

The pathology overlaps to a great extent, and antimicrosomal and antithyroglobulin antibodies are present in high titer in both disorders. However, patients with Hashimoto's thyroiditis have more severe histologic changes with greater fibrosis, more frequent oxyphilic changes, and the presence of germinal centers in higher frequency. Hashimoto's thyroiditis has a greater propensity for progression to frank hypothyroidism, it tends to be more familial, and there is a much higher prevalence of involvement in women. Furthermore, except for end-stage disease causing permanent hypothyroidism, the ^{131}I uptake is not depressed. Although hyperthyroidism may develop in the setting of Hashimoto's thyroiditis (hashitoxicosis), the ^{131}I uptake is elevated and the hyperthyroidism does not remit (155,160).

The reports of a few patients with acute painful exacerbations of Hashimoto's thyroiditis (137) may cause confusion. Like patients with subacute thyroiditis, they present with pain and tenderness that involves some or all of the gland and lasts for 1 to 28 days. They may be febrile and have elevated white blood cell counts and erythrocyte sedimentation rates, but titers of thyroglobulin and microsomal antibodies are low. In contrast, thyroid function tests may be high, low, or normal, and technetium (Tc)-99m pertechnetate scintigrams demonstrate heterogeneous trapping in most cases. Pathologic examination of the gland reveals destruction of follicles with lymphocytic infiltration and loose arrangement of fibrosis. Patients may require steroid treatment and relapses are quite common. Persistent goiter with or without hypothyroidism is the rule.

The separation of lymphocytic thyroiditis from Graves' disease is generally straightforward in the nonpregnant patient. Although there have been scattered reports of patients having both conditions, the differentiation is readily made. Lymphocytic thyroiditis is never associated with exophthalmos or pretibial myxedema. The ^{131}I uptake is always depressed and the development of the hyperthyroidism is not insidious. In patients with Graves' disease, iodine administration may lower the ^{131}I uptake, but it is rarely as depressed as in lymphocytic thyroiditis (161).

The etiology of postpartum thyrotoxicosis, however, may be confusing (53,65). Graves' disease frequently ameliorates during pregnancy, with relapse quite frequent in the early postpartum period (65). In a study of 41 patients with Graves' disease in remission, Amino and coworkers found that 32 patients relapsed within 2 to 4 months of delivery and that the thyrotoxicosis fell into one of three types (65) (see Fig. 2): ten women had persistent hyperthyroidism with elevated ^{131}I uptakes, ten women had transient thyrotoxicosis with high or normal radioactive iodine uptakes, and the remaining patients had transient hyperthyroidism with low radioiodine up-

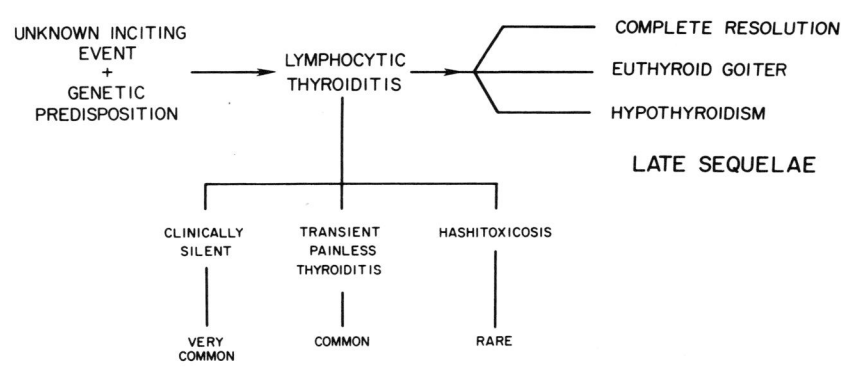

FIG. 4. A proposed scheme that indicates the various modes of presentation and the possible late sequelae of lymphocytic thyroiditis. (From ref. 18, with permission.)

takes. Patients in the last category had higher titers of antimicrosomal antibodies and a longer euthyroid interval prior to pregnancy, whereas the first two groups had a higher free T_4 index earlier in pregnancy. In women who are unable to have ^{131}I studies, the use of the T_3 to T_4 ratio has been proposed to separate lymphocytic thyroiditis from Graves' disease (162), but other workers have not found this parameter to be useful (23). In these women, a trial of antithyroid drug may be indicated.

ACKNOWLEDGMENT

The author wishes to thank Mrs. Elizabeth Skelton for her secretarial assistance.

REFERENCES

1. Hamburger JI. The various presentations of thyroiditis: diagnostic considerations. *Ann Intern Med* 1986;104:219–224.
2. Berger SA, Zonszein J, Villamena P, Mittman N. Infectious diseases of the thyroid gland. *Rev Infect Dis* 1983;5:108–122.
3. Rich EJ, Mendelman PM. Acute suppurative thyroiditis in pediatric patients. *Pediatr Infect Dis J* 1987;6:936–940.
4. Kodama T, Ito Y, Obara T, Fujimoto Y. Acute suppurative thyroiditis in appearance of unusual neck mass. *Endocrinol Jpn* 1987;34:427–430.
5. Miyvauchi A, Matsuzuka F, Kuma K, Takai S. Piriform sinus fistula: an underlying abnormality common in patients with acute suppurative thyroiditis. *World J Surg* 1990;14:400–405.
6. Falchuk SC, Ahlgren JD, Holt RW. Acute thyroiditis as a complication of chemotherapy administration through a Hickman catheter. *Cancer Treat Rep* 1987;71:788–790.
7. von Graevenitz A, Colla F. Thyroiditis due to *Brucella melitensis*—report of two cases. *Infection* 1990;18:179–180.
8. Goudreau E, Comtois R, Bavardelle P, Beauregard H, Larochelle D. *Capnocytophaga ochracea* and group F beta-hemolytic streptococcus suppurative thyroiditis. *J Otolaryngol* 1986;15:59–61.
9. Queen JS, Clegg HW, Council JC, Morton D. Acute suppurative thyroiditis caused by *Eikenella corrodens*. *J Pediatr Surg* 1988;23:359–361.
10. Stevenson, J. Acute bacterial thyroiditis presenting as otalgia. *J Laryngol Otol* 1991;105:788–789.
11. Sudar JM, Alleman MJ, Jonkers GJ, de Groot R, Jongejan C. Acute thyroiditis caused by *Moraxella nonliquefaciens*. *Neth J Med* 1994;45:170–173.
12. Dall SM, Chopra P, Nayak NC. Thyroiditis in adenomatous goitre and adenoma of thyroid. *Indian J Med Res* 1984;80:670–676.
13. Reichling JJ, Rose DN, Mendelson MH, Hirschman SZ. Acute suppurative thyroiditis caused by *Serratia marcescens*. *J Infect Dis* 1984;149:281.
14. Vaidya KP, Lomvardias S. Cryptococcal thyroiditis: report of a case diagnosed by fine-needle aspiration cytology. *Diagn Cytopathol* 1991;7:415–416.
15. Khan EM, Hague I, Pandey R, Mishra SK, Sharma AK. Tuberculosis of the thyroid gland: a clinicopathological profile of four cases and review of the literature. *Aust N Z J Surg* 1993;63:807–810.
16. Schofield PM, Keal EE. Subacute thyroiditis associated with *Chlamydia psittaci* infection. *Postgrad Med J* 1986;62:33–34.
17. Guttler R, Singer PA. *Pneumocystis carinii* thyroiditis: report of three cases and review of the literature. *Arch Intern Med* 1993;153:393–396.
18. Woolf PD. Transient painless thyroiditis with hyperthyroidism: a variant of lymphocytic thyroiditis? *Endocr Rev* 1980;1:411–420.
19. Schorr AB, Miller JL, Shtasel P, Rose LI. Low incidence of painless thyroiditis in the Philadelphia area. *Clin Nucl Med* 1986;11:379–380.
20. Vitug AC, Goldman JM. Silent (painless) thyroiditis: evidence of a geographic variation in frequency. *Arch Intern Med* 1985;145:473–475.
21. Woolf PD, Daly R. Thyrotoxicosis with painless thyroiditis. *Am J Med* 1976;60:73–79.
22. Dorfman SG, Cooperman MT, Nelson RL, Depuy H, Peake RL, Young RL. Painless thyroiditis and transient hyperthyroidism without goiter. *Ann Intern Med* 1977;86:24–28.
23. Nikolai TF, Brosseau J, Kettrick MA, Roberts R, Beltaos E. Lymphocytic thyroiditis with spontaneously resolving hyperthyroidism (silent thyroiditis). *Arch Intern Med* 1980;140:478–482.
24. Jansson R, Dahlberg PA, Karlsson FA. Postpartum thyroiditis. In: *Bailliere's clinical endocrinology and metabolism*, vol 2. Kent, England: Bailliere Tindale, 1988;619–635.
25. Rasmussen NG, Hansen JM, Hegedus L. Frequency of thyroiditis and postpartum thyroiditis in a 10-year consecutive hyperthyroid Danish population. *Thyroidology* 1989;3:143–147.
26. Amino N, Mori H, Iwatani Y, et al. High prevalence of transient postpartum thyrotoxicosis and hypothyroidism. *N Engl J Med* 1982;306:849–852.
27. Jansson R, Bernander S, Karlsson A, Levin K, Nilsson G. Autoimmune thyroid dysfunction in the postpartum period. *J Clin Endocrinol Metab* 1984;53:681–687.
28. Freeman R, Rosen H, Thysen B. Incidence of thyroid dysfunction in an unselected postpartum population. *Arch Intern Med* 1986;146:1361–1364.
29. Nikolai TF, Turney SL, Roberts RC. Postpartum lymphocytic thyroiditis: prevalence, clinical course, and long-term follow-up. *Arch Intern Med* 1987;147:222–224.
30. Jansson R, Dahlberg PA, Karlsson FA. Postpartum thyroiditis. *Thyroidology* 1989;1:143–147.
31. Fung HYM, Kologlu M, Collison K, et al. Postpartum thyroid dysfunction in mid Glamorgan. *Br Med J (Clin Res Ed)* 1988;296:241–296.
32. Rajatanavin R, Chailurkit L-O, Tirarungsikul K, Chalayondeja W, Jittivanich U, Puapradit W. Postpartum thyroid dysfunction in Bangkok: a geographical variation in the prevalence. *Acta Endocrinol* 1990;122:283–287.
33. Walfish PG, Meyerson J, Provias JP, Vargas MI, Papsin FR. Prevalence and characteristics of post-partum thyroid dysfunction: results of a survey from Toronto, Canada. *J Endocrinol Invest* 1992;15:265–272.
34. Sulimani RA, Ba'Aqeel HA, al-Nuaim AR, al-Meshari AA, Haleem K. Post partum thyroiditis in Saudi women. *East Afr Med J* 1993;70:556–557.
35. Nikolai TF, Coombs GJ, McKenzie AK, Miller RW, Weir CJ Jr. Treatment of lymphocytic thyroiditis with spontaneously resolving hyperthyroidism (silent thyroiditis). *Arch Intern Med* 1982;142:2281–2283.
36. Shigemasa C, Abe K, Taniguchi S-I, et al. Lower serum free thyroxine (T4) levels in painless thyroiditis compared with Graves' disease despite similar serum total T4 levels. *J Clin Endocrinol Metab* 1987;65:359–363.
37. Smallridge RC, De Keyser FM, Van Herle AJ, Butkus NE, Wartofsky L. Thyroid iodine content and serum thyroglobulin: clues to the natural history of destruction-induced thyroiditis. *J Clin Endocrinol Metab* 1986;62:1213–1219.
38. Sugimoto I, Momotani N, Lino S, Ito K. Clinical significance of the measurement of the urinary concentration of iodine in differentiating silent thyroiditis from Graves' disease. *Folia Endocrinol Jpn* 1994;70:1083–1092.
39. Momotani N, Noh J, Ishikawa N, Ito K. Relationship between silent thyroiditis and recurrent Graves' disease in the postpartum period. *J Clin Endocrinol Metab* 1994;79:285–289.
40. Nikolai TF, Coombs GJ, McKenzie AK. Lymphocytic thyroiditis with spontaneously resolving hyperthyroidism and subacute thyroiditis: long-term follow-up. *Arch Intern Med* 1981;141:1455–1458.
41. Amino N. Commentary in Chapter 2: Are silent thyroiditis and postpartum silent thyroiditis forms of chronic thyroiditis or different (new) forms of viral thyroiditis? In: Hamburger JI, Meier DA, eds. *Clinical thyroidology*. New York: Springer-Verlag, 1981;31–36.
42. Yamamoto M, Sakurada T, Yoshida K, et al. Thyroid function and antimicrosomal antibody during the course of silent thyroiditis. *Endocrinol Jpn* 1987;34:357–363.
43. Hamburger JI, Meier DA. Are silent thyroiditis and postpartum silent thyroiditis forms of chronic thyroiditis or different (new) forms of viral thyroiditis? In: Hamburger JI, Meier DA, eds. *Clinical thyroidology*. New York: Springer-Verlag, 1981;21–67.
44. Choe W, McDougall IR. Ablation of thyroid function with radioactive iodine after recurrent episodes of silent thyroiditis. *Thyroid* 1993;3:311–313.

45. Hedberg CW, Fishbein DB, Janssen RS, et al. An outbreak of thyrotoxicosis caused by the consumption of bovine thyroid gland in ground beef. *N Engl J Med* 1987;316:993–998.
46. Kinney JS, Hurwitz ES, Fishbein DB, et al. Community outbreak of thyrotoxicosis: epidemiology, immunogenetic characteristics, and long-term outcome. *Am J Med* 1988;84:10–18.
47. Ogura T, Hirakawa S, Suzuki S, Ota Z, Togawa T, Nogami I. Five patients with painless thyroiditis simultaneously developed in a nursery school. *Endocrinol Jpn* 1988;35:225–230.
48. Morrison J, Caplan RH. Typical and atypical ("silent") subacute thyroiditis in a wife and husband. *Arch Intern Med* 1978;138:45–48.
49. Fein HG, Goldman JM, Weintraub BD. Postpartum lymphocytic thyroiditis in American women: a spectrum of thyroid dysfunction. *Am J Obstet Gynecol* 1980;138:504–510.
50. Taylor HC, Sheeler LR. Recurrence and heterogeneity in painless thyrotoxic lymphocytic thyroiditis. *JAMA* 1982;248:1085–1088.
51. Singer PA, Gorsky JE. Familial postpartum transient hyperthyroidism. *Arch Intern Med* 1985;145:240–242.
52. Amino N, Miyai K, Kuro R, et al. Transient postpartum hypothyroidism: fourteen cases with autoimmune thyroiditis. *Ann Intern Med* 1977;87:155–159.
53. Jansson R. Autoimmune thyroiditis: a clinical, epidemiological and immunological study with special reference to transient aggravation in the postpartum period. *Acta Univ Uppsaliensis*. Abstracts of Uppsala dissertations from the Faculty of Medicine, Uppsala, Sweden 1984;492:1–73.
54. Stewart DE, Addison AM, Robinson GE, Joffe R, Burrow GN, Olmsted MP. Thyroid function in psychosis following childbirth. *Am J Psychiatry* 1988;145:1579–1581.
55. Vargas MT, Briones-Urbina R, Gladman D, et al. Autoimmune pathogenesis for post partum thyroid dysfunction. *J Clin Endocrinol Metab* 1988;67:327–333.
56. Hayslip CC, Fein HG, O'Donnell VM, Friedman DS, Klein TA, Smallridge RC. The value of serum antimicrosomal antibody testing in screening for symptomatic postpartum thyroid dysfunction. *Am J Obstet Gynecol* 1988;159:203–209.
57. Parkes AB, Othman S, Hall R, John R, Richards CJ, Lazarus JH. The role of complement in the pathogenesis of postpartum thyroiditis. *J Clin Endocrinol Metab* 1994;79:395–400.
58. Kampe O, Jansson R, Karlsson FA. Effects of L-thyroxine and iodide on the development of autoimmune postpartum thyroiditis. *J Clin Endocrinol Metab* 1990;70:1014–1018.
59. Amino N, Miyai K. Postpartum autoimmune endocrine syndromes. In: Davies TF, ed. *Autoimmune endocrine disease*. New York: John Wiley & Sons, 1983;247–272.
60. Walfish PG, Chan JYC. Post-partum hyperthyroidism. In: Dunton N, ed. *Clinical endocrinology metabolism: hyperthyroidism*. Philadelphia: WB Saunders, 1985;14:417–447.
61. Tachi J, Amino N, Tamaki H, Aozasa M, Iwatani Y, Miyai K. Long term follow-up and HLA association in patients with postpartum hypothyroidism. *J Clin Endocrinol Metab* 1988;66:480–484.
62. Othman S, Phillips DIW, Parkes AB, Richards CJ, Harris B. A long-term follow-up of postpartum thyroiditis. *Clin Endocrinol* 1990;32:559–564.
63. Roti E, Minelli R, Gardini E, et al. Impaired intrathyroidal iodine organification and iodine-induced hypothyroidism in euthyroid women with a previous episode of postpartum thyroiditis. *J Clin Endocrinol Metab* 1991;73:958–963.
64. Bech K, Hertel J, Rasmussen NG, et al. Effect of maternal thyroid autoantibodies and post-partum thyroiditis on the fetus and neonate. *Acta Endocrinol* 1991;125:146–149.
65. Amino N, Tanizawa O, Mori H, et al. Aggravation of thyrotoxicosis in early pregnancy and after delivery in Graves' disease. *J Clin Endocrinol Metab* 1982;55:108–112.
66. Nakamura S, Kosaka J, Sugimoto M, Watanabe H, Shima H, Takuno H. Silent thyroiditis following rubella. *Endocrinol Jpn* 1990;37:79–85.
67. Blitzer JB, Paolozzi FP, Gottlieb AJ, Zamkoff KW, Chung CT. Thyrotoxic thyroiditis after radiotherapy for Hodgkin's disease. *Arch Intern Med* 1985;145:1734–1735.
68. Walfish PG, Caplan D, Rosen IB. Postparathyroidectomy transient thyrotoxicosis. *J Clin Endocrinol Metab* 1992;75:224–227.
69. Calle RA, Cohen KL. Transient thyroiditis due to surgical trauma. *Am J Med* 1993;95:546–548.
70. Faird NR, Bear JC. Autoimmune endocrine disorders and the major histocompatibility complex. In: Davies TF, ed. *Autoimmune endocrine disease*. New York: John Wiley & Sons, 1983:59–91.
71. Gerstein HC. Incidence of postpartum thyroid dysfunction in patients with type I diabetes mellitus. *Ann Intern Med* 1993;118:419–423.
72. Tajiri J, Higashi K, Morita M, Ohishi S, Umeda T, Sato T. Elevation of anti-DNA antibody titer during thyrotoxic phase of silent thyroiditis. *Arch Intern Med* 1986;146:1623–1624.
73. Tachi J, Amino N, Iwatani Y, et al. Increase in antideoxyribonucleic acid antibody titer in postpartum aggravation of autoimmune thyroid disease. *J Clin Endocrinol Metab* 1988;67:1049–1053.
74. Farid NR, Hawe BS, Walfish PG. Increased frequency of HLA-DR3 and 5 in the syndromes of painless thyroiditis with transient thyrotoxicosis: evidence for an autoimmune aetiology. *Clin Endocrinol (Oxf)* 1983;19:699–704.
75. Jansson R, Safwenberg J, Dahlberg PA. Influence of the HLA-DR4 antigen and iodine status on the development of autoimmune postpartum thyroiditis. *J Clin Endocrinol Metab* 1985;60:168–173.
76. Mizukami Y, Michigishi T, Hashimoto T, et al. Silent thyroiditis: a histologic and immunohistochemical study. *Hum Pathol* 1988;19:423–431.
77. Mizukami Y, Michigishi T, Nonomura A, et al. Postpartum thyroiditis: a clinical, histologic, and immunopathologic study of 15 cases. *Am J Clin Pathol* 1993;100:200–205.
78. Jansson R, Totterman TH, Sallstrom J, Dahlberg PA. Intrathyroidal and circulating lymphocyte subsets in different stages of autoimmune postpartum thyroiditis. *J Clin Endocrinol Metab* 1984;58:942–946.
79. Hayslip CC, Baker JR Jr, Wartofsky L, Klein TA, Opsahl MS, Burman KD. Natural killer cell activity and serum autoantibodies in women with postpartum thyroiditis. *J Clin Endocrinol Metab* 1988;66:1089–1093.
80. Kushima K, Ban Y, Taniyama M, Itoh K. Circulating activated T lymphocyte subsets in patients with silent thyroiditis. *Endocr J* 1994;41:663–669.
81. Vassilopoulou-Sellin R, Sella A, Dexeus FH, Theriaulr RL, Pololoff DA. Acute thyroid dysfunction (thyroiditis) after therapy with interleukin-2. *Horm Metab Res* 1992;24:434–438.
82. Atkins MB, Mier JW, Parkinson DR, Gould JA, Berkman EM, Kaplan MM. Hypothyroidism after treatment with interleukin-2 and lymphokine-activated killer cells. *N Engl J Med* 1988;318:1557–1563.
83. Pichert G, Jost LM, Zobeli L, Odermatt B, Pedio G, Stahel RA. Thyroiditis after treatment with interleukin-2 and interferon α-2a. *Br J Cancer* 1990;62:100–104.
84. Kodama T, Katabami S, Kamijo K, et al. Development of transient thyroid disease and reaction during treatment of chronic hepatitis C with interferon. *J Gastroenterol* 1994;29:289–292.
85. Kamikubo K, Takami R, Suwa T, et al. Case report: silent thyroiditis developed during alpha-interferon therapy. *Am J Med Sci* 1993;306:174–176.
86. Hoekman K, von Blomberg-van der Flier BM, Wagstaff J, Drexhage HA, Pinedo HM. Reversible thyroid dysfunction during treatment with GM-CSF. *Lancet* 1991;338(8766):541–542.
87. Vagenakis AG, Wang C, Burger A, Maloof F, Braverman LE, Ingbar SH. Iodine-induced thyrotoxicosis in Boston. *N Engl J Med* 1972;287:523.
88. Savoie JC, Massin JP, Thomopoulous P, Leger F. Iodine-induced thyrotoxicosis in apparently normal thyroid glands. *J Clin Endocrinol Metab* 1975;41:685–691.
89. Mariotti S, Martino E, Cupini C, et al. Low serum thyroglobulin as a clue to the diagnosis of thyrotoxicosis factitia. *N Engl J Med* 1982;307:410–412.
90. Dymling J-F, Becker DV. Occurrence of hyperthyroidism in patients receiving thyroid hormone. *J Clin Endocrinol Metab* 1967;27:1487–1491.
91. McMillin JM. Hamburger thyrotoxicosis: the endocrinologist as sleuth. *Thyroid Today* 1988;11:1–9.
92. Greene JN. Subacute thyroiditis. *Am J Med* 1971;51:97–108.
93. Hamburger JI. Subacute thyroiditis: diagnostic difficulties and simple treatment. *J Nucl Med* 1974;15:81–89.
94. Shibutani Y, Inoue D, Koshiyama H, Mori T. Thyroid hemiagenesis with subacute thyroiditis. *Thyroid* 1995;5:133–135.
95. Sanders LR, Moreno AJ, Pittman DL, Jones JD, Spicer MJ, Tracy KP. Painless giant cell thyroiditis diagnosed by fine needle aspiration and associated with intense thyroidal uptake of gallium. *Am J Med* 1986;80:971–975.

96. Coolens JL, Sprengers D, Van Parys G, De Roo M. Subacute thyroiditis detected by 67 gallium-citrate scintigraphy. *Acta Clin Belg* 1986;41:328–332.
97. Kimura M, Amino N, Takada K, Miyai K. Subacute thyroiditis associated with systemic multi-organ disorders. *Endocrinol Jpn* 1989;36:859–864.
98. Rotenberg Z, Weinberger I, Fuchs J, Maller S, Agmon J. Euthyroid atypical subacute thyroiditis simulating systemic or malignant disease. *Arch Intern Med* 1986;146:105–107.
99. Tajima K, Mashita K, Yamane T, et al. Thyrotoxic myopathy associated with subacute thyroiditis. *Clin Endocrinol* 1984;20:307–312.
100. Kallmeyer JC, Hackmann R. Vocal cord paralysis associated with subacute thyroiditis. A case report. *S Afr Med J* 1985;67:1064.
101. Sakata S, Nagal K, Maekawa H, et al. Serum ferritin concentration in subacute thyroiditis. *Metab Clin Exp* 1991;40:683–688.
102. Volpe R, Johnston MAW, Huber N. Thyroid function in subacute thyroiditis. *J Clin Endocrinol Metab* 1958;18:65–78.
103. Izumi M, Larsen PR. Correlation of sequential changes in serum thyroglobulin, triiodothyronine, and thyroxine in patients with Graves' disease and subacute thyroiditis. *Metabolism* 1978;27:449–460.
104. Madeddu G, Casu AR, Costanza C, et al. Serum thyroglobulin levels in the diagnosis and follow-up of subacute painful thyroiditis: a sequential study. *Arch Intern Med* 1985;145:243–247.
105. Fragu P, Rougier P, Schlumberger M, Tubiana M. Evolution of thyroid ^{127}I stores measured by x-ray fluorescence in subacute thyroiditis. *J Clin Endocrinol Metab* 1982;54:162–166.
106. Volpe R. Subacute (de Quervain's) thyroiditis. *Baillieres Clin Endocrinol Metab* 1979;8:81–95.
107. Kamio N, Kobayashi I, Mori M, et al. Permissive role of thyrotropin on thyroid radioiodine uptake during the recovery phase of subacute thyroiditis. *Metabolism* 1977;26:295–299.
108. Yamamoto M, Saito S, Sakurada T, et al. Recurrence of subacute thyroiditis over 10 years after the first attack in three cases. *Endocrinol Jpn* 1988;35:833–839.
109. Roti E, Minelli R, Gardini E, Bianconi L, Braverman LE. Iodine-induced hypothyroidism in euthyroid subjects with a previous episode of subacute thyroiditis. *J Clin Endocrinol Metab* 1990;70:1581–1585.
110. Mizukami Y, Michigishi T, Kawato M, Matsubara F. Immunohistochemical and ultrastructural study of subacute thyroiditis, with special reference to multinucleated giant cells. *Hum Pathol* 1987;18:929–935.
111. Schmid KW, Ofner C, Ramsauer T, et al. CA 19-9 expression in subacute (de Quervain's) thyroiditis: an immunohistochemical study. *Mod Pathol* 1992;5:268–272.
112. Yamamoto M, Saito S, Sakurada T, et al. Effect of prednisone and salicylate on serum thyroglobulin level in patients with subacute thyroiditis. *Clin Endocrinol (Oxf)* 1987;27:339–344.
113. Wartofsky L, Schaaf M. Graves' disease with thyrotoxicosis following subacute thyroiditis. *Am J Med* 1987;83:761–764.
114. Fukata S, Matsuzuka F, Kobayashi I, Hirai K, Kuma K, Sugawara M. Development of Graves' disease after subacute thyroiditis: two unusual cases. *Acta Endocrinol* 1992;126:495–496.
115. Singer PA. Thyroiditis: acute, subacute and chronic. *Med Clin North Am* 1991;75:61–77.
116. Blum M, Schloss MF. Martial-arts thyroiditis. *N Engl J Med* 1984;311:199–200.
117. Leckie RG, Buckner AB, Bornemann M. Seat belt-related thyroiditis documented with thyroid Tc-99m pertechnetate scans. *Clin Nucl Med* 1992;17:859–860.
118. Volpe R. Subacute thyroiditis. In: Soto RJ, De Nicola A, Blaquier J, eds. *Physiopathology of endocrine diseases and mechanisms of hormone action*, vol 84. New York: Alan R. Liss, 1981;115–134.
119. Bliddal H, Bech K, Feldt-Rasmussen U, Hoier-Madsen M, Thomsen B, Nielsen H. Humoral autoimmune manifestation in subacute thyroiditis. *Allergy* 1985;40:599–604.
120. Volpe R, Row VV, Ezrin C. Circulating viral and thyroid antibodies in subacute thyroiditis. *J Clin Endocrinol* 1967;27:1275–1284.
121. Weetman AP, Smallridge RC, Nutman TB, Burman KD. Persistent thyroid autoimmunity after subacute thyroiditis. *J Clin Lab Immunol* 1987;23:1–6.
122. Ikenoue H, Okamura K, Kuroda T, Sato K, Yoshinari M, Fujishima M. Thyroid amyloidosis with recurrent subacute thyroiditis-like syndrome. *J Clin Endocrinol Metab* 1988;67:41–45.
123. Martino E, Buratti L, Bartalena L, Cupini C, Aghini-Lombardi F, Pinchera A. High prevalence of subacute thyroiditis during summer season in Italy. *J Endocrinol Invest* 1987;10:321–323.
124. Eylan E, Zmucky R, Sheba CH. Mumps virus and subacute thyroiditis: evidence of a causal association. *Lancet* 1957;1:1062–1063.
125. Rubin RA, Guay AT. Susceptibility to subacute thyroiditis is genetically influenced: familial occurrence in identical twins. *Thyroid* 1991;1:157–161.
126. de Bruin TWA, Riekhoff FPM, de Boer JJ. An outbreak of thyrotoxicosis due to atypical subacute thyroiditis. *J Clin Endocrinol Metab* 1990;70:396–402.
127. Levine SN. Current concepts of thyroiditis. *Arch Intern Med* 1983;143:1952–1956.
128. McGregor AM, Hall R. Thyroiditis. In: DeGroot LJ, Besser GM, Cahill GF Jr, Marshall JC, Nelson DH, Odell WD, Potts JT Jr, Rubenstein AH, Steinberger E, eds. *Endocrinology*, 2nd ed, vol 1. Philadelphia: WB Saunders, 1989;683–701.
129. Weetman AP. Autoimmune thyroiditis: predisposition and pathogenesis. *Clin Endocrinol* 1992;36:307–323.
130. Tomer Y, Davies TF. Infection, thyroid disease, and autoimmunity. *Endocr Rev* 1993;14:107–120.
131. DeGroot LJ, Quintans J. The causes of autoimmune thyroid disease. *Endocr Rev* 1989;10:537–562.
132. Baker JR. Immunologic aspects of endocrine diseases. *Ann Intern Med* 1988;108:26–30.
133. Baker BA, Gharib H, Markowitz H. Correlation of thyroid antibodies and cytologic features in suspected autoimmune thyroid disease. *Am J Med* 1983;74:941–944.
134. Drexhage HA, Bottazzo GF, Doniach D, Bitensky L, Chayen J. Evidence for thyroid-growth-stimulating immunoglobulins in some goitrous thyroid diseases. *Lancet* 1980;2:287–291.
135. Holm L-E, Blomgren H, Lowhagen T. Cancer risks in patients with chronic lymphocytic thyroiditis. *N Engl J Med* 1985;312:601–604.
136. Matsuzuka F, Kuma K, Tominaga S. Chronic thyroiditis as a risk factor of B-cell lymphoma in the thyroid gland. *Jpn J Cancer Res* 1985;76:1085–1090.
137. Ishihara T, Mori T, Waseda N, Ikekubo K, Akamizu T, Imura H. Histological, clinical and laboratory findings of acute exacerbation of Hashimoto's thyroiditis—comparison with those of subacute granulomatous thyroiditis. *Endocrinol Jpn* 1987;34:831–841.
138. Shigemasa C, Ueta Y, Mitani Y, et al. Chronic thyroiditis with painful tender thyroid enlargement and transient thyrotoxicosis. *J Clin Endocrinol Metab* 1990;70:385–390.
139. Hayashi Y, Tamai H, Fukata S, et al. A long term clinical, immunological, and histological follow-up study of patients with goitrous chronic lymphocytic thyroiditis. *J Clin Endocrinol Metab* 1985;61:1172–1178.
140. Kinney J, Fishbein DB, Hurwitz ES, et al. A long-term follow up of patients with autoimmune thyroid disease. *Clin Endocrinol (Oxf)* 1977;6:41–48.
141. Turnbridge WMG. The epidemiology of hyperthyroidism. *Baillieres Clin Endocrinol Metab* 1979;8:21–27.
142. Maenpaa J, Raatikka M, Rasanen J, Taskinen E, Wager O. Natural course of juvenile autoimmune thyroiditis. *J Pediatr* 1985;107:898–904.
143. Dugan JM, Atkinson BF, Avitabile A, Schimmel M, LiVolsi VA. Psammoma bodies in fine needle aspirate of the thyroid in lymphocytic thyroiditis. *Acta Cytol* 1987;31:330–334.
144. Guarda LA, Baskin HJ. Inflammatory and lymphoid lesions of the thyroid gland: cytopathology by fine-needle aspiration. *Am J Clin Pathol* 1987;87 14–22.
145. Nguyen G, Ginsberg J, Crockford PM. Fine needle aspiration biopsy cytology of the thyroid. *Pathol Ann* 1991;26:63–91.
146. Mizukami Y, Michigishi T, Kawato M, et al. Chronic thyroiditis: thyroid function and histologic correlations in 601 cases. *Hum Pathol* 1992;23:980–988.
147. Marks AD, Channick BJ, Adlin EV, Kessler RK, Braitman LE, Denenberg BS. Chronic thyroiditis and mitral valve prolapse. *Ann Intern Med* 1985;102:479–483.
148. Brauman A, Rosenberg T, Gilboa Y, Algom L, Fuchs L, Schlesinger Z. Prevalence of mitral valve prolapse in chronic lymphocytic thyroiditis and nongoitrous hypothyroidism. *Cardiology* 1988;75:269–273.
149. Hamburger JI, Miller JM, Kini SR. Lymphoma of the thyroid. *Ann Intern Med* 1983;99:685–693.
150. Matsubayashi S, Tamai H, Nagai K, Kuma K, Nakagawa T. Mono-

clonal gammopathy in Hashimoto's thyroiditis and malignant lymphoma of the thyroid. *J Clin Endocrinol Metab* 1986;63:1136–1139.
151. Timsit J, Karsenty G, Monteiro R, et al. Hashimoto's thyroiditis with a monoclonal antithyroglobulin autoantibody: disappearance of the monoclonal antibody after thyroidectomy. *J Clin Endocrinol Metab* 1988;66:880–884.
152. Comings DE, Skubi KB, Van Eyes J, Motulsky AG. Familial multifocal fibrosclerosis. *Ann Intern Med* 1967;66:844–892.
153. Hay ID. Thyroiditis: a clinical update. *Mayo Clin Proc* 1985;60:836–843.
154. Schwaegerle SM, Bauer TW, Esselstyn Jr. CB. Riedel's thyroiditis. *Am J Clin Pathol* 1988;90:715–722.
155. Fatourechi V, McConahey WM, Woolner LB. Hyperthyroidism associated with histologic Hashimoto's thyroiditis. *Mayo Clin Proc* 1971;46:682–689.
156. Woolner LB, McConahey WM, Beahrs OH. Invasive fibrous thyroiditis (Riedel's struma). *J Clin Endocrinol Metab* 1957;17:201–220.
157. Taubenberger JK, Marino MJ, Medeiros LJ. A thyroid biopsy with histologic features of both Riedel's thyroiditis and the fibrosing variant of Hashimoto's thyroiditis. *Hum Pathol* 1992;23:1072–1075.
158. Zimmerman-Belsing T, Feldt-Rasmussen U. Riedel's thyroiditis: an autoimmune or primary fibrotic disease? *J Intern Med* 1994;235:271–274.
159. Laitt RD, Hubscher SG, Buckels JA, Darby S, Elias E. Sclerosing cholangitis associated with multifocal fibrosis: a case report. *Gut* 1992;3:1430–1432.
160. McConahey WM. Hashimoto's thyroiditis. *Med Clin North Am* 1972;56:885–896.
161. Fradkin JE, Wolff J. Iodide-induced thyrotoxicosis. *Medicine (Baltimore)* 1983;62:1–20.
162. Amino N, Yabu Y, Mike T, et al. Serum ratio of triiodothyronine to thyroxine, and thyroxine-binding globulin and calcitonin concentrations in Graves' disease and destruction-induced thyrotoxicosis. *J Clin Endocrinol Metab* 1981;53:113–116.

CHAPTER 22

Solitary Thyroid Nodule: Concepts in Diagnosis and Treatment

George L. A. From and Victor G. Lawson

The finding of a solitary nodule on clinical examination of the thyroid gland is a common experience. In the often cited Framingham study (1), nontoxic nodules were found in 3.9% of persons between 30 and 50 years of age, with a further 0.3% having had nodules excised at some previous time. Seventy-two percent of these nodules were considered to be solitary, suggesting an overall prevalence of approximately 3% of the population, with a 5:1 preponderance of women over men. Recent experience with ultrasound studies has revealed nodules in up to 50% of the population beyond the fifth decade of life (2), and more widespread use of these types of diagnostic aids could lead to a substantial increase in patients referred for evaluation. It is important, therefore, to find a way to determine the need for further evaluation and therapy for the patient with a thyroid nodule. Some conditions that may present clinically as solitary nodules in the thyroid gland are listed in Table 1.

The most important consideration in deciding the need for therapy of a thyroid nodule is the possibility of malignancy. Occult cancer is seen in approximately 6% of thyroid glands examined at autopsy, and it may be multicentric and even metastatic to regional lymph nodes without apparent clinical significance (3,4). Most of these occult carcinomas are between 4 and 10 mm in diameter, with the larger ones being at about the threshold for clinical detection. With the possible exception of patients in whom there is a suspicion of medullary carcinoma, delay in diagnosis until the lesion is palpable probably does not affect prognosis. We do not therefore recommend any intervention or further investigation of nodules discovered accidentally by imaging techniques unless they are palpable, or at least exceed 10 mm in their largest dimension. However, once a follicular or papillary carcinoma exceeds 15 mm in size, the possibility of cancer-related death increases, and timely and appropriate therapy may alter the ultimate outcome (5).

CLINICAL CONSIDERATIONS

The history and physical examination of the patient may be of value in determining the direction of subsequent evaluation. Evidence of hyperthyroidism would suggest a hyperfunctioning, or "toxic," adenoma. It is important, however, to realize that in some patients with Graves' disease, the thyroid may enlarge asymmetrically, and the large lobe may be mistaken for a nodule. The radionuclide scan in this situation will show bilateral activity and lead to the correct diagnosis. In the euthyroid patient, the clinical presentation will not usually distinguish between functioning and nonfunctioning nodules.

Sex

The finding of a solitary nodule in an adult woman is common, and the majority of these are benign and often part of a benign nodular goiter, at any age. Thyroid carcinoma is more common in women, but the incidence of malignancy in thyroid nodules in most surgical specimens is somewhat greater in men (6–8). The number of men with carcinoma in each series is small, and the difference is of doubtful statistical significance in any individual report. However, it is a consistent finding and, therefore, it must be assumed that a nodule in a man's thyroid is somewhat more likely to be malignant than one in

---

G. L. A. From: Department of Medicine, University of Toronto, The Toronto Hospital, Toronto, Ontario, Canada M5G 2C4.
V. G. Lawson: Central Kentucky Otolaryngology—Head and Neck Surgical Associates, Bluegrass Medical Center, Paris, Kentucky 40361.

TABLE 1. *Some conditions presenting as solitary thyroid nodule*

Common
Colloid nodule
Thyroid adenoma
Thyroid cyst
Thyroid carcinoma
Thyroiditis
Asymmetrical thyroid enlargement
Uncommon
Thyroid lymphoma
Parathyroid enlargement or cyst
Abscess or infection (including fungal)
Agenesis of contralateral lobe
Hamartoma
Neurofibroma
Amyloid
Metastatic carcinoma

a woman's. It is unclear if this means that the sex of the patient should be a major factor in arriving at a therapeutic decision, because even in men the cumulative experience suggests that the majority of nodules are benign.

Age

Solitary nodules of the thyroid occur infrequently in children, and the incidence of carcinoma in early studies was about 40%, representing about a three- to fourfold increase over the incidence in adults. This has led to the recommendation that biopsy, at least, is indicated in every child (9), and some clinicians would excise all solitary nodules. The prognosis of differentiated thyroid carcinoma in childhood is quite favorable, even with local metastases, and some doubts have been raised about the frequency and importance of malignant lesions in nodular thyroids in children (10,11). In older patients, thyroid nodules are more common and the proportion of malignant nodules is lower (6). However, thyroid cancer diagnosed in men over the age of 40 and women over the age of 50 is more aggressive and has a considerably poorer prognosis (12). It is not clear whether this difference in tumor aggressiveness is related to the appearance of new lesions in older patients, to delay in instituting therapy, or to changes in biologic behavior of longstanding indolent carcinomas. Age alone should not be the sole factor in deciding which therapy is the most appropriate, but it may be of some prognostic significance if a malignancy is found.

History of Radiation Exposure

External irradiation of the thyroid area commonly occurred as a consequence of radiotherapy for enlarged tonsils, thymus, and adenoid tissue in children, and for the treatment of facial acne in adolescents and young adults. The possible relationship between neck irradiation and thyroid carcinoma was suggested by Duffy and Fitzgerald (13) in 1950. They found that nine of a series of 28 children with thyroid carcinoma had a history of thymic irradiation. As attention was focused on this phenomenon, it became apparent that a significant proportion of adults with thyroid carcinoma gave a history of head and neck irradiation during childhood (14). The resulting publicity and recall campaigns have led to many studies to determine if head and neck irradiation is indeed a risk factor. Thyroid carcinomas were found in about 30% (15) to 50% (16) of patients with abnormalities detected by palpation or radionuclide scanning in some studies. But other reports (17,18) failed to substantiate this, finding that carcinoma did not occur any more commonly in these patients than in nonirradiated persons.

It should be noted that in some patients with benign nodules, malignancies detected in surgical specimens were clinically undetectable (carcinoma *in situ*) and at sites other than in the clinically apparent abnormality (16), a situation that under ordinary circumstances (i.e., without another reason for surgery such as palpable nodule) would have been undiscovered or ignored. It is impossible to say if a carcinoma *in situ* in an irradiated patient carries a less favorable prognosis than it does in the general population, except that they are found in younger persons than those in whom these incidental microscopic lesions are usually discovered. Fortunately, radiotherapy for benign conditions of the head and neck is no longer prevalent, so the problem may gradually disappear with the passage of time. However, thyroid abnormalities have been found in adults many years after childhood irradiation of the area (19), so it may be many years before the issue is settled or disappears as a clinical problem.

Radiation exposure of children after the nuclear reactor explosion at Chernobyl (in the Ukraine in 1986) was followed by a marked increase in thyroid carcinoma within a few years. The tumors were predominantly papillary (often follicular variant) and fairly aggressive in their behavior (20,21). The radiation source in these cases was most likely internal in the form of isotopes of iodine rather than external. Thus it appears that both external and internal radiation of the thyroid in children may increase the risk of the subsequent development of differentiated thyroid carcinoma, and this risk may persist for many years.

Physical Characteristics

The findings on physical examination that most reliably suggest a need for surgical therapy are signs of local invasion or metastatic spread. Associated involvement of the vocal cords or respiratory passages by nodules that are not extremely large suggests malignancy, as does enlargement of local lymph nodes. The consistency and texture of the nodule itself is less reliable. Although carcinomas may be stony hard and irregular, so may benign nodules, and some malignant lesions may be rubbery or even softer. Recent increase in size is also unreliable. A painful nodule with a rapid increase in size suggests bleeding into a benign cyst, which is easily evacuated with relief of symptoms. Tenderness may suggest inflammation or infection of the thyroid gland as well as hemorrhage, but it may also occur with anaplastic carcinoma. Finally, a nodule that does not move with swallowing, unless it is firmly fixed to local structures, is likely to be extrathyroidal in origin.

DIAGNOSTIC IMAGING

Ultrasonography

Ultrasound examination is a relatively inexpensive, rapid, and noninvasive technique for the evaluation of a thyroid nodule. As noted previously, it is extremely sensitive and will identify abnormalities in many thyroid glands in which there is no palpable abnormality on clinical examination. In the majority of cases, we disregard these incidental abnormalities even though they may represent occult malignancy. With the exception of familial medullary carcinoma, there is no evidence to suggest that identification or excision of carcinoma *in situ* has any beneficial effect in terms of eventual outcome, and even fine-needle aspiration of these lesions for the purpose of decision-making regarding therapy cannot be recommended. The major role of ultrasound is to determine if the nodule is solid or cystic, and to evaluate the remainder of the thyroid gland. The finding of a multinodular thyroid in which the major nodule is the only one palpable is quite common and often favors a benign diagnosis, although it does not exclude the possibility of carcinoma in any or all of the nodules. Absence of thyroid tissue on the contralateral side suggests that the palpable nodule represents hypertrophic tissue with agenesis of the other lobe.

Ultrasound-assisted fine-needle aspiration can help ensure that the sample for cytologic examination is taken from the most appropriate area. Finally, the accuracy and reproducibility of ultrasonographic measurement is a useful aid in evaluating the progression or regression of the nodule.

Radionuclide Scintigraphy

The radionuclide scan was once the cornerstone of investigation of thyroid nodules, but it has to some extent been superseded by a combination of fine-needle aspiration biopsy (FNAB), ultrasonography, and the ability to detect subclinical hyperthyroidism with reliable assays of thyroid stimulating hormone (TSH). This technique may still, however, sometimes offer useful adjunctive information in certain situations. We do not recommend routine radionuclide scanning of nodules found to be cystic on ultrasound. The scan will show reduced uptake in the cyst, but no further information will be obtained. It is sometimes useful to scan solid nodules to see if there is any associated alteration in radionuclide uptake.

The preliminary scan is usually performed using pertechnetate, and iodine isotopes are reserved for those few patients in whom the nodule concentrates pertechnetate (i.e., it appears warm), but in whom there is still a strong suspicion of malignancy. Most thyroid carcinomas and many benign nodules have defective iodine transport and will concentrate neither pertechnetate nor iodine, and thus they appear as areas of reduced uptake (i.e., cold) on the scan.

The ability to concentrate radionuclide strongly favors a benign process. However, some well-differentiated thyroid malignancies will concentrate iodine and pertechnetate, and they may appear to be warm on early scanning. It is unusual for these tumors to organify iodine, however, and scanning with iodine at 24 hr will show a cold area (22).

The radionuclide scan may show the nodule to be isofunctioning (warm), or hyperfunctioning (hot). The latter situation, especially if accompanied by reduced or absent uptake in normal thyroid tissue, suggests a toxic adenoma that may eventually secrete sufficient thyroid hormone to render the patient thyrotoxic. It is the hot nodule that can be diagnosed correctly only with a radionuclide scan, and that may be indistinguishable from a cellular follicular neoplasm on aspiration cytology. For this reason, a thyroid scan is essential in any patient in whom the TSH is suppressed to below the normal level. In other patients routine radionuclide scanning is not mandatory but may occasionally be useful.

Radiography

Examination of the thyroid area using classic x-ray imaging is of limited value because the extent of the gland can be better visualized by other means. However, simple x-rays may show the extent of tracheal deviation, and the presence of flecks of calcification in the nodule area is suggestive of calcospherites (psammoma bodies) of well-differentiated carcinoma.

Computerized Tomography and Magnetic Resonance Imaging

The thyroid gland is well visualized on computerized tomography (CT) (23). The resolution of nodules is no better than with ultrasonography, however, and the radiation dose is significant. Magnetic resonance imaging (MRI) is a relatively new technique, and the experience is more limited, as is the availability of equipment. Imaging with high-field-strength surface-coil MRI can be useful in detecting malignant lesions because of the ability to detect irregular margins of the carcinomas, as compared to benign lesions, and to identify cervical lymph nodes that may be the site of metastases (24). Although at this time these techniques do not offer any major diagnostic advantage over ultrasonography, they do provide superior anatomic images that may be of value to the surgeon.

FINE-NEEDLE ASPIRATION BIOPSY

Fine-needle aspiration biopsy with cytologic examination of the aspirate has become a widespread diagnostic aid. Large-needle biopsy has not gained wide acceptance because of the expertise required to perform the procedure safely, and the (largely unfounded) fear of spreading carcinoma along the needle track. Fine-needle aspiration is much easier to learn, and, in collaboration with an experienced cytopathologist, can give very useful information and reduce the need for more costly and more elaborate diagnostic tests. We prefer to use a 22- or 23-gauge needle; a finer needle may yield a good specimen for cytopathology, but it may be too fine to drain a thyroid cyst, whereas a larger needle often results in a bloody aspirate. The highly viscous contents of a colloid goiter cannot be drained with even these larger needles, but sufficient material can be aspirated to make the diagnosis obvious immediately, and more liquid contents can often be removed almost completely, with resolution of the nodule.

Thin, straw-colored fluid is nearly always associated with a benign cyst, and although it may reaccumulate and require further aspiration or excision, it allows the physician to give the patient a more favorable prognosis immediately. Clear watery fluid suggests a parathyroid cyst, and parathyroid hormone assay of the fluid will confirm the diagnosis. The finding of hemorrhagic fluid may carry a somewhat higher risk of malignancy, and the patient is told that the initial impression is favorable, but the final answer must await interpretation of the cytology and repeat aspiration if the initial results are unsatisfactory. Residual nodularity after aspiration of fluid contents requires further evaluation such as ultrasonography, and possibly further FNAB under ultrasonographic control. Indeed, ultrasonographic guidance improves needle placement for FNAB in lesions that are inhomogeneous or difficult to palpate (25,26). Lesions as small as 5 mm may be biopsied, which can prove useful if multicentric metastatic disease is suspected. However, because the clinical significance of differentiated carcinoma *in situ* is questionable (4), we do not recommend routine biopsy of nodules found by ultrasonography alone if they are smaller than 10 mm.

Diagnostic accuracy is quite high if the cytology is positive for malignancy (27–29), and surgery is recommended in the majority of cases. A positive diagnosis of an inflammatory or infective process also alters the course of further investigation. Unfortunately, in the case of differentiated follicular cell neoplasms, distinction between benign and malignant lesions is impossible on cytologic examination of fine-needle aspirate, and cellular follicular aspirates are considered suspicious for malignancy (unless hyperfunctioning), usually resulting in excision for definitive pathological examination.

There is some evidence that proton magnetic spectroscopy may distinguish benign from malignant tissue, and application of this technique on fine-needle aspirates may obviate the need for surgery for purely diagnostic purposes (30). Lesions that are nondiagnostic but clinically suspicious may require multiple aspirations and ultimately surgical exploration based on other criteria before a diagnosis is finally established. Nevertheless, if properly carried out and interpreted, fine-needle aspiration is a very useful diagnostic modality that can improve the selection of patients for further investigation or treatment.

LABORATORY EVALUATION

Assessment of Thyroid Function

The presence of hyperthyroidism or hypothyroidism in a patient with a thyroid nodule is of major importance, in terms of both defining the diagnostic probabilities and determining the form of therapy. Although the clinical assessment is of major importance in the evaluation of thyroid status, the final diagnosis rests on finding abnormal levels of thyroid hormones in the serum. We recommend routine assessment of TSH. The finding of hypothyroidism suggests that the nodule may be part of a more generalized thyroid disorder that must be characterized. The nodule itself, however, still requires independent assessment, because malignancy may coexist with other forms of thyroid pathology. Suppressed levels of TSH with or without elevated levels of thyroid hormones may be seen in patients with autonomously functioning adenomas, or in whom more diffusely affected thyroid glands (e.g., Graves' disease) have enlarged irregularly or asymmetrically. Radionuclide scintigraphy is recommended in patients with increased or decreased thyroid function, and, if the nodule is hypofunctioning, cytologic examination should be carried out. In either situation, the attainment of a euthyroid state becomes the primary concern, for even if surgical intervention is decided upon, it is seldom so urgent that it cannot be postponed until after abnormalities of function have been corrected.

Antibody Studies

Tests for thyroid autoantibodies should also be performed. Hashimoto's thyroiditis may present with unilateral enlargement. The appearance of a new nodule, or thyroid enlargement, in a patient with Hashimoto's disease should also alert the physician to the possibility of lymphoma of the thyroid gland (31,32).

Serum Thyroglobulin

Increased levels of thyroglobulin in the serum are commonly encountered in patients with differentiated thyroid carcinoma. However, this finding is not specific, because elevated levels may be seen in a variety of benign thyroid disorders, including goiters, adenomas, inflammatory conditions, and hyperthyroidism (33). Patients with undifferentiated thyroid carcinoma and medullary carcinoma usually have normal levels. Measurement of serum thyroglobulin is of limited value in the diagnostic workup of a thyroid nodule, and it is not useful as a routine procedure to detect malignancy. A suppression of serum thyroglobulin in response to levothyroxine administration may be a useful indicator of the efficacy of this form of therapy in reducing the size of thyroid nodules (34).

Serum Calcitonin

Serum calcitonin is a useful marker for medullary thyroid carcinoma. Routine measurement of calcitonin is not recommended except in situations where there is a family history of this disorder or related features of multiple endocrine neoplasia. If medullary carcinoma is found, serum calcitonin measurement with provocative stimulation, if necessary, is carried out in family members for screening purposes, and in the patient to determine adequacy of therapy, or recurrence.

THYROID CYSTS

Purely or partially cystic thyroid nodules account for between 6% and 25% of solitary thyroid nodules (35). The majority of purely cystic lesions are benign, although some thyroid carcinomas may have cystic components or even be purely cystic (35). Symptoms may be produced acutely by hemorrhage into a cyst that results in painful enlargement, or more gradually by growth and pressure.

Aspiration of cyst contents may be followed by complete resolution, or gradual or rapid reaccumulation of fluid. We routinely aspirate thyroid cystic lesions for therapeutic and diagnostic (cytology) purposes. Residual tissue after aspiration is viewed as any other thyroid nodule, and reassessed and treated as necessary. Recurrent cysts may be reaspirated or excised. Some authors have found that instillation of tetracycline as a sclerosing agent may be beneficial in preventing recurrence (36). Whether or not thyroxine administration reduces the reaccumulation of cyst contents is questionable (35), and its use is optional. Follow-up is important, however, because the occasional cystic lesion may prove to be malignant.

AUTONOMOUSLY FUNCTIONING THYROID NODULES

The autonomously functioning thyroid nodule is a functioning nodule that is independent of pituitary function and unrelated to the function of the remaining thyroid tissue (37). It may produce sufficient thyroid hormone to render the patient thyrotoxic, or at least to suppress TSH, in which case the remaining normal thyroid tissue may become atrophic and fail to concentrate radionuclide, and thus the nodule appears hot on scanning. Rarely, it may appear to be isofunctioning on initial scan, and autonomy of function is established only when it fails to suppress after administration of thyroid hormones.

Functioning thyroid nodules are very unlikely to be malignant (38), and the main indication for therapy is the presence of, or potential for development of, hyperthyroidism. Hyperthyroidism, sometimes with only an increased triiodothyronine level (T_3 toxicosis), is usually associated with nodules larger than 3 cm. Those smaller than 2 cm seldom change much in size or function when followed for up to 10 years (39).

Occasionally, a unilateral thyroid gland may be mistaken for a hot nodule on radionuclide scanning, and for this reason ultrasonographic identification of the contralateral lobe is recommended. Normal thyroid tissue that has been suppressed and thus rendered invisible on the usual radionuclide scan using iodine, or pertechnetate, may be stimulated by TSH and identified by a repeat scan. This technique, however, is potentially hazardous, because it may result in additional thyroid hormone secretion; it should be avoided in patients who are hyperthyroid and in the elderly. Suppressed thyroid tissue has been shown to concentrate thallium-201 sufficiently to be seen on a scan using this agent, thus eliminating the need for TSH stimulation (40).

Identification of suppressed thyroid tissue is of less importance in the hyperthyroid patient, because radioablation or excision of the hyperfunctioning tissue is still necessary. If the nodule is warm (i.e., it is not associated with suppression of the remainder of the gland) and the patient is euthyroid, administration of 75 to 100 μg of triiodothyronine, or 150 to 200 μg of sodium levothyroxine for 7 to 10 days, followed by rescanning, will show tissue that is autonomously functioning. This procedure may produce symptomatic hyperthyroidism in the occasional patient, and is best avoided in the elderly.

Suppressed levels of TSH, or lack of TSH response to thyrotropin-releasing hormone (TRH), also suggests autonomy of function. The hyperthyroid patient with a solitary autonomously functioning nodule requires therapy, and our method of choice in younger patients is surgical excision after a euthyroid state is achieved with antithyroid medication (41). In older patients, the nodule may be ablated with iodine-131. The radiation dose required is relatively high, because the iodine uptake is often in the normal range, and in spite of the apparent suppression of normal thyroid tissue, hypothyroidism may follow in some cases (42), and the palpable nodule, although often smaller, tends to remain, and becomes cold.

In the euthyroid patient with an autonomous nodule, the necessity for therapy remains controversial. Although some nodules become hyperfunctioning, and cause symptoms, most of the small ones will change little over many years. We favor removal, or radioablation, of nodules over 3 cm in size, and follow-up of smaller lesions. Percutaneous ethanol injection (43) has been used successfully in some patients with small autonomously functioning thyroid nodules. The absence of radiation exposure and scarring make this procedure an attractive alternative to surgery or radioiodine therapy in some patients. We have had no personal experience with this technique. Thyroxine suppression is of no value in this disorder and may produce iatrogenic thyrotoxicosis. It is essential that if no definitive therapy is carried out, lifelong follow-up should be maintained.

SOLID OR MIXED CYSTIC/SOLID NONFUNCTIONING (COLD) NODULES

The management of the patient with a thyroid nodule that is not purely cystic, and nonfunctioning, remains one of the more controversial areas in clinical medicine. If the nodule is symptomatic, because of mechanical interference with local structures such as respiratory passages, laryngeal function, or the pharynx, attempts at mass reduction or excision are necessary. Cystic degeneration with recurrent hemorrhages with pain and enlargement of the nodule are also good reasons for its removal. If a nodule is a cosmetic nuisance, surgical therapy is probably justified if thyroxine administration fails to reduce its size. It is the identification of the patient harboring a malignancy, and the effect of therapy on the prognosis of the malignancy, that remain controversial. Cancerphobia is prevalent among both physicians and patients, and in the absence of evidence that observation or conservative therapy is superior, nodules that are highly suspicious, on either clinical or cytologic grounds, are usually excised, unless there is a definite contraindication for surgery. This is not to imply that there is evidence that significant numbers of lives will be saved by this approach.

The true incidence of malignancy in thyroid nodules is difficult to assess. Most of the published data refer to surgical series, and the number of malignancies found will depend on the selection criteria used for referral and subsequent surgery, as well as the pathologist's impression of lesions that are difficult to interpret. It is of interest that in the Framingham study (1), no malignant lesions were identified in 64 nodules excised, before or during the study period. A review of various reports shows the probability of malignancy in thyroid nodules to be about 11% of all nodules and 17% of cold nodules (44), but individual reports vary from between 0% and 1.5% (1,45) to over 30% (46), which may reflect variable criteria in patient selection or referral for surgery.

Thyroxine Suppression

The administration of oral thyroid hormone to reduce the size of thyroid nodules and goiters has been popular for 30 years. It is based on the assumption that thyroid tissue, which is dependent on TSH, will regress if TSH is suppressed. The efficacy of this form of therapy is difficult to assess, because criteria for TSH suppression and methods of assessing response have been so variable. Historically, about 30% of thyroid nodules may be suppressed with thyroid feeding (44), but individual reports are highly variable and more recent studies are less optimistic.

Unfortunately, suppressibility does not distinguish between benign and malignant nodules sufficiently to be useful for diagnostic purposes, with about 16% of malignant and 21% of benign nodules being suppressible in studies that correlate with the final diagnosis (44). The ultrasensitive TSH assays and ultrasonography that are now available offer more objective criteria for efficacy of therapy on which future recommendations may be based. Using these criteria, several studies suggest that thyroxine suppression is less effective than previously believed (47,48). Suppression may cause the occasional nodule to shrink, and if the patient is otherwise healthy this form of therapy may be attempted. If there is no reduction in the size of the nodule after 2 to 3 months, the thyroxine may be stopped and the patient simply followed clinically and ultrasonographically. If the nodule increases in size, surgical removal may be considered.

MANAGEMENT REGIMEN FOR THE EUTHYROID PATIENT WITH AN ASYMPTOMATIC THYROID NODULE

The ideal management regimen would identify a high proportion of lesions that should be surgically excised in a convenient, cost-effective manner, avoiding unnecessary surgery or other forms of therapeutic or diagnostic intervention in patients who do not require them. There is probably no single best approach to the problem, but we have been able to formulate certain useful guidelines (Fig. 1). We do not generally single out any group of patients for surgical therapy, except those in whom there is suspicion of familial forms of thyroid cancer. There is some justification to being more aggressive with male patients and patients exposed to external radiation, but not enough to consider routine surgical excision.

Clinical suspicion of malignancy, such as fixation, invasion, or lymphadenopathy, is an indication for surgery. The recommended initial investigative procedure in the

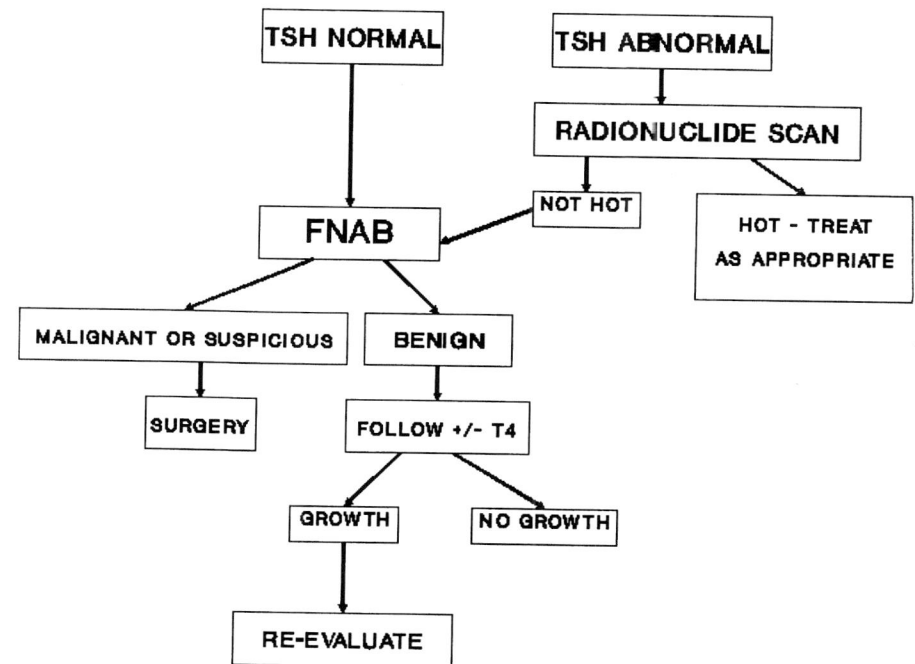

FIG. 1. Suggested sequence for the investigation of a patient with a thyroid nodule. Fine-needle aspiration biopsy (FNAB) is the usual initial procedure if the TSH is normal, with radionuclide scanning recommended if TSH is abnormal (especially if suppressed). Levothyroxine (T_4) suppression may be attempted in some cases, but has been disappointing. Assessment of size, both initially and subsequently, is usually done by ultrasonography.

euthyroid patient of lesions larger than 10 mm is the FNAB. Smaller lesions, if discovered accidentally are followed to see if they progress. Malignant or suspicious cytology is indication for surgical excision, as are lesions that are troublesome to the patient, such as recurrent or painful cysts or nodules that are a cosmetic nuisance. Radionuclide scanning is done routinely if the TSH is abnormal. Scanning of nodules routinely if the TSH is normal is optional; we find that the distinction between cold and warm nodules, at least with pertechnetate scans, is of limited diagnostic value. Iodine-123 scans may be more useful, but the added expense must be considered in the light of additional information obtained.

Most patients who do not have suppressed levels of TSH and have benign cytology may be given a trial of suppression therapy with levothyroxine, or simply followed after initial ultrasound assessment of size and, if the lesion remains stable or regresses, followed indefinitely. Nodules that continue to grow are usually removed surgically, or at least rebiopsied, and many of those that fail to decrease in size during suppression therapy will eventually be removed for a variety of reasons, including a desire by the patient to be rid of the nodule, or to get a tissue diagnosis. This approach leads to a high yield of thyroid carcinomas in those patients who are treated surgically on the basis of initial investigation, and a low yield in those who are operated on at a later time. There may be occasional patients who continue to harbor low-grade malignancies, but there is no evidence that their health or life expectancies have been compromised by this approach.

SURGICAL CONSIDERATIONS AND PREOPERATIVE CONCEPTS

Indications

The recommendation to advise surgery for a solitary nodule should come jointly from the endocrinologist and surgeon, with the concurrence of the referring physician. The patient is told that surgery is being recommended, and for clearly stated reasons. If malignancy is suspected, the incidence of such disease should be put into perspective for the patient. If the nodule is being removed because of a pressure sensation in the neck, for functional reasons, or for cosmetic reasons, the patient should clearly understand the reason as well as the change in symptomatology that can be expected once the nodule is removed.

Clinical Examination

Although the patient may have already been examined by at least three physicians, it is important to remember that a detailed preoperative clinical examination immediately prior to surgery is essential. This should be undertaken by the surgeon or his or her designate. It should include a careful examination of the thyroid gland, and complete palpation of both sides of the neck. The size of the thyroid nodule, its consistency, and its mobility should be carefully documented.

Similarly, any nodal enlargement is noted and recorded. The movement of the cervical spine is examined. Loss of extension or flexion resulting from abnormalities in the cervical spine may impair adequate positioning of the patient during surgery or may result in unusual postoperative neck discomfort. The upper aerodigestive tract is examined for evidence of ectopic thyroid tissue involving the mucosa; displacement, compression, or infiltration of the larynx or trachea; impairment of recurrent or superior laryngeal nerve function; and pooling of secretions in the hypopharynx. A description of the voice is recorded, and any coincidental findings that might affect voice production, such as smoker's laryngitis, vocal nodules, or hypertrophy of the false vocal cords, is noted. If a wheeze or stridor (inspiratory, biphasic, or expiratory) is present, it should be accurately described and evaluated.

The thyroid function must be documented biochemically prior to surgery. If the patient is hyperthyroid or hypothyroid, the functional abnormality is corrected prior to surgery. Preoperative calcium assessment is also necessary, not only as it will relate to postoperative management, but also for the purpose of screening for coexistent parathyroid disease. The incidence of parathyroid disorders in surgery for thyroid disease is reported at 0.43%, compared with 0.1% in the general population (49). Although this is statistically low, it is important to have a calcium level done preoperatively so that a detailed investigation can be undertaken prior to surgery, if indicated. If the patient is hypercalcemic, it is important to know if the patient has symptoms caused by the hypercalcemia and to prepare the patient properly for a possible combined thyroid/parathyroid surgical procedure. If medullary carcinoma is suspected, serum calcitonin levels are obtained. Thyroid antibody levels are obtained in all patients with solitary nodules. A study by Ott et al. (50) suggests that there is a higher incidence of carcinoma in coexistent Hashimoto's thyroiditis. Although a lymphoma may arise as a primary tumor in the thyroid gland, it too is more common with coexistent Hashimoto's thyroiditis. Antibody screening may alert the surgeon to the presence of Hashimoto's thyroiditis.

Imaging

As a function of usefulness and cost-effectiveness, ultrasound and CT scanning provide the most information from a surgical management perspective. Ultrasound provides a detailed image of the thyroid gland. CT scanning will give complementary imaging of the thyroid gland, along with detailed information regarding the contiguous airway, blood vessels, and lymph nodes (Fig. 2). It is now our practice to use these two modalities routinely with all solitary thyroid nodules. Also, occult thyroid disease may be identified on CT and ultrasound imaging (Fig. 3). If esophageal disease is suspected, a contrast study is obtained. If aberrant vasculature is suspected, angiography must be done. If the imaging suggests involvement of the upper aerodigestive tract, an endoscopic examination is indicated prior to the definitive operative procedure.

Patient Preparation

Once surgery has been recommended, the surgical strategy and the nature of the procedure should be fully explained to the patient. With solitary nodules, the patient is told that the procedure will be performed under a general anesthesia. An incision measuring 4 to 8 cm in length, placed in the root of the neck, is used for the average-sized neck, and the average type of thyroid nodule.

Initially, a hemithyroidectomy or a subtotal thyroidectomy is performed for diagnostic and therapeutic purposes. The tissue is then submitted to the pathologist for frozen section examination. If the frozen section examination indicates benign disease, the procedure is terminated. However, there is a small chance (approximately 5%) of a different final report, which may result in the need for a later completion thyroidectomy. This is particularly so if a follicular tumor is present. If the pathologist reports a carcinoma, the usual strategy is to do a completion thyroidectomy immediately. If a lymphoma is present, the surgical procedure is generally discontinued af-

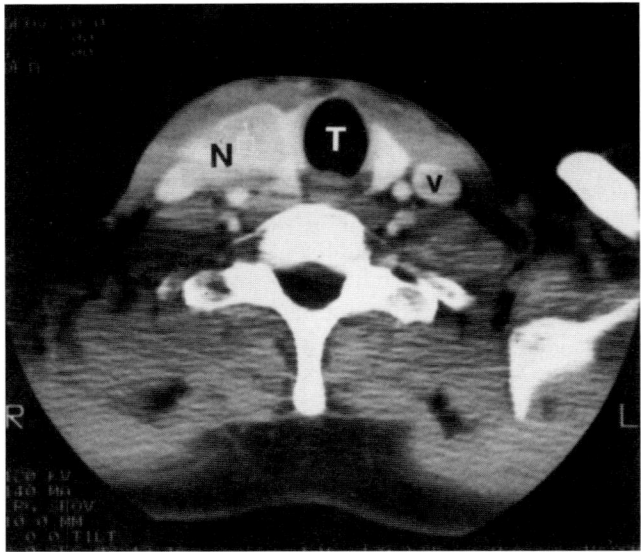

FIG. 2. Computerized tomography (CT) scan of the neck. N, solitary thyroid nodule; T, trachea; V, internal jugular vein.

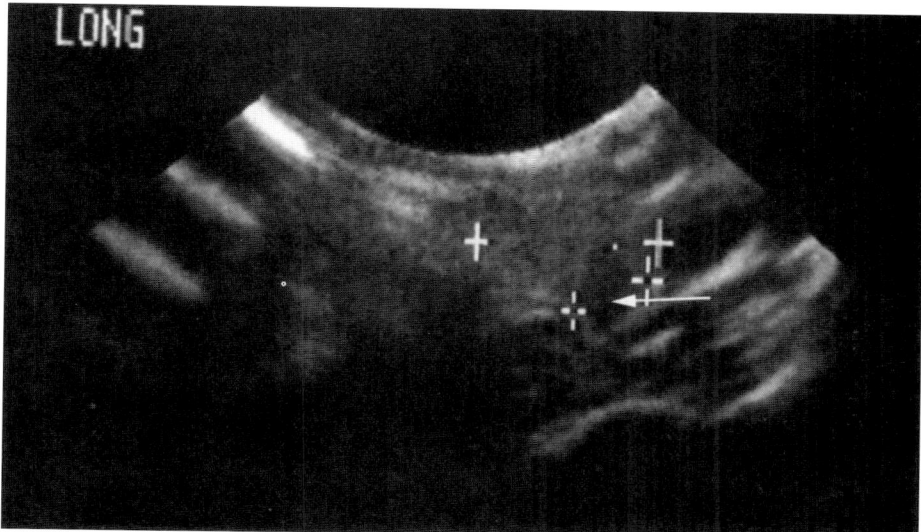

FIG. 3. Ultrasound examination of thyroid gland. *Arrow* points to a 5-mm hypoechoic area that was found to be an occult (nonpalpable) focus of medullary carcinoma on histopathologic examination of the thyroidectomy specimen from a patient with the familial form of the disease.

ter the diagnosis is made or debulking is achieved. If there is infiltrative disease, involving strap muscles, nodes, or other soft tissues, a functional, modified, or radical neck dissection is performed depending on the specific extent of the disease. If the airway is infiltrated, an airway resection is usually done *en bloc* with the thyroid and neck resection, followed by immediate airway reconstruction. Surgery for airway infiltration would entail the use of a defunctioning tracheostomy in most instances.

The patient is told that the recurrent laryngeal nerves and superior laryngeal nerves are at risk with all thyroid procedures. Although the risks are extremely small, impairment of function can result. If the recurrent laryngeal nerves are damaged, the disability may range from changes in the voice, such as hoarseness, breathiness, and weakness, to airway distress. If the superior laryngeal nerves are damaged, there may be a change in the pitch of the voice.

The parathyroid glands are also at risk in thyroid surgery. The patient is told that the glands usually need to be repositioned during the thyroid procedure, and that they may sustain vascular damage during this process. The patient is also told that the location, the size, and the number of glands (ranging from two to six glands) are variable, so there is a small risk that the glands may be taken out inadvertently during the procedure. Occasionally, it is necessary to transplant the parathyroid glands into adjoining or distant muscle in order to conserve parathyroid function. However, if parathyroid function should fail, despite all of the precautions that are taken to conserve it, the patient will require calcium and vitamin D supplements temporarily or permanently. The incidence of parathyroid gland dysfunction in primary surgery for solitary thyroid nodules is extremely low. However, the incidence becomes somewhat greater at reoperation.

The patient is also advised that there is a small risk of postoperative hemorrhage. If a hematoma results, reopening of the wound is necessary and the patient may also require blood replacement. Ordinarily, one would not expect to replace blood during resection of a solitary thyroid nodule. There is also a small risk of wound infection. Such an occurrence would require antibiotic treatment.

The patient is told that he will be hospitalized for 1 day with a routine thyroid nodule, and up to 3 days with a complex thyroid nodule requiring extensive surgery and/or a neck dissection. The patient will have a suction drain (usually a small Argyle drain connected to an Emmerson pump at negative pressure 30) for 1 to 2 days postoperatively. Negative pressure suctioning reduces the incidence of postoperative hematoma formation. The patient is advised to remain off work from 10 to 14 days after surgery for a routine thyroid nodule.

If a malignant thyroid disorder is diagnosed, the patient will be advised to remain off thyroid replacement therapy for 4 to 6 weeks so that a whole-body radioisotope scan can be done to assess for metastatic disease. The patient may then require a therapeutic dose of radioactive iodine, and in rare instances the postoperative therapy may also include external beam irradiation of the neck. Such additional treatment could prolong the patient's morbidity.

Finally, the patient is told that in most instances it is advised that exogenous thyroxine be taken indefinitely after a partial thyroidectomy to reduce the risk of new disease developing in the remaining thyroid tissue. If a total thyroidectomy is performed, the patient will require thyroid replacement medication for physiologic purposes.

Informed Consent

After the standard preparation, the patient is asked if he or she requires any further explanation or has any questions. If the patient understands the proposed operative procedure and the inherent (albeit small) risks, as well as the potential benefits to be achieved, a consent is obtained for thyroidectomy, and, if necessary, endoscopy, neck dissection, and laryngotracheal resection. Such careful preparation and informed consent will optimize results and lessen the chance of patient management problems postoperatively.

INTRAOPERATIVE CONCEPTS

Anesthesia

Ordinarily, a thyroidectomy is performed under general anesthesia. Having chosen a suitably sized endotracheal tube, the anesthetist must be prepared to down-size the endotracheal tube if the airway is significantly distorted or infiltrated by the nodule. In those situations, the endotracheal tube must be introduced more carefully than usual in an effort to avoid mucosal trauma. The endotracheal tube and circuitry are carried over the superior part of the face. It is carefully secured to the middle third of the face with proper protection of the eyes. Extra length circuitry is used. The circuitry is then carried around the left side of the head and down the left side of the operating table to an anesthesia machine placed at the midportion of the operating table on the left side. Such an arrangement allows the surgeon and the team full access to the head and neck. Esophageal stethoscopes and temperature monitors should not be placed in the esophagus, as they tend to displace the cervical esophagus and make it more difficult to locate the recurrent laryngeal nerves in the tracheoesophageal groove.

Endoscopy

If there is a history of hoarseness or hemoptysis, or if the clinical examination or imaging studies show significant displacement, compression, or infiltration of the larynx, trachea, or esophagus, an endoscopic examination is indicated. Generally, rigid laryngoscopes, bronchoscopes, and esophagoscopes are used. The procedure is done immediately after induction of the anesthetic. Venturi jet ventilation is used for the laryngoscopic and bronchoscopic components of the examination. The patient is then intubated; in the case of a particularly difficult intubation, this is often best done by the surgeon who has already inspected the upper airway. The esophagoscopic examination is then completed with the endotracheal tube in place.

Positioning

It is essential that the patient be properly positioned on the operating table to optimize the surgical procedure and the therapeutic, functional, and cosmetic end result. The patient must be positioned symmetrically, with the proper amount of head and neck extension so that the head is supported and so that the incisions can be planned accurately. Full surgical access is necessary, not only in the region of the thyroid gland, but also to both sides of the neck, and possibly the upper chest. If the patient is properly positioned and draped, incisions can be extended as necessary.

Technique

There are many important technical considerations that will allow the surgeon to optimize the therapeutic and functional result. The skin incision should be planned carefully, not only in terms of length, but also in terms of neck topography. If the neck is long with the cricoid at the midportion of the neck, and 6 to 7 cm of cervical trachea in the neck, the incision must be placed higher than usual. Ordinarily, one would place a thyroidectomy incision 1 cm above the sternoclavicular joints, in a lower neck crease (Fig. 4). However, with a longer neck, the incision might require placement 3 or even 4 cm above that point (Fig. 5). If the incision is placed too low, it can be difficult to ligate the superior vascular pedicles or to remove a long pyramidal lobe (Fig. 6). In a small neck, the incision can be 4 cm in length. In a larger neck with a larger gland or nodule, it may need to be 8 cm in length. If the thyroid nodule is large and predominantly unilateral, one must adjust the incision to compensate for the asymmetrical distortion of the skin of the neck by the nodule (Figs. 7,8). Failure to do this will result in an asymmetric scar that may be quite unsightly. The skin flap should include subcutaneous tissue and platysma unless tumor extends into those sites. All pen markouts that are not used for incisions should be erased at the end of the operative procedure.

After the flaps are elevated, the sternomastoid muscles should be mobilized on both sides of the neck, with resultant exposure of the omohyoid muscles and the carotid sheaths. It is important to identify the deep carotid, internal jugular, and omohyoid lymph nodes that are most proximal to the thyroid nodule. If the nodes are enlarged, they require sampling and frozen section analysis. After the sternomastoid muscles are mobilized and the perithyroid tissues are examined, the strap muscles are incised in the midline and divided on the ipsilateral side, if the nodule is large or impacted in the inlet (Fig. 9). However, if the nodule is small, the strap muscles may be retracted, rather than divided, for adequate exposure. Preferably, the strap muscles should be divided above or below the level of the skin incision, rather than at the level of the skin incision, to avoid overlying

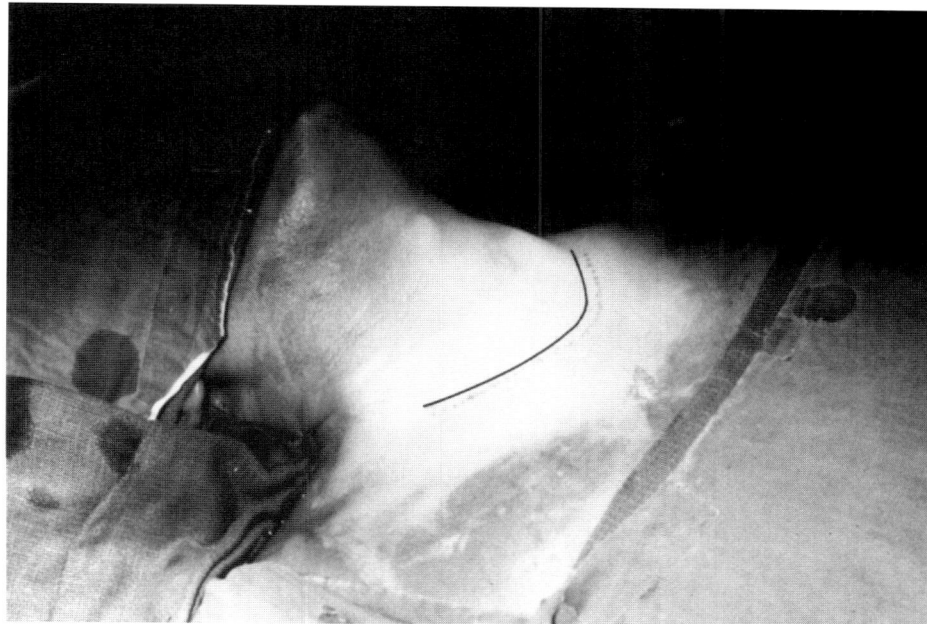

FIG. 4. Usual placement of a thyroid incision 1 cm above sternoclavicular joints and clavicles. *Solid line* indicates the incision. *Dotted line* indicates the sternoclavicular joints and clavicles.

skin and muscle incisions that might result in scar contracture and tenting of the skin postoperatively.

The usual surgical strategy is to mobilize the involved lobe by clearing, ligating, and dividing the inferior and middle thyroid veins. The thyroid gland is carefully retracted using finger retraction, and the ispilateral recurrent laryngeal nerve is identified prior to division of branches of the inferior thyroid artery to the thyroid gland. However, with large or impacted nodules, it may be necessary to mobilize the superior pole of the thyroid gland by dividing the superior vascular pedicle. This results in increased mobility of the gland and better access

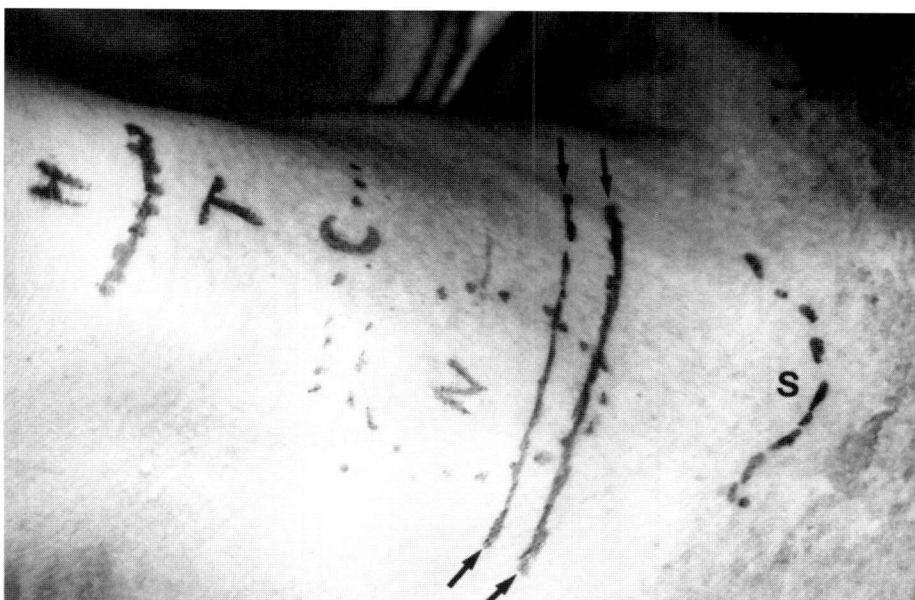

FIG. 5. Long neck with incision planned 3 to 4 cm above the sternoclavicular joint. *Arrows* are placed on possible incisions. The uppermost incision was chosen because of a fine skin crease at that level. H, hyoid; T, thyroid alae; C, cricoid; N, solitary nodule; S, suprasterna notch.

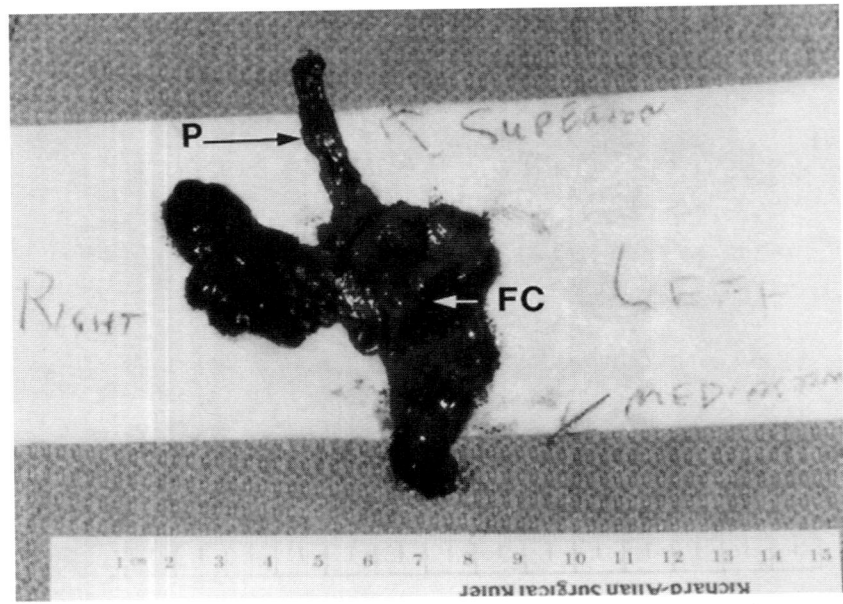

FIG. 6. The importance of accurate incision placement. There is a long pyramidal lobe (P) that extended superiorly to the level of the hyoid bone, and a pathological left lobe (follicular carcinoma, FC) that extended inferiorly into the thoracic inlet.

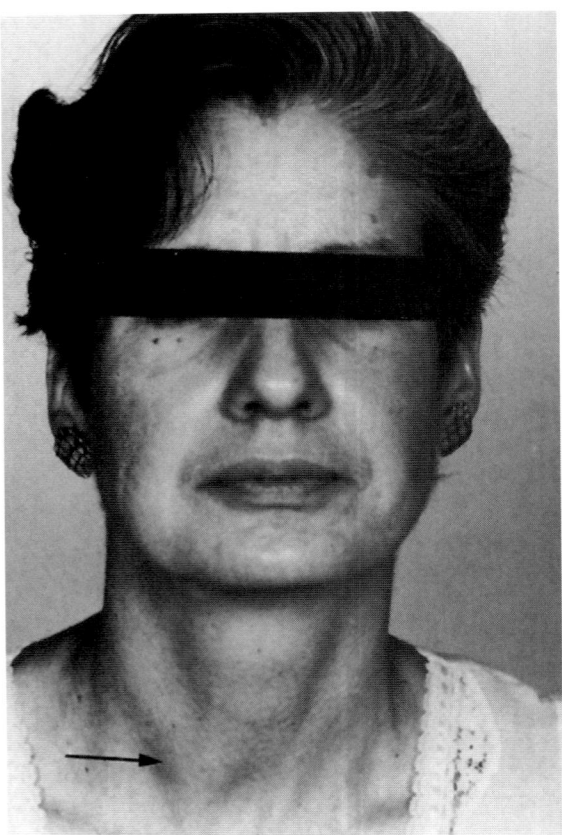

FIG. 7. Anterior view of neck showing distortion of the neck skin and right sternocleidomastoid muscle by a moderately large unilateral solitary thyroid nodule *(arrow)*.

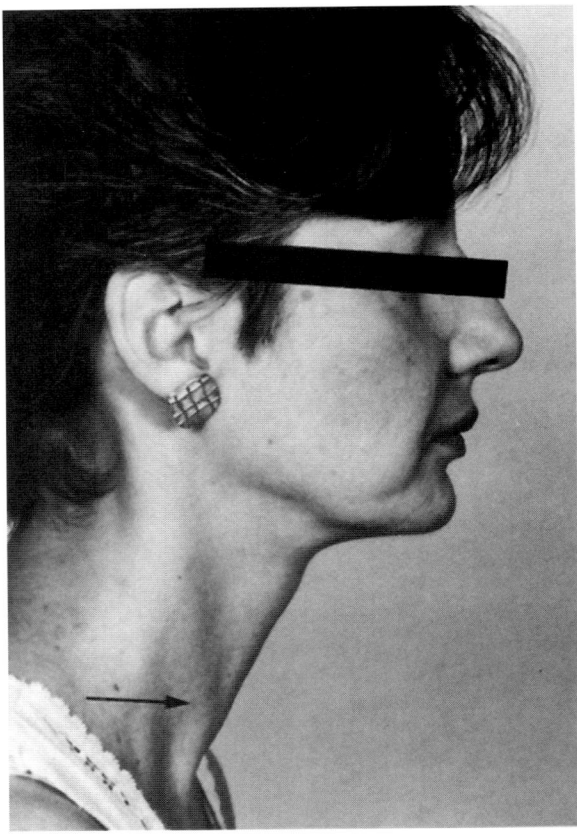

FIG. 8. Lateral view of neck showing distortion of neck skin and right sternocleidomastoid muscle by a moderately large solitary thyroid nodule *(arrow)*.

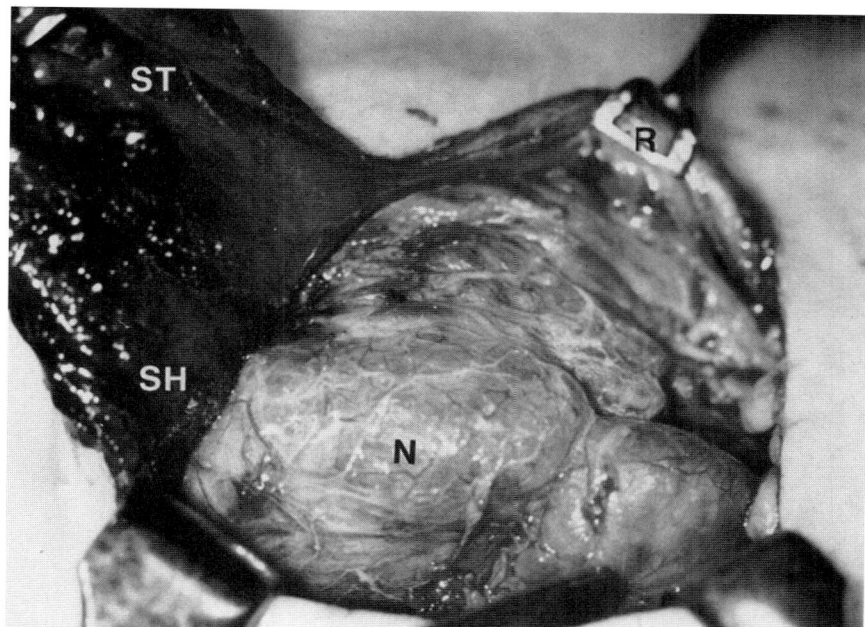

FIG. 9. The divided right sternothyroid (ST) and right sternchyoid (SH) muscles, as well as the retracted left strap muscles (R). A large right solitary thyroid nodule (N) is evident.

to the recurrent laryngeal nerve. During the mobilization process, the surgeon must always be on the lookout for parathyroid glands (Fig. 10). If the glands are identified, they are best preserved *in situ*. If that is not possible, they can be removed and placed into cool Ringer's solution for later reimplantation after the thyroid gland has been resected.

Histopathological confirmation of parathyroid tissue may be necessary. This is done by taking a 2-mm incisional biopsy of the parathyroid gland. Fine vascular forceps (Cooley's) are used to do such a biopsy as atraumatically as possible.

If the nodule is well placed laterally in the affected lobe of the thyroid gland, a hemithyroidectomy is done to

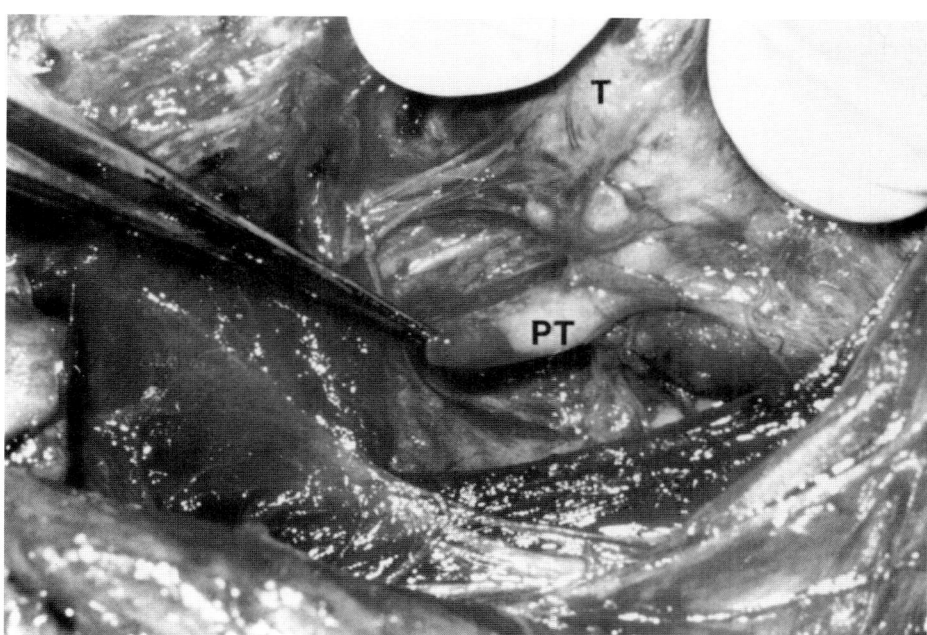

FIG. 10. The thyroid gland (T) is retracted medially to expose a hyperplastic parathyroid gland (PT).

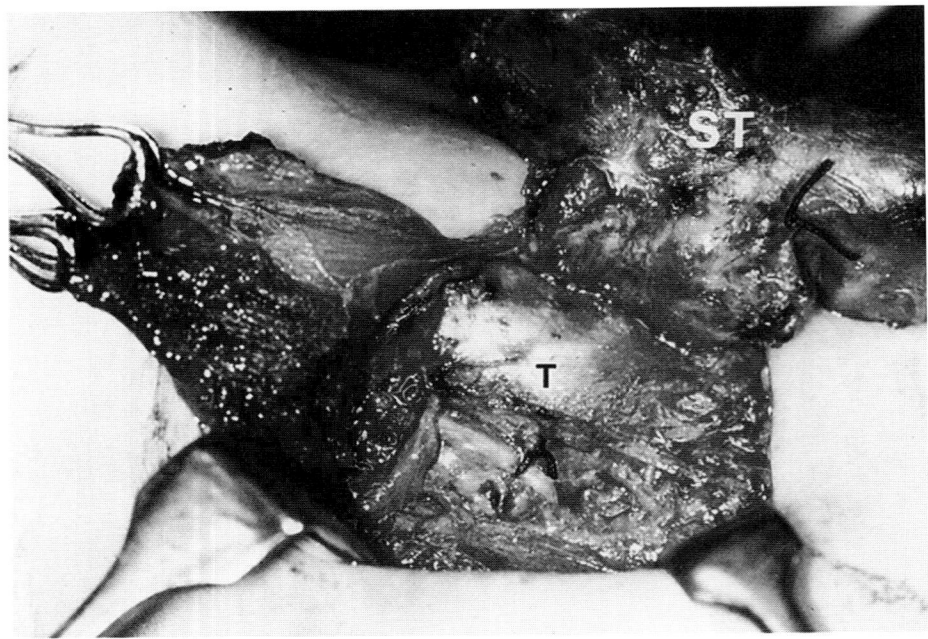

FIG. 11. The mobilization of a large solitary nodule prior to a subtotal thyroidectomy. ST, subtotal thyroid mobilization; T, trachea.

include all of the isthmus. It is best to include the isthmus with the ipsilateral lobe so as to avoid the development of palpable thickening in the pretracheal region postoperatively. Such a finding might confuse subsequent clinical examiners. However, if the nodule is very large or extends into the midline, a subtotal thyroidectomy should be done. This would include the medial aspect of the contralateral lobe (Figs. 11,12).

If there is macroscopic evidence of extracapsular spread of the tumor from the thyroid gland to adjacent soft tissues, the involved soft tissue should be resected *en bloc* with the thyroid nodule. If there is nodal involvement in the cervical or mediastinal regions, the thyroid incision can be extended laterally as far as the anterior border of the trapezius muscle. A second parallel upper cervical (McPhee) incision is often added (Fig. 13). Gen-

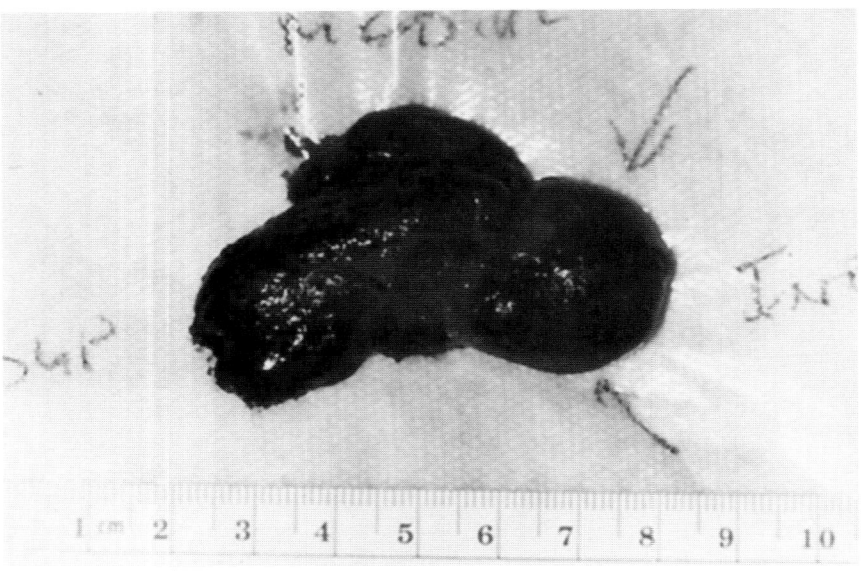

FIG. 12. Subtotal thyroidectomy specimen oriented for pathologic examination.

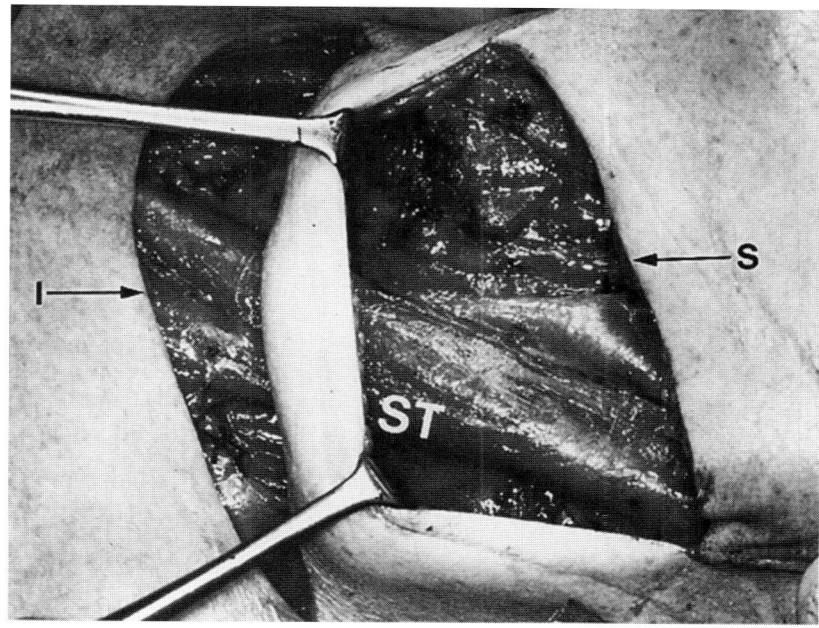

FIG. 13. McPhee incision left neck with flat elevation for left functional neck dissection. I, interior skin incision; S, superior skin incision; ST, sternocleidomastoid muscle.

erally, a functional type of neck dissection is performed, but a modified or radical neck dissection may be necessary if muscle or other soft tissues are involved. It is important to include the pretracheal and superior mediastinal nodes in that dissection.

Rarely, a sternotomy is necessary when the thyroid nodule is entrapped in the mediastinum, when there is aberrant mediastinal vasculature, or when mediastinal node disease is extensive. If the airway is involved, an appropriate *en bloc* resection and reconstruction is carried out at the time of the initial surgery.

If the strap muscles or large amounts of soft tissue are resected, particularly from the anterior neck, a myogenous flap may be fashioned by splitting the sternomastoid muscle and folding it over on its anterior border. This provides a source of muscle for reconstruction of anterior neck muscle deficits. This reconstructive procedure will result in improved bulk in the anterior neck and less postoperative sensitivity, with subsequent improved cosmesis.

If coexistent parathyroid disease is present, it may require concurrent management. Ideally, the preoperative evaluation of the patient will have identified the hypercalcemic problem and allowed for preparation of both the patient and the surgeon. It is imperative that all of the standard principles of management of parathyroid disease apply when treating coexistent parathyroid disorders during thyroid surgery. In particular, no parathyroid tissue should be removed, other than for incisional biopsy purposes, without a thorough siting and assessment of all of the parathyroid glands. The number of glands present and the nature of the pathological disorder must be established before any parathyroid tissue is removed for ablative purposes.

The recurrent laryngeal nerves must be identified and tracked meticulously to the cricothyroid membrane during the course of surgery for thyroid nodules. Frequently, the recurrent laryngeal nerve has extralaryngeal branches. At times, as many as five branches may be found prior to the nerve entering the cricothyroid membrane (Fig. 14). There may also be tiny motor branches to the esophagus. All of these branches should be preserved. At times, the recurrent nerve does not recur but comes directly off the vagus nerve at the level of the thyroid gland (Fig. 15). Also, the recurrent laryngeal nerve may be intertwined with the inferior thyroid artery (Fig. 16). In those instances, the recurrent laryngeal nerve is at greater risk than usual. It should not be resected except where the perineurium is involved by tumor. In that case, there is generally evidence of recurrent nerve malfunction preoperatively.

During neck closure, the divided strap muscles are repaired, and the anterior strap muscle diastasis should be opposed with one or two sutures in the upper part of the separation. However, a tight closure of the strap muscles in the anterior midline is avoided, as such closure is potentially dangerous if a postoperative hemorrhage occurs. The platysma and subcutaneous tissues are repaired accurately. A continuous subcuticular suture or histoacryl glue is used for skin closure. A negative pressure drain of the Argyle chest drain type attached to an Emmerson pump is generally used for suction drainage upon completion of the surgery (Fig. 17).

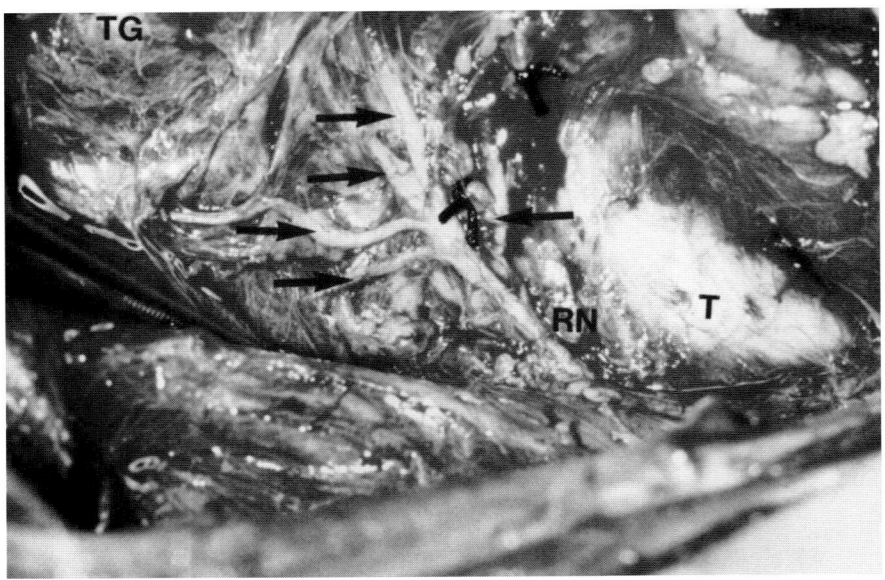

FIG. 14. Right recurrent laryngeal nerve (RN) with five extralaryngeal branches *(arrows)*. T, trachea; TG, thyroid gland.

POSTOPERATIVE CONSIDERATIONS

Postanesthetic

Ordinarily, the patient is capable of spontaneous respirations at the end of the operative procedure. The extubation should be as smooth as possible to avoid straining on the endotracheal tube that may result in laryngospasm or venous congestion in the neck. If the patient has not been reversed satisfactorily at the completion of the operative procedure, extubation can be done later in the recovery room or in the intensive care unit. If the patient has undergone an associated neck dissection or laryngotracheal resection, postanesthetic ventilation, either through the endotracheal tube or through a tracheotomy, may be advisable for 24 hr to defunction the upper airway, thereby reducing the strain on the operative site. The patient also may require postanesthetic ventilation for chronic lower respiratory tract disease or other systemic problems. If postanesthetic ventilation is necessary, the patient should be properly paralyzed to avoid endolaryngeal and endotracheal irritation with the associated straining, coughing,

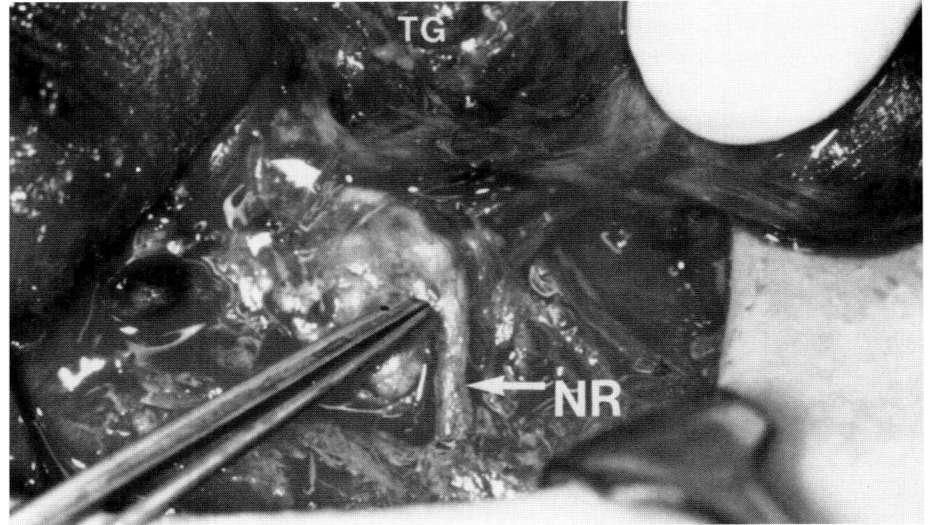

FIG. 15. "Nonrecurrent" right recurrent laryngeal nerve (NR). TG, thyroid gland.

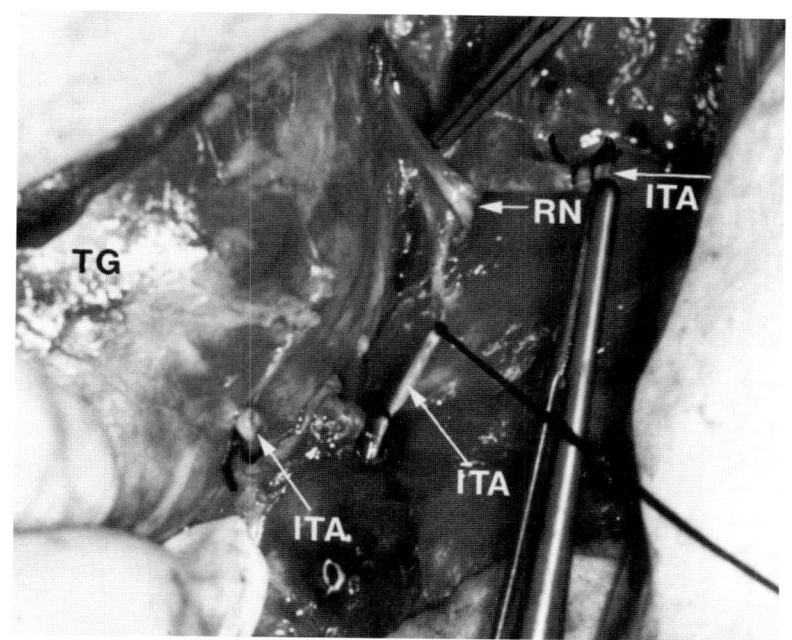

FIG. 16. Recurrent laryngeal nerve (RN) intertwined with inferior thyroid artery (ITA). One branch of the artery has been ligated and divided. TG, thyroid gland.

venous congestion, and possible mucosal trauma. The patient who does not require extraordinary postanesthetic support is sent to the recovery room. However, if more intensive postanesthetic support, or ventilation, is required, the patient is sent to the surgical intensive care unit.

Routine immediate postoperative inspection of the larynx or trachea is generally not indicated, nor is it advisable, because such an examination may, of necessity, be done under less than optimum conditions. However, if such an examination is deemed necessary by the surgeon, it is best carried out using an anterior commissure laryngoscope, or a rigid or flexible bronchoscope, rather than the anesthetist's laryngoscope. The Magill type of anesthetist's laryngoscope is not designed for inspection of the endolarynx or upper trachea. Instead, it is designed for introduction of endotracheal tubes. If postoperative endoscopy is necessary, it should be performed by a properly trained endoscopist. The examination is commenced with the patient fully relaxed, and topical anesthesia (10% endotracheal lidocaine) should be introduced to diminish the airway reflexes as the anesthetic is lightened, so that motor function of the vocal cords can be assessed. To do this, the patient must be fully reversed from the muscle-relaxing portion of the anesthetic so that spontaneous respiratory activity returns and the abduction/adduction function of the vocal cords can be evaluated. Finally, it should be noted that the anesthetist must not hesitate to inspect the pharynx and larynx for accumulated secretions, which should be removed prior to extubation.

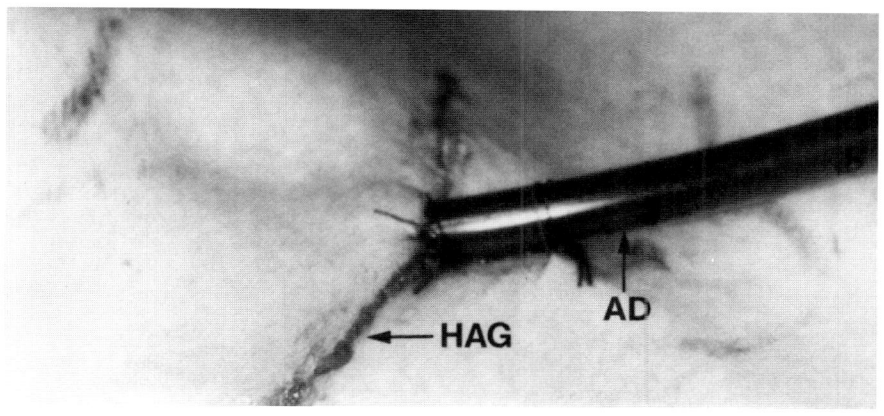

FIG. 17. Argyle drain (AD) and histoacryl glue closure of skin incision (HAG).

Calcium

Serum calcium is monitored, both biochemically and clinically, on a regular basis after the removal of a thyroid nodule, until calcium metabolism has stabilized. A serum calcium level is obtained immediately postoperatively, 6 hr later, and then on a daily basis. Chvostek's and Trousseau's tests are done every 4 hr in this initial postoperative period to determine if increased neuromuscular irritability is present. Even with a hemithyroidectomy, there may be a transient (24- to 72-hr) drop in serum calcium. As the magnitude of the resective procedure increases, the risk of malfunction of calcium metabolism increases. If serum calcium levels are significantly reduced and signs of neuromuscular irritability develop, calcium is given by intravenous infusion. If the serum calcium is still low after 72 hr, it is generally best to start the patient on supplemental calcium and vitamin D even if it is only necessary to do so on a temporary basis.

Voice

All patients will have at least a mild degree of hoarseness on a transient basis after removal of a thyroid nodule. Some may be aphonic because of the neck pain, surgical manipulation, and endotracheal intubation in the early postoperative phase. These symptoms are not alarming and the surgeon should reassure the patient and the family. However, if there is excessive breathiness or weakness of the voice and a weak cough, recurrent nerve damage or endolaryngeal trauma such as submucosal hematoma or cricoarytenoid joint damage must be considered. Appropriate mirror or fiberoptic examinations are carried out. In any case, all patients who have undergone thyroid surgery should have a mirror or fiberoptic examination of the larynx and upper trachea before discharge from the hospital and on the first postoperative visit.

Other Considerations

The drains are removed on the first or second postoperative day, depending on the amount of drainage present. Neck movement is encouraged immediately, but such movements should be gentle for the first few days. The patient is ambulated and oral feedings are started on the day of surgery. Prophylactic antibiotics are not used. Postoperative visits are scheduled with both the surgeon and the endocrinologist. Thyroxine is prescribed as indicated.

REFERENCES

1. Vander JB, Gaston EA, Dawber TR. The significance of nontoxic thyroid nodules. Final report of a 15-year study of the incidence of thyroid malignancy. *Ann Intern Med* 1968;69:537–540.
2. Horlocker TT, Hay ID, James EM, et al. Prevalence of incidental nodular thyroid disease detected by high resolution parathyroid ultrasonography. In: Medeiros-Neto G, Gaitan E, eds. *Frontiers in thyroidology*, vol. 1. New York: Plenum Press, 1986;1309–1312.
3. Sampson RJ. Prevalence and significance of occult thyroid cancer. In: DeGroot L, Frohman LA, Kaplan EL, et al, eds. *Radiation-associated thyroid carcinoma*. New York: Grune & Stratton, 1977;137–153.
4. Lang W, Borrusch H, Bauer L. Occult carcinomas of the thyroid. Evaluation of 1020 sequential autopsies. *Am J Clin Pathol* 1988;90:72–76.
5. Mazzaferri EL. Longterm impact of initial surgical and medical therapy or papillary and follicular thyroid cancer. *Am J Med* 1994;97:418–428.
6. Veith FJ, Brooks JR, Grigsby WP, Selenkow H. The nodular thyroid gland and cancer. A practical approach to the problem. *N Engl J Med* 1964;270:431–436.
7. Cady B. Surgery of thyroid cancer. *World J Surg* 1981;5:3–14.
8. Burrow GN, Mujtaba Q, LiVolsi V, Cornog J. The incidence of carcinoma in solitary "cold" thyroid nodules. *Yale J Biol Med* 1978;51:13–17.
9. Kirkland RT, Kirkland JL, Rosenberg HS, et al. Solitary thyroid nodules in 30 children and report of a child with a thyroid abscess. *Pediatrics* 1973;51:85–90.
10. Rallison ML, Dobyns BM, Keating FR. Thyroid nodularity in children. *JAMA* 1975;233:1069–1972.
11. Scott MD, Crawford JD. Solitary thyroid nodules in childhood. Is the incidence of thyroid carcinoma declining? *Pediatrics* 1976;58:521–525.
12. Cady B, Rossi R. An expanded view of risk group definition in differentiated thyroid carcinoma. *Surgery* 1988;104:947–953.
13. Duffy BJ, Fitzgerald PJ. Cancer of the thyroid in children: a report of 28 cases. *J Clin Endocrinol* 1950;10:1296–1308.
14. DeGroot L, Paloyan E. Thyroid carcinoma and radiation: a Chicago endemic. *JAMA* 1973;225:487–491.
15. Favus MJ, Schneider AB, Stachura ME, et al. Thyroid cancer occurring as a late consequence of head and neck irradiation—evaluation of 1056 patients. *N Engl J Med* 1976;294:1019–1025.
16. Becker FO, Economou SG, Wouthwick HW, et al. Adult thyroid cancer after head and neck irradiation in infancy and childhood. *Ann Intern Med* 1975;83:347–351.
17. Royce PG, MacKay BR, DiSabella PM. Value of postirradiation screening for thyroid nodules. *JAMA* 1979;242:2675–2678.
18. Hamburger JI, Miller JM, Garcia M. Do all nodules appearing in patients subsequent to radiation therapy to the head and neck area require excision? In: Hamburger JI, Miller JM, eds. *Controversies in clinical thyroidology*. New York: Springer-Verlag, 1981;217–244.
19. Refetoff S, Harrison J, Karanfilski BT, et al. Continuing occurrence of thyroid carcinoma after irradiation to the head and neck in infancy and childhood. *N Engl J Med* 1975;292:171–175.
20. Baschieri L, Antonelli A, Ferdeghini M, et al. Thyroid cancer in children after Chernobyl nuclear disaster *[Abstr 60]*. *Thyroid* 1995;5:(suppl),S30.
21. Bogdanova T, Bragarnik M, Tronko ND, et al. Thyroid cancer in the Ukraine post-Chernobyl *[Abstr 56]*. *Thyroid* 1995;5(suppl):S28.
22. Keyes JW Jr, Thrall JH, Carey JE. Technical considerations in in vivo thyroid studies. *Semin Nucl Med* 1978;8:43–57.
23. Reede DI, Bergeron RT, McCauley DI. CT of the thyroid and of other thoracic inlet disorders. *J Otolaryngol* 1982;11:349–357.
24. Gefter WB, Spritzer CE, Eisenberg B, et al. Thyroid imaging with high-field-strength surface-coil MR. *Radiology* 1987;164:483–490.
25. Sanchez RB, Shank T, Oglevie S, et al. Ultrasound-guided biopsy of nonpalpable and difficult to palpate thyroid masses. *J Am Coll Surg* 1994;178:33–37.
26. Yokozawa T, Miyauchi A, Kuma K, et al. Accurate and simple method of diagnosing thyroid nodules by the modified technique of ultrasound-guided fine needle aspiration biopsy. *Thyroid* 1995;5:141–145.
27. Walfish PG, Hazani E, Strawbridge HTG, et al. Combined ultrasound and needle aspiration cytology in the assessment and management of hypofunctioning thyroid nodule. *Ann Intern Med* 1977;87:270–274.
28. Bugis SP, Young JEM, Archibald SD, et al. Diagnostic accuracy of fine-needle aspiration biopsy versus frozen section in solitary thyroid nodules. *Am J Surg* 1986;152:411–416.
29. Irish JC, Van Nostrand AWP, Asa SL, et al. Accuracy of pathologic diagnosis in thyroid lesions. *Arch Otolaryngol Head Neck Surg* 1992;118:918–922.
30. Lean CL, Delbridge L, Russel P, et al. Diagnosis of follicular thyroid lesions by proton magnetic resonance on fine needle biopsy. *J Clin Endocrinol Metab* 1995;80:1306–1311.
31. Hamburger JI, Miller JM, Kini SR. Lymphoma of the thyroid. *Ann Intern Med* 1983;99:685–693.
32. Holm L-E, Blomgren H, Lowhagen T. Cancer risks in patients with chronic lymphocytic thyroiditis. *N Engl J Med* 1985;312:601–604.

33. Van Herle AJ, Vassart G, Dumont JE. Control of thyroglobulin synthesis and secretion (second of two parts). *N Engl J Med* 1979;301:307–314.
34. Morita T, Tamai H, Oshima A, et al. Change in serum thyroid hormone, thyrotropin and thyroglobulin concentrations during thyroxine therapy in patients with solitary thyroid nodules. *J Clin Endocrinol Metab* 1989;69:227–230.
35. Miller JM, Hamburger JI, Taylor CI. Is needle aspiration of the cystic thyroid nodule effective and safe treatment? In: Hamburger JI, Miller JM, eds. *Controversies in clinical thyroidology.* New York: Springer-Verlag, 1981;210–236.
36. DeYoung JP, Kahn A, Lerman S, et al. Tetracycline instillation for recurrent cystic thyroid nodules. *Can J Surg* 1986;29:118–119.
37. Hamburger JI. Solitary autonomously functioning thyroid lesion: diagnosis, clinical features and pathogenetic considerations. *Am J Med* 1975;58:740–748.
38. Alderson PO, Sumner HW, Siegel BA. The single palpable thyroid nodule. Evaluation by 99mTc-pertechnetate imaging. *Cancer* 1976;37:258–265.
39. Hamburger JI. Evaluation of toxicity in solitary nontoxic autonomously functioning thyroid nodules. *J Clin Endocrinol Metabol* 1980;50:1089–1093.
40. Iida Y, Kasagi K, Misaki T, et al. Visualization of suppressed normal thyroid tissue by thallium-201 in patients with toxic nodular goiter. *Clin Nucl Med* 1988;13:283–285.
41. David E, Rosen IB, Bain J, et al. Management of the hot thyroid nodule. *Am J Surg* 1995;170:481–483.
42. Goldstein R, Hart IR. Followup of solitary autonomous thyroid nodules treated with 131-I. *N Engl J Med* 1983;309:1473–1476.
43. Papini E, Pacella CM, Verde G. Percutaneous ethanol injection (PEI): What is its role in the treatment of benign thyroid nodules? *Thyroid* 1995;5:147–150.
44. Molitch ME, Beck JR, Dreisman M, et al. The cold thyroid nodule: an analysis of diagnostic and therapeutic options. *Endocr Rev* 1984;5:185–199.
45. Kambal A. Carcinoma of solitary thyroid nodules. *Br J Surg* 1969;56:434–436.
46. Thomas CG Jr, Buckwalter JA, Staab EV, et al. Evaluation of dominant thyroid masses. *Ann Surg* 1976;183:463–469.
47. Gharib H, James EM, Charboneau JW, et al. Suppressive therapy with levothyroxine for solitary thyroid nodules. A double blind clinical study. *N Engl J Med* 1987;317:70–75.
48. Reverter JL, Lucas A, Audi L, et al. Suppression therapy with levothyroxine for solitary nodules. *Clin Endocrinol* 1992;36:25–28.
49. Lever EG, Refetroff S, Straus FH, et al. Coexisting thyroid and parathyroid disease—are they related? *Surgery* 1983;94:893–900.
50. Ott RA, Calandra DB, McCall A, et al. The incidence of thyroid carcinoma in patients with Hashimoto's thyroiditis and solitary cold nodules. *Surgery* 1985;98:1202–1206.

CHAPTER 23

Multinodular Goiter

George L. A. From and Victor G. Lawson

Goiter [guttur (L.), throat] has been chronicled by practitioners of the healing arts since ancient times. Goiter occurs with varying incidence in almost every country of the world, independent of climate, season, or weather, and it makes no distinctions of race, color, or creed. Some of the most notorious goiter areas are located in the high mountain regions such as the Alps, the Himalayas, the Pyrenees, and the Andes, but low-lying and coastal areas are not immune (1). In many parts of the world, goiter occurs sporadically. But elsewhere, in the absence of prophylactic measures such as sanitation or increasing the amount of iodine available to the population, goiter may be found in the majority of inhabitants. The significance of nodular goiters in any given area appears to be inverse to their prevalence. Where they are plentiful, they may be accepted as normal or even ornamental, with their main importance being as a marker for possible iodine deficiency and cretinism. When they are less frequently seen, they may be viewed as a disability, or as a potentially dangerous condition.

Speculation surrounding environmental factors in the pathogenesis of goiter and the use of iodine-rich substances for therapy are chronicled in ancient writings. Pliny the Elder, in the first century A.D., considered the cause of thyroid enlargement thus: "Guttur homini tantum et suibus intumescit aquarum quae potantur plerumque vitio" (Swelling of the throat occurs only in men and swine, caused mostly by the water they drink), an observation that may have considerable merit. Ancient Chinese writings mention the use of seaweed and preparations of animal thyroid glands in the treatment of goiter (2,3). The first clinical use of iodine in the treatment of goiter is usually attributed to Jean François Coindet (1774 to 1834), within a decade of the discovery of this element by Bernard Courtois. Coindet had been aware that certain plants and sponges were used successfully in the treatment of goiters, and he reasoned that the active ingredient may be iodine. Using a tincture of iodine, he observed virtual disappearance of goiters in a number of patients within 6 to 10 weeks, and thus he established the importance of this element in medicine (3).

DEFINITION AND CLASSIFICATION OF GOITER

The normal lobes of the adult thyroid gland are stated to be about the size of "lima beans with the isthmus appearing as a thin connecting strand" (4). The mean volume of the thyroid, as estimated by ultrasonography, is approximately 11 mL, with a range of about 4.9 to 19.1 mL (5). This wide variation in normal thyroid size is further compounded by the variability in the size and physical characteristics of the neck, which makes it difficult to accurately assess minimal enlargement of the thyroid gland by clinical examination. For the purpose of epidemiologic studies, at least, where sophisticated techniques such as ultrasonography are impractical, guidelines have been suggested based on clinical findings. Minor degrees of thyroid enlargement are not considered goitrous until the lateral lobes of the thyroid have a volume equal to that of the terminal phalanges of the thumbs of the person being examined. From this palpable but not visible enlargement, the thyroid may enlarge until it is of huge proportions, being visible at a great distance, and capable of creating respiratory as well as cosmetic embarrassment. Classification based on size divides goiter into four broad categories (4):

Grade 0—Persons without goiter (see preceding)
Grade I—Persons with palpable goiter

G. L. A. From: Department of Medicine, University of Toronto, The Toronto Hospital, Toronto, Ontario, Canada M5G 2C4.
V. G. Lawson: Central Kentucky Otolaryngology—Head and Neck Surgical Associates, Bluegrass Medical Center, Paris, Kentucky 40361.

Grade II—Persons with visible goiter (with head in normal position)

Grade III—Persons with very large goiter (visible at a distance)

Goiter may also be classified as being endemic (i.e., present in over 10% of the population) or sporadic in nature.

Congenital goitrous hypothyroidism may be produced by a defect in hormonogenesis. These familial syndromes are inherited as mendelian autosomal recessives, and several forms have been recognized (6):

1. Thyroglobulin synthesis defect (abnormal or diminished)
2. Thyroid hormone unresponsiveness
3. Iodine-trapping defect
4. Iodine organification (peroxidase) defect
5. Iodine organification defect with sensorineural deafness (Pendred's syndrome)
6. Iodotyrosine coupling defect
7. Iodotyrosine dehalogenase defect

Endemic Goiter

Endemic goiter has been the subject of intensive investigation on the part of epidemiologists and health workers around the world. The distribution and prevalence has been exhaustively outlined by Kelly and Snedden (1). The most well-known areas of endemia are located in mountainous regions mentioned previously. Endemic goiters are also seen, however, in many low-lying countries, and in coastal areas. Although iodine deficiency is probably the most common environmental factor in goiter formation, many other goitrogenic influences have been implicated in certain parts of the world, and they may act in the presence of iodine deficiency or as independent etiologic factors.

Iodine Deficiency

Iodine is an essential element for thyroid hormone synthesis. Most dietary iodine comes from food and, although the iodine content of meats is higher than that of terrestrial plants, the major determinant of dietary iodine is the soil. Iodine is continually leached from soil by snow and rain, and returned by rainfall. In general, glaciated areas (such as the mountain ranges of the northern hemisphere) are poorer in iodine than nonglaciated areas, and areas that are subject to heavy rainfall and floodings have reduced iodine content (7). Iodine-deficient diets are more likely to be seen in populations that depend strictly on locally grown food for nutrition and rely on vegetable rather than animal or fish protein. Urban dwellers, especially in wealthier nations where importation of foods is more usual, are less likely to be affected. Similarly, people who can afford a more varied diet are more protected from goiter formation.

Factors Other Than Iodine

Because goiter is not a universal finding in iodine-poor parts of the world, and because endemic goiter sometimes occurs where iodine supplies are not deficient, other factors must be considered in pathogenesis. Epidemiologic studies have suggested that malnutrition may be important. In southern Senegal, for example, where iodine deficiency is prevalent, there are discrepancies in thyroid swelling related to sex, age, and social status, suggesting that nutritional factors may play a role (8,9).

Goitrogenic substances such as cyanogenic glycosides, cyanates, and thiocyanates are found in many vegetables that form staple foods in many parts of the world, such as cassava in Nigeria or millet in Sudan. These compounds interfere with iodine trapping and may create functional iodine deficiency where ordinarily adequate iodine intake is seen. In Tasmania and Finland, goitrogens are found in weeds and grasses, and they are transmitted to people in the milk of animals grazing on them. Contamination of water supplies with organic matter from coal and shale or bacterial *(E. coli)* products has also been found to be goitrogenic in several regions, and several chemicals found in water from goitrous regions have been implicated (10). In addition, immunologic factors and genetic factors can obviously operate in an endemic goiter area as in any other, and they may preselect a portion of the population destined to develop goiter.

Endemic Goiter Resulting from Iodine Excess

Although sporadic iodine-induced goiter is occasionally seen, usually secondary to therapy for respiratory disorders or to kelp ingestion as a health supplement, endemic goiter resulting from iodine excess is unusual. High intake of iodine-rich kelp in the form of a soup or side dish is seen in Hokkaido, the northern island of Japan. Patients with iodine-induced goiters in these regions are euthyroid, and goiter resolves upon cessation of kelp intake (11).

Prevention of Endemic Goiter

Although improvements in nutrition and sanitation have played a role in goiter prevention, iodine supplementation is still the most important factor in goiter prophylaxis (with the obvious exception of goiter caused by iodine excess). The addition of iodine to salt and bread as a public health measure in many jurisdictions has led to a significant reduction in goiter incidence, and to virtual elimination of endemic cretinism (12). In underdeveloped nations, where the use of iodized salt is impractical for a variety of economic and geographic reasons, iodized oil, given either by injection or orally, is an inexpensive and efficacious method of iodine administration, with one injection providing correction of iodine deficiency for about 5 years (13), and an oral dose for about 1 year (14). Allergic reactions to iodine are occasionally encountered after iodized oil administration, but these are rare with the small amount administered by iodization of salt. The most frequently encountered side effect is iodine-induced hyperthyroidism (Jod-Basedow phenomenon) (15,16), which has occurred in several jurisdictions after the introduction of goiter prophylaxis. The benefits of iodine supplementation, however, appear to far outweigh any disadvantages.

Sporadic Goiter

Sporadic goiter may be defined as thyroid enlargement in the euthyroid individual, occurring in areas in which goiter is not endemic. In some cases, genetic disorders of thyroid function may be present or exposure to goitrogens elicited, but in the majority the etiology remains obscure. As in most other thyroid disorders, there is a strong female preponderance. In iodine deficiency, or in the presence of inhibitors of thyroid function, the stimulus for thyroid growth is thought to be thyroid stimulating hormone (TSH) (17), secreted in excess to overcome inadequate thyroid hormone production. In many sporadic goiters, especially those that grow in spite of thyroxine therapy, this is probably not the case (18). Thyroid follicular cells in hypophysectomized and thyroid hormone–treated experimental animals are still capable of spontaneous growth (19) (presumably in the complete absence of TSH). In addition to TSH, thyroid cells may respond to a variety of growth-promoting stimuli such as epidermal and fibroblast growth factors (20), or immune globulins. Antibody-mediated alterations in thyroid function are widely accepted as being implicated in the pathogenesis of Graves' disease and Hashimoto's disease, and it is attractive to speculate that growth of thyroid cells, without alteration in hormone production, may also be induced by immune mechanisms. Distinct immunoglobulins, capable of inducing growth of thyroid epithelial cells, have been detected in the serum of some patients with goitrous thyroid dysfunction and euthyroid nodular goiter (21,22) under some experimental conditions, but the role of immunoglobulin in the formation of simple goiter, whether endemic or sporadic, is not fully established (23).

GROWTH AND NODULAR TRANSFORMATION

The initial enlargement of the thyroid in response to trophic stimulation appears to be diffuse, but, with long-standing stimulation, nodular transformation occurs whether the stimulus is TSH or immune globulin (24,25). It is also apparent that even in minimally enlarged thyroid glands and in the absence of any known intrinsic stimulation, nodularity may frequently be seen; indeed, multiple clinically unapparent nodules may be detected on ultrasonography during investigation of either presumed solitary nodules, or during neck imaging for nonthyroid disease. Some of these will be hyperplastic, some neoplastic, some hyperfunctioning, and some hypofunctioning, with no evidence of abnormality in unaffected tissue to indicate hyperstimulation. Rather, there is the suggestion that a wide variability for growth potential among different components of the thyroid is an intrinsic characteristic of the gland, or, if trophic stimulation initiated the process, that it was unnecessary for growth and replication of cells to continue. It is probable that follicular epithelial cells are of polyclonal origin, and that weak stimulation to grow and replicate may affect different cells in different ways (26). Grafts of goiter tissue into mice show that cells from differently functioning or growing portions of multinodular human thyroids maintain their original characteristics, with some replicating in the absence of TSH, and others doing so only after prolonged stimulation (27). Functional characteristics of thyroid cells, such as iodinating activity in the presence or absence of TSH, is also variable between follicles and among cells within follicles (27). Prolonged low-level stimulation of growth, whether it be caused by mild elevations of TSH due to goitrogenic factors, or by other extrinsic or intrinsic growth-promoting factors, may lead to follicles being formed that may differ substantially in their characteristics, depending on which cell within the mother follicle gave rise to the daughter follicles. In addition, some thyroid nodules appear to be polyclonal or hyperplastic in nature, whereas others seem to be monoclonal, and both types may be present within a single thyroid gland, blurring the distinction between hyperplasia and neoplasia (28). Thus, with the passage of time, a thyroid gland may develop in which some follicles are small, some large, some hypofunctioning, some autonomous or hyperfunctioning, some hyperplastic, some neoplastic, and some with greater or smaller amounts of colloid formation. Growth, degeneration, hemorrhage, colloid accumulation, and shrinking of stromal tissue, occurring over many years, eventually lead to the characteristic appearance of the familiar large multinodular goiter, with different areas within the goiter exhibiting wide variation of morphologic and functional features (Fig. 1).

MULTINODULAR GOITER AND CARCINOMA OF THE THYROID

The possible relationship of carcinoma of the thyroid and multinodular goiter has engendered much debate, with no definite conclusion being reached. There have been some reports of increased incidence of thyroid carcinomas in patients from endemic goiter regions such as Colombia (29), but not from goitrous regions of the United States or Italy (30,31). Indeed, iodine deficiency may be associated with a lower risk of malignancy both

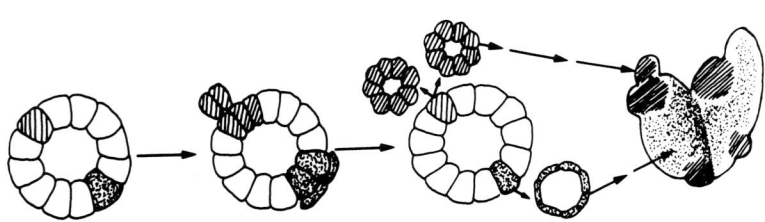

FIG. 1. Many thyroid follicles are heterogeneous structures composed of cells with different potentials for growth and function. Chronic mild stimulation induces some cells to form new follicles with increased, and relatively autonomous, capacity for hormone formation *(hatched)*, whereas other cells may form follicles that grow to a large size but have a reduced capacity for iodine metabolism *(stippled)*. Ultimately, the thyroid will be composed of large and small follicles or nodules that vary considerably in structural and functional characteristics.

in solitary thyroid nodules and multinodular glands. The protective effect of iodine deficiency seems to apply only to papillary carcinoma, and follicular or anaplastic tumors occur with about equal frequency in iodine-rich or iodine-deficient areas (31). It has been suggested that carcinomas of more malignant potential are seen in patients with multinodular goiters (32). Whether this represents a truly different neoplastic potential of goitrous tissue or merely reflects the selection of patients for surgery on the basis of changes in the character of their basic goiter is unclear. Low-grade malignancies that do not cause rapid development of symptoms (and usually carry a good prognosis) are more likely to be ignored and undiagnosed in the presence of a longstanding goiter, excluding patients with such lesions from surgical series.

On the basis of available evidence, at least in nonendemic areas, multinodular goiter does not appear to be a major risk factor in the development of thyroid cancer, but thyroid cancer certainly can develop in a multinodular goiter, and the possibility of malignancy in a goiter that is changing must be entertained. Fixation of the goiter, vocal cord involvement, or evidence of metastatic spread are indications for a more aggressive approach to diagnosis and therapy.

Clinical Approach to Multinodular Goiter

In the initial assessment of the patient with a nodular goiter, consideration should be given to factors that will dictate the need for therapeutic intervention. Multinodular goiters, even those that are very large in size, are often well tolerated by the patient. Therefore, the simple presence of a goiter is not in itself a reason to intervene, especially because the therapy may carry risks of its own. Indications for therapy may vary considerably: in some patients the goiter may pose a serious threat to life, whereas in others the goiter is only a cosmetic nuisance. A healthy patient with a large uncomplicated goiter may be a good candidate for surgical reduction, whereas the frail elderly patient with compromised cardiac function may be actively treated only if the goiter is responsible for respiratory obstruction, harbors a malignancy, or is associated with a disturbance in thyroid function.

The initial presentation may show obvious clinical or biochemical evidence of hyperthyroidism or hypothyroidism, either of which will dictate the subsequent course of events. In the majority of cases, however, the patient will be euthyroid and probably without symptoms of any kind. A careful history should elucidate whether the goiter is recent or longstanding, and whether or not the patient comes from an endemic goiter area. Since the advent of rapid and relatively inexpensive travel, it is not unusual to see patients from endemic goiter areas living or visiting in many other parts of the world. Evidence of exposure to goitrogens should be sought, most commonly lithium and iodine. The latter is often ingested in the form of kelp as a health food supplement, or it may have been prescribed as a liquefying agent for some forms of respiratory or breast disorders. Elimination of the goitrogen may result in resolution of the goiter, but if this is impractical, as in the case of lithium-dependent psychiatric illness, replacement thyroid hormone therapy may be instituted. A strong family history of thyroid disease may suggest one of the congenital forms of goiter, or an autoimmune thyroid disorder. Some patients are content to live with goiter, once they have become accustomed to the cosmetic nuisance. Many large goiters will cause significant deviation of the trachea, which can be seen radiologically, but dyspnea is unusual. Abnormalities on tests of respiratory function, such as inspiratory or expiratory flow rates, can be detected frequently (33), but they are of dubious clinical significance. However, in some cases, respiratory compromise can occur and may be severe or even life threatening. This may be precipitated by a respiratory infection, occur simply with changes in neck position, or be associated with thoracic inlet compression with a retrosternal goiter. Clinical evaluation of respiratory distress on neck flexion or arm raising is an important part of the physical examination. Similarly, dysphagia, venous obstruction, or dysphonia resulting from involvement of laryngeal innervation is rare in benign goiters. Painful enlargement may occur occasionally with hemorrhage into a degenerated or cystic nodule. Any of these symptoms should be a warning that the goiter is unusual and requires further investigation. Goiters associated with severe respiratory compromise carry a significant risk of harboring carcinoma (34). If a decision has not been made to proceed with surgical therapy in the patient with a symptomatic goiter or an enlarging dominant nodule, fine-needle aspiration biopsy of several portions of the goiter should be carried out (see Chapter 22, Solitary Thyroid Nodule), which may establish a malignant diagnosis.

ASSESSMENT OF THYROID FUNCTION

All patients with nodular goiters should have routine measurement of their serum TSH, with assay of thyroid hormones carried out should the TSH be abnormal. Subnormal levels of TSH may be seen in euthyroid patients with some autonomy of thyroid function, and this does not necessarily imply either hyperthyroidism or need for therapy. The finding of a low TSH does, however, suggest that attempting to shrink the goiter with thyroid hormone is unlikely to succeed, and the patient may be rendered thyrotoxic instead.

The radioactive iodine uptake test is of limited usefulness except in the patient who is a candidate for radioiodine therapy, or occasionally to determine the degree of suppression of thyroid function with thyroid hormone therapy. Serial measurement of serum thyroglobulin may give similar information. Radionuclide scanning does not need to be done routinely, but it may be of value to detect autonomously functioning nodules in nonsuppressible goiters, or hypofunction areas that may need biopsy in the changing goiter.

We usually measure antithyroid antibodies, although their presence does not often alter management in patients with large goiters. In patients with lesser enlargement of the thyroid gland, the presence of antibodies may establish a positive diagnosis of Hashimoto's disease, with the potential for future development of hypothyroidism, and a reasonable probability of goiter reduction with thyroid hormone feeding (35).

ASSESSMENT OF THYROID SIZE

Because many patients with goiters will be followed or treated with thyroid hormone replacement, some estimate of thyroid size and extent is necessary to determine the degree of regression or progression of the lesion. Crude estimates based on the experienced clinician's assessment of thyroid weight become unreliable once the thyroid enlarges to more than 4 or 5 times normal size. Measurement of neck circumference is also unreliable and difficult to standardize. Measurement of individual nodules in one or more areas may be carried out with slightly better precision. All of the foregoing methods, in spite of their limitations, can be very useful if the changes in thyroid size are large over a period of time, but if more precise estimates are necessary to detect subtle changes, such as slow growth of a goiter or a nodule within a goiter, or to eliminate discrepancies among multiple observers, more objective techniques such as ultrasonography (5), computerized tomography (CT) (36), or magnetic resonance imaging (37) may be employed. We employ ultrasonography most frequently, although the other techniques are more useful if retrosternal extension is present.

HYPERTHYROIDISM IN MULTINODULAR GOITER

The longstanding multinodular goiter is composed of nodules and follicles of variable functional and growth potential. In some of these follicles, function appears to be independent of TSH stimulation (27), and iodine turnover and hormone production continue autonomously even when TSH is suppressed. The appearance of thyrotoxicosis may occur insidiously over many years (Plummer's disease), or it may be precipitated by an increase in iodine intake (Jod-Basedow phenomenon). A transient rise in hormone secretion is a normal response to an exogenous iodine load (38), and it is rapidly compensated for by autoregulation in the normal thyroid. Some autonomous nodules may lack this ability to compensate and continue to produce increased amounts of thyroid hormone, leading to thyrotoxicosis in some patients. Iodine-induced thyrotoxicosis sometimes occurs as a complication of endemic goiter prophylaxis with iodized salt or oil (15,16), but this has also been observed in sporadic goiter, where iodine deficiency is not a factor (39).

Continued growth of autonomously functioning portions of a nodular goiter, whether initiated by TSH or other factors, may ultimately lead to excessive production of thyroid hormone and thyrotoxicosis. This complication tends to occur in older patients with longstanding large goiters, and it may occur gradually over many years. In some patients, the clinical examination and laboratory investigation readily establish the diagnosis. In others, clinical features may be subtle or nonspecific, and the diagnosis may be extremely difficult to establish with certainty, especially in the elderly patient who may have other concurrent illness. Unfortunately, laboratory diagnosis may also be difficult, and repeated testing and skillful interpretation of the clinical situation and test results may be necessary to establish the diagnosis.

Elevated levels of serum thyroxine may be seen in a variety of illnesses (40,41), and they must be interpreted with caution unless the triiodothyronine is also elevated. Nonsuppressed TSH levels or a rise in TSH following TRH administration makes the diagnosis of thyrotoxicosis unlikely, but a low TSH and nonresponsiveness to TRH are not sufficiently specific to establish the diagnosis, especially in the presence of other illnesses. Often, observation and repetition of thyroid function tests will clarify the issue, but occasionally an empirical trial of antithyroid medication is warranted, with further investigation done at a later time if the patient improves.

TREATMENT OF EUTHYROID GOITER WITH THYROID HORMONES

It must be emphasized again that many patients tolerate goiters well, and unless definite indications for therapy exist, they may be left alone and simply followed. The use of thyroid tissue or extracts to shrink goiters goes back to antiquity and is referred to in ancient writings. Interest in this form of therapy was revived as the concepts of pituitary–thyroid interrelationship became established, and it was reasoned that TSH suppression with thyroid hormones should cause the goiter to shrink. Initially, desiccated thyroid was used (42) with gratifying results, and later, thyroxine or liothyronine was substituted. Although thyroxine is more commonly employed, there is some evidence that liothyronine may be somewhat more effective (43). Many goiters have some reduction in size with thyroid hormone therapy (44), and a few undergo complete resolution (45). A trial of thyroid hormone therapy is warranted in most patients with nontoxic nodular goiters who are otherwise in good health, but this is best avoided in the elderly or those with cardiac disease. The presence of large amounts of autonomously functioning tissue that may continue to secrete thyroid hormone even when TSH is fully suppressed may result in the production of thyrotoxicosis, so careful clinical follow-up and chemical monitoring of thyroid hormone levels are necessary. Patients in whom TSH is suppressed initially (or who do not respond to TRH) are not considered to be good candidates for thyroid hormone therapy. If there is no significant reduction of goiter size after about 6 months of thyroxine administration, it is unlikely that this form of therapy will be of much value, and it may be discontinued. Regrowth of goitrous tissue after surgical removal is not predictably preventable, but regrowth may be somewhat reduced by postoperative administration of thyroid hormone (46,47).

RADIOACTIVE IODINE THERAPY

Reduction of goiter size with iodine-131 in the absence of hyperthyroidism is not a common form of therapy, but it has been employed with good results (48,49), and it may be useful for patients whose goiters do not shrink with thyroxine feeding and in whom surgery is contraindicated. In spite of the need to use fairly large doses (25 to 50 mCi or greater), in most cases, side effects such as radiation-induced thyroiditis and thyrotoxicosis are uncommon and are easily managed with propranolol. Subsequent development of hypothyroidism is uncommon and, if it does occur, is satisfactorily treated with thyroid hormone replacement.

Because the major indication for radioablation is to treat or prevent obstructive symptoms, patients must be observed carefully for acute thyroid swelling for the first week or two after therapy, and treated with high doses of corticosteroids if necessary. Fortunately, this complication is not commonly observed (49).

SURGICAL MANAGEMENT

Patient Selection

Despite sufficient iodine supply, multinodular goiter continues to be of considerable surgical significance on both the endemic and sporadic areas. Because of the continuing prevalence of multinodular goiter, and considering health care resource limitations, selection criteria need to be developed for patients seeking surgical treatment. Recent studies of the pathogenesis of multinodular goiter indicate three basic pathogenetic concepts: goiter heterogeneity, autonomy of growth and function, and dissociation of growth and function in human goiter tissue (50). Hence the growth patterns that are seen in multinodular goiter are somewhat unpredictable in a given case, have a variable response to thyroxine treatment, and can be modified by coexistent cystic formation, spontaneous hemorrhage, and concurrent neoplasia. These multifactorial issues make patient selection for surgery somewhat difficult, particularly in resource-poor endemic countries. Surgical treatment of sporadic goiter may be influenced more by medical practice customs in a given area than by resource availability. In many communities and medical jurisdictions, multinodular goiter is considered to be of little clinical significance. Clearly, multinodular goiter can and does produce significant mechanical, cosmetic, and dysfunctional symptoms that often require definitive and sometimes aggressive surgical treatment. Hence, in an enlightened context, multinodular goiter is now recognized as a potentially significant life-threatening disorder.

Surgical Indications

The Changing Goiter

Because of the multifactorial etiology of both endemic and sporadic goiters, as well as as the increased propensity of follicular cells to proliferate in goiters as opposed to that in a normal gland, multinodular goiter is a relatively dynamic pathological process. Accordingly, change within a multinodular goiter may be viewed as less alarming by some clinicians than change occurring in a thyroid gland with other pathology. Nevertheless, changes within a multinodular goiter can have significant surgical implications. Clinically, the changes are monitored by inspection, palpation, neck measurements, and clinical photography. However, imaging studies, particularly ultrasonography and CT scanning, are the most accurate and precise methods of monitoring change within a multinodular goiter.

Selective fine-needle aspiration biopsy (FNAB) is useful in identifying foci of neoplasia. Fine-needle aspiration biopsy alone or in conjuction with large-needle aspiration biopsy (LNAB) is useful in identifying and decompressing cystic or hemorrhagic areas within a multinodular goiter. Changes in a multinodular goiter owing to recurrent cystic formation, recurrent spontaneous hemorrhage, progressive follicular hyperplasia, cellular atypia, or cellular neoplasia are indications for surgical intervention. Although it has been reported that the incidence of carcinoma in patients with multinodular goiter is considerably lower in patients with a single cold nodule, a retrospective study by McCall et al. (51) found no significant difference in the incidence of carcinoma in patients with multinodular goiters compared with patients with a solitary cold nodule.

Mechanical Symptoms

Because of their mass effect, multinodular goiters produce mechanical symptoms that may include a sensation of a lump or pressure in the throat, odynophagia, dysphagia, and a feeling of suffocation and airway distress (Figs. 2–6). The symptoms may be intermittent, persistent, or progressive. Intermittent symptoms may be related to changes in head or neck position such as one might see between the upright and recumbent positions. Persistent symptoms occur when a critical mass effect is reached, often in conjunction with reduced mobility of the thyroid gland. Reduced mobility occurs when the multinodular goiter is entrapped in the inlet, or when strong strap muscles resist the expansion of the goiter resulting in persistent displacement (Fig. 7), compression, or displacement-compression of the usually mobile upper aerodigestive tract. Whether intermittent or persistent, mechanical symptoms that are progressively more severe will require sugical intervention, occasionally on an urgent basis.

Cosmetic Symptoms

Because the head and neck area is one of the most visible areas of the human body, and because cosmesis is an important issue in our society, multinodular goiters with obvious neck lumpiness or prominence in neck girth may not be pleasing in the eye of the beholder. For this reason, many patients seek treatment for this indication alone.

Dysfunctional Symptoms

Although the majority of patients with multinodular goiters are euthyroid, some may be hyperthyroid and others may be hypothyroid. Patients with hyperthyroid or hypothyroid dysfunctional goiters have the same surgical indications as patients with euthyroid goiters, with the additional indication of surgically correctable hyperthyroidism. Accordingly, the surgical strategies are the same regardless of the functional status.

Nevertheless, the functional status is an important consideration relative to the timing of the surgical procedure. Generally, the patient must be rendered euthyroid prior to surgical intervention. Patients that are hyperthyroid owing to an autonomous nodule within a multinodular goiter will usually require surgical treatment for management of their metabolic dysfunction.

Fear of Cancer

In a society that has been properly educated to be aware of the malignant potential of any lump, as well as in the

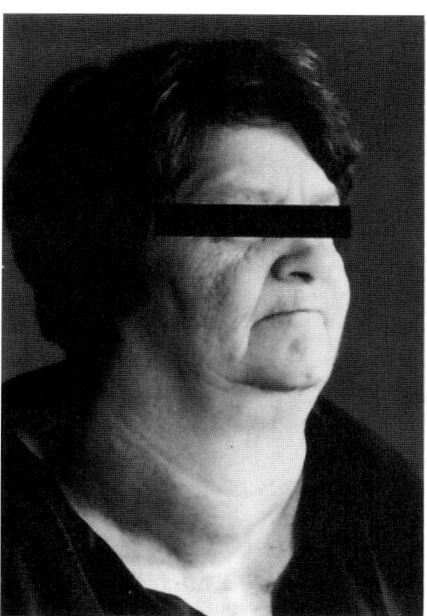
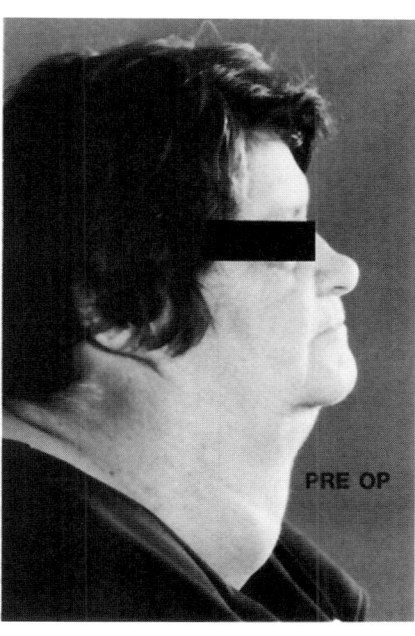

FIG. 2. Preoperative photograph of patient showing the mass effect of a 598 gm goiter filling the neck and inlet.

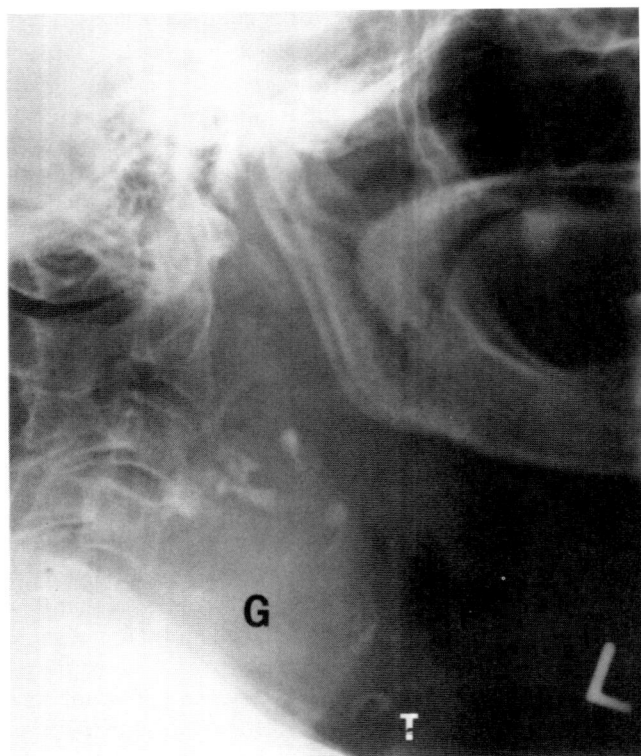

FIG. 3. Lateral view radiograph showing goiter (G) in prevertebral space, trachea (T), and calcifications in the goiter (psammoma bodies).

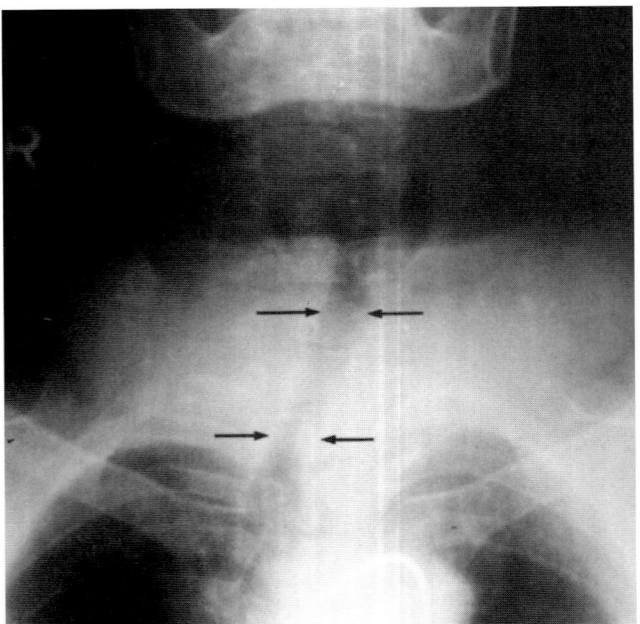

FIG. 4. A-P radiograph showing airway displacement and compression by 598 gm multinodular goiter.

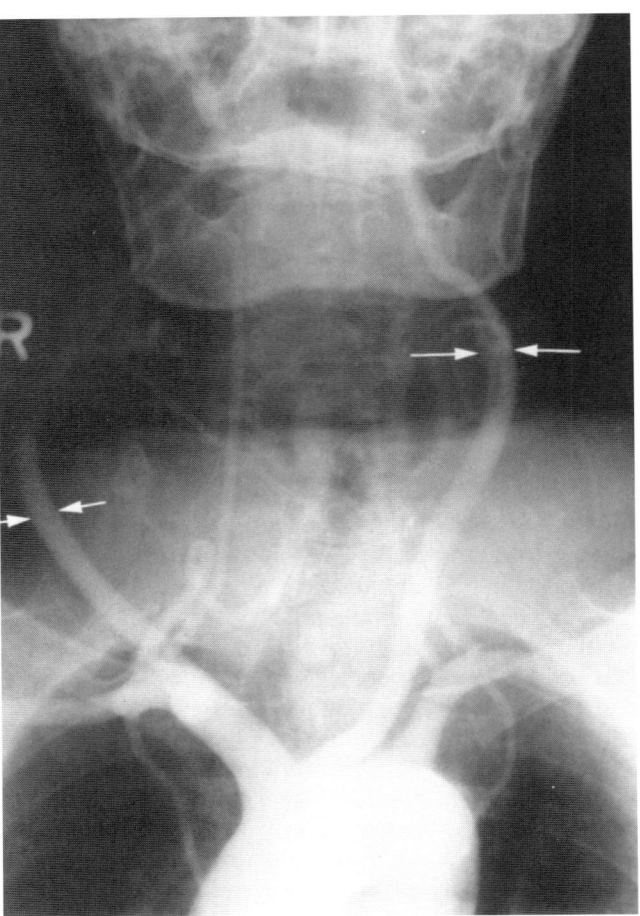

FIG. 5. Angiogram showing lateral displacement of common carotid arteries (arrows) by mass effect of 598 gm multinodular goiter.

technique of self-examination for the identification of lumps, the very presence of a multinodular goiter may be an indication for surgical removal in some patients regardless of any selection criteria that have been developed. Patients that have a high degree of normal concern and awareness of lumps in their thyroid gland will often favor early surgical removal rather than the long-term observation and removal when selection criteria are met. Other patients may have an unusually high anxiety level pertaining to their multinodular goiter, and still others may have a pathological preoccupation or fear of neoplasia rather than a logical understanding and acceptance of their multinodular goiter. In these instances, surgical intervention is reasonable, expeditious, cost-effective, and advisable. Usually, it is not possible to reassess a multinodular goiter on a monthly basis simply to allay a patient's anxiety.

Surgical Anatomy

The surgical anatomy of a multinodular goiter is quite different from the surgical anatomy of a solitary nodule, a

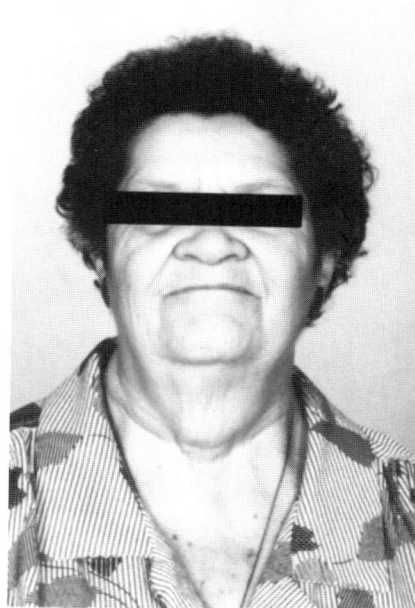 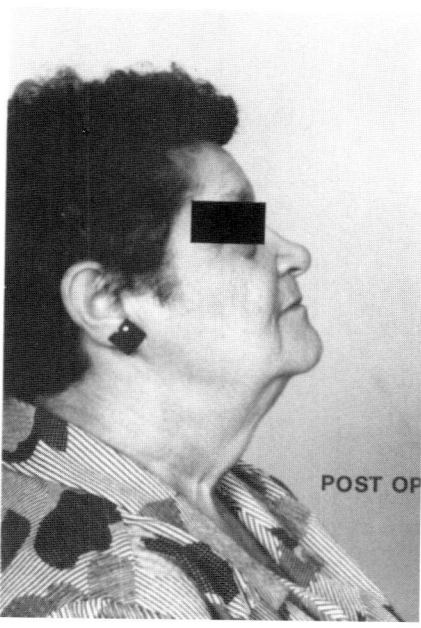

FIG. 6. Postoperative photographs of patient showing marked reduction of neck size following total thyroidectomy and removal of 598 gm goiter.

diffuse toxic goiter, or a malignant process occurring in an otherwise normal thyroid gland (Figs. 8–10). Generally, the multinodular goiter is large with an irregular nodular surface. Because of the gross enlargement of the gland, the strap muscles are often attenuated and displaced. Similarly, the gland may extend into the prevertebral space between the trachea and esophagus or into the mediastinum. The gland may be entrapped in the inlet with resultant displacement and/or compression of the trachea and esophagus. The goiter may significantly displace and separate the contents of the carotid sheaths. The recurrent laryngeal nerves may be carried laterally and elongated by the goiter. Vascular pedicles to the thyroid gland and the parathyroid glands may be elongated and unusually tortuous (Fig. 11). Aberrant vessels, particularly a thyroid ima artery, are of concern with substernal multinodular goiters (52). The

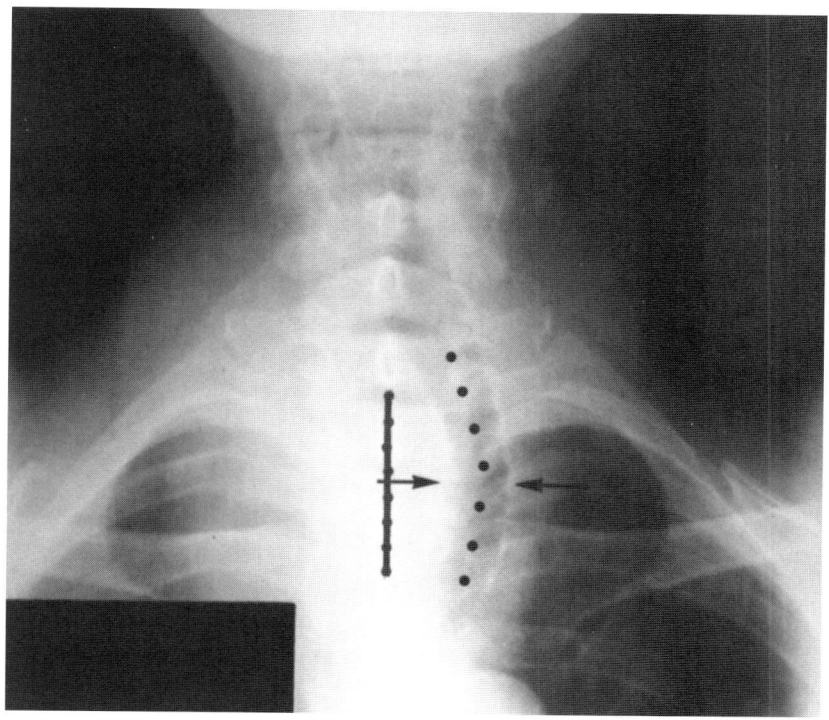

FIG. 7. A-P radiograph showing significant displacement *(dotted lines)* of trachea *(arrows)*. Midline of vertebral bodies is marked by a solid line.

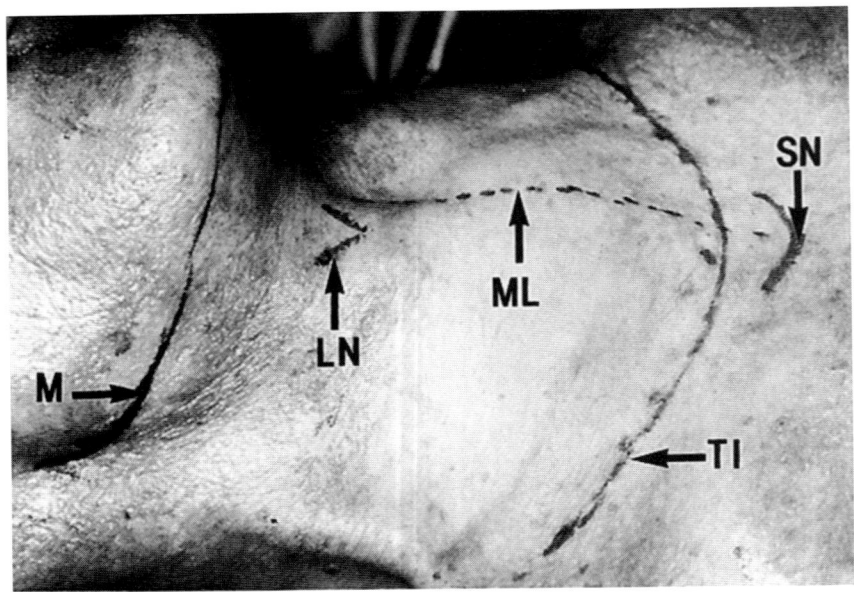

FIG. 8. Surgical anatomy of a 340 gm multinodular goiter with an irregular surface. Mandible (M), laryngeal notch (LN), midline (ML), thyroid incision (TI), suprasternal notch (SN).

parathyroid glands may be significantly displaced from their usual locations by a multinodular goiter. Also, they are more difficult to locate because of the irregular multinodular surface of the goiter.

Long-standing pressure on the airway may result in significant distortion of the cartilaginous components of the airway. This sometimes is interpreted as tracheomalacia. Although pressure on the tracheal rings may lead to significant tracheal cartilaginous deformities, pressure alone rarely causes tracheomalacia. Perichondritis, chondritis, or iatrogenic trauma to the trachea are more frequent etiological factors resulting in tracheomalacia.

Despite the gross changes in surgical anatomy seen with a multinodular goiter, goiters are generally easier to mobilize at surgery than a small thryoid gland with carcinoma or a small gland containing a solitary nodule.

Surgical Technique

In managing large multinodular goiters, standard thyroid surgical techniques are modified to enhance intraoperative safety and efficiency. The attenuated and displaced strap muscles and the contents of both carotid sheaths are clearly and extensively delineated early in the procedure. Once that is done, the sternohyoid and sternothyroid muscles can be incised safely on both sides, thereby enhancing the mobility of the goiter so that it can be retracted more effectively allowing for exposure of vital structures. Finger dissection may be used to disimpact a multinodular goiter that is entrapped in the inlet or in the superior mediastinum. However, it may be necessary to divide the superior vascular pedicles bilaterally in order to enhance the mobilization of the goiter. The carotid

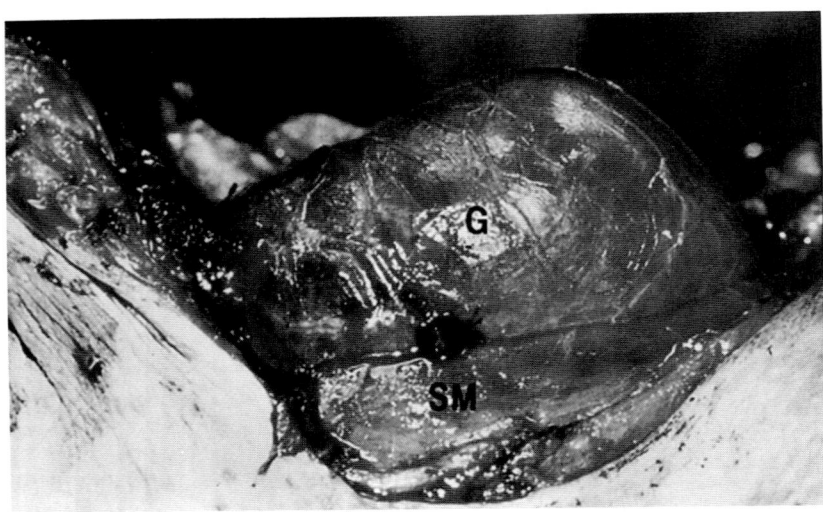

FIG. 9. Exposure of goiter (G) and sternomastoid muscle (SM) after elevation of skin flaps and division of strap muscles in patient illustrated in Fig. 8.

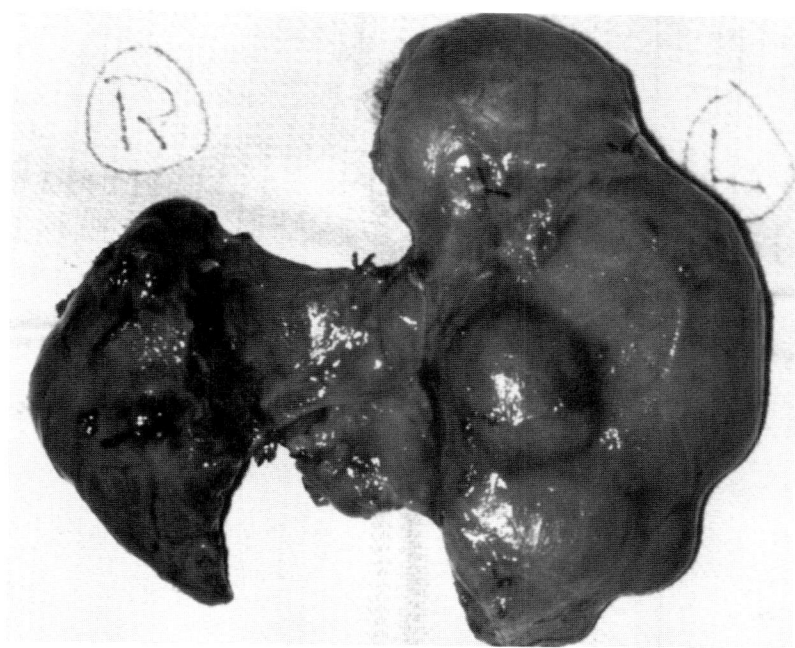

FIG. 10. Total thyroidectomy specimen from patient illustrated in Fig. 8, showing irregular nodular surface of the multinodular goiter.

sheaths are carefully separated from the goiter. If the contents are splayed over the goiter (Fig. 12), each component of the carotid sheath must be carefully separated from the gland and preserved.

It may not be possible to commence the search for the recurrent laryngeal nerves until the gland is disimpacted and elevated into the anterior neck. Accordingly, ligation of the inferior or middle thyroid veins should be done as close to the multinodular goiter as possible to avoid inadvertent trauma to a malpositioned or elongated recurrent laryngeal nerve. Ordinarily, the inferior thyroid artery should not be divided until the recurrent laryngeal nerve is identified. However, on occasion, this may not be possible with a very large multinodular goiter, and so ligation and division of the inferior thyroid artery are done with the realization that the recurrent nerve may be put at greater risk than normally.

With large multinodular goiters, the parathyroid glands may be displaced from their usual locations and the glands may be on longer and more tenuous vascular pedicles. Accordingly, it is more difficult to locate and preserve the parathyroid glands during surgery for multi-

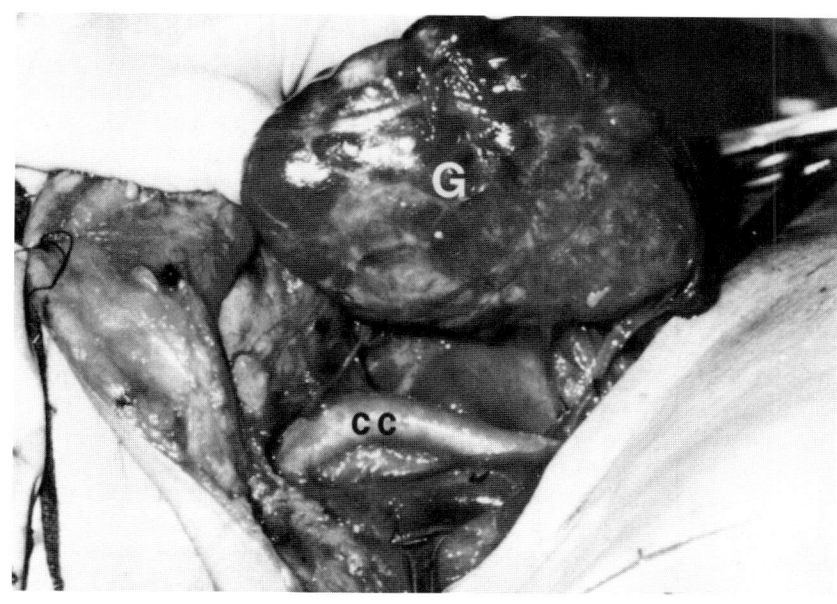

FIG. 11. Elongation and tortuosity of the right common carotid artery (CC) by a large multinodular goiter (G).

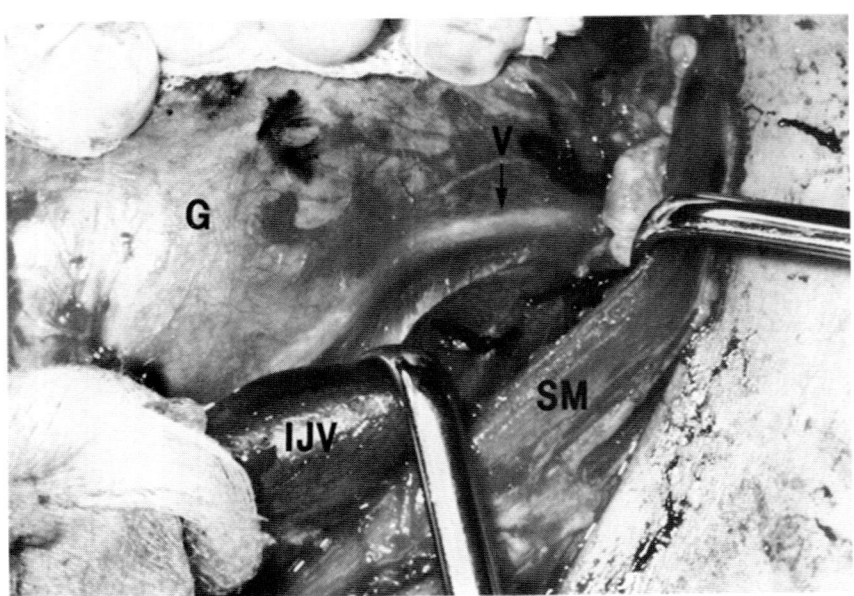

FIG. 12. The splaying of the contents of the right carotid sheath, i.e., vagus nerve (V) and internal jugular vein (IJV), by pressure from a large multinodular goiter (G), with a 280 gm right lobe. SM, sternomastoid muscle.

nodular goiters. As many parathyroid glands as possible should be identified before the goiter is removed from the neck. Those glands that can be preserved *in situ* should be. However, in those instances where the parathyroid glands cannot be preserved *in situ,* because the vascular pedicle to the parathyroid gland is compromised during surgery, the gland should be removed and placed in Ringer's solution for later autotransplantation. Because all of the parathyroid glands are at greater risk for avascular necrosis in surgery for large multinodular goiters, all glands that cannot be preserved *in situ* should be reimplanted. The parathyroid glands that require reimplantation should be divided into segments of 2 mm and then implanted into a suitable muscle, usually the sternomastoid muscle. The implantation requires a meticulous technique to prevent hematoma formation within the recipient muscle, and also to avoid extrusion of the parathyroid fragments from the recipient muscle before the fascia overlying the muscle is closed. The site of implantation into the recipient muscle should be marked with a nonabsorbable suture. Hence, the parathyroid glands require even more meticulous attention than usual when surgery is undertaken for management of multinodular goiters because of the increased difficulties encountered in localization of the parathyroid glands as well as the increased risk of avascular necrosis with both *in situ* preservation and autotransplantation.

Because of the increased risks to the recurrent laryngeal nerves and to the parathyroid glands when surgery of large multinodular goiters is done, several surgical techniques have been proposed to reduce the inherent risks. These techniques range from a hemithyroidectomy to a subtotal thyroidectomy to a near-total thyroidectomy to a subcapsular thyroidectomy. Yet, the most common procedure and probably the safest and most effective procedure done for treatment of multinodular goiter is a total thyroidectomy.

A hemithyroidectomy or subtotal thyroidectomy can be performed when normal thyroid tissue is present in a position that is remote to the main pathological process. Generally, these procedures put the contralateral recurrent laryngeal nerve and parathyroid glands at less risk. However, one can never be certain of the actual number of parathyroid glands present in a given patient. Hence, it is imprudent to assume that parathyroid glands will be present adjoining the normal thyroid tissue that will not be excised in some form of a partial thyroidectomy procedure. Therefore, the surgeon must carefully search for

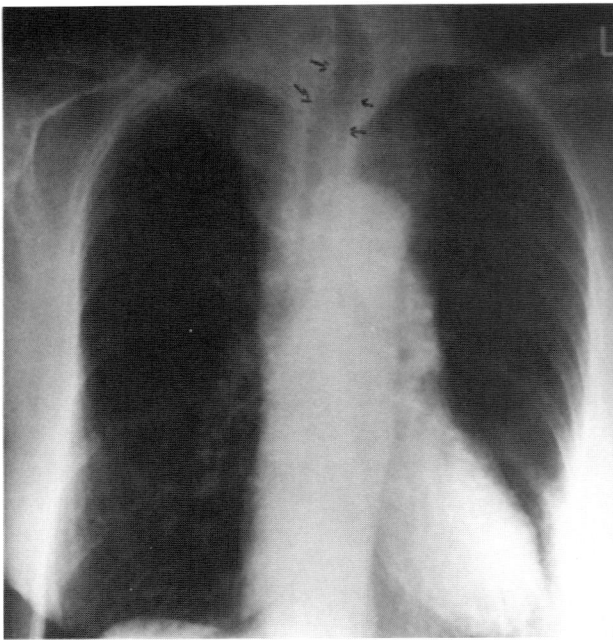

FIG. 13. A-P chest radiograph showing mediastinal tracheal displacement (arrows) and a soft tissue density in the superior mediastinum.

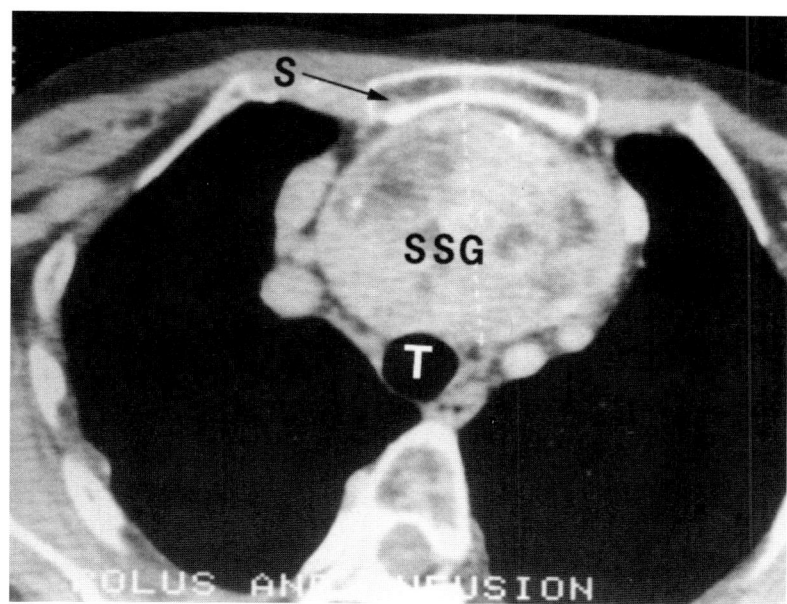

FIG. 14. Computerized tomography (CT) scan showing substernal goiter (SSG), sternum (S), and posterior displacement of the thoracic portion of the trachea (T).

all of the parathyroid tissue regardless of whether or not a modified thyroidectomy is done. Apparently normal thyroid tissue left behind during a hemithyroidectomy or a subtotal thyroidectomy for multinodular goiter may in fact have an increased propensity to develop into a goiter even if the patient is on thyroxine.

Near-total thyroidectomies and subcapsular thyroidectomies are designed to remove as much thyroid tissue as possible, yet reduce the increased risk to the recurrent laryngeal nerves and parathyroid glands that is perceived to be present with a total thyroidectomy. In fact, in our opinion these techniques actually increase the risk to the recurrent nerves and parathyroid glands.

The surgical procedure of choice in the management of large multinodular goiters is a total thyroidectomy. If performed in a meticulous fashion with the knowledge of the altered surgical anatomy, and using the modifications in surgical technique that have already been described, the risks to the recurrent laryngeal nerves and parathyroid glands can be kept to a minimum. Better hemostasis can be maintained with a total thyroidectomy than with a near-total or subcapsular thyroidectomy, thereby reducing intraoperative risks to vital structures. If neoplasia is present, a total thyroidectomy is the most effective treatment.

If aberrant vasculature such as a thyroid ima artery is present, or if there is a larger substernal component to the multinodular goiter, a sternotomy is necessary to expose the lesion adequately and remove it safely (Figs. 13–19).

The surgical wound resulting from a large multinodular goiter is much more extensive than that seen following the removal of a relatively normal-sized thyroid gland. There is usually extensive dissection of the tissue planes into the superior mediastinum, prevertebral space, and into both sides of the neck. Accordingly, spe-

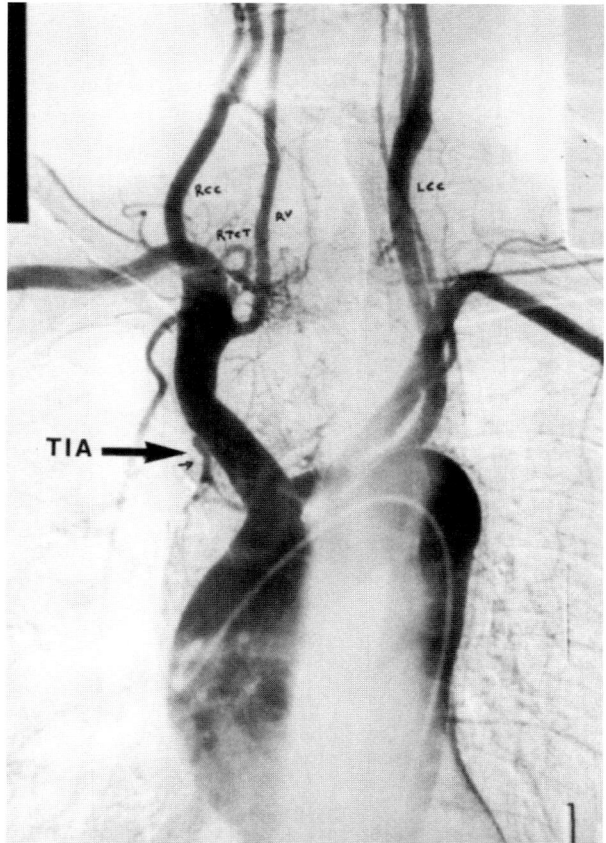

FIG. 15. A superselective angiogram (arterial phase), in a patient with a cervical/mediastinal multinodular goiter, demonstrating a thyroid ima artery (TIA) supplying the mediastinal component of the lesion.

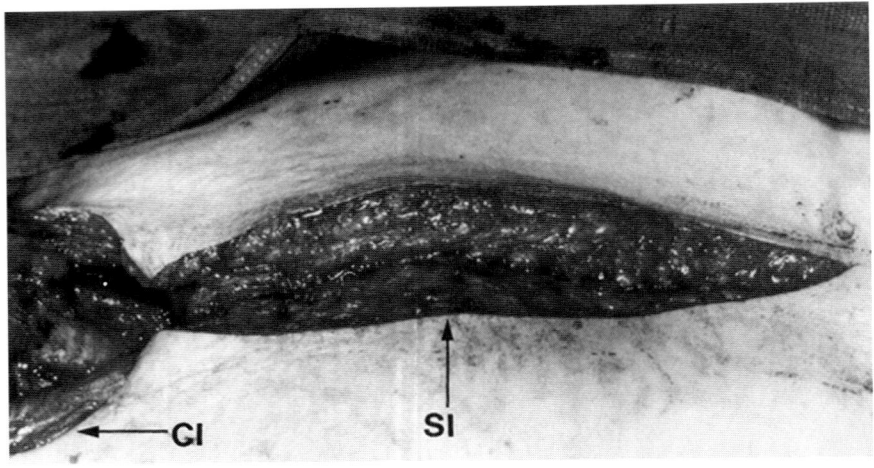

FIG. 16. Incision for a large cervical/mediastinal goiter with a thyroid ima artery. Cervical incision (CI), sternotomy incision (SI).

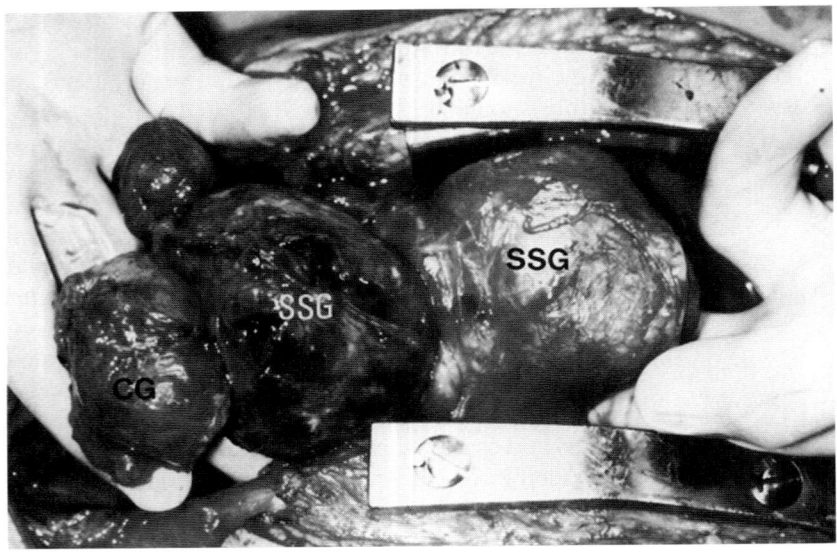

FIG. 17. Sternal split for removal of large cervical (CG) and substernal (SSG) goiter weighing 425 gm.

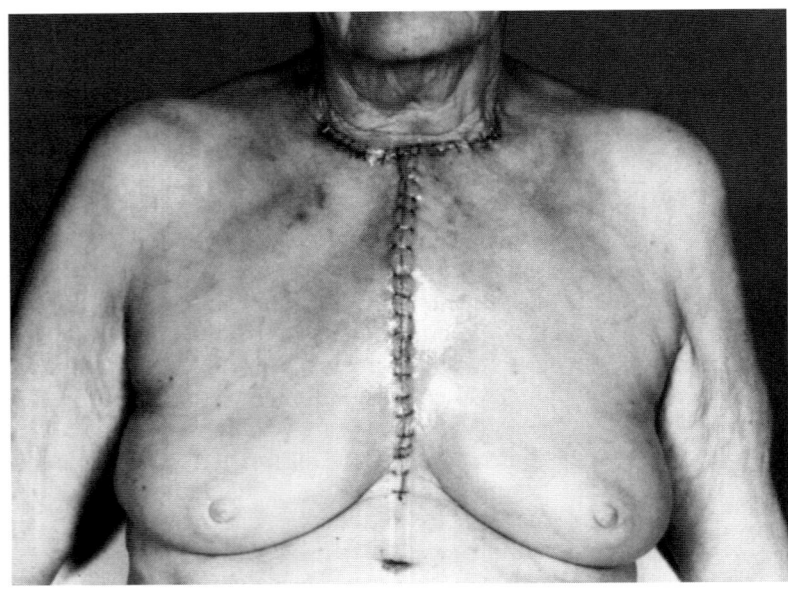

FIG. 18. Cervical and sternotomy incisions on the fifth postoperative day.

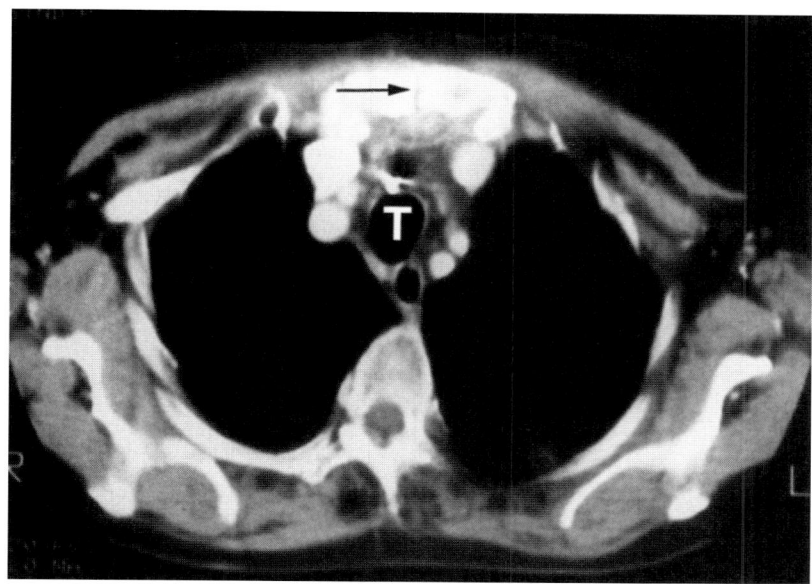

FIG. 19. CT scan taken one month following removal of a cervical/mediastinal 425 gm multinodular goiter with arrow on sternotomy incision. T, trachea.

cial attention is paid to intraoperative hemostasis. This is best accomplished by using bipolar cautery, ligatures, and, on occasion, fine-suture ligatures or surgical hemostatic agents (Surgicel). The wound is thoroughly drained using an Argyle chest type of drain connected to an Emmerson pump. Finally, if there is significant deformation of the trachea by long-standing pressure from a massive goiter, the surgeon should mold the trachea back into position in the open neck, or have an assistant place a rigid bronchoscope transorally into the tracheal lumen to restore the shape of the lumen (Fig. 20). Ordinarily, most distortion of the tracheal cartilages caused by pressure from a multinodular goiter can be corrected using these techniques. If the trachea remains significantly distorted, endotracheal intubation may be necessary for 24 to 48 hr postoperatively. The patient should be ventilated during that time. When possible, a tracheostomy should be avoided as it may result in further weakening of the trachea and tracheomalacia.

Postoperative Care

In most instances the patient is extubated at the end of the operative procedure. However, if the surgical wound is larger than usual, intensive care management is usually advisable for the first 24 hr.

If the airway has been decompressed or if there was extensive dissection in the neck or superior mediastinum, postoperative ventilation with an oral endotracheal tube for the first 24 hr is recommended.

The surgical drains are usually left in place for a minimum of 48 hr, longer if the drainage is copious. Calcium metabolism is monitored carefully, both clinically and biochemically, until it has stabilized. With large surgical wounds, this may take 4 to 5 days.

The majority of patients will have had enough thyroid tissue removed to render them hypothyroid, and thyroxine replacement therapy is usually started upon discharge from the hospital. If hypothyroidism is not present, the use of thyroxine is optional. Patients whose goiters were not originally suppressible may not derive any further benefit from this therapy, since the use of the medication

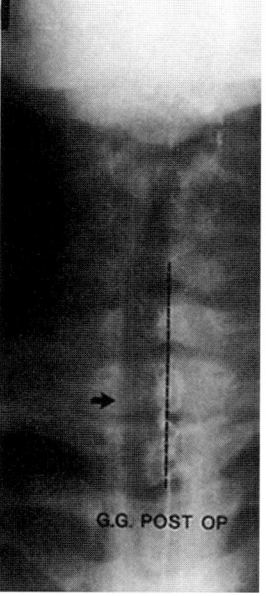

FIG. 20. Preoperative (PRE OP) A-P tomogram shows severe tracheal deformation to a 2 mm diameter (arrow) by a 280 gm right-sided multinodular goiter. Dotted line illustrates midline of neck. Following removal of the goiter, the trachea was molded back into position with resultant normal airway function. Postoperative (POST OP) A-P tomogram at 1 year shows a normal trachea, slightly to the right of midline (dotted line) because of a residual left lobe of thyroid gland.

postoperatively is of dubious value in the prevention of recurrence (53). If carcinoma is present, thyroxine may be withheld in preparation for a total body iodine scan to search for residual or metastatic disease.

REFERENCES

1. Kelly FC, Snedden WW. Prevalence and geographic distribution of endemic goitre. In: *Endemic goitre, World Health Organization monograph series no. 44*. Geneva: WHO, 1960;27–233.
2. Langer P. History of goitre. In: *Endemic goitre, World Health Organization monograph series no. 44*. Geneva: WHO, 1960;9–25.
3. Medvei VC. *A history of endocrinology*. Boston: M.T.P. Press, 1982.
4. Perez C, Scrimshaw NS, Munoz JA. Technique of endemic goitre surveys. In: *Endemic goitre, World Health Organization monograph series no. 44*. Geneva: WHO, 1960;369–383.
5. Berghout A, Wiersinga WM, Smits NJ, et al. The value of thyroid volume measured by ultrasonography in the diagnosis of goitre. *Clin Endocrinol (Oxf)* 1988;28:409–414.
6. McKusick VA. *Mendelian inheritance in man*, 5th ed. Baltimore: Johns Hopkins University Press, 1978;685–688.
7. Koutras DA, Matavinovic J, Vought R. The ecology of iodine. In: Stanbury JB, Hetzel BS, eds. *Endemic goiter and endemic cretinism*. New York: John Wiley & Sons, 1980;185–195.
8. Ingebleek Y, DeVischer M. Hormonal and nutritional status: critical conditions for endemic goiter epidemiology? *Metabolism* 1979;28:9–19.
9. Ingebleek Y, Luypaert B, DeNayer PH. Nutritional status and endemic goitre. *Lancet* 1980;1:388–392.
10. Gaitan E. Goitrogens in food and water. *Annu Rev Nutr* 1990;10:21–39.
11. Suzuki H, Higuchi T, Sawa K, et al. Endemic coast goitre in Hokkaido Japan. *Acta Endocrinol (Copenh)* 1965;50:161–176.
12. Stanbury JB, Ermans AM, Hetzel BS, et al. Endemic goitre and cretinism: public health significance and presentation. *WHO Chronicle* 1974;28:220–228.
13. Hetzel BS, Thilly CH, Fierro-Benitez R, et al. Iodized oil in the prevention of endemic goiter and cretinism. In: Stanbury JB, Hetzel BS, eds. *Endemic goiter and endemic cretinism*. New York: John Wiley & Sons, 1980;513–532.
14. Tonglet R, Bourdoux P, Minga T, et al. Efficacy of low oral doses of iodized oil in the control of iodine deficiency in Zaire. *N Engl J Med* 1992;326:236–241.
15. Maberly GF, Corcoran JM, Eastman CJ. The effect of iodized oil on goitre size, thyroid function and the development of the Jod Basedow phenomenon. *Clin Endocrinol (Oxf)* 1982;17:253–259.
16. Eastman CJ, Phillips DIW. Endemic goitre and iodine deficiency disorders—aetiology, epidemiology and treatment. *Ballieres Clin Endocrinol Metab* 1988;2:719–735.
17. Chopra IJ, Hershman JM, Hornabrook RW. Serum thyroid hormone and thyrotrophin levels in subjects from endemic goiter regions of New Guinea. *J Clin Endocrinol Metab* 1975;40:326–333.
18. Elte JWF, Hoak A, Frolich M, et al. Autonomously functioning euthyroid multinodular goitre. *Neth J Med* 1977;20:1–4.
19. Williams ED, Doniach I. Thyroid autographs in hypophysectomized and in thyroxine treated rats. *J Endocrinol* 1963;26:479–488.
20. Roger PP, Dumont JE. Factors controlling proliferation and differentiation of canine thyroid cells cultured in reduced serum conditions: effects of thyrotropin, cyclic AMP and growth factors. *Mol Cell Endocrinol* 1984;36:79–93.
21. Drexhage HA, Bottazzo GF, Doniach D. Evidence for thyroid growth stimulating immunoglobulins in some goitrous thyroid diseases. *Lancet* 1980;2:287–292.
22. Smyth PPA, McMullan NM, Grubeck-Loebenstein B, et al. Thyroid growth-stimulating immunoglobulins in goitrous disease: relationship to thyroid stimulating immunoglobulins. *Acta Endocrinol (Copenh)* 1986;111:321–330.
23. Brown RS. Immunoglobulins affecting thyroid growth: a continuing controversy [editorial]. *J Clin Endocrinol Metab* 1995;80:1506–1508.
24. Struder H, Peter HJ, Gerber H. Nature of heterogeneity of thyroid cells: the basis for understanding thyroid function and nodular goitre growth. *Endocr Rev* 1989;10:125–135.
25. Struder H, Derwahl M. Mechanisms of non-neoplastic endocrine hyperplasia—a changing concept: a review focused on the thyroid gland. *Endocr Rev* 1995;16:411–426.
26. Struder H, Ramelli F. Simple goiter and its variants: euthyroid and hyperthyroid multinodular goiters. *Endocr Rev* 1982;3:40–61.
27. Peter HJ, Gerter H, Struder H, et al. Pathogenesis of heterogeneity in human multinodular goiter. A study on growth and function of thyroid tissue transplanted onto nude mice. *J Clin Invest* 1985;76:1992–2002.
28. Kopp P, Aeschimann S, Tobler A, et al. Polyclonal and clonal nodules may co-exist within multinodular goiters. *J Clin Endocrinol Metab* 1994;79:134–139.
29. Wahner HW, Cuello C, Correa P, et al. Thyroid carcinoma in an endemic goiter area, Cali, Colombia. *Am J Med* 1966;40:58–66.
30. Pendergrast WJ, Milmore BK, Marcus BS. Thyroid cancer and thyrotoxicosis in the United States: their relation to endemic goiter. *J Chronic Dis* 1961;13:22–38.
31. Belfiore A, LaRosa G, LaPorta G, et al. Cancer risk in patients with cold thyroid nodules: relevance of iodine intake, sex, age and multinodularity. *Am J Med* 1992;93:363–369.
32. Veith FJ, Brooks JR, Grigsby WP. The nodular thyroid gland and cancer. A practical approach to the problem. *N Engl J Med* 1964;270:431–436.
33. Jauregui R, Lilker ES, Bayley A. Upper airway obstruction in euthyroid goiter. *JAMA* 1977;238:2163–2166.
34. Melliere D, Saada F, Etienne G, et al. Goiter with severe respiratory compromise: evaluation and treatment. *Surgery* 1988;103:367–373.
35. Hegedus L, Hanse JM, Feldt-Rasmussen U. Influence of thyroxine treatment on thyroid size and anti-thyroid peroxidase antibodies in Hashimoto's thyroiditis. *Clin Endocrinol* 1991;35:235–238.
36. Reede DI, Bergeron RT, McCauley DI. CT of the thyroid and of other thoracic inlet disorders. *J Otolaryngol* 1982;11:349–357.
37. Mountz JM, Glazer GM, Dmuchowski C, et al. MR imaging of the thyroid: comparison with scintigraphy in the normal and diseased gland. *J Comput Assist Tomogr* 1987;11:612–619.
38. Struder H, Bungi H, Kohler H, et al. A transient rise of hormone secretion: a response of the stimulated rat thyroid gland to small increments of iodide supply. *Acta Endocrinol (Copenh)* 1976;81:507–515.
39. Vagenakis AG, Wang C, Burger A, et al. Iodine induced thyrotoxicosis in Boston. *N Engl J Med* 1972;287:523–526.
40. Gavin LA, Rosenthal M, Cavalieri R. The diagnostic dilemma of isolated hyperthyroxinemia in acute illness. *JAMA* 1979;242:251–253.
41. Britton KE, Quinn V, Ellis SM, et al. Is "T4 toxicosis" a normal biochemical finding in elderly women? *Lancet* 1975;2:141–142.
42. Grier MA, Astwood EB. Treatment of simple goiter with thyroid. *J Clin Endocrinol Metab* 1953;13:1312–1331.
43. Shimaoka K, Sokal JE. Suppressive therapy of nontoxic goiter. *Am J Med* 1974;57:576–583.
44. Berghout A, Wiersinga WM, Drexhage HA, et al. Comparison of placebo with L-thyroxine alone or with carbimazole for the treatment of sporadic non-toxic goiter. *Lancet* 1990;336:193–197.
45. Astwood EB, Cassidy CE, Aurbach GD. Treatment of goiter and thyroid nodules with thyroid. *JAMA* 1960;174:459–464.
46. Berghout A, Wiersinga WM, Drexhage HA, et al. The long term outcome of thyroidectomy for sporadic non-toxic goiter. *Clin Endocrinol* 1989;31:193–199.
47. Miccoli P, Antonelli A, Iacconi P. Prospective, randomized double blind study about effectiveness of levothyroxine suppressive therapy in prevention of recurrence after operation: result at the third year of follow-up. *Surgery* 1993;114:1097–1102.
48. Kiederling W, Enrich D, Hanzwalki C, et al. Ergebnisse der radiojodverkleinerungstherapie euthyreoter strumen. *Dtsch Med Wochenschr* 1964;89:453–457.
49. Kay TWH, d'Emden MC, Andrews JT, et al. Treatment of nontoxic multinodular goiter with radioactive iodine. *Am J Med* 1988;84:19–22.
50. Teuscher J, Hans-Jakob P, Gerber H, et al. Pathogenesis of nodular goiter and its implications for surgical management. *Surgery* 1988;103(1):87–93.
51. McCall A, Jarosz H, Lawrence AM, et al. The incidence of thyroid carcinoma in solitary cold nodules and in multinodular goiters. *Surgery* 1986;100(6):1128–1131.
52. Shana AR, Alfonso AE, Jaffe BM. Operative treatment of substernal goiters. *Head Neck Surg* 1989;11:325–330.
53. Peter C, Persson A, Johansson H, et al. Nodular goiter—is thyroxine medication of any value? *World J Surg* 1982;6:391–396.

CHAPTER 24

Management of Substernal Thyroid Disease

William Lawson, Anthony J. Reino, and Hugh F. Biller

ETIOLOGY

The proposed pathogenesis of substernal goiters has been by inferior extension of the cervical thyroid gland, or by origination from aberrant mediastinal thyroid tissue. The majority of studies favor the former explanation (1–5).

After continued cervical growth, a goiter may extend downward into the thoracic inlet. Several factors favor the passage of goiter into the mediastinum: downward traction caused by normal deglutition, negative intrathoracic pressure, and the pull of gravity. Once the mediastinal component has enlarged sufficiently to become trapped in the chest, unlimited growth is possible because of minimal intrathoracic resistance. The communication to the neck may then become tenuous, leaving only the cervical vascular pedicle.

In support of the concept of a thyroid origin is the finding of Ellis et al. (6) that the blood supply of the mediastinal goiter is principally from the inferior thyroid artery. In an occasional aberrant case, the mass is vascularized from the aorta, subclavian artery, internal mammary artery, or thyroid ima. Sweet (7) found that posterior mediastinal goiters maintained a connection with the cervical thyroid. However, in support of the primary intrathoracic origin hypothesis, Falor et al. (8,9) observed seven patients in whom the mediastinal goiter had a completely intrathoracic blood supply. Nevertheless, mediastinal thyroid lesions with a seemingly aberrant development are exceptional and the majority have an attenuated pedicle to the neck.

INCIDENCE

Goiters arise from inadequate thyroid hormone production by the thyroid gland, inducing increased thyroid stimulating hormone (TSH) secretion and compensatory thyromegaly. The reported incidence of substernal goiters varies widely and ranges from 0.1% to 21% (Table 1). Factors responsible for these diverse data include the reporting of cases from endemic goiter areas, series published before the introduction of the use of iodized salt and thyroid hormone for TSH suppression, delayed surgical management of thyroid disease, and classification differences in reporting substernal goiters. The first three factors have resulted in an increased frequency of large multinodular goiters, some of which may extend substernally. Exemplifying this are the publications of Lahey and Swinton in 1934 (10) and Lahey in 1936 (11), which describe operating on 1300 goiters that extend to or beyond the aortic arch. The occurrence rate in recent series has been more moderate.

In the series of 872 thyroidectomies performed at the University of Michigan (1972 to 1982) and reported by Allo and Thompson (12), there were 50 patients (5.7%) with substernal disease. Most patients had a long history of goiter, with four patients having undergone previous thyroidectomy and two having received radioactive iodine for thyrotoxicosis. Katlic et al. (5) reported that their 80 cases represented 8% of the thyroid resections performed at the Massachusetts General Hospital in the period from 1976 to 1982.

The occurrence rate of intrathoracic thyroid within the general population is difficult to estimate. Based on screening chest x-rays for tuberculosis, Rundle (13) found 194 cases (0.02% rate) in the United States among 1 million patients surveyed, and Reeve et al. (14) noted 5040 cases among 967,759 adults surveyed in Australia.

CLASSIFICATION

Thyroid tissue within the chest has variously been described anatomically as substernal, retrosternal, mediasti-

---

W. Lawson, A. J. Reino, and H. F. Biller: Department of Otolaryngology—Head and Neck Surgery, Mt. Sinai Medical Center, New York, New York 10023.

TABLE 1. *Incidence of substernal thyroid disease*

Author (ref.)	Year	Total no. thyroidectomies	No. substernal	Incidence (%)
Lahey and Swinton (10)	1934	5131	1086	21.2
DeAndrade (3)	1977	9100	1300	14.3
Pemberton (33)	1921	4006	542	13.5
Wakely and Mulvany (38)	1940	1265	111	8.8
Reeve (86)	1972	2000	173	8.6
Allo and Thompson (12)	1983	872	50	5.7
Dundas (20)	1964	1003	49	4.9
Sand et al. (26)	1983	750	31	4.1
McCort (40)	1949	908	28	3.1
Georgiadis et al. (2)	1970	1600	34	2.1
Crile (59)	1939	11,800	97	0.1
Singh et al. (89)	1994	370	72	19
Wax and Briant (90)	1991	938	24	2.6
Sanders et al. (28)	1992	646	52	8
Total		40,389	3,649	
Mean		2885	261	9.0

astinal, and mediastinal aberrant. Lesions within the mediastinum lacking a connection with the cervical thyroid gland have also been termed sequestered goiters (15).

Falor et al. (8,9) proposed a system of classification based on the site of origin of the vascular pedicle. Secondary intrathoracic goiters that had descended from the neck received their blood supply by a cervical pedicle from the inferior thyroid artery. The primary intrathoracic goiter arising from ectopic thyroid tissue in the mediastinum was vascularized from short intrathoracic arteries and drained into intrathoracic veins. Both groups were subclassified into anterior and posterior mediastinal goiters not contiguous with the cervical thyroid and were described by Falor et al. (8,9). Other instances of intrathoracic thyroid lacking a connection to the cervical gland were also reported by Adams (16), Pitt (17), Fogelfeld et al. (18), Sussman et al. (19), Dundas (20), Rives (21), Ziter (22), and Salomon and Levy (23). Based on their system of classification, Falor et al. (8,9) concluded that all secondary anterior and most secondary posterior intrathoracic goiters could be removed safely through a cervical approach. Almost all primary intrathoracic goiters required a thoracotomy. Generally, a right posterolateral approach was employed, but occasionally a sternotomy was used. However, in a study of 128 posterior mediastinal goiters by DeAndrade (3), the blood supply in the vast majority of the cases was found to be from the inferior thyroid artery.

Mediastinal goiters have also been subdivided according to their anatomic location. Sweet (7) characterized anterior mediastinal goiters as arising anteriorly from the lateral lobes or isthmus of the thyroid, with displacement of the trachea and esophagus posteriorly, and situated in front of the recurrent laryngeal nerves, innominate and subclavian blood vessels, common carotid artery, and inferior thyroid arteries. Posterior mediastinal goiters arose from the posterior aspect of the gland and descended behind all of these structures.

Higgins (24) subclassified intrathoracic goiters by extent, into (a) completely intrathoracic (more than 80%) with a barely detectable or no cervical component; (b) partially intrathoracic (more than 50%); and (c) substernal, which has both mediastinal and cervical components (50% or more in the neck). By these criteria, among the 70 cases of Cho et al. (25), 54.3% were substernal, 34.3% were partially intrathoracic, and 11.4% were completely intrathoracic, and in the series of Sand et al. (26), 20 (64.5%) were substernal, 10 (32.3%) were partially intrathoracic, and 1 (3.2%) was completely intrathoracic.

PATHOLOGY

The histopathology of substernal goiter is generally benign, the majority of cases being multinodular goiters (Fig. 1), followed by follicular adenomas and thyroiditis. Among the 80 cases of Katlic et al. (5), multinodular goiters were encountered in 51%, follicular adenomas in 45%, and Hashimoto's thyroiditis in 5% of the patients. In two patients, occult papillary carcinoma was found.

In the series of 70 cases of Cho et al. (25), 90% of the lesions were benign and 10% were malignant. The benign group included 44 multinodular goiters, 18 follicular adenomas, and 1 thyroiditis; the malignant tumors consisted of 3 follicular carcinomas, 2 histiocytic lymphomas, and 2 anaplastic carcinomas.

In the series of Allo and Thompson (12), there were 42 benign lesions and 8 malignant tumors. The latter group consisted of 3 histiocytic lymphomas and 1 each of papillary carcinoma, follicular carcinoma, Hürthle cell carcinoma, medullary carcinoma, and anaplastic carcinoma.

Among the 28 cases with pathology of Lamke et al. (27), there were 22 multinodular goiters, 5 adenomas, and 1 follicular carcinoma. Among the 31 cases reported by Sand et al. (26), 29 were multinodular goiters and 2 were Hashimoto's disease.

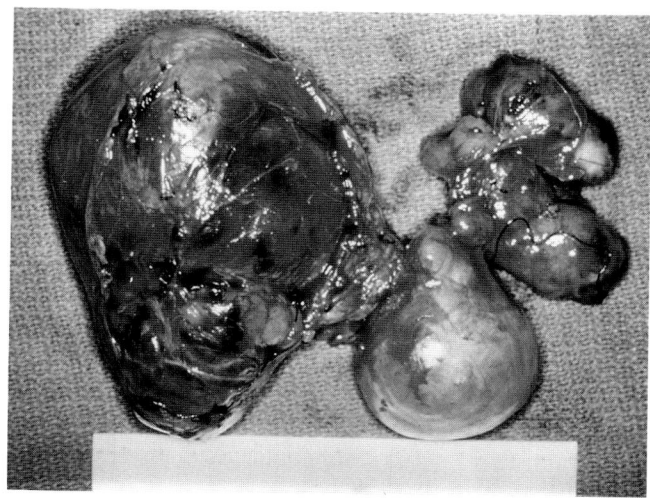

FIG. 1. Surgical specimen of a multinodular goiter with the substernal component attached.

Sanders et al. (28) retrospectively reviewed the pathology of 52 patients with substernal goiter. They noted a 17% incidence of malignancy; moreover, 21% of specimens showed incidental papillary carcinoma. The development of malignancy in these cases could not be correlated and/or identified through either the duration of goiter, patient symptomatology, or fine-needle aspiration.

Other studies have also identified a small number of patients manifesting occult carcinoma within a substernal goiter (29,30). Carcinoma was noted in 3 of the 31 cases of Sand et al. (26), 1 of the 29 cases of Lamke et al. (27), 1 of the 34 cases of Georgiadis et al. (2), and 1 of the 112 cases of Judd et al. (31). In the series of Katlic et al. (5), the mean goiter weight was 104 g with an average specimen width of 9 cm. Among the patients of Cho et al. (25), the average weight was 216 g with the largest specimen weighing 2100 g and measuring 30 cm in diameter. Johnston and Twente (32) also describe excising a massive intrathoracic goiter weighing 1730 g.

CLINICAL FEATURES

Location

The reported laterality of substernal goiters varies in different series. Among 542 substernal goiters studied by Pemberton (33), 158 were right lobe, 299 left lobe, 56 bilateral, 8 isthmic, and 21 not specified. In the series of 70 cases of Cho et al. (25), 43% were right-sided, 50% were left-sided, and 7% were bilateral. Sand et al. (26) reported 22 left, 8 right, and 1 bilateral goiter in their 31 patients.

However, Ellis et al. (6) reported a predilection of intrathoracic goiters for the right side, especially when they were in the posterior mediastinum. This occurred in 18 of their 24 cases. All 12 of the posterior mediastinal goiters reported by Rietz and Werner (34) were right-sided. A right-sided prevalence of substernal goiter was also noted by Johnston and Twente (32), Falor et al. (8), Lindskog and Goldberg (35), and Sherman and Shahbahrami (36). However, Katlic et al. (5) noted no preferential laterality in their 80 cases, with 12 being bilateral.

The great majority of intrathoracic goiters rest in the anterior mediastinum. DeAndrade (3) found 128 posterior mediastinal tumors (9.9%) among 1300 intrathoracic goiters. In smaller series, 2 of the 34 cases (6%) of Georgiadis et al. (2), 4 of the 70 cases (6%) of Cho et al. (25), 4 of the 31 cases (13%) of Sand et al. (26), and 12 of the 48 cases (25%) of Rietz and Werner (34) were posterior.

The preferred location of the mass in the right mediastinum is behind the superior vena cava and azygos vein, resting on the bodies of the vertebrae. Gourin et al. (37) noted that left-sided tumors were generally high and anterior in the mediastinum because of the oblique position of the ascending aorta, making it difficult for nodules to extend posteriorly. Rietz and Werner (34) postulated that the innominate vein and vessels from the aortic arch served to deflect posterior goiters to the right.

Age and Sex

Substernal goiters generally occur in later life and have a peak incidence in the sixth decade (26,27). Most authors report a preponderance of women, varying from an extreme of 9:1 (38) to the more common ratios of 3:1 to 4:1 (2,3,26,37,39). However, an equal ratio (34,35,40) and even a slight increase among men (27) have been noted.

In the series of 50 cases of Allo and Thompson (12), the age range was 39 to 87 years, with a mean age of 66 years. There was a sexual predilection for women in the ratio of 3.2 to 1 (38 women and 12 men).

Among the 80 cases from the Massachusetts General Hospital (1976 to 1982) reported by Katlic et al. (5), the age range was from 22 to 78 years, with a mean of 56 years. There was no sex predilection. In the series of 70 cases of Cho et al. (25), the age range was 21 to 80 years, with the majority of patients being over 50 years of age; 84% were women. In a study of 128 posterior mediastinal tumors by DeAndrade (3), all patients were older than 50 years, with a 4:1 prevalence of women.

Signs and Symptoms

The great majority of patients with substernal goiters show both objective findings and subjective complaints. However, 28% of the 29 cases of Lamke et al. (27) and 41% of the 70 cases of Cho et al. (25) were asymptomatic. The clinical manifestations of substernal goiters are related to compression or displacement of the adjacent aerodigestive tract and mediastinal great vessels.

Although a majority of patients with substernal goiters have a palpable neck mass, it is not invariably present. It was absent in as many as 10% of the cases of Katlic et al. (5), 23% of the cases of Lindskog and Goldberg (35), and 35% of those of Sand et al. (26). Rarely, a "goiter plongeont" is observed, wherein the neck mass disappears into the thoracic cavity, appearing again on swallowing or coughing (40).

In 58 patients with goiters causing severe airway compromise reviewed by Melliere et al. (41), a substernal component was present in 23 patients (7 of 15 with malignant tumors, 16 of 43 with benign lesions). The intrathoracic component served to compress the trachea between two rigid bony structures, the vertebral column and the sternum. Early compression became manifest as nocturnal choking, cough, dyspnea, asthma, and obstructive pulmonary disease.

Acute airway compression may develop secondary to hemorrhage within the tumor, which may require emergency tracheostomy (41). This occurred in 2 of the 50 cases of Allo and Thompson (12) and 2 of the 70 cases of Cho et al. (25).

The incidence of a paralyzed or paretic vocal cord appears to be greater with substernal goiters, presumably secondary to stretching and ischemia of the recurrent laryngeal nerve. In our experience, this occurs more often with right-sided lesions. However, this finding may be reversible with surgery. In 2 of the 3 patients with vocal cord weakness from benign disease operated upon by Cho et al. (25), there was return of function within 3 months postoperatively. We have made similar observations in two patients.

Extrinsic pressure on the esophagus produces dysphagia, which often accompanies the respiratory symptoms.

Obstruction of the superior vena cava and/or subclavian vein may also be produced by bulky intrathoracic goiters (43–50). Venous compression will result in the development of collateral venous drainage with the presence of facial flushing or edema, and dilated neck and upper thoracic vessels (3,27). The entity of downhill esophageal varices secondary to superior vena cava obstruction has also been reported with substernal goiter by Fleig et al. (51), Kelly et al. (52), and Sorokin et al. (53). These varices bypass the superior vena cava through the azygos vein, or drain into the portal vein when the azygos vein is also obstructed. Patients with this entity may present with gastrointestinal tract bleeding in the absence of other signs of portal hypertension.

In some cases, the symptoms are positional, with facial flushing or dyspnea developing when the patient turns his neck or raises his arms, by the goiter being pulled into the thoracic inlet (3,33). McCort (40) also described the occurrence of dyspnea when the patient lay down, especially on turning the head toward the side of the goiter.

Pain is a relatively uncommon symptom of substernal goiters. In the patients of Karadeniz et al. (54), it was an indication of abscess formation. However, pain or pressure in the head, neck, chest, and shoulders was reported in 7 of the 31 cases of Sand et al. (26), presumably from pressure on the cervical cutaneous nerves. Another unusual sign is the development of Horner's syndrome from compression of the sympathetic chain (27). Karlin (55) and Fernandez-Cruz et al. (56) reported the rare development of chylothorax from thoracic duct occlusion. Gadisseux et al. (57) reported transient ischemic attacks with cerebral dysfunction in a patient with a massive retrotracheal goiter that they attributed to a "steal" syndrome. A similar case was reported by Lesoin et al. (58), in which the patient had an anomaly of the carotid artery.

Although the above signs and symptoms are commonly present, their relative incidence varies widely in reported series of operated cases.

Forty-eight out of 50 cases of substernal goiter reviewed by Allo and Thompson (12) were symptomatic. All had symptoms of airway impingement that appeared clinically as cough, wheezing, and nocturnal dyspnea. Twenty-two patients had tracheal compression, 13 had dysphagia, 4 had hoarseness, 3 had weight loss, 10 had thyrotoxicosis from a toxic nodular goiter, and 5 had a superior vena cava syndrome.

Among the 80 patients of Katlic et al. (5), 33% complained of dysphagia, 28% of dyspnea, 16% of stridor, and 8% of cough, with 13% being asymptomatic. Objectively, tracheal deviation was present in 35%, hoarseness in 4%, wheezing in 3%, and facial flushing in 1%. A cervical mass was present in 90% of the cases.

In the 70 cases of Cho et al. (25), 41% were asymptomatic, 41% had respiratory distress, 33% had dysphagia, 7% had vascular compression, 1.4% had stridor, and one patient (1.4%) had paraplegia from a vertebral metastasis. Objectively, tracheal deviation was present in 100% of the cases, a neck mass in 89%, tracheal compression in 26%, and a vocal cord paralysis in 7%. In 2 of the 5 patients with vocal cord paralysis, it was secondary to a malignant tumor.

Functional Activity

The majority of patients with substernal goiters are euthyroid. None of the 52 patients reviewed by Katlic et al. (5) or any of the 31 patients of Sand et al. (26) in whom thyroid function tests were performed was hyperthyroid. All 70 of the patients of Cho et al. (25) were euthyroid. However, a small number of patients with large multinodular goiters may become hyperthyroid from multiple autonomous hot nodules, or by diffuse enlargement of the thyroid whereby an excessive amount of thyroid hormone is produced. Allo and Thompson (12) noted that 20% of their patients with a long history of substernal thyroid eventually developed thyrotoxicosis. Three of the 29 cases (10%) of Lamke et al. (27), 7 of the 111 cases (6%)

of Wakely and Mulvany (38), and 1 of the 34 cases (3%) of Georgiadis et al. (2) had toxic symptoms. The significance of the report by Crile in 1939 (59) that 50% of his cases were hyperthyroid is unclear.

Rare instances of hyperthyroidism caused by toxic intrathoracic goiters in patients with normal-sized and functioning cervical thyroid glands have been reported by Prakash et al. (60), Fogelfeld et al. (18), and Fui et al. (61).

Although it is theoretically possible for patients to develop overt hyperthyroidism clinically from the use of iodine-containing contrast material and from the administration of thyroid hormone to suppress a large gland in patients with mild thyrotoxicosis, this occurs infrequently. However, it was observed to develop in several cases of Allo and Thompson (12), resulting in congestive heart failure and cardiac arrhythmias, especially in older patients.

DIAGNOSTIC EVALUATION

The differential diagnosis of an anterior mediastinal mass includes thymoma, lymphoma, substernal goiter, teratoma, vascular lesion, metastatic carcinoma, dermoid cyst, neurogenic tumor, and bronchiogenic cysts. Thyroid tumors possess certain properties that facilitate diagnosis by specialized radiologic methods.

Imaging studies performed to diagnose mediastinal thyroid lesions include conventional (plain) chest radiographs, computerized tomography (CT) scanning, magnetic resonance imaging (MRI), radionuclide scintigraphy, and esophagography.

Indirect or fiberoptic laryngoscopy should be performed on all patients with thyroid enlargement. This examination will help to delineate the presence of airway compression, laryngeal deviation, and/or impaired vocal cord mobility.

Chest X-Ray

Plain films taken in the lateral and posteroanterior projections may reveal the presence of an intrathoracic goiter and serve to localize it within the mediastinum. The goiter may be manifested by tracheal displacement, tracheal compression, the presence of a smooth or nodular superior mediastinal paratracheal mass, or reflection of the mediastinal pleura over the lesion (Fig. 2).

A goiter was demonstrated by routine chest films in 7 of the 9 cases of Shih et al. (62), 20 of 31 cases of Sand et al. (26), and 27 of the 28 cases of McCort (40). Among the 80 patients of Katlic et al. (5), 79% had tracheal deviation, 56% had a soft-tissue mass, and 2% showed calcification.

The posteroanterior (PA) view reveals lateral deviation of the trachea when it is present. This typically begins high in the neck adjacent to the larynx, a finding of differential diagnostic importance. Posterior goiters may produce displacement of the trachea anteriorly in the lateral view. With fluoroscopic monitoring the mass would be seen to move on swallowing.

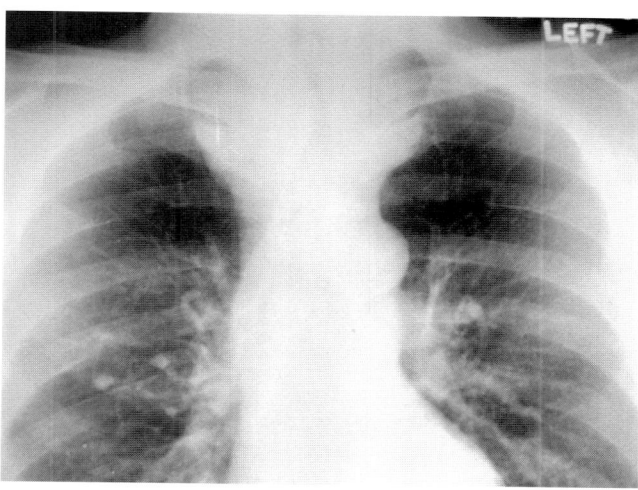

FIG. 2. Plain chest radiograph revealing a right substernal goiter partially obstructing and deviating the trachea.

Computerized Tomographic Scanning

Computerized tomographic scanning is of great diagnostic value with intrathoracic goiters because (a) it demonstrates continuity with cervical thyroid in almost all cases; (b) precontrast attenuation of thyroid is higher than adjacent muscle; (c) prolonged contrast enhancement is often present; (d) it shows well-defined borders of the lesion; (e) it may enable visualization of areas of focal calcification; and (f) the mass is nonhomogeneous with regions of low density (63–67).

Calcifications within the mass are generally punctate and have a coarse or ringlike configuration. The high iodine content of thyroid tissue is responsible for its precontrast attenuation of 15 Hounsfield units (HU) greater than muscle, which rises to 25 HU after contrast enhancement (63). The resultant prolonged enhancement after the administration of the contrast material varies with the area. The goiter is nonhomogeneous because of the presence of areas of degeneration.

Computerized tomographic scanning also gives information on the position of the goiter relative to the trachea, esophagus, and great vessels, which helps in differential diagnosis and in choosing the appropriate operative approach (Fig. 3). Typically, the goiter is paratracheal, less often retrotracheal, and rarely separate in the posterior mediastinum. Intrathoracic goiters with no connection to the cervical thyroid have been demonstrated by CT scanning by Sussman et al. (19). In addition, CT scanning may help to visualize the presence of adhesions that may make the transcervical approach hazardous.

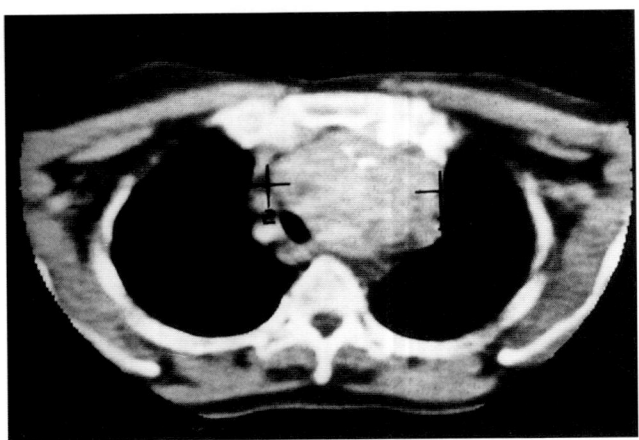

FIG. 3. Computerized tomographic scan showing an enhancing substernal mass markedly displacing the trachea.

Ultrasound, which is an important diagnostic modality with cervical thyroid lesions, is of little value with substernal goiters. However, CT scanning fills this void by providing information about lesion density. In a comparative study of 48 patients with thyroid disease by ultrasound and CT scanning performed by Radecki et al. (68), unsuspected substernal disease was detected in five cases with CT.

Magnetic Resonance Imaging

Magnetic resonance imaging has the advantages of producing high resolution tomographic images without the use of ionizing radiation or the need for a contrast agent. Using MRI, Sandler et al. (69) reported an intrathoracic goiter having the same proton density as the thyroid gland but without a physical connection with it.

Radionuclide Scintigraphy

The reported efficacy of radionuclide scanning in visualizing substernal goiters varies widely. Scintigraphy may fail to detect mediastinal thyroid because of diminished uptake of the radionuclide. Shih et al. (62) noted uptake of iodine-131 (^{131}I) in only 3 of 7 patients (43%) scanned. Sand et al. (26) found the thyroid scan to be positive in 14 of 24 patients (58%) with substernal goiters, but they did not specify the radionuclide used. Park et al. (70) noted scintigraphy with iodine-123 (^{123}I), ^{131}I, and technetium-99m (^{99m}Tc) pertechnetate to have an accuracy of 94% (51 of 54 cases). Irwin et al. (71) noted positive scans in all 24 cases of mediastinal goiter with ^{131}I. Toxic intrathoracic goiters in patients with normal cervical thyroid glands have been demonstrated scintigraphically with ^{131}I and ^{99m}Tc by Prakash et al. (60), Fui et al. (61), and Fogelfeld et al. (18).

Radionuclide scintigraphy was also used by Sy et al. (46) to evaluate four patients with the superior vena cava syndrome secondary to mediastinal thyroid. They described a characteristic appearance of these substernal goiters in which the gland was outlined by dilated thyroidal veins produced by their compression by the lesion. Vincken et al. (72) showed with radionuclide superior cavagraphy that neck flexion resulted in descent of the substernal goiter and further venous compression in a patient in whom the syndrome was intermittent.

The use of ^{131}I is considered superior to ^{99m}Tc pertechnetate because the proximity of the cardiovascular blood pool interferes with scan quality and may result in an intrathoracic goiter not being detected with the latter substance. The brighter photon energy of ^{131}I provides better imaging by compensating for the attenuation caused by the overlying bony thoracic structures. However, Park et al. (70) noted photon attenuation by bone to be a problem only with iodine-125 (^{125}I) and not with ^{131}I, ^{123}I, or ^{99m}Tc.

If the scan is performed with ^{99m}Tc pertechnetate, care must also be taken that isotope concentrated in the salivary glands, excreted in the saliva, and then swallowed and retained in the esophagus may stimulate an intrathoracic goiter (73). A parallax error has been noted by McKitrick et al. (74) and Park et al. (70) with pinhole scintigraphy in detecting substernal goiters, especially in the posterior mediastinum. Care must also be taken that ^{131}I scanning be performed before CT scanning, as the injection of contrast material with the latter will increase the body pool of iodine and interfere with thyroid gland uptake of the radionuclide (75).

In summary, although scintigraphy may identify a mediastinal mass as being of thyroid origin, lack of uptake does not eliminate the possibility of its being a goiter.

Esophagram

The esophagram is a supplemental diagnostic study providing collateral information on the presence of extrinsic compression and the displacement of the esophagus. This may be detected in patients lacking the complaint of dysphagia. Posterior mediastinal tumors almost invariably produce esophageal displacement (34). Displacement of the trachea generally accompanies esophageal deviation, with posterior goiters also producing separation.

TREATMENT

Surgery is generally deemed the treatment of choice for substernal goiter, as there is no effective alternative mode of therapy. Some studies consider the presence of a substernal goiter as an automatic indication for surgery (5,12,25,41).

The reasons for resection of substernal goiters include (a) the ineffectiveness of suppressive therapy, (b) the risk of malignancy and the unavailability of the lesion to needle biopsy, (c) the danger of hyperthyroidism, (d) the possible development of an obstructive syndrome involving the airway as well as the esophagus and great vessels, and (e) the ability to perform the surgery through a cervical incision, which carries a low operative morbidity, with only few lesions requiring sternotomy.

The natural history of this lesion is that of progressive enlargement, with patients becoming continuously more symptomatic. Treatment with thyroid hormone has generally been shown to be ineffective. Katlic et al. (5) reported that the majority of the 80 patients in their series who had received a trial of suppression with levothyroxine noted the goiter symptoms to remain and even progress. In the series of Cho et al. (25), 33% had received levothyroxine without any effect. Similarly, the treatment of hyperfunctional goiters with radioactive iodine may be ineffective or require a long period of time before a clinical response is noted. Even when the symptoms of thyrotoxicosis disappear, tracheal deviation and compression may still persist (76). The use of radioactive iodine also carries the risk of radiation thyroiditis and may precipitate acute airway obstruction (12).

Excision of a substernal goiter is generally accomplished through a cervical incision (Fig. 4), with a direct mediastinal approach reserved for exceptional cases (1, 31,33,35,38,59).

All but 1 of the 50 cases of Allo and Thompson (12) and 2 of the 80 cases of Katlic et al. (5) could be removed by a cervical approach through a low transverse incision. The remaining patients required a sternotomy and had massive goiters or adhesions from previous thyroidectomy. All of the 70 cases of Cho et al. (25) were removed from a cervical approach alone. Among the 29 cases of Lamke et al. (27) a thoracic approach was employed in 7 (6 transsternal and 1 lateral thoracotomy). In their series of 34 cases, Georgiadis et al. (2) used a cervical approach in 32 patients and a cervical and sternotomy approach in 2 patients having posterior mediastinal disease.

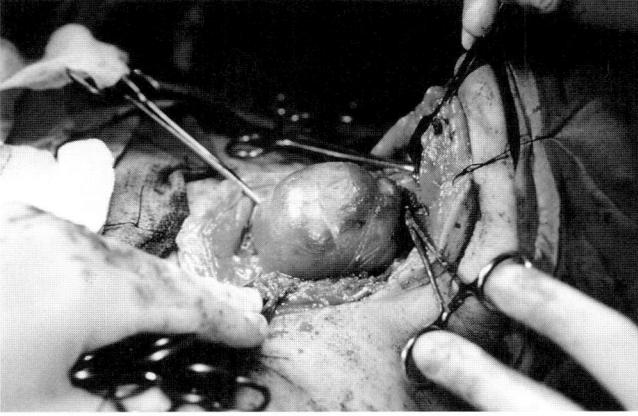

FIG. 4. Operative view of a substernal goiter being delivered through a cervical approach.

However, there is a group of surgeons who rely on a direct thoracic approach to these lesions, especially those with posterior extension (77,78), whereas Sherman and Shahbahrami (36) employed a full median sternotomy for lesions that were primarily mediastinal, Gourin et al. (37) used a combined cervical-mediastinal approach in all cases. Johnston and Twente (32) resected anterior goiters through a cervical and sternotomy incision, and posterior goiters through a cervical and anterior thoracotomy approach. However, Katlic et al. (5) noted that these posterior goiters could usually be removed through a cervical incision alone. Falor et al. (8,9) used a right thoracotomy for their primary intrathoracic cases. In an extensive study of posterior mediastinal goiters by DeAndrade (3), it was found that small lesions could be resected through a cervical approach, with thoracotomy reserved for larger ones. Among the 128 cases, 122 received a cervical procedure, with only 6 requiring a combined neck and thoracotomy approach.

With regard to the use of a thoracotomy for the removal of large posterior mediastinal tumors, DeAndrade (3) believed that an anterior approach through the second or third intercostal space facilitated a combined cervicothoracic removal and was superior to the posterolateral approach. He cited as benefits of the anterior approach the elimination of the need for repositioning the patient, the ability to perform bimanual extraction, and the removal of the cervical component with better exposure and protection of the recurrent laryngeal nerves and inferior thyroid arteries. These difficulties with the posterolateral approach were also noted in other studies (6,32). Ellis et al. (6) reported three recurrent laryngeal nerve injuries in 11 posterolateral thoracotomies.

Joyce (79) widened the thoracic inlet to permit delivery of a large mediastinal goiter by performing sternoclavicular disarticulation.

The use of the median sternotomy dates back to 1915 when Lilienthal (80) applied it to thoracic goiter surgery. Adams (81) cited the following criteria for the use of a sternotomy: (a) a very large substernal goiter, (b) the presence of a carcinoma, (c) the existence of a superior vena cava syndrome, and (d) the need for exploration and differentiation from other thoracic lesions. Sand et al. (26) added these criteria: (a) the recurrent intrathoracic goiter; (b) instances where traction endangers the recurrent laryngeal nerve, inferior thyroid blood vessels, or parathyroids; (c) cases where the lowermost border of the mass cannot be palpated; and (d) patients with emergency airway obstruction.

The size of the lesion alone does not dictate the choice of operative approach; the surgeon's personal preference plays a part. Sand et al. (26) reported an average weight of 222 g for goiters removed through a sternotomy, as compared with 130 g for those resected through a low collar incision. However, Judd et al. (31) noted in their series that the size of the goiters removed by a cervical approach was comparable to those resected through a thoracotomy.

The nature of the thyroid surgery performed depends on the extent and histopathology of the disease. With benign lesions, the hypertrophic and often obstructing portions of the gland are removed. This may require unilateral or bilateral lobectomy or subtotal resection. With malignant lesions, total thyroidectomy is generally performed.

Allo and Thompson (12) employed lobectomy and isthmusectomy in patients with small goiters that had unilateral and substernal extension. Bilateral subtotal thyroidectomy was performed with larger tumors having bilateral mediastinal extension, and total thyroidectomy was reserved for malignant tumors. In the series of Katlic et al. (5), a unilateral lobectomy was performed in 75% of the cases, lobectomy with subtotal contralateral resection in 16%, bilateral subtotal lobectomy in 6%, and total thyroidectomy in 3%. Cho et al. (25) utilized hemithyroidectomy in 69% of their cases, subtotal thyroidectomy in 24%, total thyroidectomy in 4%, and two patients (3%) had debulking of unresectable malignancies.

OPERATIVE TECHNIQUE

In patients with massive goiters, intubation may be difficult because of displacement and compression of the trachea. In some cases, it may be necessary to pass a nasoendotracheal tube over a flexible fiberoptic bronchoscope for access to the lower airway. Tracheotomy is generally of little value, as the deformed segment in the mediastinum may be distal to the tube. A low collar incision is made transversely above the sternum and clavicle, the platysma is divided, and flaps are elevated superiorly and inferiorly. The strap muscles are separated in the midline and a plane is created between the capsule of the thyroid and the overlying muscle. The muscle at times is markedly attenuated and adherent to the capsule and may require sharp dissection for adequate separation and retraction. Occasionally, the goiter is so large that it may be necessary to divide the strap muscles on one or both sides for adequate exposure.

The middle thyroid vein is isolated, divided, and ligated. The inferior thyroid artery is identified next. It is dissected onto the capsule of the thyroid gland, tracing its branches to the parathyroid glands. The artery is then ligated distally to maintain the vascularization of the parathyroid glands. It is important to identify and preserve the superior parathyroid glands in case the inferior glands are injured or devascularized in the process of mobilizing the goiter or its substernal component.

Visualization of the recurrent laryngeal nerves is mandatory. The mass may displace the nerve markedly from its normal position. Initially, the anterior aspect of the goiter is carefully inspected while dissecting out the inferior thyroid artery for the presence of the nerve. In 4 of the 50 cases of Allo and Thompson (12), the left laryngeal nerve was stretched over the anterior aspect of the goiter. The posterior surface of the goiter is next examined.

The massive size of a thyroid gland often presents difficulties in delivering it into the operative field. This is facilitated by dividing the attachments of the superior pole to increase mobilization of the tumor. This is performed close to the thyroid capsule to prevent the external branch of the superior laryngeal nerve from being injured and to maintain the blood supply to the superior parathyroid.

The substernal portion of the goiter may next require mobilization to detect a nerve displaced posteriorly. Melliere et al. (41) considered the danger of recurrent laryngeal nerve injury to be greater on the right side because of the variable relationship between the goiter and the nerve. The goiter may so markedly displace the recurrent laryngeal nerve that identification of it within the tracheoesophageal groove may be impossible (Fig. 5). In such instances, the nerve is identified as it passes through the thyrocricoid articulation and is then dissected retrograde toward the mediastinum.

The substernal component can generally be mobilized and delivered by finger dissection along the capsule of the mass, proceeding from the thoracic inlet into the superior mediastinum, carefully palpating for the great vessels. If dense adhesions are present from previous surgery, it may be necessary to perform a median sternotomy for direct access to the fixed segment.

In cases where the substernal goiter is so large that it cannot be delivered through the thoracic inlet, Lahey (1) suggested fragmentation or morcellation of the mass to facilitate removal without sternotomy. However, this maneuver carries the danger of hemorrhage and the potential spillage of malignant cells and is generally not performed. Johnston and Twente (32) reported mediastinal hematoma and death following morcellation of a large posterior mediastinal goiter. Nevertheless, Sand et al. (26) used this method in one patient, Cho et al. (25) in

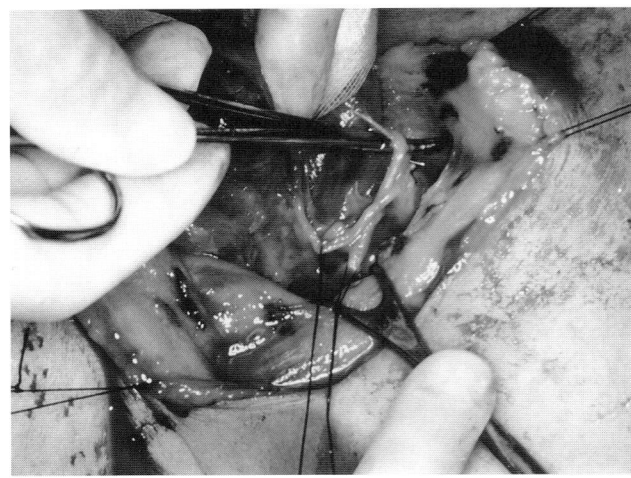

FIG. 5. Operative view of a patient with a substernal goiter having right vocal cord paralysis. The clamp is elevating a stretched recurrent laryngeal nerve.

two patients, and Allo and Thompson (12) in three cases without difficulties. Allo and Thompson (12) also reported the insertion of a soup spoon to break up the negative mediastinal pressure of large goiters when the surgeon's fingers were unable to reach the caudal extent of the lesion. Instruments have been devised to facilitate goiter extraction (82,83).

In cases with elongation of the trachea from marked deviation, Allo and Thompson (12) recommended suturing of the trachea to the strap muscles in the midline to prevent postoperative kinking. The phenomenon of tracheal collapse from tracheomalacia produced by large goiters has also been treated by suturing the trachea to the soft tissues of the neck by Green et al. (84). The wound is closed in layers after suction catheter drains are placed in the mediastinum to evacuate the dead space. A chest radiograph is taken in the recovery room. However, Karlin (55) cautioned that the mediastinum may appear widened 6 to 12 weeks postoperatively.

All postoperative patients are placed on levothyroxine; however, it is unclear if this actually prevents recurrent disease. Watt-Boolsen et al. (85) followed 15 patients for a median of 10 years and found all to have normal thyroid function tests and no elevation of the serum TSH level. They concluded that thyroid replacement was unnecessary.

COMPLICATIONS

The complications of surgery for substernal goiter vary widely in reported series and reflect differences in technical operative expertise, extent of disease, and the surgical approach used. In addition to anesthetic dangers and general medical complications, all the regional cervical and mediastinal structures, including the parathyroids, recurrent laryngeal nerves, trachea, esophagus, great vessels, and pleura, are at risk for injury.

Allo and Thompson (12) reported one unilateral vocal cord paralysis, one hematoma, two transient hypocalcemias, one pneumonia, one cardiac arrhythmia, and two late deaths from malignant neoplasms among their 50 cases. Katlic et al. (5) noted nine minor complications among their 80 patients, for a complication rate of 11%. This included three accidental excisions of parathyroids, two transient hypocalcemias, one seroma, one halothane hepatitis, and one patient with cardiac arrhythmia. Cho et al. (25) noted three complications in their series of 70 cases (4%). One patient each developed an esophageal laceration, a pneumothorax, and a vocal cord paralysis.

Sand et al. (26) had complications in 18 of 31 cases. This included dysphagia in five, hoarseness in five, transient hypocalcemia in six, fever in four, pleural effusion in two, vocal cord paralysis in one, and a transient phrenic nerve palsy in one. A low collar incision was employed in all 31 cases, with six patients also receiving a median sternotomy; these authors found no significant difference in the morbidity or length of hospitalization between the two groups. However, Judd et al. (31) noted a 37% complication rate (including one death) with thoracotomy as compared to an 11% incidence with a cervical approach.

Although the operative mortality of substernal goiter surgery is low, Georgiadis et al. (2) had one cardiac death in 34 cases. DeAndrade (3) observed one death from a malignant tumor in his series of 128 cases. Lamke et al. (27) had two fatalities in their series of 29 cases, one occurring at the time of anesthetic induction and the other 6 days postoperatively from a pulmonary embolus. They also reported two hematomas and a transient recurrent laryngeal nerve paresis. Watt-Boolsen et al. (85) also noted one of their 29 patients died postoperatively of a pulmonary embolus.

Operative injury to the trachea or postoperative kinking of a stretched trachea after goiter excision may require tracheostomy (79,86). Other reported complications are air embolism (32), chyle fistula (11), chylothorax (87), and fatal hematemesis secondary to complete esophageal erosion (88). Blood loss is generally low and none of the 50 cases of Allo and Thompson (12) required blood transfusion.

REFERENCES

1. Lahey RH. Intrathoracic goiters. *Surg Clin North Am* 1945;25:609–618.
2. Georgiadis N, Katsas A, Leoutsakos B. Substernal goiter. *Int Surg* 1970;54:116–121.
3. DeAndrade MA. A review of 128 cases of posterior mediastinal goiter. *World J Surg* 1977;1:789–797.
4. Katlic MR, Wang C, Grillo HC. Substernal goiter. *Ann Thorac Surg* 1985;39:391–399.
5. Katlic MR, Grillo HC, Wang CA. Substernal goiter: analysis of eighty Massachusetts General Hospital cases. *Am J Surg* 1985;149:283–287.
6. Ellis FH, Good CA, Seybold WD. Intrathoracic goiter. *Ann Surg* 1952;135:79–90.
7. Sweet RH. Intrathoracic goiter located in the posterior mediastinum. *Surg Gynecol Obstet* 1949;89:57–66.
8. Falor WH, Kelly TR, Krabill WS. Intrathoracic goiter. *Ann Surg* 1955;142:238–247.
9. Falor WH, Kelly TR, Jackson JB. Intrathoracic goiter. *Surg Gynecol Obstet* 1963;117:604–610.
10. Lahey FH, Swinton NW. Intrathoracic goiter. *Surg Gynecol Obstet* 1934;59:627–637.
11. Lahey FH. Intrathoracic goiter. *Surg Clin North Am* 1936;16:1613–1629.
12. Allo MD, Thompson NW. Rationale for the operative management of substernal goiters. *Surgery* 1983;94:967–977.
13. Rundle FF. Intrathoracic goiter. *West J Surg Obstet Gynecol* 1959;67:213–215.
14. Reeve TS, Rubenstein C, Rundle FF. Intrathoracic goitre: its prevalence in Sydney metropolitan mass x-ray surveys. *Med J Aust* 1957;2:149–151.
15. Ladenson PW, Vineyard GL, Pinkus GS, Ridgway EL. Sequestered substernal goiter. *Arch Intern Med* 1983;143:1015–1017.
16. Adams HD. Transthoracic thyroidectomy. *J Thorac Surg* 1950;19:741–754.
17. Pitt LP. Aberrant posterior mediastinal goiter. A review of the literature and report of a case. *Am J Surg* 1962;103:397–399.
18. Fogelfeld L, Rubinstein U, Bar On J, Feigl D. Severe thyrotoxicosis caused by an ectopic intrathoracic goiter. *Clin Nucl Med* 1986;11:20–22.
19. Sussman SK, Silverman PM, Donnal JF. CT demonstration of isolated mediastinal goiter. *J Comput Assist Tomogr* 1986;10:863–864.
20. Dundas P. Intrathoracic aberrant goitre. *Acta Chir Scand* 1964;128:729–736.
21. Rives JD. Mediastinal aberrant goiter. *Ann Surg* 1947;126:797.
22. Ziter FMH. Ectopic mediastinal thyroid. *Dis Chest* 1966;49:641–642.
23. Salomon J, Levy MJ. Mediastinal aberrant goiter: report of two cases. *Dis Chest* 1967;52:413–416.

24. Higgins CC. Intrathoracic goiter. *Arch Surg* 1927;15:895–912.
25. Cho AT, Cohen JP, Som ML. Management of substernal and intrathoracic goiters. *Otolaryngol Head Neck Surg* 1986;94:282–287.
26. Sand ME, Laws HL, McElvein RB. Substernal and intrathoracic goiter. *Am Surg* 1983;49:196–202.
27. Lamke LO, Bergdahl L, Lamke B. Intrathoracic goiter: a review of 29 cases. *Acta Chir Scand* 1979;145:83–86.
28. Sanders LE, Rossi RL, Shahian DM, et al. Mediastinal goiters: the need for an aggressive approach. *Arch Surg* 1992;127:609–613.
29. Lichtenstein IL, Rabwin M, Jaffe HL. So-called "posterior mediastinal goiter." *N Engl J Med* 1954;250:875–877.
30. DeSouza FM, Smith PE. Retrosternal goiter. *J Otolaryngol* 1983;12:393–396.
31. Judd ES, Beahrs OH, Bowes DE. A consideration of the proper surgical approach for substernal goiter. *Surg Gynecol Obstet* 1960;110:90–98.
32. Johnston JH, Twente GE. Surgical approach to intrathoracic (mediastinal) goiter. *Ann Surg* 1956;143:572–579.
33. Pemberton J. Surgery of substernal and intrathoracic goiters. *Arch Surg* 1921;2:1–21.
34. Rietz KA, Werner B. Intrathoracic goiter. *Acta Chir Scand* 1960;119:379–388.
35. Lindskog GE, Goldberg IS. Differential diagnosis, pathology, and treatment of substernal goiter. *JAMA* 1957;163:327–329.
36. Sherman PH, Shahbrami F. Mediastinal goiters: review of ten cases. *Am Surg* 1966;32:137–142.
37. Gourin A, Garzon AA, Karlson KE. The cervicomediastinal approach to intrathoracic goiter. *Surgery* 1971;69:651–654.
38. Wakeley CPG, Mulvany JH. Intrathoracic goiter. *Surg Gynecol Obstet* 1940;70:702–710.
39. Ehrenhaft JL, Buckwalter JA. Mediastinal tumors of thyroid origin. *Arch Surg* 1955;71:347–356.
40. McCort JL. Intrathoracic goiter: its incidence, symptomology and roentgen diagnosis. *Radiology* 1949;53:227–236.
41. Melliere D, Saada F, Etienne G, Becquemin JP, Bonnet F. Goiter with severe respiratory compromise: evaluation and treatment. *Surgery* 1988;103:367–373.
42. Torres A, Arroyo J, Kastanos N, et al. Acute respiratory failure and tracheal obstruction in patients with intrathoracic goiter. *Crit Care Med* 1983;11:265–266.
43. Aasted A, Bertelsen S. Superior vena cava syndrome in benign mediastinal goiter. *Acta Chir Scand* 1981;147:405–408.
44. Gomes MN, Hufnagel CA. Superior vena cava obstruction: a review of the literature and report of 2 cases due to benign intrathoracic tumors. *Ann Thorac Surg* 1975;20:344.
45. Lesavoy MA, Norberg HP, Kaplan EL. Substernal goiter with superior vena cava obstruction. *Surgery* 1975;77:325–329.
46. Sy WM, Lao RS, Seo IS. Scintigraphic features of superior vena caval obstruction due to substernal nontoxic goitre. *Br J Radiol* 1982;55:301–303.
47. Ulreich S, Lowman RM, Stern H. Intrathoracic goiter: a cause of the superior vena cava syndrome. *Clin Radiol* 1977;28:663–665.
48. Fragomeni LS, Ceratti de Azambuja P. Intrathoracic goitre in the posterior mediastinum. *Thorax* 1980;35:638–639.
49. Steenerson RL, Barton RT. Mediastinal goiter and superior vena cava syndrome. *Laryngoscope* 1978;88:1688–1690.
50. Santos GH, Ghalili K. Axillosubclavian vein thrombosis produced by retrosternal thyroid. *Chest* 1990;98:1281–1283.
51. Fleig WE, Stange EF, Ditschuneit H. Upper gastrointestinal hemorrhage from downhill esophageal varices. *Dig Dis Sci* 1982;27:23–27.
52. Kelly TR, Mayors DJ, Bontsicaris RS. "Downhill" varices: a cause of upper gastrointestinal hemorrhage. *Am Surg* 1982;48:35–38.
53. Sorokin JJ, Levine SM, Moss EG, Biddle CM. "Downhill" varices: report of a case 29 years after resection of a substernal thyroid gland. *Gastroenterology* 1977;73:345–348.
54. Karadeniz A, Hacihanefioglu U. Abscess formation in an intrathoracic goitre. *Thorax* 1982;37:556–557.
55. Karlin S. Intrathoracic goiters. *Am Surg* 1963;29:499–505.
56. Fernandez-Cruz L, Serra-Batlles J, Picado C. Retrosternal goiter and chylothorax: case report. *Respiration* 1986;50:70–71.
57. Gadisseux P, Minette P, Trigaux JP, Michel L. Cerebrovascular circulation "steal" syndrome secondary to a voluminous retrotracheal goiter. *Int Surg* 1986;71:107–109.
58. Lesoin F, Bousquet C, Thomas CE, et al. Transient ischemic attacks in patient with endothoracic goitre and congenital anomaly of the carotid artery. *Lancet* 1982;2:98.
59. Crile G. Intrathoracic goiter. *Cleve Clin Q* 1939;6:313–322.
60. Prakash R, Lakshmipathi N, Jena A, Behari V, Chopra MK. Hyperthyroidism caused by a toxic intrathoracic goiter with a normal-sized cervical thyroid gland. *J Nucl Med* 1986;27:1423–1427.
61. Fui SNT, Prior J, Saunders AJ, Maisey MN. Posterior intrathoracic goitre as a cause of thyrotoxicosis. *Br J Radiol* 1979;52:995–997.
62. Shih WJ, Cho SR, Purcell M, Tsung YH, Domstad PA, Liu GI, Deland FH. Diagnostic imaging in mediastinal thyroid tumor. *Clin Nucl Med* 1984;9:702–707.
63. Bashist B, Ellis K, Gold RP. Computerized tomography of intrathoracic goiters. *Am J Roentgenol* 1983;140:455–460.
64. Glazer GM, Axel L, Moss KA. CT diagnosis of mediastinal thyroid. *Am J Roentgenol* 1982;138:495–498.
65. Shepard JO. Computed tomography of the mediastinum. *Clin Chest Med* 1984;5:291–305.
66. Binder RE, Pugatch RD, Faling LJ, Kanter RA, Sawin CT. Diagnosis of posterior mediastinal goiter by computed tomography. *J Comput Assist Tomogr* 1980;4:550–552.
67. Morris UL, Colletti PM, Ralls PW, Boswell WD, Lapin SA, Quinn M, Halls JM. CT demonstration of intrathoracic thyroid tissue. *J Comput Assist Tomogr* 1982;6:821–824.
68. Radecki PD, Arger PH, Arenson RL, Jennings AS, Coleman BG, Mintz MG, Kressel HY. Thyroid imaging: comparison of high-resolution real-time ultrasound and computerized tomography. *Radiology* 1984;153:145–147.
69. Sandler MP, Patton JA, Sacks GA, Shaff MI, Kulkarni MV, Partain CL. Evaluation of intrathoracic goiter with I-123 scintigraphy and nuclear magnetic resonance imaging. *J Nucl Med* 1984;25:874–876.
70. Park HM, Tarver RD, Siddiqui AR, Schauwecker DS, Wellman HN. Efficacy of thyroid scintigraphy in the diagnosis of intrathoracic goiter. *Am J Roentgenol* 1987;148:527–529.
71. Irwin RS, Braman SS, Arvantidis AN, Hamolsky MW. 131 iodine thyroid scanning in preoperative diagnosis of mediastinal goiter. *Ann Intern Med* 1978;89:73–74.
72. Vincken W, Roels P, Sonstabo R, DeGreve J, Bossuyt A, Jonckheer M. Effect of neck position during radionuclide superior vena cava obstruction due to retrosternal goiter. *Clin Nucl Med* 1983;8:424–426.
73. Rajguru HL, Poulose KP, Reba RC. Esophageal tracer retention simulating substernal goiter. *J Nucl Med* 1977;18:404–405.
74. McKitrick WL, Park HM, Kosegi JE. Parallax error in pinhole thyroid scintigraphy: a critical consideration in the evaluation of substernal goiters. *J Nucl Med* 1985;26:418.
75. Nejatheim M, Strashun AM. CT versus iodine scanning in diagnosis of mediastinal thyroid [letter]. *Am J Roentgenol* 1982;139:834.
76. Beierwalter WH. The treatment of hyperthyroidism with iodine 131. *Semin Nucl Med* 1978;8:95–103.
77. Maurer ER. The surgical treatment of retrotracheal intrathoracic goiter. *Arch Surg* 1955;71:357–364.
78. Hilton HD, Griffin WT. Posterior mediastinal goiter. *Am J Surg* 1968;116:891–895.
79. Joyce TM. Incidence of substernal and intrathoracic goiters. *Arch Surg* 1940;41:364–369.
80. Lilienthal H. A case of mediastinal thyroid removed by transsternal mediastinotomy. *Surg Gynecol Obstet* 1915;20:589–593.
81. Adams HD. Transsternal thyroidectomy. *Surg Clin North Am* 1961;41:655–663.
82. Simon MM. Preservation of the airway in surgery for goiter. A useful forceps for the delivery of substernal and intrathoracic goiters. *Am J Surg* 1960;100:85–90.
83. Sacre R. A new instrument: the goiter extractor. *Head Neck Surg* 1984;6:1059–1060.
84. Green WER, Shepperd HWH, Stevenson HM, Wilson W. Tracheal collapse after thyroidectomy. *Br J Surg* 1979;66:554–557.
85. Watt-Boolsen S, Blichert-Toft M, Folke K, Christiansen C, Boberg A. Surgical treatment of benign nontoxic intrathoracic goiter: a long term observation. *Am J Surg* 1981;141:721–722.
86. Reeve TS. *Intrathoracic goiter: investigation and management.* Proceedings of the first Asian Congress of Thoracic and Cardiovascular Surgery, Manila, 1972;78–82.
87. Delgado C, Martin M, de la Portilla F. Retrosternal goiter associated with chylothorax. *Chest* 1994;106:1924–1925.
88. Parker DR, El-Shaboury A. Fatal haematemesis due to benign retrosternal goitre. *Postgrad Med J* 1992;68:756–757.
89. Singh B, Lucente FE, Shaha AR. Substernal goiter: a clinical review. *Am J Otolaryngol* 1994;15:409–416.
90. Wax MK, Briant TDR. Management of substernal goitre. *J Otolaryngol* 1992;21:165–170.

CHAPTER 25

Management of Thyroid Disorders Involving the Airway

Victor G. Lawson

Although developmentally the thyroid gland begins as an outpouching of the primitive pharynx (1), the embryologic track and the mature thyroid gland are closely related to the laryngeal and tracheal portions of the airway. The initial site of embryologic development in the foramen cecum at the base of the tongue adjoins the vallecula and lingual surface of the epiglottis. The developmental path of descent of the thyroid gland passes through the pre-epiglottic space and either through the body of the hyoid bone or deep to the periosteum of the hyoid bone, before descending to the adult anatomic position on the anterolateral aspect of the laryngopharynx, cervical trachea, and esophagus. The isthmus of the thyroid gland overlies the second and third tracheal rings.

If the tract fails to obliterate completely during development of the fetus, thyroid remnants may be found anywhere along the track of descent of the thyroid gland. Remnants of thyroid tissue may occur along the recurrent laryngeal nerves as they pass through the cricothyroid membrane into the subglottic larynx, or remnants may be present in the inlet if the thyroid gland has descended into the mediastinum. Isolated or discontinuous remnants (rests) of normal thyroid tissue occur within the airway or neck. If isolated remnants are present within lymph nodes, they almost certainly represent a neoplastic process rather than normal ectopic thyroid tissue.

These intimate developmental and anatomic relationships between the upper respiratory tract and the thyroid gland may result in variable degrees of pathological involvement of the airway by a variety of thyroid disorders. The incidence of thyroid disorders involving the airway may be as high as 35%, depending on the degree of detail in the clinical and imaging examinations (2). Such airway involvement may be either asymptomatic or symptomatic. Asymptomatic involvement is usually detected on imaging studies. Symptomatic involvement may result in cough, excessive mucus in the throat, hemoptysis, hoarseness, stridor, acute or chronic airway dysfunction, or merely a sensation of a lump in the throat.

Acute symptoms may occur because of progressive changes in the underlying pathological process that is producing the symptoms resulting in a critical-mass effect, or because of a sudden acute event occurring in preexistent pathology. Examples of such acute events include sudden cystic degeneration, spontaneous hemorrhage, and inflammation.

SURGICAL PATHOLOGY

The airway may be involved by thyroid disorders in a direct or in an indirect fashion.

Direct Process

Displacement with Compression

Displacement with compression is the most common type of airway involvement. It usually occurs with a dominant unilateral multinodular goiter (Fig. 1), but it may be seen with a solitary nodule, Hashimoto's thyroiditis, a neoplastic process, or a thyroglossal duct remnant (Fig. 2).

Displacement without Compression

Displacement without compression usually occurs with a solitary thyroid nodule, particularly if the nodule

---

V. G. Lawson: Central Kentucky Otolaryngology—Head and Neck Surgical Associates, Bluegrass Medical Center, Paris, Kentucky 40361.

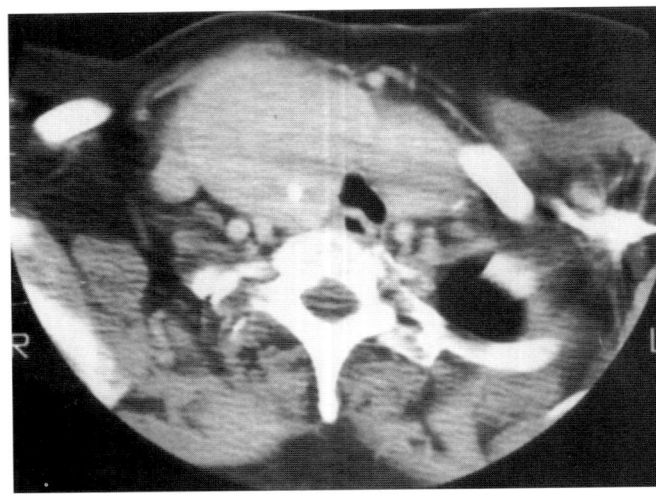

FIG. 1. A: Computerized tomography (CT) scan shows displacement of trachea to the left, with compression of the trachea, by a multinodular goiter. **B:** Plain soft-tissue radiograph of the neck in the same patient illustrates the same point, but less obviously.

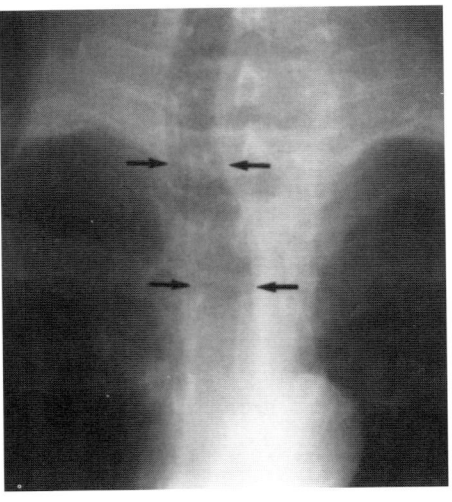

FIG. 2. Thyroglossal duct remnant (R) extending into vallecula (V) with resultant posterior displacement of the epiglottis and compression of the airway. (Xerogram.)

is not entrapped in the inlet. It may also occur with dominant unilateral multinodular goiters, Hashimoto's thyroiditis, or neoplasia (Fig. 3).

Infiltration with Displacement and/or Compression

Infiltration with displacement and/or compression is relatively rare. It most commonly occurs with a carcinoma of the thyroid gland extending into the cervical trachea or subglottic larynx. Very rarely, it may occur with a pathologically benign process extending along a recurrent laryngeal nerve through the cricothyroid membrane and hence into the airway (Figs. 4–6).

Compression

Airway compression without displacement is extremely rare. This may occur with symmetric enlargement of both lobes of the thyroid gland, resulting in bilateral symmetric pressure and compression on the trachea (Fig. 7). Usually, this form of airway involvement is the result of a benign pathological process, such as a diffuse toxic goiter, the result of bilateral adenomata (Fig. 8).

Infiltration

Infiltration without displacement of the airway is extremely rare. It can occur with a carcinoma of low volume that infiltrates the airway but lacks the mass effect to displace or compress the airway. It may occur also when a neoplastic process develops in an intralaryngeal or intratracheal extension of normal thyroid tissue.

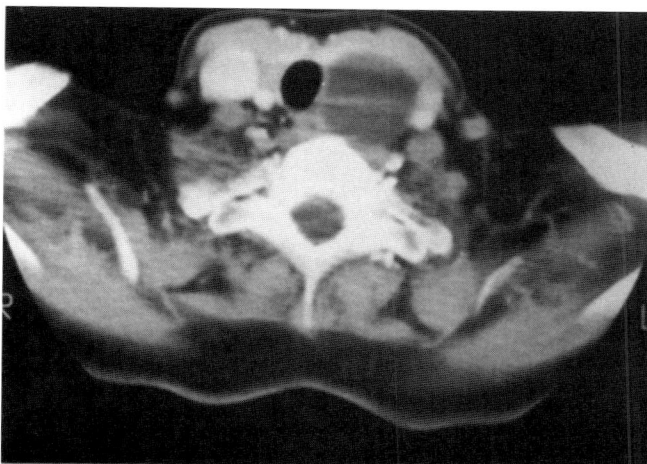
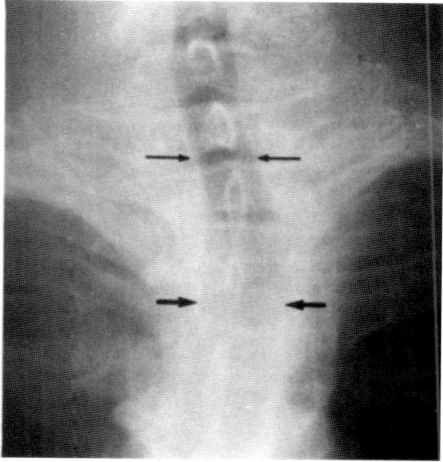

FIG. 3. CT scan (left) and plain radiograph (right) of the neck illustrate displacement of the trachea to the right by a solitary left thyroid nodule at the inlet level without compression of the trachea.

Indirect Process

The airway may also be involved by thyroid disorders in an indirect fashion through unilateral or bilateral impairment of recurrent nerve function. This usually occurs with a malignant process that results in perineural infiltration of the recurrent laryngeal nerve or nerves in the neck. Also, metastatic disease in the mediastinum or direct spread of a malignant tumor from the thyroid gland to the mediastinum can produce recurrent laryngeal nerve dysfunction. Occasionally, a large goiter may cause a traction neuropraxia of one recurrent laryngeal nerve. Similarly, an inflammatory process in the thyroid gland may result in a secondary neuritis involving one or both of the recurrent laryngeal nerves. If one recurrent laryngeal nerve is involved, the patient will develop a hoarse, weak, and breathy voice and a weak cough. If both recurrent laryngeal nerves are involved, the patient may have some mild weakness and hoarseness of the voice but will have dominant respiratory symptoms characterized by inspiratory stridor and hypoxia, rather than vocal problems.

In rare instances, other mechanisms, such as longstanding compression of the trachea by a solitary nodule or a multinodular goiter, with associated perichondritis or chondritis of the tracheal cartilages, may result in intrinsic weakening of the tracheal wall (tracheomalacia), producing collapse of the airway. This mechanism is somewhat different from a direct increasing tracheal compression resulting from increasing mass effect, as tracheomalacia implies dissolution of supporting tracheal cartilages with loss of tracheal lumen (3). Injudicious use of tracheostomy in a trachea already deformed by longstanding compression but without loss of tracheal cartilage may lead to chondritis, loss of tracheal cartilage support, and subsequent collapse.

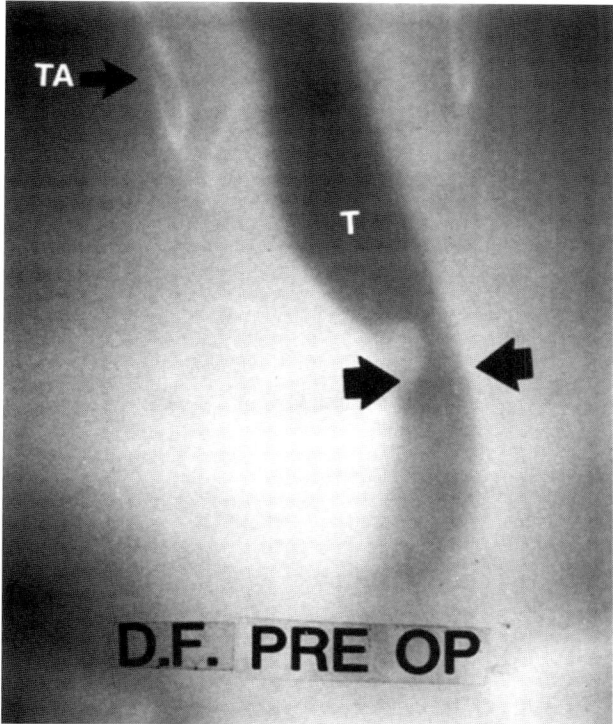

FIG. 4. Tomogram of the trachea illustrates infiltration, displacement, and compression of the airway by a papillary carcinoma involving the right lobe of the thyroid gland with invasion of the tracheal lumen. TA, thyroid ala; T, tracheal lumen.

MANAGEMENT OF AIRWAY DYSFUNCTION

If a patient is symptomatic because of a thyroid disorder involving the airway, the severity of the symptoms

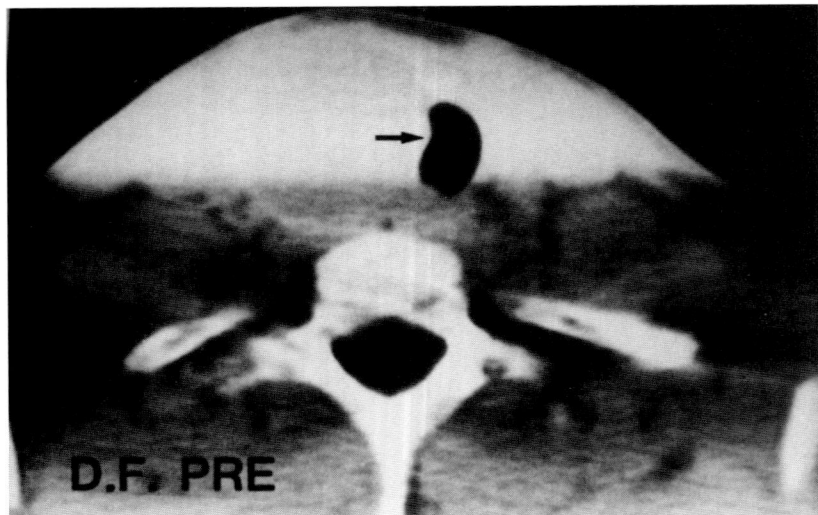

FIG. 5. CT scan of trachea illustrates the same points as the tomogram in Figure 4.

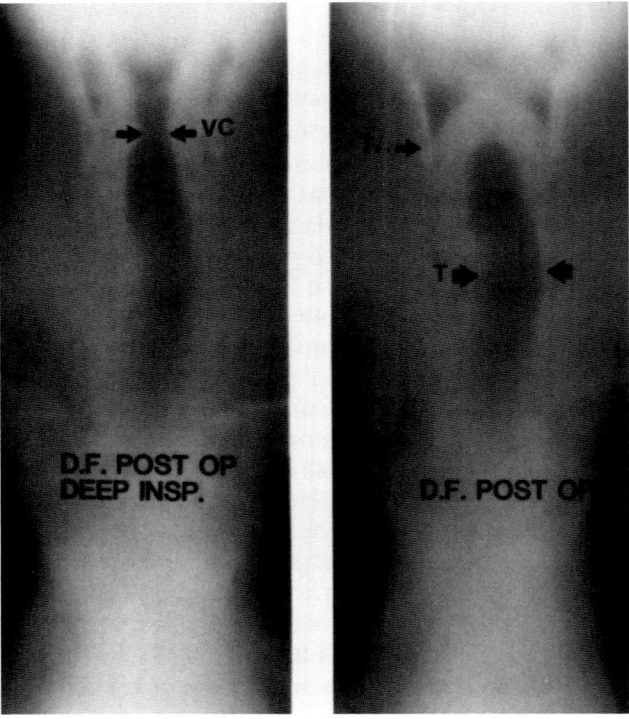

FIG. 6. Postoperative tomogram of the trachea following *en bloc* total thyroidectomy and partial three-ring trachiectomy with an end-to-end angulated asymmetric reconstruction of the trachea in the same patient illustrated in the radiographs in Figures 4 and 5. VC, abducted vocal cords with deep inspiration; TA, thyroid ala; T, tracheal lumen at site of anastomosis showing normal lumen size, with slight angulation.

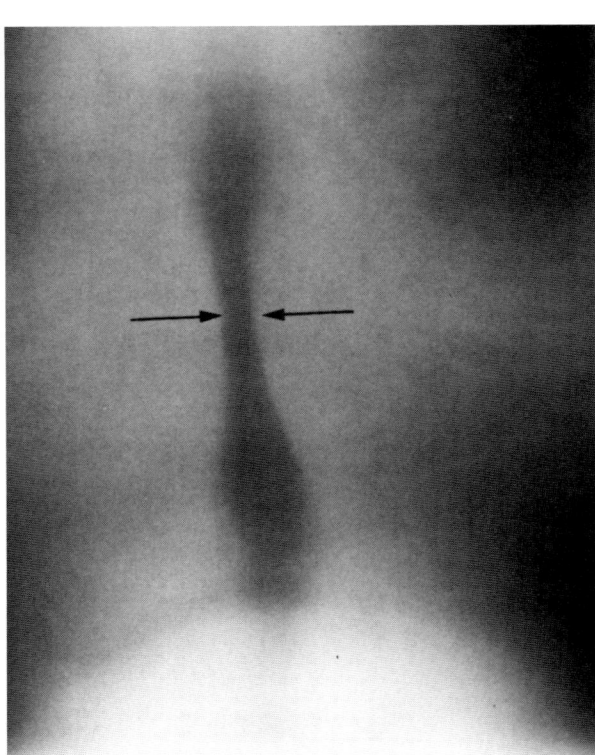

FIG. 7. Tracheal compression to 6 mm by bilateral symmetric follicular adenomata.

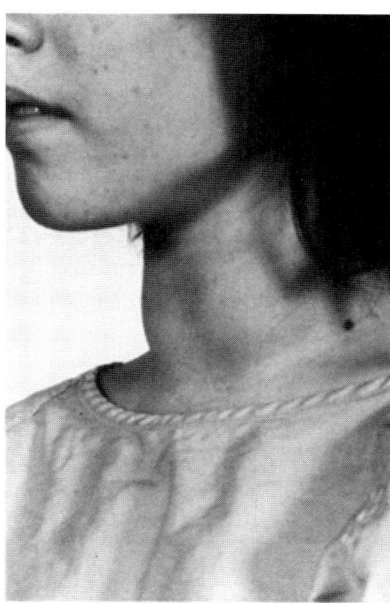 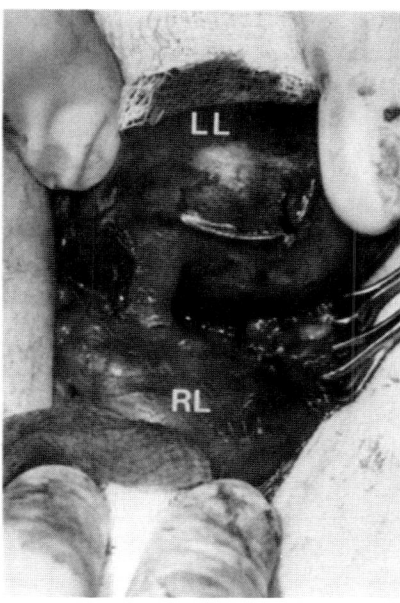

FIG. 8. Patient illustrated in the radiograph in Figure 7, showing enlargement of the right lobe (RL) and left lobe (LL) of the thyroid gland by bilateral symmetric follicular adenomata. The only normal thyroid tissue present was in the isthmus.

must be evaluated urgently and the degree of airway dysfunction determined. If there is significant airway decompensation with resultant hypoxia, stabilization of the airway becomes a priority. The respiratory rate and the characteristics of the stridor should be noted and monitored. If the stridor is inspiratory, the obstruction is at the supraglottic or glottic portion of the airway. If the stridor is biphasic, the obstruction is in the subglottic larynx or cervical trachea. If there is an expiratory wheeze, then the patient has a peripheral pulmonary disorder.

If the patient is hypoxic, supportive measures, including oxygen or a helium–oxygen mixture, must be instituted immediately. The patient must be properly hydrated with intravenous fluids. If there is superimposed upper airway inflammation, intravenous antibiotics and corticosteroids are often administered.

The nature and degree of the airway obstruction must be determined quickly by clinical examination of the neck and chest, and by mirror or fiberoptic examination of the upper airway. Blood gases and plain films of the neck and chest are obtained if there is time. However, if the respiratory impairment is critical, then an airway must be established immediately. Preferably, this should be done by using endotracheal intubation or rigid bronchoscopy. A cricothyrotomy or an emergency tracheostomy is usually extremely difficult because of the intrinsic thyroid pathology and the associated distortion of the airway. Also, an emergency surgical opening of the airway may preclude later definitive surgery with optimal end results. Hence, the airway is best secured by intubation so that surgery can proceed in an orderly fashion. If emergency surgery is indicated after the airway has been secured by intubation, a definitive resective procedure, rather than a tracheostomy alone, should be undertaken as a primary approach if the lesion is resectable. Usually, however, the airway can be stabilized using supportive measures, so immediate surgery is not necessary. If that is accomplished, treatment can best proceed on an elective basis after detailed imaging investigations are done to determine the extent of the pathological process (4).

INVESTIGATIONS

The investigations that are undertaken for assessment of thyroid disorders involving the airway are essentially the same investigations that would be done in the preoperative assessment of any potentially surgical thyroid disorder. These would include assessment of thyroid function and calcium metabolism, a fine-needle-aspiration biopsy, and various imaging tests. The imaging tests that are most useful in assessing the extent of the airway involvement are soft-tissue radiographs of the neck, a chest x-ray, and a high-resolution computerized tomography (CT) scan with enhancement.

Angiography, polytomography, magnetic resonance imaging (MRI), ultrasound, and nuclear scan are done if indicated. Blood gases, flow volume loops, and pulmonary function tests are useful in determining the extent of impairment of respiratory function. Endoscopic examination (laryngoscopy, bronchoscopy, and esophagoscopy) is essential immediately preoperatively to determine if there is mucosal involvement and to assess the actual configuration of the involved airway. A precise understanding of the nature of the airway compromise will allow for safer placement of the endotracheal tube. If there is infiltrative disease or mucosal change, biopsy and frozen-section analy-

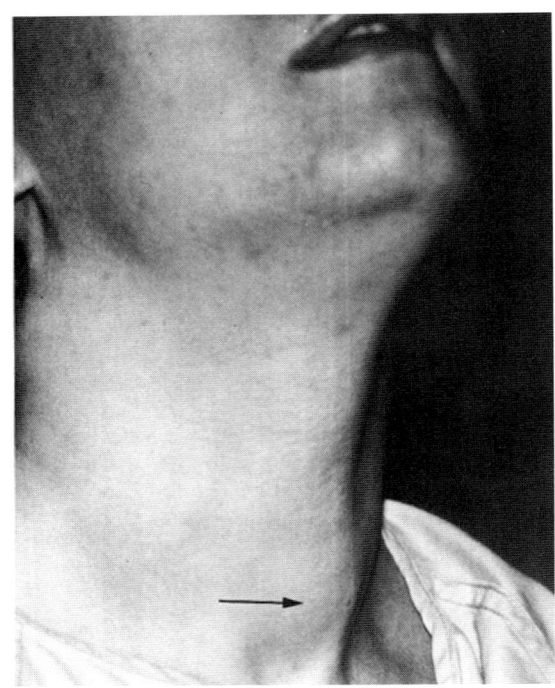

FIG. 9. *Arrow* points to a right thyroid nodule in a patient with papillary carcinoma infiltrating the trachea.

sis are useful in assessing the histopathology of the thyroid disease and in planning the extent of the airway resection.

SURGICAL CONCEPTS

Medications and Surgical Strategies

All patients with airway encroachment, whether asymptomatic or symptomatic, are best managed by reducing the pressure on the airway. With benign disease and no respiratory compromise, medical means can be tried initially. However, after the gland is suppressed with thyroid hormone and the airway does not improve, surgery should follow. In patients with malignant disease or impairment of airway function, surgery is indicated initially. The surgical procedure is best carried out in an elective fashion after detailed investigations. If there is no evidence of infiltrative disease, the standard thyroidectomy procedures are done depending on specific pathology and indications. However, if there is infiltrative disease, a one-stage thyroidectomy, airway resection, and airway reconstruction are recommended. The recurrent laryngeal nerves should be conserved unless they are directly involved by tumor (Figs. 9–15). (See also Chapter 34, Management of Thyroid Carcinoma Invading the Upper Aerodigestive System.)

Anesthesia

It is important that both the surgeon and the anesthetist understand fully the nature of the airway encroachment and that they have agreed on a plan of action. Rigid laryngoscopy and bronchoscopy can be done safely even with the most extensive airway pathology. Venturi ventilation techniques must be available. When necessary, the airway can be established using a rigid bronchoscope quickly, and then the patient can be oxygenated. If the patient's oxygen saturation is satisfactory, endoscopy is used to determine the extent of the disease as well as the specific nature of the airway deformity. Detailed understanding of the airway deformity will allow for safer introduction of the endotracheal tube. Generally, the endoscopist is the best person to in-

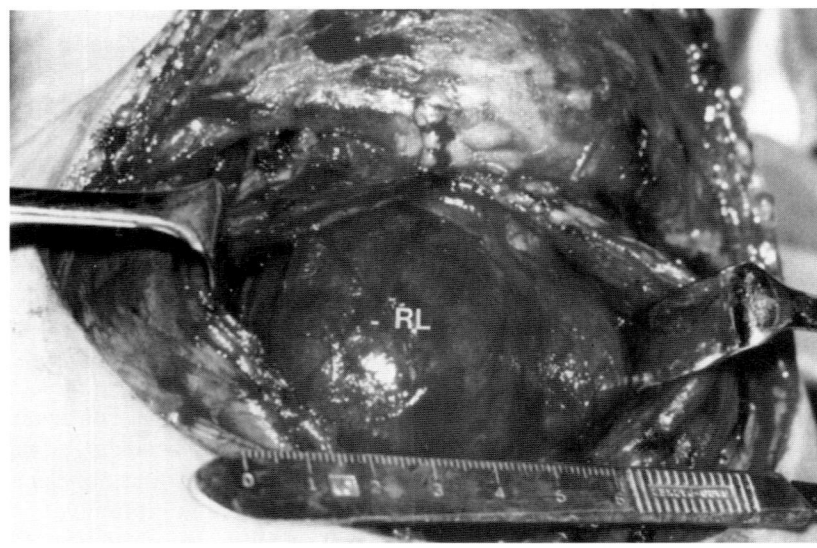

FIG. 10. Exposed right lobe (RL) of thyroid gland in a patient with papillary carcinoma.

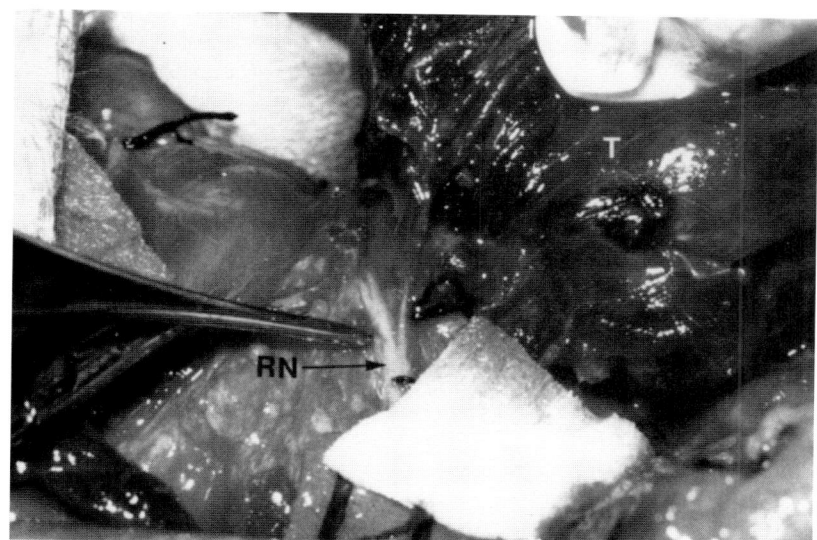

FIG. 11. Conservation of the right recurrent laryngeal nerve (RN) in a patient with papillary carcinoma of the right lobe of the thyroid gland (T), infiltrating the trachea. The recurrent nerve, in this case, has three extralaryngeal branches.

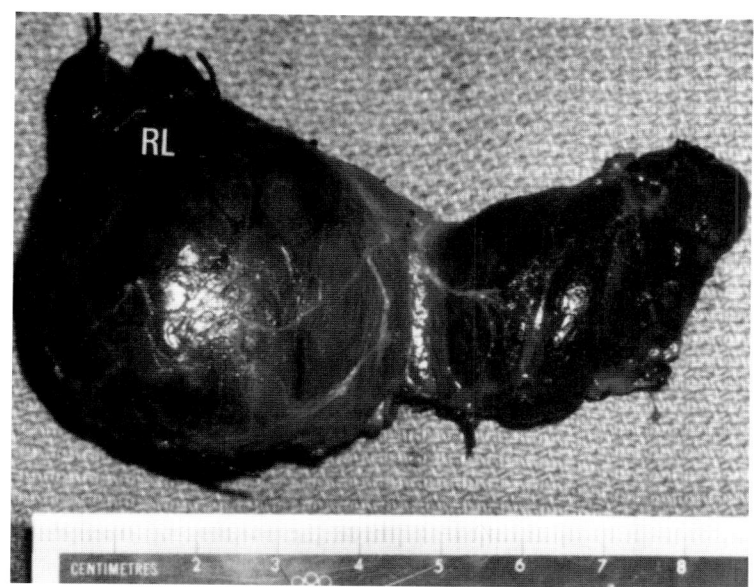

FIG. 12. Anterior view of an *en bloc* total thyroidectomy and tracheal resection in a patient with papillary carcinoma of the right lobe (RL) infiltrating the trachea.

troduce the endotracheal tube when there is significant airway deformity. Once the airway is inspected and secured, the anesthetist can proceed in the usual fashion as for any major head and neck procedure.

Postoperatively, the patient should not be extubated until there are strong spontaneous respirations. If there was a significant degree of deformity of the airway preoperatively, postoperative intubation and ventilation are maintained for 24 to 48 hr following the surgery. If an airway resection and reconstruction has been performed, a defunctioning tracheostomy is usually done, although, on occasion, postoperative endolaryngeal intubation can be maintained as an alternative. If there is loss of tracheal cartilage (tracheomalacia), a tracheostomy should be avoided if at all possible. Postoperative endolaryngeal intubation is used, at least initially.

Surgical Techniques

If the airway disorder is a result of displacement with compression, displacement without compression, or compression, the surgical techniques employed are the same as those for comparable thyroid pathology without airway

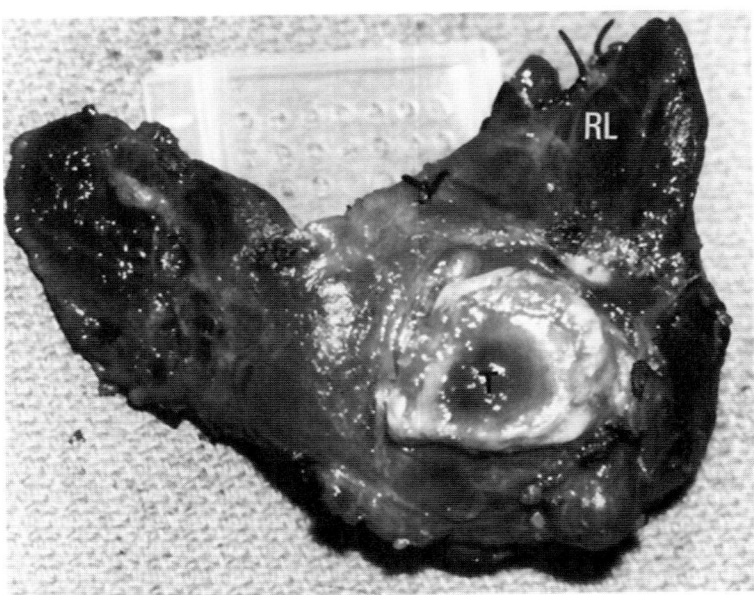

FIG. 13. Posterior view of specimen illustrated in Figure 12. T, tracheal resection with papillary carcinoma; RL, right lobe of thyroid gland.

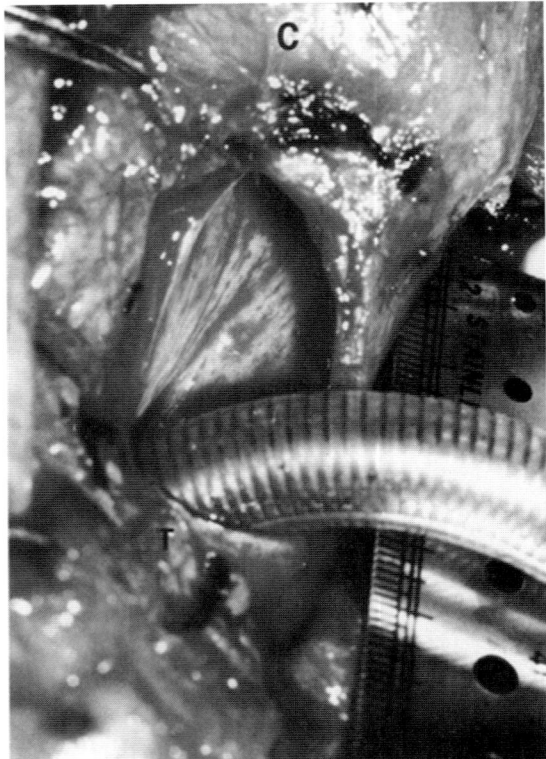

FIG. 14. Tracheal defect in patient described in Figures 9–13. C, cricoid cartilage; t, trachea.

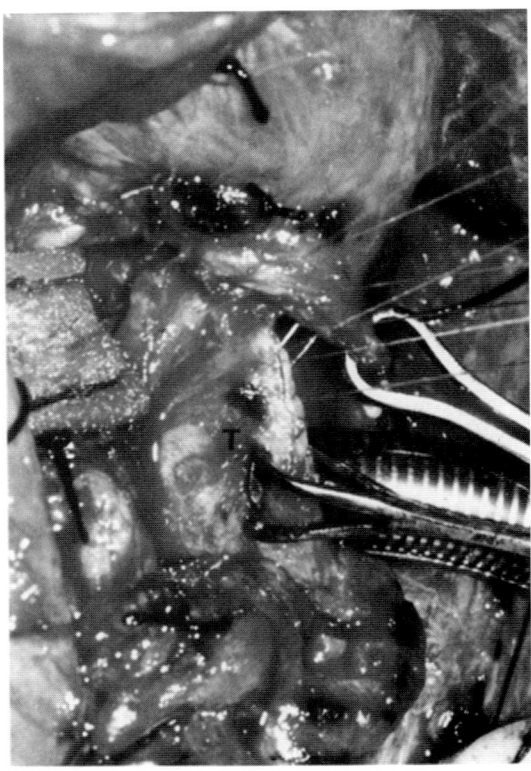

FIG. 15. The method of reconstructing the trachea (end-to-end anastomosis) in the patient described in Figures 9–14. T, trachea.

involvement. However, special attention is paid to the trachea and, if necessary, the trachea is molded back into position surgically in the neck field, or endoscopically with a bronchoscope inside the trachea.

If there is infiltrative disease, an *en bloc* total thyroidectomy with appropriate tracheal and/or laryngeal resection and immediate airway reconstruction is done. Usually, a laryngeal drop procedure is necessary to reconstruct the airway.

Depending on anatomic factors such as the length and mobility of the neck, and on the degree of calcification of the trachea, as many as six tracheal rings have been resected circumferentially, along with 50% of the subglottic larynx. The airway can be reconstructed primarily. An end-to-end anastomosis is the best form of reconstruction. If a portion of the subglottic larynx is resected, leaving a larger defect on one side of the airway than the other, the trachea can be advanced asymmetrically by dividing the anterior tracheal rings below the level of the tracheal resection, so that the trachea can be advanced more on one side than on the other (Figs. 16–18). This results in a slightly angulated airway. The technique is referred to as an asymmetric angulated anastomosis (2) (Fig. 19).

Various other types of airway reconstruction can be undertaken, ranging from a hyoid interposition graft (5) to the "trough" method of laryngotracheal reconstruction (6). If, however, the disease extends beyond six tra-

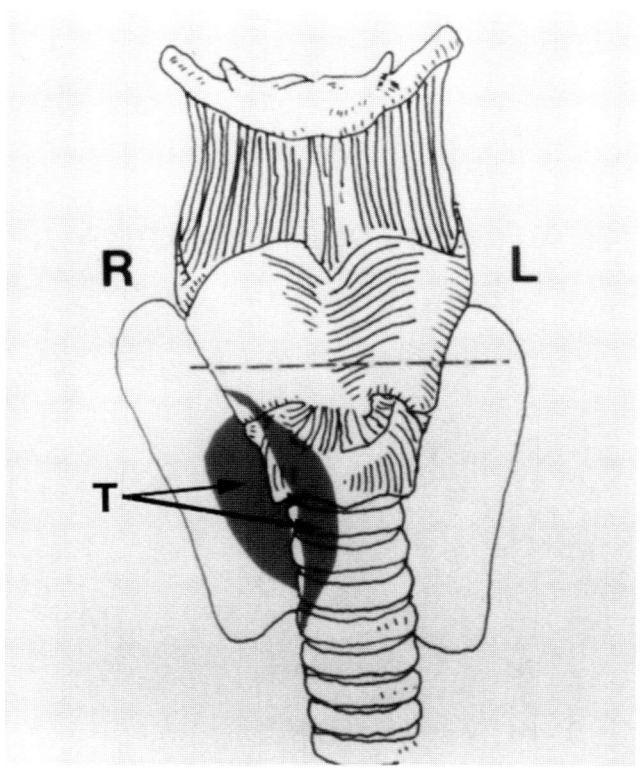

FIG. 16. The extent of a papillary tumor (T) that required a composite resection of the thyroid gland, one half of the subglottic larynx, and six tracheal rings. The *horizontal line* indicates the level of the true vocal cords.

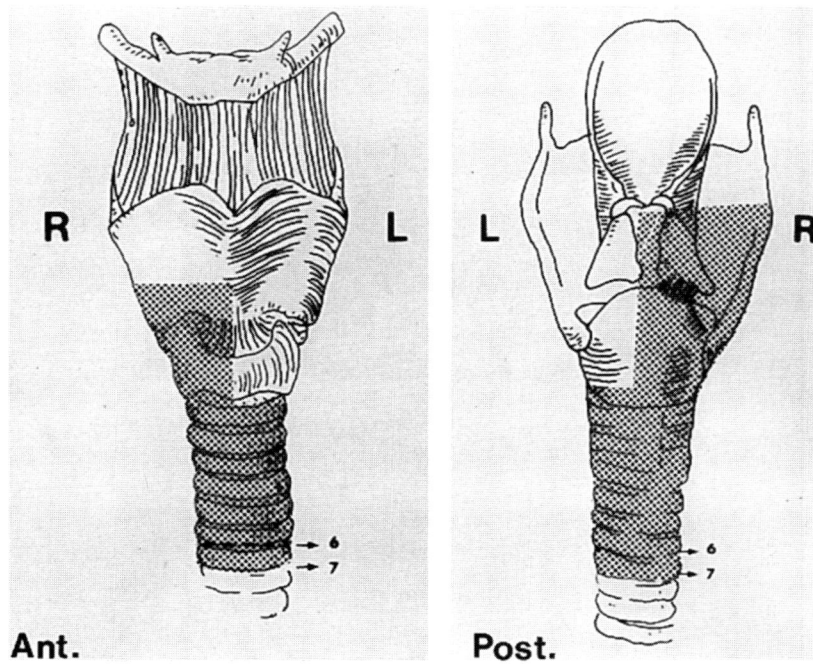

FIG. 17. The resultant airway defect (anterior and posterior views) in the patient with the tumor illustrated in Figure 16.

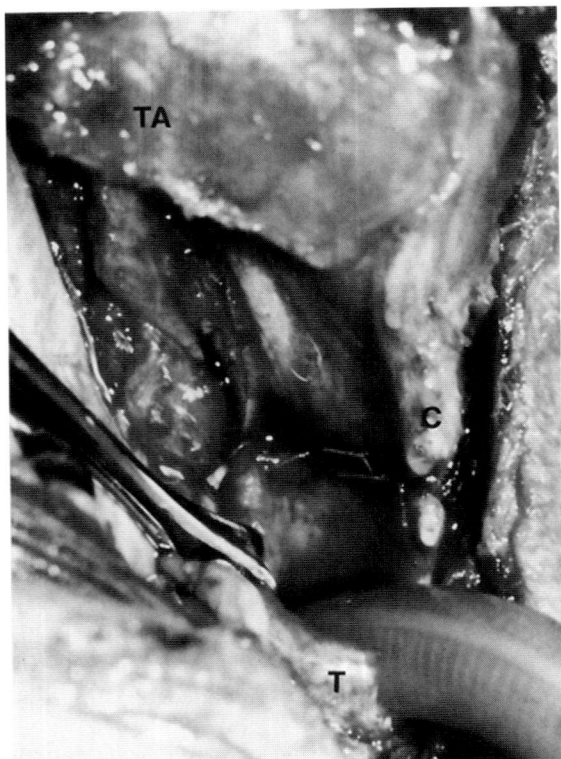

FIG. 18. The reconstruction that is under way in the patient whose tumor and surgical defect was shown in the schematics of Figures 16 and 17. Sutures are located on the left side of the cricoid (C)–tracheal anastomosis. The right side of the trachea (T) will be anastomosed to the right thyroid ala (TA) after the residual tracheal rings are divided anteriorly in the midline, so that the trachea can be advanced higher on the right side of the defect than on the left side.

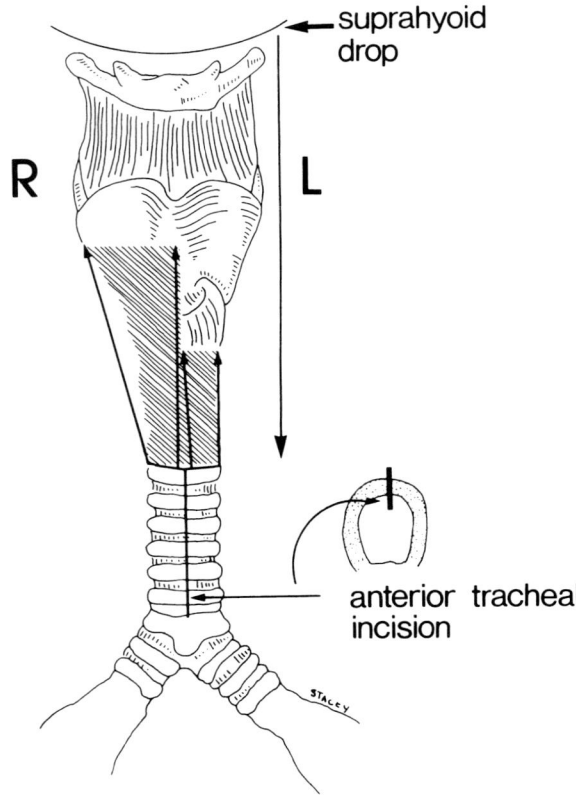

method of asymmetric angulated anastomosis

FIG. 19. The method of asymmetric angulated reconstruction used to anastomose the airway in the patient with the defect illustrated in Figure 17 and shown with the reconstruction under way in Figure 18.

cheal rings and 2 cm of the subglottic larynx on one side, a trachiectomy procedure with a permanent tracheostome or a trachiectomy–laryngectomy procedure may be necessary.

A one-stage *en bloc* thyroidectomy and airway resection with immediate airway reconstruction offers the best opportunity for long-term control of localized airway infiltrative thyroid disease. Restoration of normal airway anatomy in patients in whom thyroid disorders have affected the airway generally results in an excellent restoration of function.

REFERENCES

1. Lawson VG, Fallis JC. Surgical treatment of thyroglossal duct remnants. *Can Med Assoc J* 1969;100:855–858.
2. Lawson VG. The management of airway involvement in thyroid tumors. *Arch Otolaryngol* 1983;109:86–90.
3. Geelhoed GW. Tracheomalacia from compressing goiter: management after thyroidectomy. *Surgery* 1988;104:1100–1108.
4. Shaha A, Alfonso A, Jaffe BM. Acute airway distress due to thyroid pathology. *Surgery* 1987;102:1068–1074.
5. Looper EZ. Use of the hyoid bone as a graft in laryngeal stenosis. *Arch Otolaryngol* 1938;28:106.
6. Bryce DP, Lawson VG. The "trough" method of laryngotracheal reconstruction. *Ann Otol Rhinol Laryngol* 1967;76:793–804.

CHAPTER 26

Congenital Thyroid Cysts and Ectopic Thyroid

Charles M. Myer, III, and Robin T. Cotton

The most uncommon thyroid disorders are those with a congenital basis. The disorders fall into two broad categories—endocrine and anatomic. In the former, enzyme deficiencies prevent the normal formation of thyroid hormone. The latter, anatomic abnormalities, the subject of this chapter, are of two general types. The first involves abnormalities of the thyroglossal duct itself, in which there may be cyst formation or thyroglossal duct remnants along the path of migration. The second type involves ectopic thyroid tissue, in which there is abnormal migration of the thyroid gland to its normal pretracheal position (1). Imaging modalities and embryology of the thyroid gland are covered in detail elsewhere in this text; this chapter focuses on their relationship to the management of anatomic abnormalities.

THYROGLOSSAL DUCT ABNORMALITIES

In order to manage appropriately abnormalities arising from thyroglossal duct remnants, one must understand certain basics of thyroid embryology. The magnitude of this subject is clear because the thyroglossal duct cyst is the most common congenital cyst in the neck. It is estimated that 7% of the overall population has persistent remnants of the thyroglossal duct. Thyroglossal duct cysts may be seen in patients of any age, though 50% usually occur before the age of 20 and approximately 70% are seen before the age of 30.

Most thyroglossal duct cysts (61%) are located in the characteristic position between the thyroid gland and the hyoid bone. The remainder are located in a suprahyoid position (24%), a suprasternal location (13%), or an intralingual location (1% to 2%) (2). Occasionally, thyroglossal duct cysts have been reported in the floor of mouth (3,4). In some cases, the masses may protrude into the pre-epiglottic space or invade the thyroid cartilage to mimic laryngeal masses (5). Several different types of epithelial lining are known to occur within a thyroglossal duct cyst. The two most common types of lining are pseudostratified ciliated columnar epithelium of the respiratory type (54%), and stratified squamous epithelium (34%). Transitional epithelium (6%) and cuboidal epithelium (6%) are seen also (2).

Although radioisotope scanning will demonstrate functional thyroid tissue in 33% of patients, serial histologic sections have found thyroid tissue within the wall of a thyroglossal duct cyst in as many as 62% (2). As noted previously, thyroglossal ducts may present at any time in a patient's life. Most commonly, one sees a cystic mass in one of the aforementioned locations that may demonstrate the rapid growth associated with an upper respiratory tract infection. This swelling may either be secondary to inflammation of the associated lymphoid tissue or result from closure of the cyst's usual drainage pattern through the foramen cecum. Though the mass is commonly in the midline, it may present in a lateral cervical location, usually within 2 cm of the midline. In addition, there may be two cysts present, located one above the other (1). Thyroglossal duct cysts may exhibit slow enlargement unaccompanied by signs of infection, but approximately 60% present with acute inflammation. Thyroglossal duct fistulae are seen in 33% of cases and may be secondary to spontaneous drainage from infection, inadequate surgery, or a prior drainage procedure. When a patient presents with inflammation of the cyst, antimicrobial (particularly antistaphylococcal) therapy is indicated. Should abscess formation occur, incision and drainage are necessary in addition to antimicrobial therapy (1,6).

DIFFERENTIAL DIAGNOSIS

A thyroglossal duct cyst generally presents as an anterior neck mass in close association with the hyoid bone

---

C. M. Myer, III, and R. T. Cotton: Department of Otolaryngology, University of Cincinnati, College of Medicine; Children's Hospital Medical Center, Cincinnati, Ohio 45229-2899.

(Fig. 1). Because the cyst may be adherent to the hyoid, protrusion of the tongue usually results in elevation of the mass. The differential diagnosis must include cervical lymphadenopathy, solid ectopic thyroid tissue, cystic hygroma, branchial cyst, lipoma, dermoid cyst, and sebaceous cyst. The congenital midline cervical cleft, though uncommon, may be mistaken for a thyroglossal duct anomaly because of its midline cervical location.

As opposed to thyroglossal duct cysts, branchial cysts are usually located in the lateral neck and are unrelated to the hyoid bone. They are usually anterior to the sternocleidomastoid muscle and lateral to the carotid artery and internal jugular vein. Many present near the angle of the mandible. A parathyroid cyst usually presents near the inferior border of the thyroid gland. It is usually off the midline and anterior to the carotid artery and internal jugular vein. Thus, its location is usually lower than that of a thyroglossal duct cyst. Another lesion that can be mistaken for a thyroglossal duct cyst is a cervical thymic cyst. However, it is usually not in the midline and is frequently located in the lower portion of the neck anterior to the great vessels. Dermoid cysts are usually located near the midline in the upper neck or submental region. If the clinician is concerned that this mass represents a thyroglossal duct cyst, it should be managed in the same way as a thyroglossal duct cyst. Cystic hygromas are usually located in the posterolateral portion of the neck, behind the great vessels and sternocleidomastoid muscle. They are usually soft and compressible and may extend into the floor of the mouth. Approximately 90% present in children under 2 years of age. Teratomas are firm masses located in the region of the thyroid gland. Distinction from a thyroglossal duct cyst may not be possible prior to surgical excision. Cervical ranulas are usually located above the hyoid bone in the region of the submental or submandibular triangles. They may extend deeply into the supraclavicular area or mediastinum or even to the skull base posteriorly. Distinction from a thyroglossal duct cyst is usually possible because of the diffuse nature of the lesion.

Cervical lymphadenopathy may be present almost anywhere in the neck in association with an inflammatory or neoplastic process. However, the enlarged glands are most frequently present in the jugulodigastric triangle or submandibular triangle, and less commonly in the pretracheal region. Again, should there be any concern that the mass is a thyroglossal duct cyst, it should be managed as if it is (7,8).

Unusual inflammatory conditions also may mimic thyroglossal duct cysts. Acute suppurative thyroiditis commonly presents after an upper respiratory infection or trauma. Differentiation from a thyroglossal duct cyst may not be possible until resolution of the process after antimicrobial therapy. Progression to a thyroid abscess may occur. In this situation, incision and drainage are necessary in addition to antimicrobials. Should an abscess be noted, a barium esophagram should be obtained to rule out a fourth branchial arch internal fistula arising from the pyriform sinus, most commonly on the left side (Fig. 2) (9).

IMAGING

Several imaging modalities may prove useful in the evaluation of patients with suspected thyroglossal duct abnormalities. Plain soft-tissue radiographs of the neck add little to the diagnosis of thyroglossal duct anomalies. In the patient who is experiencing upper airway obstructive phenomenon, a lateral neck radiograph may demonstrate anterior tracheal compression. Similarly, other concurrent anatomic abnormalities may be noted on the film

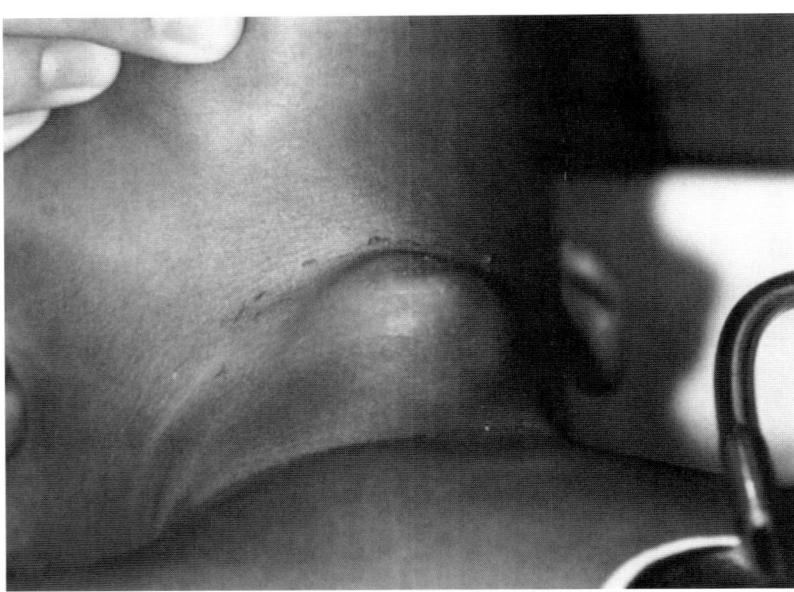

FIG. 1. An inflammatory anterior neck mass inferior to the hyoid bone that proved to be an infected thyroglossal duct cyst.

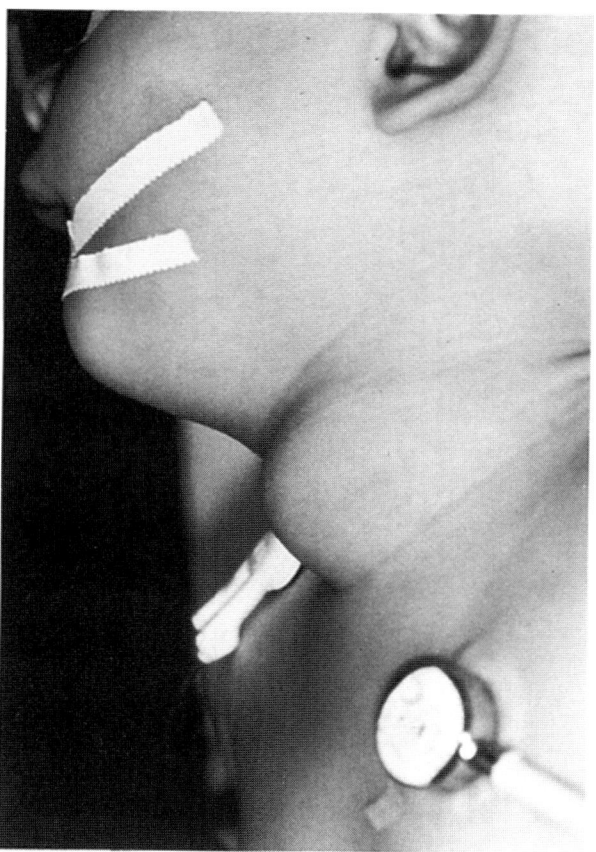

FIG. 2. A thyroid abscess secondary to a pyriform sinus fistula must be considered in the differential diagnosis of a thyroglossal duct cyst.

as potential etiologies for the patient's symptomatology. A barium esophagram may be useful in the patient who is experiencing dysphagia, because this may demonstrate other causes for the patient's complaints.

B-mode ultrasound scanning is another useful device for evaluation of the thyroid. Specifically, this instrument may be used to distinguish solid from cystic lesions in the thyroid as well as surrounding structures. Although ultrasound is certainly not specific for thyroid tissue, it may identify a cystic lesion in the neck such as a thyroglossal duct cyst, and demonstrate thyroid tissue in the normal location (1).

Computed tomography (CT) also may be useful in the evaluation of the thyroid gland. Thyroglossal duct cysts typically appear as well-circumscribed masses with an enhancing capsule and a lucent center. This imaging modality provides an accurate determination of the size and character of the cyst, as well as its relationship to other structures in the neck. In addition, CT may provide an excellent mechanism for differentiating masses such as thymic cysts that may mimic thyroglossal duct cysts (Figs. 3,4) (1,10,11).

Radioactive iodide (I-131, I-123) and pertechnetate scanning are well-known modalities for evaluating the size, distribution, and activity of thyroid tissue, and for differentiating thyroid disease from other masses in the head and neck and superior mediastinum that are not of thyroid origin. In children, technetium-99m-labeled sodium pertechnetate is generally used, because it is trapped by the thyroid gland but not organified. In addition, it is thought to be safer than I-131 because it is a pure gamma emitter as opposed to a beta emitter, and it has a half-life of only 6 hr. Whereas the other modalities of imaging are effective in defining the size and location of a cervical mass that may be thyroid in origin, only thyroid scanning enables the clinician to positively identify a mass as thyroid in origin (1).

It is important to document the presence of functional thyroid tissue before removing a thyroglossal duct cyst. In the face of recurrent infections, removal of the cyst will be necessary even if this is the only functioning thyroid tissue in the patient. It is important to make this determination preoperatively in order to counsel parents and patients regarding the implications of surgery (12). Although documentation of normally functioning thyroid tissue is appropriate (13), some authors have offered alternatives to the routine preoperative thyroid scan. Because an ectopic thyroid gland is almost always dysgenetic, there is frequently abnormal thyroid hormone production. In a patient who is clinically euthyroid with a mass suggestive of a thyroglossal duct cyst, thyroid function tests, including the thyroid stimulating hormone (TSH) level, can be obtained prior to surgery. If these are normal, excision of the cyst can be accomplished without a preoperative scan. However, if the excised mass demonstrates thyroid tissue or colloid follicles without the presence of a cystic structure, a thyroid scan should be obtained in the postoperative period.

In contradistinction to this scenario, a thyroid scan should be obtained before surgery when there are signs of hypothyroidism (chronic constipation, developmental and growth delay, excessive somnolence, weight gain despite poor eating habits) or abnormal thyroid function tests, especially an elevated TSH (14). Almost 90% of cases of ectopic thyroid are located in the tongue base, and 10% are found in the anterior neck. In this light, a thyroid scan would seem appropriate prior to removing a suspected internal thyroglossal duct cyst, because it may in fact be ectopic thyroid tissue (15).

TREATMENT

Although some authors have advocated observation of small thyroglossal duct cysts that have not become infected, we feel that removal of all suspected thyroglossal duct cysts is the treatment of choice. In essence, one is treating a neck mass of unknown etiology, and surgical removal is appropriate if there is no resolution of the mass following an adequate trial of medical therapy, in-

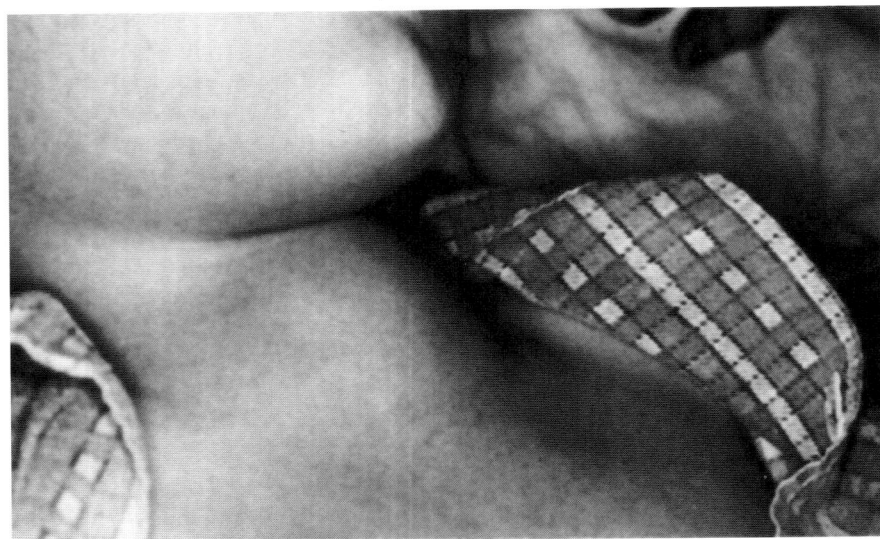

FIG. 3. A large cyst in the lower anterior neck is evaluated best by a computerized tomography (CT) scan.

cluding at least a 2-week course of oral antimicrobial therapy with antistaphylococcal coverage. As mentioned previously, should the cyst contain the patient's only functioning thyroid tissue, observation is appropriate if the mass has not been infected previously. If recurrent infections have been a problem, removal of the cyst is necessary regardless of the status of the patient's thyroid gland function. Patients should be cautioned, however, that the recurrence rate is higher when definitive surgical excision follows an episode of infection.

Surgical technique has evolved in the management of thyroglossal duct cysts. Prior to 1893, the treatment of choice was simple excision. However, recurrence rates as high as 50% were reported. In 1893, Schlange advocated removal of the cyst as well as the central portion of the hyoid bone and any portion of the duct cephalad to this. When this was accomplished, the recurrence rate dropped to 20%. Sistrunk further expanded the procedure in 1920 when he advocated the additional removal of a core of tissue at the base of the tongue. When this maneuver was added to the procedure developed by Schlange, the recurrence rate dropped to 3%. Although it is difficult to positively identify a midline neck mass as a thyroglossal duct cyst preoperatively, all masses in this location should be treated in the same manner to avoid an unnecessarily high recurrence rate. Every effort should be made to minimize acute inflammation at the time of definitive surgery in order to make dissection easier and reduce recurrence (1,2,6,12).

During the actual surgical procedure, the thyroglossal duct cyst and its attached duct should be followed cephalad to the hyoid bone. No attempt should be made to separate the duct from the hyoid bone. Rather, a block of tissue should be excised to include the central portion of the hyoid bone, because the duct may run above, below, or through the hyoid bone (Fig. 5). It has been advocated that the minimum amount of hyoid bone removed be 10 mm and that 15 mm would be preferable (16). This will prevent accidental transection of the duct as it is followed to the base of the tongue. The oral cavity is frequently entered to ensure complete removal of the tract and then sutured, generally without consequence. Horisawa et al. (16) report that there is no need to enter the oral cavity. Rather, depth of the core-out should be less than 5 mm to avoid disruption of the branched ducts near the foramen cecum, which would increase the risk of recurrence. Sometimes, a small tract extends inferiorly from the cyst toward the thyroid cartilage. It is not necessary to follow this structure, which can be transected. The wound is closed over a drain without repair of the hyoid bone. A skin resection is not needed unless there is a draining sinus tract (Fig. 6). When this tract is present, the draining sinus should be included with an ellipse of skin and excised in continuity with the thyroglossal duct cyst (1,2,6,12).

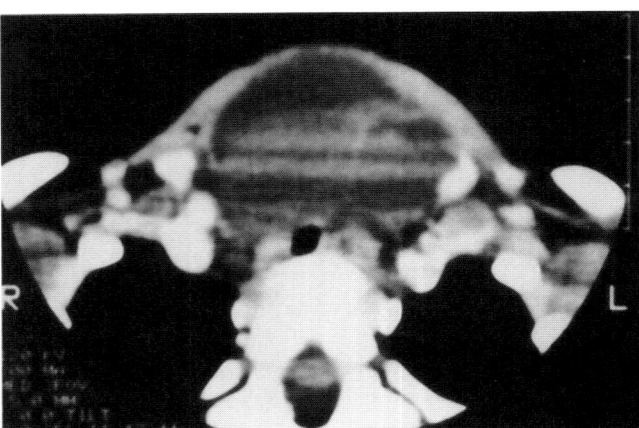

FIG. 4. A CT scan of the patient in Figure 3 confirms a large thymic cyst.

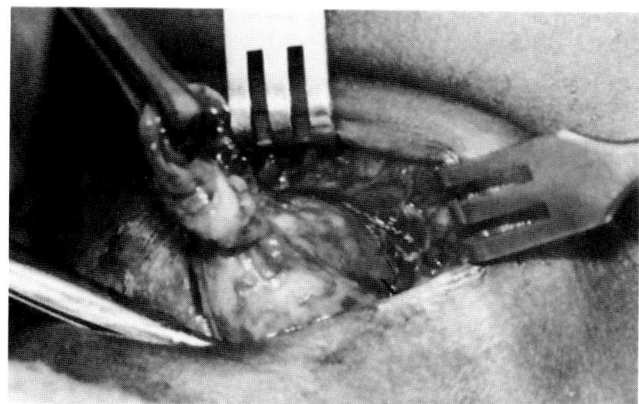

FIG. 5. A large core of tissue should be included during a Sistrunk procedure to avoid transection of the tract.

Recurrent thyroglossal duct cysts can be a challenge for the clinician. They are uncommon, and their removal can be fraught with disaster. Care must be taken to include a large core of tissue in the surgical specimen to ensure removal of the recurrent cyst and thyroglossal duct remnant. Because of prior scarring in the surgical field, certain normal structures are at risk during the removal of a recurrent cyst. Specifically, one must be cognizant of the location of the hypoglossal nerve, the lingual nerve, the superior laryngeal nerve, and the submandibular duct. In addition, the medial portion of the dissection must be done carefully to avoid inadvertent entrance into the larynx or pharynx. Should this occur, a pharyngocutaneous or laryngocutaneous fistula may result. Laryngeal inflammation may also occur with subsequent interarytenoid scarring resulting in airway or voice abnormalities, or both.

Recurrence of a thyroglossal duct cyst is rare if a Sistrunk procedure is done at the initial operation. When a patient has a draining sinus at the time of the initial procedure, the chance of recurrence is increased because the infection may obliterate the tract and surrounding landmarks. Recurrence rates may be higher also when there are multiple cysts or cysts that arise lateral to the midline. In these situations, even the inclusion of a wide core of tissue with the surgical specimen may not allow complete excision of a thyroglossal duct remnant (17,18).

CARCINOMA IN THYROGLOSSAL DUCT CYST

A related topic is the management of carcinoma that arises in a thyroglossal duct cyst. Approximately 150 cases have been reported in the literature, and only four are in children younger than 10 years of age. Although most cases have been papillary carcinoma, there have also been cases of follicular carcinoma, mixed papillary–follicular carcinoma, nonthyroid adenocarcinoma, anaplastic carcinoma, and squamous cell carcinoma (19).

There is controversy regarding the origin of these tumors, which influences recommendations for therapy. Some authors feel that these tumors represent spread of an occult thyroid carcinoma and they therefore advocate total thyroidectomy, neck dissection, and postoperative radioactive iodine, in addition to a Sistrunk procedure. Others, however, believe these tumors arise within ectopic thyroid tissue contained within the thyroglossal duct cyst, and they feel the Sistrunk operation is curative, assuming that the thyroid gland is normal on palpation and scanning (20–22).

In a child, total thyroidectomy should be considered also because of the possibility of carcinoma within the thyroid gland and the child's long life expectancy. If total thyroidectomy is performed, the child can be followed with thyroglobulin assays in an effort to detect recurrence or metastases. This is an improvement over the previous method of following patients with I-131 scans. Even though these scans could be performed on an annual basis without requiring a thyroidectomy, tumor identification was sometimes difficult because the normal residual thyroid tissue would absorb the radioisotope preferentially. A radioisotope scan may be useful, however, to determine the location of recurrences or metastases if the thyroglobulin level is equivocal or rising (19).

The type of tumor that is present also influences surgical decisions. Cervical metastases associated with a squamous cell carcinoma within a thyroglossal duct cyst require radical neck dissection and, if positive, postoperative radiation therapy. On the other hand, a modified neck dissection is appropriate in patients with papillary or follicular carcinoma and cervical metastases. A total thyroidectomy is generally appropriate with any type of thyroid carcinoma if the thyroid scan is positive or if a palpable mass is noted within the gland. Regardless of the surgical procedure chosen, all patients with carcinoma arising in a thyroglossal duct remnant should receive thyroid suppression with exogenous thyroxine (22).

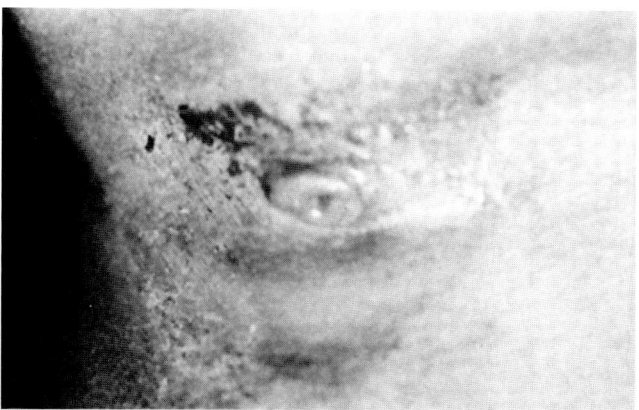

FIG. 6. Skin resection is necessary during a Sistrunk procedure when there is cutaneous granulation tissue or a fistula present.

ECTOPIC THYROID

Embryology and Pathophysiology

As noted elsewhere in this text (Chapter 2), the thyroid develops as a midline structure extending caudally from the foramen cecum. The thyroglossal duct eventually divides into the right and left thyroid lobes prior to atrophy. Colloid formation appears by the third month, and by the end of the first trimester thyroid hormone production has begun. This remains low until the end of the second trimester, when T_4 output increases secondary to TSH secretion from the pituitary.

Any thyroid tissue not located anterior to the upper trachea in the anterior midline of the neck is considered ectopic. It appears that the primary factor influencing the presence of ectopic thyroid tissue is hypoplasia of the gland. When there is abnormal development of the thyroid gland, descent of the gland to its normal position is often adversely affected. As a result, ectopic thyroid may be located anywhere along the thyroglossal duct tract between the foramen cecum at the base of the tongue and the normal location of the thyroid in the neck. Alternatively, hereditary factors may influence abnormal descent of the thyroid gland. The abnormal collection of thyroid tissue may be localized at one site or present at several different locations. In 70% of the patients with ectopic thyroid tissue present, this is the only thyroid tissue that can be found.

Hypothyroidism is common in patients with ectopic thyroid tissue. In fact, ectopic thyroid tissue is believed to be responsible for up to 75% of primary nongoitrous hypothyroidism in pediatric patients. In the first few months of life, an ectopic thyroid gland may function sufficiently to ensure normal body growth and mental development. However, as an individual ages, the ectopic tissue is unable to meet the demands of the developing individual. In such cases, hypothyroidism may develop. Depending on the amount of thyroid hormone produced, the signs and symptoms of hypothyroidism may be masked and diagnosis delayed. In various series, between 37% and 57% of the diagnoses of hypothyroidism secondary to ectopic thyroid tissue were made within the first year of life. Thus, whereas retardation of growth and development is common in patients with ectopic thyroid, the characteristic features of cretinism are absent because an appropriate amount of thyroid hormone is produced for a period of time. In some patients, delayed bone age and irregular calcification are noted secondary to hypothyroidism. Delayed bone age noted at birth is a sign of intrauterine hypothyroidism. When the bone age is less than 7 fetal months at birth, mental retardation is believed to be universal, regardless of the institution of early treatment.

Infants who are born with inadequate thyroid tissue present with diminished levels of T_4 and high TSH concentrations. In those rare cases where there is no functional thyroid tissue present, there is absent T_4 with elevated TSH concentrations. Although the signs and symptoms of hypothyroidism may be present in the neonatal period, the diagnosis is rarely made before the child is several months of age. This delay is significant because congenital hypothyroidism leads to brain dysfunction with intellectual abnormalities if therapy is not begun before the child reaches 3 months of age. In the same vein, 80% of infants begun on therapy before 3 months of age will develop normal intellectual function. However, this figure falls to 10% or less when therapy is delayed beyond 1 year (23).

Clinical Presentation

The signs and symptoms of hypothyroidism that are seen in the newborn period are nonspecific and include a large posterior fontanel, prolonged "physiologic" hyperbilirubinemia, mild myxedema of the face and neck, persistent respiratory distress in a full-term infant, hypothermia (less than 35.5°C rectal), bradycardia (rate less than 100), constipation, lethargy, poor feeding, stridor, and persistent nasal congestion. The more classic signs and symptoms of hypothyroidism usually occur later in infancy as a result of prolonged hypothyroidism. These include macroglossia, abdominal distention, umbilical hernia, hypotonia, dry hair and skin, puffy facies, and a hoarse cry. In the older child, delayed growth, delayed skeletal maturation, and delayed dental development are seen also (24).

Any mass located at the base of the tongue or in the midline of the neck in a child may potentially be ectopic thyroid tissue. Alternatively, ectopic thyroid tissue may be located within the larynx or trachea and, more rarely, within the pericardium or esophagus. Conditions to consider in the differential diagnosis include thyroglossal duct cyst, tumor, epidermal cyst, and vascular malformations.

Vallecular cysts are common at the base of the tongue and are usually yellowish or white with a thin wall. Mucous retention cysts are frequently smaller and off the midline and may be blue in color. Hypertrophic lingual tonsils are verrucous, superficially located, and usually posterior to the foramen cecum. When such a mass is noted, thyroid scanning is appropriate to ascertain if the mass contains thyroid tissue and if there is a normally situated thyroid gland (25). In some patients, a goiter may be noted because of increased TSH production resulting in secondary hypertrophy of the thyroid gland. This increase in TSH production results from failure of the ectopic thyroid tissue to produce an adequate amount of thyroid hormone. This commonly occurs during late childhood and puberty (23).

The symptoms produced by ectopic thyroid tissue are the result of the site of the ectopic tissue and the size. Approximately 90% of ectopic thyroid tissue is found at the base of the tongue. It is 4 times more common in female than male patients. Depending on the size of the ectopic thyroid tissue, upper aerodigestive tract obstruction may occur (23,26,27).

Treatment

In asymptomatic euthyroid patients whose sole thyroid tissue is located at the base of the tongue or in the region of the hyoid, no therapy is necessary. However, those patients who develop obstructive symptoms secondary to hypertrophy of the ectopic tissue because of TSH production require supplemental thyroid hormone. As long as the ectopic tissue shrinks and the obstructive symptoms abort, no surgical therapy will be needed. Occasionally, the ectopic thyroid mass will need to be removed. In the case of a lingual thyroid, this can be accomplished through several approaches, including a median pharyngotomy, a transoral approach, and a lateral pharyngeal approach. In all cases, permanent thyroid suppression is mandatory following surgical treatment (23,26,27).

Autotransplantation has been successful in some patients after resection of ectopic thyroid tissue. The tissue has been placed in major muscles of the neck, chest, abdomen, or extremities. This technique appears best suited for children with obstructive symptoms but with no evidence of hypothyroidism, and for those whose glands show no degeneration or cystic changes. In addition, it is still recommended that supplemental thyroxine therapy be used when autotransplantation is performed (23,26). Because there is some risk of carcinoma arising in ectopic thyroid tissue (20), we would discourage the practice of autotransplantation.

Two other types of ectopic thyroid tissue have been categorized as sublingual and thyroglossal. Patients with these conditions generally present with a progressively enlarging midline cervical mass, usually noted since birth. Other than the obvious mass, patients are generally asymptomatic. Thyroid scanning is extremely important in these patients prior to the removal of the mass in order to document the presence of other functional thyroid tissue. Therapeutic intervention is usually not necessary (27).

Ectopic thyroid tissue may also cause airway obstruction when located within the larynx or trachea. Most reports are of adult women and only rarely have pediatric patients been identified with this condition. Two major theories have been developed in an attempt to explain intralaryngotracheal thyroid tissue. The malformation theory was developed by Von Bruns (28); he related the presence of the thyroid tissue to sequestration of embryonic thyroid within the tracheal lumen. In contradistinction, Paltauf (29) developed the ingrowth theory; he felt there was direct invasion of the tracheal lumen by mature thyroid tissue. Once the diagnosis is made, either by biopsy or thyroid scanning, thyroid suppression is appropriate to reduce the intraluminal mass and avoid airway obstruction (27).

CONGENITAL THYROID CYST

True cysts of the thyroid are unusual lesions that may be confused with thyroglossal duct cysts and should be differentiated from goiters, adenomas, or necroses within the thyroid gland. Cells derived from the ultimobranchial bodies (UBB) are found throughout the substance of the thyroid gland as C cells. These cells are present in neonates and are responsible for the production of calcitonin. Congenital intrathyroidal cysts may result from the persistence of the UBB as a cystic structure, or they may be secondary to the intrathyroidal persistence of the thyroglossal duct (30,31).

In a patient who presents with a large cystic mass in the region of the thyroid gland, radiographic evaluation is appropriate prior to surgical resection. Because congenital cysts of the thyroid will usually present in a young patient, both a CT scan of the neck and a thyroid scan are appropriate preoperative measures. Differentiation of this lesion from a parathyroidal abscess is important. An abscess in the tissues surrounding the thyroid gland may present in a child under 2 years of age, the age at which one might see a patient affected with a congenital cyst of the thyroid. Abscesses surrounding the thyroid gland often result from fistulas arising in the pyriform sinus. Because of this a barium esophagram may be useful in the evaluation of patients with suspicious lesions (9). Any cystic lesion of the thyroid gland may be aspirated as an attempted curative measure. However, this maneuver is infrequently successful in terms of definitive therapy. Should the cyst reaccumulate, surgical excision is appropriate. In general, a thyroid lobectomy is the minimal surgical procedure necessary to remove the cyst completely while minimizing risk to the recurrent laryngeal nerve.

REFERENCES

1. Noyek AM, Friedberg J. Thyroglossal duct and ectopic thyroid disorders. *Otolaryngol Clin North Am* 1981;14:187–201.
2. Topf P, Fried MP, Strome M. Vagaries of thyroglossal duct cysts. *Laryngoscope* 1988;98:740–742.
3. Dolata J. Thyroglossal duct cyst in the mouth floor: an unusual location. *Otolaryngol Head Neck Surg* 1994;110:580–583.
4. Drucker C, Gerson CR. Sublingual contiguous thyroglossal and dermoid cysts in a neonate. *Int J Pediatr Otorhinolaryngol* 1992;23:181–186.
5. Slotnick D, Som PM, Giebfried J, Biller HF. Thyroglossal duct cysts that mimic laryngeal masses. *Laryngoscope* 1987;97:742–745.
6. Bennett KG, Organ CH Jr, Williams GR. Is the treatment for thyroglossal duct cysts too extensive? *Am J Surg* 1986;152:602–605.
7. Batsakis JG, McClatchey KD. Pathology consultation. Cervical ranulas. *Ann Otol Rhinol Laryngol* 1988;97:561–562.
8. Friedberg J. Clinical diagnosis of neck lumps. A practical guide. *Pediatr Ann* 1988 17:620–628.
9. Taylor WE, Myer III CM, Hays LL, Cotton RT. Acute suppurative thyroiditis in children. *Laryngoscope* 1982;92:1269–1273.
10. Ward RF, Selfe RW, St Louis L, Bowling D. Computed tomography and the thyroglossal duct cyst. *Otolaryngol Head Neck Surg* 1986;95:93–98.

11. Bourjat P, Cartier J, Woerther JP. Thyroglossal duct cyst in hyoid bone: CT confirmation. *J Comput Assist Tomogr* 1988;12:740–742.
12. Hawkins DB, Jacobsen BE, Klatt EC. Cysts of the thyroglossal duct. *Laryngoscope* 1982;92:1254–1258.
13. Pinczowler E, Crockett DM, Atkinson JB, Kun S. Preoperative thyroid scanning in presumed thyroglossal duct cysts. *Arch Otolaryngol Head Neck Surg* 1992;118:985–988.
14. Radkowski D, Arnold J, Healy GB, McGill T, Treves ST, Paltiel H, Fredman EM. Thyroglossal duct remnants: preoperative evaluation and management. *Arch Otolaryngol Head Neck Surg* 1991;117:1378–1381.
15. Stevens MH, Gray S. Preoperative thyroid scanning in presumed thyroglossal duct systs [letter]. *Arch Otolaryngol Head Neck Surg* 1994; 120:113.
15a. Schlange H. Über die fistula colli congenita. *Arch Klin Surg* 1893;46: 390–392.
15b. Sistrank WE. The surgical treatment of cysts of the thyroglossal tract. *Ann Surg* 1920;71:121–122.
16. Horisawa M, Niinomi N, Ito T. What is the optimal depth for core-out toward the foramen cecum in a thyroglossal duct cyst operation? *J Pediatr Surg* 1992;27:710–713.
17. Mickel RA, Calcaterra TC. Management of recurrent thyroglossal duct cysts. *Arch Otolaryngol* 1983;109:34–36.
18. Ein SH, Shandling B, Stephens CA, Mancer K. The problem of recurrent thyroglossal duct remnants. *J Pediatr Surg* 1984;19:437–439.
19. McNicoll MP, Hawkins DB, England K, Penny R, Maceri DR. Papillary carcinoma arising in a thyroglossal duct cyst. *Otolaryngol Head Neck Surg* 1988;99:50–54.
20. Borger JA, Bercu BB. Papillary-follicular carcinoma arising in a thyroglossal duct cyst in a 12-year-old child. *J Pediatr Surg* 1988;23: 362–363.
21. Katergiannakis V, Manouras A, Izardis P, Papdimitriou C, Apostolidis N. Thyroglossal duct cyst carcinoma (report of two cases). *Am Surg* 1988;54:315–317.
22. LaRouere MJ, Drake AF, Baker SR, Richter HJ, Magielski JE. Evaluation and management of a carcinoma arising in a thyroglossal duct cyst. *Am J Otolaryngol* 1987;8:351–355.
23. Kaplan M, Kauli R, Lubin E, Grunebaum M, Laron Z. Ectopic thyroid gland. A clinical study of 30 children and review. *J Pediatr* 1978;92: 205–209.
24. Fisher DA. Thyroid dysgenesis. In: Bergsma D, ed. *Birth defects compendium,* 2nd ed. New York: Alan R. Liss, 1979;1021–1022.
25. Santiago W, Rybak LP, Bass RM. Thyroglossal duct cyst of the tongue. *J Otolaryngol* 1985;14:261–264.
26. Hazzrika P, Murty PS, Nooruddin SM, Zachariah J, Rao NR. Lingual thyroid. *Ear Nose Throat J* 1988;67:161–165.
27. Chanin LR, Greenberg LM. Pediatric upper airway obstruction due to ectopic thyroid: classification and care reports. *Laryngoscope* 1988;98: 422–427.
28. Von Bruns P. Über kropfgesch-wuelste und langen des kehlkopfs und der luftroehre und ihrer entgernung. *Beitr Klin Chir* 1873;41:1903–1904.
29. Paltauf FR. Zur kenntriss der schilddreusen tumera im innern des kehlkopfs und der luftroehre. *Beitr Path Anat* 1892;11:71.
30. Roediger WEW, Spitz L. Congenital cyst of the thyroid. *S Afr Med J* 1973;47:1120–1122.
31. Roediger WE, Kalk F, Spitz L, Schmaman A. Congenital thyroid cyst of ultimobranchial gland origin. *J Pediatr Surg* 1977;12:575–576.

CHAPTER 27

Replacement and Suppressive Treatment with Thyroid Hormone

Sheldon S. Waldstein

HISTORY OF THYROID HORMONE THERAPY

Recognition of the clinical consequences of loss of thyroid function evolved during the latter half of the 19th century. Gull (1) described adult hypothyroidism in 1874 but had no idea of how to treat it. Four years later, Ord (2) proposed the term *myxedema* for the condition, and 10 years later (1888), the landmark report of the Committee of the Clinical Society of London concluded that myxedema, endemic cretinism, and cachexia strumipriva were closely related diseases and caused by destructive changes in the thyroid gland (3).

In 1891, Murray (4) was the first to attempt to overcome the thyroid deficiency of myxedema, using the subcutaneous injection of a glycerine extract of sheep thyroid glands; by 1893, successful treatment of 100 cases by this method was reported (5). Feeding of fresh sheep thyroid glands prepared by mincing or frying, or of aqueous or glycerine extracts of these glands, quickly followed, with gratifying results (6,7); an extract of sheep thyroid gland in tablet form was introduced by the Burroughs and Wellcome pharmaceutical company in 1893 (8). Thus, in a relatively few years following the Clinical Society's report, therapy of this devastating condition had evolved to the point where Osler, in 1909, could hail it as one of the most remarkable achievements of medicine (8). It was the first specific therapy for a hormone deficiency.

The next advance in thyroid therapy occurred during 1914 and 1915, when Kendall (9) succeeded in isolating and crystallizing from the thyroid an iodine-containing compound, shown to be effective calorigenically, that he later named "thyroxin." By 1927, Harrington and Barger (10) had succeeded in synthesizing the hormone, but remarkably, the administration of synthetic thyroxine for treatment of hypothyroidism was not introduced until Hart and Maclagen (11) reported their successful clinical trials in 1950. By 1954, a practical commercial method of thyroxine synthesis had been developed and the hormone became readily available for clinical purposes (12). At about the same time, Gross and Pitt-Rivers (13,14) identified triiodothyronine in the circulation, isolated it from the thyroid, and synthesized it. It, too, soon became commercially available for clinical use.

Meanwhile, basing his work on occasional earlier reports of regression of thyroid carcinoma after the feeding of desiccated thyroid, Crile (15) began to use thyroid hormone regularly in patients with metastatic thyroid carcinoma. His success with this treatment (16), along with comparable reports from others (17,18), established a role for suppressive therapy in the management of some types of thyroid carcinomas.

Today, replacement therapy for thyroid hormone deficiency is readily accomplished, and suppressive therapy for the most frequently occurring types of thyroid carcinomas is commonplace. Suppressive therapy is used also for diagnostic and therapeutic purposes in nonmalignant thyroid disease. This chapter will examine the current use of thyroid hormone preparations in clinical medicine.

AVAILABLE THYROID HORMONE PREPARATIONS

Thyroid hormone preparations are marketed today under a variety of registered trademarks (19) and in generic form (Table 1). These are available largely as tablets for oral administration, but thyroxine and triiodothyronine for parenteral injection are also available.

Both thyroxine [T_4, or levothyroxine sodium, United States Pharmacopeia (U.S.P.)] and triiodothyronine (T_3,

---

S. S. Waldstein: Division of Medicine, The National Center for Advanced Medical Education, Chicago, Illinois 60611-3319.

TABLE 1. Commercially available thyroid hormone preparations

Trademark name (manufacturer)	Synthetic origin, μg/tablet, color													
Levothyroxine sodium USP (T$_4$)[a]	25	50	75	88	100	112	125	137	150	175	200	300		
Synthroid (Knoll)[b]	orange	white	violet	olive	yellow	rose	brown	n.a.	lt. blue	lilac	pink	green		
Levothroid (Forest)	"	"	gray	mint grn.	"	"	purple	dk. blue	"	turquoise	"	"		
Levoxyl (Daniels)	"	"	purple	olive	"	"	brown	"	"	"	"	"		
Eltroxin (Roberts)	"	"	n.a.	n.a.	"	n.a.	n.a.	n.a.	"	n.a.	"	"		

	μg/tablet, color				
Liothyronine sodium USP (T$_3$)[a,c]	5	25	50		
Cytomel (SmithKline Beecham)	off white	off white	off white		

	Tablet designation				
Liotrix USP (T$_4$/T$_3$)	1/4	1/2	1	2	3
Thyrolar (Forest) μgT$_4$/μgT$_3$	12.5/3.1	25/6.25	50/12.5	100/25	150/37.5
white/with:	violet	peach	pink	green	yellow

	Animal origin				
	Grains/tablet, color				
Thyroid USP[a]	1/4	1/2	1	2	3	4	5
Armour thyroid [36μgT$_4$/9μgT$_3$ per grain (60 mg)] (Forest)	white	white	white	white	white	white	white

[a]Available as generic preparation from many manufacturers and suppliers.
[b]Parenteral form available in 10-mL vials containing 200 μg or 500 μg lyophilized hormone per vial for reconstitution.
[c]Intravenous form available as Triostat (SmithKline Beecham) in 1-mL vials containing 10 μg/ml hormone.

or liothyronine sodium, U.S.P.) are produced synthetically. Each is available in tablets of different potencies (μg per tablet); two manufacturers market tablets of thyroxine in 12 separate potencies. Potencies of tablets of thyroxine formerly were stated in fractional milligrams (e.g., 0.2 mg), but presently potency is stated in micrograms (e.g., 200 μg), thus eliminating the decimal point and the attendant confusion regarding dosage on the part of patient, physician, and pharmacist. Additionally, a mixture of both synthetic thyroxine and triiodothyronine in a fixed ratio of (T_4 to T_3) of 4:1 (liotrix, U.S.P.) is marketed in tablets of five different potencies. Finally, thyroid hormone preparations derived from beef or porcine thyroid glands are marketed in tablets of different potencies as desiccated thyroid (thyroid, U.S.P.).

Synthetic Thyroid Hormone Preparations

Most often, thyroxine tablets are color-coded so that potency is recognizable at a glance. A degree of consistency exists among three major trademarked brands of thyroxine (Synthroid, Levothroid, and Levoxyl) and many of the generic preparations of the hormone, in that orange designates 25 μg; white, 50 μg; yellow, 100 μg; rose, 112 μg; blue, 150 μg; pink, 200 μg; and green, 300 μg tablets. However, as seen in Table 1, as tablets of intermediate potencies have been marketed, a uniform color scheme has not been followed. Furthermore, the profusion of color can lead to confusion of dose. Pink can be mistaken for rose or orange, as can lilac for violet, and purple for gray. It is fortunate, then, that most manufacturers also impress the microgram amount upon the tablet as an additional means of identifying its potency.

When liotrix was conceived, it was the intention to make available a mixture of thyroxine and triiodothyronine that would mimic thyroid hormone secretion and would result in normal blood levels of both T_4 and T_3 in appropriately replaced athyreotic individuals (20). To designate the potency of each mixture, the manufacturer uses a fraction or a whole number that implies a metabolic activity corresponding to that number of apothecary grains of desiccated thyroid. Thus, Thyrolar-$1/4$ is designated to be the equivalent of $1/4$ grain of desiccated thyroid therapeutically, and Thyrolar- the equivalent of 2 grains of desiccated thyroid. Liotrix tablets are also color-coded, but there is no color correspondence to tablets containing metabolically equivalent doses of thyroxine.

Animal-Derived Thyroid Hormone Preparations

Thyroid hormone preparations derived from animals are marketed in tablets that usually are not color-coded; instead, tablet size varies directly with potency, and the supposed content of the tablet is indicated by numerals stamped on its face stating the number of apothecary grains. These preparations may not contain uniform amounts of T_4 and T_3 even among different batches prepared from the same species by the same manufacturer, making for variability in metabolic response and in circulating blood levels of T_4 and T_3 (21–23). Hog thyroid usually contains more T_3 relative to its T_4 content than does beef or sheep thyroid, accounting for its greater biologic potency (24,25). The total content of active hormone may vary considerably among different batches of commercially available desiccated thyroid. In one bioassay study, among batches conforming to U.S.P. requirements for total iodine content tested, one contained as little as 9.4% and one as much as 197% of stated potency (26). Low potency can be explained by an unusually high content of inactive monoiodotyrosine and diiodotyrosine (27). The content of T_3 and T_4 in some generic desiccated thyroid preparations has differed markedly from that found in a commonly used brand name preparation (28). The inadvertent use of an inactive preparation has led to hypothyroid symptoms and findings in patients under treatment (29).

Recommended Preparations for Clinical Use

With the above considerations in mind, it is recommended that thyroxine be the primary agent of choice for replacement and suppressive therapy, with triiodothyronine being reserved for selected applications.

There is little merit in using synthetic T_4:T_3 mixtures. Eighty percent of T_3 produced daily is derived from extrathyroidal deiodination of T_4 (30); feeding a mixture is not necessary to maintain blood T_3 levels. Because of the disparity in turnover rates of T_4 and T_3, smooth metabolic response is difficult to achieve with such mixtures. The T_3 component produces an immediate metabolic response after ingestion that dissipates in several hours (31,32). Patients with angina may be unduly sensitive to such metabolic fluctuation. Peripheral levels of T_3 vary throughout the day after the ingestion of a T_4:T_3 mixture, whereas when thyroxine is given alone, peripheral blood levels of both T_4 and T_3 remain steady once equilibrium is attained (31–33).

The uneven results of using triiodothyronine in mixtures are exaggerated when it is used as the sole hormone for replacement therapy. Because of the wide swings in blood level after ingestion of single daily doses (33), the hormone must be administered on a twice or thrice daily basis to achieve any sort of a steady blood concentration. Should the patient omit therapy for 1 or 2 days, blood levels drop drastically or disappear, resulting in complete loss of metabolic effect. As a result, chronic replacement therapy with triiodothyronine is unsatisfactory and its therapeutic use should be limited to the specific circumstances discussed later.

There is no merit whatsoever in using thyroid hormone prepared from animal sources. Such preparations have no unique therapeutic advantage and do not contain anything, other than T_4 and T_3, that is necessary for thyroid hormone economy in the human. Although many patients express a preference for hormone derived from "natural" sources, they should be made to understand that the only active materials in these preparations are T_4 and T_3 and that therapy is better accomplished by consistent and uniform administration of pure hormone than by variable mixtures of the two, admixed with inactive hormone precursors, and all contained in a matrix of cellular debris.

It also behooves the clinician to limit his choice of an oral thyroxine preparation to one source, so that he can become familiar with its color-coding and verify the dose being used by asking the patient the color of the tablet. In making the selection of source, it must be borne in mind that some generic preparations have been found to contain significantly less than labeled quantities of thyroxine, although many generics are fully potent (34). If generic prescribing is done, one should make certain that the pharmacy uses the same source consistently. If brand-name prescribing is done, care should be taken that a generic substitution is not made and mislabeled as the brand-name product (35). It has been reported (36), and the author himself has encountered a few patients in whom an unexpected loss of metabolic and biochemical response to a seemingly regular daily dose of thyroxine was explained by the substitution of a generic preparation for the prescribed brand-name preparation.

Clinical Pharmacokinetics of Thyroid Hormone Therapy

Both T_4 and T_3 are readily absorbed from the bowel as the sodium salts, the free acids being not well absorbed (37). There is no absorption from the stomach. The proximal and mid jejunum appear to be the most active sites of absorption in the human; the colon is not an active absorption site unless it has been sterilized with antibiotics (38). Absorption of T_3 is rapid and nearly complete (39). Absorption of T_4 is more variable, being reported to be as low as 48% (40,41) and as high as 93% (42). Older studies may have been distorted by an incorrect estimate of the administered dose resulting from the overstated content of Synthroid prior to 1982 (41); recent studies indicate that on the average, absorption is 81% (42). There is no evidence that malabsorption of T_4 occurs *per se* without other explanation (43). Absorption is normal in renal failure and after renal transplantation (44). Unexplained "low" absorption usually implies noncompliance or use of a tablet with less potency than labeled. Thyroid hormone absorption is enhanced by fasting (45) and by hypothyroidism (46). There appears to be a modest reduction in absorption in subjects over the age of 70 (47). Absorption is reduced in malabsorption syndromes, such as sprue, celiac-sprue, and pancreatic diseases (48,49), in short-bowel syndromes following small-bowel resection (50), and in intestinal jejunal–ileal bypass operations for treatment of obesity (51). In patients taking T_4 for replacement or suppression therapy, such conditions may necessitate a substantially greater than usual oral daily dose and careful monitoring of blood levels at frequent intervals. Thyroxine and triiodothyronine are bound by cholestyramine resin (52) and other bile sequestrants (38). In the circumstance of a hypothyroid patient taking both thyroxine and cholestyramine resin, care must be taken that at least 4 to 5 hr, and preferably 12 hr, separates the ingestion of one and the other drug. Otherwise, even small amounts of the resin will adsorb the hormone and prevent sufficient amounts from being absorbed to maintain effective blood concentrations. In cases of T_4 overdosage, the deliberate use of this resin may be helpful to enhance clearance of the hormone (53). In like manner, soybean protein interferes with absorption of thyroxine. A case has been recorded wherein an athyreotic cretin fed a soybean formula as a milk substitute developed what appeared to be thyroid "refractoriness" because of impaired hormone absorption (54). Other foodstuffs, such as cottonseed meal and walnuts, may impair absorption of T_4 (38). Likewise, ferrous sulfate (55), activated charcoal (56), aluminum hydroxide (57), and Kayexalate (58) ingested simultaneously with T_4 may bind it and reduce its absorption; ingestion of any of these drugs and T_4 should be separated by several hours whenever possible. Although it has been proposed that sucralfate interferes with T_4 absorption (59), a recent double-blind, placebo-controlled study could not confirm this (60).

Thyroxine administered orally is absorbed rapidly, reaching maximum plasma levels in 2 to 4 hr (61). Its onset of action is within 1 day, its peak metabolic effects are seen in 9 days, and its duration of action is about 15 days (62). The T_4 turnover rate is only 10% per day (63), thus accounting for the clinical observation that hypothyroid individuals on full replacement therapy with thyroxine can omit several days of therapy without visible clinical consequences. By contrast, T_3 is turned over much more rapidly, at a rate of about 75% per day (63). This accounts for the difficulty in maintaining steady blood concentrations with once-daily oral administration and why clinical manifestations of hormone deficiency quickly become evident if a hypothyroid patient treated with this agent omits more than 2 days of therapy.

As a consequence of its slow turnover time, thyroxine need not be administered more than once daily and may even be given intermittently. It has been shown that a once-weekly dose of 1.0 to 1.1 mg/m^2 maintains normal blood levels of T_4 for most of the week, as do once-weekly standard doses of 1.5 to 2.5 mg (61,64,65). Such a schedule is not desirable for most patients, but in selected instances (e.g., children not supervised regularly, recalcitrant adults, psychiatric patients), it is possible to employ it successfully. On the other hand, a limited degree of intermittence may be used when it is necessary to adjust the dose of therapy. Suppose that a patient is found to have a high blood concentration of T_4 while taking 150 µg thyroxine daily, and a decrease in the daily dose to 125 µg is desired. The patient, however, having a large supply of 150-µg tablets, would like to avoid the expense of discarding them. Here, advantage can be taken of the slow turnover of T_4. By taking the 150-µg tablet for 6 days and omitting therapy 1 day each week, the weekly dose will be 900 µg instead of 1050 µg; the average daily dose will approximate 129 µg. If an even lower average daily dose is desired, medication can be omitted twice weekly; the weekly ingestion of 750 µg (five doses per week at 150 µg/dose) will average 107 µg/day and approximate the metabolic activity of a daily dose of 100 µg. Conversely, should it be desirable to increase the daily dose, an extra tablet can be taken 1 or 2 days each week. When the on-hand supply is consumed, a prescription for the precise daily dose can usually be written, because tablets of 12 separate potencies are available commercially (see Table 1). Table 2 presents a schedule of the approximate average daily dose that will result from taking tablets of different potencies in weekly amounts of 3½ [i.e., every other day (qod)] to 9 tablets.

Minor amounts of thyroxine are excreted in breast milk. The amount is insufficient to treat adequately an athyreotic cretin who is nursing, but it may be sufficient to mask the manifestations of the disease and delay its clinical recognition (66). Care should be taken always to assess the thyroid function of newborns, but this is especially true of newborns who will be breast-fed.

REPLACEMENT THERAPY

The many causes of primary and central hypothyroidism for which thyroxine replacement therapy is indicated are listed in Table 3. In most cases, replacement therapy will be required permanently. However, in some cases, such as postpartum hypothyroidism and posttherapeutic hypothyroidism, spontaneous recovery of thyroid function may ensue within a matter of months, so that replacement should be considered temporary until the occurrence of permanent hypothyroidism is confirmed. Similarly, hypothyroidism induced by drug therapy (e.g., lithium) needs to be treated only as long as the chemical blockade to thyroid hormone secretion is maintained. Thyroxine replacement therapy may also be used in subclinical hypothyroidism and in the "euthyroid sick" syndrome, although there is not universal agreement as to the merits of doing so (see later).

Average Daily Requirements for Replacement Therapy

Prior to initiating thyroxine therapy, it is helpful to bear in mind the daily requirement to be expected for the particular patient being treated. In a careful study of patients with hypothyroidism, Stock et al. (67), in 1974, reported that the average maintenance dose for adult hypothyroidism is 169 ± 66 µg/day or 2.25 ± 0.67 µg/kg per day. The study was redone after it was discovered that Synthroid tablets prior to 1982 were not as potent as labeled. Using the current Synthroid formulation, the daily maintenance dose for adults with hypothyroidism is found to be significantly lower, namely 112 ± 19 µg/day or 1.63 ± 0.42 µg/kg per day (42). A similar study from another laboratory determined the daily maintenance dose to be 127 ± 39 µg/day or 1.72 ± 0.36 µg/kg per day (68). Although maintenance doses have been quantified in these and other studies on a µg/kg per day basis, in clinical practice such dose by weight formulas have little practical utility. Maintenance doses may vary considerably among individuals of comparable size and may be comparable between individuals of greatly different size. What does emerge from these studies, however, is that the daily maintenance dose of thyroxine in adults is likely to be between 90 and 130 µg/day, close to the daily production rate of T_4 by the normal thyroid (69). This finding contrasts sharply with the 200 to 400 µg/day doses that were commonly employed after thyroxine was first available (70,71), and it is of particular importance in light of recent evidence that subclinical thyrotoxicosis is a risk factor for osteoporosis, cardiovascular abnormalities, and other undesired metabolic consequences (see later).

TABLE 2. *Average daily equivalent dose of thyroxine taken on different weekly schedules*

Tablet potency (µg)	Standard dose 1 tablet daily	Schedule					
		Decrease daily dose				Increase daily dose	
		1 tablet 6 day/wk	1 tablet 5 day/wk	1 tablet 4 day/wk	1 tablet qod	1 tablet 6 day/wk + 2 tablets 1 day/wk	1 tablet 5 day/wk + 2 tablets 2 day/wk
200	200	171	143	114	100	229	257
150	150	129	107	86	75	171	193
100	100	86	71	57	50	114	129
50	50	43	36	29	25	57	64

TABLE 3. *Thyroxine replacement therapy*

Primary hypothyroidism
    Idiopathic (juvenile, adult)
    Cretinism (athyreotic, goitrous)
    Posttherapeutic (resection, radioiodine)
    Chronic lymphocytic thyroiditis
    Postpartum thyroiditis
    Drugs (lithium, cobalt, iodides)
Central hypothyroidism
    Panhypopituitarism
    Isolated pituitary TSH deficiency
    Secretion of abnormal TSH
    Hypothalamic disease with TRH deficiency
Subclinical hypothyroidism
Nonthyroidal illness

TRH, thyrotropin releasing hormone; TSH, thyroid stimulating hormone.

Age modifies the requirement for thyroxine. In the elderly, more so in men than women, requirements are significantly reduced, often to less than 1 µg/kg per day (72) and the daily maintenance dose is usually between 50 and 100 µg/day (73,74). Because there is a narrow range in older persons between replacement and suppressive doses of T_4, close monitoring is advisable to avoid overtreatment (75). On the other hand, the requirement in children appears to be much higher relative to weight, up to 4 µg/kg per day (72). Recommended daily doses in children on a µg/kg basis decline gradually over time, but they are still higher than 2 µg/kg per day until the early teens, when adult requirements are reached (19).

Initiating Replacement Therapy

Keeping in mind the range of maintenance doses, therapy is initiated with about one-half the expected equilibrium dose, and it is titrated over time to the final dose. Little is gained by trying to achieve maintenance rapidly or in only one or two steps. Different organ systems may respond at different rates to the exhibition of thyroxine; it is not unusual to see bradycardia disappear earlier than constipation, puffy skin, and the abnormal deep-tendon reflex pattern. Because it takes time for the full response to a given dose of thyroxine to be evident clinically, it is advisable to allow 6 to 8 weeks to pass before initiating the next higher titration step. This will give the patient time to accommodate to each new metabolic level. It is common for serum T_4 levels to overshoot the normal range if thyroxine therapy is initiated with the full expected maintenance dose, and subsequently to recede to normal even though the dose is not changed (76). It is thought that this phenomenon is caused by the initial slow metabolic clearance of thyroxine (because of the hypothyroid state) and then an increase to a normal rate of clearance as eumetabolism is achieved. It may not be necessary, therefore, to adjust the dose until it is certain that a steady state exists, which may take 6 months. However, by titrating replacement therapy stepwise, with long intervals between steps, thyroxine clearance will be increased at a rate consonant with the metabolic response, and overshoot will be less likely to confound the replacement requirement. At each titration step, it is useful to determine the serum T_4 and thyroid stimulating hormone (TSH) levels to obtain a biochemical, as well as a clinical, assessment of the progress that has been made. In end-stage renal disease, reliance should be placed on the latter because T_4 levels tend to be low (44). Further, when such patients are treated with continuous ambulatory peritoneal dialysis (CAPD), T_4 losses in the peritoneal fluid may be considerable (44) and may require higher than usual replacement doses.

In otherwise healthy young and middle-aged adults with mild to moderate clinical evidence of hypothyroidism, it is appropriate to begin therapy with 100 µg T_4 daily and to add 25 µg to the daily dose every 6 to 8 weeks until the full clinical response and normalization of the blood chemistry has been achieved. In patients with profound or longstanding hypothyroidism, the initial dose is more appropriately 50 µg/day, and in the elderly hypothyroid patient, an initial dose as low as 25 µg/day is warranted (77). Regardless of age, should the patient have a compromised cardiac status or other serious disease that might be affected adversely by too intense a metabolic or adrenergic response to therapy, it is wise to initiate T_4 therapy with as little as 25 µg/daily. It is rare, however, for patients to be so fragile as to require less than this amount for the initial dose. Hypothyroid patients have a higher incidence of severe coronary atherosclerosis, and replacement therapy may so exacerbate angina or arrhythmias as to limit its use (75,78). Such patients require coronary artery revascularization surgery. It appears to be safe, and even prudent, to operate after only partial replacement therapy has been instituted, or even before replacement therapy has begun, and then to institute T_4 or titrate it up to the full maintenance level after coronary artery blood flow has been improved (78). Untreated hypothyroid patients appear to tolerate noncardiac surgery when necessary quite well (79).

Concomitant Adrenal Insufficiency

Care must be taken to distinguish primary from central hypothyroidism. Patients with central hypothyroidism are likely to have adrenal insufficiency as well as thyroid insufficiency. On clinical grounds, one cannot distinguish central from primary hypothyroidism. If the signs of adrenal insufficiency are occult, as they often are in hypopituitarism, it is possible to treat the patient inappropriately with T_4 alone, and thereby precipitate adrenal crisis. In hypopituitarism, the thyroid hormone deficiency results in slow clearance not only of T_4 and T_3, but of cortisol and other hormones as well. The patient is able to tolerate low cortisol secretion because of its slow clearance. When T_4 is exhibited, however, cortisol clearance increases sharply; because of the adrenocorticotropic hormone (ACTH) deficiency, cortisol secretion cannot be increased to meet the demands of the tissues, and adrenal crisis ensues. Fortunately, central hypothyroidism can be readily distinguished from primary hypothyroidism by measurement of the blood level of TSH: it is high in primary, but inappropriately low in central, hypothyroidism. If hypopituitarism is the cause of the hypothyroidism, the patient must be given cortisol replacement before T_4 treatment is instituted. On rare occasion, a patient presenting with primary hypothyroidism will also have primary adrenal insufficiency, the so-called Schmidt syndrome (88), and can develop an adrenal crisis if treated with T_4 alone. The possibility of the coexistence of these two primary endocrine insufficiencies should always be borne in mind when initiating treatment for primary hypothyroidism. If there is any reason clinically to suspect an adrenal abnormality, it is wise to add cortisol until adrenal function can be carefully assessed by appropriate testing. Consideration should also be given to treating any profound pre-coma primary hypothyroidism with cortisol during the initial phases of T_4 replacement. The adrenals tend to be atrophic in myxedema, and cortisol secretion is decreased. Because of slow cortisol turnover, serum levels remain normal, although free cortisol may be decreased (80). The acceleration of cortisol clearance upon treatment of the myxedema may not effect a pituitary ACTH secretory response promptly and sufficiently enough to maintain adequate cortisol secretion. The potential for a transient, but nonetheless threatening, deficiency of cortisol secretion thereby exists (81). This can be obviated by initiating T_4 therapy together with cortisol in all pre-coma myxedema patients until the metabolic adjustment to T_4 is sufficient to assure normal responsiveness of the pituitary–adrenal axis.

Myxedema Coma

Regardless of its etiology, untreated hypothyroidism may eventuate into myxedema coma. The condition is quite rare, and presents many difficult problems in management, including hypothermia, hypoventilation, hypercapnia, hypoxia, and hypotension, in addition to the thyroid hormone deficiency (82,83). Immediate steps should be taken to support the patient and restore adequate ventilation. Although there is no conclusive evidence for overt adrenal insufficiency in myxedema coma, most experienced clinicians advocate the use of steroids early in the treatment of this condition (81–83). Thyroid hormone replacement therapy should be undertaken by the intravenous administration of T_4. Intramuscular injection of thyroid hormone is less desirable, because T_3 (and presumably T_4) has been shown to be bound to muscle protein, thus delaying its absorption and inactivating a portion of the dose by deiodination at the injection site (84). Triiodothyronine for intravenous injection is commercially available, but T_4 is preferred because the outcome appears to be better in patients so treated, perhaps because of the ease with which toxic levels of T_3 are reached when it is administered intravenously (85). Thyroxine for intravenous administration is available in vials containing either 200 or 500 µg lyophilized hormone (see Table 1). It is reconstituted with 5 mL normal saline and should not be added to other intravenous fluids. It can be given as a bolus, for it is immediately bound to thyroxine-binding globulin (TBG) upon entering the bloodstream. Metabolic effects are seen within a matter of hours (82), the T_4 concentration is increased at 24 hr, and the T_3 concentration is increased at 72 hr (81). Intravenous therapy should be repeated daily until the patient has responded sufficiently to resume oral medication. The selection of dose is somewhat empiric. Myxedema coma is the result of longstanding hormone deficiency, so one must replenish the extrathyroidal pool, which normally is approximately 800 µg in size (63). A 50% reconstitution of the pool seems reasonable as an initial therapeutic goal; a first dose of 300 or 400 µg should suffice. There is no need to attempt to replenish T_4 stores more than partly in order to achieve significant metabolic effects. Should long-term maintenance by the intravenous route be necessary, it is appropriate to administer 100 µg daily, which approximates the average normal thyroid T_4 production rate (69).

Maintaining Replacement Therapy

In determining if the correct maintenance dose has been established in treatment of either primary or central hypothyroidism, careful clinical assessment and appropriate laboratory determinations should be made 6 months after the last titration step and at yearly intervals thereafter. Symptoms of hypothyroidism or thyrotoxicity should be absent. One of the subtle symptoms of toxicity is sleeplessness. Weight gain surprisingly may occur if appetite stimulation is greater than increased caloric utilization. A sense of warmth, a degree of irritability, and an increase in bowel frequency are easily overlooked symptoms that should be sought. Minimal lid retraction, a pulse rate above 90/min, and brisk reflexes are signs that point to mild toxicity, whereas persistent eyelid ptosis, hyperkeratosis of the elbows, and slight delay in the relaxation phase of the deep tendon reflexes indicate that replacement therapy is incomplete. If the patient is pregnant, is on estrogen therapy, or has other causes of altered binding of T_4 to its carrier proteins, the resin T_3 uptake or TBG level should also be measured, so that the apparent T_4 level can be corrected for the altered binding (free thyroxine index, FT_4I). Otherwise, the blood T_4 concentration suffices for assessment of circulating thyroid hormone. Rarely will direct measurement of free T_4 by equilibrium dialysis or other means be necessary. Likewise, it is not often necessary to measure T_3 levels in following a patient on replacement therapy. On occasion, discrepant results between T_4 and T_3 are found; in these instances, the T_4 level tends to be slightly elevated, whereas the T_3 level is within the normal range. This has been interpreted to indicate that a slight excess of T_4 is needed in these patients to maintain normal T_3 levels, the latter being the determinant of the metabolic status and pituitary TSH secretion (86). However, the adequacy of replacement therapy should not be judged by circulating T_4 alone.

Measurement of TSH by a sensitive, third-generation assay (87) is of prime importance. In primary hypothyroidism, T_4 replacement should be titrated to bring the TSH level back into the normal range, while at the same time avoiding its suppression. (In central hypothyroidism, reliance must be placed solely on T_4 or FT_4 blood levels, or the FT_4I, because endogenous TSH is markedly deficient, absent, or biologically inactive to begin with.) Formerly, TSH assays could not distinguish a physiologically low from a suppressed TSH level. With the introduction between 1982 and 1985 of newer, highly sensitive immunometric assays for TSH, it became possible to distinguish normal from both increased and suppressed TSH secretion (88). By titrating therapy to a normal TSH level, one confirms that excessive thyroid hormone is not circulating and that the patient is receiving a replacement and not a suppressive dose. It is important that this be done, because it has been shown that long-term subclinical thyrotoxicosis, wherein T_4 and T_3 are normal but TSH is suppressed, is a risk factor for development of osteoporosis (89,90). This occurs particularly in postmenopausal women (91). Even premenopausal women on physiologic replacement doses (111 ± 6 μg/day) have shown reduced bone mineral density (BMD) of the femoral neck and trochanter, but not the lumbar spine (92). However, there is little evidence that actual fracture rates are increased in women taking replacement therapy (93). If the dose of T_4 used for replacement is monitored carefully, especially using sensitive TSH assays, clinically significant bone disease is not likely to occur (94). In addition, abnormal systolic time intervals (95,96), increased average 24-hr heart rate, increased numbers of atrial premature beats, and increased left ventricular mass index (97) have been shown to occur regularly in subclinical thyrotoxicosis. Although the clinical significance of these findings is as yet unclear, one would like to avoid cardiac abnormalities (98), especially since overt thyrotoxicosis is known to aggravate existing heart disease and to lead to atrial fibrillation, congestive heart failure, and angina pectoris (99). Finally, a number of hepatic enzyme and protein abnormalities (100) have been described in subclinical thyrotoxicosis. Thus, when a patient on replacement therapy is found to have a suppressed TSH by a sensitive assay method, it is appropriate to reduce the replacement dose and reassess the patient clinically and biochemically after a new equilibrium has been established (101). If results again show a suppressed TSH level, it seems prudent to repeat it. Thyrotropin-releasing hormone (TRH) testing is unlikely to add additional information (102). On retesting, if the TSH remains suppressed, a trial of an even lower maintenance dose should be undertaken. [Of course, these considerations do not apply to deliberate suppressive therapy (see later).] On the other hand, in hypothyroid patients on constant replacement doses of T_4, TSH secretion has been shown to increase during the winter (103). This phenomenon should be taken into account if TSH is found to be higher than on the previous determination. It does not require change in the usual replacement dose.

Autoantibodies against thyroid hormones are found occasionally, but they seem not to alter replacement requirements (104). Rare examples of hypersensitivity to these hormones also have been reported (105,106). Some patients are sensitive to the dyes used to color-code T_4 tablets; in such an unusual event, 50-μg tablets that contain no dye can be used and the appropriate number of tablets taken together as a single daily dose.

Thyroxine–Drug Interactions

During maintenance therapy with T_4, it is important to reassess the replacement dose whenever concurrent unrelated therapy is introduced. Estrogen therapy will increase TBG and the total T_4 and T_3 concentrations, but it will not affect metabolic status or free hormone concentrations if there is residual thyroid to compensate. In an athyreotic individual, the maintenance dose may need to be adjusted upward to keep free hormone and TSH concentrations within normal limits. Conversely, androgen therapy in women with breast cancer will reduce TBG, and in those patients receiving a fixed replacement T_4 dose, free T_4 levels will rise and necessitate a reduction in dose (107). Introduction of amiodarone may cause elevation of TSH levels and hypothyroid symptoms in previously adequately maintained primary hypothyroid patients (108). Rifampin increases thyroid hormone clearance and thereby increases replacement requirements significantly (109). Phenytoin impairs T_4 binding to TBG and accelerates T_4 clearance, likewise increasing replacement requirements (110). Similar findings have been reported to occur with carbamazepine therapy (111) and lovastatin (112).

Because T_4 accelerates the metabolic disposal of many drugs, when a hypothyroid patient being treated for another disease is begun on T_4 therapy, it may be necessary to adjust the dosage of the other medications. This is particularly true of anticoagulants, insulin, and oral hypoglycemic agents. On the other hand, hypothyroid patients on appropriate maintenance therapy with T_4 are eumetabolic and anticoagulation or diabetic management is no different than in euthyroid patients. Should T_4 therapy inadvertently be stopped, insulin requirements will decrease. Sensitivity to catecholamines is not abnormal as long as the patient is eumetabolic. The patient need not avoid nasal decongestants; therefore, the conventional warning against use in thyroid conditions really is applicable only to thyrotoxic states.

Changes in Thyroxine Requirements

If, during long-term maintenance therapy, a hypothyroid patient inexplicably becomes hypometabolic, TSH levels rise, and T_4 levels drop, the physician should first look for a lapse in treatment, a change from a fully potent preparation to one with lesser potency, or the introduction of a second drug that has interfered with T_4's absorption, metabolism, or excretion. Otherwise, the phenomenon is the result of some change in the underlying thyroid status. A partial thyroid deficiency (e.g., Hashimoto's thyroiditis) or partial T_4 secretion block (e.g., lithium therapy) may have advanced to a complete deficiency state. This usually will not influence therapy, because full replacement is usually instituted at the outset. There are, however, many reports of hypothyroidism going into remission and no longer requiring therapy. This may occur in autoimmune thyroiditis wherein the hypothyroidism was caused by TSH-blocking antibodies (113), or iodine ingestion (114).

Postpartum thyroiditis, well known to cause transient thyrotoxicosis, also may cause transient hypothyroidism, particularly between 3 and 7 months after delivery (115,116). Should recovery occur, as it does in most (116), and not be recognized, the patient will be taking replacement therapy unnecessarily. Therefore, it is recommended that when patients are treated for postpartum hypothyroidism, they be assessed at 6-month intervals to determine if recovery of intrinsic thyroid function has occurred in the interim. The patient need not be withdrawn completely from therapy, for if the patient in fact does have permanent hypothyroidism, she will become symptomatic during the trial of observation. If the replacement dose is dropped by only 50%, sufficient T_4 will still be taken to prevent overt clinical symptoms, but not to prevent a fall in T_4 and a rise in TSH levels when these are determined weeks later. If thyroid function has not recovered, the prior replacement dose can be reinstituted. If thyroid function has indeed recovered, replacement therapy can be discontinued completely and euthyroidism confirmed 2 to 3 months later by the persistence of normal clinical and laboratory findings.

A similar plan can be followed if it is necessary to determine if a patient on thyroid hormone therapy for many years really has underlying hypothyroidism. Testing after only a partial reduction of dosage avoids overt clinical manifestations in the event that the original diagnosis was correct and the patient has authentic hypothyroidism. Alternatively, T_3 can be substituted for T_4 for 1 month. At the end of this period, serum T_4 will be less than 0.6 μg/dL if the patient is hypothyroid, and higher than 1.2 μg/dL if the patient is intrinsically euthyroid (117). In like manner, hypothyroidism following treatment of Graves' disease may be transient (118). This is particularly true in patients treated with radioiodine. It is not uncommon, after such therapy, for T_4 and T_3 levels to fall to normal values within a matter of weeks and reach hypothyroid values in 3 to 4 months. Unless the patient has clinical manifestations, however, it may be worthwhile to withhold replacement therapy for a period of continued observation. It is not unusual for recovery of full function and normalization of laboratory findings to occur within a few months of treatment (118). Nevertheless, permanent hypothyroidism sooner or later occurs (119,120), and permanent replacement therapy is required.

Replacement Therapy in Posttherapeutic Hypothyroidism

The common practice of administering full T_4 replacement doses "prophylactically" after treatment of Graves' disease is to be avoided because of the possibility of inducing overt thyrotoxicosis. After treatment, the underlying mechanism controlling T_4 secretion by the thyroid remnant may remain the thyrotropin receptor autoantibodies (TRAb), and not TSH, as shown by the persistence of abnormal T_3 suppression tests (121) and significantly elevated TRAb titers (122), and the lower requirement for T_4 replacement in post-Graves' hypothyroidism than in idiopathic hypothyroidism, implying autonomous secretion from the thyroid remnant under the influence of persisting TRAb (123). The interval between treatment and the onset of hypothyroidism may be short, a matter of months, or quite long, a matter of years (119,120). This is as true after subtotal thyroidectomy as after radioiodine therapy (120). During the eumetabolic interval, should the thyroid remain insuppressible, exogenous hormone will be additive to endogenous hormone secretion and T_4 concentrations will reach toxic levels. Thyroxine should therefore be withheld until the thyroid remnant is unable to meet metabolic demands and hypothyroidism appears. When hypothyroidism begins to appear, replacement should be given gradually. Beginning with perhaps one third of the anticipated final replacement dose, each titration step should be taken only when clinical and biochemical evidence indicates further loss of endogenous thyroid hormone secretion and the need to increase the replacement dose. This titration may be completed in months to years, depending on the rate at which loss of thyroid remnant function occurs.

In some patients, however, destruction of the thyroid remnant does not occur, and physiologic control of the thyroid by TSH returns. This is particularly likely to occur in patients whose remission was induced by antithyroid drugs (124). When it occurs, replacement therapy may be unnecessary, but if used, partial replacement doses will be supplemented by an appropriate amount of TSH-regulated endogenous secretion, whereas full replacement doses will suppress TSH and inhibit endogenous secretion. After treatment of Graves' disease, therefore, it is necessary to follow the patient at regular intervals for many years, with the expectation that replacement therapy will sooner or later have to be initiated and then adjusted until the permanent maintenance requirement is attained.

Replacement Therapy in Pregnancy

The requirement for T_4 in many hypothyroid women increases significantly during pregnancy for reasons that are uncertain. This is shown by an increase in serum TSH concentration and a fall in the serum free T_4 index. In one series, the daily average T_4 requirement increased from 102 µg before pregnancy to 148 µg during pregnancy, and it reverted to 117 µg in the postpartum period (125). Care must be taken, therefore, to assess the patient's clinical and laboratory status at least once in each trimester. Avoid concomitant administration of T_4 and prenatal iron preparations (55). Thyroid function tests should be interpreted in light of the altered TBG levels that pregnancy induces. TSH levels serve as the most precise guide to replacement therapy. Particular care should be taken to avoid thyrotoxicity because of its adverse effect on the mother. Because the placenta allows only small amounts of T_4 to cross (126), the pregnant hypothyroid woman can be reassured that any increase in her daily T_4 intake will not affect the fetus adversely.

Cretinism and Juvenile Myxedema

If intrauterine cretinism, of whatever etiology, is diagnosed, it is possible to treat the fetus by transuterine, intramuscular injection (127), or by weekly intra-amniotic injection of T_4 because the fetus ingests amniotic fluid continuously (128). This maneuver may not be necessary, however, because the prompt (within 14 days) institution of high dose T_4 therapy (10 to 15 µg/kg per day) for cretinism at birth, even when first discovered by a neonatal screening program, prevents significant psychomotor and other developmental problems (129–131).

The therapeutic goal for inborn errors of thyroid hormone synthesis with goitrous cretinism is to induce goiter regression, or at least prevent goiter progression, in addition to replacing the hormone deficiency. Thyroxine should be given, therefore, in doses sufficient to suppress TSH, rather than simply to return it to the normal range. After arrest of goiter growth, or its regression, the dose of T_4 should be reduced to the point where TSH is normalized but not suppressed, to avoid chronic subclinical thyrotoxicosis in what will be, of necessity, lifelong replacement therapy.

Cretinism and juvenile hypothyroidism respond well to T_4 replacement therapy, but growth may not be completely normalized and the final attained height may be significantly below that of normal siblings (132). It is essential that continuous therapy be given, with close parental supervision at least until development is completed. If it appears that therapy is not being taken in a regular fashion, consideration should be given to using intermittent therapy with larger, but less frequent, individual doses (see p. 478). Particular attention should be paid to growth velocity and skeletal maturation (133). The level of replacement therapy for congenital hypothyroidism should be monitored at regular intervals by measurement of TSH and FT_4 levels (every few weeks, then every 2 to 3 months, then every 6 months), keeping FT_4 in the upper half of the normal range for age, and TSH within normal (134). These tests should be reassessed particularly at any indication of slowing of the growth curve or interruption of other indices of development. Initiation of therapy in juvenile hypothyroidism has been reported to be associated with the occurrence of pseudotumor cerebri, which disappears spontaneously when treatment is continued (135). Juvenile hypothyroidism characteristically presents with growth of hair across the upper back, which sheds when adequate replacement therapy is given (136). In males, prepubertal thyroid failure is associated with precocious testicular enlargement without virilization, the so-called macro-orchidism of hypothyroidism. With T_4 therapy, the testes usually decrease in size, but they may remain macro-orchid (137).

Subclinical Hypothyroidism

Whereas the above section has addressed clear indications for thyroid hormone replacement therapy, there remain circumstances in which the indication for its use is less well defined, but in which the clinician may nonetheless wish to undertake its trial. Patients will be encountered who have limited thyroid reserve [subclinical, preclinical, or partial hypothyroidism (138)]. Most often, the underlying pathology will be that of chronic thyroiditis, but drugs or ingestion of goitrogenic substances in food will occasionally induce partial blockade of hormonogenesis. In such patients, circulating T_4 and T_3 concentrations will be normal, yet TSH will be high. A goiter may be present as a compensatory phenomenon. Although not all observers agree, many believe it is worthwhile to treat such patients even though normal T_4 and T_3 blood levels are maintained (139,140). An elevated TSH implies that hormonogenesis and hormone secretion are impaired and, unless a clearly transient cause is identified, such impairment may progress to complete thyroid failure and overt hypothyroidism. Institution of replacement therapy precludes hormone deficiency, prevents progression of goiter, and may even reverse extant goiter. Women with euthyroid autoimmune thyroid disease when not pregnant, are at increasing risk for developing subclinical or clinical hypothyroidism during a pregnancy or postpartum, and they benefit by treatment with T_4 (141). Patients with type I diabetes mellitus have a high incidence of postpartum subclinical hypothyroidism, which may go on to permanent hypothyroidism (142). In women who smoke, subclinical hypothyroidism is associated with diminished T_4 action, which is reversed by exogenous hormone administration, arguing for treatment of subclinical hypothyroidism in smokers (143). In the elderly, it is quite unclear whether subclinical hypothyroidism should be treated, because symptoms are usually minimal or absent, there may be no recognizable clinical benefit, and the risks of overtreatment are great (144). For younger adults, however, there seems to be no advantage in allowing a pathologic condition to progress to clinical significance, especially when the therapy employs a physiologic substance administered in a physiologic manner.

Replacement Therapy in Nonthyroidal Illness

In severe nonthyroidal illness, the so-called euthyroid sick, low circulating T_3 (and often T_4) levels lead to the consideration of an underlying hypothyroidism (63). Diminished extrathyroidal conversion of T_4 to T_3, decreased T_4 binding as a result of inhibitors or of decreased concentrations of carrier proteins, and increased T_4 clearance account for the low T_3 and T_4 levels; these usually are not compensated for by an increase in TSH secretion. Quite the contrary, TSH concentrations are often low or undetectable. The findings therefore resemble central hypothyroidism and may be a mechanism for adapting to severe illness (63). Empiric trials of T_4 therapy in such circumstances have usually proven to be without benefit (145). In coronary artery by-pass surgery, serum T_3 declines; intravenous T_3 has been safely administered during and after the surgery, but it seems to confer no special benefit (146,147); its use as a routine inotropic agent during surgery is not recommended (147). Nevertheless, in situations where the certain distinction between true hypothyroidism and the nonspecific effect of nonthyroidal illness cannot be made, the clinician may wish to try replacement T_4 therapy. When doing so, it is prudent to use a low dose of T_4, which should induce significant metabolic improvement if the patient is truly hypothyroid, but will add only a small metabolic increment if the patient is intrinsically euthyroid.

Finally, over the years, desiccated thyroid, T_4, T_3, and thyroid hormone analogs have been used empirically for a number of clinical conditions and nonspecific syndromes for which convincing evidence of thyroid hormone deficiency is lacking and in which the reputed therapeutic effects in controlled studies cannot be distinguished from the effects of placebo. The use of these hormones for treatment of obesity, menstrual disorders, infertility, the "metabolic insufficiency syndrome," and other nonthyroidal conditions is now largely abandoned. Recently, interest has arisen in the use of T_3 for the treatment of depression. There is little evidence to support the use of this drug as a sole treatment, but some suggest that it may augment the response to antidepressant drugs in refractory cases (148).

SUPPRESSIVE THERAPY WITH THYROID HORMONES

Physiologic Basis for Suppression

Pituitary thyrotropin (TSH) regulates thyroid hormone synthesis and secretion and maintains thyroid size. Excess TSH secretion induces thyroid enlargement (goiter) by causing hyperplasia and hypertrophy; other growth factors may play a role in the pathogenesis of goiter (149). When TSH secretion is inhibited (suppressed), the thyroid ceases to secrete T_4 and T_3 and, over time, will shrink in size. TSH secretion, in turn, is regulated by the concentration of free T_4 and T_3: circulating levels of these hormones above the physiologic set-point inhibit TSH secretion, and levels below this point do not restrain secretion. Manipulation of this negative feedback servomechanism is possible by administering T_4 or T_3, raising their concentrations above the set-point, and thereby inhibiting TSH secretion. In the pituitary thyrotroph cell, inhibition of TSH secretion depends on the binding of T_3 to its nuclear receptor, regardless of whether it is derived directly from the plasma or is produced within the cell by conversion of T_4 (86). In the management of thyroid disease, exogenous administration of thyroid hormone is used deliberately to suppress TSH secretion for diagnostic and therapeutic purposes (Table 4). There are few diagnostic applications of this maneuver; it is used mainly in the management of goiter, benign nodules, and thyroid carcinoma.

Diagnostic Thyroid Suppression to Demonstrate Thyroid Autonomy

Soon after introduction of the 24-hr radioiodine uptake as a diagnostic test of thyroid function, it was discovered that not all patients with elevated uptake had hyperthyroidism. In 1954, Greer and Smith (150) introduced a diagnostic thyroid suppression test to distinguish the high uptake of hyperthyroidism from other causes of high uptake. Desiccated thyroid, administered in daily doses of 180 to 540 mg for 4 weeks, fails to decrease radioiodine uptake significantly in true hyperthyroidism because the

TABLE 4. *Thyroid suppression*

Diagnostic (agent: T_3)
    Impaired hormonogenesis with high uptake
    Autonomy in isofunctional nodules and goiter
Therapeutic (agent: T_4)
    Goiter
        Nontoxic diffuse and multinodular
        Chronic lymphocytic thyroiditis
        Goitrous cretinism
        Drug-induced
    Lingual thyroid
    Solitary, nontoxic benign nodules
    Metastatic thyroid carcinoma
        Papillary
        Papillary-follicular
        Follicular (unless hyperfunctioning)
Prophylactic (agent: T_4)
    Postresection benign nodule
    Postresection goiter in generalized resistance to thyroid hormone syndrome
    Postresection/radioablation of thyroid carcinoma
    Thyroid protective in radioablation of isofunctional nodule
    Post–medically induced remission of Graves' disease (?)

thyroid is not under TSH control (i.e., it is autonomous), whereas in nonhyperthyroid causes of high uptake, the thyroid remains physiologically regulated by TSH and the second uptake is decreased to less than 20% in most patients. Werner and Spooner (151) modified the test in 1955 by using 75 μg T_3 daily as the suppressant instead of T_4. By so doing, the time necessary to secure adequate suppression was reduced from 4 weeks to 1. Subsequent studies have shown that a minimum daily dose of 100 μg T_3 is necessary for best discrimination (152). Yet another modification was made in 1970 with the demonstration that a single dose of 3 mg T_4 orally followed by a radioiodine uptake 7 days later gives comparable separation of hyperthyroidism from euthyroidism (153). However, such suppression testing for the differential diagnosis of hyperthyroidism is not indicated today. It is hazardous and unnecessary; demonstration of a suppressed level of TSH by a sensitive assay is equivalent and sufficient.

On the other hand, it is not uncommon to encounter a patient with a high 24-hr radioiodine uptake in the absence of any manifestation of hyperthyroidism, clinical or biochemical; often the evidence points to diminished thyroid function. The uptake study in these instances usually has been obtained to investigate a goiter, and when uptake is found to be elevated, one is led to consider occult hyperthyroidism. In the author's experience, rarely is this the explanation. Instead, these findings usually prove to be a result of an acquired impairment of thyroid hormone synthesis, as in chronic thyroiditis. An elevated TSH level often can be demonstrated, reflecting the compensatory attempt to overcome the deficit in hormonogenesis. That such is the case can be confirmed by a suppression test. Decrease of the uptake to very low values indicates that the thyroid remains under physiologic regulation. These patients, of course, have limited thyroid reserve and should be treated with T_4, in order that the goiter regress and that overt hypothyroidism be prevented.

One other use for diagnostic suppression is to determine whether function of a solitary nodule or multinodular goiter is autonomous. Autonomous function in follicular adenoma is readily recognized when the scan demonstrates uptake by the nodule and suppression (absence) of uptake in the remainder of the gland. However, some readily palpable nodules are not delineated on initial scanning, being isofunctional with the normal thyroid tissue. After suppression, autonomous isofunctional nodules show persistent uptake despite absence of uptake in the remainder of the gland. TSH-regulated isofunctional nodules, by contrast, are suppressed along with the remainder of the gland. Autonomous nodules do not respond to chronic suppressive therapy, whereas nonautonomous, TSH-regulated nodules may do so. Multinodular goiters may show one to several autonomous nodules upon suppression testing. If only a small number of such nodules are demonstrated, therapeutic suppression may yet be warranted; if a large number of autonomous nodules are seen, chronic suppression is likely to fail.

Suppressive Therapy for Nontoxic Goiter

Since the pathogenesis of many goiters includes intermittent or continuous stimulation of the thyroid by TSH (149), it is reasonable to attempt to reverse the process by chronic inhibition of TSH secretion. Thyroxine is the agent of choice for chronic treatment, for reasons cited before, and it is given orally daily in doses sufficient to suppress TSH levels completely. When the patient is eumetabolic to begin with, as is the case in most nontoxic goiters, titration to full suppressive doses need not be as slow or in as many steps as for hypothyroidism. Therapy can be initiated with the average replacement dose and adjusted depending on the clinical and biochemical findings after several months of therapy. Of course, if the patient shows concurrent reasons for more cautious titration (e.g., cardiovascular disease), a smaller dose should be chosen to initiate therapy. The dose should be titrated to the point where TSH is suppressed below the normal range as assessed by a sensitive, third-generation TSH assay. Full suppression takes up to 6 months and the dose required is, on the average, higher than for replacement (154). The suppressive dose should be maintained until the goiter has regressed completely, or no further response is seen. Maximum response often is not seen in less than 1 or 2 years of treatment. After 1 year of treatment, partial or complete regression is seen in about two thirds of nontoxic diffuse goiters (155), goitrous cretinism, and chronic thyroiditis (156,157). Goiters resulting from chronic thyroiditis, and multinodular goiters, although showing a good initial response, may take years to regress completely or may never do so (157). Lingual thyroid responds to suppression, which must be lifelong (158). Once maximal regression of goiter has occurred, the dose of T_4 should be lowered for chronic maintenance, keeping TSH levels within the normal range, neither oversuppressed (to avoid subclinical thyrotoxicosis) nor undersuppressed (to prevent recurrent goiter). Thereafter, the patient should be examined annually or biennially and blood tests obtained to assure that both T_4 and TSH levels are being maintained in the appropriate range. Nontoxic goiters tend to recur if suppressive therapy is discontinued. Many patients, particularly children and teenagers, are reluctant to accept the need for lifelong suppressive therapy. In these cases, it is acceptable to interrupt therapy once thyroid size has regressed to normal. Should the goiter recur, suppressive therapy can be reinstituted, this time with the likelihood that the patient will be reconciled to the need for permanent treatment. Reappearance of goiter should raise the question of adherence to the therapeutic regimen. Appearance of toxic symptoms, signs, or biochemistry should raise concerns about the evolution of autonomous thyroid function or T_4 abuse. In the majority of patients on chronic suppressive therapy for goiter, no alteration of the regimen is required once it is established appropriately.

Generalized resistance to thyroid hormone (GRTH) is a genetic syndrome characterized by high levels of circulatory T_4, FT_4, and T_3 (despite a euthyroid or hypothyroid metabolic status), high TSH levels, and goiter (159). The goiter is usually unresponsive to T_4, but it may respond to supraphysiologic doses of T_3 (160), although not invariably (161). Not all patients require therapy, but those who have mistakenly had goiter resection or ablative radioiodine therapy should be given enough T_4 to suppress TSH (as much as 1000 µg/day), which therapy will also help prevent goiter recurrence (159).

Patients with pituitary resistance to thyroid hormone (PRTH) require treatment to overcome the peripheral thyrotoxicosis that is induced by the poorly suppressed TSH. In these patients, T_4 therapy will only aggravate the thyrotoxicity. Instead, agents acting on the pituitary, such as bromocriptine (162), or thyroid hormone analogs that have preferential TSH suppressive activity, such as triac (3,5,3'-triiodothyroacetic acid) (163), have been used with some reported success. Recent evidence points to triac having some ability to improve thyroid hormone receptor function directly (164), and thus it may be useful in GRTH, as well.

Suppressive Therapy for Benign Thyroid Nodules

A second indication for therapeutic suppression of the thyroid is the management of nontoxic solitary thyroid nodules. Detailed consideration of the pathology, course, and surgical and radioablative treatment of solitary nodules is given in Chapters 16, 17, and 22. Before undertaking a trial of suppression for such a nodule, its cytopathologic diagnosis should be established by fine-needle-aspiration biopsy. Only benign nodules are considered for suppressive therapy. Then its functional status should be assessed by isotope scanning. Hyperfunctional ("hot") or isofunctional autonomous nodules do not respond to, and are not suitable for, suppressive therapy. Nonautonomous isofunctional nodules and hypofunctional ("cold") nodules are suitable for a trial of such therapy and may or may not be responsive to it.

The premise behind suppressive therapy for solitary benign nodules is that they may show a degree of TSH dependence, even though structure and function are abnormal and factors other than TSH may have been implicated in their pathogenesis. If this be the case, inhibition of TSH secretion and withdrawal of its trophic effects may be sufficient to induce significant regression of nodule size or at least prevent its further growth (165). There is much disagreement over whether such suppression is effective. Some studies show no significant response to T_4 compared to placebo (166), although in other series, the suppression rate has varied between 9% and 69% (167). Published guidelines recommend individualized clinical judgment in this decision (168). If a trial of suppression is undertaken, it is worthwhile to use a fully suppressive dose from the onset, so that a lack of response will not be the result of an ineffective dose. Such trials should use 150 to 200 µg of T_4 daily for a period of 3 to 6 months. The dose need be reduced only if not tolerated; by limiting the time of complete suppression, there is only small potential for significant complications from subclinical toxicity. When suppression is successful and the nodule regresses in size by at least 50%, the serum thyroglobulin level falls (169). Once this occurs, the daily dose of T_4 should be titrated downward, with the goal of keeping indefinitely the TSH level at the low end of the normal range, or slightly lower, but not below 0.1 µU/ml (170). Especially in postmenopausal women, one should avoid keeping TSH suppressed to very low levels and thereby risking bone disease for an otherwise benign disorder (171). If the initial trial of suppression fails, T_4 should be stopped and the patient followed without suppressive therapy. If the nodule subsequently enlarges, it should be rebiopsied or resected (171).

After a benign thyroid nodule has been resected, it may be worthwhile to undertake continuous thyroid suppression in an attempt to prevent recurrence of nodular disease (prophylactic suppression). Although several clinical studies have questioned the efficacy of such therapy (171), a study of 511 patients followed for up to 40 years has demonstrated a sharp reduction in recurrence rate in patients treated with continuous suppressive therapy after resection of the initial benign nodule (172).

Finally, suppressive therapy can be used temporarily in the management of those autonomous, isofunctional nodules for which radioiodine therapy is elected for definitive treatment. Thyroxine or triiodothyronine can be given in advance in order to suppress function of the normal tissue and prevent it from accumulating radioiodine. There is no need for such a maneuver in treatment of an autonomous, hyperfunctioning nodule, because function of the uninvolved thyroid tissue is already suppressed.

Suppressive Therapy to Prevent Recurrence of Graves' Disease

In 1991 it was reported that the concurrent administration of T_4 during antithyroid drug therapy of Graves' disease markedly decreases the frequency of recurrence once a remission has been induced (173). The same group next reported that treatment of Graves' disease in pregnancy with T_4, after antithyroid drugs were stopped in the 5th or 6th month, and continuing it for 1 year after delivery sharply decreases the frequency of recurrence of hyperthyroidism in the postpartum period (174). The premises behind such regimens are that hyperthyroidism in Graves' disease is the result of stimulation of the follicular cells by TRAbs; that release of thyroid antigens that perpetuate the production of TRAb is stimulated by TSH secreted during antithyroid therapy; and that administration of T_4 suppresses TSH release and decreases the production of autoantibodies. TRAb levels in both these studies were shown to decline significantly in the T_4-treated study groups.

However, two subsequent studies using slightly different protocols have been unable to confirm these findings (175,176). Additional studies will be necessary to determine the usefulness of suppressive therapy in the prevention of recurrent Graves' disease.

Suppressive Therapy for Thyroid Carcinoma

The most important application of chronic suppressive therapy is in the management of thyroid carcinoma. After Crile (15,16) pointed out that metastases of papillary carcinoma of the thyroid regress with suppressive therapy, this form of adjunctive therapy gained widespread acceptance and now is employed regularly, not only for treatment of evident metastases of papillary and follicular carcinomas, but also for the prevention of tumor recurrence and the emergence of occult metastases (177). The rationale behind such therapy is that thyroid carcinoma retains TSH receptors (178,179), that its metastases are TSH dependent (180), and that TSH inhibition creates an unfavorable environment for their survival and growth. Not all metastatic thyroid carcinoma is suitable for suppressive therapy (177). Metastases of thyroid follicular carcinoma may be functional and autonomous and may produce thyrotoxicosis if the tumor burden is large enough (181). Such metastases may secrete T_3 preferentially (182). Attempts to suppress functioning metastases by exogenous T_4 will be futile if TSH is already suppressed; in such cases, it will be hazardous as well, because circulating thyroid hormone concentrations will be increased to toxic levels. Anaplastic thyroid carcinoma, medullary carcinoma of the thyroid, and thyroid lymphoma are not TSH dependent. Although not likely to be successful, a trial of suppressive therapy can be undertaken safely in these types of nonfunctioning thyroid malignancy without risk of toxicity, and occasionally the therapy appears to be beneficial (183).

The most frequent reason for the use of suppressive therapy in thyroid carcinoma is to impede progress of the disease. The routine postoperative use of suppressive therapy is recommended by most observers of thyroid carcinoma because of compelling clinical evidence of a favorable influence on longevity, and on prevention or inhibition of recurrent disease *in situ* and the appearance of metastases (184–188).

Prior to the introduction of sensitive TSH assays, complete suppression of TSH could be recognized by its failure to increase in response to the intravenous injection of TRH (189). From experience with TRH testing, it was clear that some patients require a dose of T_4 considerably above usual replacement doses to achieve complete suppression of TSH secretion (154). In a study utilizing a sensitive TSH assay, it was also found that higher doses of T_4 are needed in thyroid cancer to bring TSH levels back to normal, or to suppress TSH, than are needed in primary hypothyroidism (123). TSH secretion has a circadian rhythm, evening and early morning values being higher than day values (190). If suppression is incomplete and TSH is detectable in the morning, a physiologic nocturnal TSH "surge" continues, whereas if TSH is undetectable in the morning, the nocturnal surge is not seen and TRH fails to stimulate any TSH secretion (190). Sensitive TSH assays have led to reconsideration of what constitutes adequate suppression for management of differentiated thyroid carcinoma. If complete inhibition of TSH secretion is the goal, some degree of thyrotoxicosis may be the price to pay to achieve it, since fourth-generation TSH assays have detected measurable TSH even in some thyrotoxic patients (191). However, such very low levels of TSH may result from constitutive release and may not be stimulative to thyroid tissue (192). Following primary ablation of thyroid carcinoma, the goals of T_4 therapy are two: to prevent the metabolic consequences of hypothyroidism (replacement) and to create an environment adverse to the growth of residual and metastatic carcinoma cells (suppression). How completely one should attempt to suppress TSH will depend on many factors, including the patient's age and sex, the type and extent of the primary carcinoma, the presence or absence of known metastases, the level of thyroglobulin on and off suppression, and the potential impact of subclinical or overt therapeutic thyrotoxicosis.

When TSH is appropriately suppressed to the desired degree as measured by a sensitive TSH assay, the patient should be evaluated for any symptoms or signs of thyrotoxicosis, and levels of T_4 and T_3 should be obtained. If the latter exceed limits of normal, it is advisable to confirm that free hormone concentrations are indeed elevated, using direct measurement (e.g., equilibrium dialysis), lest a reduction in the suppressive dose be undertaken needlessly. When there is no metastatic disease recognized by radiographic and tracer studies, suppression therapy to the point of overt toxicity is considered not warranted. On the other hand, subclinical thyrotoxicosis or even mild toxicity may be the price paid in overt metastatic thyroid carcinoma, because of the seriousness of the disease and the importance of such adjuvant therapy. Here, it may be advisable to continue therapy and control cardiac manifestations with beta-adrenergic blockade. Such therapy has been shown to improve cardiac symptoms, function, and the quality of life (193,194).

Suppressive doses of T_4 for thyroid carcinoma put both pre- and postmenopausal women at risk for osteoporosis (195). Estrogen therapy in conjunction with suppression may overcome bone loss in postmenopausal women (196); bisphosphonates may be useful in younger women to prevent osteopenia from the onset (197). Some have questioned whether the degree of osteopenia found on measurement in women on suppressive T_4 therapy (for 3 to 27 years) has clinical relevance (198).

Diagnostic Imaging in the Course of Chronic Suppression

During chronic suppressive therapy for thyroid carcinoma, periodic scanning of the entire body should be accomplished in a search for metastases. Since these are largely TSH-dependent, and TSH must be present for uptake to occur, the goal of management during the test is to interrupt suppression and have TSH in the system for the shortest period of time possible, to encourage the least possible stimulation of growth of any metastases that are present. Some years ago, uptake of tracer in the face of endogenous TSH suppression was achieved by using one to three injections of bovine TSH (bTSH) prior to administration of the tracer. However, it was shown that bTSH injection does not effect a maximal stimulus of radioiodine uptake (199) and may provoke allergic reactions in a high percentage of people (200). Further, bTSH soon becomes ineffective as antibody to it is developed, so that repeated testing is limited to a small number of examinations (201). TRH, administered orally, is effective in augmenting radioiodine uptake, which is not augmented further by injection of bTSH (202). However, TRH must be given in large doses orally and it is expensive. Recently, injection of recombinant human TSH has been shown to be a safe and effective way to stimulate radioiodine uptake and thyroglobulin secretion by metastases in patients on long-term T_4 treatment, without having to interrupt therapy and have the patient become hypothyroid with high endogenous TSH secretion for a protracted period of time (203). Until this new agent becomes available commercially, most centers will continue to interrupt exogenous suppressive therapy for a period of time to allow endogenous TSH secretion to resume and stimulate tracer uptake.

After its protracted administration, withdrawal of exogenous desiccated thyroid is followed by return of thyroid function in a matter of 1 to 3 months (204). Although a protracted period of inhibition of TRH secretion may occur in some persons (205), pituitary TSH secretion usually resumes within 2 to 3 weeks, but it may take up to 6 weeks to do so when suppression has been accomplished with desiccated thyroid or T_4 (206). On the other hand, recovery of TSH secretion takes no more than 10 days after withdrawal of T_3 as the suppressant (206). Scans obtained 2 weeks after withdrawal of T_3 are as good as those obtained 4 weeks after its withdrawal (207), so there is no advantage in withholding suppression for longer than 2 weeks. Therefore, the following plan is used by many centers to accomplish diagnostic body scans, while at the same time limiting the length of time suppressive therapy is interrupted. Thyroxine is stopped 6 weeks prior to the scan. In its place, a 25-μg dose of T_3 is given two or three times daily until 2 weeks prior to testing. This allows T_4 to decay and be eliminated while at least partial TSH suppression is maintained, as is the eumetabolic state. When T_3 is discontinued abruptly, TSH secretion recovers in no more than 10 days and is at a level satisfactory for effective tracer studies by the time of the test. The patient is usually asymptomatic the first week off medication but is noticeably hypothyroid by the time of the scan. If the scan demonstrates metastases, a treatment dose of radioiodine is given and suppressive therapy reinstituted 72 hr later. If the scan is negative, suppressive therapy with T_4 is reinstituted immediately using the previously established daily dose. Supplemental T_3 can be given initially until T_4 has equilibrated and exerts its full metabolic activity.

Other than for scanning purposes and for the administration of radioiodine therapy, there is no indication to interrupt T_4 suppressive therapy in the management of thyroid carcinoma. Measurement of thyroglobulin (Tg) concentration, which serves as an effective tumor marker, can be done at intervals during suppression and whenever suppression is interrupted for tracer study purposes. In this way, the function of metastatic tumor can be assessed on and off suppression. During suppression, low and steady levels of Tg give some assurance that metastases are in check. If Tg levels rise and exceed 10 μg/mL during suppression, search for metastases can begin (208). Measurement of the Tg level, combined with the scan while the patient is off suppression, appears to be a most reliable means of detecting metastases of thyroid carcinoma (209,210). Thus, when chronic suppressive therapy is employed and is interrupted only at intervals for tracer studies, Tg measurement and the administration of radioiodine, if indicated, the most common types of thyroid carcinoma ordinarily can be so well contained that the prognosis for a useful, comfortable, and protracted survival is excellent (184–188). (See also Chapters 30 and 31.)

SUMMARY

Thyroid hormone has been used to replace thyroid gland secretory deficiency for over a century. Extracts of animal thyroid glands, although usually effective, contain variable amounts of the active hormones T_4 and T_3, and are not optimal for therapy. Synthetic levothyroxine in appropriate dosage maintains normal extrathyroidal concentrations of both T_4 and T_3, so that T_3 need not be administered separately or in combination with T_4 for adequate replacement therapy. The average daily dose of T_4 needed to correct thyroid deficiency is lower than was estimated when the synthetic hormone was first introduced into clinical practice. It is now recognized to approximate the T_4 secretion rate of the normal gland. Measurement of blood TSH concentration by a sensitive immunometric assay method, in conjunction with measurement of blood thyroid hormone concentrations, permits T_4 replacement therapy to be adjusted precisely, so that the individual is neither under- nor overreplaced.

Thyroid hormones are also used clinically for the deliberate inhibition of TSH secretion, thereby suppressing intrinsic thyroid function and growth. Because of the rapidity of its action, T_3 is used when suppression is induced for diagnostic purposes. For therapeutic purposes, thyroid suppression is accomplished by the chronic administration of T_4. Long-term therapeutic thyroid suppression is used in the management of goiter and both benign and malignant neoplasms of the thyroid. Such therapy also is monitored by measurement of TSH and thyroid hormone concentrations and should be individualized to achieve an effective degree of thyroid suppression without attendant thyrotoxicosis, insofar as is possible.

ACKNOWLEDGMENTS

I am indebted to Ms. Susan Fuger of the National Center for Advanced Medical Education, Chicago, Illinois, for her invaluable assistance in the preparation of this manuscript.

REFERENCES

1. Gull WW. On a cretinoid state supervening in adult life in women. *Trans Clin Soc Lond* 1874;7:180.
2. Ord WM. On myxoedema, a term proposed to be applied to an essential condition in the "cretinoid" affection occasionally observed in middle-aged women. *Medico-Chir Trans* 1878;61:57–78.
3. Report of a committee of the Clinical Society of London, nominated December 14, 1883 to investigate the subject of myxoedema. *Trans Clin Soc Lond* 1888;21(suppl).
4. Murray GR. Note on the treatment of myxoedema by hypodermic injections of an extract of the thyroid gland of a sheep. *Br Med J* 1891;2:796–797.
5. Beadles CF. The treatment of myxedema and cretinism, being a review of the treatment of the diseases with the thyroid gland, with a table of 100 published cases. *J Ment Sci* 1893;39:343–355,509–536.
6. Mackenzie HWG. A case of myxedema treated with great benefit by feeding with fresh thyroid glands. *Br Med J* 1892;2:940–941.
7. Fox EL. A case of myxedema treated by taking extract of thyroid by the mouth. *Br Med J* 1892;2:941.
8. Aikawa JK. *Myxedema*. Springfield, Illinois: Charles C. Thomas, 1961.
9. Kendall EC. The isolation in crystalline form of the compound containing iodin, which occurs in the thyroid. Its chemical nature and physiologic activity. *JAMA* 1915;64:2402–2403.
10. Harrington CR, Barger G. Chemistry of thyroxine. III. Constitution and synthesis of thyroxine. *Biochem J* 1927;21:169–183.
11. Hart FD, Maclagen NF. Oral thyroxine in treatment of myxoedema. *Br Med J* 1950;1:512–518.
12. Starr P, Liebhold-Schueck R. Treatment of hypothyroidism with sodium levo-thyroxine given orally. *JAMA* 1954;155:732–736.
13. Gross J, Pitt-Rivers R. The identification of 3:5:3'-L-triiodothyronine in human plasma. *Lancet* 1952;1:439–441.
14. Gross J, Pitt-Rivers R. 3:5:3'-Triiodothyronine. I. Isolation from thyroid gland and synthesis. *Biochem J* 1953;53:645–650.
15. Crile G Jr. Treatment of cancer of thyroid with desiccated thyroid. *Cleve Clin Q* 1955;22:161–163.
16. Crile G Jr. Endocrine dependency of papillary carcinomas of the thyroid. *JAMA* 1966;195:721–724.
17. Thomas CG Jr. Hormonal treatment of thyroid cancer. *J Clin Endocrinol Metab* 1957;17:232–237.
18. Starr P. Pulmonary metastases of papillary cancer of the thyroid gland. Regression after nine years' observation. *JAMA* 1962;180:978.
19. *Physicians' desk reference*, 50th ed. Montvale, New Jersey: Medical Economics Company, 1996.
20. Selenkow HA, Wool MS. A new synthetic thyroid hormone combination for clinical therapy. *Ann Intern Med* 1967;67:90–99.
21. Braverman LE, Ingbar SH. Anomalous effects of certain desiccated thyroid on serum protein bound iodine. *N Engl J Med* 1964;270:439–442.
22. Pileggi VJ, Golub OJ, Lee ND. Determination of thyroxine and triiodothyronine in commercial preparations of desiccated thyroid and thyroid extract. *J Clin Endocrinol Metab* 1965;25:949–956.
23. Rees-Jones RW, Larsen PR. Triiodothyronine and thyroxine content of desiccated thyroid tablets. *Metabolism* 1977;26:1213–1218.
24. Brennan MD. Thyroid hormones. *Mayo Clin Proc* 1980;55:33–44.
25. Stasilli NR, Kroc RL. Biologic activity of pork and beef thyroid preparations. *J Clin Endocrinol Metab* 1956;16:1595–1606.
26. Mangieri CN, Lund MH. Potency of United States Pharmacopeia desiccated thyroid tablets as determined by the antigoitrogenic assay in rats. *J Clin Endocrinol Metab* 1970;30:102–104.
27. Kologlu S, Schwartz HL, Carter AC. Quantitative determination of the thyroxine, triiodothyronine, monoiodotyrosine and diiodotyrosine content of desiccated thyroid. *Endocrinology* 1966;78:231–239.
28. Rees-Jones RW, Rolla AR, Larsen PR. Hormonal content of thyroid replacement preparations. *JAMA* 1980;243:549–550.
29. Catz B, Ginsberg E, Salenger S. Clinically inactive thyroid USP: a preliminary report. *N Engl J Med* 1962;266:136–137.
30. Engler D, Burger AG. The deiodination of the iodothyronines and of their derivatives in man. *Endocr Rev* 1984;5:151–184.
31. Saberi M, Utiger RD. Serum thyroid hormone and thyrotropin concentrations during thyroxine and triiodothyronine therapy. *J Clin Endocrinol Metab* 1974;39:923–927.
32. Surks MI, Shadlow AR, Oppenheimer JH. A new radioimmunoassay for plasma L-triiodothyronine: measurements in thyroid disease and in patients maintained on hormonal replacement. *J Clin Invest* 1972;51:3104–3113.
33. Surks MI. Treatment of adult hypothyroidism. *Thyroid Clin* 1981;1:1–6.
34. Stoffer SS, Szpunar WE. Potency of brand name and generic levothyroxine products. *JAMA* 1980;244:1704–1705.

35. Stoffer SS, Szpunar WE. Letter to the editor. *JAMA* 1988;259:1945.
36. Dong BJ, Harmon-Brown C. Hypothyroidism resulting from generic levothyroxine failure. *J Am Board Fam Pract* 1991;4:167–170.
37. Sawin CT. Edward C Kendall (1886-1972) and thyroxine. *Endocrinologist* 1991;1:291–293.
38. Choe W, Hays MT. Absorption of oral thyroxine. *Endocrinologist* 1995;5:222–228.
39. Hays MT. Absorption of triiodothyronine in man. *J Clin Endocrinol Metab* 1970;30:675–677.
40. Hays MT. Absorption of oral thyroxine in man. *J Clin Endocrinol Metab* 1968;28:749–756.
41. Surks MI, Schadlow AR, Stock JM, Oppenheimer JH. Determination of iodothyronine absorption and conversion of L-thyroxine (T_4) to L-triiodothyronine (T_3) using turnover rate techniques. *J Clin Invest* 1973;52:805–811.
42. Fish LH, Schwartz HL, Cavanaugh J, Steffes MW, Bantle JP, Oppenheimer JH. Replacement dose, metabolism, and bioavailability of levothyroxine in the treatment of hypothyroidism. Role of triiodothyronine in pituitary feedback in humans. *N Engl J Med* 1987;316:764–770.
43. Ain KB, Refetoff S, Fein HG, Weintraub BD. Pseudomalabsorption of levothyroxine. *JAMA* 1991;266:2118–2120.
44. Kaptein EM. Thyroid hormone metabolism and thyroid diseases in chronic renal failure. *Endocr Rev* 1996;17:45–63.
45. Wenzel KW, Kirschsieper HE. Aspects of the absorption of oral L-thyroxine in normal man. *Metabolism* 1977;26:1–8.
46. Read DG, Hays MT, Hershman JM. Absorption of oral thyroxine in hypothyroid and normal man. *J Clin Endocrinol Metab* 1970;30:798–799.
47. Hays, MT, Nielsen KRK. Human thyroxine absorption: age effects and methodological analyses. *Thyroid* 1994;4:55–64.
48. Hiss JM Jr, Dowling JT. Thyroxine metabolism in untreated and treated pancreatic steatorrhea. *J Clin Invest* 1962;41:988–995.
49. Grinspoon SK, Daniels GH. Case report: increased levothyroxine requirement in a patient with cryptic celiac-sprue disease. *Endocr Pract* 1995;1:88–90.
50. Stone E, Leiter A, Lambert JR, Silverberg JDH, Jeejeebhoy KN, Burrow GN. L-thyroxine absorption in patients with short bowel. *J Clin Endocrinol Metab* 1984;59:139–141.
51. Azizi F, Belur R, Albano J. Malabsorption of thyroid hormones after jejunoileal bypass for obesity. *Ann Intern Med* 1979;90:941–942.
52. Northcutt RC, Stiel JN, Hollifield JW, Stant EG Jr. The influence of cholestyramine on thyroxine absorption. *JAMA* 1969;208:1857–1861.
53. Shakir KMM, Michaels RD, Hays JH, Potter BB. The use of bile acid sequestrants to lower serum thyroid hormones in iatrogenic hyperthyroidism. *Ann Intern Med* 1993;118:112–113.
54. Pinchera A, MacGillivray MH, Crawford JD, Freeman AG. Thyroid refractoriness in an athyreotic cretin fed soybean formula. *N Engl J Med* 1965;273:83–87.
55. Campbell NRC, Hasinoff BB, Stalts H, Rao B, Wong NCW. Ferrous sulfate reduces thyroxine efficacy in patients with hypothyroidism. *Ann Intern Med* 1992;117:1010–1013.
56. Bergman F, Halvorsen P, Van der Linden W. Increased excretion of thyroxine by feeding activated charcoal to Syrian hamsters. *Acta Endocrinol* 1967;56:521–524.
57. Sperber AD, Liel Y. Evidence for interference with the intestinal absorption of levothyroxine sodium by aluminum hydroxide. *Arch Intern Med* 1992;152:183–184.
58. McLean M, Kirkwood I, Epstein M, Jones B, Hall C. Cation-exchange resin and inhibition of intestinal absorption of thyroxine. *Lancet* 1993;341:1286.
59. Havrankova J, Lahaie R. Levothyroxine binding by sucralfate. *Ann Intern Med* 1992;117:445–446.
60. Campbell JA, Schmidt BA, Bantle JP. Sucralfate and the absorption of L-thyroxine. *Ann Intern Med* 1994;121:152.
61. Sekadde CB, Slaunwhite WR Jr, Aceto T Jr, Murray K. Administration of thyroxin once a week. *J Clin Endocrinol Metab* 1974;39:759–764.
62. Blackburn CM, McConahey WM, Keating FR Jr, Albert A. Caloriginic effects of single intravenous doses of L-triiodothyronine and L-thyroxine in myxedematous persons. *J Clin Invest* 1954;33:819–824.
63. Utiger RD. The thyroid: physiology, hyperthyroidism, hypothyroidism, and the painful thyroid. In: Felig P, Baxter JD, Broadus AE, Frohman LA, eds. *Endocrinology and metabolism,* 2nd ed. New York: McGraw-Hill, 1987;389–472.
64. Bernstein RS, Robbins J. Intermittent therapy with L-thyroxine. *N Engl J Med* 1969;281:1444–1448.
65. Thein-Wai W, Larsen PR. Effects of weekly thyroxine administration on serum thyroxine, 3,5,3'-triiodothyronine, thyrotropin, and the thyrotropin response to thyrotropin-releasing hormone. *J Clin Endocrinol Metab* 1980;50:560–564.
66. Sack J, Amado O, Lunenfeld B. Thyroxine concentration in human milk. *J Clin Endocrinol Metab* 1977;45:171–173.
67. Stock JM, Surks MI, Oppenheimer JH. Replacement dosage of L-thyroxine in hypothyroidism. A reevaluation. *N Engl J Med* 1974;290:529–533.
68. Hennessey JV, Evaul JE, Tseng Y-C, Burman KD, Wartofsky L. L-thyroxine dosage: a reevaluation of therapy with contemporary preparations. *Ann Intern Med* 1986;105:11–15.
69. Ladenson PW, Goldenheim PD, Cooper DS, Miller MA, Ridgway EC. Early peripheral responses to intravenous L-thyroxine in primary hypothyroidism. *Am J Med* 1982;73:467–474.
70. Robertson JD, Kirkpatrick HFW. Changes in basal metabolism, serum protein-bound iodine, and cholesterol during treatment of hypothyroidism with oral thyroid and L-thyroxine sodium. *Br Med J* 1952;1:624–628.
71. Salter WT, Rosenblum I. Oral sodium L-thyroxine in the treatment of myxedema and cretinism. *Am J Med Sci* 1952;224:628–631.
72. Singer PA, Cooper DS, Levy EG, Ladenson PW, Braverman LE, Daniels G, Greenspan FS, McDougall IR, Nikolai TF. Treatment guidelines for patients with hyperthyroidism and hypothyroidism. *JAMA* 1995;273:808–812.
73. Sawin CT, Herman T, Molitch ME, London MH, Kramer SM. Aging and the thyroid. Decreased requirement for thyroid hormone in older hypothyroid patients. *Am J Med* 1983;75:206–209.
74. Davis FB, LaMantia RS, Spaulding SW, Wehmann RE, Davis PJ. Estimation of a physiological replacement dose of levothyroxine in elderly patients with hypothyroidism. *Arch Intern Med* 1984;144:1752–1754.
75. Mariotti S, Franceschi C, Cossarizza A, Pinchera A. The aging thyroid. *Endocr Rev* 1995;16:686–715.
76. Brown ME, Refetoff S. Transient elevation of serum thyroid hormone concentration after initiation of replacement therapy in myxedema. *Ann Intern Med* 1980;92:491–495.
77. Spaulding SW. Age and the thyroid. *Endocrinol Metab Clin North Am* 1987;16:1013–1025.
78. Becker C. Hypothyroidism and atherosclerotic heart disease: pathogenesis, medical management, and the role of coronary artery bypass surgery. *Endocr Rev* 1985;6:432–440.
79. Sherman SI, Ladenson PW. Complications of surgery in hypothyroid patients. *Am J Med* 1991;90:367–370.
80. DeGroot LJ, Stanbury JB, eds. *The thyroid and its diseases,* 4th ed. New York: John Wiley & Sons, 1975;405–471.
81. Ridgway EC, McCammon JA, Benotti J, Maloof F. Acute metabolic responses in myxedema to large doses of intravenous L-thyroxine. *Ann Intern Med* 1972;77:549–555.
82. Holvey DN, Goodner CJ, Nicoloff JT, Dowling JT. Treatment of myxedema coma with intravenous thyroxine. *Arch Intern Med* 1964;113:89–96.
83. Jordan RM. Myxedema coma: the prognosis is improving. *Endocrinologist* 1993;3:149–153.
84. DeGroot LJ, Pretell E, Garcia ME. Absorption of intramuscularly administered tri-iodothyronine. *N Engl J Med* 1966;274:133–135.
85. Hylander B, Rosenqvist U. Treatment of myxoedema coma: factors associated with fatal outcome. *Acta Endocrinol (Copenh)* 1985;108:65–71.
86. Larsen PR. Thyroid-pituitary interaction. Feedback regulation of thyrotropin secretion by thyroid hormones. *N Engl J Med* 1982;306:23–32.
87. Nicoloff JT, Spencer CA. Clinical review 12. The use and misuse of the sensitive thyrotropin assays. *J Clin Endocrinol Metab* 1990;71:553–558.
88. Ridgway EC. Thyrotropin radioimmunoassays: birth, life and demise. *Mayo Clin Proc* 1988;63:1028–1034.
89. Ross DS, Neer RM, Ridgway EC, Daniels GH. Subclinical hyperthyroidism and reduced bone density as a possible result of prolonged suppression of the pituitary-thyroid axis with L-thyroxine. *Am J Med* 1987;82:1167–1170.
90. Paul TL, Kerrigan J, Kelly AM, Braverman LE, Baran DT. Long-term L-thyroxine therapy is associated with decreased hip bone density in premenopausal women. *JAMA* 1988;259:3137–3141.
91. Adlin EV, Maurer AH, Marks AD. Bone mineral density in postmenopausal women treated with L-thyroxine. *Am J Med* 1991;90:360–366.
92. Kung AWC, Pun KK. Bone mineral density in premenopausal women

receiving long-term physiological doses of levothyroxine. *JAMA* 1991;265:2688–2691.
93. Gupta KL, Rolla AR. Endocrine causes of bone disease. *Endocrinol Metab Clin North Am* 1995;24:373–393.
94. Cobin RH. Thyroid hormone excess and bone—a clinical review. *Endocr Pract* 1995;1:404–409.
95. Ross DS. Subclinical hyperthyroidism: possible danger of overzealous thyroxine replacement therapy. *Mayo Clin Proc* 1988;63:1223–1229.
96. Banovac K, Papic M, Bilsker MS, Zakarija M, McKenzie JM. Evidence of hyperthyroidism in apparently euthyroid patients treated with levothyroxine. *Arch Intern Med* 1989;149:809–812.
97. Biondi B, Fazio S, Carella C, Amato G, Cittadini A, Lupoli G, Sacca L, Bellastella A, Lombardi G. Cardiac effects of long-term thyrotropin-suppressive therapy with levothyroxine. *J Clin Endocrinol Metab* 1993;77:334–338.
98. Ladenson PW. Thyrotoxicosis and the heart: something old and something new [editorial]. *J Clin Endocrinol Metab* 1993;77:332–333.
99. Woeber KA. Thyrotoxicosis and the heart. *N Engl J Med* 1992;327:94–98.
100. Gow SM, Caldwell G, Toft AD, Seth J, Hussey AJ, Sweeting VM, Beckett GJ. Relationship between pituitary and other target organ responsiveness in hypothyroid patients receiving thyroxine replacement. *J Clin Endocrinol Metab* 1987;64:364–370.
101. Helfand M, Crapo LM. Monitoring therapy in patients taking levothyroxine. *Ann Intern Med* 1990;113:450–454.
102. Utiger RD. Thyrotropin measurements: past, present and future. *Mayo Clin Proc* 1988;63:1053–1056.
103. Konno N, Morikawa K. Seasonal variation of serum thyrotropin concentration and thyrotropin response to thyrotropin-releasing hormone in patients with primary hypothyroidism on constant replacement dosage of thyroxine. *J Clin Endocrinol Metab* 1982;54:1118–1124.
104. Sakata S, Nakamura S, Miura K. Autoantibodies against thyroid hormones or iodothyronine. Implications in diagnosis, thyroid function, treatment, and pathogenesis. *Ann Intern Med* 1985;103:579–589.
105. Lahat N, Sheinfeld M, Baron E, Glaser B. L-thyroxine-induced leukopenia in a patient with Hashimoto's disease: involvement of suppressor-cytotoxic T cells. *J Clin Endocrinol Metab* 1985;61:980–982.
106. Shibata H, Hayakawa H, Hirukawa M, Tadokoro K, Ogata E. Hypersensitivity caused by synthetic thyroid hormones in a hypothyroid patient with Hashimoto's thyroiditis. *Arch Intern Med* 1986;146:1624–1625.
107. Arafah BM. Decreased levothyroxine requirement in women with hypothyroidism during androgen therapy for breast cancer. *Ann Intern Med* 1994;121:247–251.
108. Figge J, Dluhy RG. Amiodarone-induced elevation of thyroid stimulation hormone in patients receiving levothyroxine for primary hypothyroidism. *Ann Intern Med* 1990;113:553–555.
109. Isley WL. Effect of rifampin therapy on thyroid function tests in a hypothyroid patient on replacement L-thyroxine. *Ann Intern Med* 1987;107:517–518.
110. Blackshear JL, Schultz AL, Napier JS, Stuart DD. Thyroxine replacement requirements in hypothyroid patients receiving phenytoin. *Ann Intern Med* 1983;99:341–342.
111. Aanderud S, Strandjord RE. Hypothyroidism induced by anti-epileptic therapy. *Acta Neurol Scand* 1980;61:330–332.
112. Demke DM. Drug interaction between thyroxine and lovastatin. *N Engl J Med* 1989;321:1341–1342.
113. Takasu N, Yamada T, Takasu M, Komiya I, Nagasawa Y, Asawa T, Shinoda T, Aizawa T, Koizumi Y. Disappearance of thyrotopin-blocking antibodies and spontaneous recovery from hypothyroidism in autoimmune thyroiditis. *N Engl J Med* 1992;326:513–518.
114. Tajiri J, Higashi K, Morita M, Umeda T, Sato J. Studies of hypothyroidism in patients with high iodine intake. *J Clin Endocrinol Metab* 1986;63:412–417.
115. Goldman JM. Postpartum thyroid dysfunction. *Arch Intern Med* 1986;146:1296–1299.
116. Mestman JH, Goodwin TM, Montoro MM. Thyroid disorders of pregnancy. *Endocrinol Metab Clin North Am* 1995;24:41–71.
117. Duick DS, Stein RB, Warren DW, Nicoloff JT. The significance of partial suppressibility of serum thyroxine by triiodothyronine administration in euthyroid man. *J Clin Endocrinol Metab* 1975;41:229–234.
118. Sawers JSA, Toft AD, Irvine WJ, Brown NS, Seth J. Transient hypothyroidism after iodine-131 treatment of thyrotoxicosis. *J Clin Endocrinol Metab* 1980;50:226–229.
119. Nofal MM, Beierwaltes WH, Patno ME. Treatment of hyperthyroidism with sodium iodide I131. *JAMA* 1966;197:605–610.
120. Bronsky D, Kiamko RT, Waldstein SS. Posttherapeutic myxedema. Relative occurrence after treatment of hyperthyroidism by radioactive iodine (^{131}I) or subtotal thyroidectomy. *Arch Intern Med* 1968;121:113–117.
121. Werner SC. Response to triiodothyronine as index of persistence of disease in the thyroid remnant of patients in remission from hyperthyroidism. *J Clin Invest* 1956;35:56–61.
122. Feldt-Rasmussen U, Schleusener H, Carayon P. Meta-analysis evaluation of the impact of thyrotopin receptor antibodies on long term remission after medical therapy of Graves' disease. *J Clin Endocrinol Metab* 1994;78:98–102.
123. Burmeister LA, Goumaz MO, Mariash CN, Oppenheimer JH. Levothyroxine dose requirements of thyrotropin suppression in the treatment of differentiated thyroid cancer. *J Clin Endocrinol Metab* 1992;75:344–350.
124. Vander Laan WP. Results of administration of desiccated thyroid to subjects in remission from hyperthyroidism after treatment with antithyroid drugs. *N Engl J Med* 1957;256:511–512.
125. Mandel SJ, Larsen PR, Seely EW, Brent GA. Increased need for thyroxine during pregnancy in women with primary hypothyroidism. *N Engl J Med* 1990;323:91–97.
126. Dussault JH. Transplacental transport of thyroid hormone: possible clinical implications. *Thyroid Today* 1992;15(2):1–7.
127. Van Herle AJ, Young RT, Fisher DA, Uller RP, Brinkman CR III. Intrauterine treatment of a hypothyroid fetus. *J Clin Endocrinol Metab* 1975;40:474–477.
128. Perelman AH, Johnson RL, Blemons RD, Finberg HJ, Clewell WH, Trujillo L. Intrauterine diagnosis and treatment of fetal goitrous hypothyroidism. *J Clin Endocrinol Metab* 1990;71:618–621.
129. Fisher DA. Clinical review 19: management of congenital hypothyroidism. *J Clin Endocrinol Metab* 1991;72:523–529.
130. LaFranchi S. Congenital hypothyroidism: a newborn screening success story? *Endocrinologist* 1994;4:477–486.
131. Dubuis JM, Glorieux J, Richer F, Deal CL, Dussault JH, Van Vliet G. Outcome of severe congenital hypothyroidism: closing the developmental gap with early high dose levothyroxine treatment. *J Clin Endocrinol Metab* 1996;81:222–227.
132. Rivkees SA, Bode HH, Crawford JD. Long-term growth in juvenile acquired hypothyroidism. The failure to achieve normal adult stature. *N Engl J Med* 1988;318:599–602.
133. Federman D, Robbins J, Rall JE. Some observations on cretinism and its treatment. *N Engl J Med* 1958;259:610–615.
134. Focarile F, Rondanini GF, Bollati A, Bartolucci A, Chiumello G. Free thyroid hormones in evaluating persistently elevated thyrotopin levels in children with congenital hypothyroidism on replacement therapy. *J Clin Endocrinol Metab* 1984;59:1211–1214.
135. Van Dop C, Conte FA, Koch TK, Clark SJ, Wilson-Davis SL, Grumbach MM. Pseudotumor cerebri associated with initiation of levothyroxine therapy for juvenile hypothyroidism. *N Engl J Med* 1983;308:1076–1080.
136. Perloff WH. Hirsutism—a manifestation of juvenile hypothyroidism. *JAMA* 1955;157:651–652.
137. Jannini EA, Ulisse S, D'Armiento M. Thyroid hormone and male gonadal function. *Endocr Rev* 1995;16:443–459.
138. Staub JJ, Noelpp B, Grani R, Gemsenjager E, Havenstein M, Girard J. The relationship of serum thyrotropin (TSH) to the thyroid hormones after oral TSH-releasing hormone in patients with preclinical hypothyroidism. *J Clin Endocrinol Metab* 1983;56:449–453.
139. Cooper DS, Halpern R, Wood LC, Levin AA, Ridgway EC. L-thyroxine therapy in subclinical hypothyroidism. A double-blind, placebo-controlled trial. *Ann Intern Med* 1984;101:18–24.
140. Tibaldi J, Barzel US. Thyroxine supplementation method for the prevention of clinical hypothyroidism. *Am J Med* 1985;79:241–244.
141. Glinoer D, Riahi M, Grün J-P, Kinthaert J. Risk of subclinical hypothyroidism in pregnant women with asymptomatic autoimmune thyroid disorders. *J Clin Endocrinol Metab* 1994;79:197–204.
142. Gerstein HC. Incidence of postpartum thyroid dysfunction in patients with type I diabetes mellitus. *Ann Intern Med* 1993;118:419–423.
143. Müller B, Zulewski H, Huber P, Ratcliffe JG, Staub JJ. Impaired action of thyroid hormone associated with smoking in women with hypothyroidism. *N Engl J Med* 1995;333:964–969.
144. Robuschi G, Safran M, Braverman LE, Gnudi A, Roti E. Hypothyroidism in the elderly. *Endocr Rev* 1987;8:142–153.

145. Brent GA, Hershman JM. Thyroxine therapy in patients with severe nonthyroidal illnesses and low serum thyroxine concentration. *J Clin Endocrinol Metab* 1986;63:1–8.
146. Klemperer JD, Klein I, Gomez M, Helm RE, Ojamaa K, Thomas SJ, Isom OW, Krieger K. Thyroid hormone treatment after coronary artery bypass surgery. *N Engl J Med* 1995;333:1522–1527.
147. Bennett-Guerrero E, Jimenez JL, White WD, D'Amico EB, Baldwin BI, Schwinn DA. Cardiovascular effects of intravenous triiodothyronine in patients undergoing coronary artery bypass graft surgery. A randomized, double-blind, placebo controlled trial. *JAMA* 1996;275:687–692.
148. Joffe RT, Sokolov STH, Singer W. Thyroid hormone treatment of depression. *Thyroid* 1995;5:235–239.
149. Burrow GN. The thyroid: nodules and neoplasia. In: Felig P, Baxter JD, Broadus AE, Frohman LA, eds. *Endocrinology and metabolism*, 2nd ed. New York: McGraw-Hill, 1987;473–507.
150. Greer MA, Smith GE. Method for increasing the accuracy of the radioiodine uptake as a test for thyroid function by use of desiccated thyroid. *J Clin Endocrinol Metab* 1954;14:1374–1384.
151. Werner SC, Spooner M. A new and simple test for hyperthyroidism employing L-triiodothyronine and the twenty-four hour I-131 uptake method. *Bull NY Acad Med* 1955;31:137–145.
152. Cotton GE, Gorman CA, Mayberry WE. Suppression of thyrotropin (h-TSH) in serums of patients with myxedema of varying etiology treated with thyroid hormones. *N Engl J Med* 1971;285:529–533.
153. Wallack MS, Adelberg HM, Nicoloff JT. A thyroid suppression test using a single dose of L-thyroxine. *N Engl J Med* 1970;283:402–405.
154. Bartalena L, Martino E, Pacchiarotti A, et al. Factors affecting suppression of endogenous thyrotropin secretion by thyroxine treatment: retrospective analysis in athyreotic and goitrous patients. *J Clin Endocrinol Metab* 1987;64:849–855.
155. Astwood EB, Cassidy CE, Aurbach GD. Treatment of goiter and thyroid nodules with thyroid. *JAMA* 1960;174:459–464.
156. Levy RP, Kelly LW Jr, Jefferies WM. The effects of thyrotropin and desiccated thyroid upon hypothyroidism with goiter. *Am J Med Sci* 1956;231:61–68.
157. Hayashi Y, Tamai H, Fukata S, et al. A long-term clinical immunological, and histological follow-up study of patients with goitrous chronic lymphocytic thyroiditis. *J Clin Endocrinol Metab* 1985;61:1172–1178.
158. Kansal P, Sakati N, Rifai A, Woodhouse N. Lingual thyroid. Diagnosis and treatment. *Arch Intern Med* 1987;147:2046–2048.
159. Refetoff S, Weiss RE, Usala SJ. The syndromes of resistance to thyroid hormone. *Endocr Rev* 1993;14:348–399.
160. Brooks MH, Barbato AL, Collins S, Garbincius J, Neidballa RG, Hoffman D. Familial thyroid hormone resistance. *Am J Med* 1981;71:414–421.
161. Gharib H, Klee GG. Familial euthyroid hyperthyroxinemia secondary to pituitary and peripheral resistance to thyroid hormones. *Mayo Clin Proc* 1985;60:9–15.
162. Dulgeroff AJ, Geffner ME, Koyal SN, Wong M, Hershman JM. Bromocriptine and triac therapy for hyperthyroidism due to pituitary resistance to thyroid hormone. *J Clin Endocrinol Metab* 1992;75:1071–1075.
163. Bracco D, Morin O, Schutz Y, Liang H, Jequier E, Burger AG. Comparison of the metabolic and endocrine effects of 3,5,3'-triiodothyroacetic acid and thyroxine. *J Clin Endocrinol Metab* 1993;77:221–228.
164. Takeda T, Suzuki S, Liu R-T, DeGroot LJ. Triiodothyroacetic acid has unique potential for therapy of resistance to thyroid hormone. *J Clin Endocrinol Metab* 1995;80:2033–2040.
165. Mazzaferri EL. Management of a solitary thyroid nodule. *N Engl J Med* 1993;328:553–559.
166. Gharib H, James EM, Charboneau JW, Naessens JM, Offord KP, Gorman CA. Suppressive therapy with levothyroxine for solitary thyroid nodules: a double-blind controlled clinical study. *N Engl J Med* 1987;317:70–75.
167. Molitch ME, Beck JR, Dreisman M, Gottlieb JE, Pauker SG. The cold thyroid nodule: an analysis of diagnostic and therapeutic options. *Endocr Rev* 1984;5:185–199.
168. AACE Clinical practice guidelines for the diagnosis and management of thyroid nodules. *Endocr Pract* 1996;2:78–84.
169. Morita T, Tamai H, Ohshima A, Komaki G, Matsubayashi S, Kuma K, Nakagawa T. Changes in serum thyroid hormone, thyrotropin and thyroglobulin concentrations during thyroxine therapy in patients with solitary thyroid nodules. *J Clin Endocrinol Metab* 1989;69:227–230.
170. Blum M. Why do clinicians continue to debate the use of levothyroxine in the diagnosis and management of thyroid nodules? *Ann Intern Med* 1995;122:63–64.
171. Cooper DS. Clinical review 66. Thyroxine suppression therapy for benign nodular disease. *J Clin Endocrinol Metab* 1995;80:331–334.
172. Fogelfeld L, Wiviott MBT, Shore-Freedman E, Blend M, Bekerman C, Pinsky S, Schneider AB. Recurrence of thyroid nodules after surgical removal in patients irradiated in childhood for benign conditions. *N Engl J Med* 1989;320:835–840.
173. Hashizume K, Ichikawa K, Sakurai A, Suzuki S, Takeda T, Kobayashi M, Miyamoto T, Arai M, Nagasawa T. Administration of thyroxine in treated Graves' disease. Effects on the level of antibodies to thyroid-stimulating hormone receptors and on the risk of recurrence of hyperthyroidism. *N Engl J Med* 1991;324:947–953.
174. Hashizume K, Ichikawa K, Nishii Y, Kobayashi M, Sakuri A, Miyamoto T, Suzuki S, Takeda T. Effects of administration of thyroxine on the risk of postpartum recurrence of hyperthyroid Graves' disease. *J Clin Endocrinol Metab* 1992;75:6–10.
175. Tamai H, Hayaki I, Kawai K, Komaki G, Matsubayashi S, Kuma K, Kumagai LF, Nagataki S. Lack of effect of thyroxine administration on elevated thyroid stimulating hormone receptor antibody levels in treated Graves' disease patients. *J Clin Endocrinol Metab* 1995;80:1481–1484.
176. McIver B, Rae P, Beckett G, Wilkinson E, Gold A, Toft A. Lack of effect of thyroxine in patients with Graves' hyperthyroidism who are treated with an antithyroid drug. *N Engl J Med* 1996:334:220–224.
177. Waldstein SS. Suppressive therapy in the management of metastatic thyroid carcinoma. *Otolaryngol Clin North Am* 1980;13:115–118.
178. Ichikawa Y, Saito E, Abe Y, Homma M, Muraki T, Ito K. Presence of TSH receptors in thyroid neoplasms. *J Clin Endocrinol Metab* 1976;42:395–398.
179. Takahashi H, Jiang N-S, Gorman CA, Lee CY. Thyrotropin receptors in normal and pathologic human thyroid tissues. *J Clin Endocrinol Metab* 1978;47:870–876.
180. Molnar GD, Colby MY Jr, Woolner LB. Demonstration of thyroid-stimulating-hormone dependence in a case of metastatic carcinoma of thyroid origin. *Mayo Clin Proc* 1963;38:280–288.
181. McLaughlin RP, Scholz DA, McConahey WM, Childs DS. Metastatic thyroid carcinoma with hyperthyroidism: two cases with functioning metastatic follicular thyroid carcinoma. *Mayo Clin Proc* 1970;45:328–335.
182. Mack RE, Hart KT, Druet D, Bauer MA. An abnormality of thyroid hormone secretion. *Am J Med* 1961;30:323–326.
183. Crile G. Desiccated thyroid for thyroid lymphoma. *Surg Gynecol Obstet* 1963;116:449–450.
184. Mazzaferri EL, Young RL. Papillary thyroid carcinoma: a 10-year follow-up report of the impact of therapy in 576 patients. *Am J Med* 1981;70:511–518.
185. Crile G Jr, Antunez AR, Esselstyn CB Jr, Hawk WA, Skillern PG. The advantages of subtotal thyroidectomy and suppression of TSH in the primary treatment of papillary carcinoma of the thyroid. *Cancer* 1985;55:2691–2697.
186. McConahey WM, Hay ID, Woolner LB, van Heerden JA, Taylor WF. Papillary thyroid cancer treated at the Mayo Clinic 1946 through 1970. Initial manifestations, pathologic findings, therapy, and outcome. *Mayo Clin Proc* 1986;61:978–996.
187. Schlumberger M, Tubiana M, De Vathaire F, et al. Long-term results of treatment of 283 patients with lung and bone metastases from differentiated thyroid carcinoma. *J Clin Endocrinol Metab* 1986;63:960–967.
188. Schlumberger M, De Vathaire F, Travagli JP, Vassal G, Lemerle J, Parmentier C, Tubiana M. Differentiated thyroid carcinoma in childhood: long-term follow-up of 72 patients. *J Clin Endocrinol Metab* 1987;65:1088–1094.
189. Hoffman DP, Surks MI, Oppenheimer JH, Weitzman ED. Response to thyrotropin releasing hormone: an objective criterion for the adequacy of thyrotropin suppression therapy. *J Clin Endocrinol Metab* 1977;44:892–901.
190. Bartelena L, Martino E, Falcone M, et al. Evaluation of the nocturnal serum thyrotropin (TSH) surge, as assessed by TSH ultrasensitive assay, in patients receiving long-term L-thyroxine suppression therapy and in patients with various thyroid disorders. *J Clin Endocrinol Metab* 1987;65:1265–1271.
191. Ross DS, Ardisson LA, Meskell MJ. Measurement of thyrotropin in clinical and subclinical hyperthyroidism using a new chemiluminescent assay. *J Clin Encocrinol Metab* 1989;69:684–688.

192. Spencer CA, LoPresti JS, Nicoloff JT, Dlott R, Schwarzbein D. Multiphasic thyrotropin responses to thyroid hormone administration in man. *J Clin Endocrinol Metab* 1995;80:854–859.
193. Biondi B, Fazio S. Carella C, Sabatini D, Amato G, Citttadini A, Bellastella A, Lombardi G, Sacca L. Control of adrenergic overactivity by β-blockade improves the quality of life in patients receiving long-term suppressive therapy with levothyroxine. *J Clin Endocrinol Metab* 1994;78:1028–1033.
194. Fazio S, Biondi B, Carella C, Sabatini D, Cittadini A, Panza N, Lombardi G, Sacca L. Diastolic dysfunction in patients on thyroid-stimulating hormone suppressive therapy with levothyroxine: beneficial effect of β-blockade. *J Clin Endocrinol Metab* 1995;80:2222–2226.
195. Diamond T, Nery L, Hales I. A therapeutic dilemma: suppressive doses of thyroxine significantly reduce bone mineral measurements in both premenopausal and postmenopausal women with thyroid carcinoma. *J Clin Endocrinol Metab* 1990;72:1184–1188.
196. Schneider DL, Barrett-Connor EL, Morton DJ. Thyroid hormone use and bone mineral density in elderly women: effects of estrogen. *JAMA* 1994;271:1245–1249.
197. Rosen HN, Moses AC, Gundberg C, Kung VT, Seyedin SM, Chen T, Holick M, Greenspan SL. Therapy with parenteral pamidronate prevents thyroid hormone-induced bone turnovers in humans. *J Clin Endocrinol Metab* 1993;77:664–669.
198. Müller CG, Bayley TA, Harrison JE, Tsang R. Possible limited bone loss with suppressive thyroxine therapy is unlikely to have clinical relevance. *Thyroid* 1995;5:81–87.
199. Schlumberger M, Charbord P, Fragu P, Gardet P, Lumbroso J, Parmentier C, Tubiana M. Relationship between thyrotropin stimulation and radioiodine uptake in lung metastates of differentiated thyroid carcinoma. *J Clin Endocrinol Metab* 1983;57:148–151.
200. Krishnamurthy GT, Blahd WH. Human reaction to bovine TSH. *J Nucl Med* 1977;18:629.
201. Melmed S, Harada A, Hershman JM, Krishnamurthy GT, Blahd WH. Neutralizing antibodies to bovine thyrotropin in immunized patients with thyroid cancer. *J Clin Endocrinol Metab* 1980;51:358–363.
202. Duick DS, Wahner HW, Edis AJ, Van Heerden JA. Effects of oral thyrotropin releasing hormone, exogenous thyroid-stimulating hormone, and withdrawal of triiodothyronine on ^{131}I uptake after subtotal thyroidectomy. *J Clin Endocrinol Metab* 1980;50:502–506.
203. Meier CA, Braverman LE, Ebner SA, Veronikis I, Daniels GH, Ross DS, Deraska DJ, Davies TF, Valentine M, DeGroot LJ, Curran P, McEllin K, Reynolds J, Robbins J, Weintraub BD. Diagnostic use of recombinant human thyrotropin in patients with thyroid carcinoma (phase I/II study). *J Clin Endocrinol Metab* 1994;78:188–196.
204. Greer MA. The effect on endogenous thyroid activity of feeding desiccated thyroid to normal human subjects. *N Engl J Med* 1951;244:385–390.
205. Singer PA, Nicoloff JT, Stein RB, Jaramilo J. Transient TRH deficiency after prolonged thyroid hormone therapy. *J Clin Endocrinol Metab* 1978;47:512–518.
206. Vagenakis AG, Braverman LE, Azizi F, Portnay GI, Ingbar SH. Recovery of pituitary thyrotropin function after withdrawal of prolonged thyroid-suppression therapy. *N Engl J Med* 1975;293:681–684.
207. Goldman JM, Line BR, Aamodt RL, Robbins J. Influence of triiodothyronine withdrawal time on ^{131}I uptake postthyroidectomy for thyroid cancer. *J Clin Endocrinol Metab* 1980;50:734–739.
208. Mazzaferri EL. Treating high thyroglobulin with radioiodine: a magic bullet or a shot in the dark? [editorial]. *J Clin Endocrinol Metab* 1995;80:1485–1487.
209. Schneider AB, Line BR, Goldman JM, Robbins J. Sequential serum thyroglobulin determinations, ^{131}I scans, and ^{131}I uptakes after triiodothyronine withdrawal in patients with thyroid cancer. *J Clin Endocrinol Metab* 1981;53:1199–1206.
210. Ozata M, Suzuki S, Miyamoto T, Liu RT, Fierro-Renoy F, DeGroot L. Serum thyroglobulin in the follow-up of patients with treated differentiated thyroid cancer. *J Clin Endocrinol Metab* 1994;79:98–105.

CHAPTER 28

Thyroid Cancer: Controversies and Etiopathogenesis

Sharon L. Collins

A chapter concerning etiopathogenesis of thyroid cancer is likely to evoke a mental, if not physical, yawn. But much of the "classic" information on thyroid cancer is not summarized in the literature in an easily accessible or readily understandable form, and there is exciting new information emerging from clinical and animal investigations, and from new technology applied at the cellular and molecular levels, that has not yet been collated in review form. This chapter attempts to correct the former deficit and introduce the reader to new research directions that may eventually provide a basis for scientific management of the clinical situation. This chapter is an introduction to thyroid cancer, and it provides a tumor biology approach to evaluating controversies in the field. None of the perennial controversies have been definitively elucidated since the first edition of this book, but references are updated at the end of each section.

To many people, the term *thyroid cancer* evokes an entity that is unique in many respects compared to solid carcinomas in other systems (breast, lung, colon): it is cancer that does not kill the patient; cancer that metastasizes frequently but the metastases have no negative effect and possibly even a positive effect on the patient's prognosis; and cancer for which prognostic factors relevant to other cancers, such as those that reflect tumor burden (TNM staging), are almost irrelevant compared with parameters such as the patient's age and sex. Other etiologic factors, such as induction by radiation, the relationship to dietary iodine, and hormone dependence, are almost unique to thyroid cancer.

These unique features and unusual etiologic factors can be studied using animal models, with the goal of elucidating underlying mechanisms of carcinogenesis. For this reason, among others, tumors of the thyroid gland have long provided a focus of interest in oncology that is out of all proportion to their clinical frequency or lethality. Because general concepts of neoplasia can be studied in this setting, they have inspired a great deal of interesting experimental work and have attracted the attention of geneticists, biochemists, statisticians, physicists, embryologists, endocrinologists, epidemiologists, immunologists, pathologists, internists, surgeons, and radiotherapists.

Nevertheless, the topic of thyroid cancer appears simple and straightforward only to those who are not familiar with the literature in detail. In fact, thyroid cancer remains enigmatic. Perusal of the voluminous literature relating to the many subtopics relevant to thyroid cancer soon frustrates the reader because of the plethora of articles on either side of each issue and the persistence of age-old controversies, reliable answers to which cannot be found.

Many studies on thyroid cancer are flawed by design, execution, or interpretation, and they may be heavily biased by the beliefs and prejudices of their authors. Statements on both the significance of prognostic variables and the effect of treatment are presented dogmatically as established fact in much of the existing literature. This does not indicate to the reader that many, if not all, areas are controversial to a greater or lesser extent, primarily because of limitations inherent in accumulating adequate data on a rare cancer with a paradoxically benign natural history.

Factual answers are not forthcoming because of the indolent overall nature of thyroid cancer and its long natural history, which preclude randomized prospective studies. In their absence, treatment controversies will inevitably persist. Attributing significance to a particular treatment is virtually impossible, although a great num-

---

S. L. Collins: Department of Otolaryngology—Head and Neck Surgery, Loyola University of Chicago Medical Center, Maywood, Illinois 60153; and Section of Otolaryngology—Head and Neck Surgery, Hines Veterans Administration Hospital, Hines, Illinois.

ber of researchers have tried. The otolaryngologist reader will appreciate similar problems in the ENT (ear, nose, and throat) literature on treatment for Bell's palsy (a condition that usually normalizes without treatment) and for Ménière's disease (which is difficult to interpret because of its fluctuating nature).

This chapter presents information on the tumor biology of thyroid cancer and a critical assessment of the problems in interpreting the literature. Clinician readers may feel inclined to proceed to subsequent chapters where the "meat" of the topic presumably lies. This chapter, however, should be read by all persons who have occasion to read the clinical thyroid cancer literature, as it provides a basis for critical assessment. Clinicians with research interests will get an up-to-date overview of current and future research directions. Basic researchers can profit from the perspective on the clinical controversies.

The term *thyroid cancer* is misleading in that it is not a homogeneous entity but rather comprises a variety of subsets demonstrating a biologic spectrum of aggressiveness, from indolent and benign to some of the most aggressive, anaplastic, and rapidly lethal tumors known to man. In this chapter, discussion is not grouped by individual histologic types. Rather, there are a number of "concept" sections that discuss relevant aspects of the various subgroups of thyroid cancer. For orientation, a brief initial section provides an overview of the subtypes of thyroid cancer, followed by a critical discussion of problems in interpreting the thyroid cancer literature, which is vital to understanding the unresolved issues presented in subsequent sections.

Because thyroid cancer is still basically a puzzle, the remainder of the chapter outlines the natural history and etiopathogenesis that have contributed clues to understanding the puzzle. These clues include factors in the macrocosm (the environment) and the microcosm (at the levels of the organism, the cell, and the molecule). This chapter does not discuss the details of treatment issues (which are covered in subsequent chapters), except as they relate to underlying tumor biology issues.

The hundreds of articles written about thyroid cancer over the years have originated in many countries and have appeared in a wide variety of journals. Those cited in this chapter are included because they are classic articles, they represent majority opinion, they review an aspect of the topic particularly well, or because they are recent contributions to the literature that reflect the new directions that studies in thyroid carcinogenesis are taking.

Caveat! In the absence of statistically compelling data, the ingenuity of authors is often manifested by justifications for their preconceived conclusions based on teleological explanations of underlying mechanisms of thyroid metabolism and growth, and frequently it results in extrapolation (albeit intuitively logical) beyond the data. The significance of the newer contributions, particularly, has usually not been solidified by broad experience and clinical or experimental confirmation and they are included primarily to indicate the directions that are being taken in thyroid cancer research.

THE TREATMENT CONTROVERSIES

A brief overview of the clinical controversies gives perspective to the upcoming topics on the natural history of thyroid cancer. Overall, the biologic nature of differentiated thyroid cancer (DTC) is benign. In the past, a few authors even suggested that patients never die of the disease. It is now realized, however, as with every other type of cancer, that a spectrum of malignancy and aggressiveness exists for DTC. The basic controversy on the treatment of DTC can be stated as follows: What is the significance and necessity of clearing disease in DTC patients? How important is it to remove every last thyroid cancer cell in the patient's body? How important is it that treatment be initiated expeditiously—does early versus late treatment affect the outcome?

Answers are clouded because reports in the literature seldom specify whether the patients died with or of disease; the site of treatment failure is usually not clearly stated. Thus, the significance of residual disease in the gland, in the neck, and distantly is unclear.

The optimal management of DTC remains controversial. There are strong proponents who emphasize just their one treatment modality, not taking into account either the natural history of the disease (which also remains controversial) or the importance of prognostic factors (which remain to a large extent uncertain, unproved, and frequently uninvestigated in an individual series). Considerable attention has been focused on the appropriate extent of surgical excision of the thyroid gland, and arguments on either side are frequently supported mainly by the strength of the surgeon's personality, verbal bombast, and reputation. Whether or not the survival of DTC patients is affected at all by treatment remains an open question, although this would be deemed a nihilistic consideration by many clinicians.

The treatment of thyroid carcinoma remains controversial, with basic philosophies of treatment ranging from radical to conservative regarding resection of the thyroid gland, excision of regional lymphatics, use of radiation therapy, and thyroid "feeding" for suppression postoperatively. The unresolved treatment questions on thyroid cancer will be settled only by prolonged prospective randomized trials which so far have not been instituted for a variety of compelling reasons (see later).

The major surgical controversy is whether cancer that is clinically confined to one lobe should be treated by total thyroidectomy or by more conservative procedures. Removal of all primary thyroid tissue decreases the competition for uptake of iodine-131 (^{131}I) by metastatic deposits elsewhere and is a necessary prerequisite if ^{131}I scans or therapy will be part of the therapeutic regimen to eradicate distant metastases and to allow thyroglobulin markers to be used to follow patients for recurrence postoperatively.

The argument for total thyroidectomy is the reported high incidence of microscopic cancer foci in the opposite lobe. Halstedian surgical oncology principles (largely outmoded—see later) dictate that every last cancer cell be removed to effect cure. The theoretical prevention of anaplastic change in small residual foci of thyroid cancer is also cited as an argument in favor of total thyroidectomy, as is the low morbidity of the procedure in experienced hands.

Advocates of a more conservative surgical approach (selective surgery with the extent depending on gross findings at the time of operation) note that treatment of metastatic disease is of little clinical importance and that the complication rate after total thyroidectomy is not negligible. The morbidity of the operation of total thyroidectomy in the hands of nonexperts can be lifelong and consists primarily of persistent hypoparathyroidism and damage to the recurrent laryngeal nerve. Such risks must be carefully weighed against the relatively benign prognosis for the individual with thyroid cancer. Also, despite multifocal primary disease, the patient with papillary cancer treated by lobectomy alone (with or without isthmusectomy) develops clinical recurrent cancer in the opposite lobe in only 5% to 10% of cases. (The incidence recorded depends to some extent on the length of follow-up in the particular series. Some series show no recurrent disease whatever on long-term follow-up.) [One recent series, however, indicates that the incidence of major postoperative complications is low even when residents are the primary surgeons, as long as there is close supervision by attending surgeons. In a series of 200 consecutive thyroidectomies of varying extents, there was one temporary palsy of the recurrent laryngeal nerve and one instance of hypoparathyroidism (1).]

Another major treatment controversy is whether or not DTC should be treated differently in young versus old patients. Less aggressive treatment is frequently recommended for the patient subgroups of children and young women with inherently good prognoses. An increasing body of evidence suggests, however, that treatment should be as aggressive in these groups as in those with risk factors that predict a poor outcome. Uncertainty concerning the significance of metastatic disease with DTC precludes an answer to this treatment controversy.

PROBLEMS WITH THE THYROID CANCER LITERATURE

The thyroid cancer literature is in many ways a hopeless muddle. Most of the current concepts were in place by 1960, and the past 30 years have witnessed persisting controversies on the same topics. There are many articles on either side of each issue, and, in the absence of a compelling scientific basis to support one or the other, pendulum swings of opinion on treatment persist. Review articles tend to be selective in the topics discussed and frequently list study results without providing perspective or a conceptual framework to assist the reader's interpretation. Particular institutions and expert authors tend to maintain positions in which they have accumulated a vested interest over the years. In these respects, the thyroid cancer literature does not significantly differ from the cancer literature on many other organ systems (2).

Ideal conditions to allow valid assessment and correct generalization about such factors as incidence, mortality, clinical signs and symptoms, the benefit of various diagnostic procedures, age and sex distribution, the effects of surgical treatment, and prognosis have been outlined by Borup Christensen et al. (3):

1. Patient series should be representative of an entire demographically defined population.
2. The treatments given should be uniform and easy to classify.
3. Follow-up should be complete, detailed, and of sufficient length.
4. All histopathologic material should be revised and reclassified in accordance with a current, generally accepted system.
5. The autopsy frequency should be high.

If these conditions are fulfilled, the possibility of comparing the findings in different areas and centers should improve. Currently, the evidence supporting one side or the other of most issues can be considered at best circumstantial.

Study Population Heterogeneity

Series that contain different proportions of patients varying in composition on age, histologic type of tumor, and sex cannot be scientifically compared because of the significant effect of these and other variables on the natural history and, therefore, outcome of thyroid cancer. Unless the populations under comparison are matched for variables relevant to thyroid cancer prognosis, conclusions concerning the significance of single parameters are probably invalid. Attributing differences in outcome to factors under study such as geographic area, diet, race, or mode of treatment could reflect a true difference but could also be simply methodological. The case-control format is sometimes used by epidemiologists to help solve this problem, but this does not take into consideration all of the relevant prognostic factors for thyroid cancer.

Including patients with varying extents of disease in one series also contributes to the heterogeneity of the population. For example, including patients with incurable disease will skew the outcome of a patient series. An attempt should be made to use a homogeneous population with respect to such factors, for example by including only patients with curable disease. Such attempts have been made in the thyroid cancer literature to some extent, attested to by papers that deal with a particular subgroup of thyroid cancer patients, such as those with locally aggressive cancer, patients who had a fatal outcome, and those with distant metastases.

Referral Bias

Another problem with many thyroid cancer studies is that in order to accumulate sufficient patient numbers, they usually originate in referral centers to which patients are often sent because their cancer has special clinical features that put them in a difficult management category. Such reports, therefore, focus on a selected population. Because of the rarity of DTC, extensive experience is usually limited to large referral centers. In such centers, patients are usually treated in a manner reflecting the experience of the attending physician and/or an institutional bias. Patients reaching the operating room (for example, for nontoxic goiter) comprise a highly selected group that is not representative of the population at large.

Series from referral centers generally include a much higher proportion of patients with a poor prognosis than is found in the general population. (In some countries with socialized medicine, all patients with a particular disease entity are sent to a specific referral center, and this does not necessarily imply the presence of ominous prognostic factors.) With this composition of patient material, the attribution of significance in outcome to different variables and treatments may be skewed. Some authors, however, note that having a high proportion of patients with a poor prognosis permits analysis of prognostic factors with greater ease and reliability than if most patients had good prognostic factors. Papers on thyroid cancer should specifically include comments as to the "drawing area" of the referral center and the nature of the population treated.

Tumor Registries

In accumulating enough patients to review, many thyroid cancer series have extended over decades, using data from tumor registries. The method of tumor registration, whether compulsory or voluntary, has significance for the completeness and composition of the patient series collected, as does the population drawing base—whether from a restricted area or from the whole country.

One question that has been addressed with tumor registry data is whether the true incidence of thyroid cancer is increasing or is an artifact of the increased awareness of the disease. Epidemiologically, an increase in the incidence of only small or early tumors is probably related to increased health awareness and to the availability of medical care.

Problems encountered in comparing thyroid cancer incidence across tumor registries include lack of standardization of data collection, lack of precise definition of causes of morbidity and mortality, difficulty in distinguishing benign from malignant lesions, and varying prevalence rates resulting from different techniques used at autopsy and in examination of surgical specimens (especially of occult carcinoma). Some of these problems of ascertainment are minimized by the quality control procedures routinely conducted by the Surveillance, Epidemiology, and End Results Program (SEER) of the National Cancer Institute (NCI) in the United States. SEER participants maintain a population-based cancer reporting system for unique population subgroups located in many geographic areas, and quality control is periodically verified by NCI field staff, who reabstract and recode samples of records and conduct audits to ensure complete coverage of the SEER area by each participant. Coding of all cases is uniform. The SEER program area covers approximately 13% of the population of the United States and yields large numbers of thyroid cancer cases.

When comparing the incidence of thyroid cancer in different countries, one must consider the varying standards, availability, and/or utilization of medical care by different segments of the populace. Differences in ethnic incidence may be artifacts of this situation—for example, there is a high incidence of thyroid cancer among Jews who are generally well educated and presumably health conscious, whereas thyroid cancer is relatively rare in blacks and Hispanics who are in lower socioeconomic groups.

Problems Resulting from Lengthy Accrual

The prognostic evaluation of thyroid cancer requires a long follow-up period because it has been found that deaths, local recurrences, and distant metastases (DMs) appear as long as 25 years after initial treatment. Thus, reports on the result of treatment for thyroid cancer need follow-up for at least 20 years if series are to be meaningful (4). Such long follow-up periods result, however, in very aged patient populations that may have a deviated composition with respect to demographic, etiologic, histopathologic, and clinical factors.

Many series report less than 10-year follow-ups, particularly those that evaluate cellular and molecular prognostic factors derived from DNA technology. In many studies of this type, the length of follow-up is either relatively short or not stated. Ideally, such studies should be derived from stored blocks of tissue in which patient follow-up of 20 years is available; however this is generally not logistically feasible. Whether or not flow cytometry studies on blocks stored for such a length of time are comparable to those evaluated from recently prepared specimens is also open to question.

The lengthy accrual periods (decades) necessary for thyroid cancer create problems because over long periods of time changes have inevitably occurred in diagnostic and treatment methods, definitions of disease, and technical capabilities. For example, in the 1950s, radical surgery was common in the United States, as was the use of radioiodine and external irradiation, whereas in subsequent decades a more conservative treatment philosophy has emerged. Yet patients treated over this entire time period are generally included in the large extended treatment series that have been reported from prominent referral institutions. Ideally, series should be reported over a period of time that reflects relative uniformity in diagnosis and treatment.

Problems in Histopathologic Interpretation

Interpretation of thyroid cancer histopathology is not straightforward (5–10). When clinical data are collected from more than one center or over a long period of time, many different pathologists have participated, and there have been changes in pathologic terminology and interpretation of the significance of various findings over the years. That there is considerable observer variation in histologic classification of thyroid cancer between pathologists is attested to by a study from Scandinavia (11). In only 58% of nearly 700 cases of thyroid cancer did five individual observers agree on the diagnosis. Observer variations occurred in the number of carcinomas diagnosed and also in the classification of tumors in various histologic categories. Not surprisingly, observer disagreement is highest for follicular carcinoma, where the differentiation between benign and malignant forms can be difficult.

For the purpose of comparative studies, it is necessary to have all cases reviewed by the same pathologist, or a small group of pathologists, to obtain reliable results. Comparison between different countries and probably between different institutions within a country is unreliable because of varying definitions of what constitutes thyroid cancer and the different histologic types represented. For example, the inclusion of "small collections of thyroid follicles with vesiculated cells with ground glass or clear nuclei without sclerosis" by Harich et al. (12) in their definition of occult thyroid cancer, a category not included in the World Health Organization (WHO) classification, contributed to the greatly increased incidence reported from Scandinavia. Because a scheme for staging cancer of the thyroid has not been generally accepted in the past, data comparison between series is of limited value. The recent 1988 staging system represents concurrence between the American Joint Committee on Cancer (AJCC) and the TNM (tumor, node, metastasis) committee of the UICC (Union Internationale Contre le Cancer) (Fig. 1)—the type of standardization necessary to establish a uniform basis for reporting.

Reporting of End Results

A problem exists in the entire cancer literature on end-results reporting—deciding what is an appropriate means of assessing treatment outcome. Commonly used end points are "control in the treated volume" and "survival." It is important to study cancer-related survival rather than absolute survival in order to obtain an adjustment for deaths unrelated to cancer.

In general, survival is a "contaminated" end point for assessing cancer treatment outcome, because it is affected by deaths from other medical and nonmedical causes. For most carcinomas that are treated by surgery and external beam radiotherapy (RT), the appropriate end result to report is "control in the treated volume" (the primary tumor and the regional nodes), because surgery and RT are local/regional treatment modalities and do not directly influence distant metastases. Evaluation of treatment outcome is complicated for DTC because both local/regional (surgery) and systemic (radioiodine, thyroid hormone) treatments are frequently given to an individual patient. Local/regional control issues are also difficult to define because of the close proximity of the primary tumor and its regional metastases (thyroid gland and cervical nodes), which clouds the issue of whether recurrent disease occurs at the primary site or in the regional nodes.

The differentiation of whether patients die with or of cancer is particularly relevant for thyroid cancer but is seldom reported. One of the few studies that attempted to define treatment outcome on this basis was the study from the University of Michigan (13). Some reports in the thyroid cancer literature are quite lamentably lacking in regard to end-results reporting. For example, one article that purported to assess the significance of distant metastatic disease was undermined because it was not possible to define the cause of death in most of the patients in the series (14).

Statistical Issues

Many different statistical methods are used to interpret thyroid cancer data in various series, and this contributes to the difficulty in comparing retrospective series. In general, clinicians lack the requisite level of biostatistical sophistication necessary to report the confusing thyroid cancer data legitimately and must rely on a biostatistician to interpret the significance of the data and to choose the appropriate statistical parameters and methods (15,16). A large number of individual statistics can be found in the thyroid cancer literature, which arouses the suspicion of many that statistics can be manipulated to prove whatever point is desired. An attempt to ensure uniformity in statistical reporting for thyroid cancer data should be made.

Definitions

Primary Tumor (T)
All categories may be subdivided: (a) solitary; (b) multifocal—measure the largest for classification

[ ] TX   Primary tumor cannot be assessed
[ ] T0   No evidence of primary tumor
[ ] T1   Tumor 1 cm or less in greatest dimension limited to the thyroid
[ ] T2   Tumor more than 1 cm but not more than 4 cm
[ ] T3   Tumor more than 4 cm in greatest dimension limited to the thyroid
[ ] T4   Tumor of any size extending beyond the thyroid capsule

Lymph Node (N)
Regional modes are the cervical and upper mediastinal lymph nodes

[ ] NX   Regional lymph nodes cannot be assessed
[ ] N0   No regional lymph node metastasis
[ ] N1   Regional lymph node metastasis
    [ ] N1a   Metastasis in ipsilateral cervical lymph nodes
    [ ] N1b   Metastasis in bilateral, midline, or contralateral cervical or mediastinal lymph nodes

Distant Metasteses (M)
[ ] MX   Presence of distant metastasis cannot be assessed
[ ] M0   No distant metastasis
[ ] M1   Distant metastasis
    Specify

Nodal Involvement
Cervical unilateral _____   Cervical bilateral _____
Delphian _____   Mediastinal _____

Indicate on diagram primary tumor and regional nodes involved

Stage Grouping
Separate stage groupings are recommended for papillary and follicular, medullary, and undifferentiated.

Papillary or Follicular

Under 45 Years
[ ] Stage I   Any T, Any N, M0
[ ] Stage II   Any T, Any N, M1

45 Years and Over
[ ] Stage I   T1, N0, M0
[ ] Stage II   T2, N0, M0
                T3, N0, M0
[ ] Stage III   T4, N0, M0
                Any T, N1, M0
[ ] Stage IV   Any T, Any N, M1

Medullary
[ ] Stage I   T1   N0   M0
[ ] Stage II   T2   N0   M0
               T3   N0   M0
               T4   N0   M0
[ ] Stage III   Any T   N1   M0
[ ] Stage IV   Any T   Any N   M1

Undifferentiated
All cases are Stage IV
[ ] Stage IV   Any T   Any N   Any M

Histopathologic Type
The World Health Organization (WHO) classification of thyroid cancer should be used, including at least four major types:
Papillary carcinoma (with or without follicular foci)
Follicular carcinoma (extent of invasion of tumor capsule should be noted)
Medullary carcinoma
Undifferentiated (anaplastic carcinoma)
Unclassified malignant tumor

FIG. 1. Staging for cancer of the thyroid gland—American Joint Committee on Cancer, 1988.

For example, Beierwaltes (17) notes that when data from the Mayo Clinic supporting the nonlethal nature of DTC was reinterpreted by biostatisticians from the School of Public Health at the University of Michigan, all of the survival curves presented in the Mayo Clinic papers actually showed subnormal survival. Survival curves must be exactly matched to the thyroid cancer population being evaluated and cannot be matched to several different populations. The Mayo Clinic authors applied their normal life-table survival curve to three different populations. The Mayo Clinic paper had been taken as weighty evidence that patients with DTC do not die of cancer. This is no longer believed in view of more recent data and reinterpretation of the statistics.

Appropriately applied statistical methods can help compensate for some of the problems inherent in recording thyroid cancer data. Using the life-table method to estimate survival rate partially compensates for the requirement for lengthy follow-up because it enables the use of all survival information on the closing date of the study. The reliability of the method, however, presupposes that the survival experience for late entries in the study after the closing date is similar to that of patients under observation for the entire period, and this is not quite true for patients with DTC and therefore may lead to slight overestimation of the survival rate.

The death rate was used as the main statistic in generating the European Organization for Research on Thyroid Cancer (EORTC) index (18) and a question has been raised about the validity of using this statistic as opposed to the duration of survival plotted on Kaplan-Meier curves. Using the total death rate as the end point is justified for tumors with a high mortality rate but not for cancers with a high survival rate where deaths from causes unrelated to the cancer become increasingly probable. Using the total death rate as the end point, one underestimates the importance of tumor-related factors and overestimates the effect of age.

Univariate Versus Multivariate Analysis

With thyroid cancer, a number of variables are relevant to prognosis and some tend to be highly correlated with others. Many studies on thyroid cancer have separately analyzed prognostic factors, whereas only a limited number of multivariate or multifactorial analyses (MFA) have been published [reviewed in Schelfhaut et al. (19)]. Univariate analysis precludes an insight into the interrelationship between factors, whereas multivariate analysis helps determine the order of importance of several prognostic factors and has been used to advantage for other cancers where many prognostic factors are relevant, such as malignant melanoma.

Series that undertake MFA on a number of variables yield somewhat more information than series that do not, but they are still limited by variation in the patient population under discussion, and conflicting views of the significance of various factors persist despite the application of MFA. The contribution of a single variable in a multivariate model is assessed while adjusting for the other variables in the model, and this may help to explain why findings from MFAs sometimes differ from studies that look at only one variable at a time in a population whose composition of parameters varies.

The general consensus of opinion on the significance of prognostic factors for DTC is that age is by far the most important, with histologic type of cancer and the sex of the patient also very important. When the patient population is matched for age and sex, however, it has sometimes been found that the significant difference in survival related to histologic subtype (papillary versus follicular) disappears. On the other hand, with appropriate matching for important variables, differences that result from other significant variables emerge. For example, in the recent study of Schelfhaut et al. (19), tumor stage was the most important factor, followed by histologic subtype, with age at diagnosis and sex of lesser importance. In some MFAs, however, age is still found to be the primary significant prognostic factor for survival. Most discrepancies between the results of various MFAs can be explained by differences in patient selection, the coding of the variables, and the statistical methods. The advantage of an MFA is that the weight of each significant factor can be quantitatively evaluated and prognostic indices calculated.

An MFA is not easily performed, however, because it requires a large collection of controlled data and a suitable statistical method. Centers unable to perform their own analyses are inclined to use results obtained by others, and the questionable validity of this practice was recently documented (20). A population of 480 patients in Reims, France, was compared to three published MFAs—the EORTC study and two from Paris (Institut Curie and Institut Gustave Roussy studies). The studies showed that even when different populations are artificially homologized and the same statistical method is applied, unresolved discrepancies between the results cannot be attributed to different biologic behavior of the tumor as long as the covariate matrices in these populations are not known and differences in treatment are not measured. This severely hampers the application of the results from one multivariate study to other populations. The overall conclusion of the study was that for thyroid carcinoma the significant factors can change from one population to another, and that one should be cautious in applying results obtained by others when calculating a prognostic index. The creation of one's own MFA seems necessary before calculating a prognostic index.

The Value of Prospective Randomized Clinical Trials

Explaining differences between MFAs that use retrospective data is always risky and it is necessary to perform prospective analyses to find accurate explanations. In the absence of randomization of treatment and in dealing with a large number of relevant variables, it is not possible to analyze in detail the impact of each variable on all others, particularly in relation to survival, because there are relatively few deaths from this disease. Only when data are sufficient can a more detailed analysis of the effect of one variable on another (such as the effect of a given mode of therapy on a specific histologic cancer type) be evaluated. (If the number of deaths is insufficient to provide survival analyses, the frequency of recurrence is another criterion of effectiveness that can be used.)

The continuing discussion of the appropriate treatment of DTC with respect to the extent of surgery on the thyroid gland, as well as other issues, can be answered only by prospective randomized (PR) studies because of the rarity and the relatively indolent biologic behavior of the disease. Without such an approach, it is not possible to say which therapy is best for patients with DTC. DTC does not lend itself to strict management guidelines, and controversies will continue until a PR trial is done. This is a Herculean logistical problem. Also, many surgeons believe that they know what is best for their patients and therefore they do not submit patients to protocol study. Treatment managers have to believe that the question under investigation is truly important in order for PR studies to work.

Because of the overall favorable prognosis of DTC, it is difficult, if not impossible, to attribute changes in outcome to treatment without PR trial format. Some patients do well for decades without treatment. Relating a favorable or unfavorable outcome to treatment or lack of treatment is an assumption rather than a fact, and the outcome may relate to endogenous and exogenous factors that have little to do with the treatment carried out.

Because of the rarity of the condition, patients would have to be directed to treatment centers, a problem in the health maintenance organization (HMO)-dominated

United States. Because there are so many apparently relevant prognostic factors for DTC, any stratification variables would be involved, resulting in small numbers of patients in each group. With the new levels of technologic investigation, the problem is further complicated by the multiple layers of possibly relevant prognostic factors, from the level of the organism to the subcellular level.

Appropriate PR studies are not likely to originate in the United States. In 1986, it was noted that there had been a 9-year attempt to begin a prospective study, but attempts to get the National Institutes of Health (NIH) to fund such a study have been unsuccessful (21).

A PR study has been started at Karolinska Institute in Stockholm in patients with papillary thyroid carcinoma, in whom preoperative DNA measurement and fine-needle aspiration shows a diploid content. Patients with a UICC clinical tumor stage of less than T2N1M0 and age at diagnosis of more than 20 years are randomized between total thyroidectomy and radioiodine ablation versus hemithyroidectomy only. (If a higher tumor stage is observed intraoperatively, the patient is treated accordingly.) In a second group, patients with tumor stages of T2N2M0 or higher (without DMs), and older than 40 years at diagnosis, are randomized between total thyroidectomy, radioiodine ablation, and external radiotherapy versus total thyroidectomy and radioiodine ablation. It is expected that there will be no difference between total thyroidectomy and hemithyroidectomy in lesions confined to one lobe, and the role of external radiation will be evaluated (22).

HISTOPATHOLOGIC OVERVIEW/STAGING CONSIDERATIONS

Overview

The term *thyroid cancer* is almost meaningless without further subdivision and definition, because malignant disease in this organ is derived from several different cell types that vary significantly in their history (see also Chapter 6). Criteria for the histologic classification of thyroid cancers are subject to individual pathologists' interpretations and are controversial. Histologic findings often vary considerably within one lesion, and a large number of sections are necessary to obtain an accurate histopathologic diagnosis. The diagnosis of malignancy in thyroid neoplasms rests on the interpretation of specific architectural and cytologic features. For years, pathologists have attempted to define histologic features for malignancy of endocrine tissues with little success, and the diagnosis of malignancy still rests in many instances on the presence of metastases.

Cancers originate from each of the two major epithelial cell types in the thyroid: the follicular cell derived from the primitive foregut, which produces thyroxine and triiodothyronine, and the parafollicular or C cell, which is derived from the neural crest and produces calcitonin. Medullary thyroid carcinomas (MTC), derived from the C cell, make up about 10% of thyroid carcinomas (discussed later). The follicular epithelial cells of the thyroid gland are the source of two major groups of malignant neoplasms with striking differences in their growth pattern and natural history: well-differentiated carcinomas, often associated with an extremely good prognosis, and undifferentiated carcinomas, with an extremely bad prognosis.

In the past 15 years, thyroid cancer has generally been divided into four main histologic groups: papillary and follicular (together comprising the DTCs), medullary, and anaplastic. The mixed papillofollicular carcinoma is commonly included in the papillary category, and Hürthle cell types (Askanazy or oxyphil carcinoma) are usually included with follicular carcinoma because the criteria for malignant diagnosis and the biologic behavior are similar. Recent overviews of thyroid cancer are given in references 23–32.

Differentiated Thyroid Carcinoma

The DTCs together comprise 80% to 90% of thyroid carcinomas. Some authors maintain that the distinction between papillary and follicular thyroid cancer is of little more than academic interest and that there is essentially no biologic difference, whereas others disagree, citing differences in the age of occurrence, apparent epidemiologic factors, and natural history (33).

Confusion exists in the literature because of the changing definition of histologic types as well as interpretations of their significance. For many years, what we now consider papillary carcinoma was thought to be a benign lesion, and the natural history of follicular carcinoma is undoubtedly obscured by the inclusion in some series of follicular adenomas, which are difficult to differentiate histologically from follicular carcinomas. In addition, some papillary carcinomas have undoubtedly been incorrectly diagnosed as follicular (34).

Papillary carcinomas are the most common thyroid malignancies, are seen mainly in young patients, and have the best prognosis of all thyroid tumors. They are typically multifocal, not encapsulated, and invade the regional lymphatics and metastasize frequently to local lymph nodes in the neck. They are prone to local infiltration, possibly related to their unencapsulated nature, and this may explain their occasional local aggressiveness. A subgroup of patients will die from local extension of the tumor into vital structures of the neck. Distant metastasis, generally to the lungs, is also common.

Follicular carcinoma is most often solitary and encapsulated, invades veins, and, when it metastasizes, often involves bone and lungs. Neck metastases are seldom seen except in the presence of extensive capsular invasion of the gland or recurrent tumor. These growth patterns have led to the general conception that follicular carcinomas metastasize almost exclusively via the bloodstream, whereas papillary carcinomas metastasize predominantly via lymphatics.

Follicular tumors have the typical cytologic hallmark of ground-glass nuclei. Differentiating follicular adenoma from follicular carcinoma is notoriously difficult and the definition of malignancy has generally required demonstration of vascular or capsular invasion or the presence of metastases. The first two criteria are not universally seen as being significant. Some authors have felt that veins are seldom invaded (35) and, therefore, venous invasion cannot be regarded as a criterion for diagnosing the disease. There is a question as to whether the penetration of veins by thyroid tissue is mechanical in origin or a result of true malignant invasion. Other evidence, however, suggests that follicular carcinomas comprise a spectrum of biologic behavior based on histopathologic classification, ranging from very slightly invasive cancers with a low metastatic potential to aggressive neoplasms having a considerable incidence of fatal results, with the angioinvasive forms tending to disseminate as DMs.

Invasion of blood vessels is generally considered the most important criterion for distinguishing benign from malignant encapsulated follicular tumors, and modern immunocytochemical techniques have been applied to this problem. Immunostaining with factor VIII–related antigen (synthesized by endothelial cells) has been extensively used for the identification of normal and neoplastic endothelial cells in many situations, but it is not reliable for follicular thyroid tumors because endothelial cells disappear in vessels that are totally occluded by carcinoma, and antigen in formalin-fixed paraffin-embedded tissue is labile. *Ulex europaeus* I lecithin is another marker of endothelial cells that has the potential to surmount these problems (36).

A recent autopsy study of 138 patients without clinical thyroid disease yielded some interesting findings on the significance of capsular and extracapsular involvement (37). The glands were grossly well encapsulated, but in 86 patients focal capsular defects were found. In these areas of incomplete capsule, thyroid follicles were found outside the thyroid gland in the perithyroid areolar tissue and frequently in the strap muscles associated with the isthmus. Extrathyroid follicle accumulations could also be found outside the capsule when it was intact. Follicles were found within the capsule in 20 cases. Therefore, gaps in the capsule and the finding of follicles outside of the gland can apparently be a normal anatomic variant, especially in the vicinity of the thyroid isthmus and pyramidal lobe—an important finding relating to the criteria for diagnosing follicular carcinoma. Change in the thickness of the capsule as well as its defects can make the evaluation of capsular invasion challenging in thyroids with follicular tumors. New research on differentiated thyroid carcinoma histopathology and variants is listed in references 38–52.

Anaplastic Thyroid Carcinoma

At the opposite end of the spectrum from DTC is anaplastic thyroid carcinoma (ATC), one of the most rapidly growing and highly fatal of all human neoplasms. It is incorrect to consider this a single entity. Anaplastic thyroid cancer is generally subdivided into spindle cell, giant cell, and small cell types. Reevaluation using modern immunohistochemical techniques has shown that many cases formerly classified as small cell are in fact lymphomas (positive for leukocyte common antigen) or, more rarely, medullary carcinomas (positive for calcitonin)—an extremely important differentiation to make because of the treatability and better prognosis of these categories. Of the remainder, some cases show positive immunohistochemical staining for thyroglobulin (Tg), indicating follicular origin, but a significant number are so undifferentiated that they show no reaction with any antibodies used in immunoperoxidase studies (53).

Anaplastic thyroid cancer has a rapidly progressive course, shows local invasion early, and metastasizes widely below the clavicles, with an average life expectancy of 4 to 6 months after diagnosis. Anaplastic carcinomas are all classified as stage IV tumors, attesting to their dismal prognosis. Fortunately, they are rare and tend to occur later in life.

Although controversial, the literature suggests that ATC represents an end-stage development from DTC. ATCs have arisen in goitrous thyroids, and careful examination of resected tissues has frequently demonstrated benign tumors or well-differentiated carcinomas in close association with the anaplastic neoplasm. Simultaneous or prior associated "precursor" lesions have included papillary, follicular, Hürthle cell, and insular carcinomas in 7% to 100% of ATCs. The rate of conversion is unknown, but it is rare because undifferentiated cancers represent a small percentage of clinical cancer and an even smaller percentage of occult cancer, estimated at occurring in less than 1% of papillary cancers.

Evidence to support this type of transformation comes from histopathologic studies (35) in which a constant association of ATC with DTC was demonstrated, as well as areas of transition between the two. In a recent series, DTC admixed with ATC was found in the metastases of three patients (54).

Because ATC is not found in children and has a mean age at presentation of nearly 60 years, and because there is an association with preexisting DTC, it is suggested that over time the likelihood of exposure to a "transforming agent" increases. It might be expected that if conversion to more aggressive forms of undifferentiated carcinoma in longstanding DTC was common, the incidence of late deaths from thyroid cancer would continue at a steady rate as long as patients were followed. Evidence from some appropriate long-term clinical studies shows that this does not occur. Although some authors maintain that all ATCs arise from preexisting DTCs, it must be remembered that only a very small proportion of DTCs will progress to ATCs, and this eventuality is of only minor significance in determining the plan of treatment for DTC. More aggressive treatment of DTC is not indicated based on the unlikely eventuality of anaplastic transformation.

Clues to the nature of the unusual malignant progression of ATC have been sought in experimental animal models. Transformation of a slow-growing thyroid epithelial tumor into a more malignant spindle and giant-cell tumor has been demonstrated in mice (55), but serial passage of a thyroid-stimulating-hormone (TSH)-induced thyroid tumor over a 7-year period was necessary before the transformation occurred.

Beierwaltes (17) notes that the clinical pattern of development of anaplastic, rapidly fatal carcinoma from DTC simulates findings in fish and rats. TSH induction and promotion of thyroid carcinoma associated with chromosomal abnormalities yield a progression from well-differentiated TSH-dependent tumors through a transitional state to TSH-autonomous undifferentiated carcinomas that kill rats in as little as 13 days after transplant, with metastases to every organ. Clinically, it has been postulated that the high incidence of anaplastic carcinoma in Switzerland compared to the United States could be related to TSH stimulation, operating via an increase in follicular carcinoma in the past or through the effect of TSH on existing differentiated tumors.

The possibly causal relationship between therapeutic radiation and unusually aggressive thyroid cancer growth (and many other cancers) has been suggested for many years because some patients with papillary thyroid cancer treated primarily with external radiation underwent rapid enlargement with metastatic dissemination and death (56,57). In such case reports, the age at which the tumor develops is much lower than for most cases of ATC. Also, the fact that ATC is rarely, if ever, found in the children who have undergone radiation in infancy can be interpreted as evidence against radiation-induced transformation of DTC to ATC. It is not possible to determine a causal relationship because reports show ATC after both external beam radiation and ^{131}I treatments, as well as in cases with no previous radiation, and because of the small number of patients and lack of a controlled population. But by inference, radiation must be a rare cause of ATC in man.

Newer diagnostic techniques have yielded information that pertains to the transformation issue. In one series, 11 of 26 (42%) anaplastic carcinomas demonstrated Tg on immunohistochemical staining, indicative of a follicular cell origin (53). On the other hand, one study using DNA flow cytometry indicated that the majority of cases of ATC arise *de novo* rather than through clonal transformation of DTC (58). Of 126 cases of giant cell anaplastic carcinoma, 13.5% contained histologically well-differentiated tumor foci (mostly papillary) within or adjacent to the high-grade malignant tumor. Anaplastic carcinomas were generally aneuploid, but seven of the associated DTCs were diploid. Thus, coexistence of ATC and well-differentiated carcinoma is rare, and when it occurs, only one third of the well-differentiated tumors contain aneuploid cells. New research on anaplastic thyroid carcinoma is listed in references 59–63.

Medullary Thyroid Carcinoma

Medullary thyroid carcinoma (see also Chapter 32) was first described in 1959 (64), but its cytologic origin was not recognized until 1966 when it was suggested to be a tumor of thyroid parafollicular cells (65). MTC can occur sporadically as a unilateral thyroid lobe lesion without associated endocrinopathy, or it can present bilaterally, associated with multiple endocrine neoplasm (MEN) syndromes. MEN type IIA is characterized by bilateral MTC, pheochromocytoma, and parathyroid hyperplasia. MEN type IIB is typified by bilateral MTC and pheochromocytoma associated with a characteristic phenotype consisting of multiple mucosal neuromas and ganglioneuromatosis of the gastrointestinal tract. Both types are inherited as autosomal dominant traits with high penetrance. MTC can also occur as an autosomal dominant trait without associated endocrinopathy, and clinically this is the least aggressive form of MTC yet described (66).

In its natural history, MTC resembles papillary carcinoma by metastasizing to regional nodes; however, this presentation is associated with lower survival rates more typical of the expected pattern with solid carcinomas in other organ systems. The survival rates of MTC fall between those of DTC and ATC, with a 50% to 80% 5-year survival and a 20% to 50% 10-year survival. It is well established that MTC in individuals with MEN type IIB (mucosal neuroma syndrome) is an extremely aggressive tumor with fewer than 20% of patients surviving 5 years, as opposed to the more benign MEN type IIA (Sipple's syndrome).

Patients with familial MTC generally have a better prognosis because of screening and early detection of small lesions. The classic marker is calcitonin. Sporadic MTC is always associated with raised calcitonin levels, which may be extremely high. Calcitonin levels tend to be lower in the familial form than in sporadic cases, and a small but significant number of patients have normal baseline levels requiring provocative tests to stimulate secretion (calcium and pentagastrin are effective calcitonin secretogogues). In familial cases, measuring the circulating levels of calcitonin can distinguish family members who bear the gene.

Serial calcitonin measurements are used postoperatively in patients who have undergone thyroidectomy, and a rise indicates recurrence of the disease and usually precedes the onset of clinical symptoms. Histaminase and carcinoembryonic antigen (CEA) have also been found to be increased in some patients with MTC, but they are not reliable for early detection of disease.

No predictably effective therapy has yet been developed for disseminated MTC, and continued investigation of prognostic indicators is under way to identify the subset of patients who might benefit from adjuvant therapy in the future. New material regarding medullary thyroid carcinoma is listed in references 67–77.

Staging of Thyroid Cancer

Although staging for cancers in other head and neck sites is based entirely on the anatomic extent of disease, it is not possible to follow this pattern for the unique group of malignant tumors that arise in the thyroid. Because both the histologic type and the age of the patient are of such importance in the behavior and prognosis of thyroid cancer, these factors have to be taken into account in any staging system.

The attempt to define prognostic factors (prognosis, from the Greek meaning toward knowing) that will predict who will do poorly and, therefore, need particularly aggressive treatment, has traditionally been addressed by the TNM staging system, which has proven inadequate in many respects. Tumor stage (the anatomic extent of the malignant disease at diagnosis) is a valuable prognosticator in many malignant diseases but has generally been considered less so in thyroid carcinoma because of the questionable significance of metastatic disease (discussed in detail below). Recent reports increasingly suggest that tumor burden is, in fact, very relevant prognostically for thyroid cancer, but no standardized staging system has existed that is practical and accepted internationally. Most commonly, thyroid tumors have been classified as occult, intrathyroidal, or extrathyroidal, but histopathologic findings such as vascular invasion and intrathyroidal dissemination have also been used in nonstandardized ways as part of the basis for a division into stages.

The third edition of the AJCC manual for staging thyroid cancer (78) is reproduced in Figure 1. This version represents concurrence between the AJCC and the UICC for the first time. Clinical staging is now amplified by permissible inclusion of the results of radioisotope, computerized tomography (CT), magnetic resonance imaging (MRI) scans, and ultrasound, as well as biopsy of the primary tumor, lymph nodes, or other areas of suspected local or distant spread. All information available prior to the first treatment can be used, and all available clinical data are combined with pathologic study of the surgically resected specimen for pathologic staging. The surgeon's evaluation of gross unresected residual tumor is also included.

The primary differences between the second and the third editions of the AJCC manual with respect to thyroid cancer are using 4 cm as a dividing measurement in the definitions of T2 and T3, and not considering an age division for medullary and undifferentiated cancers.

In addition to the new AJCC staging system, a second edition of the WHO Histological Classification of Thyroid Tumors has been published, reflecting "important changes in our understanding of thyroid pathology" (78a). The first WHO histological classification was generated by an international committee of thyroid pathologists in 1974.

The separation of differentiated thyroid cancers into papillary and follicular has been amply justified and has been continued. The distinction between follicular adenoma and carcinoma is still based on identification of invasion or metastasis, with recognition that minimally and widely invasive subgroups should be separated. Another significant change recognizes that the majority of tumors previously diagnosed as "small cell carcinomas of the thyroid" are malignant lymphomas or small cell medullary or follicular carcinomas, and that these types should be excluded before the diagnosis of "small cell undifferentiated thyroid carcinoma" is entertained. In practice, this requires the use of immunohistochemistry in many cases.

In the new classification, immunocytochemistry is recommended as a useful adjunct but is not the prime basis of classification. In the future, a number of the subcellular methods of characterizing thyroid tumors may be included, such as DNA flow cytometry. This second edition should serve for at least the next decade. The epidemiology of cancer and the treatment of patients require a solid diagnostic foundation that must respond to change, but not so often that studies are frustrated by changing the rules in the middle of the game.

THE SIGNIFICANCE OF PROGNOSTIC FACTORS

The main reason treatment controversies persist is because methods cannot be compared without considering the relevant prognostic factors for thyroid cancer: age, sex, and tumor histology. These are in contradistinction to the usual factors considered prognostic for solid carcinomas reflected in TNM staging systems, which quantitate tumor burden.

Almost every one of the numerous articles written about treatment of thyroid cancer considers various combinations of the factors listed in Table 1 as being prog-

TABLE 1. *Factors that have been implicated in thyroid cancer prognosis*

Age
Sex
Histologic subtype
Histologic features
    Extent of capsular involvement
    Multifocal disease
    Marked atypia
    Loss of "ground glass" nuclei
    Tall-cell variant of papillary
    Oxyphilic metaplasia
    Solid, trabecular, scirrhous patterns
    Presence of vascular invasion
Tumor burden
    Primary tumor size/extent
        intra/extraglandular
    Lymph node involvement
    Distant metastases
Response to treatment
    Extent of primary surgery
    Extent of radioiodine uptake
Cellular-molecular-genetic factors
    HLA phenotype
    Oncogene composition
    Nuclear DNA pattern (ploidy)
    Receptor content
        Thyroglobulin
        Epidermal growth factor
        Nerve growth factor
        Vasoactive intestinal polypeptide
        Platelet-derived growth factor
        Adenylate cyclase
        Hormones (estrogen, androgen)

nostically significant. Almost every study looks at a slightly different combination of factors that have been deemed significant by the authors for reasons pertaining to the population under study. An exhaustive discussion of each of the prognostic variables listed in Tables 1 and 2 is beyond the scope of this chapter. Studies assessing the prognostic significance of individual variables in a univariate manner can be found to support the significance or insignificance of each item. Combinations of ranked prognosticators vary in significance between multifactorial analyses.

The situation is further complicated because, with modern technology, the prognostic significance of new parameters can be assessed. Traditionally, the prognostic factors that have been examined in thyroid cancer are those that are clinically significant or relate to morphologic features of primary or metastatic lesions detectable at the light microscope level. A current trend is to biochemically phenotype individual tumors and relate cellular and molecular parameters to individual tumor aggressiveness. In short, it is now possible to investigate whether macroscopic parameters are simply "epigenetic" manifestations of processes at the cellular and molecular levels, which are in fact the real determinants of the expression of carcinogenesis in the individual. Many and perhaps all manifestations of oncogenesis detectable in the organism are determined at the molecular level. For example, it is possible that the significance of age and sex for DTC relate to the underlying sex hormone status of the tumor host (see later). Similarly, the significance of the age factor has been attributed recently to an underlying increase in aneuploidy (80). However, the addition of subcellular parameters, and attempting to correlate them with macroscopic or clinical parameters, complicates the attribution of prognostic significance.

Because a number of prognostic factors are of significance for thyroid carcinoma patients, using one or more of them to attempt to predict survival in a single case or to define groups of patients with similar survival probabilities is difficult, and conclusions as to which variables are important and their rank order of importance varies among series. The variable significance of individual prognostic factors among series probably relates to different compositions of the population studied with respect to age, stage, and histologic type. (See previous section, Problems with the Thyroid Cancer Literature.) Large series with long-term follow-up have emerged in the United States from the Lahey Clinic, the Mayo Clinic, and the University of Michigan. Initial reports

TABLE 2. *Factors that have been implicated in the etiology of thyroid cancer*

Radiation (proven)
Dietary iodine
Goitrogens (chemical or dietary)
Preexisting benign thyroid disease
    Hashimoto's thyroiditis
    Graves' disease
    Goiter
Age
Sex
Ethnicity (Jewish)
Antecedent breast cancer
Gardner's syndrome
Partial thyroidectomy
Tonsillectomy
Allergy and skin conditions
Parathyroid adenoma
Alcohol consumption
Dietary calcium and vitamin D
Common drugs
    Phenobarbital
    Diphenoxylate
    Griseofulvin
    Bisacodyl
    Senna
    Spironolactone
Obesity
Multiparity
Oral contraceptives
Lactation suppressants
Estrogens

from the Lahey and Mayo Clinics generated risk-group definitions for DTC based primarily on age, and they led to the widespread belief that thyroid cancer grows more rapidly, metastasizes more widely, and kills more frequently in men past 40 years of age or women past 50 years of age. The age-based risk-group definition for DTC has been extended at the Mayo Clinic (81) to include the grade, extent, and size of the primary tumor as significant prognostic factors. The Lahey Clinic's updated series attributes significance to age, the presence of DMs, and the size and extent of the primary cancer, and it sets up a multifactorial system that defines high- and low-risk groups with a mortality rate ratio of 26:1 (82). Low-risk cases made up almost 90% of patients seen between 1961 and 1980, and the associated death rate was 1.8%. The high-risk group constituted 11% of cases and had a 46% mortality rate.

The low-risk group was composed of patients without DMs, men under 41 years, women under 51 years, and older patients with intrathyroidal papillary cancer or minor tumor capsule involvement from follicular carcinoma, and primary cancers less than 5 cm in diameter with no DMs. The high-risk group consisted of all patients with DMs and all older patients with extrathyroidal papillary cancer or major tumor capsule involvement by follicular carcinoma and primary cancers 5 cm in diameter or larger, regardless of the extent of disease.

One notable attempt to organize prognostic data for DTC was presented in 1979 by the European Organization for Research on Thyroid Cancer (EORTC) cooperative group (18). Because therapy was nonstandard and administered according to the practices at the participating centers, therapy was not considered as a variable in the analysis. (Strictly speaking, therapy can be ignored in studying prognostic factors only if it is known that therapy has no effect on the natural history of the disease. Most authors feel that this is probably not the case for DTC, because for some cell types it is quite likely that surgery, radiation, radioiodine, and hormone treatment are effective therapies even though their precise roles have not been documented in properly designed prospective randomized trials.) With DTC, incorrect conclusions can easily be drawn if outcome is attributed to treatment, unless particularly close attention is paid to prognostic factors.

In the EORTC study, the cell types were grouped as papillary, follicular (well-differentiated and less well-differentiated), medullary, epidermoid, and anaplastic. The median follow-up in the analysis was only 40 months, but it was possible to construct survival curves up to 6 years. Of 1183 patients from 23 hospitals in various European countries, a restricted sample of 507 patients was used for multivariate analysis, because it was only this number in whom follow-up data was adequate on all the variables needed. Unfortunately, survival curves were based on all causes of death rather than cancer-specific deaths, because information on the cause of death was unavailable.

The following variables were sufficient to predict survival: age at diagnosis, sex, principal cell type, presence of anaplastic carcinoma, T category (from TNM category, see following section, Tumor Burden), and number of metastatic sites. Lymph node status could be omitted because, with its correlation with the other variables, it did not add significantly to the ability to predict survival.

Based on regression coefficients from the model, a "simple" scoring system was devised for assigning patients to prognostic risk groups (Tables 3–5, Fig. 2). This process was putatively successful in defining groups of patients with widely differing survival probabilities. The observed 5-year survival rates ranged from 95% for risk group 1, to 5% in risk group 5. The separation of the survival curves in the study, based on the risk groups as defined, was so great that the authors considered it likely that any additional prognostic factors would be correlated with those already studied rather than on independent importance. Rationalizing the exclusion of therapy as a variable was also justifiable on this basis; the survival differences demonstrated with the variables chosen were so great that they were likely to overshadow any changes caused by therapy, unless such improvements were studied in well-designed randomized clinical trials.

TABLE 3. *Characteristics of risk groups*

Risk group	Number of patients	Patients' age (range)	% male	% MED or FLD	% ANAP	% T3	% single mets	% multiple mets	Observed 5-yr survival (%)[a]
1	173	29.6 (6–47)	22.5	5.8	0.0	4.0	1.2	0.0	95
2	102	49.6 (20–65)	33.3	33.3	0.0	4.9	5.9	0.0	80
3	96	59.7 (29–79)	35.4	41.7	1.0	19.8	22.9	0.0	51
4	68	64.3 (40–90)	44.1	50.0	17.6	45.6	45.6	1.5	33
5	68	66.6 (37–87)	41.2	4.4	94.1	64.7	25.0	10.3	5
All	507	48.9 (6–90)	32.5	23.9	15.2	20.9	15.4	1.6	64

[a]Calculated by the actuarial method (see ref. 21).
MED, medullary cell type; FLD, follicular less-differentiated principal cell type; ANAP, anaplastic cell type, principal or associated; mets, metastatic sites.

TABLE 4. *Prognostic index (EORTC) for thyroid carcinoma*

Age at diagnosis (yr)
  +12 if male
  +10 if medullary
    or
    if principal cell type is follicular less differentiated, provided that the associated cell type is not anaplastic
  +45 if the principal or associated cell type is anaplastic
  +10 if T-category is T3
  +15 if there is at least one distant metastatic site
  +15 in addition to above if there are multiple distant metastatic sites
  = Total score

This study developed a summary prognostic index that could be used to predict survival of individual patients, as a single stratifying variable in designing prospective randomized clinical trials, or as an adjustment variable in comparing uncontrolled series with other sets of data or historical controls. The institution of burdensome randomized clinical trials was considered potentially useful only in comparisons of risk groups 3 through 5, where appreciable mortality may be expected.

The EORTC study generated a numerical score for each of the prognostic factors identified, but this was not validated in a different group of patients (83). This study also noted that it was so cumbersome that widespread use was unlikely. Elsewhere, however, the EORTC prognostic index has begun to be used in determining the extent of surgery at the primary site and in prescribing postoperative radioiodine (84).

Tumor Burden

The controversy of whether or not young and old patients with DTC should be treated in an equally aggressive manner centers on the significance of tumor burden as manifested by the extent of disease at the primary site and in metastatic areas. Historically, tumor burden has been a less important factor in DTC than age, sex, and histologic type. Long-term follow-up of patients with DTC indicates that prognosis is less favorable than had been generally perceived in the past, and a number of multivariate studies have identified tumor stage as one of the most important prognostic parameters (19).

Updates of both the Mayo and Lahey Clinic series indicate the importance of tumor burden—in the former by extent and size of the primary tumor, and in the latter by size of the primary tumor and presence or absence of DMs. In a comparison of many prognostic variables in 113 patients from the Netherlands (85), the presence of DMs at diagnosis was the most important prognostic factor. A recent multifactorial analysis on 1055 cases of DTC from Norway collected in 1970 to 1979 showed that stage and age were the only significant prognostic factors (86). The impact of age on survival was clearly dependent on tumor stage, indicating biologic differences between tumors presenting in various stages.

Extrathyroidal invasion at the primary site is becoming increasingly recognized as a prognosticator of a poor outcome, although in some series it is not found to be a predictor of recurrence. Patients with this factor frequently have other ominous prognostic factors, such as

TABLE 5. *Risk groups based on total scores, with observed survival rates*

Variable	Levels	Number of patients	Number of deaths	Total months follow-up[a]	Death rate[b]
Age	0–30	91	4	5077.5	0.79
	31–40	79	9	4176.5	2.15
	41–50	84	25	3746.0	6.67
	51–60	87	30	3666.5	8.18
	61–70	119	69	3637.5	18.97
	71+	47	38	933.5	40.71
Sex	female	342	103	15428.0	6.68
	male	165	72	5809.5	12.39
Cell type	Anaplastic[c]	77	68	760.5	89.41
	MED[d] or FLD[e]	121	45	4769.5	9.43
	All other	309	62	15707.5	3.95
T-category	T0,T1,T2	401	106	18242.5	5.81
	T3	106	69	2995.0	23.04
Metastatic	none	421	122	19041.5	6.41
	single	78	46	2142.0	21.48
	multiple	8	7	54.0	129.63
All patients		507	175	21237.5	8.24

[a]Because only completed months were recorded, 0.5 has been added to all follow-up times.
[b]Death rates expressed in deaths/1000 patient months.
[c]Whether principal or associated.
[d]Medullary.
[e]Principal cell type follicular less-differentiated, provided associated type is not anaplastic.

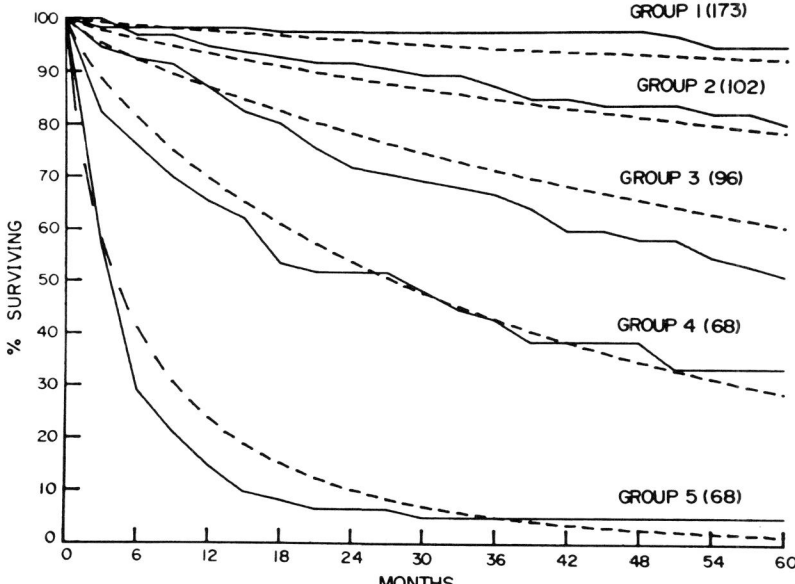

FIG. 2. Observed and predicted survival curves for the five risk groups.

large primary tumor size, older age, and more frequent metastases.

In the EORTC study (18), individual analysis of TNM factors revealed a significant decrease in prognosis as the extent of disease increased at the primary site. The survival curves for patients with T0, T1, T2, and T3 lesions (intrathyroidal) were similar and significantly more favorable than those with T4 (extrathyroidal) lesions. The condition of the regional nodes did correlate with survival, but the regional node status did not add to the ability to predict survival in the presence of the other variables included in the model. Patients with homolateral, contralateral, or bilateral mobile nodes did not differ significantly in survival, although both groups differed from that for N0 lesions "approaching" the $p = .05$ level of significance. All three of these categories differed significantly from that for fixed nodes. For DMs (assessed clinically or by radiologic methods), survival was significantly worse in patients presenting with metastases regardless of single or multiple sites.

Overall, the importance of tumor burden in many recent multifactorial analyses is superseding the sex factor, formerly considered the second most important prognostic factor for DTC (87).

The Age Factor

Although many human cancers have a worse prognosis in older patients, none shows as sharply defined an age separation between high and low mortality groups as DTC. The significance of the age factor generally attributed to the landmark Lahey Clinic publication (88) was first reported by William V. McDermott, Jr., of Massachusetts General Hospital in 1954, based on a study of 190 patients treated from 1913 to 1951. He found "the older the patient is, the poorer the outcome of the treatment; the younger the patient is, the better the prognosis."

There are a number of puzzling features about the age incidence of thyroid cancer that differ from cancers at other sites. There is a remarkable spread of age incidence of papillary carcinoma from the first year of life to extreme old age. Follicular carcinomas are seen in comparatively young as well as older adults. The peak incidence of thyroid carcinoma lies between 40 and 50 years of age, younger than the peak incidence of cancers in most other organs. The mortality of thyroid cancer is very much higher in patients over 40 years of age. Cancers tend to become more aggressive when the patient is nearing the age of 40, apparently unassociated with any concomitant alteration in histology and related primarily to the age of the patient.

It has been pointed out that the life expectancy of a person less than 21 years of age at the time of diagnosis of a DTC is the same as that of the normal population in spite of typically more advanced disease stage in this age group. (This truism is undergoing some alteration in interpretation based on results of long-term studies.) Because of the likely significance of sex hormones in the development of thyroid cancer (see later section, Studies on Sex Hormones and Their Receptors), it may be more relevant to place patients into subsets in the childhood category based on age: 0 to 8 years versus older than 8 years, rather than speaking of outcome in "children" versus "adults" (89,90).

Should DTC in Young Patients be Treated Equally or Less Aggressively Than in Older Patients?

The philosophy that advocates conservative surgical procedures for low-risk patients (primarily young) has achieved widespread support over the years, but controversy is reappearing (91).

Many studies indicated that in the good prognosis groups (young and female) treatment can be less aggressive than in patients with poor prognostic factors. Exemplary of this attitude is the Mayo Clinic's recent update (81), which found that children in general had more neck node metastases at diagnosis, less extrathyroidal invasion at the primary site, more DMs, and more frequent recurrence of nodal disease postoperatively, but not local neck recurrences. Significantly fewer children died with DMs than adults (14% versus 68%). Even though DTC in children was more often metastatic to neck nodes and lungs before initial surgery and more often recurrent in neck nodes postoperatively, it tended to be less fatal than in adults.

Similarly, Cady (92) at the Lahey Clinic found that there are a few patients in the younger age group who have bad features but that they can almost always be recognized on clinical grounds. Evaluation of a series of patients with bad features (unresectable or gross residual disease at initial presentation) found 92% of young persons to be alive and free of disease 5 years later, whereas only 31% in the high-risk group with comparable disease features were alive. Other recent studies also support the conservative approach to low-risk groups (93,94) and the increased risk of lifelong complications in children relating to total or subtotal thyroidectomy is emphasized. A counterpoint from an experienced thyroid cancer surgeon (95) is that there is considerable emotional trauma to both children and parents when reoperation over a 10- to 15-year period is required. This presumably can be avoided if adequately aggressive surgery is performed initially.

Opinion in the recent literature is numerically weighted toward recommending surgical treatment for children and adolescents that is equally aggressive, if not more so, to that performed in adults. Predicating treatment on the basis of clinical prognostic factors should be done with caution, especially when a less aggressive approach is advocated in younger patients.

According to the advocates of aggressive treatment for young DTC patients, reliance on the age factor alone to define a low-risk group is dangerous and can lead to a false sense of security. If younger patients are treated more conservatively than older patients, then some of the younger patients are undertreated, and DTC should be considered as a potentially lethal disease in the young (19). In one recent study, 72 children were followed for a median of 13 years (96). Despite relatively favorable long-term survival (90% at 20 years) excessive mortality caused by cancer was significant and the mortality ratio was in fact higher than that reported for older patients.

Some papers relate poor results to "a permissive surgical policy of incomplete cancer clearance" (97). Again, relating the issue of individual tumor aggressiveness to the treatment that the patient receives has not been proven to be valid in DTC, and such arguments relate mainly to Halstedian surgical oncology concepts.

Some findings suggest that DMs in young patients with DTC can be treated more effectively than in older patients, supporting a more radical treatment approach in younger age groups (13,98).

Prognostic Factors for MTC

A recent study looking at prognostic factors for MTC suggests that although this type of cancer arises from a different thyroid cell anlage, many of the same prognostic factors are as relevant as for DTC (99). For example, women do better than men, and patients under 40 better than those over 40. Patients with cervical soft-tissue invasion, regional lymph node metastases, and DMs did significantly worse than those without such disease extent. There was no apparent relationship between survival and tumor histology, histologic architecture, cytologic type, presence of amyloid, or intensity of calcitonin staining. Patients with the inherited form of the disease tended to have a better prognosis than those with the sporadic form, but the difference was not significant.

The distribution of CEA and calcitonin with biochemical phenotyping was studied for a variety of MTCs, some of which were early and localized and others late and diffuse (100). Results indicated that retention of CEA (a marker for early epithelial differentiation) and loss of calcitonin (a marker for terminal differentiation or cellular maturity) may reflect a degree of maturation block in tumor from patients with aggressive disease. Additional follow-up, confirmation, and clinicopathologic correlation are needed to assess the significance of such prognosticators.

Biochemical Phenotyping Prognosticators

The new era of subcellular technology enables the definition of a large number of parameters that are being investigated for prognostic significance. The inevitable tendency to attribute responses at the level of the organism to subcellular factors is seen with thyroid carcinoma. Several of the recent multifactorial clinical series refer to ploidy in explaining their results. The Mayo Clinic's update (81) suggests that the decreased incidence of fatality seen in children with DTC may be related to the infrequency of nondiploid DNA content in childhood tumors. Hamming et al. (85) studied patients without DMs in the Netherlands and found multiploidy was the only significant prognostic factor for overall survival (the analysis evaluated histology, tumor grade, extrathyroidal growth, nodal involvement, nuclear DNA content, age at diagnosis, and sex). For disease-free survival, multiploidy was second only to the age factor. Thus, it seems that nuclear DNA content is a prognostic factor in patients with DTC without DMs at diagnosis. The Lahey Clinic's update (82) suggested that in the future ploidy might become as relevant, if not more so, than histologic grade for prognostication, and that it was necessary to determine if DNA ploidy status represented an independent prognostic variable in papillary thyroid cancer. These studies show the current tendency to relate clinical processes to cellular and molecular mechanisms.

NATURAL HISTORY

The "natural history" of a disease process generally refers to its pattern of progression and outcome without treatment, and it serves as a baseline against which to measure putative treatment effects. Many long-term favorable outcomes are documented for DTC without treatment of any kind. Unlike many other entities, the natural history of thyroid cancer (emphasis on DTC) can also be deduced from treated patients, because the overall progression of the disease is indolent and the overall outcome is benign. In such a context, controversies over the efficacy of various types of treatment inevitably persist. Before examining the natural history of thyroid cancer in detail, it is helpful to review some recent principles of relevant tumor biology.

Tumor Heterogeneity

Tumor heterogeneity applies to tumor–host interactions from the organism to molecular levels. At the organism level, as outlined previously, thyroid cancer subtypes span the spectrum of malignancy from extremely slow-growing types compatible with an almost normal life expectancy despite metastases, through those with extremely aggressive behavior, with death following diagnosis often in a matter of weeks or months. Within this general classification, the aggressiveness of a particular histologic type of neoplasm remains unpredictable in the individual case. The multitude of relevant prognostic parameters confuse the issue further for DTC and the hope that studying them may guide more effective therapy tailor-made for the individual patients has not been realized yet.

It is hoped that modern cytogenetic techniques may reveal the critical features that determine the individual tumor-host interaction. A cellular and molecular basis for the variation in individual cancer behavior patterns seen at the clinical level is provided by the concept of tumor cell heterogeneity pioneered by the work of Fidler and Hart (101) and others (102,103). The original concept of a tumor population as the monoclonal expansion of identical cells frozen in a particular state of differentiation is no longer valid. It is now known that cells populating a primary neoplasm, as well as those in metastases, are not uniform but are biologically diverse and heterogeneous. Tumor heterogeneity exists for a number of biologic characteristics, including morphologic features, cell cycle–dependent phenomena, immunogenicity, tumorigenicity, sensitivity to treatment modalities, ploidy, cell surface receptors, enzyme markers, hormone receptors, growth rate, metabolic characteristics, platelet production, and metastatic potential. Clonal subpopulations within individual cancers have been detected.

Intratumoral heterogeneity is a dynamic phenomenon with a more or less continual emergence of new variant subpopulations that may differ in many characteristics and can also interact with each other to influence growth of metastases and sensitivity to treatment. Tumor cells tend to stabilize their varying proportions and impose an equilibrium on the conglomerate population. Removal of a major clone by some treatment modality can permit the other subpopulations to proliferate unchecked and become dominant. The diversified resurgent population is likely to be resistant to the treatment modality that killed the dominant clones(s) initially. In addition, the tumor cell population may contain intrinsically resistant cells and the mechanisms of their resistance may differ from those of acquired resistance.

This concept has important implications for treatment strategies. Certain therapies such as radiation and chemotherapy can act as selective agents on a heterogeneous tumor cell population by selecting out resistant clones that, when removed from intratumoral influences, can act in a particularly malignant manner. Such treatment modalities kill some, but not all, cells in a heterogeneous population, and residual tumor cells can then "take off." In some ways, surgery avoids this problem more than other treatment modalities because the entire tumor mass is removed at one time.

Metastatic potential in the past has generally been correlated with gross features of the primary tumor, such as site, size, and histologic differentiation. The concept of tumor heterogeneity as applied to metastasis suggests that the successful establishment of metastases represents the selective emergence of preexisting subpopulations of cells that are endowed with special properties that allow them to survive to complete the arduous, multistaged, and highly selective process of metastasis which contains a number of potentially lethal steps. There is evidence that this selection process is not random, which is fortunate because a random process cannot be manipulated therapeutically, whereas a selective process can be altered once the mechanisms that regulate it are discovered.

Historically, a poor patient outcome has usually been attributed to inadequate cancer treatment in some way. Based on our emerging understanding of events at the cellular and molecular levels, in combination with multifactorial clinical prognostic factors, the complexity of the tumor–host interaction can be imagined, and attributing a particular outcome only to the treatment the patient receives is somewhat naive. In many situations, but particularly in the case of DTC, it is almost impossible to attribute a clinical result to a particular treatment. The outcome may relate to poorly understood tumor–host interactions and may in fact be independent of treatment altogether. Oncologists in various clinical specialties have all seen "biologic survivors" who seem to do well despite an ominous TNM prognosis, regardless of the treatment that they receive. The converse is also observed—an inexorable downhill course with a putatively favorable situation despite heroic treatment efforts. Attempts, to date, to predict cancer behavior in the individual patient based on clinical parameters have been unsuccessful. Elucidation of underlying mechanisms with modern cytogenetic technology may be more successful.

Pathogenesis

Evidence from animal models of thyroid carcinoma suggests a transformation or progression through discrete stages from a benign to a malignant state (see later). Although various types of clinically benign and malignant thyroid lesions can be found in the same gland, accumulated evidence favors origin of carcinomas *de novo* in the human. In a careful histologic study of 80 serially sectioned thyroid glands, none of the primary carcinomas was associated with any pathologic change suggestive of a previously existing adenoma (35). If follicular carcinomas arose by malignant change in adenomas, one would expect the average age of the patients to be higher in the carcinoma group, but in several series there has been no significant age difference in patients who came to surgery for removal of a solitary nodule that proved to be either adenoma or follicular carcinoma.

It is postulated that neoplasia begins in MTC, with an abnormal stimulus or an abnormal response to a normal stimulus leading to diffuse hyperplasia of the C cells, which in turn leads to the development of carcinoma. No other significant factors are known to influence the development of MTC in man, although radiation has been reported to precede the development of MTC in an animal model.

Despite its rarity, MTC has attracted considerable interest during the past few decades, focusing on clinical, pathologic, and biologic aspects, and the tumor serves as a valuable model for studying tumor evolution and progression. It is popular as a target for study of neoplasia because the parent C cell has been clearly identified, the tumor cells produce a number of specific and nonspecific marker proteins that can be used to track the course of the disease, and familial cases occur in which a progression can be traced from preneoplastic C cell hyperplasia to MTC. The varied clinical behavior allows comparison of indolent tumors at one end of the spectrum with virulent tumors at the other.

Natural History of DTC

A classic study from the Lahey Clinic (88) illustrates well the natural history of DTC because it records changing patterns of disease occurrence over 40 years, an adequate period of time. In this series, the most remote first recurrence occurred within 25 years after operation and the most delayed death occurred within 30 years. Therefore, presumably all cancer-related events will have occurred by approximately 25 years postdiagnosis. Patients need lifelong follow-up.

The majority of early deaths occurred in the 6% of patients presenting initially with "incurable" disease, technically unresectable or metastatic. Even in these patients with presumably the worst prognosis, long-term survival could be seen, demonstrating that this is possible in some patients with DTC regardless of the extent of disease. Of these patients, 15 of 17 with DMs were dead of disease within 5 years, but two patients were alive and free of apparent disease 9 and 15 years after treatment. Twenty patients had locally unresectable disease and the only surgery consisted of biopsy for pathologic confirmation. Of these, 11 patients died of disease by 15 years after treatment (eight within 5 years). Eight of the patients, however, were living free of apparent disease from 17 to 26 years later. Of the 37 patients with "incurable" carcinoma, 26 died of disease but almost 60% of patients who were less than 41 years of age at diagnosis survived. Only 13% of patients 49 years or older survived. There are many anecdotal reports in the thyroid cancer literature of patients who were, for one reason or another, not treated, and who nevertheless lived for 20 or more years following diagnosis.

A 40-year follow-up of the Mayo Clinic series (104) on 859 patients with papillary cancer showed 6.5% of patients dying from the cancer. Death was associated with age greater than 50, male sex, large tumor size, tumor grade, initial extent of disease, and the absence of Hashimoto's disease. The mean time of death following operative treatment was 8 years (range of 1 month to 31 years). When DMs appeared, 36% of patients died within 5 years and 65% within 20 years. Large tumors greater than 4 cm were associated with the development of either local recurrence or DMs, and increased risk of death. Recent advances in diagnostic methods to detect recurrent and metastatic disease are discussed in references 105–122.

Death from DTC

The literature during at least the first half of the 20th century promulgated the view that patients rarely, if ever, die of disease. In fact, early on, papillary carcinoma was considered a benign rather than a malignant entity. In the

1960s and 1970s, however, studies began to appear that documented the occurrence of thyroid cancer-related deaths and the existence of a particularly aggressive subgroup of DTC. In fact, cases have been reported of clinically occult carcinoma that presented with large metastases and caused death (see later).

The generally indolent course of DTC is inferred from the disease process in untreated patients and from a local/regional failure much lower than expected from the known incidence of subclinical disease in neck nodes and the multifocal pattern in the thyroid gland. Patients who do not undergo elective lymph node dissection or who have less than total thyroidectomy require reoperation for recurrent nodal or primary disease in only 10% to 20% of cases. Multiple operations are sometimes necessary over time and the salvage rate is high.

The proportion of patients dying of DTC is difficult to assess because of inaccuracies in reporting sites of failure and because reports on this topic are not often expressed as the percentage of total patients treated. In one recent study (123), patients who died of DTC comprised 12% of the patients undergoing their initial treatment at M. D. Anderson Hospital between 1968 and 1977.

Several papers from state-of-the-art institutions have attempted to address the issue of how significant it is to clear a DTC patient of cancer (124). One study from the University of Michigan (13) evaluated the effect of persistent thyroid cancer in the patient on survival. The causes of death were carefully documented in order to categorize patients as being with or without DTC. The series reported on 51 patients with and 52 without disease who at some time in their course had metastases outside of the neck. In this series, 60% of the metastases were detected at the time of the first operation, and the remainder after an average of about 8 years. For papillary cancer, patients alive without disease survived 50% longer than those alive with disease—17 versus 11 years. Those who died without thyroid carcinoma survived 2.5 times longer than those who died with carcinoma—15 versus 6 years ($p < .0005$). Those alive and free of disease were half the age of those alive with disease—22 versus 40 years. For patients with follicular carcinoma without disease, survival was about 2.5 times longer than in patients with disease—17.5 versus 7.2 years. The patients without disease were younger than those with persistent disease—36 versus 57 years of age. (When patients were weighted by age and sex, no significant survival differences were found between the papillary and follicular histologic subtypes.) Overall, patients who could be rendered free of metastatic disease with ^{131}I survived 3 times longer than those who had persistent disease.

Prognosis

A recent update of the Michigan experience with 46-year follow-up, consisting of nearly 800 patients with DTC treated from 1940 to 1986, showed that 24% of patients died from thyroid cancer, 8% from other causes with extensive thyroid cancer present, 44% without thyroid cancer, and 24% with an unknown status of thyroid cancer.

Of the 42 patients dying because of thyroid cancer, 15 were men and 27 women. The mean age at diagnosis was 48 (+/-18) years, with one third of the dying patients presenting at age 45 or younger. The primary tumors were large, greater than 4 cm; 60% of the patients had local invasion and/or cervical metastases, and DMs were present in 21% of the patients at the time of diagnosis. The survival time and disease-free interval were significantly shorter for follicular than papillary neoplasms. However, the survival and disease-free intervals were often very long in both types prior to death. It was emphasized that onset of DTC before the age of 40 does not preclude serious sequelae and death, and that no known histopathologic features can consistently predict outcome.

The studies discussing this disease pattern have correlated poor outcome with various prognostic factors in an attempt to define high-risk patients, but they have been uniformly unsuccessful in accomplishing this goal. In general, deaths resulting from papillary cancer have been related to older age at diagnosis, a large primary tumor, angioinvasiveness of the tumor, local aggressiveness manifested as local recurrence in the neck, and the presence of DMs. The impression emerges that the single most important prognosticator is age at presentation, with death from cancer being very rare in young people. In older patients, papillary carcinoma of the thyroid, although histologically the same, may not be the same tumor or the same disease because of a highly undifferentiated component and/or propensity for invasiveness.

Although it is generally accepted that in patients with papillary thyroid cancer who die of disease, uncontrolled local cancer is usually the contributing factor (involvement of larynx, trachea, recurrent nerve, cervical esophagus, and major neck and mediastinal vessels), a tumor can locally attain a large size and be present for many years, with some degree of direct invasion of neighboring structures, without progressing to a fatal outcome. Also, local recurrences can be cured by further treatment in a significant proportion of cases (40%), with the pattern of curability of first recrudescence unaltered by the time of appearance of the recurrence or metastases [the percentage of patients with extraglandular disease progressively decreased over the years, from 67% in 1931 to 1940 to 11% in 1961 to 1980 at the Lahey Clinic (88)].

A recent update of the Lahey Clinic series (82) addresses the significance of incomplete removal of cancer. In the subgroup of patients in whom all apparent disease could not be removed with surgery because of massive unresectable neck disease, gross residual disease left in the neck postoperatively, or DMs, death owing to cancer was related to risk-group classification (low versus high as defined by age and sex) rather than to extent of disease or management. Patients in the low-risk group could overcome massive negative factors such as tracheal wall invasion and DMs. Patients in the low-risk group with "incurable" neck disease died of local (30%) or metastatic (3%) disease; patients in the high-risk group died of these causes more frequently (26% and 31%, respectively). Thus, the risk of death from disease in the low-risk group was low even when resection was incomplete. Local recurrence is not synonymous with lack of survival for DTC because the situation can be salvaged frequently.

Thus, we see that opinion differs on the significance of cancer clearance to the DTC patient. In the Michigan series, emphasis is placed on the importance of clearing the patient of disease, whereas in the Lahey Clinic series, details of the disease presentation and management were subordinate to the risk factors of age and sex. New information on the prognosis of DTC is discussed in references 125–132.

The Significance of Metastatic Disease with DTC

Metastasis is a very complicated multistage cascade process involving many different interactions between tumor and host, and it is influenced by humoral, cellular, endocrine, nutritional, metabolic, and chronobiologic factors that currently are largely undefined. Complex factors, including tumor growth rate, degree of differentiation, the presence or absence of barriers to spread, blood supply, tumor–host immunologic interactions, and cancer treatment modalities, have an impact on the tumor–host relationship in ways that are poorly understood. For carcinomas in other organs, cancer spread to regional lymph nodes (RLNs) is generally conceded to be the most significant prognosticator of patient outcome because this predicts distant spread with a uniformly fatal outcome. The traditional and modern view of cancer spread from solid carcinomas and their implications for treatment strategy (Table 6) are beyond the scope of this chapter [see Collins (133) for an in-depth discussion]. For most solid carcinomas (head and neck, lung, breast, colon, genitourinary) the modern era has seen better local/regional control of disease achieved with combinations of conventional therapy, but patients are not surviving longer because the cause of death is changing. They now succumb to DMs more often, and this is a major limiting factor in the ultimate cure of these patients.

The situation with DTC is generally considered to be almost completely different from the typically dismal prognosis associated with metastatic disease for other solid carcinomas. We shall see if it really is. The presence of metastatic disease in DTC patients has historically been considered so trivial as to be inconsequential in treatment strategy. In some cases, metastatic disease has been stated to convey a survival advantage to the patient! The basis for such an interpretation of metastatic disease in DTC is reviewed below including some of the unusual, if not bizarre, observations and interpretations that have been applied. Opinion is beginning to acknowledge that at least the process of distant, if not regional, metastasis is in fact quite ominous for the DTC patient.

Neck Metastases

The primary lymphatic drainage from the thyroid to the mid and lower jugular chain is depicted in Figure 3. Mediastinal nodes are one of the principal drainage routes of the thyroid gland and undoubtedly harbor many occult lymph node metastases, although there are reports that the anterior/superior mediastinum is involved only in

TABLE 6. *Two divergent hypotheses of tumor biology*

Halstedian	Alternative
Tumors spread in an orderly defined manner based on mechanical consideration	There is no orderly pattern of tumor cell dissemination
Tumor cells traverse lymphatics to lymph nodes by direct extension supporting *en bloc* dissection	Tumor cells traverse lymphatics by embolization challenging the merit of *en bloc* dissection
The positive lymph node is an indicator of tumor spread and is the instigator of distant disease	The positive lymph node is an indicator of a host tumor relationship, which permits development of metastases rather than being the instigator of distant disease
Regional lymph nodes (RLNs) are barriers to the passage of tumor cells	RLNs are ineffective as barriers to tumor cell spread
RLNs are of anatomic importance	RLNs are of biologic importance
The bloodstream is of little significance as a route of tumor dissemination	The bloodstream is of considerable importance in tumor dissemination
A tumor is autonomous of its host	Complex host tumor interrelationships affect every facet of the disease
Operable breast cancer is a local/regional disease[a]	Operable breast cancer is a systemic disease[a]
The extent and nuances of operation are the dominant factors influencing patient outcome	Variations in local/regional therapy are unlikely to substantially affect survival

[a] May apply to other solid carcinomas as well, but can not extrapolate between organ systems without confirmatory data.
Modified from ref. 427.

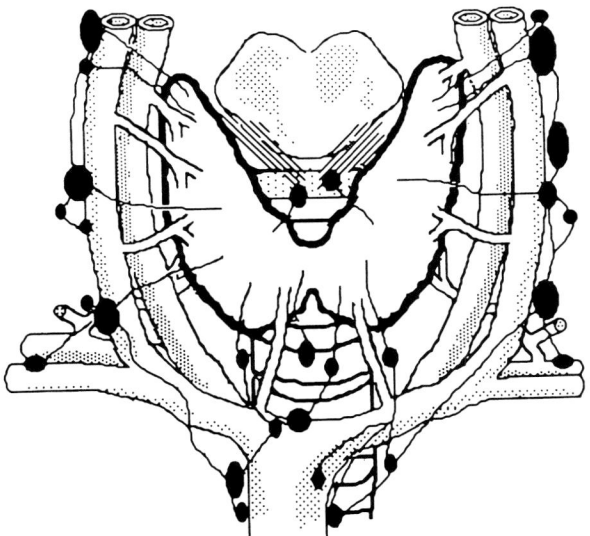

FIG. 3. Lymphatics of the thyroid gland. (Modified from ref. 139.)

patients with tumors in the recurrent laryngeal nerve chain. Submental and submandibular areas are not typical drainage routes for thyroid cancer, and it is generally acknowledged that in the absence of palpable disease dissection in this area is not necessary for DTC. In fact, the third edition (1988) of the AJCC staging of thyroid cancer states that "metastases to submandibular and submental nodes are considered distant spread." Metastatic nodes may undergo cystic degeneration and be misdiagnosed clinically as branchial cleft cysts.

When elective neck dissections are performed systematically, up to 90% of all patients with papillary thyroid cancer have metastases in regional nodes, and an enlarged lymph node is not infrequently the first clinical manifestation of papillary thyroid carcinoma. If no neck dissection is performed, nodes develop later in 7% to 15% of cases with a mean delay of 4.5 years (with a range of 7 months to 7 years) (134).

In the 1960s, the finding of apparently benign thyroid follicles in lateral cervical lymph nodes (found incidentally in neck dissection specimens done for malignant tumors of nonthyroidal origin) suggested that these deposits had developed through a process of benign lymphatic transport in a manner analogous to endometriosis (135,136). The concept of "lateral aberrant thyroid" was quickly challenged when concurrent small primary carcinomas of the thyroid were demonstrated.

Metastases to cervical nodes are found in a greater proportion of younger than older patients. The frequency of regional metastases is not directly related to the size of the primary tumor.

In follicular cancer, lymph node metastases are far less common but have a more negative implication for prognosis. In one series (137), 12% of patients with nodal disease had follicular carcinoma primaries.

With anaplastic carcinoma, neck nodes are usually involved, although the primary tumor and involvement of the soft tissues of the neck are frequently so extensive that regional node status is difficult to assess. In contrast to the mobile nodes associated with differentiated lesions, those associated with anaplastic carcinoma are often "fixed." Cured patients (who are rare) have disease confined to the gland and regional nodes, without extension into the soft tissues of the neck.

Medullary carcinoma is associated with palpable lymph nodes at presentation in 25% of the patients, and 50% to 75% of all patients have positive nodes at operation. Involvement of mediastinal nodes is also common. For MTC, positive nodes have the usual relationship to survival found with other carcinomas—prognosis is decreased by 50% in patients with positive nodes. In a Mayo Clinic series (138), clinically apparent tumor recurrences following resection with curative intent in 128 patients were noted in almost two thirds of the patients with positive nodes, and in about 10% in those with negative nodes. The majority of recurrences were local or regional (neck and mediastinum). Therefore, surgical treatment of MTC generally includes total thyroidectomy and bilateral neck dissection because of the high incidence of occult metastases and because of permeation of the soft tissues of the neck. Postoperative external beam radiation is also recommended. Medullary carcinomas do not concentrate radioiodine or suppress with thyroid hormone. Adjuvant chemotherapy is considered more frequently now as an additional treatment to attempt to control local/regional disease.

The biologic significance of cervical metastases from DTC is not entirely clear. Some authors feel that nodal disease can be a serious factor in survival, and others suggest that positive nodes have a paradoxically favorable influence. Extracting valid illuminating data to help resolve this controversy is difficult because the literature is usually based on patients in whom positive nodes have been identified and treated, and thereby it incorporates treatment bias. The discovery of nodes at surgery may have been an alarming sign to the clinician, prompting more extensive treatment that otherwise might have been delayed or not instituted. Also, because the primary tumor and neck node metastases are in close proximity, it can be difficult to separately evaluate the significance of extrathyroidal invasion from the gland and the presence of nodal metastases. The concurrence of another poor prognosticator such as advanced age or extrathyroidal invasion has undoubtedly influenced the results of many reports on the significance of nodal metastases. The general consensus is that survival for DTC appears unaffected by nodal involvement or the extent of its treatment.

Nodes involved by DTC are usually discrete and mobile for many years without extracapsular spread (ECS).

Sometimes enlargement after as long as 30 years of dormancy has been observed. In one author's experience (139), cancerous peritracheal nodes have a greater tendency to invade neighboring structures than do the jugular nodes.

At least one study claimed that invasion through the nodal capsule was of significant prognostic value (80). In another study (87), when patients with and without nodal involvement were compared, there was no significant survival difference for DTC, but when patients with and without extranodal invasion were analyzed, nodal involvement demonstrated a deleterious influence. Another recent report (140), however, compared the survival of 25 patients with ECS to 63 controls and showed no statistically significant difference in regional recurrence, DMs, death from cancer, or recurrence-free survival between the two groups.

More than 30 years ago, George Crile, Jr., pointed out that patients with thyroid cancer die from invasion by the primary tumor or from remote metastasis, and not from uncontrolled cervical node metastasis. Excluding anaplastic carcinoma, papillary carcinoma is the most common histologic type to extend through the thyroid capsule. Interestingly, extracapsular extension at the primary site appears to correlate with extension through the capsule of the regional nodes. It is generally considered that extrathyroidal extension into the soft tissues of the neck from the primary site influences survival negatively to a much greater extent than does the presence of nodal metastases. Although some authors observe an increased rate of neck recurrence in patients with positive nodes, this is generally observed in the older age group and has no adverse affect on survival as an independent factor. Some do not even find more recurrences. Other reports suggest, however, that extracapsular/extranodal extension does not affect survival unless it precludes surgical excision and even in this context, the Lahey Clinic data on technically unresectable cancer (see preceding) show that prolonged survival is possible. In one study, survival or recurrence did not significantly differ between patients with disease in the gland only and those with disease in the gland plus neck nodes.

The unusual "insignificance" of lymph node metastasis in papillary thyroid cancer derives from the 1976 Lahey Clinic report (88) in which lymph node metastases were interpreted to exert a protective effect in all categories of disease. This was directly related to the number of lymph node metastases—no deaths occurred in patients with more than ten positive nodes. Even patients with local recurrence did better if nodal metastases were present at the time of recurrence. The apparent protective effect of positive lymph nodes was related to their putative role as biologic depots for antitumor immunosurveillance [the significance of the RLN in this context has been widely debated for many years (133)], or because they called attention to the presence of the primary tumor when it was small and amenable to complete surgical removal. The series was not weighted with respect to age, now considered to be the flaw that invalidates the conclusion concerning the "insignificance" of positive cervical nodes in DTC. Because the age of the patient is known to affect the prognosis of DTC so strongly, the prognostic significance of metastases to the RLNs (or any other prognostic factor) can be determined with certainty only if the patients are matched by age.

In a counterpoint series, (137) the recurrence rate and mortality of patients with and without metastases to the RLNs were compared on age, sex, pathologic findings, and the extent of nodal involvement. Mean follow-up was 17 years. The mortality of thyroid cancer in age-matched patients with and without metastases to nodes showed a worse prognosis for patients with metastases ($p < .05$), although age influenced survival to a greater extent than did the number of involved nodes. In patients without nodes, only 8% died of thyroid cancer and all were older than 40 at the time of operation. With nodes, patients dying of disease increased with age from 11% to 50%. The conclusion was that nodal disease does have an adverse effect on prognosis, especially in older patients—41% of patients over 40 with involved nodes died of thyroid carcinoma. Thus, this study placed an entirely different perspective on the significance of positive nodes with DTC than did the Lahey Clinic series.

A lively discussion followed this study, attesting to the difficulty surgeons have in reconciling this new finding with the negative findings of a number of other large series. The conclusion was defended by Dunphy (137), who thought that if patients were carefully matched by age, it would be found that DTC behaves as do carcinomas in other sites, but that is a more benign disease in younger patients. It was pointed out that the adverse effect of RLN involvement is masked if the patient series includes relatively few elderly patients. The matched series in Harwood et al. (137), reported previously, dealt with a predominantly older age group, and this probably accounts for the dire prognostic significance attributed to nodal involvement.

Thus, the issue is still cloudy because of the difficulty of comparing series resulting from unmatched populations differing presumably in other significant factors, such as age and concurrent presence of extrathyroidal cancer extension. It does not seem, however, that the presence of positive node metastases confers a protective advantage to the DTC patient, and cancer in neck nodes seems to be better tolerated in young patients than in old.

The influence of the type of operation for RLNs is also difficult to assess. Treatment of neck nodes has been guided by extant surgical oncology concepts that change over time. For example, radical neck dissection was generally performed through the 1950s, consistent with the Halstedian principles applied to all solid carcinomas. Halstedian surgical oncology postulated that if every cancer cell could be surgically removed from the patient's body by performing a large enough operation, then the patient would be cured. The fact that solid carcinomas are systemic from a time preceding clinical detection of the primary tumor negates the validity of this concept in the modern era (see Table 6).

But traditional surgical paradigms die hard and modified "Halstedianism" persists in the literature (141). Routine node sampling of the ipsilateral lower jugular chains in thyroid cancer cases is recommended to satisfy the need for completing a formal modified neck dissection. Although the authors concede the usually successful outcome for DTC regardless of neck treatment, they are uncomfortable about leaving residual disease in the neck based on the known high incidence of occult spread to the nodes, and they advocate complete cancer clearance of occult disease to "prevent the emergence of future malignant disease in at least some patients." In the 1960s, neck operations for DTC switched to the opposite end of the spectrum, with no operation or "node plucking" being considered adequate, a heretical deviation from Halstedian principles, championed by George Crile, Jr. (his father had performed the first modern radical neck dissection in a patient with thyroid cancer). Simple removal of individually involved nodes could result in long-term disease-free survival (30 years), although repeated excisions might be necessary. In one of Crile's patients, 22 procedures were necessary over time to render the patient disease free (142).

This policy is also advocated in the recent literature. One series shows that for limited nodal involvement, modified neck dissection is not superior to node plucking combined with an ablative dose of ^{131}I, except when metastases are lateral to the carotid artery (143).

The surgical controversies concerning the extent of operation required both at the primary site and in the neck persist because those who die of papillary thyroid cancer have uncontrolled local/regional growth that presumably might have been prevented if the source had been removed early. The issue is confused by the frequently noted observation that although recurrence rate in the neck is higher in patients with positive nodes (and increases as the patient ages), survival does not appear to be adversely affected because recurrent disease is salvageable (144). Similarly, the extent of neck recurrence has been correlated with the magnitude of surgery, but a corresponding correlation with survival is not found (145).

Generally accepted principles for management of neck disease with DTC include the following:

1. There is no need for *en bloc* dissection, because lymph node metastases from DTC rarely implant in the surgical field and seldom extend beyond the lymph node capsule.

2. There is no place for radical neck dissection for DTC, because modified neck dissection with preservation of important structures (internal jugular vein, spinal accessory nerve, sternocleidomastoid muscle) is all that is necessary.

3. There is no evidence that prophylactic node resections in the absence of gross nodal enlargement play any role in management despite the high incidence of occult nodal metastases. Postponement of neck dissection until nodes become palpable does not compromise prognosis.

4. Control of regional metastases is unlikely to influence the overall length of survival, although generally a higher recurrence rate in the neck is seen in patients with positive nodes, and there may be a small group of patients saved by controlling the neck disease. This can be accomplished secondarily in many cases.

5. Nodal metastases or nodal or primary tumor recurrences do not lessen the curability in any stage of disease.

6. The extent of surgery for similar stages of disease seems not to be a major determinant of survival.

7. Lymph node involvement is more important with respect to local recurrence than survival, but, in general, soft-tissue involvement of the neck from the primary tumor seems to carry a worse prognosis than nodal involvement. Nodal involvement is a predictor of tumor recurrence but seems unimportant with respect to survival, which further suggests that management of nodal recurrence is successful (134,138,146,147).

New material regarding neck metastases is listed in references 148–158.

The Relationship Between Positive Regional Lymph Nodes and Distant Metastases in DTC

Whereas for most solid carcinomas the presence of regional metastases predicts the eventual development of DMs, the relationship between the two is difficult to define for DTC. Clinical conclusions are hampered because the incidence and location of metastatic disease is related to the histologic cancer type and the thoroughness of the search. It appears that for papillary cancer, the involvement of lymph nodes does not necessarily increase the risk of DMs (159). On rare occasions, papillary cancer will spread via the bloodstream in the apparent absence of nodal involvement. Follicular carcinoma usually spreads to bone or lung without first (or ever) invading the lymph nodes.

A direct pathway of disease extension from neck to lung has sometimes been suggested because ^{131}I scans can show tracts of uptake between the thyroid bed and the lungs, especially behind the sternoclavicular joints. In some series, lung metastases are more frequently found in patients with involvement of the recurrent laryngeal nerve node chain, suggesting dissemination via permeation of regional lymphatics (96,160). One study maintained that mediastinal lymph node involvement represented secondary metastasis from pulmonary metastases instead of direct invasion from involved cervical nodes (14). The conjecture that pulmonary metastases arise by permeation from neck lymphatics is a remnant of Halstedian surgical anatomy principles and ignores the fact that metastatic spread of solid carcinomas is now generally conceded to be embolic in vascular channels and to occur simultaneously in lymph and blood.

The permeation theory is supposedly supported by indirect evidence such as the hematogenous dissemination responsible for bone metastases, which occurs more frequently in the absence of cervical lymph node involvement. This more likely reflects the histology of the primary tumor—follicular versus papillary. To assume that papillary and follicular carcinomas spread by strictly separate channels (lymphatic versus hematogenous) is naive, based on modern knowledge of lymphaticohematogenous communications in metastatic spread. Because the thyroid is an endocrine organ with a luxurious blood supply, access for hematogenous metastatic dissemination is readily available and attested to by the occurrence of occasional fatal DMs resulting from occult thyroid primaries.

The Significance of Distant Metastases in DTC

With most solid carcinomas, the diagnosis of DMs is a harbinger of fatality in an average of 9 months. With DTC, however, the presence of metastases has traditionally been considered more of a confirmation of the malignant nature of the lesion, a sometimes difficult distinction based on histopathology of the primary tumor. The bizarre natural history of DTC is manifested most obviously in the absence of survival disadvantage for patients who develop metastatic disease.

Relatively few papers in the literature shed light on the true significance of DMs, because of inadequate reporting of sites of failure at the time of death and the cause of death in retrospective series accumulated over a long time. For example, one paper that purported to discuss the significance of pulmonary metastases in DTC failed in its objective because the cause of death could not be established for most of the patients (14).

Knowing the true significance of DMs for DTC has implications for treatment of the primary tumor. The controversy over total versus subtotal thyroidectomy versus lobectomy is related in large part to the need to remove all primary thyroid tissue—a competing source of uptake of ^{131}I, which is used in the treatment of concurrent or subsequent DMs. If untreated DMs have no survival disadvantage to the patient, then this surgical controversy loses its impact.

This issue is further confused because treatment of DMs varies between decades and countries. Over the years, DMs have been increasingly treated with ^{131}I at certain institutions in the United States. However, in earlier times and currently in most foreign countries, ^{131}I therapy for DMs is rarely used. The controversy over the benefit of treatment for DMs is also clouded by studies attributing a favorable outcome to treatment when other important prognostic variables such as age and sex are not controlled.

The incidence of DMs varies significantly in the literature because of heterogeneous study populations (see earlier section, Problems with the Thyroid Cancer Literature). The highest rates seem to occur in young people, and in European series in contrast to lower values observed in American series. Clearly, the incidence of subclinical metastases detected depends on the aggressiveness with which such disease is diagnostically sought, the length of follow-up, and the method of treatment of the primary tumor. If significant thyroid tissue remains in the neck, radioiodine scans will have decreased ability to detect DMs because thyroid tissue anywhere in the body successfully competes for uptake.

For DTC, the incidence of metastasis outside of the neck is 10% to 50% as reported in the literature as a whole. In several large series from referral centers in the United States and elsewhere, the incidence is approximately 7% to 12% (14,161,162). In general, the incidence of DMs increases to some extent based on histologic type: papillary least, follicular intermediate, and Hürthle cell most frequent [9%, 13%, 25%, respectively, in one recent series (161).] In the aggregate, fewer than 1% of all patients with papillary carcinomas and 3% to 5% of those with follicular cancers have DMs at the time of diagnosis. DMs developed subsequently in 4% to 20% of all well-differentiated tumors.

The amount of time to occurrence of DMs depends on the extent of surgery at the primary site, according to some authors, and the aggressiveness with which the diagnosis is sought. In the University of Michigan series (13), 40% of patients with DMs were first given this diagnosis on an average of almost 8 years after the initial operation (patients were treated with ^{131}I after near-total thyroidectomy). In another series (162), 45% of the cases were diagnosed within 1 year of the primary diagnosis or simultaneously; however, they continued to occur as long as 17 years after the initial diagnosis was made. Similarly, in another series (163), DMs were discovered with a maximum frequency during the first 6 months after treatment of the thyroid tumor. Although the annual recurrence rate decreased, DMs could be discovered as long as 41 years after the initial treatment. Therefore, follow-up should be most intensive early on but is needed indefinitely.

It is generally thought that DMs are less important in patients with papillary than follicular cancer. This is probably because of the relative treatability of the metastases in papillary carcinoma, which are typically in the lung, as opposed to the relative untreatability of metastases from follicular carcinoma, which are frequently skeletal. In the University of Michigan series (13), however, survival time was the same for patients with papillary or follicular carcinoma and metastases outside the neck when patients were matched for age and sex.

In contradistinction to past studies, a number of recent ones suggest that DTC patients with metastases outside of the neck have a significantly decreased survival rate when compared with patients without metastases or with a control population. Mortality in DTC is primarily related to the presence of DMs, a phenomenon independent of the size of the primary lesion or the presence of neck metastases, as distinct from other solid carcinomas.

A look at the natural history of DMs can be obtained from a report from Norway (162). At this referral center, postoperative ^{131}I treatment was rarely used. More than 50% of patients died within 1 year of the diagnosis of DMs and 70% within 2 years. Three patients survived for more than 10 years after the diagnosis, two with pulmonary and one with skeletal metastases. The location of the metastases seems unrelated to the length of survival.

A 1974 review of the literature indicated that more than 75% of patients with thyroid cancer and DMs die within 5 years of diagnosis. Other summaries found that 27% to 75% of patients with DMs die within the first 5 years. From another viewpoint, it has been reported that in patients who died from any type of thyroid cancer, the prevalence of pulmonary, hepatic, and bone metastases was 65%, 60%, and 35%, respectively (164).

In a series of patients with treated pulmonary metastases from M. D. Anderson Hospital (161), overall 5-year survival was 69% and 10-year survival was 44%. Another study reporting the long-term results of treatment in almost 300 patients with lung and bone metastases from DTC (163) showed survival rates from the time of discovery of metastases of 53% at 5 years, 38% at 10 years, and 30% at 15 years. In the recent Lahey Clinic series update (165) of patients with disease metastatic to the lung at presentation, 60% were alive 5 years later in the young age group, but only 9% in the older group were alive. Four of ten patients who presented with pulmonary metastases survived, but all patients with metastases to the liver, bone, and brain died of the disease. In a Czechoslovakian series, the 10-year survival rate in patients with pulmonary metastases was 20% (166).

Lung metastases occur more frequently among patients with papillary cancer, whereas bone metastases are diagnosed mainly in older patients, especially those with follicular carcinoma. Even without specific treatment, pulmonary metastases may follow a very slow course. Although the effect of treatment is difficult to define for any manifestation of thyroid cancer, lung disease in particular seems to be favorably affected by radioiodine (and mediastinal disease even more so). The occurrence of bone disease, either alone or in combination with other sites, significantly worsens the prognosis of patients with DMs, presumably because of the reduced sensitivity of this form of disease to radioiodine, resulting from the lower capacity to absorb it.

Pulmonary Metastases

Two forms of pulmonary metastases (PMs) (see also Chapter 31) are categorized in the literature: (a) miliary or micronodular disease, consisting of multiple parenchymatous lesions that are granular or nodular and known as "fine types"; and (b) localized pulmonary infiltrations often associated with hilar and mediastinal enlargement and pleural effusion, known as "coarse types." Whether these two forms of lung disease constitute a continuum is unknown. The former is much more treatable than the latter.

The reported incidence of metastases that take up radioiodine affects the treatment of the primary tumor and the diagnostic aggressiveness used in the search for them. In general, radioiodine uptake is positive in approximately 50% of pulmonary metastases. In an M. D. Anderson series (161) radioiodine uptake was positive in 60% of patients with papillary carcinoma, in 64% of patients with follicular carcinoma, and in 36% of patients with Hürthle cell.

^{131}I is not uniformly taken up by biometastases. Patients with both lung and bone disease can show uptake in one or the other. The degree of uptake on diagnostic scan does not always predict the response to ^{131}I, because uptake varies with the tumor mass. Uptake correlates with young age of patients, histologic well-differentiated tumors, and immunohistochemical demonstration of thyroxine and triiodothyronine in the tumor tissue (although uptake cannot be predicted in the absence of this phenomenon) (167).

Some patients who initially show good uptake of radioiodine later have little or no uptake as the disease progresses, possibly because of the differentiation of the tumor. Based on the concept of tumor heterogeneity, the lack of radioiodine uptake progressively over time may also be an effect of treatment on a heterogeneous tumor cell population.

In general, PMs can be eradicated by radioiodine if the tumor burden is not great and the tumor concentrates radioiodine well. Patients with ^{131}I-accumulating metastases apparently have a far better prognosis than patients with metastases lacking such uptake, and the literature indicates that survival even correlates with the dose of ^{131}I needed for tumor ablation. If the tumor burden is great or the tumor does not concentrate radioiodine well, sometimes symptoms can be relieved temporarily but survival may not be prolonged significantly. Even when gross tumor disappears completely on clinical, radiologic, and radioisotopic study, the tumor will recur eventually in most patients, except when microscopic.

Long-term survival rarely occurs with metastatic carcinoma to the lung without treatment. In a Norwegian study (64), the results of the treatment when PMs became clinically apparent (without routine postoperative use of ^{131}I) showed that only 5 of 91 patients were "cured" after ^{131}I treatment, and all of these had miliary micronodular PMs.

One study reporting the long-term results of treatment of almost 300 patients with lung and bone metastases showed overall survival at 15 years of 30% (163). This related, however, to the quantity of disease present: 55% in patients with micronodular PMs (radiologically smaller than 1 cm) and 95% in patients with a normal chest x-ray (CXR). Complete response after treatment of metastases sometimes occurred very slowly, probably owing to the long doubling time of DTC. Serum thyroglobulin (Tg) levels remained detectable in 66% of patients and lung computed axial tomographic scan showed micronodules in two thirds of patients who had detectable serum Tg levels.

A number of reports indicated that treating PMs early improves rates of survival. Radioiodine uptake is a favorable prognostic factor, especially in patients with normal CXRs. Patients treated with ^{131}I for occult disease have a longer survival than those not treated ($p < .002$) (161). Some patients survive more than 20 years. The most favorable prognosis is associated with micronodular or miliary metastases, whereas the lowest survival is associated with large isolated parenchymal lesions or mediastinal lymph node involvement (77% versus 9%, 8-year survival) (14).

Because PMs with DTC can be treated more effectively in young patients than in old (71% versus 16% survival, $p < .01$) (161) a more radical treatment approach is indicated in younger age groups. In the University of Michigan series (13), patients who could be rendered free of metastatic disease with ^{131}I survived 8 times longer than those who had persistent disease. Schlumberger et al. (163) showed that the prognosis for survival was greatly increased if metastatic disease was treated before a CXR showed evidence of disease; 64% of patients had complete responses at 5 years when they had normal CXRs at the time of discovering metastatic disease, in contrast to an 8% remission rate at 5 years in patients with an initially abnormal CXR. The only predictive factor for 5-year disease-free survival after treatment of metastases was the initial extent of the disease, suggesting that metastases should be detected and treated in patients with thyroid cancer as early as possible—when CXRs are still normal. (In this series, CXR was normal in one third of the patients with metastatic lung disease.) Lung CT was more sensitive than CXR in detecting disease. In one third of the patients with a normal CXR, lung uptake was documented on total body scintigraphy only after an extra-large dose of ^{131}I was administered (100 mCi). Because thyroid remnants decrease the detecting capacity of these diagnostic procedures, thyroid ablation is advocated in the initial treatment of the gland especially in patients with high risk of metastases (Table 7).

In a recent discussion among thyroid surgeons, however, Cady (168) maintained that in low-risk patients, PMs that appeared clinically could be cured as effectively as PMs that were occult and detected by scans. High-risk patients with PMs who have metastases anywhere except the lungs will all die of disease. This philosophy represents the opposite side of the controversy on PMs: the low-risk patients can almost all be cured later and the high-risk patients are going to die anyway.

Table 7. *Population and clinical characteristics and the 5- and 10- yr survival rates of 101 patients with pulmonary metastasis*

	Total no. of patients	No. of patients who died	5-yr survival rate (%)	10-yr survival rate (%)
Sex				
Male	48	30	73	40
Female	53	37	66	47
Age at diagnosis of thyroid cancer				
0–20	16	2	94	88
21–40	19	8	84	53
41–60	42	35	69	24
61–80	23	21	43	9
>80	1	1		
Histology				
Papillary	68	44	69	49
Follicular	22	17	68	36
Hürthle	11	6	73	36
Extent of disease at diagnosis				
Glands only	25	20	96	84
Glands and nodes	33	21	73	45
Pulmonary metastatic sites	31	16	55	26
Pulmonary and other metastatic sites	12	10	42	8
Surgery				
Total	70	42	71	43
Subtotal	12	9	75	42
Lobectomy	13	10	62	54
<Lobectomy	6	6	50	50
Radioactive iodine				
-uptake	59	31	61	31
-uptake	42	36	29	7

From ref. (161) with permission.

Overall, the results indicate that disseminated DTC can be cured in a significant proportion of patients. In others, durable palliation can be achieved and the presence of PMs can be compatible with decades of survival. Patients with disseminated DTC are among the few with widespread tumors who benefit from intensive therapy and close follow-up. It appears to be easier to cure micrometastases than to palliate macrometastases. Hence, initial and subsequent cancer management should probably facilitate detection and treatment of metastases as early as possible. New references on pulmonary metastases are 169–171.

Bone metastases are of ominous prognostic significance (172) especially when they are visible on x-ray, as they generally are. These metastatic tumors have a tendency to invade bone by growing in an expansile manner, eroding the bony cortex and giving a radiographic picture similar to osteolytic sarcoma or giant-cell tumor. The bone metastases are frequently pulsatile and occasionally enlarge during menstruation and pregnancy, possibly related to a hormone-dependency effect.

There is some evidence that the location of bone metastases affects treatability. In one series, patients with bone metastases at the base of the skull were much more frequently cured than patients with skeletal metastases in other locations (163). It was suggested that enhanced curability was a result of the limited extent of these metastases, which were systemically sought during isotope scans and often discovered before being visible on x-rays. Their detection was made possible by frontal and lateral scintigrams, which allowed differentiation between uptake in the salivary glands and that in skull metastases.

Metastases exhibiting no radioiodine uptake or requiring palliation are indications for surgical removal, which can have a favorable effect in some cases (146,163,173). When the patient's condition permits, an aggressive surgical approach to solitary metastases can be considered, particularly in the skeletal system, to palliate excruciating pain and problems with pathologic fractures. Metastatic thyroid cancer is typically extremely vascular, however, and surgical excision is not always a straightforward process. Embolization of vascular bony tumors has been anecdotally reported to be of great value (174).

Chemotherapy has not been found useful in the treatment of uncontrolled DMs from DTC with either single agents or combined regimens (doxorubicin, cisplatin, bleomycin, methotrexate) (163). As a treatment modality, chemotherapy is reserved for patients with uncontrolled disease in phase II or III clinical trials (174a).

The Significance of Occult Disease

At the opposite end of the biologic spectrum of DTC from patients presenting with locally unresectable disease or distant metastases (the groups in whom the majority of deaths from thyroid cancer occur) is the process of occult thyroid cancer, a type of "microcarcinoma" (a concept proposed in 1947 by G. Mestwerdt), also known as "incipient" or "minimal" neoplasia, which typically never becomes clinically significant during the patient's lifetime (175,176). The confusion surrounding the significance of this disease presentation illustrates the importance of differentiating what represents cancer to the pathologist, to the surgeon, and to the patient.

Occult thyroid carcinoma (OTC) is detected when it presents as metastasis to the cervical nodes (common) or distantly (rare), or when it is incidentally noted in a resected thyroid specimen or at autopsy. Careful histologic examination of the thyroid (as with the prostate) reveals an incidence of thyroid carcinoma far in excess of its clinical prevalence.

Minimal thyroid carcinoma is almost synonymous with minimal papillary carcinoma. Only one case of occult medullary cancer was found in a series of 138 autopsies (37), and in a Swedish autopsy study five occult medullary carcinomas were found in 500 thyroids (177).

Although generally acknowledged to be of almost no clinical significance, the topic of occult or minimal thyroid cancer has generated controversy, in part because of varying definitions. Originally, a 1.5-cm diameter was suggested for the upper size limit. Some authors have included tumors with diameters of up to 3 cm. However, because tumors of this size can frequently be palpated (therefore are not inconsequential to many surgeons) and are easily detected by other diagnostic methods, upper limits of both 1 cm and 0.5 cm have since been recommended. An upper limit of 0.5 cm falls more often within the range acceptable to surgeons. The new WHO Histological Classification of Thyroid Tumors (79) acknowledges the phenomenon of OTC by recommending that the term *papillary microcarcinoma* replace the former term *occult papillary carcinoma* for lesions 1 cm or less in diameter. It was felt that separating lesions of this size from large clinically evident tumors was justified because of evidence that the former are of low malignancy, whereas the latter, especially if associated with gross extrathyroidal invasion, have the potential to be relatively aggressive.

Data on the prevalence and significance of OTC is clouded by methodologic problems. *Prevalence* refers to the fraction of the population affected by occult thyroid tumors, which cannot be measured directly in any living intact population and can only be inferred from thyroid specimens obtained either at operation or at autopsy. Nonuniformity occurs in both the numerator of the prevalence fraction (the tumor) and its denominator (the sample population). Valid conclusions are difficult to draw because of nonuniformity in the method of pathologic processing of specimens, and surgical histopathology reports studied retrospectively are notoriously inadequate in this regard.

Problems in interpretation of the significance of OTC are related to the representativeness of the sample populations derived from hospital autopsy series. It is questionable if any autopsy series can be regarded as representative of the general living population. Sampson (178) believes that for OTC (as opposed to most other diseases), the autopsy data can be considered a valid sample of the underlying general population because:

1. The prevalence does not increase with age.
2. OTC does not cause death.
3. There is no significant shortening of the lifespan of patients with OTC.
4. There is no association between OTC and other malignancy or any other specific fatal disease.

For thyroid cancer, the composition of the population autopsied is of significance with respect to age, the cause of death (frequently difficult to ascertain), and the presence of associated thyroid pathology.

To ensure sectioning the smallest known tumor (0.1 mm in diameter), microscopic slides must be prepared at intervals no wider than that—about 300 per block, or 300 to 900 per gland. In one case, 1375 sections of a gland were cut to identify an occult carcinoma 0.3×0.6 mm in size that was associated with a small cervical node metastasis (179). A less extensive examination of any thyroid gland will miss some of the smaller tumors. Some studies have included only grossly visible lesions, whereas others have microscopically examined frequent sections from apparently normal thyroid tissue. The most careful recent studies have generally looked at only one histologic slide per block—about $\frac{1}{30}$ the number needed for certain detection of the smallest known lesions. It is therefore certain that all of the prevalence figures in the literature are profound underestimates of the actual numbers of OTCs present (Tables 8,9).

When the same population was examined using different methods, greatly differing rates were found, as documented by the Atomic Bomb Casualty Commission (ABCC) study. Two populations can be compared only if the examination methods are similar. Sampson (178) believes that the "one block—one slide" method used in recent studies should be standardized as the method of choice because it is logistically feasible and easily duplicated. Typically, each gland is cut into 10 to 30 histologic blocks, each about 3 mm thick.

Reports from various countries on the prevalence of OTC at autopsy have shown that there are geographical differences in the occurrence of these tumors. In one valid study, glands from patients in several countries were serially sectioned and examined microscopically using identical techniques and diagnostic criteria (180). The prevalence of OTC in Japan was 28%, in Hawaiian Japanese 24%, in Poland 9%, in Canada 6%, and in Colombia 5.6%. Although the Japanese have a significantly higher rate of OTC than most others, some other populations also have fairly high rates, with the highest in the world reported from Finland 36.6% (12). This high incidence may, however, be an artifact caused by the inclusion of an expanded spectrum of histopathological lesions. OTCs were present in 7.5% to 13% of recent American autopsy studies, which translates to 10 to 30 million Americans having small OTCs (181). A recent autopsy study shows the highest incidence yet reported of OTC in thyroid glands. Although the glands were not totally sectioned, occult carcinomas were found in 62% (182).

One possible explanation of the geographic incidence is that the Japanese are exposed to a carcinogen more than others or are more susceptible to the carcinogen. The lack of increased clinical cancer in the Japanese suggests that they lack or have decreased quantities of the host factor that promotes the growth of the initiated thyroid car-

TABLE 8. *Prevalence of occult thyroid carcinoma in people aged 20 to 40 years*

Investigators	Location	Population studied			Cancer			% with cancer	Papillary	Totally embedded
		Men	Women	Total	Men	Women	Total			
Bondeson and Ljungberg	Sweden	79	38	117	4	4	8	6.8	8	No
Farooki	Philadelphia	5	4	9	0	0	0	0.0	0	No
Franssila and Harich	Finland	26	9	35	8	2	10	28.6	10	Yes
Fukunaga and Yatani	Worldwide	272	124	396	11	12	23	5.8	23	Yes
Hanson and Komorowski	Milwaukee	33	23	56	1	0	1	1.8	1	Yes
Harich, Fransilla, and Wasenius	Finland	2	2	4	0	1	1	25.0	1	Yes
Oertel and Klinck	USA	134	0	134	1	0	1	0.75	1	No
Nishiyami, Ludwig, and Thompson	Michigan	*	*	22	*	*	1	4.5	1	Yes
Sampson, Woolner, Bahn, and Karland	USA	4	1	5	0	0	0	0.0	0	No
Sobrinko-Simoes, Sambade, and Goncalves	Portugal	55	47	102	1	2	3	2.9	3	No
Komorowski and Hanson	Milwaukee	86	52	138	3	2	5	3.6	4	Yes
TOTALS	—	696	300	1018	29	23	53	5.2	52	—

*Study did not separate population by sex.
From ref. 37 with permission.

TABLE 9. *Prevalence of occult thyroid carcinoma in adults*

Age group) (years)	Men		Women		Total*	
	No. of thyroids examined	No. with cancer	No. of thyroids examined	No. with cancer	No. of thyroids examined	No. with cancer (%)
20 to 40	696	29	300	23	1018	53 (5.2)
≥41	1277	117	880	124	2230	253 (11.3)

*One study did not separate population by sex.
From ref. 37 with permission.

cinoma. There is some evidence from the Hiroshima/Nagasaki study that exposure to radiation may initiate some OTCs, but such lesions are not believed to differ in their biologic behavior from their naturally occurring counterparts (183). A modest but statistically significant association was found between exposure to ionizing radiation and prevalence of OTC. Tumors associated with 50 rads of exposure are larger in women, but smaller in men, than those not associated with radiation exposure, which implies that tumor growth is not enhanced by radiation exposure, and this is consistent with the interpretation that radiation acts as an initiating but not as a promoting factor in thyroid carcinogenesis. Also, the rate of metastases to the cervical lymph nodes is no different in the exposed and unexposed groups.

Histologically, OTCs can be found in either thyroid lobe with about equal frequency, and 8% to 10% are found in the isthmus. There is no predilection for location within the lobe, except that almost half are found adjacent to and involving the capsule of the gland. The tumors have a marked tendency to be multifocal, and secondary foci are frequently present in ipsilateral and/or contralateral lobes; 32% of the ABCC survivors had more than one tumor present.

Histologically, occult tumors can show invasive properties. In one series of 141 microcarcinomas of less than 0.1 cm, 55 were invasive (184). In the series of Lang et al. (182), 65% of OTCs had an invasive pattern and 46% were multifocal; two thirds of these were bilateral. Small thyroid carcinomas were subdivided and classified as minute (less than or equal to 5 mm) or tiny (5 to 10 mm) in a recent Japanese study (185). Minute carcinomas were of the follicular type significantly more often than were tiny carcinomas ($p < .005$), suggesting to the authors that the ratio of papillary to follicular carcinoma increases as the size of the carcinoma increases, and that follicular carcinoma is the "seed" or initial form of thyroid cancer (possibly extrapolating beyond the data?). Extrathyroidal invasion was found in one patient with minute carcinoma and in five patients with tiny carcinomas.

It is well established that small, clinically undetected thyroid carcinomas can produce extensive lymphatic metastases. OTC can also present as blood-borne metastases with the potential for death, but this presentation is distinctly uncommon (186). The process known as "benign metastasizing goiter of Cohnheim," described in 1876, is now generally considered an example of this phenomenon of small, clinically unrelated thyroid carcinomas producing extensive lymphatic metastases. At the time, this was thought to be a bizarre natural process because the metastatic "deposits," when they could be found, were more differentiated than the primary tumors (187,188).

The incidence of metastatic carcinoma has been underestimated because of the minimal amount of lymph node–bearing material available in many autopsy series. In Lang's study of 1020 sequential autopsies, periglandular lymph node metastases were found in 14% of the carcinomas (182). All but one of the carcinomas that metastasized was multifocal. Kafai and Sakamoto (185) found the incidence of cervical lymph node metastases was 13% in minute carcinomas and 59% in tiny carcinomas ($p < .01$). This was interpreted (overinterpreted?) by the authors to indicate that there is a threshold size of the primary tumor that must be reached before the process of lymphatic metastasis occurs. In the ABCC study, cervical metastases were generally small, with no noticeable enlargement of the lymph node, and they were widely distributed on either side of the neck and in the mediastinum. Microscopic metastases from the thyroid gland have been found in 0.1% of 1500 specimens on routine sectioning of cervical nodes removed for unrelated head and neck cancer (189).

Occult thyroid carcinoma manifesting as blood-borne metastasis without clinically detectable node involvement is rare and, by 1984, only ten cases had been reported (186). Thyroglobulin staining helped to indicate the thyroidal origin of the metastatic deposits (the lack of staining does not necessarily exclude a primary thyroid source, however).

Most studies of OTC have shown no significant sex or age prevalence. The equal incidence between the sexes implies no sex difference in carcinogenesis (induction). The prominent sex difference in clinical DTC indicates a differential effect of promoting factors between the sexes. Clinical expression, therefore, may relate to hormonal influences.

The literature generally reports that the prevalence of OTC does not increase with age after adulthood, that there is a slight tendency for decreasing prevalence with increasing age, and that there is a decrease in multifocality and tumor size with advancing age. This gives the impression that some of the tumors are actually shrinking away. In fact, the concept of spontaneous OTC as a disease that spares the young is probably an artifact of results from autopsy series that have had few young subjects. Until recently, the prevalence in people under 40 years of age had not fully been evaluated in any adequately performed autopsy series.

Two studies have looked at a young reference population and shed light on the baseline prevalence of OTC. In 1965, Oertel and Klinck (190) carefully sectioned the thyroids of 137 male military personnel between the ages of 18 and 39 who died suddenly. Only one OTC was found, in a 24-year-old man, representing an incidence of less than 1%. In a recent study, thyroid glands from autopsies of 20- to 40-year-olds (causes of death not stated) without clinical thyroid disease were "serially sectioned" at 2-mm intervals (37). Whole glands with adjacent tissue were included. Five patients (4%) had OTC, three men and two women. The average size was 0.2 cm. This was significantly less than in patients older than 40 ($p < .001$) (see Table 9). The increasing incidence of OTC with advancing age in this study presumably reflects a lifetime accumulation of carcinogenic influences.

There is little direct information on the prognosis of patients with untreated proven occult papillary cancer (191). One anecdotal report described long-term survival of 20 to 32 years without evidence of local recurrence or DMs in six patients who had resection of cervical metastases but no thyroid tissue removed. All received radiation to the neck postoperatively, however. The general assumption is that OTC is present in a significant percentage of the population and probably results in no increased morbidity or mortality. In the series of Woolner et al. (138) from the Mayo Clinic, no patient with a primary tumor of less than 1.5 cm died of carcinoma. The autopsy series of 518 OTCs from Japan attributed only one death to occult papillary adenocarcinoma of the thyroid (193). In this study, the prevalence-to-mortality ratio was 107:1, indicating that for each fatality caused by thyroid carcinoma, more than 100 persons with this neoplasm died from other causes. Such data suggest that almost all occult papillary carcinomas of the thyroid remain occult until death. Table 10 gives an indication of the probability of a given occult tumor having a fatal outcome.

TABLE 10. *Follow-up results of Atomic Bomb Casualty Commission (ABCC) Study*

Study/result	Number of cases
In the JNIH-ABCC life span study	100,000
Occult thyroid carcinomas	28,400
Surgically excised tumors in 15 years	90
Deaths from thyroid cancer in 15 years	5

From ref. 178 with permission.

In interpreting the clinical significance of OTC, Sampson points out that the increased prevalence of the finding is not correlated with an increase in the death rate from thyroid carcinoma. The death rate for thyroid carcinoma in Japan is the lowest among 24 countries studied, although it has almost the highest incidence of OTC. It is necessary to resist the interpretation that having a higher prevalence of OTC somehow protects the population from deaths from overt thyroid carcinoma. Sampson notes that the dissociation between the prevalence rate of OTC and the mortality from overt tumors may be a reflection of the two-stage theory of carcinogenesis demonstrated in experimental animals (initiation/promotion). An increase in prevalence of the smaller occult carcinomas may reflect an increase in initiating factors, including various environmental carcinogens and spontaneous radiation exposure, whereas larger thyroid tumors associated with mortality may result from rare individual differences in endogenous or exogenous promoting factors.

Controversy has arisen in recent years on the clinical significance of OTC, as reports have appeared of cases of OTC acting aggressively with a poor prognosis. Evidence suggests that, with longer follow-up, an increasing incidence of unfavorable disease progression is seen. Sampson's data show that about 90 of 28,400 occult carcinomas became clinically evident (and were surgically excised), and 5 of 28,400 occult carcinomas eventually caused death (193). In a longer follow-up of the Mayo Clinic series, six patients with tumors less than 1.5 cm have now died of metastatic thyroid carcinoma (104). This has been extrapolated to show "significant morbidity and mortality" in the recent literature (192).

Surgical studies show unsuspected microscopic foci of occult papillary cancer in almost 90% of apparently uninvolved contralateral lobes removed at surgery for an obvious papillary carcinoma. Presumably, these microscopic tumors are left behind whenever less than a total thyroidectomy is performed. Predictably, the diffuse nature of such occult disease has stimulated some surgeons (stuck in the Halstedian paradigm) to want to initiate aggressive treatment. However, clinical data indicate that it is most unusual for patients treated with less than total thyroidectomy to subsequently develop clinical evidence of recurrent cancer in the remaining lobe or portion of the lobe.

For example, in a series of patients treated by conservative thyroid resection at the Mayo Clinic who underwent less than total thyroidectomy between 1926 and 1960, there were no deaths attributable to thyroid cancer during a 40-year follow-up (138). In cases not undergoing total thyroidectomy at the time of original surgery, no recurrence of tumor was noted in the thyroid region and not a single instance of subsequent cervical node or distant metastasis was demonstrated. Twelve subsequent operations were necessary, among the 95 cases of OTC with metastases to cervical nodes, for recurrent lateral neck nodes, but none showed midline recurrence of the tumor.

DMs were not noted in a single patient. Either residual cancers grow so slowly as to be of no consequence, or they involute spontaneously or as a result of growth suppression by thyroid hormone, which is frequently prescribed postoperatively for these patients.

Thus, there is evidence that OTC with or without regional metastases can be cured by conservative surgical treatment (less than total thyroidectomy) and that once surgically removed, would almost never recur or metastasize. Clearly, all clinically evident and eventually fatal tumors were at one time occult, but it is to be hoped that until significant sequelae from OTC are more widely documented, surgeons will not jump on this new bandwagon and start recommending aggressive surgical treatment. Sampson points out that to remove all occult cancer, a total thyroidectomy as well as dissection of both sides of the neck and mediastinum is necessary. Such radical therapy cannot be advocated because the treatment is worse than the disease, based on the significant risk of permanent postoperative hypoparathyroidism and the potential for damage to the recurrent laryngeal nerve.

Already, however, a more aggressive interpretation of the significance of OTC is appearing in the surgical literature (193). It has been recommended that papillary carcinomas smaller than 1.5 cm should be judged by invasiveness, multifocality, and metastatic potential rather than by size alone, and that one should not fail to treat small lesions just because they are small. The choice of operation should not be predicated on size but rather on degree of certainty that the tumor is unifocal and known to be on one side or the other of the thyroid gland (how this could be ascertained without total gland removal is unclear). "In some cases because location of the primary tumor may not be obvious, one can argue that there may be a need for a more extensive surgical ablation than lobectomy alone" (193). Surgeons are so predictable.

The phenomenon of OTC has the potential to shed light on the genesis of malignant tumors, which is currently viewed as a multistaged phenomenon from the viewpoint of both molecular biology and morphology. That OTCs neither progress to the clinically detectable stage nor frequently metastasize provides a useful situation to study for understanding and controlling neoplasia. Studies of serum factors such as TSH, prolactin, thyroxine, and inorganic iodine are in progress to look for a clue to explain the high prevalence of occult carcinoma without increased incidence of clinical cancer in the Japanese. New data on occult and small primary tumors can be found in references 194–197.

ETIOPATHOGENESIS

Etiology

A variety of possible factors in the causation of thyroid cancer have come to light through epidemiology surveys, clinical searches for antecedent factors, and pathologic and experimental investigations. The issue is clouded because each of the major pathologic subtypes is likely to originate by different mechanisms.

The origin of thyroid tumors appeared at one time to be straightforward (198), a simple example of failure of feedback control. A thyroid gland failing to put out enough thyroxine was under constant pressure from the pituitary to do better, and sooner or later it gave way under the strain, producing irregular overgrowth. This failure might be the result of an inadequate supply of raw material (especially in regions of the world where the soil was depleted of iodine during the last ice age), or a metabolic defect that prevented the proper production of pituitary-affecting thyroid hormone, or reduced reproductive capacity of the gland itself (whether congenital or induced by infection or radiation), or thyroid-suppressing substances either in the diet or medically administered (goitrogens). The common denominator in tumor development seemed to be prolonged TSH stimulation, the most frequent predisposing factor was endemic goiter, and the best preventive measure was iodized table salt.

Several case-controlled studies in women showed a high risk of thyroid cancer in patients with a history of thyroid nodules or goiter (199). Because the experimental induction of goiter and thyroid tumors in animals is dependent on maintained excess secretion of TSH, a similar mechanism was proposed for the development of human thyroid cancer. Presumably, dietary iodine deficiency leads to compensatory increased secretion of TSH with resultant goiter formation and, in time, adenoma production with eventual malignant change. Experimental studies indicate that chronic iodine-deficient diets may lead to thyroid cancer in animals through stages including follicular hyperplasia, nodule formation, and adenoma formation. Currently, the progression of benign lesions to cancer in humans is doubtful, as is the whole concept of dependency of human thyroid neoplasia.

In Doniach's 1970 review (200), it was concluded that among all the postulated etiologic factors relative to thyroid cancer, ionizing radiation in childhood was the least disputed. There was a slight association of follicular carcinoma with endemic goiter, but no association of goiter with papillary carcinoma. The only definite example of TSH-induced tumors in humans occurred in dyshormonogenetic goiters, but the carcinomas produced were nonfatal and totally hormone dependent. It was postulated that TSH and other growth factors could promote tumor formation in thyroid cells in which malignant change had already been initiated, in particular by radiation.

Doniach's 1970 review is in large part still timely 26 years later. Over the years, especially with the recent increase in the number of population-based case control studies, a large number of factors possibly associated with thyroid cancer have been enumerated (see Table 2). The significance of all suspected risk factors with the exception of radiation remain to be confirmed and documented with respect to the etiology of thyroid cancer (199).

Incidence, Mortality, and Ethnicity

Thyroid cancer constitutes about 1% of all malignant tumors and the highly differentiated types account for 0.8% of all human malignancies. Official statistics cite an annual incidence of 0.3 to 10 cases per 100,000 persons. The Third National Cancer Survey in 1975 cited annual rates of newly diagnosed cases of thyroid carcinoma of 2.1 per 100,000 men and 5.2 per 100,000 women (201). In the United States, the 1989 estimated new thyroid cancer cases total 11,300 (8300 female and 3000 male). The estimated 1989 cancer deaths are 1025 (650 female and 375 male) (202). Trends in survival by cancer site and race in the first 3 years of each decade between 1960 and 1984, show relative 5-year survival rates in whites with thyroid cancer of 83%, 86%, 92%, and 93%. Data for blacks are available for the last two periods—88% and 95%. Thyroid cancer ranks among the five most frequent cancers in the 15-to-40 age group. For 5-year survivors, the relative survival for years 5 to 10 is in the range of 99% (203). Survival rates have improved over time with prominent decreases in mortality, especially for women and among middle-aged groups (204), presumably owing to earlier detection and possibly because of more effective treatment.

The role of racial and genetic factors in the genesis of papillary carcinoma is ill defined, and it is not possible to disentangle these from environmental factors in studies of geographic distribution in the incidence of thyroid cancer. Because of heterogeneous populations, such studies are seldom comparable and they use different techniques and diagnostic criteria in their formulation. Population surveys of thyroid cancer show geographic variation in incidence from over 6 cases per 100,000 women per year in Iceland and Hawaii to less than 1.5 in Denmark and England.

Descriptive epidemiologic findings for 7696 patients with newly diagnosed thyroid cancer reported to the SEER program for the years 1973 to 1981 show the preponderance of thyroid cancer in women and the papillary subtype documented (205). Previously reported increases in the incidence of thyroid cancer among whites leveled off in the late 1970s. Differences in the incidence of cancer among ethnic groups was striking. Puerto Ricans, Hispanics, and blacks had significantly lower thyroid cancer rates than whites. New Mexicans, Hispanic men, and Chinese, Japanese, Hawaiian, and Filipino men and women had significantly higher rates. The elevated rates for residents of Hawaii, regardless of ethnic group, were confirmed, although the significance of this finding is still unclear. It was concluded that thyroid cancer risk according to ethnic group and geographical residence may reflect socioeconomic or local environmental influences.

In general, neoplasms etiologically related to reproductive and endocrinologic functions are said to occur less frequently in ethnic minorities in the United States and in these ethnic groups in their native countries. The diversity in incidence of thyroid cancer among ethnic groups in the United States seems to bear a direct relationship to census indicators of socioeconomic status. Blacks, American Indians, and Hispanics have the lowest mean income and years of schooling and the highest percentages of families living below the poverty level, concomitant with the largest family sizes. Japanese and Chinese, on the other hand, exhibit the highest socioeconomic levels and achieve higher educational levels than do whites. It is also possible that easier access to the health care system results in the diagnosis of greater numbers of occult cancers that might otherwise remain undetected. It is not likely that genetic susceptibility could account for the increased risk among Orientals, because Japanese, Chinese, and Filipino residents of the United States all exhibit rates more than twice as high as in their native countries.

The high incidence in Hawaii, irrespective of ethnicity, cannot be attributed to either hormonal or socioeconomic factors. It has been related to the location of active volcanoes—the "Ring of Fire"—which follows the margins of continents surrounding the Pacific Ocean. Of the populations and countries bordering the "Ring of Fire," Colombians, Filipinos, and Polynesians of New Zealand exhibit high incidence rate of thyroid cancer, as do female Alaskan natives and Melanesians of New Caledonia. It has been suggested that the frequent volcanic eruptions disperse great volumes of dust and gases composed of an array of chemicals, and a release of hydrocarbons as well as radon "daughters" and possible consumption of carcinogenic agents in lava (volcanic ash) and fish products may be relevant. (It is always admitted that an artifact of the data cannot be ruled out to explain the high incidence in Hawaii.)

Comparison of the incidence of thyroid cancer in Iceland with other localities (including other areas of Scandinavia) revealed an exceedingly high overall incidence rate, especially in women (4 per 100,000 per year for men and 12 per 100,000 for women). The incidence of disease varies significantly in different years, which suggests the importance of environmental factors in causation. Many factors have been investigated, including the presence of active volcanoes producing lava, which has been sought as a common denominator in the high incidence in Iceland and Hawaii. However, because the natural history of thyroid cancer is unknown, it is not possible to show any correlation between changes in the incidence of this disease and the volcanic activity in Iceland (206).

Increasingly, reports on familial occurrence of papillary thyroid cancer are appearing, indicating that genetic factors may be important determinants of the geographic distribution of this disease. This may be particularly relevant in Iceland because of the isolation of the small population over a long period of time. High iodine intake may also be relevant. It has also been suggested that the high incidence of thyroid cancer in Icelanders is an artifact of easy detection. There is no endemic goiter in Iceland and the thyroid gland is normally very small as a result of the high intake of iodine from seafood. It is, therefore, easy for physicians to find thyroid tumors in the typically small glands, and this is a plausible explanation for the high incidence of this disease in Iceland.

From the late 1940s to the mid 1970s, the incidence of thyroid cancer increased, both nationally and internationally (207). Proposed explanations for the increase included exposure to carcinogenic agents such as chemicals, drugs, and ionizing radiation. The practice of irradiating benign childhood conditions existed from 1930 through 1960. Some authorities have maintained that the apparent epidemic increase in thyroid cancer incidence was really a result of greater clinical vigilance and better diagnostic procedures. The prevalence of thyroid cancer is considerably higher than it would appear from the annual incidence figures, suggesting that the number of patients with the clinical diagnosis is dependent on the frequency and quality of clinical examinations and health-screening procedures, as well as on the accuracy of the histopathologic examination of surgically excised thyroid glands.

Association of Thyroid Cancer with Other Types of Thyroid Pathology

A spectrum of benign and malignant diseases can occur in the thyroid gland of both radiated and nonradiated individuals, either simultaneously or sequentially. Different antibodies against human thyroid antigens produce a variety of clinical disorders ranging from the stimulation of Graves' disease to the glandular destruction of Hashimoto's autoimmune thyroiditis. The former is typically associated with hyperthyroidism and the latter with hypothyroidism. An extensive literature has arisen, putatively relating thyroid cancer to several types of basically coincidental nonmalignant thyroid pathology—Graves' disease, Hashimoto's thyroiditis, and goiter. Depending on the method of study, some associations appear compelling, but none has been proven to be etiologic. Most nonneoplastic diseases of the thyroid do not seem to be precursors of malignant diseases, with the exception of autoimmune thyroiditis, which may predispose to malignant lymphoma.

The opportunity to examine the thyroid gland has usually arisen as a result of thyroidectomy undertaken for the disease originally diagnosed and the discovery of occult carcinoma results. As we have seen, this is not equivalent to clinically significant cancer. Also, the presence of pathology in a thyroid gland draws clinical attention to it, which makes it more likely that patients receive scrupulous attention and surgery than those without thyroid pathology, at least in countries where there is access to sophisticated medical diagnosis and treatment. For example, in Hashimoto's thyroiditis, asymmetry of the gland or failure of response to thyroid hormone raises the clinical suspicion of malignancy, which encourages extirpation. On the other hand, the presence of pathology such as goiter might make it difficult to detect an emerging neoplasm and lead to underdiagnosis of cancer, especially in endemic areas, where the level of concern on the part of the patient is low, and in areas that lack access to medical facilities.

In the literature, thyroid cancer has been found in 0% to 11% of goitrous patients with multiple nodules, in 3% to 35% of cases of solitary thyroid nodules, and in 2% to 20% of cases of cold nodules. Of course, the incidence in each of these categories varies greatly with technique, the scrupulousness of pathologic examination, and the characteristics of the population that was operated or autopsied. These factors explain the wide percentage ranges and make data on associations almost uninterpretable. Appropriate follow-up protocols for patients with benign thyroid pathology is important for determining their likelihood of developing cancer.

To define the clinical significance of any of these associations, it is necessary to prospectively follow both a large group of patients with benign pathology and a control group of patients without it, and to record the incidence of thyroid cancer development in each group. It is intuitively logical that benign conditions that stimulate hyperplasia of adult thyroid epithelial cells might lead to malignant transformation, and this accounts in large part for the continuing interest in these conditions. But because of the endogenous occurrence of occult thyroid carcinomas (which are found in a comparable incidence in both normal thyroid glands and those with associated benign pathology), it is impossible to infer a causal association from histopathologic studies showing more than one type of benign and/or malignant thyroid pathology in an individual gland (208–211).

Thyroiditis

Doniach (200) reviewed the many reports in the literature that favor or oppose an association of thyroid cancer with focal or diffuse thyroiditis. The frequency of focal thyroiditis is probably higher in patients with thyroid cancer than in the general population. Cancer immune surveillance mechanisms have inevitably been evoked when cancer and thyroiditis are seen together, and it has been suggested that a presumably improved prognosis in papillary carcinomas accompanied by thyroiditis is related to reduced growth of metastases as a result of immunological factors. The observed thyroiditis has been assumed to be an immune response to the tumor, but it could as well be the result of local tissue damage produced by the tumor. The role of immunological factors in the pathogenesis of thyroid cancer is complex and poorly understood. Thyroiditis as a predisposing factor for lymphoma of the thyroid has been suggested by analogy with comparable reactions in the parotid gland and thymus, which are associated with the lymphomas of Sjögren's syndrome and the thymomas of myasthenia gravis, respectively.

Hashimoto's autoimmune thyroiditis could provide a fertile soil for malignant change on theoretical grounds. Proliferation of thyroid cells occurs in Hashimoto's thyroiditis, partly as a reparative response to cell destruction and possibly as a result of increased TSH secretion in response to diminished output of thyroid hormone. Hypothyroidism develops insidiously in patients with Hashimoto's thyroiditis, and their thyroid glands are subject to prolonged periods of TSH stimulation. [In animals (see later), endogenous stimulation of the thyroid by TSH is associated with an increase in the incidence of thyroid cancer. In humans, however, the situation is much less clear-cut.] It is also known that several classes of antibodies are produced against thyroid antigens in Hashimoto's thyroiditis. Some destroy thyroid tissue and others promote growth. In the latter category, thyroid-stimulating immunoglobulins promote the synthesis and secretion of thyroid hormone by activation of adenyl cyclase. This growth-promoting process could activate microscopic thyroid cancer foci and thereby produce clinically detectable lesions.

Reports of the association between Hashimoto's thyroiditis and thyroid cancer based on histopathologic study prior to the use of serologic testing for thyroid autoantibodies are of dubious significance. Autoimmune thyroiditis is currently thought to represent a defect in immune surveillance because of an abnormal population of suppressor T lymphocytes. In many reports, Hashimoto's thyroiditis has not been adequately confirmed as an entity immunologically, and so it can be confused with common nonspecific cellular lymphocytic thyroiditis, which can appear adjacent to a thyroid neoplasm. The histologic diagnosis of Hashimoto's thyroiditis also requires oxyphilia of epithelium and diffuse lymphocytic infiltrations.

Controversy continues in the recent literature. Reports variously conclude that true Hashimoto's autoimmune thyroiditis carries with it no increased risk of associated thyroid malignancy (212), that there is a highly statistically significant degree of correlation between the two, with Hashimoto's being a predisposing factor in the development of thyroid carcinoma (213), and that an association between the two is relative at best (214). Ott's series (213) purported to circumvent problems seen with earlier reports—patients were analyzed with Hashimoto's or with thyroid carcinoma, but not with both. This series included 800 patients consecutively operated for thyroid nodules not associated with a radiation history. Of 161 patients with thyroid carcinoma, 38% had coexistent Hashimoto's thyroiditis, and of 267 patients with Hashimoto's thyroiditis, 23% had coexistent carcinoma. The incidence of these occurrences in age- and sex-matched patients with noncancerous thyroid abnormalities was much lower. The conclusion was that patients with Hashimoto's thyroiditis should undergo an aggressive search for associated carcinoma, and specific treatment guidelines were discussed. (This series has been criticized on the basis that using colloid nodules as an internal control for benign disease with which to compare the incidence of Hashimoto's and cancer may not be appropriate.)

How to identify patients with the goiter of Hashimoto's thyroiditis who are presumably at high risk for associated thyroid malignancy continues to be of concern. Most authors agree that the majority of cases at high risk have a clinically apparent nodule or a cold nodule on thyroid scan. Thyroid ultrasonography can also help detect a nodule buried in a firm goiter. Soft-tissue x-ray of the neck revealing psammomatous or coarse calcific deposits characteristic of DTC can also be helpful, as can fine-needle aspiration (FNA) (215). New references for this section are 216 and 217.

Graves' Disease

Four decades ago the association of thyroid cancer with Graves' disease was thought to be very rare. Indeed, it was thought that thyrotoxicosis (and Hashimoto's thyroiditis) might actually confer a protective influence against thyroid neoplasia. A change in opinion has taken place over time, because a number of reports showed a significant incidence of malignant change in thyroid glands resected for hyperthyroidism (218,219). Most neoplasias are clinically unsuspected and are microcarcinomas of the occult type. Once again, because this represents an underlying baseline, an etiologic association (1% to 8% incidence of cancer) is not compelling (218,220,221).

The significance of investigating various benign hyperplastic thyroid conditions may relate, more interestingly, to the information that can be shed on the processes regulating thyroid growth in general. In earlier decades, it seemed that neither the stimulation resulting from long-acting thyroid stimulator (LATS) in primary hyperthyroidism, nor the additional stimulation by TSH in antithyroid drug-treated cases, led to a higher incidence of thyroid cancer despite a presumably favorable autonomous soil. Recently, the possibility that thyroid-stimulating antibodies (TSAs) may play a part in the pathogenesis and progression of thyroid neoplasia has been reinvestigated. The circulating thyroid-stimulating immunoglobulins characteristic of Graves' disease are presumably antibodies against the thyrotropin receptor and, like thyrotropin, they activate thyroid adenyl cyclase and cause the development in the intrinsically normal thyroid of the hyperfunction and hyperplasia characteristic of this disease. *In vitro* studies with IgG isolated from the serum of three patients with concurrent Graves' disease and metastatic thyroid cancer demonstrated that thyroid carcinoma cells respond to TSAs as they do to thyrotropin (222).

The suggestion that TSAs can act as promoters in thyroid carcinogenesis, in a manner similar to thyrotropin, has therapeutic implications. Currently, suppressive therapy with exogenous thyroid hormone is a keystone in the management of thyroid cancer (predicated on the ability of such treatment to inhibit thyrotropin secretion and its resultant thyroid hyperplasia, which presumably provides a fertile soil for neoplastic transformation—see later). Thyroid hormone, however, does not inhibit and may enhance the synthesis of TSAs. Therefore, suppression of thyrotropin secretion would be ineffective in patients with Graves' disease, in whom stimulatory antibodies (rather than thyrotropin) support the growth and function of the cancer. In patients with Graves' disease who can be shown to possess thyrotropin receptor antibodies and in whom metastatic thyroid tumors are progressing despite suppressive therapy and periodic treatment with radioiodine (admittedly, a small number of patients fit this description), attempts to inhibit the synthesis of TSAs would seem justified. This might include administration of high doses of glucocorticoid, which can alleviate hyperthyroidism and decrease levels of TSAs in patients with Graves' disease (222).

A critique of this concept notes that the postulation that thyroid-stimulating immunoglobulins may act as tumor promoters is far from established, because the incidence of thyroid cancer among patients with Graves' disease does not exceed that of thyroid cancer among patients who have Graves' disease but are negative for thyroid-stimulating immunoglobulin (223). To show that thyroid-stimulating immunoglobulins are possible tumor promoters in human thyroid cancer cells, one must prove that these cells become adenosine $3',5'$-cyclic monophosphate (cyclic AMP) dependent in growth. Therefore, convincing evidence that thyroid-stimulating immunoglobulins act as tumor promoters in DTC is still lacking.

Thyroid Lymphoma

The observation that the great majority of malignant thyroid lymphomas (224–228) show evidence of severe thyroiditis, often of the Hashimoto's type, is subject to the same criticisms cited above. It has been generally concluded, however, that the presence of thyroiditis in malignant lymphoma of the thyroid is not a response to the tumor, but rather that the lymphoma arises from a preexisting thyroiditis. However, whereas most cases of malignant lymphoma show evidence of preexisting thyroiditis, only a minute proportion of patients with thyroiditis develop malignant lymphoma (229). By analogy with the malignant lymphoma occurring in association with Sjögren's syndrome, it has been suggested that there may be a general association of organ-specific malignant lymphoma with organ-specific autoimmune disease.

Goiter

The commonest thyroid disease is simple nontoxic goiter. At one time, simple goiter was regarded as a common precursor of thyroid cancer, and the older studies often suggested that in goitrous areas, frequently known to be iodine deficient, the incidence of thyroid carcinoma was substantially higher than in nongoitrous areas. A swing in opinion has taken place over the past five decades, however, and currently the relationship between thyroid cancer and endemic goiter or dietary iodine is not entirely clear. Although it is widely believed that goiter, both the endemic and sporadic types, is a precancerous lesion, much of the old evidence was accumulated at a time when papillary tumors were classified as benign rather than malignant, making comparisons between old and new evidence difficult.

The suggestion that endemic goiter predisposes to thyroid cancer was based on four main arguments:

1. There was a clinical impression of a strong correlation supported by the pathologist Wegelin who, in 1928, noted that thyroid cancer was found 10 times more frequently in autopsies in Bern, Switzerland, than in Berlin, Germany, the former being an area of endemic goiter and iodine deficiency. In general, in areas of the world where goiter is endemic, the incidence of thyroid cancer is usually elevated. Reports from Cali, Colombia, clearly indicated an association of follicular and anaplastic thyroid carcinoma with endemic nodular goiters. [A puzzling feature of the Cali findings is the absolute increase in all types of thyroid cancer as compared to nongoitrous regions. The absolute increase in papillary carcinomas suggests the existence in Cali of an additional thyroid carcinogenic factor separate from endemic goiter (230).]

2. Surgeons in widely distributed clinics reported an incidence varying from 5% to 25% of primary thyroid carcinoma in thyroidectomy specimens done for nodular goiter.

3. A coincidental fall in prevalence of both goiter and thyroid carcinoma in Switzerland as a result of the introduction of iodized table salt was reported in 1952.

4. Diet—The maintenance of a goitrogenic regimen in experimental rats leads to the development of thyroid adenomas and metastasizing carcinomas. Goitrogens are chemical compounds that inhibit thyroid hormone synthesis, secretion, and metabolism. By virtue of their abil-

ity to inhibit hormone synthesis and indirectly stimulate TSH secretion, they induce goiter formation. Examples are perchlorate and thiocyanate ions. In large quantities, goitrogens cause thyroid cancer in laboratory animals by blocking iodine uptake in the synthesis of thyroid hormones, thus causing the pituitary to increase TSH secretion. Cabbage, Brussels sprouts, and broccoli are known to contain goitrogens. These cruciferous vegetables contain indole components, isothiocyanates, and phenols that may actually inhibit the development of certain cancers.

Salmon collected during the 1976 spawning runs from the Great Lakes had spontaneous goiters in 6% to 80% of animals, with no correlation between serum thyroid hormone levels or iodine content of the water. The apparent increase in goiter frequency in salmon was taken to reflect an increase in the concentration of environmental goitrogens because the Great Lakes have been polluted with a vast array of chemicals that have been reported to alter thyroid activity in fish, birds, and mammals. This may mean increased goitrogenic activity in humans because the fish are eaten and the lake water is increasingly used for drinking (231).

Counterevidence that goiter does *not* predispose to thyroid cancer includes the following:

1. Some studies have found no difference in the incidence of thyroid cancer in goitrous and nongoitrous regions, and analysis of the geographical distribution of mortality figures for thyroid cancer showed no relation to goiter incidence.

2. Recent reports from Switzerland do not substantiate the findings of a reduction in thyroid malignancy resulting from the introduction of iodized salt in 1923 (232). A decreased incidence of malignant thyroid disease has been seen in people under 35 years of age since the introduction of iodine, but that was countered by an increased incidence in older age groups. Comparisons between World Wars I and II suggest that the introduction of iodized salt, although effective in reducing the prevalence of goiter in some areas, has not significantly reduced thyroid malignancy, which has apparently increased slightly.

3. Aggregate studies in the United States have not supported an association between goiter and thyroid cancer. The frequency of carcinoma in surgical thyroidectomy specimens of nodular goiter rose from less than 2% before 1929 to an average of 10% three decades later, and this coincided with a three- to fourfold drop in the absolute incidence of nodular goiters. Also, the annual total death rate from thyroid cancer has remained remarkably constant in the United States at about 1 in 200,000 over the past three decades despite the fall in the incidence of nodular goiter.

4. Surgical thyroidectomy specimens of nodular goiter are not representative because they come from a highly selected group of patients who attracted medical attention for reasons such as unusual symptoms, malaise, increased growth rate, or pain. Confusion exists as a result of the endogenous presence of occult thyroid carcinoma in surgical specimens. Moreover, single nodules are most likely to prove malignant; this is contrary to the correlation with endemic goiter which is usually multinodular.

Overall, the conflicting evidence cannot be completely resolved. It appears that endemic goiter plays no part in the inception of papillary or medullary carcinoma, but follicular and anaplastic carcinomas occur more frequently in some areas of endemic goiter than elsewhere. However, these latter two types also arise in otherwise normal thyroid glands. The facts that there are estimated to be over 200 million people suffering from endemic goiter, and that follicular carcinoma is a comparative rarity, have cast doubt on the once generally held belief that endemic goiters cause thyroid cancer. In the Cali, Colombia, study, the authors stated that they could not establish any etiologic relationship between nodular goiter and thyroid carcinoma. Foci of carcinoma were found more frequently in extranodular tissue than within thyroid nodules, supporting the concept that goitrous nodules cannot be considered forerunners of thyroid carcinoma. Similarly, the great prevalence of thyroid nodules and the rarity of thyroid carcinoma have dispelled the belief that most thyroid carcinomas in humans arise from malignant change in adenomas.

Because many DTCs grow very slowly, a history of the presence of a nodule for many years is compatible with the view that the nodule was malignant from the outset. Doubt has also been cast on the theory that excess TSH secretion is an etiologic factor in the majority of cases of human thyroid carcinoma, because in nonendemic goiter areas most of the thyroids containing a primary carcinoma show no evidence of parenchymatous hyperplasia. Also, follicular carcinoma in nongoitrous regions is most often found in otherwise normal glands, indicating that prolonged excessive TSH secretion is not an essential etiologic factor. More recent discussions of goiter and thyroid cancer are in references 233 and 234.

Relationship to Diet

Although prolonged iodine deficiency is seen to lead both to thyroid hyperplasia and to high levels of TSH in the blood of man, its direct connection with malignant tumors of the thyroid has been much harder to establish than was at one time expected. In general, follicular carcinoma appears to be more common in areas of iodine deficiency and endemic goiter, whereas papillary carcinoma is more common in areas that have a high dietary iodine content and are nonendemic for goiter (235). There is a high incidence of papillary carcinoma in the fishing communities of northern Norway where the diet is high in iodine because of the consumption of shellfish. A positive correlation has been found between the incidence of endemic goiter and follicular thyroid carcinoma in Cali, Colombia. It has also been found, however, that the consumption of shellfish seems to increase the risk of follicular thyroid cancer, whereas consumption of goitrogen-containing cruciferous vegetables appears to reduce the risk of thyroid cancer. Confusion of this sort demonstrates the difficulty of assigning significance to individual factors in a situation with multifactorial etiology. With iodine supplementation of the diet in iodine-deficient regions, the incidence of follicular carcinoma decreases and the incidence of papillary carcinoma increases within 5 years based on Swiss studies (236,237). This phenomenon remains unexplained.

The underlying assumption is that because the highest rates of fatal thyroid cancer are found in iodine-deficient countries (Austria and Switzerland), which are areas of endemic goiter, differences in TSH levels reflecting iodine deficiency-induced hyperplasia may be of importance in determining whether a tumor behaves in malignant fashion.

Radiation-Induced Cancer

The one undisputed etiologic factor for DTC is a history of prior radiation, whether therapeutically applied or environmentally acquired from fallout or from natural radioactivity in the soil. Knowledge about radiation-induced thyroid neoplasia comes largely from two sources: (a) studies of children exposed to gamma radiation for benign disease in the head and neck; and (b) studies of survivors exposed to gamma radiation from nuclear fallout at Hiroshima and Nagasaki, in the Marshall Islands, and more recently, at Chernobyl.

Forty years have elapsed since the association was demonstrated between radiation of the neck in infancy and the development of thyroid tumors in later life (238). Ten of 28 children with carcinoma of the thyroid had been given radiotherapy (RT) to the thymus in infancy. The magnitude of the problem was not appreciated until studies from the University of Chicago indicated the high prevalence, not only of benign but also of malignant thyroid lesions in the groups at risk (239,240). The original observation has now been confirmed many times with studies that have been both prospective (following children known to have received radiation to the head and neck in infancy or early childhood, and their unirradiated siblings) and retrospective (searching for a history of previous RT in children who develop cancer).

External radiation was given in the past for a wide variety of conditions and over a wide dose range for enlarged thymus, enlarged tonsils and adenoids (241), cervical lymphadenopathy related to tuberculosis or Hodgkin's disease, whooping cough, cerebral tumors, and a variety of skin conditions including angioma, keloid, acne, and tinea capitis. Irradiation to the thymus in infancy was done on the grounds that an enlarged thymus indicated an increased risk of upper respiratory infections and even carried the risk of unexpected death from "status thymicolymphaticus" (242). (It was not fully appreciated that filling of the upper mediastinum on anteroposterior chest x-ray can be a normal finding resulting from distension of the veins in a crying infant and not indicative of thymic enlargement.) On these grounds, thousands of infants, mostly in the United States, were given RT in doses of 75 to over 600 rads from the 1920s to the 1950s. In many cases, the port used was 10 cm^2, so that the neck as well as the thymus lay in the primary x-ray beam. During the mass immigration to Israel from 1944 to 1960, about 17,000 children were treated for ringworm of the scalp (tinea capitis) with doses in the range of 350 to 400 rads.

Much of the information on this topic has emerged from the Chicago area, where there has been persistent interest in the problem and a large number of patients with radiation-associated thyroid cancers (RATC) have been treated and followed. The University of Chicago population provides a group in which to study the natural history of RATC. The control population for most of these studies consisted of patients with DTC, under 55 years of age, who had not received radiation and who received their primary care at that institution. The radiated group, composed of both primary-care and referred patients, appeared similar in other factors thought to influence prognosis. [Chicago's Michael Reese study also had a high proportion, 75% to 90%, of Jewish patients (see later).]

Irradiated subjects tended to have more advanced disease at diagnosis, a higher incidence of recurrence, and a higher incidence of multifocal or widely disseminated intrathyroidal primary tumors. The majority of the patients had papillary tumors, and no medullary or anaplastics were described.

In general, the follow-up studies so far reveal no evidence that RATC has any unusual features in its biologic behavior: there is no conclusive evidence that RATC is any more or less lethal than its naturally occurring counterpart or that its histopathology is different. The patients tend to be young, female, and have papillary cancer. A series from M. D. Anderson Hospital comparing radiated and nonradiated patient groups (matched for age, sex, and extent of disease) showed little difference in disease-free interval or survival (243).

In radiated children, there is a higher prevalence of benign thyroid nodules, but there is no evidence that the thyroid in infants and children is more susceptible to radiation carcinogenesis than is the adult gland. It is suggested that tumor formation results from summation of radiation effects, with the subsequent proliferation of thyroid cells that takes place during the normal growth of the thyroid from infancy to puberty. Radiation can be carcinogenic to the adult thyroid, too, providing the dose is nonsterilizing. The paucity of reported cases of RATC in adults is a result of the difficulty of proving a direct correlation in the presence of numerous other etiologic factors. The thyroid gland has ceased growing in the adult and the promoting factor of growth is, therefore, absent.

Other events leading to proliferation in an adult thyroid (partial thyroidectomy, endemic goiter, Graves' disease, and treatment with goitrogenic antithyroid drugs) after therapeutic radiation (500 to 1500 rads) could result in cancer. Some adult patients who underwent therapeutic irradiation to the supraclavicular nodes in the treatment of breast carcinoma, and subsequently developed Graves' disease, have developed RATC.

Information on exposure to nuclear fallout is available from two events with long-term follow-up. Survivors of Hiroshima and Nagasaki have been studied in the ABCC study, which found an increased risk of thyroid cancer, not only in young subjects, but in subjects who were adults at the time of radiation exposure.

Radiation exposure to the thyroid gland occurred to 251 inhabitants of islands in the Marshall group from planned exposure to fallout from the first hydrogen bomb exploded by the United States on the Bikini atoll in 1954. Radiation exposure included external gamma irradiation and beta radiation from internally absorbed mixtures of radionuclides I-131, I-132, I-133, and I-135 (244,245). Two days after the thermonuclear explosion, the inhabitants were removed. They had received 175 rads of whole-body gamma radiation and an additional 100 rads to adult thyroids and 1000 rads to infant thyroids from ingestion of radioactive isotopes of iodine (the dose from radioiodine varied with the age of the subject because of the low mass of the thyroid in the younger age groups).

Because all of the resultant thyroid cancers have occurred in women (see later), this indicates that the female thyroid gland is more sensitive to radiation than the male gland. Cancers have occurred through a wide range of thyroid doses, and there is no correlation between dose and latency period and no evidence for a higher sensitivity to radiation among younger persons.

After a nuclear reactor accident, the population of the contaminated area will have a rapid uptake of released radioactivity by inhalation of airborne radionuclides as well as a prolonged uptake from the food. Therefore, measurable activity in the thyroid remains for a much longer period than could be expected from the effective half-life of I-131 (5 to 7 days).

The worst accident in the history of nuclear power occurred at Chernobyl in the Soviet Union on April 26, 1986, at 1:23 AM (Swedish time). Two time periods with winds directed from Chernobyl to Sweden happened to coincide with the two peaks in radionuclide emission from the reactor. Continuous measurement of airborne particular activity by the Swedish Defense Institute and the autopsy of a person who died on April 27 showed immediate uptake within a maximum of 18 to 26 days after the accident and no measurable levels after 93 days (246).

Histologic Changes

Within the range of carcinogenic radiation doses, the thyroid can respond with a variety of disorders including focal hyperplasia, thyroiditis, fibrosis, and adenomas that may be associated with carcinoma. The type of pathology expressed depends on the type of radiation exposure, time since exposure, and other factors such as age, sex, and heredity.

Thyroid nodules, including malignant ones, have occurred in more than one third of patients with thyroid cancer and in more than 10% of the individuals who received childhood RT to the head and neck area. Factors previously found to correlate with an increased risk of developing nodules are higher treatment dose, younger age at treatment, and female sex.

Almost all RATCs are well differentiated. Most are papillary, although follicular RATCs also occur. Case reports of anaplastic thyroid cancer related to radiation have appeared, but there is no evidence that well-differentiated thyroid cancers found in patients who receive radiation are more likely to undergo transition to a more aggressive or less differentiated form. Medullary carcinoma of the thyroid has not been associated with radiation.

Dose

Thyroid carcinoma has been reported after exposure to as little as 6.5 rads and as much as 2500 rads. There appears to be a linear relationship between radiation dose and the incidence of thyroid carcinoma. An increase in thyroid cancer is seen with doses between 100 and 600 rads, and a dose over 300 rads places the patient in an especially high-risk group. Above 1500 rads, the incidence declines, presumably because higher doses achieve total or near-total destruction of viable thyroid tissue and there is no living tissue left to undergo malignant transformation. Thus, hypothyroidism rather than neoplasia is the long-term effect of such high doses. There is no evidence that hypothyroidism, subclinical thyroid failure, or hyperthyroidism results from the levels of radiation used to treat benign childhood conditions. It is postulated that the small initiating dose of radiation summates with the promoting effect of the normal mitotic growth of the thyroid from infancy through puberty.

Latency

The usual latency period from delivery of radiation to the discovery of thyroid cancer is 10 to 20 years (means in various series are 12 to 18 years). RATC has been diagnosed at as early as 6 years of age and as late as 71 years, the average being between 35 and 40 years. In one series of irradiated patients undergoing thyroidectomy over a 20 year period, the average duration between radiation exposure and operation was 27 years (247). A recent Swedish study points out that the risk of cancer development exists for the remainder of the patient's life; the mean time from radiation treatment to diagnosis of a malignancy was 46 years, with a range of 26 to 56 years (248). (The time period to discovery of cancer is determined in part by the intensity of the search.)

A 5-year minimum latency period is assumed for the development of thyroid cancer. It appears that there may be a somewhat longer minimum induction for benign nodules than for thyroid cancer—10 versus 5 years (249). There is little information on the pattern of increased risk with time elapsed from exposure, so excess risk is usually assumed to be constant for the entire period of increased risk. There is some evidence that persons exposed during childhood experience higher subsequent risk of thyroid cancer than those exposed at later ages; however, the evidence is not solid.

Incidence

The units used to describe the increased risk of RATC are somewhat unintelligible to the clinician: "excess radiothyroid carcinoma per million person-year-rad" is difficult for the nonstatistician to interpret. Overall, it is stated that the risk of RATC is on the order of two to five cases per million children exposed per rad per year. In other words, the risk per rad estimates for thyroid cancer from studies using external low-dose radiation in most populations are not more than four per million per rad in women and not more than one per million in men. The increased or absolute risk of radiation exposure has also been expressed as three cases of cancer per year per million people, each with a thyroid dose of 1 rad, or (to bring dose units in line with the exposure doses actually used in x-ray treatments) there are nine cases of cancer per year per 10,000 people, each with a thyroid dose of 300 rads.

The risk of developing palpable thyroid nodules is said to be about 4 times the risk of developing cancer, or 12 cases per year, for ages 44 to 47, per million people with a thyroid dose of 1 rad. One author attempted to express these factors with a practical example: if 25 years ago the thyroid glands of 100 people were exposed to 300 rads each, the above risk formula predicts that about two people will have developed thyroid cancer and nine will have benign nodules.

Risk: How Lethal is Radiation-Associated Thyroid Cancer?

The 1977 SEER report identified four deaths (2.8%) in 142 cases of RATC at a mean of 24 years after exposure (250). In the thymic-irradiated patients from Rochester, New York, with thyroid cancer, two (7%) of 28 excess cancers resulted in death over a mean period of 35 years (151).

In the more than 10,000 children irradiated for tinea capitis in Israel who have been followed between 12 and 23 years, six thyroid cancers have developed. (The mean dose to the thyroid from this treatment was in the range of 5 to 17 rads.) The risk in this group has also been stated to be about 14 excess cases per million per rad per year (252).

Of 2872 persons radiated for enlarged thymus in early infancy with an average dose to the thyroid of 119 rads, 24 cancers developed during a follow-up period of almost 40 years. The risk in women was 2.3 times that in men. Only one death attributed to thyroid cancer has occurred in this group (253).

When the results of several large studies from the United States are combined, an excess was found of 109 thyroid cancers in almost 8000 subjects representing about 43 million person-rads at risk. The composite risk is about 2.5 excess cancers per million persons per rad-year (250).

Through 1980 at the University of Chicago Hospital, 416 patients with a history of radiation to the head and neck were examined and 113 were operated. The incidence of carcinoma was 36% in these patients, or about 10% of all patients examined (254). (A cancer incidence of 30 to 55% is found in near-total thyroidectomy specimens if a meticulous, detailed histopathologic examination is performed.)

The incidence of thyroid cancer in the ABCC Japanese atomic bomb survivors (people in the study are examined biannually) has shown 40 thyroid cancers identified in the group of about 20,000 people originally in the study, 29 papillary and 11 follicular (255). Only one death has occurred in the 40 diagnosed cancers. At autopsy, 34 more cancers were diagnosed. A 1963 report on about 19,000 Hiroshima and Nagasaki subjects who had been heavily or moderately radiated or not exposed showed 21 histologically confirmed thyroid cancers: 14 in the heaviest radiation group, 5 in those with moderate radiation, and 2 in the nonexposed group. This prevalence did not significantly differ from that elsewhere in Japan, but the age at diagnosis was significantly younger. This was interpreted to be the result of a deliberate search for thyroid disease (256).

In the Marshall Islanders, seven tumors were demonstrated from a group of 243 at risk.

In the above-mentioned groups, the risk coefficient of thyroid cancer (per million rads) is 20 for the Japanese, 70 for those undergoing neck irradiation, 92 for those with tinea capitis, and 134 for the Marshall Islanders.

After the Chernobyl incident, it was predicted that the increase in dose-equivalents to the thyroid for the population of southern Sweden may lead to an increase in the incidence of thyroid cancer of 0.1% during a 25-year period (246). This estimate has been challenged (257) on the basis that it is unlikely that any increased risk of thyroid cancer would result. The study used in counterpoint was one that had previously been questioned by other epidemiologists, however (258).

Mechanisms of Action

The mechanisms by which radiation causes thyroid changes are not certain, but several hypotheses have been put forward, primarily relating to the TSH-dependent hypothesis of thyroid carcinogenesis in animal models. Experimental thyroid carcinogenesis by x-ray shows that the optimal dose in rats is between 500 and 2500 rads and this effect is potentiated by TSH-induced proliferation of radiated cells. The classic early study giving evidence for development of thyroid neoplasia through a sequence of hyperplasia progressing to adenoma formation and eventuating in carcinoma was performed in irradiated rats (259).

External beam radiation or ^{131}I may act on the thyroid gland as an inducer of hyperplasia—a fertile soil for cancer development. The radiation delivered to the gland is indirect via a scatter effect, which results in the loss of only some functioning thyroid parenchyma. The pituitary, in an attempt to overcome the failure of its target organ, increases thyrotropin output. No response to the TSH ensues, however, in the degenerated portion of the thyroid gland. Therefore, unaffected tissue tends to compensate, leading to islands of hyperplasia. Hypophysectomy in laboratory animals reduces the incidence of RATC and one can postulate that interrupting the thyroid–pituitary axis interferes with the reflex arm leading to compensatory thyroid gland hyperplasia and incipient neoplasia. Radiated lab animals that undergo hypophysectomy do not show thyroid neoplasm formation, whereas those with a functioning pituitary developed a 96% incidence of follicular carcinoma in one study (260).

In addition, irradiation may directly cause genetic alterations in chromosomes, followed by the appearance of errors in cell replication leading to the development of mutant and neoplastic, or at least altered, cells. This process may occur alone or in an additive manner with underlying hyperplasia. It may be a separate process because RATC has been diagnosed in euthyroid patients with no evidence of excess TSH stimulation or thyroiditis. Also, it has been noted that chromosome changes can be induced experimentally in animal thyroids by exposure to radiation (261). It is well established in animals that after chromosome changes are induced by radiation, thyrotropin stimulation of hyperplasia then acts as a promoter for the induced thyroid cancer.

Many of the irradiated individuals have one or more siblings who were also irradiated, and this provides the opportunity to study the influence of genetics on the phenomenon of RATC—whether or not some individuals are more susceptible than others to the effects of radiation (262). [There is ample precedent for genetic factors influencing radiation sensitivity, as demonstrated in studies in patients with ataxia-telangiectasia (263).] A University of Cincinnati study compared almost 10,000 family members of irradiated and nonirradiated cohorts and revealed no evidence of a familial bias toward thyroid disease in the irradiated group (264).

A genetic factor is suggested by a University of Rochester study that showed the relative risk for Jews when compared with non-Jews was about 3.5, after adjustment for sex, time since irradiation, and irradiation dose (253). The risk for the development of RATC seems to be especially high in young Jewish women.

Surveys in New York City and Los Angeles County have also indicated that the risk of thyroid cancer is increased among Jews, and irradiated individuals of this subgroup are at an especially high risk. Because this population was exposed to a larger dose of radiation, ethnic background does not entirely account for the increased risk (253).

Other Radiation-Associated Conditions

The thyroid is more radiosensitive than other organs in the head and neck, but tumors in other head and neck sites can arise in relationship to childhood irradiation, which is termed postirradiation polyglandular neoplasia syndrome of the head and neck (265). Areas affected by neoplasia include the salivary glands, parathyroids, facial skin, and nerves. Even the most common of these associated tumors—salivary gland tumors—are over 20 times less frequent than thyroid tumors. In patients who have received tonsillar and nasopharyngeal irradiation, salivary gland tumors most commonly occur in the parotid area. In the population treated for tinea capitis by radiation epilation, more malignant brain tumors occurred than in the control group. Benign tumors such as neurilemomas and acoustic tumors have developed in these individuals, and it has also been reported that those who develop radiation-related salivary or benign neural tumors are more likely to develop thyroid neoplasms (266). The time course for the development of these tumors is similar to the time course of those that occur in the thyroid. They can arise many years after the initial RT and continue to occur almost indefinitely after induction.

The development of parathyroid adenomas late after radiation therapy has also been considered to be a complication of such therapy. The average interval to diagnosis of parathyroid adenoma is 33 years and was just beginning to be noticed in 1970. Postradiation hyperparathyroidism has also been reported (267).

Although the indications for benign childhood conditions are no longer in effect, thyroid cancer has more recently been reported after prophylactic cranial radiation for acute lymphoblastic leukemia (268) and after cervical radiation for Hodgkin's disease (269). Although this does not seem to be a numerically significant problem, it has been suggested that iodine compound or thyroid hormone extract be administered to such patients prophylactically (270), because theoretically T_4 may block TSH secretion and hyperplastic stimulation of damaged cells to undergo malignant transformation, when instituted soon after radiation exposure.

It has been suggested that thyrotropic stimulation resulting from radiation injury to the thyroid may promote the growth of occult carcinoma (271). The possibility that radiation can induce such lesions or promote the transformation of biologically benign cancers into clinically significant disease cannot be established by existing data (see also ref. 217).

Conclusions

A flowchart useful in conceptualizing diagnostic and therapeutic action in patients with a history of childhood irradiation is shown in Figure 4. Controversies in screening, diagnosis, and surgical treatment are summarized by August and Seiko (270).

A recent report demonstrates interesting changes in RATC features over time. In a series of irradiated patients undergoing thyroidectomy over a 20-year period (206 patients operated from 1965 to 1985), the average time between radiation exposure and operation was 27 years. The indication for operation was the presence of a nodular thyroid, and pathology revealed 42% carcinoma (73 papillary, 13 follicular, 1 undifferentiated), 45% follicular adenoma, and 13% thyroiditis. A comparison of the first 100 patients operated, with the last 106, demonstrated that the incidence of carcinoma had dropped from 48% to 37%, the incidence of lymph node metastases had decreased from 35% to 26%, and the incidence of bilaterality had fallen from 75% to 54%. Based on the trends for decreasing incidence, bilaterality, and metastatic disease, the recommendation for near-total thyroidectomy for RATC might have to be reevaluated (247).

Because the practice of irradiating children ended 40 years ago, the majority of patients who will develop RATC have already appeared or will shortly. It seems reasonable, therefore, that the emphasis in etiologic studies on thyroid cancer should shift now to other factors and issues (see later), such as the sex hormones. Recent research on radiation induced cancer is listed in references 272–285.

Radioiodine: Relationship to Thyroid Cancer

The known radiation-associated etiology of thyroid cancer has raised concern about the evolution of this condition in patients who receive various types of therapeutic radiation, specifically those who undergo therapeutic ^{131}I administration (typically administered for thyrotoxicosis related to Graves' disease).

Since a 1952 report that administration of radioiodine to rats produced thyroid carcinoma, many animal models have included ^{131}I induction in their carcinogenesis (286).

As of 1970, of the estimated 50,000 people treated since 1948 with therapeutic doses of radioiodine for primary hyperthyroidism, no case report had appeared on the development of a metastasizing thyroid carcinoma. The mean dose to the thyroid of 5 to 15,000 rads from therapeutic ^{131}I seems to sterilize the gland, leading to loss of any potentially malignant cells. The typically nonuniform distribution of ^{131}I within thyroid tissue, compared with gamma radiation, results in localized hot spots and a lower dose to the remaining thyroid tissue. The rising incidence of hypothyroidism after this therapy is of more concern than the development of cancer and it has been suggested that the dose of ^{131}I be reduced. If a nonsterilizing dose is given, however, it will carry the theoretical danger of initiating thyroid-stimulating antibody-related hyperplasia.

It appears that the large doses of radioiodine used to treat hyperthyroidism are associated with a lower incidence of thyroid cancer than that after antithyroid drugs (see later) or surgical thyroidectomy. In one series of more than 16,000 patients with Graves' disease who underwent ^{131}I therapy, 86 subsequently came to operation and were found to have nodules; 77 were benign and 9 were cancerous. On this basis, the prevalence of thyroid cancer in Graves' disease treated with ^{131}I would be about 0.06% compared with the spontaneous prevalence in Graves' disease of about 0.1% (287). As with any nonselected surgical series, especially for Graves' disease where the indication for surgery may be persistent thyrotoxicosis rather than the presence of palpable abnormalities, some of the cancers found were occult.

In a Swedish study of about 4500 patients with hyperthyroidism treated with ^{131}I, four cancers were found, all in women with previous toxic nodular goiters (288). This was an insignificant excess of two cases over the predicted number in a similar nonirradiated group. Thus, in these two populations with a total of more than 20,000 patients followed for 8 to 10 years, there was no evidence of ^{131}I-induced thyroid carcinogenesis at doses higher than 2000 rads in adults.

Exposure to ^{131}I in radioactive fallout has occurred not only in the Marshall Islands (see preceding), but also in the western United States, in the area of the Nevada test sites. One investigation of this population failed to find significant differences between irradiated and nonirradiated subjects in the presence of benign or malignant thyroid nodules at an average follow-up time of 14 years (289). Overall, experience with mean thyroidal doses from ^{131}I of less than 200 rads does not indicate that hu-

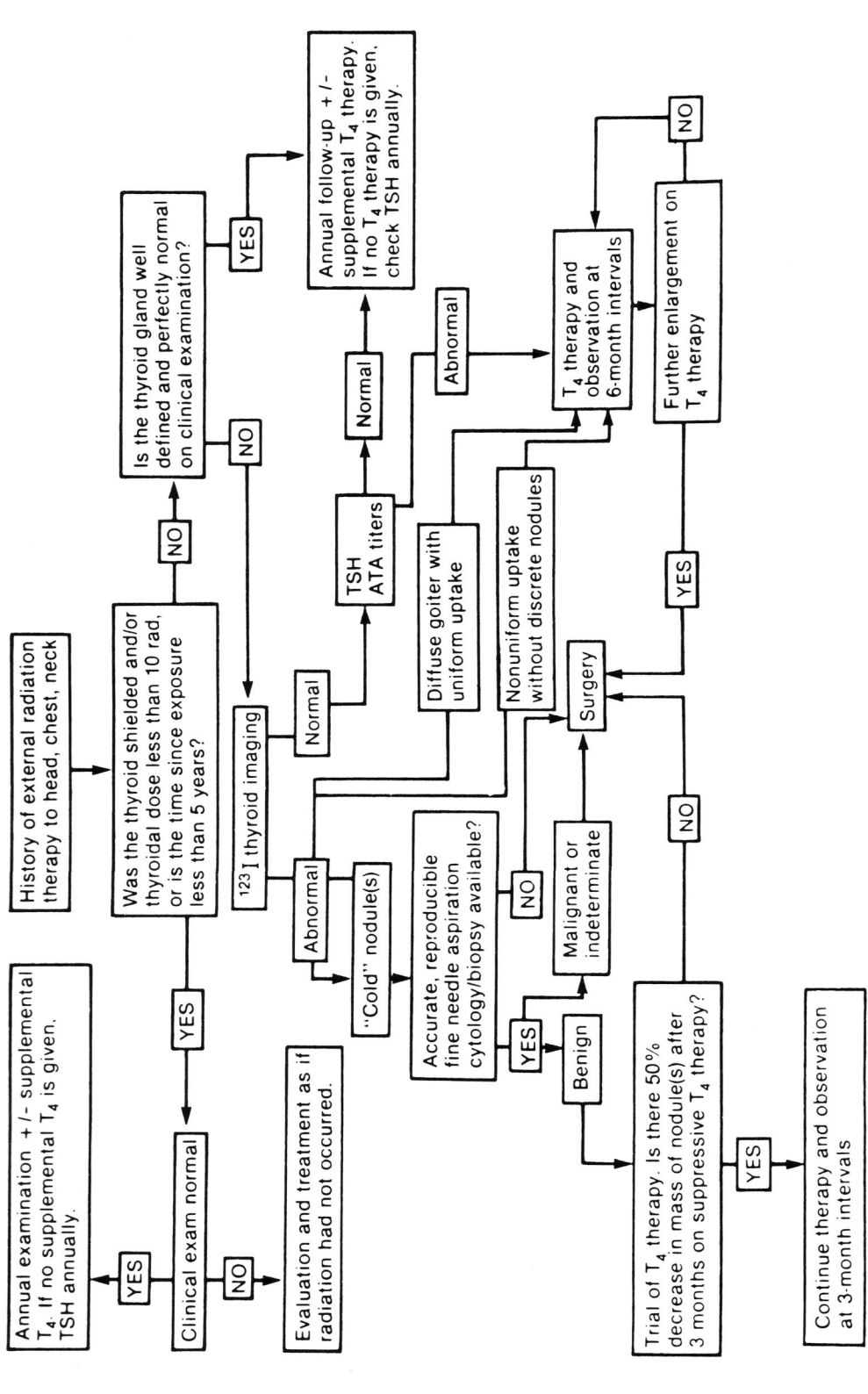

FIG. 4. Diagnostic and therapeutic approach for the management of patients exposed to external radiation to the thyroid area. ATA, antithyroid antibodies. (From ref. 250.)

man radiation carcinogenesis occurs after exposure to ^{131}I. This agent is apparently less carcinogenic on a rad-for-rad basis than external gamma radiation in humans ($\frac{1}{50}$ to $\frac{1}{20}$ as effective), although the two sources are equally effective in causing cancer in rats. Some maintain that a range of from $\frac{1}{10}$ as effective to equal effectiveness is necessary to span the possibilities (290), although the preponderance of animal and human studies indicates that it is unlikely that the two are equally effective. An increased risk from doses of ^{131}I below 400 or 500 rads has not been established in either human or animal studies.

The administration of ^{131}I in a diagnostic context (less than 1 mCi) has also been evaluated for thyroid carcinogenesis. In one report from Sweden, the incidence of thyroid cancer was evaluated in more than 35,000 patients examined for suspected thyroid disorders between 1951 and 1969 (258). The conclusions are difficult to interpret because the test was administered for suspected thyroid disease. The overall conclusion was that the incidence of thyroid cancer was insignificantly greater than that expected in the general population, and this supported the notion that the carcinogenic potential of internal ^{131}I beta particles might be as low as 4 times less than external x-rays or gamma rays (258). [The standard incidence ratio of other cancers, however, has significantly increased on follow-up study in this population, including endocrine cancers other than thyroid, lymphomas, leukemias, and nervous system tumors (291).] This study has been criticized because of inappropriate epidemiologic comparisons. A rebuttal and response are illuminating as examples of how thyroid cancer studies can be intelligently criticized by persons knowledgeable in epidemiologic/statistical analysis at a level that most clinicians cannot hope to approximate (292).

Public health applications apply to populations that may be exposed to short-lived radioiodines from fallout that may occur during nuclear reactor accidents. It appears that these isotopes (the high-energy beta emitters, I-132, I-133, and I-135) are effective inducers of thyroid nodules, and the absolute risk coefficient is almost the same as that estimated for gamma radiation. Populations exposed to radioiodine fallout should not only be considered for potassium iodide prophylaxis at the time of contamination but should also be carefully followed for late development of thyroid nodules.

The role of ^{131}I as an inducer of thyroid neoplasia remains controversial. Any dose of radioiodine over 1000 mCi is associated with an increased risk of leukemia induction. A dose of 1500 mCi has a 10% risk of associated leukemia (293).

Antithyroid Drugs

The possibility that antithyroid drugs may be carcinogenic should also be considered. There are publications based on studies in experimental animals, usually rats, that suggest that goiters induced by antithyroid drugs may develop into metastasizing tumors if treated with carcinogens or radioiodine (200). An essential feature of the successful induction of these experimental thyroid cancers is the creation of conditions in which excess pituitary TSH is secreted

Although there are a few reports of carcinoma of the human thyroid associated with exposure to thiouracil, this cannot be common because drugs of this type have been used extensively for many years. It seems likely that there are significant species differences.

Association of Thyroid Cancer with Other Cancers

At Memorial Sloan-Kettering Cancer Center, 50% of patients in whom an autopsy found a history of, or the presence of, thyroid cancer had a second and entirely separate and different cancer—in an exceedingly high incidence (294). Several reports have indicated a unique association between a first primary tumor in the thyroid or salivary gland and increased incidence of subsequent breast cancer (295). Others have shown either an insignificant slight excess or none at all. A recent series from Johns Hopkins showed an increased risk of developing a second cancer in men and women with a first thyroid malignancy, and the reported association between cancers of the thyroid and breast was confirmed for both sexes (296). The histologic composition of the thyroid cancers was not mentioned; however, some were medullary carcinomas. The adrenal, brain, lymphatic system, and breasts were the most common sites after a first thyroid cancer.

Several pieces of evidence suggest that breast and thyroid cancer have some etiologic factors in common. Both occur more commonly in women than in men, and a geographic correlation between the incidences of goiter and breast cancer as well as between breast cancer and thyroid cancer has been observed in several populations. Women with breast cancer have a 2- to 4-times-higher risk of developing thyroid cancer than women in the general population, and women with thyroid cancer are also more likely to develop breast cancer. It is unlikely that breast cancer per se increases a woman's risk of thyroid cancer, but rather that the two cancers share some etiologic factors (297). It has been observed in laboratory animals that diets low in iodine increase susceptibility to breast carcinogenesis (298).

Although cancers of the breast and thyroid are epidemiologically similar in some ways, there are important differences in a number of their risk factors. Factors that increase the risk of breast cancer (maternal history of breast cancer, nulliparous state, late age of first birth, late menopause, early menarche, abortion or oral contraceptive use prior to first full-term pregnancy) have not been found to increase the risk of thyroid cancer and may actually decrease the risk of thyroid cancer. This makes sense for nonpregnancy-related events. Pregnancy increases the risk of thyroid cancer, presumably because of increased circulating levels of TSH, whereas it decreases the risk of breast cancer if it occurs early in reproductive life.

Heavy radiation exposure to the breast has been found to increase the risk of breast cancer by a factor of four, depending on the dose of radiation, the woman's age at the time of exposure, and the number of years from radiation exposure. It appears that both the breast and thyroid are highly sensitive to the carcinogenic effects of radiation, possibly related to their growth and development.

NEW DIRECTIONS IN CLINICAL AND BASIC RESEARCH

During the past decade, new technologies at the cellular and molecular levels have opened avenues for productive exploration of the mechanisms of carcinogenesis. The following sections summarize the application of these explorations to thyroid neoplasia. In general, this work is still preliminary, but some authors extrapolate beyond the data to potential clinical applications. An update of this chapter 5 or 10 years from now would put these issues in better perspective.

Genetic Studies

Whereas MTC shows genetic inheritance patterns, no definite inheritance has been observed for DTC other than a possible association of papillary thyroid carcinoma with Gardner's syndrome (familial adenomatous polyposis of the colon associated with multiple osteomas, epidermoid cysts, and fibromas of cutaneous and subcutaneous origin), which was described in 1953 (299). Carcinoma of the thyroid gland has been reported sporadically in patients with adenomatous polyposis, and a recent paper based on a review of the polyposis registry from London indicated that young women under 35 years of age are particularly at risk of developing thyroid cancer, mainly of the papillary type (300). Their chances of being affected were approximately 160 times that of the normal population, and it was therefore suggested that all patients with Gardner's syndrome should have regular thyroid examinations. Many other malignancies have been reported in association with adenomatous polyposis (in the central nervous system, bladder, and liver), although it is unclear whether these are coincidental or genetically determined.

There have been reports of thyroid carcinomas occurring in multiple members of the same family with no evidence of prior irradiation. Because papillary cancers have occurred both in father/son and mother/daughter pedigrees, it is possible that both environmental and genetic factors operate. One recent case report notes the occurrence of papillary thyroid cancer in identical twins (301), and MTC has also been reported in twins (302).

Earlier indications that genetic factors may be involved in the susceptibility to thyroid cancer have recently been emphasized by the finding of an association of differentiated epithelial thyroid cancer with human leukocyte antigens (HLA) and immunoglobulin G heavy-chain markers. The HLA-DR group has been particularly studied. The interest in the association of HLA antigens with DTC was triggered by a pilot study where HLA-DR1 was found to be increased among 20 Italian patients with thyroid cancer (303). This was confirmed in a larger patient group from eastern Hungary, and HLA-DR7 was reported to be increased in patients with thyroid carcinoma from the American Midwest. On the other hand, a study from Newfoundland found no association of HLA with DTC markers in 45 patients. It has been conjectured that because both southern Italy and eastern Hungary are iodide-deficient areas, this may predispose HLA-DR1-positive individuals to thyroid cell transformation, whereas iodine sufficiency apparently negates such an influence (as seen in Newfoundland) unless some other environmental factors supervene (304).

A recent report purporting to document familial occurrence of differentiated nonmedullary thyroid carcinoma (305) had the significance of its conclusions expertly questioned in an accompanying discussion (306). Apparently the associations reported between the HLA allele and thyroid cancer did not retain their significance "after allowing for the Bonferroni inequality." As scientific methodology increases in complexity, it requires correspondingly sophisticated analysis of methods and statistics to assess the validity of contributions to the literature, and this level of sophistication is lacking in many clinicians.

Immunogenetic and immunologic studies of DTC are ongoing, and theories incriminating somatic mutation or an immunological defect in the etiology of thyroid tumors have had adherents for a long time. Certainly, chromosomal abnormalities in antigen-deficient cells abound in thyroid tumors, but their role in tumor induction or behavior has not been fully characterized. They may be the results of disorder and overgrowth rather than the cause. Interest in these areas initially developed in the late 1960s and early 1970s and has undergone a resurgence with the application of modern techniques to the immune response that facilitate studies at the cellular, molecular, and genetic levels (307).

For example, evidence indicates that an increased H_2 antigen expression is directly related to increased metastatic potential. The opposing host response in this case is apparently related to natural killer (NK) cell activity which operates best in the absence of H_2 antigens on the target cells. The correlation between metastatic potential and the increased expression of all or some major histocompatibility complex (MHC) class I alleles, observed for several tumors, could be ascribed to selection of certain phenotypes that are able to escape NK cell surveillance. On the other hand, in a variety of virally or chemically induced tumors, a selective absence of MHC class I molecules has repeatedly been reported to be associated with enhanced tumor growth and metastasis. These controversies need to be clarified by study of additional epithelial and mesenchymal cell lines infected with a variety of retroviruses carrying different oncogenes.

One study suggested that transformation in rat thyroid epithelial cells is strongly associated with the modulation of MHC class I antigen expression (308). This study (in undifferentiated transformed cell lines rather than a differentiated cell line) purported to show that this modulation occurs *in vivo* and is not a consequence of establishing cells in culture. The absence of MHC class I antigens on the surface of cells from different tumors suggests a general mechanism by which tumor cells escape immunosurveillance. This study also suggests that tumor cells may escape control by mechanisms not triggered by reduced or absent expression of MHC class I antigens. This view is further supported by the finding that normal human thyroid tissues express low levels of MHC class I antigens, whereas over 50% of thyroid carcinomas show an increased expression of such antigens (309,310).

Oncogene Studies

A recent major thrust of molecular oncology is the attempt to predict clinical behavior based on various patterns of oncogene activation: in other words, to define prognosticators of individual tumor biology at the genetic level (see also Chapter 13). Activation and mutation of cellular oncogenes is thought to be an important event in tumor initiation, promotion, and progression.

Nucleotide sequences present in the genome of mammalian cells that are homologous to sequences of certain RNA tumor viruses are called proto-oncogenes, and proteins encoded by these sequences are thought to be important in normal cell differentiation and growth. When enhanced proto-oncogene expression is present, the genes are referred to as oncogenes, and they appear to be integrally responsible for neoplastic differentiation. Strong evidence has accumulated supporting the hypothesis that abnormalities in either the structure or activity of proto-oncogenes contribute to the development and/or maintenance of the malignant phenotype, and a unified concept of neoplastic transformation and normal growth stimulation is emerging. Oncogenes are viewed as representing altered versions of normal cellular genes (proto-oncogenes) that encode proteins that operate along the mitogenic pathway. Oncogenes are, therefore, thought to transform the cell by generating an abnormal growth stimulus that causes a short-circuit in the mitogenic pathway. Thus, an unscheduled synthesis of a growth factor in cells that carry the cognate receptor (autocrine growth stimulation) is generally thought to be one of several mechanisms of transformation (311–313).

By 1987, approximately 25 to 30 oncogenes had been identified, isolated, and characterized from mammalian tissue, and their gene products can be grouped into functional classes as affecting levels of second messenger molecules, modulating transcription, or encoding growth factors or their receptors (314).

There is great interest in this area and correspondingly rapid evolution of new data and technology. For the majority of known neoplasms, no specific genomic alterations have yet been defined. In some cases, however, tumor aggressivity and state of differentiation have been correlated with the expression of certain oncogenes.

Thyroid cancer provides an attractive model to investigate the role of oncogene activation in different stages of neoplasia because of the spectrum of growth abnormalities that occur in the gland, both hyperplastic and neoplastic (varying from slowly progressive well-differentiated tumors to anaplastic highly malignant neoplasms). Other attractions are that thyroid cancer is related to rather well-defined factors (radiation) and displays nonrandom geographic distribution. Investigating the possible involvement of oncogenes in the trophic hormone control of the thyroid is also of interest. MTC is an important human cancer for the study of molecular abnormalities that underlie initiation and progression of neoplasia (315). The tumor occurs in different inherited forms, each mediated by autosomal dominant genetic events. (Germ line abnormalities on chromosome 10 are linked by MEN type II.)

Such studies are facilitated by the availability of animal models and cell lines of both DTC (316) and MTC (317). In cell culture, chemical modulation of gene insertion can lead to partial correction of defects in differentiation capacity by activating cellular signaling processes. The successful establishment of both normal and neoplastic thyroid cells in culture provides a useful arena for genetic technology.

The molecular basis of thyroid disease is only beginning to be explored by oncogene studies. Enhanced oncogene expression observed in lymphocytes from patients with systemic lupus erythematosus has suggested the importance of studying oncogene expression and regulation in autoimmune thyroid diseases.

Thyroid tumors have only recently been included in surveys of oncogene expression in humans, probably because of their low incidence and low mortality. The current directions in oncogene studies on thyroid cancer are indicated below. Detailed discussion is not warranted at this point, because these studies require confirmation and amplification.

Evidence for the existence of a new transforming gene in thyroid papillary carcinomas and their lymph node metastases was first presented in 1987 (318). The same oncogene was activated in five papillary carcinomas and in two of their respective metastases, strongly suggesting tissue-specific activation. This was the first report of a transforming gene associated with thyroid cancer present in both primary tumor and metastases, and also one of the few cases in which a new oncogene had been isolated from specimens obtained from several patients carrying the same histologic type of tumor. The authors presumed that the transforming gene was somatically activated in the tumor cells because they did not observe transforming activity in human DNA extracted from normal thyroid and lymphoid tissues obtained from the same patients. The activation of the oncogene in 5 of the 12 patients with papillary carcinoma and the fact that the oncogene did not cross-hybridize with a broad range of cloned viral and human oncogenes indicated the activation of a new transforming gene in these carcinomas designated papillary thyroid carcinoma (PTC). It was frequently activated in the primary tumors and lymph node metastases of the same patients. Molecular cloning of PTC shows that this oncogene is located on chromosome 10, and work is in progress to isolate a full-length cDNA of PTC and to obtain sequence data of the coding regions that have been identified.

This group of investigators is also cloning another activated oncogene detected in a sixth patient harboring PTC. The gene is not homologous to PTC and does not cross-hybridize with the *ras* gene family (319). Investigations are ongoing to ascertain whether the activation of thyroid-related oncogenes is a common feature of thyroid cancer or specific to the histologic subtype.

In most transfection studies of human tumor material, transforming activity has been found to be caused by a member of the *ras* oncogene family, which has been studied more intensively than any other group of cellular oncogenes. The *ras* oncogenes encode a 21-kilodalton protein termed P-21, which interacts with cellular plasma membranes, binds guanyl nucleotide specifically, and possesses guanosine triphosphatase (GTPase) activity. Thus, *ras* P-21 is thought to participate in the control of cell proliferation, possibly as a signal transducer from the extracellular environment to the nucleus. Transformation of some mammalian cells occurs if P-21 is expressed at an abnormally high level or if a point mutation on the *ras* gene alters the P-21 primary structure. Controversy persists over whether or not *ras* activation is necessary in carcinogenesis or tumor progression. Both enhanced and normal levels of *ras* expression have been found in various human malignant neoplasms based on immunohistochemical studies using monoclonal antibodies (MoAbs) to the *ras* P-21 product.

Recently, *ras* P-21 has been detected in normal, benign, and malignant human thyroid tissue (320). Elevated apical surface expression of *ras* product in papillary carcinoma suggests that it is the site of reception of environmental stimuli and may be necessary in neoplastic proliferation of follicular epithelium. The regular presence of apical surface staining in carcinomas as opposed to adenomas may become useful in differential diagnosis.

Activation of *ras* oncogenes has also been detected in human anaplastic thyroid carcinomas (321). This study suggested that H-*ras* activation could predispose a papillary carcinoma to become anaplastic, which could prove to be a useful prognosticator for the development of malignant progression in thyroid cancers.

In another study, DNA transfection analysis of five follicular and ten papillary thyroid cancers showed a statistically significant difference in the pattern of gene activation between the two histologic types (322). Activated *ras* oncogenes were found in 80% of follicular tumors but in only 20% of papillary tumors. In addition, activation of all three oncogenes (H-*ras*, K-*ras*, and N-*ras*) was found in follicular cancers, the first time that this had been demonstrated in a primary human tumor as opposed to cell lines. It should be noted that oncogene technology is not standardized, and different rates of transforming activity reported for the same histologic entities can be explained by technical differences such as the greater sensitivity of particular assays at various institutions. In this study, the detection of serially transmissible transforming activity in 100% of the follicular cancer DNAs and in 90% of the papillary cancer DNAs was unexpectedly high, because previous studies had shown only 10% to 20% of randomly selected human tumors contained transforming genes detectable by transfection assays.

The marked difference in the frequency of activated *ras* oncogenes in papillary versus follicular cancers was interpreted by the authors to represent an oncogene manifestation of the marked difference seen clinically in the biologic behavior of these tumor types. Transfection experiments have shown that the metastatic potential of tumor cells may be modified by introduction of an activated *ras* oncogene, and it has been suggested that the *ras* gene product may trigger a program of metastasis that is specific for the particular cell type. In some animal models, preferential hematogenous metastasis has been shown after introduction of the activated *ras* oncogene into carcinoma cells, and this may relate to the almost exclusively hematogenous metastatic pattern seen with follicular thyroid cancers (which in this study were associated with a very high frequency of *ras* oncogene activation).

The oncogene c-*myc* is thought to play a role in the cellular proliferation of solid and hematopoietic human tumors and may also be important in the pathogenesis of autoimmune disorders. The expression of c-*myc* has been studied in normal, adenomatous, and cancerous thyroid tissue (323) as well as in thyrocytes and lymphocytes from patients with autoimmune thyroid disease (324). In the thyroid, TSH (presumably acting through its receptor) can activate c-*myc* expression, and interleukin-1 can also stimulate c-*myc* RNA expression in thyroid follicular cells in culture, as can dibuteryl cyclic AMP. Expression of c-*myc* oncogene is comparable in normal thyrocytes and in thyroid nodules or thyroid cancer samples and, therefore, may have a role in both normal and neoplastic thyrocyte growth. The oncogene c-*fos* can also be induced by TSH, dibuteryl cyclic AMP, and interleukin-1 in cultured rat or dog thyroid cells.

Recently, oncogene expression was studied in fresh biopsies from eight patients with different types of thyroid tumors and in biopsies from a diffuse toxic goiter and a lymphoma of the thyroid (325). Oncogene c-*erb* B, which encodes the receptor for epidermal growth factor (EGF) and transforming growth factor alpha, as well as the closely related c-*erb* B2/neu, were expressed in papillary thyroid carcinomas. These receptor-type oncogenes have been found amplified and/or overexpressed in a number of human tumors of epithelial origin, such as squamous carcinoma, and in brain tumors. Because it has recently been shown by several groups that EGF induces proliferation and dedifferentiation of normal thyroid epithelial cells in culture (326), the authors conjectured that elevated expression of EGF receptors or other ligands for the c-*erb* B and c-*erb* B2/neu receptors may contribute to the development of a malignant phenotype of thyroid cancer by increasing proliferation and dedifferentiation. Because one anaplastic carcinoma exhibited a markedly different pattern of oncogene expression when compared to the papillary carcinomas (c-*myc* and N-*ras* oncogenes were expressed at high levels as well as RNA specific for the alpha and beta chains of platelet-derived growth factor), it was suggested that these differences might reflect the varying clinical aggressiveness of these two types of tumors.

Medullary thyroid carcinoma naturally lends itself to oncogene analysis, because these tumors produce multiple regulatory peptide products. Structural characterization of these peptides has provided insight into the pathways of posttranslational processing of prohormones in the tumor cells. Preliminary work needs to be amplified using more tumor samples to determine if certain pathways are generally followed in MTCs (327).

In patients with MTC, there is a distinct relationship between the degree of cellular differentiation and clinical behavior. Diminished calcitonin production is a constant feature of tumor tissues in patients dying of metastases, whereas retention of high calcitonin content is seen in patients with more indolent tumors. Presumably, the loss of critical genes that maintain normal differentiation accompanies cell transformation and/or tumor progression. The genes responsible for maintenance of proper endocrine cell differentiation and regulation of calcitonin production in thyroid C cells (and whose expression might be impaired in tumor cells, preventing proper maturation) are not known.

Introduction of the viral Harvey *ras* (v-Ha-*ras*) oncogene into cultured human MTC cells can reverse the changes in gene expression associated with the loss of differentiation that leads to decreased calcitonin content. A return of endocrine differentiation of the tumor cells can be induced (328). Such work is potentially very exciting for redifferentiation or preventing dedifferentiation in neoplasia.

Activation of the proto-oncogene N-*myc* has been implicated in the pathogenesis of neuroendocrine neoplasia such as small-cell lung cancer, retinoblastoma, and Wilms' tumor. N-*myc* expression has recently been demonstrated in several MTC samples, strengthening the hypothesis that *myc* oncogene activation plays a role in neuroendocrine neoplasia (329). N-*myc* was present in about 30% of thyroid C cell tumors but was undetectable in normal adult C cells and was, therefore, considered to be a specific feature of C cell tumors and not merely a differentiation marker representing their cell of origin. The mechanism of the increase in N-*myc* messenger RNA (mRNA) in the tumor cells remains to be investigated, as well as whether the increase is a cause or consequence of the neoplastic phenotype.

Studies indicating that the c-*erb* A gene encodes a thyroid hormone receptor have suggested a relationship between oncogenes and hormonal receptors not previously recognized (330). Application of this approach to thyroid tissue could determine whether the TSH receptor is a constitutive oncogene protein and whether other thyroid cell growth factors also interact with oncogene proteins.

The utility of assessing RNA as well as DNA in patients with thyroid and other diseases is being recognized. Studies are now being performed to assess whether neoplastic cells express oncogenic RNA either in excessive amounts or in abnormal forms.

These are examples of the use of subcellular technology to dissect the molecular events that regulate endocrine cell differentiation. It is hoped that it will be possible to determine the precise abnormalities that underlie the initiation and tumor progression events in MTC, DTC, and related cancers and, thereby, to identify new targets for therapeutic intervention. Continued studies on the molecular control of differentiation may identify new target points for design of "biomodifier" agents that can contribute to cancer therapy by inducing maturation of cancer cells in patients. The idea of redifferentiating dedifferentiated cancer cells has been around for a long time, but with the new genetic engineering techniques, theory emerges into the realm of possibility. The ability to differentiate MTC cells *in vitro* suggests that some phenotypic consequences of genetic alteration in cancer cells can be overcome through manipulation of cell signaling processes. These and similar findings in other tumor systems have raised hopes for the use of such manipulations *in vivo* for therapeutic purposes (315). Oncogenes in thyroid cancer are also discussed in references 331–341.

Tumor Markers

New methods in immunocytochemistry and hybridization techniques now enable the pathologist to clarify problems in the classification and prognosis of tumors. The study of tumor markers includes the identification of biologic products secreted by cells that are specific for the cell or origin. Aspects of the topic have recently been reviewed in general (342) and as they relate to thyroid cancer (343,344). Metabolic processes and their products are compared and contrasted between normal and neoplastic cells. The study systems include animal models and in vitro systems. Monoclonal antibody techniques are being applied not only to thyroid surgical specimens and to tissues in culture, but to thyroid needle aspiration specimens that aid cytologic interpretation (345).

It is hoped that in the future such studies can be exploited as mechanisms for understanding, diagnosing, and managing many tumors, including those of the thyroid. For example, the aggressive approach to thyroid tumors currently advocated by many surgeons will undoubtedly continue in the absence of a biologic marker that will allow the identification of patients whose disease is ultimately fatal. Because clinical prognosticators as reflected by the TNM tumor staging system have not proven to be sufficiently accurate to accomplish this objective, the search has progressed, with the aid of recent technological advances, to the cellular and subcellular level, where it is hoped that accurate prognostic parameters will be identified.

As in many other fields of tumor pathology, application of immunohistochemical techniques to thyroid lesions has provided new insight into histogenesis and has proved to be of considerable diagnostic help. Poorly differentiated neoplasms in the thyroid gland and metastatic lesions associated with "unknown primary tumor" site can frequently be categorized by their degree of differentiation and/or thyroidal origin with the application of tumor markers. Thyroglobulin, intermediate filaments, and calcitonin are the most useful. The T_3, T_4, and Tg markers are typically found in tumors with follicular differentiation, and there is coexpression of cytokeratins and vimentin in approximately 50% of follicular and in virtually all papillary carcinomas. Tumor cells with epithelial differentiation can be defined by immunocytochemical localization of cytokeratins; this has aided in the documentation of the epithelial origin of most undifferentiated (anaplastic) thyroid carcinomas.

Anaplastic thyroid carcinoma (ATC) is subdivided into three categories: giant cell, spindle cell, and small cell. Immunohistochemistry has proven invaluable in defining variants in the small cell category. Nearly all tumors formerly known as anaplastic small cell carcinoma are either malignant lymphomas, small cell types of medullary carcinomas, or poorly differentiated "insular" carcinomas, a tumor of follicular cell origin with morphologic and behavioral features intermediate between well-differentiated and anaplastic carcinoma and uniformly positive for Tg (346). Most of the lymphomas are B cell, non-Hodgkin's type.

A variety of neuroendocrine hormones originate from membrane-bound neurosecretory granules in MTC including calcitonin, somatostatin, bombesin, gastrin-releasing peptide, substance P, L-dopa decarboxylase, histaminase, neuron-specific enolase, chromogranin, calcitonin gene-related peptide, and CEA. (CEA has also been detected in undifferentiated carcinomas with a squamoid growth pattern and in Hürthle cell carcinomas.)

With the exception of rare anaplastic variants, the prognosis of MTC cannot be predicted on a histologic basis alone, and it is hoped that correlation with various products identifiable by immunohistochemistry will solve this problem. Attempts have been made to correlate CEA and calcitonin patterns with tumor virulence. One study showed that in early disease, both markers have a similar distribution and are present in virtually every cell whether disease is diffuse or localized (100). In the case of virulent disseminated disease, however, CEA expression persists in cells that have poor or no staining for calcitonin. This suggests that in MTC, expression of CEA (a marker for early epithelial differentiation) in the face of loss of calcitonin (a marker for terminal differentiation/cellular maturity) may reflect a degree of maturation block in patients with aggressive disease, and that persistently high or increasing CEA levels in the face of falling or stable calcitonin levels might predict aggressive clinical behavior. A more recent study, however, indicates that poor or heterogeneous staining for calcitonin does not always predict aggressive behavior, nor does homogeneous staining guarantee a favorable outcome (347).

Immunohistochemical techniques also have the potential of offering a more precise classification of thyroid carcinomas than is available by light microscopy. Recently, immunohistochemical studies using a broad library of antibodies to polypeptide hormone products have identified tumors with combined follicular and C cell differentiation, suggesting a mixed medullary–follicular type of carcinoma not definable at the light microscope level without marker technology.

An increasing number of tumor- and thyroid-associated antigens have been demonstrated in the spectrum of thyroid carcinoma subtypes. Many of the modern tumor markers defined by MoAbs represent carbohydrate antigens derived from blood group determinants or blood group precursor substances. Recently, tumor-associated carbohydrate antigens (defined by the MoAbs CA50 and CA19-9) were found to be significantly expressed in carcinoma tissue as opposed to normal and hyperplastic thyroid tissue (348). It has been suggested that expression of tumor-associated carbohydrate antigens may be essential for tumor cells to maintain their transformed phenotype.

The ability to express blood-group antigens is widespread in most embryonic tissue and is lost with differentiation. Reexpression is gained in some tissues under pathological conditions. In some studies, epithelial expression of blood group isoantigens was not observed in normal thyroid tissue, but was reexpressed upon neoplastic transformation, more frequently in papillary than in follicular tumors. Medullary carcinomas have not been found to express ABO blood group isoantigens in some studies. Besides MoAbs, lectins are the major analysis tools for studying glycoconjugates. Studies of the lectin reactivity of normal, adenomatous, and carcinomatous thyroid tissues have revealed differences in binding properties between these entities. Interestingly, many of the lectins whose binding properties differ in normal and neoplastic thyroid tissue possess blood group specificity. This suggests that at least some of the different lectin-binding properties distinguishing normal follicular from neoplastic differentiated thyroid cancer cells may be a result of their reaction with blood group isoantigens reexpressed in the carcinomas.

Thyroglobulin Markers (See also Chapters 30 and 31)

Thyroglobulin is one of the most important thyroid cell proteins because of its fundamental role in the synthesis, secretion, and accumulation of thyroid hormones. This glycoprotein is situated in the thyroid cells and gains access to the peripheral circulation only after damage to cell membranes. A very small amount is detectable under physiologic conditions. Most tumors with histologically recognizable follicular or papillary differentiation produce Tg, whereas undifferentiated (anaplastic) thyroid carcinoma and pure medullary carcinomas are negative for Tg, although undifferentiated tumors having a residual well-differentiated component can show positivity in these areas. The subject is not completely clear in the literature, because nonneoplastic follicles entrapped by the tumor react strongly, and diffusion of Tg can occur immediately around these entrapped follicles, causing spurious staining of cancer cells.

Biochemical study of Tg secretion by thyroid tumors has been slow to develop, largely as a result of the complexity of this macromolecule. Interestingly, the Tg produced by thyroid carcinoma may exhibit some structural differences in chemical composition and configuration from that of the normal gland. If confirmed, this alteration may be exploited as an additional tool for the understanding and diagnosis of thyroid tumors. Synthesis of Tg by well-differentiated thyroid carcinomas has been demonstrated by direct extraction of the protein from the neoplastic tissue, by its presence in the serum of patients, by its immunohistochemical detection in primary and metastatic tumors, and by the identification of Tg messenger-RNA with *in situ* hybridization. Pathologically increased Tg production returns to normal or subnormal levels after removal of the thyroid tumor, and in the presence of local recurrence or metastatic disease, the Tg level may rise significantly. These factors allow it to be used as a marker for disease persistence or progression.

Thyroglobulin measurements have been used to determine the probability of a thyroid nodule occurring in the population that underwent childhood radiation. A normal Tg level initially, followed by a rise, has been shown to be associated with the development of thyroid nodules. If the initial serum Tg level is above normal, the chance of developing a nodule is increased. Similarly, a change in serum Tg is significant: an increase of more than 10 ng/mL during less than 10 years indicates an increased chance that a nodule has developed (249). Most individuals with nodular thyroid disease have an increased Tg level, but when thyroid nodular disease is detected, the serum Tg level is unable to distinguish between malignant and benign disease, so it is not sufficient for complete evaluation. In general, serum Tg does not have good predictive value as a screening test for thyroid malignancy because of its low specificity and the low prevalence of the disease.

With thyroid cancer, it has been demonstrated that in patients with metastases from an unknown primary site, a high level of serum Tg helps point to the thyroid as the source. Lower levels do not rule out thyroid origin, however (350).

Serum Tg is useful for detection of metastatic disease in the majority of patients with DTC who have been totally thyroidectomized by either surgery alone or surgery and radioiodine ablation. If the serum Tg level rises above the normal range in follow-up, it indicates recurrent or metastatic disease, and it is best used now in conjunction with the standard ^{131}I scan (see later).

Serum Tg levels in patients with metastatic disease increase after withdrawal of hormonal replacement as a result of a rise in TSH secretion. The normal Tg level ranges from 5 to 60 ng/mL in different studies, and its sensitivity in detecting recurrent thyroid DTC in follow-up ranges from 85% to 90%. In some patients with verified metastases, a normal Tg level is found and this is associated with the presence of anti-Tg antibody, at least in some cases. The level of Tg should be nearly zero after total thyroidectomy when there is no residual tumor. When thyroid hormone is discontinued to perform a thyroid scan with radioiodine, patients with metastatic disease will often show increased Tg levels. This Tg increase suggests not only that residual thyroid tumor is present, but also that this residual tumor responds to TSH stimulation.

A high degree of correlation exists between ^{131}I uptake and Tg synthesis by metastatic foci; however, not all Tg-synthesizing carcinomas concentrate iodine well, and scintigraphy is sometimes unable to detect micrometastases except with a megadose of radioiodine. The Tg level, however, is a suitable indicator in this context. Also, because Tg measurement requires only a serum sample and there is no need for transient hypothyroidism (in order to assure appropriate iodine uptake in detection of metastases the patient must be in a hypothyroid state, which induces an overproduction of TSH), studies have evaluated whether or not Tg is adequate alone as a substitute for scintigraphy in follow-up of thyroid cancer patients. The hypothyroid state is at least theoretically dangerous based on growth-controlling mechanisms relating to induction of thyroid cancer (see later).

Both serum Tg and ^{131}I total body scans are recommended now to detect recurrence (351), because there is not a one-to-one correspondence in all studies comparing these two methods of follow-up. In one study, Tg synthesis and concomitant ^{131}I uptake were observed in only two thirds of the patients, so serum Tg concentration cannot be used as a parameter for the prediction of ^{131}I uptake by metastases. [Considering the sequential steps of thyroid hormone biosynthesis, the presence of T_3 or T_4 in carcinomatous tissue would be expected to reflect the ability of metastatic lesions to take up ^{131}I more exactly than does the presence of Tg (352,353).]

Thyroglobulin measurement could substitute for whole-body radioiodine scans only if all primary thyroid tissue has been eliminated during the patient's initial treatment. If not, remaining thyroid tissue will by itself generate near-normal serum Tg levels and recurrence/metastasis-induced Tg stimulations will, therefore, merely elevate this level, whereas in athyreotic patients, nondetectable Tg levels will rise to significant levels.

In some cases, Tg positivity precedes the development of metastases on scan. (The absence of TSH receptors is presumably the mechanism accounting for lack of uptake of iodine by some DTCs.) The opposite pattern can also be seen. In one recent case report in a patient with papillary thyroid carcinoma with lung metastases, a normal Tg level was found and metastases were demonstrated on total-body ^{131}I scan. Hypothetical explanations for this situation include presence of immunologically altered Tg not detected by the standard assay, of Tg antibodies, or of thyroid cancer whose cells have lost their ability to synthesize Tg.

T_4 therapy can nearly completely suppress Tg production. One recent study suggested that in high-risk patients, both tests (Tg measurement and scintigraphy) should be performed to document that low Tg levels on T_4 therapy correspond to negative scan findings off T_4 therapy before continuing to follow patients with serum Tg levels alone (354).

In short, a normal Tg level does not always preclude the possibility of metastatic disease, but serum Tg measurements are now considered routine in follow-up of DTC patients. A detectable Tg level while the patient is receiving thyroid supplementation warrants further investigation, beginning with a total-body scan. A negative scan does not preclude the existence of metastases, and additional attempts to localize thyroid tissue should be made, especially if the serum Tg level is higher than 10 ng/mL while the patient is receiving thyroid treatment, or if it increases above this level after thyroid hormone withdrawal. Additional tests may include neck ultrasound, neck and thoracic CT scans, and administration of high-dose ^{131}I (100 mCi) followed by a total-body scan 5 days later (163).

Until recently, little has been known about the role of Tg and TSH in the preclinical phase of thyroid cancer. In an interesting recent study, the pathobiologic understanding of carcinogenesis in the thyroid was enhanced when Tg levels were compared between individuals who later developed cancer and healthy persons (355). This was made possible by using the biologic serum bank obtained from 100,000 Norwegians in combination with the nationwide cancer registry of Norway. It was possible to compare Tg and TSH levels in sera taken several years before clinical appearance of thyroid tumors, and comparison with matched healthy controls was made from the same geographic area. The main findings were that in papillary and follicular carcinomas, there is no fundamental change in serum Tg levels from the preclinical stage to the clinical stage developing years later, and that there was a highly significant difference between serum Tg levels in blood samples between patients and controls.

The prolonged latency period from serum Tg elevation to clinical tumor manifestation suggested a continued release from dormant tumor cells rather than from destruction of adjacent thyroid follicles being actively invaded by growing tumor. The authors postulated that the presence of subclinical tumors for several years was responsible for the relatively large leakage of Tg into the peripheral blood, and that the early elevation of serum Tg is not a tumor secretory cell product as such, but rather a leakage phenomenon caused by some destructive carcinogenic factor relating to altered histologic architecture in the tumor and abnormal Tg release into the extracellular fluid and lymphatics. Alternatively, serum Tg leakage might open the gland to the influence of circulating carcinogens.

This series has implications concerning hypothetical mechanisms of thyroid carcinogenesis mentioned in other sections of this chapter. Because serum Tg tends to be increased years before the clinical appearance of thyroid cancer, whereas serum TSH is not elevated, the initiating carcinogenic factors might not act by inhibition of thyroid hormone production with secondary TSH stimulation leading to tumor promotion and progression. New references on Tg markers are 356–358.

Ploidy as a Tumor Marker

To date, no single microscopic or ultrastructural feature has emerged as a reliable means of predicting a fatal outcome in any cancer patient, although a prominent focus is the attempt to identify subcellular and molecular prognosticators. One methodology touted as having considerable promise in this regard is DNA flow cytometry, which assesses cellular ploidy. In general, over the past few years, aggregate results suggest that patients with aneuploid tumors do more poorly than those with diploid tumors; however, there are many dissenting series that indicate the opposite conclusion as well.

In attributing prognostic significance to cytomorphometric parameters, such as mitotic activity, nuclear area, nuclear diameter, and DNA content, conclusions are limited, especially for thyroid cancer, by short follow-up, loss of patients to follow-up, and lack of correlation with other presumably significant clinical prognostic factors, such as sex and age.

An objective quantitative analysis of cellular DNA content in solid tissues has become possible during the past decade with the advent of flow cytometry and appropriate tissue disaggregation techniques. Difficulty in producing a single-cell tumor suspension has been a major stumbling block. Single-cell technique is advantageous in that individual cells can be identified and selected prior to measurement, and irrelevant cells can be eliminated. This process does lead to sampling errors, however, and single cell measurements are comparatively time consuming currently. Discrepancies between reports are largely a result of differing methods of DNA determination or of different criteria for histologic classification. Other problems arise because the effects of preoperative therapeutic modalities, such as hormone suppression and radioiodine or external irradiation on flow cytometric analysis of thyroid neoplasms, are unknown.

Histologic changes often vary considerably within the lesions, especially with thyroid cancer, and a large number of sections are therefore necessary to obtain a correct histopathologic diagnosis. For thyroid malignancy, quantitative histopathology is merely an adjunct to the scrupulous examination that must be conducted at the light microscope level to differentiate malignancy from benignancy. Both ploidy and proliferative activity of thyroid lesions have been studied (some suggest that a high proliferative activity may be of greater prognostic importance than the nuclear DNA content), and comparisons have been made between primary and metastatic thyroid cancers.

Thyroid tumors have been found to be both euploid and aneuploid and, in general, increased and/or highly variable DNA amounts (aneuploidy) are associated with markedly atypical cells of poorly differentiated histologic pattern and more aggressive biologic behavior than tumors exhibiting euploid DNA values, which are associated with a more differentiated growth pattern and better clinical outcome. The situation is still not clear cut. Some benign lesions with extensive hyperplasia have DNA contents characteristic of malignancy, whereas some cancers do not display the DNA content typical of malignant tumors.

As of 1983, an abnormal nuclear DNA content (aneuploidy) as determined by flow cytometry was found to occur in about 75% of human solid cancers (359). With thyroid cancers, 0% to 40% of papillary, 65% of follicular, and about 50% of medullary carcinomas are aneuploid. The 35 references in a recent review article provide a good up-to-date bibliography on this topic (360).

Some of the more interesting examples of utilization of DNA studies on controversial issues in thyroid neoplasia are summarized below. As noted before, these data should be considered preliminary and should not be accepted as fact until considerably more extensive experience accumulates.

DNA analysis has been applied to the knotty and persistent problem of differentiating follicular adenomas from carcinomas. In one study, the size of nuclei increased from normal thyroid to adenoma to carcinomatous tissue (361). One study claims a reliable differentiation between benign and malignant tumors of thyroid follicular origin based on DNA content (362), but Cady lends perspective to this claim pointing out that distinguishing microinvasive follicular adenocarcinomas from follicular adenoma is extremely difficult and requires extensive capsular sampling and pathologic evaluation, so it is unlikely that the DNA content of cells in the center of such lesions would allow separation of these two entities.

A German study of 53 thyroid carcinomas examined the prognostic information obtained by DNA cytophotometry for clinical outcome, although the median follow-up on patients was only 4 years (363). In general, euploid carcinomas had a good prognosis, whereas aneuploid tumors had a bad prognosis and a generally shortened life span. Interestingly, the encapsulated variants of DTC with their generally excellent prognosis exhibited DNA histograms similar to those of their widely invasive counterparts. This suggested that the favorable prognosis of these minimally invasive subtypes was primarily caused by the tumor's encapsulation rather than to a particular DNA content.

Another recent study showed that DNA nuclear content correlated significantly with histologic type and, for papillary cancers, with tumor grade (85). In a comparison of many prognostic variables in 113 patients from the Netherlands, the presence of DMs at diagnosis was the most important prognostic factor, but in the patient group without DMs, multiploidy was the only significant prognostic factor for overall survival (including histology, tumor grade, extrathyroidal growth, nodal involvement, nuclear DNA content, age at diagnosis, and sex). For indicating disease-free survival, multiploidy was second only to the age factor. The conclusion was that DNA content is a prognostic factor in patients with DTC without DMs at diagnosis.

Similarly, in another study, tumor cell DNA that could be studied both preoperatively in needle aspiration smears and postoperatively in tissue sections was found to have great predictive power and to give significant additional prognostic information when added to other factors such as sex, age, tumor size, and TNM classification (364). Nuclear DNA content alone had a predictive power equivalent to, and in papillary carcinoma significantly greater than, all other prognostic factors combined (age, sex, tumor size, extent of primary tumor, lymph node involvement, the presence of DMs), and DNA assessment significantly added to statistical predictive power for all three kinds of thyroid carcinomas. The authors noted, however, that they were dealing with a selected young population of patients, which would bias an analysis of the prognostic power for age but would not influence the conclusions concerning the additional value of DNA measurement. Another study of DTC showed age at diagnosis to be more strongly associated with a poor outcome than DNA aneuploidy, however (80).

One of the few flow cytometric studies comparing the ploidy of primary thyroid carcinomas and their metastases indicated clonal heterogeneity for DTC (360). In several cases, diploid metastatic tissue was found to originate from a primary tumor with DNA aneuploidy, and in several primary tumors two stem lines of tumor cells with different DNA indices could be demonstrated. In general, however, the DNA content of regional metastases for DTC was similar to that found in the primary tumor. Because patients with aneuploid tumors were on the average 9 years older than those with diploid tumors, age is an additional possibly significant factor affecting the conclusions of this study. The study did show, however, that diploid carcinomas can metastasize and that the spread of thyroid cancer is not dependent on an aneuploid state of the primary.

In another study, it was shown that the nuclear DNA pattern in thyroid tumor cells is stable over time (365). Sixty-eight primary DTCs were compared with 84 metastases and/or recurrences up to 22 years later. In all but one of the recurrences, the DNA distribution pattern showed the same ploidy level as the corresponding primary tumor, and this was found even when many years had elapsed. Ten-year survivors had tumors with diploid nuclear content, whereas patients who died of thyroid carcinoma had tumors showing increased and scattered DNA values.

Recent studies have supported the possibility of clonal transformation of low-grade DTCs into anaplastic tumors. In one study comparing anaplastic and DTC, similar nuclear DNA patterns were found in 4 of 11 cases, suggesting that clonal transformation to a more malignant type had occurred (366). However, in the seven other cases, it was more likely that the anaplastic and well-differentiated euploid tumor populations represented two different tumor stem lines as measured by DNA content.

Another interesting finding arises from a study comparing radiation-association thyroid cancers (RATC) to those from patients who did not undergo prior radiation. Unexpectedly, all 16 RATCs were diploid, whereas of 37 nonradiation-associated tumors, 10 were aneuploid. This suggested that if the initiating radiation causes a DNA aberration, this is not reflected in DNA content as measured by flow cytometry (367).

Quantitative cytology with DNA measurements is being more widely applied to fine-needle aspirates with the goal of determining to what extent it can reduce the rate of false negatives (to exclude the benign condition) (368).

If the true biologic behavior of DTC, or even better, of the adenomatous nodule of the thyroid, could be accurately and reliably predicted by analysis of DNA content from cells aspirated by needle before surgery, some of the areas of treatment controversy might be modified. Preoperative determination of the degree of aneuploidy from cytologic smears or punch biopsies possibly could be used to guide surgical treatment; surgery could be restricted to hemithyroidectomy in cases with good prognosis or at least a conservative surgical approach could be considered (364).

Future studies combining multiple parameters such as DNA-RNA indices, or DNA-thyroglobulin or DNA-calcitonin assessment may yield a more precise and objective insight into the differentiation and pathophysiology of endocrine-derived neoplasms whose malignant potential cannot be determined by routine histopathologic examination (369).

In conclusion, it is likely that the extensive presence of aneuploidy in a thyroid neoplasm can prove the malignant potential of the tumor, whereas its absence does not finally exclude it. The detection of vascular and/or capsular invasion is still required to indicate malignancy, and this cannot currently be assessed at the suborgan level. In cases of proven malignancy, however, the cellular DNA content allows better tumor grading, with the diploid or aneuploid pattern predicting lesser or greater aggressiveness, respectively. Because cytology is remarkably accurate in the analysis of malignant papillary lesions, the DNA measurement contributes to tumor grading.

Receptor Studies

Because hormone-sensitive cancers contain receptors, the measurement of receptor levels in surgically removed tumors might be of prognostic and therapeutic value; this is currently under intensive study.

Although thyrotropin (TSH) is considered to be the main regulator of the thyroid cell, it has become increasingly evident that other factors are involved as well. Recent studies suggest several candidates that may eventually be shown to be of importance equal to or greater than that of TSH.

Studies generally report either the presence of a particular factor in the serum of patients with a particular thyroid neoplastic condition, or they report quantitative comparisons of the content of receptors and growth factors in various types of preparations from thyroid neoplasms (adenomas and carcinomas) and from normal thyroid tissue. Differing results in similar types of studies result from variations in the technology used [e.g., measuring high-affinity versus low-affinity receptors and using different *in vitro* cell systems, including established cell lines, primary cultured cells, and membrane preparations (the latter can be affected by a number of nonspecific factors)]. Additional studies on more material (patient and *in vitro*) with standardized techniques are necessary before the significance of these types of investigations can be assessed, but the following is a brief summary of the current status.

Thyroid Stimulating Hormone and TSH-Receptor

Thyroid stimulating hormone is known to act through the TSH receptor (TSH-R) adenyl cyclase (AC) system (see also Chapter 11). When TSH-R is activated by the binding of TSH, stimulatory G protein is activated. This protein in turn activates AC, an enzyme that converts adenosine triphosphate (ATP) to cyclic AMP (cAMP), which serves as a second messenger to activate a number of intracellular processes involved in thyroid growth and secretion. The cAMP activates practically all of the specific enzyme systems of the thyroid follicular cell.

In the past, the AC/cAMP system has been more closely linked to the functional responses of the thyroid cell to TSH (such as iodine uptake, organification, and Tg synthesis) rather than to growth response. It has recently been demonstrated that TSH induces cell proliferation of human thyroid cells in culture, acting through cAMP.

The cell membranes of normal follicular cells contain TSH-R, which has also been documented in the cells of well-differentiated thyroid carcinomas but not in undifferentiated or medullary carcinomas. Thus, DTCs appear to have an intact receptor-AC system. The response of well-differentiated carcinomas to TSH stimulation appears to vary greatly in individual cases. Increased, normal, and decreased levels of AC activity have all been reported. Thus, the data concerning the mediation of thyroid cell growth by cAMP are controversial. There are only slight differences in the capacity and affinity of TSH-R in thyroid neoplasms when compared to histologically normal thyroid from the same patients, but AC responsiveness is greater in most neoplastic thyroid tissue than in normal thyroid tissue.

Why tumors have a greater AC response to TSH than does normal thyroid tissue is under investigation. The responsiveness of AC to TSH is presumably a way of quantitating the level of TSH-R activity. The relationship has been attributed by Clark's group to an altered guanyl nucleotide regulatory protein (GNRP) (370,371). An alteration was shown in the ratio of inhibiting to stimulating GNRPs in thyroid neoplasms. There are more stimulating and less inhibiting GNRPs in DTCs of follicular origin than in normal thyroid tissue. This appears to be responsible for the greater AC response to TSH that occurs in most thyroid neoplasms when compared to normal thyroid tissue, and it may be an important stimulus to aberrant cell growth. Although no specific mention was made of the difference between benign and malignant neoplasms in Clark's report, the comparison of the ratio of regulatory proteins with nuclear DNA content is worthy of further research and would be facilitated by the development of MoAbs to both inhibitory and stimulatory proteins (372). New references on TSH and its receptor are 373–378.

New Prognostic Factors

Another study from Clark's group attempted to correlate an intracellular second-messenger event with the histologic type of thyroid neoplasm and clinical behavior. AC activity showed a consistent inverse correlation to tumor stage or aggressiveness. The cyclase responsiveness decreased progressively in lesions varying from benign through stage I to IV carcinoma and medullary carcinoma.

Other biochemical processes relating to the AC-cAMP system have been studied with respect to thyroid cancer. Prostaglandins (PGs) take part in cellular growth and are associated with the activation of the AC-cAMP system through specific membrane-bound receptors that have been demonstrated in several tissue fractions or at cell surface membranes. The effects of PGs and their synthesis inhibitors, aspirin and indomethacin, have not been reported for thyroid cancer. PGs of the E series are known to stimulate intracellular thyroid processes through interaction with specific surface membrane-bound receptors. In a recent study, PG binding to normal thyroid tissue was compared with benign thyroid adenomas and well-differentiated and less-differentiated cancers. Thyroid neoplasms showed different binding capacities of prostacyclin (PGI_2) high affinity binding sites depending on their differentiation status. The cancer state was associated with a significant loss of specific binding sites for PGI_2 (379).

Numerous clinical studies have demonstrated that treatment of patients with benign thyroid tumors with thyroid hormone causes about one half of these tumors to decrease significantly in size. Similarly, some DTCs will decrease in size in response to such treatment, although thyroid neoplasms can grow despite TSH deprivation, and recurrent thyroid cancer seems less common and survival somewhat better. These responses are presumably a result of the fact that benign tumors and DTCs have TSH-R and increase their AC activity in response to TSH, whereas undifferentiated medullary tumors and other tumors of nonthyroidal origin lack TSH-R and fail to respond in such a manner to TSH.

Epidermal Growth Factor

Epidermal growth factor is a set of diverse polypeptide growth factors involved in the regulation of cell growth and differentiation (380). It stimulates cell proliferation, and in some cells it is accompanied by a stimulation of differentiation, whereas in other cells, such as thyroid follicular cells, it is associated with the inhibition of differentiated function, in particular the synthesis of tissue-specific protein (381,382). In contrast to the endocrine action of TSH, EGF probably acts in a paracrine or autocrine manner to stimulate thyroid growth. EGF binds to specific receptors (EGF-R) on the cell membrane of its target organs.

EGF-R is thought to be an oncogene because there exists a homology between it and the v-*erb* B transforming oncogene of avian erythroblastosis virus. EGF-R has been found in some tumors of the esophagus, stomach, breast, bladder, lung, brain, ovary, and uterus, and the existence of EGF-R is being correlated with tumorigenicity or malignant grade. EGF-R has also been demonstrated in both normal and neoplastic thyroid tissue. EGF-R has been reported in animal and human thyroid cells to be a growth stimulator, while at the same time inhibiting differentiated functions such as iodide metabolism. Both EGF and EGF-R have been found in normal and neoplastic thyroid tissues. Generally speaking, neoplastic thyroid tissue is reported to have higher EGF binding levels than the normal thyroid tissue. EGF receptors have been detected on the cell surface of well-differentiated and undifferentiated thyroid carcinomas of follicular origin. In other studies, EGF-R content has been found to be very low in medullary carcinomas.

It has been shown that thyroid growth is regulated by an interplay between EGF and TSH, but the physiologic role of EGF and thyroid growth remains to be precisely elucidated, as does the relationship between EGF receptors and TSH receptors. *In vitro* studies of normal follicular cells suggest that the effects of EGF are opposite to those of TSH: EGF markedly inhibits the differentiation induced by TSH and results in reduction of Tg and peroxidase synthesis.

A recent study looked at EGF and TSH receptors in neoplastic thyroid and adjacent normal tissues with the aim of clarifying the role of TSH and EGF in the regulation of malignant thyroid cell growth (383). The amount of EGF-R in papillary and anaplastic thyroid carcinomas differed significantly from that in follicular and medullary carcinomas, and alterations in EGF-R content in malignant thyroid tissues were independent of TSH-R content. Interestingly, in the cell system under study, no correlation was found between the EGF-R amount and the patient's age or the EORTC prognostic index, suggesting that EGF-R content is not a determinant of the degree of malignancy. A previous study had concluded that thyroid tumors with a poor prognosis appeared to have higher EGF binding than tumors with a better prognosis (384). TSH treatment of porcine thyroid cells increases EGF-R capacity by threefold (385).

In a study using human thyroid cells in primary culture, there was a significant decrease in EGF affinity in thyroid carcinoma cells compared with that in nonneoplastic and adenoma cells, although the binding capacities and mitogenic response to EGF were almost the same in all three groups (386). It was also found that TSH and EGF cooperatively stimulated adenoma cell proliferation, and mechanisms of this action were hypothesized.

Another recent study evaluated the presence of morphologically detectable EGF-R in more than 30 thyroid neoplasms of various histologic types (387). Both normal and benign adenomas showed no apparent immunoreactive staining; however, the reaction was especially positive on medullary and anaplastic carcinomas that stained more intensively than DTCs. EGF-R staining in papillary carcinomas, when correlated with the UICC classification of thyroid tumors, showed a higher frequency of positive staining in cases with multifocal metastases. (In this study, the demonstration of EGF-R in some limited areas of tissues of adenomatous goiters was adduced by the authors to suggest that adenomatous goiter may possess some malignant potential.) New material on growth factors is provided in references 388 and 389.

Nerve Growth Factor

Nerve growth factor (NGF) presumably maintains sympathetic nerve growth, and increased levels of the factor have been demonstrated in children with neuroblastoma and patients with disseminated neurofibromatosis. The factor is being studied in MTC, which is considered to result from a defect in the neuroectodermal cell system (familial MTC is often associated with mucosal neuromas, diffuse ganglioneuromatosis, and neurofibromatosis).

One case report showed that the serum of a patient with familial MTC who died of progressive metastatic disease had an unusually high level of sympathetic nerve growth–promoting factor (390). It was hypothesized that the NGF-like substance might be a biologically active product of the thyroid tumor or, alternatively, that an excess of NGF could precede thyroid tumor growth and could explain the generalized abnormalities of the neuroectodermal cell system usually found in the MTC syndrome. This latter possibility was favored because of the increased NGF activity in the serum of the elder son of the patient, who still had normal calcitonin secretion. Reports of a diffuse C cell hyperplasia at an early stage of the disease and the high NGF level found in disseminated neurofibromatosis gives further support to this hypothesis.

Detection of NGF may be of importance in the future diagnosis and follow-up of MTC (391). Residual postoperative MTC is a continuing problem and low remission rates are seen only with chemotherapy. This may be explained by cell heterogeneity of tumors, which leads to increasing drug resistance. A preliminary report suggests that NGF sensitizes human MTC cells for cytostatic therapy *in vitro* (392) and has the potential, therefore, to improve the response rate of these tumors to chemotherapy. Stimulation of C cells with growth factors is postulated to increase the number of cells in the S and M phases and to decrease the number in the G_0 phase. It remains to be seen if these *in vitro* findings reflect a corresponding physiologic behavior of MTC to chemotherapeutic drugs *in vivo*.

Vasoactive Intestinal Polypeptide

Vasoactive intestinal polypeptide (VIP) is present in nerves that innervate thyroid blood vessels and follicles. Independent of its action on blood flow, VIP also causes the release of thyroid hormone from slices of thyroid tissue or thyroid cells in culture and, *in vivo*, may be a major locally produced regulator of thyroid hormone secretion.

It has been documented that VIP stimulates AC activity in cultured normal and hyperplastic (Graves') thyroid tissue, thus increasing intracellular cAMP concentration. When VIP is released from nerve endings in the thyroid gland, it activates a distinct receptor, which is coupled through the same stimulatory G protein as TSH, to turn on AC. VIP is a potent stimulator of AC in both normal and neoplastic human thyroid tissues, with a magnitude similar to that produced by TSH, implying that VIP plays a physiologically important role in the regulation of the secretion and growth of normal and neoplastic thyroid tissues (393).

Platelet-Derived Growth Factor

In a recent study platelet-derived growth factor (PDGF) receptors were found in an anaplastic carcinoma cell line (394). Receptors for PDGF had previously been found only on cells of mesenchymal and glial origin. Various types of epithelial cells, including thyroid follicle cells, lack PDGF receptors and do not respond to the factor. Therefore, finding a structurally altered PDGF receptor in human epithelial-derived cells (anaplastic thyroid carcinoma in cell culture) that also expressed thyroglobin mRNA is noteworthy. It was postulated to be crucial in tumor development by conferring a selective growth advantage to the cancer cells.

Studies on Sex Hormones and Their Receptors

The relevance of hormonal factors to thyroid cancer has long been suspected because of the high incidence rates in women and the peak occurrence in women at ages 15 to 29, when hormonal activity is enhanced. The underlying hypothesis is that individual hormones, which usually control normal growth of target organs, can cause neoplastic growth when hormone levels are excessive. The higher incidence of thyroid cancer in women suggests that an endogenous rather than an environmental factor should be sought for a better understanding of the disease etiology. Because the preponderance of thyroid carcinoma in women seems to exist worldwide, it is unlikely that this is an artifact resulting from some other factor (e.g., that women seek medical attention more frequently and are therefore likely to have thyroid abnormalities detected).

That sex hormones influence development of thyroid neoplasms is supported by several facts. Spontaneous thyroid tumors predominate in women by ratios as high as 4:1. The mortality rates from thyroid carcinoma in humans are reportedly higher in men than women. There have been anecdotal reports of regression of thyroid cancers in response to treatment with testosterone or estrogens. Animal experiments also provide further support.

Data from cancer registries throughout the world show that thyroid cancer incidence is consistently 2 to 3 times higher in women than in men, and that the incidence is similar in girls and boys under age 10 and changes to a female preponderance (3:1 over men) between ages 10 and 19. It stays at this ratio until women reach menopause, and then it declines steadily to a ratio of 1:5 at age 62 (207). Speculation as to the nature of the survival impairment beginning at age 50 in a disease that largely affects women must center on the role of sex hormone changes that occur at menopause. The relationship between age and mortality in men is more linear and without such a sharp age-related break in the death rate. If endogenous estrogen production ameliorates the effects of the disease, there must be other reasons why men under the age of 40 have a prognosis comparable to that of women of the same age.

Further study is needed on the interrelationships of age, sex, and risk of death. Variations in urinary steroids could account for these relationships (395). Epidemiologic data suggest that the benignity of thyroid cancer depends on the presence of adequate levels of sex steroids, by extrapolation from the survival rate for all types of thyroid cancer (best documented for papillary), which is better when these cancers are diagnosed in patients between 8 and 40 years of age, the period of time when urinary estrogens and 17-ketosteroids are highest.

Changes with age in estrogens and androgens, when compared with mortality from thyroid cancer, suggest that benign behavior of this entity between ages 7 and 45 might be influenced by sex hormones. The biologic behavior of thyroid tumors can be correlated to age and to the presence or absence of sex steroids. Children diagnosed with thyroid cancer before age 7 have a mortality rate of about 60%, whereas when diagnosed from ages 8 to 15, the rate is about 13%. At age 7 or 8, children have a slight but significant increase in urinary estrogen and 17-ketosteroids. Thyroid cancer is also more aggressive and lethal after age 40, a time associated with a decrease in urinary estradiol, estriol, and estrone in women and decreased estradiol, estrone, and androgens in men, but with a moderate increase in excretion of estriol.

Recently, clinical studies have been directed at the young female population to test the hypothesis that development of thyroid cancer is related to endogenous hormones, because the only known cause of thyroid cancer—ionizing radiation—does not account for the striking female predominance of this disease (396), which does not obtain in the population of men and women exposed to head and neck irradiation in infancy or youth. Presumably, elevated levels of endogenous female sex hormones lead to an increase in TSH, which promotes hyperplasia of the thyroid and in turn increases the risk of thyroid cancer. Because TSH increases in pregnancy, and hormonal changes accompany other menstrual and reproductive events, it would be expected that pregnancy would increase the risk of thyroid cancer and other events might also be relevant.

Thyroid nodular disease in pregnancy is usually ascribed to physiologic or functional causes rather than to neoplasia, but the latter should be considered in the differential diagnosis. There is a 50% increase in thyroxine-binding globulin (TBG) and in TSH during early pregnancy. Changes in the size and activity of the thyroid during a normal menstrual cycle have also been observed and are probably a result of transient elevations in TSH. In one recent series on pregnancy as a predisposing factor in thyroid neoplasia, 26 operations were performed on pregnant women for thyroid abnormalities (397). A 43% incidence of cancer and a 37% incidence of adenoma was found for a total neoplasia rate of 80%. One-fifth of the patients showed marked increase in nodular growth during pregnancy. Based on what we know of the incidence of occult thyroid, these findings are difficult to interpret.

Other growth factors that might relate to thyroid neoplasia during pregnancy include growth hormone, human placental lactogen, somatomedins, insulin growth factor, epidermal growth factor, and growth-stimulating immunoglobulins. Because pregnancy represents a state of altered immunologic tolerance to permit survival of a nonself placental allograft, it may theoretically be a permissive state for malignancy based on traditional (and outmoded?) concepts of immune surveillance.

Many reproduction-related events have been studied epidemiologically for an association with thyroid cancer, including parity and use of menopausal estrogens. In one study in women under age 35, risk factors included a history of miscarriage, and parity seemed to potentiate the radiation risks after childhood exposure (199). A history of pregnancy has been associated with an elevated risk of thyroid cancer in several recent studies. Others have found an increased risk of thyroid cancer correlated with the use of oral contraceptives and lactation suppressants among young women. In one study, admittedly with short follow-up (6 to 7 years), relating thyroid disease to pregnancy history in the population of white women at ages 15 to 40 from Los Angeles County, a comparison with neighboring controls showed major associations with a history of benign hyperplastic thyroid disease. The second strongest association was with miscarriage, an event suspected of reflecting abnormal thyroid physiology. An independent and increased risk was observed with an increase in the total number of pregnancies (after excluding women with benign hyperplastic thyroid disease and a history of miscarriages). Prior exposure to RT was not an important factor in this study.

Estrogen receptors (ER) and more recently androgen receptors have been found in normal and neoplastic thyroid glands. Well-differentiated carcinomas seem to contain more ERs than the adjacent normal tissues. The hypothesis that normal tissue cells contain ER and that the transformed cells retain the ability to synthesize the receptor proteins is the generally accepted explanation for the presence of ER in tumors that derive from established target tissues for estrogens (such as breast and endometrial cancers). That tissue cells can acquire ER during the process of malignant transformation presumably explains the presence of ER in tumors that are not traditionally considered hormonally sensitive (lung, pancreas, colon, bone, kidney, melanoma, lymphoma). The presence of ER in both normal and neoplastic tissue outside the reproductive tract suggests that such tissues may be hormonally responsive and may therefore be susceptible to endocrine manipulation.

In a recent study, both estrogen and TSH receptors were demonstrable in human neoplastic and nonneoplastic thyroid tissue, but there was no evident correlation between the number of sex hormone receptors and TSH receptors in both types of tissue (398).

Estrogen growth stimulation and tamoxifen growth inhibition of a tumor cell line derived from human MTC has been recently demonstrated (399). Responsiveness to tamoxifen is encouraging. A combination of hormonal therapy with chemotherapy (and NGF?) might be of future benefit in the treatment of residual MTC. The cytotoxic efficacy of chemotherapeutic drugs can be enhanced by concomitant treatment with estrogens and antiestrogens in breast cancers. It is possible that the presence of functional ER in thyroid cancers may provide the basis for a response to hormonal therapy.

Elucidation of the effects of sex hormones on thyroid carcinoma is also being studied in animal models. The results are contradictory. Estrogen treatment has been shown to inhibit goitrogen-induced thyroid tumors in rats of both sexes, but opposite results have also been found.

In one animal study, the incidence of radiation-induced thyroid follicular tumors in male rats was markedly reduced by castration of the animals prior to irradiation (400). The high incidence of thyroid follicular tumors could be restored in castrated male rats when testosterone replacement was delivered, either continuously or during early life, but not when administered later. Alteration of serum TSH levels by testosterone treatment was more apparent in young than in old animals. It was postulated that growth modification of thyroid tumors could involve (a) an action of steroid hormones directly on thyroid tissue via specific cellular receptors for androgens and/or estrogens, which have both been demonstrated in thyroid lesions (401), or (b) an indirect effect by increasing TSH production via altered hypothalamic or pituitary function.

Further prospective clinical studies are necessary to determine if estrogen and TSH receptors can be useful prognostic indicators for patients with thyroid cancer, and whether or not they will prove useful in selecting patients for adjuvant therapy with sex hormones or their antagonists remains to be seen. There has been one brief experimental trial of estrogen administration in recurrent and metastatic thyroid carcinoma (402). In the future, sex hormones and their antagonists might be useful adjuvant therapy for metastases in operatively treated thyroid cancer patients. If, however, sex steroid hormones act indirectly via TSH to influence thyroid tumor growth, the postsurgical treatment of choice may still be the standard thyroxine administration with its associated TSH suppression (403,404).

Growth-Controlling Mechanisms in Thyroid Neoplasia

Hormone Dependency

Whereas in most organ systems the factors governing cellular metabolism are relatively obscure, the endocrine system is unique because of the known regulatory influence of trophic hormones on normal cellular growth and function and possibly also on neoplastic growth arising in target organs, a quantitative rather than qualitative difference. A relationship between tumors of the endocrine system and their trophic hormones is recognized for cancers of the breast, prostate, adrenal, thyroid, and uterus. Such tumors have been termed dependent or conditioned, because their growth may be enhanced or modified by their hormonal environment (405). A transition from dependency to increasing autonomy has been noted repeatedly in endocrine tumors in man. Similarly, in experimental animals following appropriate hormonal stimuli, transition from normal to hyperplastic to conditioned and finally to autonomous growth can occur (see later).

These concepts are enumerated in a classic study that provided a basis for hormone manipulation in the treatment of thyroid cancer (406). Attention was focused on the apparent dependency of certain thyroid neoplasms upon thyroid stimulating hormone (TSH). The underlying principle is that thyroid tumors exhibit varying degrees of dependency during their development and growth. Both function and growth of thyroid cancer, either primary or metastatic, may be inhibited or stimulated according to the relative level of TSH. This was the basis of the suggestion in the 1940s of Purves and Griesbach (407) that "it may, therefore, be possible to influence the course of malignant thyroid disease in human beings by the therapeutic administration of desiccated thyroid."

The major controversy is over the possibility that human thyroid cancer results from the growth-promoting effect of excessive TSH secretion. On the other hand, there is evidence that excess TSH is not the cause of clinical thyroid carcinoma, although it is considered etiologic in animal models (see later).

The analogy between thyroid carcinogenesis in experimental animals and man is supported by the many instances in which the development of thyroid cancer in children has been preceded by the administration of roentgen therapy. The effects of x-rays might simulate their initiating role in the experimental animal. The increasing malignancy of human thyroid cancer with age is also somewhat comparable to experimentally induced thyroid neoplasms which, although initially dependent, may finally become autonomous. Clinically, the supervention of autonomous behavior in TSH-responsive thyroid carcinoma is not rare. Increased growth of existing thyroid cancer has also been noted when patients are prepared for treatment with radioiodine, which involves increasing the level of TSH either by way of the anterior pituitary or by direct administration. During such a period of stimulation, metastases have been observed to increase in size, and the reverse has also been noted after the coincidental development of hyperthyroidism. Metastases may show a growth spurt in spite of continuation of treatment with thyroid hormone that has previously kept them in check. A similar change occurs experimentally after serial transplantation of dependent thyroid tumors. Thus, the metastasizing TSH-dependent thyroid carcinoma may be regarded as a slow-growing cancer of low-grade malignancy, with a growth rate that is responsive to stimulation by TSH and is reduced as a result of depression of TSH secretion.

The putatively high incidence of thyroid cancer in regions of endemic goiter is also cited to reinforce similarities between human and animal thyroid neoplasia. As has been discussed earlier, however, in a number of goitrous regions there is no evidence of maintained excess TSH secretion, or diffuse hypertrophy or hyperplasia of the parenchyma of glands in thyroid cancer patients. In one recent study, however, the history of goiter was strongly associated with subsequent thyroid cancer, especially follicular (408). Women who had ever had thyroid nodules had a 12 times greater risk of developing thyroid cancer than women without such a history.

Excess TSH does not appear to be the cause of clinical thyroid carcinoma, but that does not imply that differentiated carcinomas are not responsive to TSH. There is clinical evidence that a proportion of follicular elements in thyroid carcinomas show a functional response to TSH.

There is one clinical condition (apart from endemic goiter) in which the thyroid is subjected to sustained extreme TSH stimulation. This is the rare condition of dyshormonogenetic goiter. In this situation, prolonged high TSH secretion is a sequel to a biochemical defect that impairs the efficiency of thyroid hormone production and regularly leads to the development of multiple benign follicular tumors. Carcinomas are rare but are usually of the follicular type, and the diagnosis of malignancy has been made in a few cases, but no case with metastases has been documented (recall the difficulty in differentiating histologically between follicular adenomas and carcinomas when considering this argument).

In addition to TSH-induced hyperplasia, other types of thyroid growth have been studied for their association with cancer (409). Embryonic growth, postnatal thyroid development, and reparative/regenerative hyperplasia (de Quervain's subacute thyroiditis) are all TSH independent, but in each case the product is responsive to the stimulus of TSH.

The same trophic stimuli may regulate neoplastic as well as normal thyroid activity in humans, as it is not unusual for DTC to arise at a much earlier age than most malignant neoplasms, presumably at a time when the physiologic demands on the thyroid are high (in the second and third decades of life). If the physiologic stimulus can serve as a promoting factor, there should be multiple foci of origin of these tumors, and this is borne out in histopathologic studies. Cells in the anterior pituitary that produce thyrotropic hormone also increase, supporting the role of a physiologic stimulus (410).

These early reports included descriptions that fit the modern definition of tumor heterogeneity. Thomas (406) studied dependency as a quantitative phenomenon with greater autonomy of growth developing over time, and noted that "this may or may not be associated with morphologic change in the neoplasm and does not affect all of the cells in a single neoplasm identically. Many times, the development of autonomy is progressive, suggesting a mosaic effect."

A recent study looked at the effects of TSH on tissue cultures derived from malignant and benign thyroid tumors; it found that many thyroid carcinomas are dependent on the growth-promoting properties of TSH (411). TSH can affect the morphology and protein synthesis of primary tissue cultures derived from benign or malignant thyroid tumor differently. When TSH was added to cultures derived from benign tumors, a reorganization of follicle-like structures of the monolayer and a reduction in protein synthesis was found. When monolayers derived from carcinomas had TSH added, however, the monolayers did not reorganize and their protein synthesis was not inhibited. Amplification of such studies using *in vitro* systems may help elucidate the mechanisms of control of thyroid neoplasia, which are still unclear.

Clinically, 0.2 to 0.4 mg of thyroxine will suppress the endogenous output of TSH by the anterior pituitary. The rationale for TSH-suppressive therapy is that the growth of many primary and metastatic thyroid carcinomas appears to be dependent on the thyroid growth-promoting properties of TSH, and the purpose of the suppressive therapy is to create, by elimination of TSH, an adverse environment for cancer growth. This theoretically could cause involution of existing tumors and could prevent the emergence of autonomous cancers. Thyroid hormone was used as an adjunct in the palliative treatment of many cases of malignant disease in the early part of the 20th century, and prophylaxis with thyroid hormone is now commonly used postoperatively and frequently as primary thyroid tumor treatment. Prophylaxis with thyroid hormone is also appropriate based on the known incidence of multifocal occult thyroid cancer. A partial thyroidectomy in a patient with occult latent cancer or other goitrogenic stimulus could result in a relative preponderance of TSH and conceivably an increasingly autonomous neoplasm. By adequate pituitary suppression in these individuals, the development of thyroid cancer might be effectively decreased.

Early recommendations for total thyroidectomy were formulated on the basis that only by this means could multifocal thyroid cancer be excluded from subsequent growth stimulus. It was recognized that once total thyroidectomy was performed, it would be mandatory to provide adequate amounts of exogenous thyroid hormone to preclude the development of hypothyroidism, for it is in the context of hypothyroidism that any remaining tumor receives its maximal growth stimulus. (This is the rationale for discontinuing thyroid supplementation several weeks prior to diagnostic scanning to detect metastatic disease.)

Information from Animal Models

A considerable amount of work with experimental thyroid carcinogenesis in animals has been performed since the early decades of this century, and understanding the findings is of more than academic interest because the interpretation of many clinical aspects of human thyroid cancer has been extrapolated from this work. Because opportunities for experimentation in human cancer patients is obviously limited, animal models give insight into the mechanisms of thyroid carcinogenesis and tumor metabolism. Animal experiments can only serve as guideposts to the study of the disease in humans, but they are advantageous because experimental conditions can be precisely controlled.

Cancer of the thyroid, although it is a relatively small percentage of human cancer, is important for the study of mechanisms of carcinogenesis, both in man and animals. The enormous capacity of normal thyroid gland tissue to concentrate iodine and to utilize that iodine in metabolic functions provides a tissue wherein not only anatomic but also extremely sensitive functional changes can be detected and studied simultaneously.

The experimental study of thyroid tumors stems from investigations of endemic goiter in dogs and rats, and from attempts to reproduce thyroid hyperplasia in healthy animals. Because of the infrequent occurrence of thyroid gland tumors in both the rat and mouse, these species are suitable subjects for use in the induction of experimental cancer of the thyroid gland. In the 1920s, the classic experiments of Marine and Leo Loeb (412) elucidated the role of dietary iodine deficiency and of partial thyroidectomy in producing compensatory hyperplasia of the thyroid gland. They established the dependence and control of thyroid function on anterior pituitary secretion.

The discovery of chemical goitrogenic compounds in the early 1940s and investigation of their mode of action confirmed the role of TSH in controlling thyroid activity. It was found that prolonged maintenance of rats and mice on goitrogens in the food or drinking water led to the development of gross thyroid hyperplasia and eventually to the development of tumors. Interest was stimulated in the experimental induction of thyroid tumors, not only by chemical goitrogens, but by other means. Many experiments were initiated. The subject has been comprehensively reviewed by Doniach (200), Oshima and Ward (413), and Morris (414).

Two general approaches have been reported for inducing thyroid tumors in rodents. The first approach aims at establishing a hormonal imbalance that will lead to tumor development. In this method, the first stage in the development of thyroid tumors is inhibition of hormone production by thyroid tissue under the influence of antithyroid substances. The second stage is a sustained intensification of synthesis and release of TSH. This approach induces thyroid tumors selectively without tumors in other organs arising, but a long time is required to obtain tumors.

The second approach is based on the use of strong chemical carcinogens. These substances induce tumors, not only in the thyroid gland, but also in a number of other organs. A combination of an antithyroid drug or goitrogen and chemical carcinogen (2-acetylaminofluorene) can result in acceleration of tumor development in the thyroid.

The classic methods used to produce experimental tumors of the thyroid gland include:

1. Chronic ingestion of a thiocarbamide-type goitrogen by both rats and mice.
2. Direct irradiation of the thyroid gland by a single massive dose of radioiodine.
3. Chronic feeding of an iodine-deficient diet to rats.
4. Combination of a goitrogen with low doses of radiation in rats.
5. Combination of a carcinogen with a goitrogen.
6. Combination of a goitrogen with low doses of ^{131}I irradiation.
7. External x-ray irradiation.
8. Subtotal thyroidectomy in rats (induces endogenously maintained excess secretion of TSH).
9. Implantation of autonomous thyrotropic hormone-secreting pituitary tumors.
10. A combination of a carcinogen, a goitrogen, and radioactive iodine (which produces the greatest incidence of experimental tumors).

Investigators interested in carcinogenesis study the rat thyroid as a model of two-stage mechanisms—initiation and promotion. In general, thyroid adenomas and carcinomas regularly develop in experimental animals that are maintained for a long period on a regimen that induces prolonged endogenous excess TSH secretion and progress through a sequence of thyroid hyperplasia, adenoma formation, and eventual formation of TSH-responsive carcinomas. Experimental thyroid tumors, benign and malignant, dependent and autonomous, have been produced in both the mouse and the rat. In the genesis of these tumors, either a carcinogen or the hereditary factor of high tumor strain can serve as an initiating factor, whereas a goitrogen, which acts by reducing circulating thyroxine, increases TSH and serves as the promoting factor.

Studies on tumor promotion or cocarcinogenesis in the thyroid gland generally use a variety of chemical goitrogens as promoters of thyroid tumors. These chemical compounds interfere with the normal processes of thyroid hormone secretion and synthesis and induce goiter formation. The inorganic ions perchlorate and thiocyanate inhibit the iodide transport mechanism and thereby reduce available substrate for hormone formation. The commonly employed antithyroid agents that are derivatives of thiourea and mercaptoimidazole exert more complex actions on pathways of hormonal biosynthesis. These agents, as well as certain aniline derivatives, inhibit the initial oxidation (organic binding) of iodide, decrease the proportion of diiodothyronine relative to monoiodothyronine, and block coupling of iodothyronines to form the hormonally active iodothyronine. Iodine-deficient diets also have goitrogenic effects in animals, although iodine itself, when given acutely in large doses, is capable of blocking the organic binding and coupling reactions. Presumably, a dietary iodine deficiency leads to compensatory increased secretion of TSH with resultant goiter formation and, in time, adenoma production with eventual malignant change (in animals).

Although there is no proof that iodine deficiency in humans is associated with a higher incidence of thyroid carcinoma, data from animal models (fish and rats) suggest that hyperplasia from iodine deficiency may be an inducer of chromosomal abnormalities that may lead to the production of thyroid cancer (415). Chromosomal abnormalities increase in frequency with the duration of iodine deficiency, and the percentage of goiter transplant "takes" increases directly with duration of iodine deficiency–induced hyperplasia. Iodine deficiency may act primarily as a potent promoter rather than as an initiator of carcinogenesis, or as a weak complete carcinogen.

As to radiation induction, it is well established in animals and humans that TSH stimulation of hyperplasia acts as a promoter for the development of thyroid cancer after chromosomal changes are induced. Irradiation from x-rays or the gamma or beta radiation from ^{131}I may induce the necessary chromosomal changes. The thyroid is particularly susceptible to the action of ionizing radiation. X-ray doses of 500 to 2000 rads to the thyroid consistently produce adenomas in most rats and carcinomas in about 20% of animals. Similarly, ^{131}I is carcinogenic to the rat thyroid. Doses of 5 to 40 mCi intraperitoneally produce adenomas and carcinomas after 1 to 2.5 years. Higher doses sterilize the thyroid gland. Apparently, radiation initiates a neoplastic process that is promoted to tumor formation by raised TSH secretion secondary to radiation damage of the thyroid gland. The latter effect is enhanced by goitrogens or a low-iodine diet.

In experimental animals, radiation exposure followed by excessive production of TSH increases the rates of thyroid tumors, as compared to animals with radiation exposure and normal TSH production (416). Experiments have shown that administration of thyroxine after exposure of the thyroid to radiation markedly reduces the incidence of subsequent thyroid neoplasia; this finding led to its prophylactic use in humans. Because the carcinogenic action of ionizing radiation is markedly reduced by subsequently maintained administration of thyroxine, it appears the TSH stimulation has an essential tumor-promoting action in radiation carcinogenesis. The tumor-promoting action of thyroid hyperplasia subsequent to radiation found experimentally has been advanced as an explanation of the susceptibility of the human infant thyroid to the carcinogenic action of small doses of radiation. It is suggested that, in this context, normal growth of the thyroid from infancy to puberty is the promoting factor.

It is generally thought that thyroid neoplasms in rodents appear to develop through a series of gradual changes, from hyperplasia, to local areas of proliferation of altered cells, to formation of adenomas, to development of carcinomas. The progression of experimental thyroid tumors through stages apparently depends on the inducing agent and genetic factors. The administration of propylthiouracil to a strain of mice with a low incidence of tumors is followed by hyperplastic nodules and so-called benign tumors of the thyroid. If a high tumor strain of mice is employed, malignant and autonomous tumors develop. In the rat, application of a goitrogen alone (antithyroid drug or iodine deficiency) may produce benign as well as malignant tumors.

Although most experimental thyroid tumors remain dependent, a progression has sometimes been demonstrated in which induced hyperplasia of the thyroid produces increasing chromosomal abnormalities, leading from dependent to transitional to autonomous tumor development. With autonomy comes the ability to metastasize and grow in the absence of elevated levels of thyrotropic hormone. Intravenous inoculation of dissociated cells from goitrogen-induced thyroid tumors in mice produces pulmonary metastases, but this occurs only in recipient mice thyroidectomized by ^{131}I or rendered thyroxine-deficient by short-term goitrogen treatment (417).

In humans, however, it is thought that most thyroid cancers are malignant from their outset without arising in a preexisting benign phase. In other aspects, applications of experimental results to humans is also questionable. The findings in experimental animals maintained for more than half their life-span on an intense goitrogenic regime do not correlate with clinical experience. Inhabitants of goitrogenic areas where iodine is deficient in the soil and is not supplemented in the diet develop large nodular thyroids, but there is no definite evidence (see preceding) of an associated increased incidence of thyroid cancer. This suggests that the intensity of TSH stimulation is, fortunately, not as marked as in animals submitted to a goitrogenic regime.

A variety of transplantation studies (418) have also been done in experimental animals. Pretreatment of an animal with thiouracil may be required for a successful thyroid tumor transplant until such time as sufficient tumor progression has taken place, when the preliminary thiouracil administration ceases to be necessary. Serial transplantation of tumors can lead to the emergence of autonomous carcinomas. It has been shown that subcutaneous implants of goitrogen-induced rat thyroid tumors grow successfully in thyroidectomized young rats or rats receiving methylthiouracil, but they do not survive in rats without thyroxine deficiency.

A possible early example of tumor heterogeneity is demonstrated by one case where a tumor produced three different histologic types on serial transplantation, one of which included anaplastic transformation with successful growth in rats without thyroxine deficiency.

Recently, the thymic dysplastic (nude) mouse has proved to be an experimental model in which human tissue can be examined under controlled reproducible conditions (419). Morphologically and functionally, viable grafted thyroid tissue can be maintained in such mice, and xenotransplantation offers possibilities for *in vivo* studies on pathogenesis, tumor biology, endocrine function, and regulation of human thyroid disorders. In one recent study, the cell kinetics of transplantable human anaplastic thyroid carcinoma were studied (420). In another recent study, tissue from 16 patients with benign thyroid lesions and from 18 patients with malignant thyroid tumors was xenografted into nude mice, and it maintained full morphologic and functional integrity for at least 4 months after transplantation. Tumor "take" rates in differentiated and medullary carcinoma were 15% and in undifferentiated carcinomas, 100%. There was a correlation between tumor growth in the patient and the length of the resting phase of the grafted tissue in the nude mouse. Tumors with a short resting phase of 3 weeks showed rapidly progressive disease in patients, leading to death within 3 months, whereas tumors with longer resting phases showed a more prolonged course of disease and survival times up 2.5 years. The patients whose tumors did not "take" in the nude mice were still alive at the time of the report without signs of progressive tumor growth 9 to 34 months after surgery. All but one patient with positive tumor "take" died within 3 months after surgery. There were identical biologic behaviors of the original tumor and its graft in this animal model, which was proposed to be suitable for predicting the clinical course of thyroid cancer (421).

The mechanism by which TSH-induced hyperplasia leads to neoplasia is unknown despite suggestive avenues from animal research, and so far experimental thyroid carcinoma has not elucidated the etiology of the majority of clinical thyroid cancers in nonendemic goiter areas in which there is no evidence of preexisting thyroid hyperplasia. Also, thyroid tumors in both animals and humans have decreased capacity to collect and bind iodine compared to the normal thyroid gland, and although the mechanisms of this remain largely unknown, it seems that the explanation may be quite similar in both situations.

Secreting cells of the thyroid gland normally have a remarkably slow turnover rate in adult life, but these organs respond to partial removal or increased functional demands by cellular hypertrophy and hyperplasia. The cellular hyperplasia is mediated by increased TSH secretion, usually in response to reduction in blood levels of thyroid hormone. The thyroid reserve (its capacity to maintain an active response to TSH stimulation) appears almost unlimited. The concept of overwork/exhaustion of thyroid cells is not borne out experimentally. It appears that the thyroid is not adapted to induced, maintained, rapid mitotic rates, as opposed to tissues with normally high cell renewal rate such as squamous epithelium, hematopoietic cells, and mucosa of the intestine. Therefore, it is likely that the rate of formation of somatic mutations is much increased. Because there is little, if any, loss of viable cells, any mutation that leads to increased growth rate will be at a selective advantage. Ionizing radiation is likely to increase the rate and range of somatic mutation in cells capable of undergoing viable mitoses after radiation. TSH is unlikely to be a direct carcinogenic agent, but the hyperplasia it induces in the thyroid appears to be a precancerous process.

CONCLUSION

This chapter has summarized the classic issues on thyroid cancer and the new directions (422–424) that clinical and basic research are taking in the late 1980s. The major debates and controversies concerning thyroid cancer have been in place since the 1950s, with the subsequent 30 years witnessing an accumulation of reports on both sides of each issue based largely on personal bias in the clinical arena, and a large number of flawed studies of the significance of various prognostic variables, most of which have contributed much heat but little light.

With the development of technical probes allowing study at the molecular, genetic, and cellular biology levels, the hope has emerged that at last a scientific basis for clinical judgments and therapeutic maneuvers may be emerging. Now controversies also exist at the subcellular level. Technical differences on immunohistochemical and cellular and molecular technology remain to be worked out, and additional studies of more patients with standardized techniques are necessary before the significance of information arising from such studies can be properly assessed.

Some insight into the origins and variable patterns of behavior of malignant disease of the thyroid gland is provided by Smithers in the older literature (425). He suggested that understanding of the apparently complex processes involved is simplified when two separate but related factors, both of which are continuously variable, are considered: progressive differences are occurring over time, both in the thyroid glands in which the tumors are arising and in the tumors themselves. The issue is determined both by the ability of the thyroid to respond and by the demands being made on it at any one time.

For example, a thyroid gland irradiated in an infant suffers an impaired capacity for replication prior to the time when the main impact of normal growth demand is made and before the extra needs of puberty or pregnancy have to be met. On the other hand, the thyroid of a child brought up under conditions of iodine deficiency may have an impaired capacity for hyperplasia despite its inability (through lack of raw material) to make sufficient thyroxine to reduce the level of circulating TSH.

The same stresses exerted on such different thyroid glands are hardly likely to produce the same effects. Moreover, male and female thyroids are not identical. For example, follicular cell height and basal metabolic rate are normally higher in the male, so that again, identical pressures may not be met with identical responses. Such factors may account for the observed sex variation in prevalence and prognosis of thyroid cancer.

Adenocarcinomas of the thyroid tend to exhibit particularly slow progression, especially in the young, and provide a good example of a combination of changing tissue and changing tumor. They are slowly advancing tumors in less and less resilient thyroids, together producing a variable long-term effect on gland structure and on tumor behavior. Progress both in understanding and in therapeutics of thyroid neoplasia may depend to a great extent on examination of this interplay between demand and response in the thyroid, and on variation with time in the capacity of each individual gland to handle a progressively disordered structure.

The management of thyroid carcinoma remains controversial because of a lack of long-term prospective controlled trials and the considerable variability in the biology and characteristics of thyroid cancer. Therefore, any technique that can reliably predict a tumor's potential for aggressive behavior should aid the clinical and pathologic assessment and facilitate the correct choice of treatment. To date, no single microscopic or ultrastructural feature has emerged as a reliable means of predicting a fatal outcome in the individual thyroid cancer patient. Certainly, a major clue in understanding the biology of thyroid carcinoma would derive from knowledge of the relationships of age, sex, and risk of death. Urinary steroid changes could account for these relationships (see preceding).

A great amount of work is under way to attempt to define subcellular and molecular prognosticators. It is important to evaluate new prognostic factors only in prospective trials to avoid the muddle that clouds the significance of clinical prognostic factors derived from uncontrolled univariate studies. These studies are steps forward in the attempt to understand the factors responsible for the growth or suppression of growth of thyroid neoplasms. The identification of specific abnormalities in the hormone-receptor-cyclase cascade may help in the future to predict the aggressiveness of certain thyroid tumors, as well as to help to explain why some thyroid neoplasms respond to TSH suppressive therapy by decreasing in size, whereas others do not.

The examination of intracellular growth signals in the thyroid follicular cell is clearly of vital importance in the further understanding of thyroid cancer. More basic research is the keystone to understanding the mechanisms of tumor growth, which will eventually lead to a consistent approach to the treatment of thyroid carcinomas. Such avenues may have a significant impact on the management of the disease clinically (372,426). In the future, it seems relevant to correlate TSH receptor-adenyl cyclase activity with DNA analysis with respect to patient survival. Because the adenyl cyclase-cAMP mechanism is only one of several intracellular systems fulfilling the role of second messenger, studies examining TSH stimulation of, for example, phosphatidylinositol, protein kinase C, and perhaps even nuclear oncogene expression, may also be relevant.

Problems with thyroid cancer studies have been outlined above. Certainly, the potential information to be gained from the new sophisticated studies underway will be diluted unless a consistent manner of reporting results is developed, at the cellular, molecular, and clinical levels. Attention should be directed by biostatisticians to codifying statistical methods appropriate for use in a biologic entity with the natural history of thyroid cancer, to assure uniformity, validity, and relevance of data-reporting in the future. Especially in the context of prospective randomized trials, validity at the statistical level is a necessary prerequisite for standardizing methods of analysis.

In the context of increasingly sophisticated cellular and molecular technology, formatting the literature with invited commentary by experts (such as is currently done in the proceedings of the Society of Endocrinologic Surgeons in the *World Journal of Surgery*) is valuable in providing perspective to the uninitiated reader and even to the expert who may not be familiar with every aspect of the technology used in research and clinical arenas.

The natural history of thyroid cancer has, in general, been permissive enough to allow the long-term persistence of clinical controversies without grave consequences to the patient. A longstanding belief that the tumor biology of thyroid cancer is almost completely different from that of other solid carcinomas and is related to unique etiologic and prognostic factors is recently giving way to a feeling that more traditional cancer parameters are, in fact, significant for DTC. Apparently, total tumor burden is significant for DTC, with survival being negatively influenced by distant metastases as in other solid human tumors.

The significance of cervical metastasis for DTC still seems to be diametrically opposed to its usual significance with other solid carcinomas—as a harbinger of eventual death from distant metastases. Specific assessment of the nature of this discrepancy could have far-reaching implications for understanding solid tumor oncology. Study in tandem of two tumor systems, both of them carcinomas of the head and neck that spread to regional nodes and distantly, which have different prognostic implications for the significance of cervical metastasis (insignificant in one case versus extremely ominous in the other), could be vitally illuminating.

What would be the underlying mechanisms of the difference between two such tumor systems? Such a study using appropriate prospective randomized clinical format and modern cytogenetic technology has the potential to elucidate important problems in the general process of metastasis—a current major limiting factor in survival for cancer patients. Systems that differ in this regard that are appropriate for such study might include (a) papillary versus follicular thyroid carcinoma, which differ primarily in their incidence of spread to the neck (common in the former and rare in the latter); and (b) a comparison of DTC and squamous cell carcinoma, both carcinomas of the head and neck that spread to regional nodes and distantly but have the requisite difference in the prognostic implications of such spread.

Whether or not treatment issues for thyroid cancer will ever move from controversy to scientifically based fact depends on the institution of a valid, multinational, prospective, randomized, clinical study. Such an undertaking is truly a monumental endeavor, considering the standardizing population entrance criteria, the technology of parameters under study, and the treatment administered. The problem of accruing sufficient patient numbers in itself would be time consuming, not to mention the necessary follow-up time required to generate a valid study—preferably at least 20 years, and ideally 30 years. Most planners of such a study would be retired or even dead by the time its results were available, which would inevitably decrease enthusiasm for participating in the project.

It is hoped that the reader now has a more adequate data base on thyroid tumor biology that will enable critical evaluation of the data in the subsequent chapters, in the literature, and in the frequently eloquent arguments of individual presenters.

REFERENCES

1. Shaha A, Jaffe BM. Complications of thyroid surgery performed by residents. *Surgery* 1988;104:1109.
2. Borup Christensen S, Ljungberg O, Tibblin S. A clinical epidemiologic study of thyroid carcinoma in Malmo, Sweden. *Curr Probl Cancer* 1984;8(14):7.
3. Harness JK, McLeod MK, Thompson NW, et al. Deaths due to differentiated thyroid carcinoma: a 46 year perspective. *World J Surg* 1988;12:632.
4. Hannequin P, Liehn JC, Delisle MJ. Multifactorial analysis of survival in thyroid cancer. Pitfalls of applying the results of published studies to another population. *Cancer* 1986;58:1749.
5. Fassina AS, et al. Histological evaluation of thyroid carcinomas: reproducibility of "WHO" classification. *Tumori* 1993;79:314.
6. Hedinger CE. The problems in classification of thyroid tumors. Their significance for prognosis and therapy. *Schweiz Med Wochenschr* 1993;123:1673 (German-Eng abstr).
7. Crowe PJ, et al. Thyroid frozen section: flawed but helpful. *Aust NZ J Surg* 1993;63:275.
8. Kingston GW, Bugiss P, Davis N. Role of frozen section and clinical parameters in distinguishing benign from malignant follicular neoplasms of the thyroid. *Am J Surg* 1992;164:603.
9. Jayaram G, et al. Cytology and the diagnosis of thyroid lesions—a review. *J Assoc Physicians India* 1993;41:164.
10. Cor A, et al. Measurement characteristics of stereological and histochemical methods in the diagnosis of thyroid tumours. *Oncology* 1994;51:426.
11. Saxen E, Franssila K, Bjarnason S, et al. Observer variation in histologic classification of thyroid carcinoma. *APMIS* 1978;86:483.
12. Harich RH, Franssila KL, Wasenius Z. Occult papillary carcinoma of the thyroid—a normal finding in Finland. A systematic autopsy study. *Cancer* 1985;56:531.
13. Beierwaltes WH, Nishiyama RH, Thompson NW, et al. Survival time and "cure" in papillary and follicular thyroid carcinoma with distant metastases: statistics following University of Michigan therapy. *J Nucl Med* 1982;23:561.
14. Massin J-P. Pulmonary metastasis in differentiated thyroid carcinoma. *Cancer* 1984;53:982.
15. Berkson J, Gage RP. Calculation of survival rates for cancer. *Mayo Clin Proc* 1950;25:270.
16. Colton T. *Statistics in medicine*. Boston: Little, Brown, 1974.
17. Beierwaltes WH. The natural history of thyroid cancer. In: DeGroot L, Frohman LA, Kaplan EL, et al., eds. *Radiation-associated thyroid carcinoma*. New York: Grune & Stratton, 1976;63.
18. Byar DP, Green SB, Dor P, et al. A prognostic index for thyroid carcinoma: a study of the EORTC thyroid cancer cooperative group. *Br J Cancer* 1979;15:1033.
19. Schelfhaut LJ, Creutzberg CL, Hamming JF, et al. Multivariate analysis of survival in differentiated thyroid carcinoma: the prognostic significance of the age factor. *Eur J Cancer Clin Oncol* 1988;24:331.
20. Hannequin P, Liehn JC, De Lisle MJ. Multifactorial analysis of survival in thyroid cancer—pitfalls of applying the results of published series to another population. *Cancer* 1986;58:1749.
21. Thompson N, Kaplan EL. Discussion. *Surgery* 1986;100:1096.
22. Backdahl M. Invited commentary. *World J Surg* 1988;12:508.
23. McGrath PC, et al. Diagnosis and management of thyroid malignancies. *Curr Opin Oncol* 1994;6:60.
24. Staunton MD, et al. Thyroid cancer in the 1980s—a decade of change. *Ann Acad Med Singapore* 1993;22:613.
25. Hay ID, et al. Predicting outcome in papillary thyroid carcinoma: development of a reliable prognostic scoring system in a cohort of 1779 patients surgically treated at one institution during 1940 through 1989. *Surgery* 1993;114:1050,1057.
26. Hay ID, et al. Thyroid cancer diagnosis and management. *Clin Lab Med* 1993;13:725.
27. Blahd WH. Management of thyroid cancer. *Compr Ther* 1993;19:197.
28. DeGroot LJ, et al. Does the method of management of papillary thyroid carcinoma make a difference in outcome? *World J Surg* 1994;18:123.
29. Hennen G. Cancer of the thyroid—explorations of clinical biology. *Acta Chir Belg* 1994;94:30.
30. Squifflet JP, et al. Incidence of thyroid carcinoma in a common surgical practice: the problems. *Acta Chir Belg* 1994;94:23.
31. Langsteger W, et al. The impact of geographical, clinical, dietary, and radiation-induced features in epidemiology of thyroid cancer. *Eur J Cancer* 1993;29A:1547.
32. O'Douherty MJ, et al. Radionuclides and therapy of thyroid cancer. *Nucl Med Commun* 1993;14:736.
33. Franssila KO. Is the differentiation between papillary and follicular thyroid carcinoma valid? *Cancer* 1973;32:853.
34. Carcangiu ML, Zampi G, Rosai J. Papillary thyroid carcinoma: a study of its many morphological expressions and clinical correlates. *Pathol Annu* 1985;20:1.
35. Russel WO, Ibanez ML, Clark RL, et al. Thyroid carcinoma: classification intraglandular dissemination and clinicopathologic study based upon whole organ sections of 80 glands. *Cancer* 1963;16:1425.
36. Ordonez NA, Batsakis JG. Comparison of *Ulex europaeus* I lectin & factor VIII-related antigen in vascular lesions. *Arch Pathol Lab Med* 1984;108:129.
37. Komorowski RA, Hanson GA. Occult thyroid pathology in the young adult: an autopsy study of 138 patients without clinical thyroid disease. *Hum Pathol* 1988;19:689.
38. Goepfert H, et al. Differentiated thyroid cancer—papillary and follicular carcinomas. *Am J Otolaryngol* 1994;15:167.
39. Damiani S, et al. Cytologic rating of aggressive and nonaggressive variants of papillary thyroid carcinoma. *Am J Clin Pathol* 1994;101:651.
40. McCaffrey TV, et al. Locally invasive papillary thyroid carcinoma: 1940–1990. *Head Neck* 1994;16:165.
41. Akslen LA. Prognostic importance of histologic gradient in papillary thyroid carcinoma. *Cancer* 1993;72:2680.
42. Oyama T, et al. Encapsulated papillary carcinoma of the thyroid gland: clinicopathological and cytofluorometric study in comparison with non-encapsulated papillary carcinoma. *Acta Pathol Jpn* 1993;43:516.
43. Wingren G, et al. Determinants of papillary cancer of the thyroid. *Am J Epidemiol* 1993;138:482.
44. Tielens ET, et al. Follicular variant of papillary thyroid carcinoma. A clinicopathologic study. *Cancer* 1994;73:424.
45. Emerick GT, et al. Diagnosis, treatment and outcome of follicular thyroid carcinoma. *Cancer* 1993;72:3287. *Cancer* 1994;74:985.

46. Collin JV. Diagnosis, treatment, and outcome of follicular thyroid carcinoma [letter, comment]. *Cancer* 1994;72:3287, 74:985.
47. Baker JR Jr, et al. Immunological aspects of cancers arising from thyroid follicular cells. *Endocr Rev* 1993;14:729.
48. Lax SF, et al. Coexistence of papillary and medullary carcinoma of the thyroid gland—mixed or collision tumour? Clinicopathological analysis of three cases. *Virchows Arch* 1994;424:441.
49. Michal M, et al. Mixed medullary-follicular and medullary-papillary carcinoma of the thyroid: one or two entities? *Zentralbl Pathol* 1993; 139:333.
50. Sobrinho-Simoes M. Mixed medullary and follicular carcinoma of the thyroid. *Histopathology* 1993;23:287.
51. Moreno Egea A, et al. Prognostic value of the tall cell variety of papillary cancer of the thyroid. *Eur J Surg Oncol* 1993;19:517.
52. Moreno Egea A, et al. Clinical pathological study of the diffuse sclerosing variety of papillary cancer of the thyroid. Presentation of four new cases and review of the literature. *Eur J Surg Oncol* 1994;20:7.
53. Shvero J, Gal G, Avidor I, et al. Anaplastic thyroid carcinoma: a clinical, histologic and immunohistochemical study. *Cancer* 1988;62: 319.
54. Spires JR, Schwartz MR, Miller RH. Anaplastic thyroid carcinoma associated with differentiated thyroid carcinoma. *Arch Otolaryngol Head Neck Surg* 1988;114:40.
55. Ueda G, Furth J. Sarcomatoid transformation of transplanted thyroid carcinoma: similarity to anaplastic human thyroid carcinomas. *Arch Pathol Lab Med* 1967;83:3.
56. Ibanez ML, Russell WO, Albores-Saavenra J, et al. Thyroid carcinoma: biological behavior and mortality. *Cancer* 1966;19:1039.
57. Tollefson HR, de Cosse JJ, Hutter RVP. Papillary carcinoma of the thyroid: a clinical and pathologic study of 70 fatal cases. *Cancer* 1964;17:1035.
58. Wallin G, Backdahl M, Tallroth-Ekman E, et al. Coexist anaplastic and well-differentiated thyroid carcinomas: nuclear DNA study. *Eur J Surg Oncol* 1989;15:43.
59. Hadar T, et al. Anaplastic carcinoma of the thyroid. *Eur J Surg Oncol* 1993;19:511.
60. Bal C, et al. "Insular" carcinoma of the thyroid. A subset of anaplastic thyroid malignancy with a less aggressive clinical course. *Clin Nucl Med* 1993;18:1056.
61. Baba M, et al. Preparation of a human monoclonal antibody derived from cervical lymph nodes of a patient with anaplastic carcinoma of the thyroid. *Hum Antibodies Hybridomas* 1993;4:181.
62. Tennvall J, et al. Combined doxorubicin, hyperfractionated radiotherapy, and surgery in anaplastic thyroid carcinoma. Report on two protocols. The Swedish Anaplastic Thyroid Cancer Group. *Cancer* 1994; 74:1348.
63. Greval RS, et al. Chemotherapy and combination therapy in anaplastic thyroid carcinoma. *Indian J Med Sci* 1993;47:269.
64. Hazard JB, Hawk WA, Crile G Jr. Medullary (solid) carcinoma of the thyroid—a clinical pathological entity. *J Clin Endocrinol Metab* 1959;19:152.
65. Williams ED. Histogenesis of medullary carcinoma of the thyroid. *J Clin Pathol* 1966;19:114.
66. Sarndon JR, Dilley WG, Baylin SB. Familial medullary thyroid carcinoma without associated endocrinopathy: a distinct clinical entity. *Br J Surg* 1986;73:273.
67. Wells SA Jr, et al. Current perspectives on the diagnosis and management of patients with multiple endocrine neoplasia type II syndromes. *Endocrinol Metab Clin North Am* 1994;23:215.
68. Dunn JT. When is a thyroid nodule a sporadic medullary carcinoma? [editorial; comment]. *J Clin Endocrinol Metab* 1994;78:824, 78:826.
69. Wells SA Jr, et al. Predictive DNA testing and prophylactic thyroidectomy in patients at risk for multiple endocrine neoplasia type II. *Ann Surg* 1994;220:237–247.
70. Nelkin DB, et al. Molecular abnormalities in tumors associated with multiple endocrine neoplasia type II. *Endocrinol Metab Clin North Am* 1994;23:187.
71. Utiger RD. Medullary thyroid carcinoma, genes, and their prevention of cancer [editorial; comment]. *N Engl J Med* 1994;331:870, 828.
72. Decker RA. Expression of papillary thyroid carcinoma in multiple endocrine neoplasia type IIA. *Surgery* 1993;114:1059.
73. Snow KJ, et al. Management of individual tumor syndromes, medullary thyroid carcinoma and hyperparathyroidism. *Endocrinol Metab Clin North Am* 1994;23:157.
74. Ellenhorn JB, et al. Impact of therapeutic regional lymph node dissection for medullary carcinoma of the thyroid gland. *Surgery* 1993;114:1078–1081.
75. Moley JS, et al. Reoperation for recurrent or persistent medullary thyroid cancer. *Surgery* 1993;114:1090–1095.
76. Fugazzola L, et al. Disappearance rate of serum calcitonin after a total thyroidectomy for medullary thyroid carcinoma. *Int J Biol Markers* 1994;9:21.
77. Girelli ME, et al. Prognostic value of early postoperative calcitonin level in medullary thyroid carcinoma. *Tumori* 1994;80:113.
78. Beahrs OH, Henson DE, Hutter RNP, et al. Manual for staging of cancer, 3rd ed. AJCC. Philadelphia: Lippincott, 1988;57.
78a. Hedinger C, et al. Histological typing of thyroid tumors. *WHO international histological classification of tumors*, 2nd ed. Berlin-New York: Springer-Verlag, 1988.
79. Hedinger C, Williams ED, Sobim LH. The WHO histological classification of thyroid tumors: a commentary on the 2nd edition. *Cancer* 1989;63:908.
80. Joensuu H, Klemi P, Eerola E, et al. Influence of cellular DNA content on survival in differentiated thyroid carcinoma. *Cancer* 1986;58:2462.
81. Zimmerman D, Hay ID, Gough IR, et al. Papillary thyroid carcinomas in children and adults: longterm follow-up of 1039 patients conservatively treated at one institution during three decades. *Surgery* 1988; 104:1157.
82. Cady B, Rossi R. An expanded view of risk-group definition in differentiated thyroid cancer. *Surgery* 1988;104:947.
83. Tennvall J, Bjorklund A, Moller T, et al. Is the EORTC prognostic index of thyroid cancer valid in differentiated thyroid cancer? *Cancer* 1986;57:1405.
84. Andry G, Chantrain G, van Glabbeke M, et al. Papillary and follicular thyroid carcinoma: individualization of the treatment according to the prognosis of the disease. *Eur J Cancer Clin Oncol* 1988;24:1641.
85. Hamming JI, Schelfhout LJDM, Cornelisse CJ. Prognostic value of nuclear DNA content in papillary and follicular cancer. *World J Surg* 1988;12:503.
86. Thoresen SO, Akslen LA, Glattre E, et al. Survival and prognostic factors in differentiated thyroid cancer—a multivariate analysis of 1055 cases. *Br J Cancer* 1989;59:231.
87. Simpson WJ, McKinney SE, Carruthers JS. Papillary and follicular thyroid cancer prognostic factors in 1578 patients. *Am J Med* 1987; 83:479.
88. Cady B, Sedgwick CE, Meissner WA, et al. Changing clinical, pathologic, therapeutic and survival patterns in differentiated thyroid carcinoma. *Ann Surg* 1976;184:341.
89. Hopwood NJ, et al. Thyroid masses: An approach to diagnosis and management in childhood and adolescence. *Pediatr Rev* 1993;14:481.
90. Newman KD. The current management of thyroid tumors in childhood. *Semin Pediatr Surg* 1993;2:69.
91. Proceedings of the American Association of Endocrine Surgeons. *Surgery* 1988;104.
92. Cady B. Discussion. *Surgery* 1987;102:1080.
93. Beenken F, Guillamondegui O, Shallenberger R, et al. Prognostic factors in patients dying of well-differentiated thyroid cancer. *Arch Otolaryngol Head Neck Surg* 1989;115:326.
94. La Quaglia MP, Corbally MT, Heller G. Recurrence and morbidity in differentiated thyroid cancer in children. *Surgery* 1988;104:1149.
95. Thompson N. Discussion following Zimmerman D, Hay ID, Gough IR, et al. Papillary thyroid carcinoma in children and adults: longterm follow-up of 1039 patients treated conservatively at one institution during 3 decades. *Surg* 1988;104:1147.
96. Schlumberger M, de Vathaire F, Dravagli JP, et al. Differentiated thyroid carcinoma in childhood: longterm follow-up of 72 patients. *J Clin Endocrinol Metab* 1987;65:1088.
97. Rosen IB, Bowden J, Luk CS, et al. Aggressive thyroid cancer in low-risk age population. *Surgery* 1987;102:1075.
98. Leeper RD. The effect of 131-iodine therapy on survival of patients with metastatic papillary or follicular thyroid carcinoma. *J Clin Endocrinol Metab* 1973;36:1143.
99. Schroeder S, Bocker W, Baisch H, et al. Prognostic factors in medullary thyroid carcinomas. *Cancer* 1988;61:806.
100. Mendelsohn G, et al. Relationship of tissue CEA and calcitonin to tumor virulence in medullary thyroid carcinoma. *Cancer* 1984;54:657.
101. Fidler IJ, Hart IR. The origin of metastatic heterogeneity in tumors. *Eur J Cancer* 1987;17:487.

102. Woodruff MFA. Tumor clonality and its biological significance. *Adv Cancer Res* 1988;50:197.
103. Schilsky RL (ed.) Tumor cell heterogeneity. *Semin Oncol* 1985;12(3):201–353.
104. McConahey WM, Hay ID, Woolner LB, et al. Papillary thyroid cancer treated at the Mayo Clinic, 1946–1970: initial manifestations, pathologic findings, therapy and outcome. *Mayo Clin Proc* 1986;61:978.
105. Ohnishi T, et al. Detection of recurrent thyroid cancer: MR versus thallium-201 scintigraphy. *Am J Neuroradiol* 1993;14:1051.
106. Russell P, et al. Proton magnetic resonance in human thyroid neoplasia. I: Discrimination between benign and malignant neoplasms. *Am J Med* 1994;96:383.
107. Bakheet SM, et al. False-positive radioiodine whole-body scan in thyroid cancer patients due to unrelated pathology. *Clin Nucl Med* 1994;19:325.
108. Tenenbaum F, et al. Usefulness of technetium-99M hydroxymethylene diphosphonate scans in localizing bone metastases of differentiated thyroid carcinoma. *Eur J Nucl Med* 1993;20:1168.
109. Lubin E, et al. Serum thyroglobulin and iodine-131 whole-body scan in the diagnosis and assessment of treatment for metastatic differentiated thyroid carcinoma. *J Nucl Med* 1994;35:257.
110. Oommen R, et al. Scintigraphic diagnosis of thyroid cancer. Correlation of thyroid scintigraphy and histopathology. *Acta Radiol* 1994;35:222.
111. Sundram FX, et al. Role of technetium-99M sestamibi in localization of thyroid cancer metastases. *Ann Acad Med Singapore* 1993;22:557.
112. Sundram FX, et al. Investigation of thyroid nodules using technetium-99M sestamibi. *Ann Acad Med Singapore* 1993;22:560.
113. Lebouthillier G, et al. TC-99m sestamibi and other agents in the detection of metastatic medullary carcinoma of the thyroid. *Clin Nucl Med* 1993;18:657. (Note: Uptake of radioiodine in normal structures such as hiatal hernia and esophageal strictures can mimic recurrence of papillary thyroid carcinoma.)
114. Willis LL, et al. Mediastinal uptake of I-131 in a hiatal hernia may mimic recurrence of papillary thyroid carcinoma. *Clin Nucl Med* 1993;18:961.
115. Sherman SI, et al. Clinical utility of posttreatment radioiodine scans in the management of patients with thyroid carcinoma. *J Clin Endocrinol Metab* 1994;78:629.
116. Langsteger W, et al. False-positive scans in papillary thyroid carcinoma [letter; comment]. *J Nucl Med* 1993;34:2280–2289.
117. Bloom AD, et al. Determination of malignancy of thyroid nodules with positron emission tomography. *Surgery* 1993;114:728–734.
118. Adler LP, et al. Positron emission tomography of thyroid masses. *Thyroid* 1993;3:195.
119. Park HM, et al. Influence of diagnostic radioiodine on the uptake of ablative doses of iodine-131. *Thyroid* 1994;4:49.
120. Arad E, et al. Ablation of remaining functioning thyroid lobe with radioiodine after hemithyroidectomy for carcinoma. *Clin Nucl Med* 1993;18:662.
121. Comtois R, et al. Assessment of the efficacy of iodine-131 for thyroid ablation. *J Nucl Med* 1993;34:1927.
122. Coburn M, et al. Recurrent thyroid cancer. Role of surgery versus radioactive iodine (I-131). *Ann Surg* 1994;219:587–593.
123. Samaan NA, Maheshwari YK, Nader S, et al. Impact of therapy for differentiated cancer of the thyroid: an analysis of 106 cases. *J Clin Endocrinol Metab* 1983;56:1131.
124. Ruiz de Almodovar JM, et al. Analysis of risk of death from differentiated thyroid cancer. *Radiother Oncol* 1994;31:207.
125. Puls T. The changing aspect of thyroid surgery: The review of 130 consecutive cases. *Acta Otorhinolaryngol Belg* 1993;47:351.
126. Shah JP, et al. Lobectomy versus total thyroidectomy for differentiated carcinoma of the thyroid: a matched-pair analysis. *Am J Surgery* 1993;166:331.
127. Goretzki PE, et al. Surgical reintervention for differentiated thyroid cancer. *Br J Surg* 1993;80:1009.
128. Mori Y, et al. Induction of discriminate function concerning postoperative local recurrence or distant metastasis in 589 patients with differentiated thyroid cancer. *Surg Today* 1993;23:777.
129. Sugino K, et al. Surgical treatment of locally advanced thyroid cancer. *Surg Today* 1993;23:791.
130. Sugino K, et al. The enucleation of thyroid tumors indeterminate before surgery as papillary thyroid carcinoma: should immediate reoperation be performed? *Surg Today* 1994;24:305.
131. Grossenbacher R, et al. Thyroidectomy and recurrent laryngeal nerve. *Laryngorhinootologie* 1994;73:179 (Ger-Eng Abstr).
132. Andersen PE, Kansella J, Loree TR, et al. Differentiated carcinoma of the thyroid with extra-thyroidal extension. *Am J Surg* 1995;170:467.
133. Collins SL. Controversies in the management of cancer in the neck. In: Thawley SE, Panje WR, eds. *Comprehensive management of head and neck tumors*, vol 2. Philadelphia: WB Saunders, 1987;1385–1443.
134. McGregor GI, Luomo A, Jackson SM. Lymph node metastases from well-differentiated thyroid cancer: a clinical review. *Am J Surg* 1985;149:610.
135. Gerard-Marchant R. Thyroid follicle inclusions in cervical lymph nodes. *Arch Pathol* 1964;77:633.
136. Roth LM. Inclusions of non-neoplastic thyroid tissue within cervical lymph nodes. *Cancer* 1965;18:105.
137. Harwood J, Clark OH, Dunphy JE. Significance of lymph node metastasis in differentiated thyroid carcinoma. *Am J Surg* 1978;136:107.
138. Woolner LB, Beahrs OH, Black BM, et al. Thyroid carcinoma: general considerations and follow-up data on 1181 cases. In: Young S, Inman DR, eds. *Thyroid neoplasia*. New York: Academic Press, 1968;51.
139. Attie JN. Modified neck dissection and treatment of thyroid cancer: a safe procedure. *Eur J Cancer Clin Oncol* 1988;24:315.
140. Spires JR, Robbins KT, Luna M, et al. Metastatic papillary carcinoma of the thyroid: the significance of extranodal extension. *Head Neck Surg* 1989;11:242.
141. Rosen EB, Maitland A. Changing the operative strategy for thyroid cancer by node sampling. *Am J Surg* 1983;146:504.
142. Crile G Jr. The fallacy of the conventional radical neck dissection for papillary carcinoma of the thyroid. *Ann Surg* 1957;145:317.
143. Hamming JF, van de Velde CJH, Fleuren JH, et al. Differentiated thyroid carcinoma: stage-adapted approach to the treatment of regional lymph node metastases. *Eur J Cancer Clin Oncol* 1988;24:325.
144. McKenzie AD. The natural history of thyroid cancer. *Arch Surg* 1971;102:273.
145. Attie JN, et al. Elective neck dissection and papillary carcinoma of the thyroid. *Am J Surg* 1971;122:464.
146. Rossi RL, Cady B, Silverman ML, et al. Surgically incurable well-differentiated thyroid carcinoma—prognostic factors and results of therapy. *Arch Surg* 1988;123:569.
147. Mazzaferri EL, Young RL, Oertel JE, et al. Papillary thyroid carcinoma: the impact of therapy in 576 patients. *Medicine (Baltimore)* 1977;56:171.
148. Proye C, et al. Recurrence of cervical lymph node involvement in surgically treated thyroid cancer. Uselessness of routine cervical lymph node excision (medullary carcinoma excluded). *Chirurgie* 1992;118:448–453 (French-Eng Abstr).
149. Sugino K, et al. Regional lymph node recurrence in patients with papillary thyroid carcinoma who did not undergo neck dissection. *Nippon Geka Gakkai Zasshi* 1993;94:1108 (Jpn-Eng abstr).
150. Dralle H, et al. Compartment-oriented microdissection of regional lymph nodes in medullary thyroid carcinoma. *Surg Today* 1994;24:112.
151. Som PM, et al. The varied presentations of papillary thyroid carcinoma cervical nodal disease: CT and MR findings. *Am J Neuroradiol* 1994;15:1123.
152. Attie JN, et al. Thyroid carcinoma presenting as an enlarged cervical lymph node. *Am J Surg* 1993;166:428.
153. Sugino K. An analysis of lymphocyte subsets in the regional lymph nodes of patients with papillary thyroid carcinoma. *Surg Today* 1994;24:323.
154. Buhr HJ, et al. Microsurgical neck dissection for occultly metastasizing medullary thyroid carcinoma: three-year results. *Cancer* 1993;72:3685.
155. McHenry CR, Rosen IB, Walfish PG. Prospective management of nodal metastases in differentiated thyroid cancer. *Am J Surg* 1991;162:353.
156. Sellers M, Beenken S, Blankenship A, et al. Prognostic significance of cervical lymph node metastases in differentiated thyroid cancer. *Am J Surg* 1992;164:578.
157. Colburn MC, Wanabo HJ. Prognostic factors and management considerations in patients with cervical metastasis of thyroid cancer. *Am J Surg* 1992;164:671.
158. Hughes CJ, Shaha AR, Shah JP, et al. Impact of lymph node metasta-

159. Hirabayashi RN, Lindsey I. Carcinoma of the thyroid gland. A statistical study of 390 patients. *J Clin Endocrinol Metab* 1961;21:1596.
160. Elias D, Schlumberger M, Treich A, et al. Repérage des parathyroids par le bleu de mèthylene aucours de la chirurgie thyroidienne. *Presse Med* 1983;12:1229.
161. Samaan NA, Schultz PN, Haynie TP, et al. Pulmonary metastasis of differentiated thyroid carcinoma: treatment results in 101 patients. *J Clin Endocrinol Metab* 1985;65:376.
162. Hoie J, Stenwig AE, Kullmann G, et al. Distant metastases in papillary thyroid cancer: a review of 91 patients. *Cancer* 1988;61:1.
163. Schlumberger M, Tubiana M, de Vathaire F, et al. Longterm results of treatment of 283 patients with lung and bone metastases from differentiated thyroid carcinoma. *J Clin Endocrinol Metab* 1986;63:960.
164. Weiss L, Gilbert HA. Pattern of pulmonary metastases: introduction. In: Weiss L, Gilbert HA, eds. *Pulmonary metastases.* Boston: Martinus Nijhoff Medical Division, 1978;100.
165. Rossi RL, Cady B, Silverman ML, et al. Current results of conservative surgery for occult thyroid carcinoma. *World J Surg* 1986;10:612.
166. Nemec J, Pohunkova D, Zamrasile A. Pulmonary metastases of thyroid carcinoma. *Czech Med* 1979;2:78.
167. Kodama T, Fugimoto Y, Obara T, et al. Histochemical demonstration of thyroxine, triiodothyronine and thyroglobulin in the primary lesions of thyroid carcinoma and its predictability for radioiodine uptake by metastatic lesions. *World J Surg* 1988;12:439.
168. Cady B. Discussion. *Surgery* 1988;104:953.
169. Powell ME, et al. Surveillance after treatment for well-differentiated thyroid cancer: audit for chest radiography. *Clin Oncol (R Coll Radiol)* 1994;6:151.
170. Ozaki O, et al. Clinicopathologic study of pulmonary metastasis of differentiated thyroid carcinoma: age-, sex-, and histology-matched case-control study. *Int Surg* 1993;78:218.
171. Casara D, et al. Different features of pulmonary metastases in differentiated thyroid cancer: natural history and multivariate statistical analysis of prognostic variables. *J Nucl Med* 1993;34:1626.
172. McCormack KR. Bone metastases from thyroid carcinoma. *Cancer* 1966;19:181.
173. Niederle B, Roka R, Schemper M, et al. Surgical treatment of distant metastases in differentiated thyroid carcinoma: indications and results. *Surgery* 1986;100:1088.
174. Reeves TS. Discussion. *Surgery* 1986;100:1096.
174a. Goletti O, et al. Inoperable thyroid carcinoma: palliation with percutaneous injection of ethanol. *Eur J Surg* 1993;159:639.
175. Bocker W, Schroder S, Dralle H. Minimal thyroid neoplasia. *Recent Results Cancer Res* 1988;106:131.
176. Bottner IG. Minimal thyroid cancer: clinical consequences. *Recent Results Cancer Res* 1988;106:139.
177. Bondeson L, Ljungberg O. Occult thyroid carcinoma at autopsy in Malmo, Sweden. *Cancer* 1981;47:319.
178. Sampson RJ. Prevalence and significance of occult thyroid carcinoma. In: DeGrott LJ, Frohman LA, Kaplan EL, et al., eds. *Radiation-associated thyroid carcinoma.* New York: Grune & Stratton, 1976.
179. Gikas PW, Labow SS, Guilo W, et al. Occult metastasis from occult papillary carcinoma of the thyroid. *Cancer* 1967;20:2100.
180. Fukanaga FH, Yatani R. Geographic pathology of occult thyroid carcinomas. *Cancer* 1975;36:1095.
181. Nishiyama RH, Ludwig GK, Thompson NW. The prevalence of small papillary thyroid carcinomas in 100 consecutive necropsies in an American population. In: DeGroot L, Frohman LA, Kaplan EL, et al., eds. *Radiation-associated thyroid carcinoma.* New York: Grune & Stratton, 1976;123.
182. Lang W, Borrusch H, Bauer L. Occult carcinomas of the thyroid: evaluation of 1020 sequential autopsies. *Am J Clin Pathol* 1988;90:72.
183. Sampson RJ, Okaki CR, et al. Metastases from occult thyroid carcinoma: an autopsy study from Hiroshima and Nagasaki, Japan. *Cancer* 1970;25:803.
184. Sampson RJ, Bruncher CR, et al. Smallest forms of papillary carcinoma of the thyroid. *Arch Pathol* 1971;91:334.
185. Kafai N, Sakamoto A. New subgrouping of small thyroid carcinomas. *Cancer* 1987;60:1767.
186. Strate FM, Lee EL, Childers JH. Occult papillary carcinoma of the thyroid with distant metastases. *Cancer* 1984;54:1093.
187. Cohnheim J. Einfacher Gallertkropf mit methasen. *Arch Pathol Physiol Anat* 1876;68:547.
188. Matovinovic J, Nishiyama RH, Lalli A, et al. "Benign metastasizing goiter" of Cohnheim: an experimental study in the transplantable thyroid tumor of the rat. *Cancer Res* 1971;31:288.
189. Clark RL, Hickey RC, Butler JJ, et al. Thyroid cancer discovered incidentally during treatment for an unrelated head and neck cancer: review of 15 cases. *Ann Surg* 1966;163:665.
190. Oertel JE, Klinck GH. Structural changes in the thyroid glands of healthy young men. *Med Annals Dist Columbia* 1965;34:75.
191. Edis AJ. Natural history of occult thyroid cancer. In: DeGroot L, Frohman LA, Kaplan EL, et al., eds. *Radiation-associated thyroid carcinoma.* New York: Grune & Stratton, 1976;155.
192. Lloyd RV, Beierwaltes WH. Occult sclerosing carcinoma of the thyroid: potential for aggressive biological behavior. *South Med J* 1983;76:437.
193. Allo MD, Christianson W, Koivunen D. Not all "occult" papillary carcinomas are "minimal." *Surgery* 1988;104:971.
194. Salvadori B, et al. "Occult" papillary carcinoma of the thyroid: a questionable entity. *Eur J Cancer* 1993;29A:1817.
195. Takami H, et al. A rapid immunoperoxidase method for pathological diagnosis of occult thyroid carcinoma. *Int Surg* 1993;78:225.
196. Miki H, et al. Diagnosis and surgical treatment of small papillary carcinomas of the thyroid gland. *J Surg Oncol* 1993;54:78–80.
197. Liaw KY, et al. Management of thyroid cancers diagnosed histologically after surgery. *J Formos Med Assoc* 1993;92:312.
198. Smithers D, ed. *Tumours of the thyroid gland.* London: Livingstone, 1970.
199. Ron E, Kleinerman RA, Boice JD Jr, et al. A population-based case control study of thyroid cancer. *J Natl Cancer Inst* 1987;79:1.
200. Doniach I. Experimental thyroid tumors. In: Smithers D, ed. *Tumours of the thyroid gland.* London: Livingstone, 1970;73.
201. Cutler SJ, Young JL Jr, eds. *Third national cancer surgery incidence data.* Washington DC: Department of Health, Education, and Welfare publication (NIH) 75, NCI Monograph #41, 1975;25.
202. Silverberg E, Lubera JA. Cancer statistics 1989. *CA Cancer J Clinic* 1989;39(1):3.
203. Myers MH, Ries L. Cancer patient survival rates: SEER program results for 10 years of follow-up. *CA Cancer J Clinic* 1989;39(1):21.
204. Devesa SS, Silverman DT, Young JL Jr. Cancer incidence and mortality trends among whites in the US; 1947–1984. *J Natl Cancer Inst* 1987;79:701.
205. Spitz MR, Sides JG, Katz RL, et al. Ethnic patterns of thyroid cancer incidence in the United States, 1973. *Int J Cancer* 1988;42:549.
206. Arnbjornsson E, Arnbjornsson A, Olaffson A. Thyroid cancer incidence in relation to volcanic activity. *Environ Health* 1986;41:36.
207. Waterhouse J, Muir C, Shanmugaratnam K, et al., eds. *Cancer incidence in five continents,* vol 4. Lyon, France: IARC Scientific Publications, 1982.
208. Olen E, Klinck GH. Hyperthyroidism and cancer. *Arch Pathol* 1966;81:531.
209. Mortensen JD, Woolner LB, Bennett WA. Gross and microscopic findings in clinically normal thyroid glands. *J Clin Endocrinol Metab* 1955;15:1270.
210. Mortenson JD, Bennett WA, Woolner LB. Incidence of carcinoma in thyroid glands removed at 1000 consecutive routine necropsies. *Surg Forum* 1955;5:569.
211. Silverberg SG, Vidone RA. Carcinoma of the thyroid in surgical and postmortem material. *Ann Surg* 1966;164:291.
212. Maceri DR, Sullivan M, McClatchney KD. Autoimmune thyroiditis: pathophysiology and relationship to thyroid cancer. *Laryngoscope* 1986;96:82.
213. Ott RO, McCall AR, McHenry C. The incidence of thyroid carcinoma and Hashimoto's thyroiditis. *Am Surg* 1987;53:442.
214. McLeod MK, East ME, Burney RE, et al. Hashimoto's thyroiditis revisited: the association with thyroid cancer remains obscure. *World J Surg* 1988;12:509.
215. Fugimoto Y. Invited commentary. *World J Surg* 1988;12:516.
216. McKee RF, et al. Thyroid neoplasia coexistent with chronic lymphocytic thyroiditis. *Br J Surg* 1993;80:1303.
217. Peyrade F, et al. Hashimoto thyroiditis, adenocarcinoma, and malignant lymphoma of the thyroid. A case of triple association [letter]. *Presse Med* 1993;22:1150.
218. Shapiro SJ, Friedman NB, Perzik SL, et al. Incidence of thyroid carcinoma in Graves' disease. *Cancer* 1970;26:1261.

219. Farbota LM, Calandra BD, Lawrence AM, et al. Thyroid carcinoma and Graves' disease. *Surgery* 1985;98:1148.
220. Dobyns BM, Sheline GE, Workman JB, et al. Malignant and benign neoplasms of the thyroid in patients treated for hyperthyroidism: a report of the cooperative thyrotoxicosis therapy follow-up study. *J Clin Endocrinol Metab* 1974;38:976.
221. Giorgiadis NJ, Leoutsakos BJ, Katsas AG. The association of thyroid cancer and hyperthyroidism. *Surgery* 1971;55:27.
222. Filetti S, Belfiore A, Amir SM, et al. The role of thyroid stimulating antibodies of Graves' disease and differentiated thyroid cancer. *N Engl J Med* 1988;318:753.
223. Roher HD, Goretzki PE, Frilling A. Thyroid stimulating antibodies of Graves' disease and thyroid cancer [letter]. *N Engl J Med* 1988;319:1669.
224. Brownlie BE, et al. Primary thyroid lymphoma. Clinical features, treatment, and outcome: a report of 8 cases. *NZ Med J* 1994;107:301.
225. Pilotti S, et al. A novel panel of antibodies that segregate immunocytochemically poorly differentiated carcinoma from undifferentiated carcinoma of the thyroid gland. *Am J Surg Pathol* 1994;18:1054.
226. Doria R, et al. Thyroid lymphoma. The case for combined modality therapy. *Cancer* 1994;73:200.
227. Das DK, et al. Fine-needle aspiration cytology diagnosis of non-Hodgkin lymphoma of the thyroid: a report of four cases. *Diagn Cytopathol* 1993;9:639.
228. Tsang RW, et al. Non-Hodgkin lymphoma of thyroid gland: prognostic factors and treatment outcome. The Princess Margaret Hospital Lymphoma Group. *Int J Radiat Oncol Biol Phys* 1993;27:599.
229. Williams ED. Pathologic and natural history. *Recent Results Cancer Res* 1980;73:487.
230. Wahner HW, Cuello C, Correa P, et al. Thyroid carcinoma in an endemic goiter area, Cali, Colombia. *Am J Med* 1966;40:58.
231. Beierwaltes WH. Natural history of thyroid cancer. In: Ingbar SH and Brauerman LE, eds. *Werner. The thyroid—a fundamental and clinical text,* 5th ed. Philadelphia: JB Lippincott, 1986;1319.
232. Kind HP. In: Smithers D, ed. *Tumours of the thyroid gland.* London: Livingstone, 1970;113.
233. Ledent C, et al. Models of thyroid goiter and tumors in transgenic mice. *Mol Cell Endocrinol* 1994;100:167.
234. Mathai V, et al. Do long-standing nodular goitres result in malignancies? *Aust NZ J Surg* 1994;64:180.
235. Williams ED, Doniach I, Bjarnason O, et al. Thyroid cancer in an iodine rich area. *Cancer* 1977;39:215.
236. Thalmann A. Die haufigkeit der struma maligna am Berne pathologischen institut von 1910–1950 urd ihre beziehung zujodprophy laxe des endemischen Kropfes. *Schweitz Med Wochenschr* 1954;84:473.
237. Heitz P, Moser H, Staub JJ. Thyroid cancer, a study of 57 thyroid tumors observed over a 30 year period. *Cancer* 1976;37:2329.
238. Duffy BJ Jr, Fitzgerald PJ. Cancer of the thyroid in children—a report of 28 cases. *J Clin Endocrinol Metab* 1950;10:1296.
239. DeGroot L, Paloyan E. Thyroid carcinoma and radiation—Chicago endemic? *JAMA* 1973;225:487.
240. Refetoff S, Harrison J, Karanfilski BT, et al. Continuing occurrence of thyroid carcinoma after irradiation to the neck in infancy and childhood. *N Engl J Med* 1975;292:171.
241. Witherbee WD, Roentgen ray treatment of tonsils and adenoids. *Am J Roentgenol* 1921;8:25.
242. Friedlander A. Status lymphaticus and enlargement of the thymus with a report of a case successfully treated by the X-ray. *Arch Radiat* 1907;24:490.
243. Samaan NA, Schultz PN, Ordonez NG, et al. A comparison of thyroid carcinoma in those who have and have not had head and neck irradiation in childhood. *J Clin Endocrinol Metab* 1987;64:219.
244. Conard RA. Summary of thyroid findings in Marshallese 2 years after exposure to radioactive fallout. In: DeGroot L, Frohman LA, Kaplan EL, et al., eds. *Radiation-associated thyroid carcinoma.* New York: Grune & Stratton, 1976.
245. Hamilton TE, van Belle G, LoGerfo JP. Thyroid neoplasia in Marshall Islanders exposed to nuclear fallout. *JAMA* 1987;258:629.
246. Strand F-E, Erlandsson K, et al. Thyroid uptake of iodine^{131} and iodine^{133} from Chernobyl and the population of southern Sweden. *J Nucl Med* 1988;29:1719.
247. Calandra DB, Shah KH, Lawrence AM, et al. Total thyroidectomy in irradiated patients—a 20 year experience in 206 patients. *Ann Surg* 1985;202:356.
248. Bergstrom B. Late complications after irradiation treatment for cervical adenitis in childhood—a 60 year follow-up study. *Acta Otolaryngol (Stockh)* 1985;100:151.
249. Shore RE. Radiation and health factors and human thyroid tumors following sinus irradiation. *Health Phys* 1980;38:451.
250. Maxon RH. Radiation-induced thyroid disease. *Med Clin North Am* 1985;69:1049.
251. Werner SC, Ingbar SH, eds. *The thyroid,* 3rd ed. New York: Harper & Row, 1971.
252. Ron E, Modan B. Thyroid cancer and other neoplasms following childhood scalp irradiation. In: Boice JD, Fraumeni JF, Fraumeni JM, eds. *Radiation carcinogenesis: epidemiology and biologic significance.* New York: Raven Press, 1984.
253. Hempelmann LH, Hall WJ, Phillips M, et al. Neoplasms of persons treated with x-rays in infancy: fourth survey in twenty years. *J Natl Cancer Inst* 1975;55:519.
254. Kaplan EL. Discussion. *Ann Surg* 1985;202:359.
255. Parker LN, Belsky JL, Yamamoto T, et al. Thyroid carcinoma after exposure to atomic radiation. *Ann Intern Med* 1974;80:600.
256. Socolow EL, Hashizume A, Neriishi S, et al. Thyroid carcinoma in man after exposure to ionizing radiation: a survey of the findings in Hiroshima and Nagasaki. *N Engl J Med* 1963;268:206.
257. Holm L-E, Lundell G. Swedish thyroid cancer risk from Chernobyl? *J Nucl Med* 1989;30:721.
258. Holm L-E, Wiklund KE, Lundell GE, et al. Thyroid cancer after diagnostic doses of I^{131}: a retrospective cohort study. *J Natl Cancer Inst* 1988;80:1132.
259. Lindsay S, Sheline GE, Potter JD, et al. Induction of neoplasms in the thyroid gland of the rat by x-irradiation of the gland. *Cancer Res* 1960;21:9.
260. Ladler J, Mandavia M, Goldberg M. The effect of hypophysectomy on the experimental production of rat thyroid neoplasms. *Cancer Res* 1970;30:1909.
261. Moore W Jr, Calvin M. Chromosomal changes in the Chinese hamster following x-irradiation in vivo. *Int J Radiat Biol* 1968;14:161.
262. Perkel ZS, Gail MA, Lubin J, et al. Radiation-induced thyroid neoplasms: evidence for familial susceptibility factors. *J Clin Endocrinol Metab* 1988;66:1316.
263. Taylor AR, Harnden DG, Arlett CS, et al. Ataxia telangiectasia: a human mutation with abnormal radiation sensitivity. *Nature* 1975;258:427.
264. Lessard ET, Peterson KR, Miltenberger RP, et al. Unpublished observations. University of Cincinnati, 1983.
265. Swelstad JA, Scanlon EF, Oviado MA, et al. Irradiation-induced polyglandular neoplasia of the head and neck. *Am J Surg* 1978;135:820.
266. Schneider AB, Shore-Freeman E, Weinstein RA. Radiation-induced thyroid and other head and neck tumors: occurrence of multiple tumors and analysis of risk factors. *J Clin Endocrinol Metab* 1986;63:107.
267. Prinz RA, Paloyan E, Lawrence AM, et al. Radiation-associated hyperparathyroidism: a new syndrome? *Surgery* 1977;92:296.
268. Tang TT, Holcenberg JS, Duck SC, et al. Thyroid carcinoma following treatment for acute lymphoblastic leukemia. *Cancer* 1980;46:1502.
269. Weshler Z, Krashokuki D, Peshin Y, et al. Thyroid carcinoma induction by irradiation for Hodgkin's disease: report of a case. *Acta Radiol Oncol* 1978;17:383.
270. Auguste LJ, Seiko K. Radiation and thyroid carcinoma. *Head Neck Surg* 1985;7:217.
271. Turrin A, Pillotti S, Basso S, et al. Characteristics of thyroid cancer following irradiation. *Int J Radiat Oncol Biol Phys* 1985;11:2149.
272. Viswanathan K, et al. Childhood thyroid cancer. Characteristics and long-term outcome in children irradiated for benign conditions of the head and neck. *Arch Pediatr Adolesc Med* 1994;148:260.
273. Sala E, et al. Thyroid cancer in the age group 0–19: time trends and temporal changes in radioactive fallout. *Eur J Cancer* 1993;29A:1443.
274. Williams ED. Radiation-induced thyroid cancer. *Histopathology* 1993;23:387.
275. Hallquist A, et al. External radiotherapy prior to thyroid cancer: a case-control study. *Int J Radiat Oncol Biol Phys* 1993;27:1085.
276. Baverstock KS. Thyroid cancer in children in Belarus after Chernobyl. *World Health Stat Q* 1993;46:204.

277. Hall P. Radiation-induced thyroid cancer. *Med Oncol Tumor Pharmacother* 1992;9:183.
278. Hallquist A, et al. Medical diagnostic and therapeutic ionizing radiation and the risk for thyroid cancer: a case-control study. *Eur J Cancer Prev* 1994;3:259.
279. Domann FE, et al. Quantifying the frequency of radiogenic thyroid cancer per clonogenic cell in vivo. *Radiat Res* 1994;137:330.
280. Poverennyi AM, et al. The probable causes of thyroid diseases in the victims of the Chernobyl accident. *Radiat Biol Radioecol* 1994;34:8 (Rus-Eng Abstr).
281. Nikiforov Y, et al. Pediatric thyroid cancer after the Chernobyl disaster. Pathomorphologic study of 84 cases (1991–1992) from the Republic of Belarus. *Cancer* 1994;74:748.
282. Bitton R, et al. Leukemia after a small dose of radioiodine for metastatic thyroid cancer. *J Clin Endocrinol Metab* 1993;77:1423.
283. Meyer MA. Cancer risk after iodine-131 therapy for hyperthyroidism [letter; comment]. *J Natl Cancer Inst* 1994;86:1026. Comment on: *J Natl Cancer Inst* 1991;83:1072.
284. Livingston GK, et al. Effect of in vivo exposure to iodine-131 on the frequency and persistence of micronuclei in human lymphocytes. *J Toxicol Environ Health* 1993;40:367.
285. Esik O, et al. Prophylactic external radiation in differentiated thyroid cancer: a retrospective study over a 30-year observation period. *Oncology* 1994;51:371.
286. Goldenberg RC, Chaikoff LL. Induction of thyroid cancer in the rat by radioiodine. *Arch Pathol* 1952;53:22.
287. DeGroot LJ, Stanbury JB. *The thyroid and its diseases.* New York: John Wiley & Sons, 1971;335.
288. Holm L-E, Dahlquist I, Israelson A, et al. Malignant thyroid tumors after I131 Therapy. *N Engl J Med* 1980;303:188.
289. Rallison ML, Dobyns BM, Keating FR. Thyroid disease: a survey of subjects potentially exposed to fallout radiation. *Am J Med* 1974;56:457.
290. Zeighami EA, Morris MD. Thyroid cancer risk in the population around the Nevada test site. *Health Phys* 1986;50:19.
291. Holm L-E, Wiklund KE, Lundell GE, et al. Cancer risk in a population examined with diagnostic doses of I131. *J Natl Cancer Inst* 1989;81:302.
292. Archer VE. Risk of thyroid cancer after doses of radioiodine. *J Natl Cancer Inst* 1989;81:713.
293. Brincker H, Hansen HS, Andersen AP. Induction of leukaemia by I^{131} treatment of thyroid cancer. *Br J Cancer* 1972;28:232.
294. Strong E. Discussion. *Ann Surg* 1976;184:553.
295. Wyse EP, Hill CS, Ibanez ML, et al. Other malignant neoplasms associated with carcinoma of the thyroid: thyroid carcinoma multiplex. *Cancer* 1969;24:701.
296. Johns ME, Shikhani AH, Kashima HK, et al. Multiple primary neoplasms in patients with salivary gland or thyroid gland tumors. *Laryngoscope* 1986;96:718.
297. McTiernan JM, Weiss S, Daling JR. Incidence of thyroid cancer in women in relation to known or suspected risk factors for breast cancer. *Cancer Res* 1987;47:292.
298. Eskin BA. Iodine and mammary cancer. *Adv Exp Med Biol* 1978;91:293.
299. Gardner EJ, Richards RC. Multiple cutaneous and subcutaneous lesions occurring simultaneously with hereditary polyposis and osteomas. *Am J Hum Genet* 1953;5:139.
300. Plail RL, Bussey HJR, Glazer G, et al. Adenomatous polyposis in association with carcinoma of the thyroid. *Br J Surg* 1987;74:77.
301. Chandler JJ, Schwartz MJ, Stahl TJ, et al. Papillary thyroid cancer in identical twins. *J Surg Oncol* 1988;37:175.
302. Galerah-Gonzales S, Campora R, Matilla A, et al. MEN type II B in twins. *Histopathology* 1982;6:111.
303. Panza N, Delvecchio L, Maio M, et al. Strong association between an HLA-DR antigen and thyroid carcinoma. *Tissue Antigens* 1982;20:155.
304. Larsen B, Thompson C, Quan A, et al. Lack of association of HLA with thyroid cancer and effect of iodine sufficiency—a safe environment? *Tissue Antigens* 1986;28:298.
305. Ozaki O, Ito K, Kobayashi K, et al. Familial occurrence of differentiated non-medullary thyroid carcinoma. *World J Surg* 1988;12:565.
306. Bernal JE. Invited commentary. *World J Surg* 1988;12:571.
307. Juhasz F, Buros P, Fzegedi G, et al. Immunogenetic and immunologic studies of differentiated thyroid carcinoma. *Cancer* 1989;63:1318.
308. Fontanas F, Delvecchio L, Racioppi L, et al. Expressions of major histocompatibility complex class I antigens in normal and transformed rat thyroid epithelial cell lines. *Cancer Res* 1987;47:4178.
309. Natali PG, Bigotti A, Nicotra MR, et al. Distribution of human class I (HLA-A,B,C) histocompatibility antigens in normal and malignant tissues of nonlymphoid origin. *Cancer Res* 1984;44:4679.
310. Milne D. Genetic tests predict thyroid cancer risk, making preventive surgery possible (news). *J Natl Cancer Inst* 1994;86:1268.
311. Bister K, Jansen HW. Oncogenes in retroviruses and cells: biochemistry and molecular genetics. *Adv Cancer Res* 1986;47:99.
312. Alitalo K, Schwab M. Oncogene amplification in tumor cells. *Adv Cancer Res* 1986;47:235.
313. Buckley I. Oncogenes and the nature of malignancy. *Adv Cancer Res* 1988;50:71.
314. Weinberg RA. The action of oncogenes in the cytoplasm and nucleus. *Science* 1985;230:770.
315. Nelkin BD, De Bustros AC, Mabry M, et al. The molecular biology of medullary thyroid carcinoma: a model for cancer development and progression. *JAMA* 1989;261:3130.
316. Miller RC, Kopecky KJ, Hiralka T. Comparison of the radiosensitivities of human autologous normal and neoplastic thyroid epithelial cells. *Br J Radiol* 1986;59:127.
317. Nakamura A, Kakudo K, Watanabi K. Establishment of a new human thyroid medullary carcinoma cell line. *Virchows Arch [B]* 1987;53:332.
318. Fusco A, Grieco M, Santoro M, et al. A new oncogene in human thyroid papillary carcinomas and in their metastases. *Nature* 1987;328:170.
319. Grieco M, Santoro M, Bertingieri MT, et al. Molecular cloning of differentiated thyroid carcinoma: a new oncogene found activated in thyroid human papillary carcinomas and their lymph node metastases. *Ann NY Acad Sci* 1988;551:380.
320. Mizukami Y, Nonamura A, Hashimoto T, et al. Immunohistochemical demonstration of ras p21 oncogene product in normal, benign and malignant human thyroid tissues. *Cancer* 1988;61:873.
321. Stringer BM, Rowson JM, Parker MH, et al. Detection of the H-ras oncogene in human thyroid anaplastic carcinoma. *Experientia* 1988;45:372.
322. Lemoine NR, Mayall ES, Wyllie FS, et al. Activated *ras* oncogenes in human thyroid cancers. *Cancer Res* 1988;48:4459.
323. Burman KD, Djuh Y-Y, LaRocca RV. C-Myc expression in the thyroid. I: Normal, adenomatous and cancerous thyroid tissue. *Horm Metab Res* 1987;17:63.
324. Nunes ME, Djuh Y-Y, LaRocca RV. C-Myc expression in the thyroid. II: Thyrocytes and peripheral and intrathyroidal lymphocytes from patients with autoimmune thyroid disease. *Horm Metab Res* 1987;17.
325. Aasland R, Lillehaug JR, Male R. Expressions of oncogenes in thyroid tumours: coexpression of C-Erb B2/Neu and C-Erb B. *Br J Cancer* 1988;37:358.
326. Waters MJ, Tweedale RC, Whys TA, et al. Differentiation of cultured thyroid cells by epidermal growth factor: some insight into the mechanism. *Mol Cell Endocrinol* 1987;49:109.
327. Conlon JM, McGregor GP, Wallin G. Molecular forms of katacalcin, calcitonin gene-related peptide and gastrin-releasing peptide in a human medullary thyroid carcinoma. *Cancer Res* 1988;48:2412.
328. Nakagawa T, Malbry M, De Bustros A, et al. Introduction of V-Ha-*ras* oncogene induces differentiation of cultured human medullary thyroid carcinoma cells. *Proc Natl Acad Sci USA* 1989;84:5923.
329. Boultwood J, Wyllie FS, Williams ED, et al. N-Myc expressions in neoplasias of human thyroid C-cells. *Cancer Res* 1988;48:4073.
330. Weinberger C, Thompson CC, Ong EG. The C-ErbA gene encodes a thyroid hormone receptor. *Nature* 1986;324:641.
331. Fagin JA. Molecular genetics of human thyroid neoplasms. *Annu Rev Med* 1994;45:45.
332. Farid NR, et al. Molecular basis of thyroid cancer. *Endocr Rev* 1994;15:202.
333. Bon JA, et al. In vitro reconstruction of tumour initiation in a human epithelium. *Oncogene* 1994;9:281.
334. Masood S, et al. Differential oncogenic expression in thyroid follicular and Hurthle cell carcinomas. *Am J Surg* 1993;166:366.
335. Yoshida A, et al. Alteration of tumorigenicity in undifferentiated thyroid carcinoma cells by introduction of normal chromosome 11. *J Surg Oncol* 1994;55:170.
336. Van Heyningen Z. Genetics. One gene-four syndromes [news; comment]. *Nature* 1994;367:319,375–380.

337. Farley DR, et al. Expression of a potential metastasis suppressor gene (nm23) in thyroid neoplasms. *World J Surg* 1993;17:615–620.
338. Yoshida A, et al. Production of cytokines by thyroid carcinoma cell lines. *J Surg Oncol* 1994;55:104.
339. Baxter JD. Advances in molecular biology. Potential impact on diagnosis and treatment of disorders of the thyroid. *Med Clin North Am* 1991;75:41.
340. Auguste L-J, Masood S, Westerband A, et al. Oncogene expression in follicular neoplasms of the thyroid. *Am J Surg* 1992;164:592.
341. Said S, et al. Oncogenes and anti-oncogenes in human epithelial thyroid tumors. *J Endocrinol Invest* 1994;17:371.
342. Seifert G, ed. Morphological tumor markers: general aspects and diagnostics relevance. *Curr Top Pathol* 1987;77:279.
343. Heitz PU. Neuroendocrine tumor markers. In: Seifert G, ed. Morphological tumor markers: general aspects and diagnostics relevance. *Curr Top Pathol* 1987;77:279.
344. Stanta G, Carcangiu ML, Rosai J. The biochemical and immunohistochemical profile of thyroid neoplasia. *Pathol Annu* 1988;23(1):129.
345. Davila RM, Bedrossian CWM, Silverberg AB. Immunocytochemistry of thyroid surgical and cytologic specimens. *Arch Pathol Lab Med* 1988;12:51.
346. Pizzolo A, Sloane G, Beverly P, et al. Differential diagnosis of malignant lymphoma and nonlymphoid tumors using monoclonal antileukocyte antibody. *Cancer* 1980;46:2640.
347. Takami H, Bessho T, Kameya T. Immunohistochemical study of medullary thyroid carcinoma: relationship of clinical features to prognostic factors in 36 patients. *World J Surg* 1988;12:572.
348. Vierbuchen M, Schroder S, Uhlenbruck G, et al. CA-50 and CA 19-9 antigen expression in normal hyperplastic and neoplastic thyroid tissue. *Lab Invest* 1989;60:726.
349. Schneider AB, Shore-Freeman E, Ryo UY. Prospective serum thyroglobulin measurements in assessing the risks of developing thyroid nodules in patients exposed to childhood neck irradiation. *J Clin Endocrinol Metab* 1985;61:547.
350. Panza N, Lombardi G, De Rosa M, et al. High serum thyroglobulin levels: diagnostic indicators in patients with metastases from unknown primary sites. *Cancer* 1987;60:2233.
351. Schlumberger M, Travagli P, Fragu P, et al. Follow-up of patients with differentiated thyroid carcinoma: experience at Institut Gustave-Roussy, Villejuif. *Eur J Cancer Clin Oncol* 1988;24:345.
352. Bottger IG. Minimal thyroid cancer: clinical consequences. *Recent Results Cancer Res* 1988;106:139.
353. Szanto J, Vincze B, Simkovics I, et al. Postoperative thyroglobulin level determination to follow-up patients with highly differentiated thyroid cancer. *Oncology* 1989;46:99.
354. Miller JH, Marcus CS. Metastatic thyroid carcinoma with normal serum thyroglobulin level. *Clin Nucl Med* 1988;13:652.
355. Thoresen SO, Myking O, Gattre E, et al. Serum thyroglobulin as a preclinical tumor marker in subgroups of thyroid cancer. *Br J Cancer* 1988;57:105.
356. Ozata M, et al. Serum thyroglobulin in the follow-up of patients with treated differentiated thyroid cancer. *J Clin Endocrinol Metab* 1994;79:98.
357. Pacini F, et al. Serum thyroglobulin in thyroid carcinoma and other thyroid disorders. *J Endocrinol Invest* 1980;3:283.
358. Ozata M, et al. Serum thyroglobulin in the follow-up of patients with treated differentiated thyroid cancer. *J Clin Endocrinol Metab* 1994;79:98.
359. Barlogie B, Raber M, Schuman J, et al. Flow cytometry and clinical cancer research. *Cancer Res* 1983;43:3982.
360. Joensuu H, Klemi P. Comparison of nuclear DNA content in primary and metastatic thyroid carcinoma. *Am J Clin Pathol* 1988;89:35.
361. Lee T-K, Myers RT, Bond NG, et al. The significance of nuclear diameter in the biological behavior of thyroid carcinomas: a retrospective study of 127 cases. *Hum Pathol* 1987;18:1252.
362. Bengtsson A, Malmaus J, Grimelius L, et al. Measurement of nuclear DNA content and thyroid diagnosis. *World J Surg* 1984;8:481.
363. Arps H, Sablotny B, Dietel M, et al. DNA cytophotometry in malignant tumors—use of different evaluation schemes for prognostic statements. *Virchows Arch [A]* 1989;413:319.
364. Backdahl M, Carstensen J, Auer G, et al. The prognostic value of nuclear DNA content in papillary, follicular and medullary. *World J Surg* 1986;10:974.
365. Backdahl M, Cohn K, Auer G, et al. Comparison of nuclear DNA content in primary & metastic papillary thyroid cancer. *Cancer Res* 1985;45:2890.
366. Wallin G, Backdahl M, Tallroth-Ekman E, Lundell G, Auer G, Lowhagen T. Co-existent anaplastic and well differentiated thyroid carcinoma: A nuclear DNA study. *Eur J Surg Oncol* 1989;15(1):43–48
367. Komorowski RA, Deaconson TF, Vetsch R. DNA content in radiation-associated thyroid carcinoma. *Surgery* 1988;104:992.
368. Liautaud-Roger F, Dufer J, Pluot M. Contributions of quantitative cytology to the cytological diagnosis of thyroid neoplasms. *Adv Cancer Res* 1989;9:231.
369. Kraemer J, Srigley R, Batsakis JG. DNA flow cytometry of the neoplasms. *Arch Otolaryngol* 1985;111:34.
370. Clark OH, Gerend PL, Nissenson RA. Mechanisms for increased adenyl cyclase responsiveness to TSH in neoplastic human thyroid tissue. *World J Surg* 1984;8:466.
371. Clark OH, Gum ET, Siperstein EC, et al. Guanylnucleotide regulatory proteins in neoplastic and normal human thyroid tissue. *World J Surg* 1988;12:538.
372. Harness JK. Invited commentary. *World J Surg* 1988;12:544.
373. Shi Y, et al. Expression of thyrotropin receptor gene in thyroid carcinoma is associated with a good prognosis. *Clin Endocrinol (Oxf)* 1993;39:269. Comment in: *Clin Endocrinol (Oxf)* 1993;39:267.
374. Maini CL, et al. Delayed thyroid-stimulating hormone suppression by L-thyroxine in the management of differentiated thyroid carcinoma [letter]. *Eur J Cancer* 1993;29A:2071.
375. Florkowski CM, et al. Bone mineral density in patients receiving suppressive doses of thyroxine for thyroid carcinoma. *NZ Med J* 1993;106:443.
376. Faber J, et al. Changes in bone mass during prolonged subclinical hyperthyroidism due to L-thyroxine treatment: a meta-analysis. *Eur J Endocrinol* 1994;130:350.
377. Sheppard MC. Thyrotrophin receptor expression: does it help in assessing the prognosis of thyroid cancer? *Clin Endocrinol (Oxf)* 1993;39:267–269.
378. Samuel AM, et al. Thyroid hormones in differentiated thyroid cancer. *Clin Nucl Med* 1994;19:49.
379. Virgolini I, Hermann M, Sinzinger H. Decrease of prostaglandin I_2 binding sites in thyroid cancer. *Br J Cancer* 1988;58:584.
380. Editorial. Growth factors in malignance. *Lancet* 1986;2:317.
381. Carpenter G, Cohen S. Epidermal growth factor. *Annu Rev Biochem* 1979;48:193.
382. Errick JE, Eggo MC, Burrow GN. Epidermal growth factor inhibits thyrotropin-mediated synthesis of tissue-specific proteins in cultured ovine thyroid cells. *Mol Cell Endocrinol* 1985;43:51.
383. Makinen T, Pekonen F, Franssila K, et al. Receptors for epidermal growth factor and thyrotropin in thyroid carcinoma. *Acta Endocrinol (Copenh)* 1988;117:45.
384. Duh Q-Y, Gum ET, Gerend PL, et al. Epidermal growth factor receptors in normal and neoplastic thyroid tissue. *Surgery* 1985;98:1000.
385. Westermark K, Karlsson FA, Westermark B. Thyrotropin-EGF receptor function in porcine thyroid follicle cells. *Molec Cell Biol Endocrinol* 1985;40:17.
386. Miyamoto M, Sugawa H, Mori T, et al. Epidermal growth factor receptors on cultured neoplastic human thyroid cells and effects of epidermal growth factor and thyroid-stimulating hormone on their growth. *Cancer Res* 1988;48:3652.
387. Masuda H, Sugenoia A, Kobayashi F, et al. Epidermal growth factor receptor in human thyroid neoplasms. *World J Surg* 1988;12:616.
388. Hoelting GT, et al. Epidermal growth factor enhances proliferation, migration, and invasion of follicular and papillary thyroid cancer in vitro and in vivo. *J Clin Endocrinol Metab* 1994;79:401.
389. Holting T, et al. Transforming growth factor-beta 1 is a negative regulator for differentiated thyroid cancer: studies of growth migration, invasion, and adhesion of cultured follicular and papillary thyroid cancer cell lines *J Clin Endocrinol Metab* 1994;79:806.
390. Bigazzi M, Revoltella R, Casciano S. High level of nerve growth factor in the serum of a patient with medullary carcinoma of the thyroid gland. In: Robbins J, Braverman L (eds.) *Thyroid research—proceedings of the Seventh International Thyroid Conference.* New York: Elsevier, 1976;558.
391. Cramer SF, Bradshaw RA, Baglan NC, et al. Nerve growth factor in medullary carcinoma of the thyroid. *Hum Pathol* 1979;6:731.
392. Goretzky PE, Wahl RA, Becker R, et al. Nerve growth factor sensi-

tizes human medullary thyroid carcinoma cells for cytostatic therapy in vitro. *Surgery* 1987;102:1035.
393. Siperstein AE, Miller RA, Clark OH. Stimulatory effect of vasoactive intestinal polypeptide on human normal and neoplastic thyroid tissue. *Surgery* 1988;104:985.
394. Heldin M-E, Gustavsson B, Claesson-Welsh L, et al. Aberrant expression of receptors for platelet-derived growth factor in an anaplastic thyroid carcinoma cell line. *Proc Natl Acad Sci USA* 1988;85:9302.
395. Pincus G, Dorfman RI, Romanoff LP, et al. Steroid metabolism in aging men and women. *Recent Results Horm Res* 1955;11:307.
396. Henderson BE, Ross RK, Pike MC, et al. Endogenous hormones as a major factor in human cancer. *Cancer Res* 1982;42:3232.
397. Rosen IB, Walfish TG. Pregnancy as a predisposing factor in thyroid neoplasia. *Arch Surg* 1986;121:1287.
398. Clark OH, Gerend PL, Davis M, et al. Estrogen and thyroid-stimulating hormone receptors in neoplastic and nonneoplastic human thyroid tissue. *J Surg Res* 1985;38:89.
399. Yang K-P, Pearson CE, Samaan NA. Estrogen receptor and hormone responsiveness of medullary thyroid carcinoma cells in continuous culture. *Cancer Res* 1988;48:2760.
400. Hofmann C, Oslapas R, Nayyar R, et al. Androgen-mediated development of radiation-induced thyroid tumors in rats: dependence on animal age during interval of androgen replacement in castrated males. *J Natl Cancer Inst* 1986;77:253.
401. Prinz RA, Sandberg L, Chaudhuri PK. Androgen receptors in human thyroid tissue. *Surgery* 1984;96:996.
402. Rawson RW, Leeper R. Factors influencing benignancy vs. malignancy of thyroid neoplasms. In: Young S, Inman DR, eds. *Thyroid neoplasia*. New York: Academic Press, 1968;159–177.
403. Bur M, et al. Estrogen and progesterone receptor detection in neoplastic and non-neoplastic thyroid tissue. *Mod Pathol* 1993;6:469.
404. Yane K, et al. Expression of the estrogen receptor in human thyroid neoplasms. *Cancer Lett* 1994;84:59.
405. Crile G Jr. Dependency of papillary carcinomas of the thyroid. *JAMA* 1966;195:721.
406. Thomas CG Jr. The dependency of thyroid cancer: a review. *Ann Surg* 1957;146:879.
407. Purves HD, Griesbach WE. Studies on experimental goiter VIII: thyroid tumors in rats, treated with thiourea. *Br J Exp Pathol* 1947;28:46.
408. McTiernan JM, Weiss NS, Daling JR. Incidence of thyroid cancer in women in relation to previous exposure to radiation and history of thyroid disease. *J Natl Cancer Inst* 1984;73:575.
409. Doniach I. Etiologic considerations of thyroid carcinomas. In: Smithers D, ed. *Tumours of the thyroid gland*. London: Livingstone, 1970;55.
410. Rushfield AB. Histology of the human hypophysis in thyroid disease, hypothyroidism, hyperthyroidism and cancer. *J Clin Endocrinol Metab* 1955;15:1393.
411. Komlos L, Shimberg R, Halbrecht I. Primary tissue culture of benign and malignant human thyroid tumors: effect of TSH. *Otolaryngol Head Neck Surg* 1988;99:1015.
412. Loeb L. Studies on compensatory hypertrophy of the thyroid gland. VII: Further investigation of the influence of iodine on hypertrophy of the gland with an interpretation of the differences of the effect of iodine on the thyroid gland under various pathological conditions. *Am J Pathol* 1926;2:19.
413. Oshima M, Ward JM. Dietary iodine deficiency as a tumor promoter and carcinogen in male rats. *Cancer Res* 1986;46:877.
414. Morris HP. The experimental development and metabolism of thyroid gland tumors. *Adv Cancer Res* 1955;3:51.
415. Al-Saadi AA, Beierwaltes WH. Sequential cytogenetic changes in the evolution of transplanted thyroid tumors to metastatic carcinoma in the fish or rat. *Cancer Res* 1967;27:1831.
416. Lindsay SL, Nichols CW, Chaikoff H. Induction of benign and malignant thyroid neoplasms in the rat. *Arch Pathol* 1966;81:308.
417. Taptiklis N. Dormancy of dissociated thyroid cells in the lungs of mice. *Eur J Cancer* 1968;4:59.
418. Hoang-Vu C, et al. Xenotransplanted thyroid tumors heterogeneously expressed differentiation markers in nude rats. *Transplant Proc* 1993;25:2799.
419. Giovanelli BC, Fogh J. The nude mouse in cancer research. *Adv Cancer Res* 1985;44:70.
420. Yoshida A, Fukazawa M, Ushio H. Study of cell kinetics in anaplastic thyroid carcinoma transplanted to nude mice. *J Surg Oncol* 1989;41:1.
421. Dralle K, Bocker W, Dohler KD, et al. Growth and function of 34 human benign and malignant thyroid xenografts in untreated nude mice. *Cancer Res* 1985;45:1239.
422. Terzioglu T, et al. Concurrent hyperthyroidism and thyroid carcinoma. *Br J Surg* 1993;80:1301.
423. Walker RP, Oslapas R, Ernst K, et al. Hyperparathyroidism induced by hypothyroidism. *Laryngoscope* 1993;103:263.
424. Fedorak IJ, et al. Increased incidence of thyroid cancer in patients with primary hyperparathyroidism: a continuing dilemma. *Am J Surg* 1994;60:427.
425. Smithers D, ed. *Tumours of the thyroid gland*. London: Livingstone, 1970.
426. Wheeler MH. Invited commentary. *World J Surg* 1988;12:53.
427. Fisher B. The contribution of recent NSABP clinical trials of primary breast cancer therapy to an understanding of tumor biology. An overview of findings. *Cancer* 1980;46:1009.
428. Farooki MA. Epidemiology and pathology of cancer of the thyroid. Part I: Material, methods and results. *Int Surg* 1969;51:232.
429. Farooki MA. Epidemiology and pathology of cancer of the thyroid. Part II: Discussion. *Int Surg* 1969;51:317.
430. Franssila KO, Haradi HR. Occult papillary carcinoma of the thyroid in children and young adults: a systematic autopsy study in Finland. *Cancer* 1986;58:715.
431. Fukunaga FH, Yatani R. Geographic pathology of occult thyroid carcinoma. *Cancer* 1975;36:1095.
432. Hanson GA, Komorowski RA, Cerletty JM, et al. Thyroid gland morphology in young adults: normal subjects versus those with prior low-dose neck irradiation in childhood. *Surg* 1983;94:984.
433. Sampson RJ, Woolner LB, Bahn RC, et al. Occult thyroid carcinoma in Olmsted County, Minnesota: prevalence at autopsy compared with that in Hiroshima and Nagasaki, Japan. *Cancer* 1974;34:2072.
434. Sobrinho-Simoes MA, Sambade MC, Goncalves V. Latent thyroid carcinoma at autopsy: a study from Oporto, Portugal. *Cancer* 1979;43:1702.

CHAPTER 29

Evaluation and Surgical Treatment of Papillary and Follicular Carcinoma

Elliot W. Strong

INCIDENCE AND EPIDEMIOLOGY

Nodular disease of the thyroid gland is a subject of concern to patients, and its management is complex and controversial for physicians. Whereas thyroid disease is common, thyroid cancer is relatively rare. In the United States, clinically apparent nodules are present in 4% to 7% of the adult population, and they are more common in women than in men. The prevalence of thyroid nodules increases linearly with age, with spontaneous nodules occurring at a rate of 0.08% per year beginning early in life and extending into the eighth decade (1). Exposure to ionizing radiation increases the incidence of both benign and malignant nodules (2,3). Palpable thyroid abnormalities occur in 20% to 30% of a radiation-exposed population. The true incidence of thyroid abnormalities is probably much higher.

In a report from the Mayo Clinic, Mortensen and associates (4) studied 821 thyroid glands at autopsy in patients having no clinical history or evidence of thyroid disease. Gross and microscopic examination of the glands revealed that 49.8% had nodules; 12.5% were uninodular and 37.3% were multinodular. Nodules varied in size from 2 mm to 7.5 cm in diameter. Nodularity increased in frequency with age in both sexes but was 10% to 20% more frequent in females. The most common nodule was nonneoplastic and involutional, with true adenomas seen in one quarter of all glands and one half the nodules detected. Thyroid cancer was detected in 4.2% of the nodular glands and varied from 0.2 to 1.5 cm in diameter.

Clinically-important thyroid cancers occur in about 40 per million patients, or 0.004 people per year (5). Fukunaga and Yatani (6), using multiple histologic sections (300 to 900 slides/gland), showed that the prevalence of occult thyroid cancer depended on the population being studied; they found prevalences of 6% in Canada, 9% in Poland, and 28.4% in Sendai, Japan. The prevalence of occult thyroid cancer increased with age (3) and with exposure to radiation (2,3,5,7,8). It is also apparent that the incidence of thyroid carcinoma found in patients with prior head and neck irradiation is directly related to the absolute number of pathologic slides examined by the pathologist (9,10). The more careful the search, the higher the incidence of thyroid pathology and of malignancy. The clinical significance of the finding of occult microscopic well-differentiated papillary thyroid cancer at autopsy is uncertain.

Harach et al. (11) carefully studied the thyroid gland harvested from 101 consecutive autopsies of patients dying with no history or findings consistent with thyroid cancer in a small community in Finland. Careful review of the glands subserially sectioned at 2 to 3 mm revealed an overall incidence of occult thyroid cancer of 34.5% (1). The rate was higher in men than in women, 43.3% versus 27.1%. Tumor diameter varied from 0.15 to 14 mm, with 67% of the tumors under 1 mm usually circumscribed and almost solely composed of follicles. The authors concluded that these micropapillary carcinomas can be regarded as a normal finding which should not be treated when incidentally found, and that small clinically occult papillary carcinomas under 5 mm in diameter should be described as occult papillary tumor rather than carcinoma. This is not to indicate that microscopic and occult tumors are entirely innocuous, because primary thyroid cancers under 1 cm in diameter have caused metastases and death (12–14).

E. W. Strong: Head and Neck Service, Memorial Sloan Kettering Cancer Center; and Cornell University Medical College, New York, New York 10021-6007.

Rosen et al. (14) recently described a series of 99 patients with tumors equal to or less than 1.5 cm in diameter, one third of whom had lymph node metastases, extrathyroidal invasion, or distant metastases. Six had residual cancer following surgery, 31 were alive without disease, 3 were living with disease, and 1 had died of thyroid cancer. They concluded that the need for treatment should not be based solely on the size of the primary tumor, but also on the clinical behavior and aggressiveness of the lesion. The second WHO histologic classification of thyroid tumors indicates that the term *papillary microcarcinoma* should replace the former term *occult papillary carcinoma*, and it should be defined as those papillary carcinomas 1 cm or less in diameter (10).

Most studies indicate that papillary thyroid carcinoma, if surrounded by adequate normal thyroid tissue without evidence of regional lymph node metastasis, is almost universally cured by conservative surgical excision (10,15). The Mayo Clinic series of papillary microcarcinoma (15) included 535 patients retrospectively analyzed. Ninety-nine percent were histologically grade 1, and 98% were not locally invasive. Thirty-two percent of patients had nodal metastases upon admission. Twenty-year tumor recurrence rate was 6%, with higher rates seen either with node-positive patients or after unilateral lobectomy. Recurrence rates did not appear to be significantly altered by total thyroidectomy or radioiodine remnant ablation in nodal positive patients. The authors concluded that "papillary microcarcinoma has an excellent prognosis if managed initially by bilateral lobar resection." Closer review of the data indicates that multiple foci were found in only 20% of patients, and the disease was bilateral in 10%. Thus, the recommendation for bilateral lobar resection is somewhat tenuous. Only 2 of the 535 patients died of thyroid carcinoma (15). The American Cancer Society estimates that a total of 15,600 new cases of thyroid cancer (4000 men versus 11,600 women) will occur in the United States in 1996, with 1210 deaths (440 men versus 770 women). This should be viewed in the overall context of 1,359,150 estimated new cancers and 554,740 deaths from tumors of all sites in the United States in 1996 (16).

The incidence of thyroid cancer is rising in many parts of the world (17,18). Carroll et al. (19), in a review of data from New York State exclusive of New York City, documented a greater-than-twofold increase in incidence in the time interval from 1941 to 1962. This incidence was largely in those patients under the age of 55, with the rate apparently doubling for each successive decade. It was postulated the most likely cause was the increased rate of exposure to ionizing radiation in the younger age population, occurring after 1900.

Pathologic examination of surgical specimens in patients with previous history of radiation exposure has documented a significantly increased incidence of thyroid abnormalities. In one series of 68 thyroid glands subjected to previous low-dose childhood irradiation, 88% showed moderate-to-severe focal hyperplasia, 51% contained single or multiple adenomas or adenomatous hyperplastic nodules, 68% exhibited chronic lymphocytic thyroiditis, 51% revealed colloid nodules, 41% presented with oxyphilic change, 25% had mild fibrosis, and 59% contained well-differentiated papillary, follicular, or mixed thyroid carcinoma averaging 1.6 cm in diameter. There were three small sclerosing carcinomas. The 34 control thyroids from age- and sex-matched autopsy cases without thyroid irradiation showed only 32% colloid nodule formation, 17% focal hyperplasia, 6% adenomatous hyperplasia, and no identifiable carcinomas (8). This study is representative of multiple other studies documenting the significant difference in the histopathologic findings in irradiated versus nonirradiated thyroid glands.

Komorowski and Hanson (20), in their study of 138 thyroid glands harvested from autopsies on patients 20 to 40 years of age without a clinical history of thyroid disease, documented other important morphologic changes. These included incomplete thyroid capsule in 62%, thyroid follicles within the capsule in 14%, follicles or nodules outside the gland in perithyroidal connective tissue in 88% of cases, and thyroid follicles in perithyroid strap muscles attached to the pyramidal lobe in 7%. Papillary microcarcinoma was found in 3% of the glands, along with a single medullary carcinoma. These morphologic changes are of great importance to surgical pathologists and indicate that unsuspected abnormal findings in otherwise normal thyroid glands must be carefully differentiated from those occurring in patients with neoplastic disease.

Geographic and racial patterns of thyroid cancer incidence vary widely. Hawaii has one of the highest incidences of thyroid cancer in the world. Within that island complex, there are dramatic variations with ethnicity. Thyroid cancer comprised 2.7% of all noncutaneous cancers in Hawaii from 1973 through 1977. This compares to the overall U.S. national estimate of only 1.2%. In Hawaii from 1960 through 1984, the overall age-adjusted incidence rates were 8.1 per 100,000 in women and 3.1 per 100,000 in men. The highest rates for women occurred in Philippinos (18.2 per 100,000), and for men and Chinese people at 6.3% per 100,000. In women during the study period, the incidence in Philippinos rose and in Chinese fell, and it remained stable in Hawaiian Caucasians and Japanese. In men, the rates rose in all ethnic groups except in Caucasians, in whom they fell. Comparison of incidence rates in similar ethnic groups living in other geographic areas showed that Hawaiian natives had much higher rates. Various etiologic factors were postulated, with environmental factors seeming to take precedence over the genetic (21).

The etiology of thyroid cancer is unknown. Implicated factors include previous radiation exposure, previous thyroid cancer, family history of thyroid cancer, certain genetic syndromes, including Gardner's syndrome (familial polyposis) and Cowden's disease (multiple hamartoma syndrome), iodine deficiency or endemic goiter (leading to increased incidence of follicular and anaplastic thyroid cancer), and previous history of breast cancer. Higher circulating levels of estrogen may minimally increase the risk of breast and thyroid cancer. Exposure to certain carcinogens, residence near volcanoes, and possibly alcohol ingestion may be also implicated. Functional thyroid disorders and smoking are not associated with thyroid carcinoma (22).

PATHOLOGY

Well-differentiated thyroid cancers comprise the overwhelming proportion of thyroid neoplasia. In a nationwide review of thyroid cancers by the American College of Surgeons during the year 1992, papillary carcinoma represented 54.8% of the total spectrum of 6423 patients. Follicular cancer represented 30.5%, medullary 2.9%, undifferentiated 0.7%, non-Hodgkin lymphomas 3.7%, and other histologies 7.5% (23). In a consecutive series of 931 previously untreated patients with differentiated thyroid cancer seen over a 50-year interval at Memorial Sloan-Kettering Cancer Center, 78.5% were papillary carcinomas, 15.5% follicular, and 6% Hürthle cell tumors (24). The differences may represent the impact of patterns of referral to a tertiary care institution. Those tumors demonstrating both follicular and papillary elements will behave as papillary tumors even though histologically follicular elements may predominate. It is important that the follicular variant of papillary carcinoma be carefully identified and segregated from follicular cancer, because its clinical behavior mirrors that of the well-differentiated papillary variety. Many of the thyroid cancers demonstrate more than one cytologic component, with the papillary element predominating.

Subvarieties of papillary carcinoma include the tall cell and columnar cell variants and diffuse sclerosing tumor. The tall cell variant comprises approximately 10% of the papillary carcinoma spectrum, tends to occur in elderly patients, is often large, and extends beyond the thyroid capsule with significant vascular invasion. The cells are twice as tall as they are wide, and the cytoplasm is often eosinophilic. The tumor frequently arises in glands showing significant chronic thyroiditis. The prognosis for this variant is worse than that of the usual papillary carcinoma, with a high propensity to local recurrence and invasion. No significant differences in DNA ploidy between tall cell and the usual papillary carcinomas have been identified (25).

The columnar variant of papillary carcinoma is rare, only four published cases having been reported. The histologic features include extreme papillarity, tall columnar cells, and nuclear stratification without clearing of the nucleus (25).

The diffuse sclerosis variant of papillary carcinoma often affects children as a more aggressive type of papillary cancer. The tumor freely permeates the gland, with tumor nests composed of papillae with associated solid areas, many psammoma bodies, and a prominent lymphocytic infiltrate. These tumors have a greater propensity to regional lymph node and pulmonary metastases, with resultant more ominous prognosis (25). The encapsulated variant of papillary carcinoma has the gross appearance of an adenoma, comprises 8% to 13% of papillary cancers, and exhibits total encapsulation but persistent cytologic features of papillary carcinoma. The overall prognosis with this group is better than that of papillary carcinoma, in general (25).

Other isolated unusual variants of papillary carcinoma have been reported, including solid variant, clear cell type, oxyphilic variant, papillary carcinoma with fatty stroma, papillary carcinoma with fasciitis-like stroma, and cribriform papillary carcinoma (25).

Spindle and giant cell metaplasia may be seen in selected papillary carcinomas, often in the older patient. These more anaplastic tumors tend to increase with increasing age and recurrence of the primary lesion, with significant worsening of the overall prognosis: a shortened disease-free interval, more frequent local recurrence, and fatal outcome (26). (See also Chapter 6 for further discussion of thyroid pathology.)

PATHOGENESIS

The thyroid gland is a single parenchymatous organ enclosed in a capsule, with rich intralobular network of lymphatics. Using *in vivo* injection of the lymphatics of the thyroid gland in dog and man, Reinhoff (27) demonstrated an anastomosing endothelial reticulum or plexus of lymphatics lying in the interfollicular spaces of the gland external to the vascular network surrounding each follicle and interconnecting with the intraglandular plexus composed of large lymphatic trunks situated on the surface of the lobule. These, in turn, connected with the extraglandular plexus on the outer surface of the gland beneath the fibrous capsule. From this external lymphatic plexus, larger lymphatic trunks emanated, accompanying the superior thyroid vessels to the internal jugular lymph nodes and inferiorly into trunks, forming a reticulum in the pretracheal fascia that drains into the mediastinum. There was no direct connection between the thyroid follicles and the bursella of the lymphatic collecting system. On the surface of the gland, the connecting network of lymphatics communicated with the capsular lymph nodes. Russell et al. (28) concluded that thyroid cancer originated at one site within the gland and metastasized from that primary site to all parts of the gland via this intraglandular lymphatic network. The lymph vessels on the capsule collected and carried the malignant cells to the pericapsular lymph nodes, and from there to more distant regional nodes.

Papillary carcinoma is not a lesion in which multiple clones of cells undergo malignant transformation at the same time, so it is not a multicentric tumor (25). The multifocality seen clinically must be a result of intrathyroidal lymphatic spread. Early reports describing random pathological sections through the thyroid gland indicated that the tumor occurred in multiple foci in about one third of the patients studied (29,30). However, it was left to Russell and his colleagues (28) to document (in an elegant study of 80 total thyroid specimens analyzed by whole-organ pathologic section) that 87.5% of specimens contained multiple histologic foci of tumor beyond the presumed primary site of origin within the gland. Subsequently, reports from the same institution indicated an incidence of 56.4% of so-called multifocal cancer within the thyroid in 218 patients, regardless of the method of study.

The significance of this multifocal intraglandular distribution of well-differentiated papillary cancer is uncertain. If most patients were to have cancer disseminated throughout the gland, it is logical to assume that, with continued progression, after less than total thyroidectomy, most, if not all, would eventually develop local recurrence within the remaining thyroid parenchyma. Such is not the case. In a series of 216 patients treated primarily by less-than-total thyroidectomy at Memorial Sloan-Kettering Cancer Center, followed for a minimum of 5 and an average of 14 years, only 4.6% developed clinical evidence of recurrence in the thyroid remnant. During the same time interval, those patients subjected to total thyroidectomy for clinical unilateral thyroid cancer had a 38% incidence of microscopic cancer in the contralateral lobe studied by routine, not subserial, pathologic examination (31). Other authors have reported recurrence rates in the remaining thyroid tissue after subtotal thyroidectomy for papillary carcinoma from 6.8% (32) to 18% (33) to 33% (34). Most authors have found that such microscopic multifocal cancer, if occult, carries no adverse prognostic impact on survival (24,33,35,36), but total thyroidectomy may lessen the incidence of local recurrence (5,22,36–40).

Total thyroidectomy will facilitate the subsequent use of radioiodine to detect and treat residual normal thyroid gland or local/distant metastases, facilitate the use of serum thyroglobulin as a sensitive tumor marker of recurrence, eliminate the risk of recurrence of subclinical metastatic disease in the contralateral lobe, lessen the incidence of local recurrence, and eliminate the risk (under 1%) of well-differentiated thyroid cancer changing to an undifferentiated tumor (22). Those advocates of less-than-total thyroidectomy indicate that fewer complications accompany the unilateral/subtotal thyroidectomy, less than 5% of recurrences occur within the residual thyroid gland, one half of local recurrences can be cured with further surgery, there is little clinical significance to the concept of multicentricity, and the prognosis is good in low-risk patients with lesser procedures (22).

In a recent report from the Mayo Clinic, Grant et al. (40) documented that survival was not influenced by the extent of thyroid resection, but that local recurrence in the thyroid remnant was lessened by bilateral subtotal/near-total thyroidectomy over unilateral resection. There was no significant difference in local recurrence in those patients undergoing near-total thyroidectomy versus those with total thyroidectomy. The risk of death from papillary thyroid cancer was significantly greater with recurrence outside the thyroid remnant than with a local "stump" remnant recurrence alone. Unilateral resection of papillary carcinoma in this series led to a small but increased risk of locally recurrent disease, all of which was cured by subsequent treatment. None of the 52 patients with recurrence confined to the thyroid remnant died of thyroid cancer, with follow-up as long as 41 years. The risk of anaplastic transformation of residual foci of well-differentiated thyroid cancer is so rare as to be insignificant (26,41). Secondary total thyroidectomy for recurrence is accompanied by a higher risk of complications than primary total thyroidectomy (42–44).

Similarly, Samaan et al. (38) documented that those patients with intrathyroidal papillary carcinoma who underwent total thyroidectomy had significantly fewer local recurrences than those patients treated with unilateral surgery. This difference was negated by the use of postoperative radioiodine. However, in the group that did not receive radioiodine, patients undergoing total thyroidectomy had a statistically significant advantage over those undergoing subtotal thyroidectomy. Among those patients with intrathyroidal follicular carcinoma, those subjected to total thyroidectomy showed fewer recurrences than those treated by unilateral surgery. Although there is no evidence that routine total thyroidectomy for all patients with well-differentiated thyroid cancer will increase survival (22,24,33,35,36,40,45), there is a selected group of patients with larger lesions and unfavorable prognostic factors who will benefit from total thyroidectomy (37–39,43).

In the absence of evidence to conclusively document the benefits of total thyroidectomy, one needs to assess its risks. The complications of total thyroidectomy include injury to recurrent laryngeal nerve and parathyroid glands. The rate of complications following total thyroidectomy clearly exceeds those following less-than-total resection of the gland (33,46–49). Postsurgical complications are increased when more extensive cancer requires more extensive resections, with reoperative surgery, and with less experienced surgeons (45,50). In one series, the total incidence of complications for partial thyroidectomy was 1.9%, compared to 23.5% for total thyroidectomy (48). The authors concluded there was no evidence to indicate benefit from routine more radical resection for nonmedullary well-differentiated thyroid cancer. In another series of patients studied after thyroidectomy, 83% were biochemically hypocalcemic. Although most required no treatment, 13% were symptomatic and 4% were permanently hypoparathyroid. Of those undergoing total thyroidectomy, 23% were symptomatically hypocalcemic and 12% suffered permanent hypoparathyroidism. When thyroidectomy was combined with modified neck dissection in this series, 50% were symptomatic and 17% were permanently hypoparathyroid (47).

Although more experienced surgeons may be more technically proficient and have fewer postoperative complications, this expertise is acquired only with long years of training, experience, and dedication to excellence and technical perfection (43,44,49,50). The experience reported by Mazzaferri et al. (33) is probably more representative of actual practice. In this series of 576 patients with papillary carcinoma treated by multiple surgeons with varied training and experience, the incidence of permanent unilateral vocal cord paralysis following total thyroidectomy was 1.6%, and of permanent hypoparathyroidism, 13.5%. Whereas near-total thyroidectomy may be a viable compromise, can we assume that any residual microscopic foci of cancer potentially remaining in the thyroid remnant will be less significant than those for which the near-total thyroidectomy was initially done? Foster (46) reviewed records of 24,108 thyroid operations done in 1970 and reported an overall mortality of 0.3%, with morbidity for surgery of thyroid cancer of 1.2%. No mortality occurred under the age of 40. The incidence of postoperative hypoparathyroidism in those undergoing total thyroidectomy for cancer was 8%; in those undergoing subtotal thyroidectomy, it was 1.3%, and 2.5% required tracheostomy and 0.9% suffered postoperative vocal cord paralysis.

How total is total thyroidectomy? Few authors have documented the completeness of their radical extirpations by postoperative documentation of absent radioisotope uptake in the thyroid bed. A notable exception is the report by Attie et al. (51), in which 140 thyroidectomy patients were studied. Seventy-five percent had less than 1.5% radioisotopic uptake in the thyroid bed, 17.8% had uptake ranging from 0.6% to 2.5%, and 7.1% had uptake greater than 2.5% of the administered dose in the neck. In Attie's 150 subsequent total thyroidectomies, there was only one instance of permanent hypoparathyroidism. Radioiodine uptake was further diminished as he gained more personal experience with the surgery, with no increase in complications.

Thus, it would appear that total thyroidectomy should be selectively rather than routinely applied in the management of well-differentiated thyroid cancer. There is no evidence to suggest that the more radical procedure adds anything to the conservative management of papillary microcarcinoma. In those patients in whom clinical and histologic evidence of disease is well confined to the thyroid capsule without evidence of extracapsular spread by either local extension or regional nodal metastases, total resection of the primary tumor with adequate margins is sufficient. Of those large tumors with extracapsular spread, as radical a surgical procedure as can be safely accomplished on the involved side is indicated. Completion of total thyroidectomy will facilitate additional adjunctive treatment, usually radioiodine, for the management of any residual/metastatic tumor. Microscopic thyroid remnants will take up the radioisotope more effectively than residual gross cancer. The higher the percentage uptake in the residual tumor, the more difficult it is to successfully ablate the tumor with radioiodine. Surgeons must aid the remnant ablation and subsequent intensive search for metastases with radioactive iodine with the best possible total thyroidectomy if effective radioisotopic treatment is to be given (22,38,53).

Thus, it seems apparent that in those patients requiring total thyroidectomy, the resection should be as anatomically complete, removing all thyroid tissue, both benign and neoplastic, as is possible without adding unduly to complications or sacrificing uninvolved structures. If the recurrent laryngeal nerve can be unequivocally identified and preserved, and the parathyroid glands lie at some distance from the thyroid capsule and their blood supply can be unequivocally preserved, then total thyroidectomy is a safe operation in competent, experienced hands. Near-total thyroidectomy may be a reasonable compromise in those patients in whom these criteria do not exist, in order to minimize complications and lessen local recurrence, especially in those patients at high risk of such recurrence (22,40,43).

CLINICAL PRESENTATION

Most patients with thyroid cancer present with a solitary, nontender, asymptomatic mass within the thyroid gland. With increasing sophistication of the public, the extent of thyroid cancer present at initial presentation is significantly less than previously reported (53,54). Occasionally, attention may be called to the mass by pain resulting from hemorrhage within it. In our experience, 20% of patients with subsequently proven papillary thyroid cancer presented with enlargement with one or more cervical lymph nodes and a clinically occult primary tumor. In most patients, such tumors could be detected on careful palpation of the ipsilateral thyroid lobe by an experienced examiner, with a high index of suspicion (31). Occasionally, patients present with no clinical abnormalities in the thyroid gland, but with bone or lung metastases that on biopsy show an atypical papillary follicular pattern, staining positively for thyroglobulin, confirming the thyroid origin of the neoplasm. It is uncommon for vocal cord dysfunction or tracheal or esophageal obstruction to be the initial symptom without clinical evidence of a primary cancer in the gland.

The primary tumor may vary greatly in size, from the clinically occult lesion to the huge obvious neck mass displacing the trachea and esophagus, usually of long-standing duration. Most patients present with tumors of intermediate size (1 to 4 cm) without evidence of extrathyroidal extension, regional nodal or distant metastases (30,33,35,54). Vocal cord dysfunction was seen in only 8% of 393 patients reported by Frazell and Foote in 1958 (30) and in only 5% in the series of McConahey et al. from the Mayo Clinic (54). Most patients have a solitary or dominant nodule, whereas a minority of 21% of the Mayo series had two or more nodules in the gland.

In the same series, 76% had no clinical evidence of regional lymph node metastases, 10% had one clinically positive node, and 14% had two or more clinically involved lymph nodes. This is in contrast to the pathologic assessment of regional lymph nodes with papillary cancer, in which the frequency of histologically positive nodes varies from 30% to 70% (55). In the series reported by Shah et al. (24), regional lymph node metastases were clinically suspected in 389 patients. Pathologic examination of the surgical specimens confirmed the presence of nodal metastatic deposits in 370. Out of 542 patients without evidence of lymph node metastases, 164 underwent elective neck dissection or biopsy; of these, 78 (or 48%) were found to have nodal metastases. Forty-eight percent of the entire study population were classified as N+, and 56% of patients with papillary carcinomas were classified as N+. In contrast, only 20% of the patients with follicular cancers had clinically apparent neck node metastases. Clinical lymph node metastases in papillary carcinoma are clinically evident or pathologically confirmed in up to 80% of patients, yet their impact on prognosis is controversial (56). Almost 80% of patients under 20 years of age have palpable nodal metastases at presentation, whereas in older patients, only 20% have clinically involved lymph nodes. The potential adverse effect of regional nodal metastases in the young may be mitigated by the improved prognosis relating to age (57). Lymph node metastases increase the incidence of regional recurrence (metastasis) in the neck but do not adversely impact survival in most series (56). Mazzaferri (37) indicated that patients with cervical lymph node metastases had a higher 30-year recurrence rate than those without such metastases (32% versus 28%, $p < .01$). In patients with follicular cancer, cancer mortality rates were higher with nodal metastases than without. Thirty-year cancer mortality rates were higher for patients with mediastinal and bilateral cervical lymph node metastases, regardless of tumor histology.

Follicular cancers demonstrate a different natural history and prognosis from that of papillary cancers. Young et al. (58) reported on 214 patients with pure follicular cancers: 85% presented with a single thyroid nodule, 70% of which were under 3 cm in diameter. Only 9% had clinically positive nodes on admission; 19% had histologically confirmed lymph node metastases and only 9.8% demonstrated distant metastases. In a report on follicular cancers by Tollefsen et al. (59), 30.4% had overall incidence of nodal metastases, most of which were apparent at the time of initial presentation. In neither of these two reports did recurrence of follicular thyroid cancer develop in the treated regional lymph node bed, nor did any patient die of uncontrolled cervical metastases in the absence of local recurrence at the primary site.

The marked difference between papillary and follicular cancers was further documented in the report by Fransilla (60), who showed that the incidence of positive lymph nodes in papillary carcinoma was 42%, versus 2% in follicular carcinoma, and the incidence of distant metastases was 14% in papillary versus 72% in follicular carcinoma. Relative 5-year survival rates for papillary carcinoma was 85% versus only 54% for follicular carcinoma. The prognostic significance of cervical nodal metastases in well-differentiated thyroid cancer is negligible in almost all reported series (24,38,53,54,56,58,59,62–64). Simpson et al. (35), on multivariate analysis of cause-specific survival rates, documented that nodal involvement was significant for follicular cancers. Harwood et al. (57) reported that when patients with and without lymph node metastases were matched by age and gender, lymph node metastases had an adverse effect on recurrence and survival. Tennvall et al. (61) reported that patients with matted lymph nodes had an appreciably worse prognosis. On the contrary, Cady et al. (53) suggested an improved prognosis in patients with 10 or more involved lymph nodes, but their data were skewed because the youngest patients (those having the best prognosis) tended to have the highest incidence of nodal metastases.

In a study from Japan, Noguchi and Murakami (65) reported their experience with papillary thyroid cancer over a 34-year interval. Of those patients undergoing modified radical neck dissection, 88.2% were found to have pathologically involved regional lymph nodes. The status of these nodes was accurately assessed intraoperatively in only 48% of patients, with 23% false negatives. Small tumors were accompanied by metastases in the tracheo-esophageal groove/paratracheal area, with larger tumors having positive nodes in both paratracheal and jugular regions. The more extensive the metastases in the paratracheal area, the greater the likelihood of internal jugular node metastases. Younger patients tended to have more metastatic cervical nodes than older patients. In the same series, in 306 women undergoing surgery from 1966 to 1983 with primary tumors less than 1 cm in diameter and no neck dissection, none had recurrence. Of 582 women with tumors of all sizes without neck dissection, only seven died of cancer, and eight had cervical metastases successfully treated by therapeutic cervical lymph adenectomy. In the authors' experience, 69% of their patients with thyroid cancers over 10 mm in diameter had histologic evidence of thyroid cancer in cervical lymph nodes. Their overall experience clearly documented that patients with numerous lymph node metastases had a worse prognosis than those with only a few involved lymph nodes. Clinical assessment of the regional nodes, even in the operating room, was frequently in error.

In 1955, Frazell and Foote (66) reviewed 182 radical neck dissection specimens for papillary thyroid cancer and documented that 84.6% contained pathologically positive lymph nodes. If the neck was clinically positive, 96% had pathologic confirmation of nodal involvement. If the neck appeared uninvolved clinically, 61.2% had histologically confirmed nodal metastases. In those patients with positive nodes, multiple levels of involvement were more common, with 75% in the jugular chain, 36% in the spinal accessory chain, 32% in the juxtathyroid nodes, and 6% in the mediastinal nodes. If the neck was clinically negative, 30% had jugular nodal metastases but only 6% had involved nodes in the posterior triangle, 13% in the juxtathyroid area, and none in the superior mediastinum. The incidence of positive nodes in the submandibular triangle was only 1.8%. Patients with clinically negative necks were 4 times more likely to have their occult metastatic disease confined to a single level in the neck than were those having clinically positive lymph nodes. This study documents the poor accuracy of clinical assessment of regional lymph nodes in patients with well-differentiated thyroid cancer. The presumed reasons for this inaccuracy relate to the relatively small size of the cervical nodal involvement and their soft consistency; these factors lead to errors in clinical assessment. The study also confirms the validity of modified neck dissection in the treatment of cervical lymph node metastases based on the location of involved nodes in the neck.

DIAGNOSIS

The diagnosis of well-differentiated thyroid carcinoma can be established only by appropriate biopsy. The index of suspicion for cancer in any thyroid mass is influenced by the history of radiation exposure, less so by the family history, and very strongly by the physical findings. Any thyroid mass may contain cancer irrespective of its clinical presentation and the results of diagnostic studies. The small, soft, ill-defined solitary nodule without other suspicious clinical characteristics is not likely to be malignant, but it could be. The solitary, hard, fixed mass adherent to adjacent structures with ipsilateral vocal cord paralysis and enlarged hard cervical lymph nodes is cancer until proven otherwise.

The importance of fine-needle aspiration biopsy (FNAB) as the one definitive diagnostic study in the assessment of any patient with thyroid mass(es) cannot be overemphasized. Sonography, radioisotopic scans, and blood tests can indicate only the more suspicious nodules, but they cannot establish a histologic diagnosis. In most instances, thyroid exploration for diagnosis alone is no longer appropriate. Although specific limitations of FNAB exist, it is the most definitive diagnostic tool currently available. The accuracy is clearly dependent on the diligence and accuracy of the aspirator, the adequacy and proper preservation of the aspirate, the appropriate communication between aspirator and cytopathologist, and, last but not least, the experience of that cytopathologist (67).

A negative FNAB should never exclude the diagnosis of cancer in a patient who has overwhelmingly suspicious findings (68) (see also Chapter 7 for further discussion of FNAB). In most instances, complete history, physical examination, and FNAB will suffice for adequate preoperative evaluation of the thyroid gland and neck. Careful assessment of the larynx with particular reference to vocal cord mobility is imperative. Tracheal displacement, if present, should be noted. History of voice change, difficulty in swallowing, respiratory difficulties, cough, hemoptysis, chest pain, weight loss, and musculoskeletal complaints (e.g., bone pain) should raise the index of suspicion for metastatic disease.

Routine general physical examination, routine hematologic and biochemical studies, and chest x-ray should be obtained prior to any surgical procedure. The euthyroid state of the patient should be biochemically documented before the patient is subjected to general anesthesia. Other more extensive diagnostic studies should usually be reserved for those patients who present with signs, symptoms, or findings suggestive of disseminated tumor.

FACTORS INFLUENCING PROGNOSIS

Recent medical literature abounds with reports concerning prognostic factors in well-differentiated thyroid cancer. Multiple clinical factors including age, gender, size of the primary tumor, presence or absence of extracapsular spread, regional and/or distant metastases, histologic grade, as well as tumor histology, DNA content, adenylate cyclase response of the tumor to thyroid stimulating hormone (TSH) stimulation, epidermal growth factor (EGF) receptor status, and the presence of oncogenes and tumor-suppressor gene mutations have been implicated in estimates of prognosis (22). Age as a prognostic factor was first described in 1954 by Sloane (29) and McDermott et al. (69). In the survey of papillary thyroid cancer by Frazell and Foote (30), there was only one death from thyroid carcinoma under the age of 40. Tollefsen et al. (70), describing 70 fatal cases of papillary thyroid cancer, documented the average age at the time of first treatment as being 52 years. Large tumors, extrathyroidal spread, and anaplastic changes were present in a significant proportion of these fatal cases. The greater the amount of spindle and giant cell metaplasia seen, the shorter the disease-free interval and the shorter the overall survival. Recurrent nerve paralysis and distant metastases clearly indicated a more ominous prognosis and the most common finding at death was uncontrolled locally recurrent cancer in the center of the neck.

In 1966, Halnan (71) reported the experience from the Christie Hospital in Manchester of 344 unselected new patients with thyroid cancer. There was a constant inverse relationship between age at diagnosis and survival, but no difference in survival between the sexes. A male-to-female ratio of 2.8:1.0 was noted, and poorly differentiated tumors occurred about 10 years later than did the well-differentiated ones.

Mazzaferri et al. (33), in their report of 576 preponderantly male patients with well-differentiated papillary carcinoma, noted a higher proportion of recurrence under the age of 30, but a significantly greater proportion of deaths in those over the age of 40. Gender, previous radiation exposure, and pregnancy did not influence prognosis. Deaths were more common in those patients having tumors greater than 2.5 cm in diameter. The presence or extent of regional lymph node metastasis and the extent of surgery on the primary and neck nodes had no impact on survival. The incidence of local/regional recurrence was higher in those patients undergoing less than total thyroidectomy or no treatment beyond surgery, but survival was not adversely effected. Only 3.3% of the patients died, five as a direct result of cancer, for a cumulative survival at 10 years of 94.9%. Seventy patients developed recurrences, only four of whom eventually died of their cancers. Other factors having no prognostic importance included tumor multicentricity (28.6% with 9% local recurrence in the thyroid after subtotal thyroidectomy) and histology. The incidence of recurrence related to the extent of thyroid resection, as did the incidence of postoperative complications. The age of the patient, the size of the primary lesion, the presence of local tumor invasion beyond the gland, the extent of thyroidectomy, and the use of iodine-131 and thyroid hormone all significantly influenced either recurrence or survival, or both.

In a subsequent report, Mazzaferri and Jhiang (37) updated the initial experience, added significantly more patients, and added those with follicular thyroid cancer treated over a 40-year interval. Median follow-up was 15.7 years. After 30 years, the survival rate was 76% overall, the recurrence rate was 30%, and the cancer death rate was 8%. Recurrences were most frequent at the extremes of age. Cancer mortality rates were lowest in patients under the age of 40 and increased successively with each subsequent decade of life. Thirty-year cancer mortality rates were greatest in those patients with adverse prognostic factors, which included older age, larger tumors, more mediastinal nodal metastases and distant metastases, and follicular histology. In a Cox's regression model that excluded patients presenting with distant metastases, the likelihood of cancer death was increased by age over 40 years, tumor size over 1.5 cm, local tumor invasion, regional lymph node metastases, and delay in therapy longer than 12 months. The likelihood of fatal outcome was reduced by female gender, surgery more extensive than lobectomy, and radioiodine plus thyroid hormone therapy postoperatively; interestingly enough, it was unaffected by tumor histologic type. In patients receiving radioiodine therapy for ablation of the remaining normal thyroid gland only, the recurrence rate was less than one third that of those who received thyroid hormone therapy alone. Similarly, the cumulative cancer rate after I-131 therapy, regardless of the reason for its use, was one third that in patients not so treated.

Cady et al. (53) reporting in 1976, studied well-differentiated papillary thyroid cancer at the Lahey Clinic and noted changing patterns of disease, with more recent patients presenting at younger age with smaller primary tumors. Low- and high-risk groups were identified, and the prognostic factors of age, sex, extraglandular extension, blood vessel invasion, major capsular invasion, and multifocal disease were correlated with higher death rates. In this series, lymph node metastasis exerted a protective effect in all categories of disease studied. Subsequent analysis of these data indicated that the age of the host was a far more significant factor. Hormone suppression lessened mortality rates in patients with papillary and mixed papillary and follicular cancers, but not those with follicular carcinoma. A subsequent report from the same group indicated that risk could be defined by age and sex alone (72). The low-risk group consisted of men 40 years of age or younger and women 50 years of age and younger, with the remainder comprising the high-risk group for differentiated thyroid cancer. Recurrence and death rates in the low-risk group were 11% and 4%, respectively, whereas those in the high-risk group 33% and 27%. Basic risk-group definition in these authors' experience was more prognostically significant than pathologic type, local extent of disease, extent of surgery, or site of recurrence or metastasis. Of those patients at low risk who developed recurrence and were treated with radioiodine, 70% were cured, but of those high-risk patients who developed recurrence, only 10% survived.

In their most recent report, Cady and Rossi (73) enlarged and updated their clinical series and reported a risk definition description, AMES, an acronym for age, metastases to distant sites other than lymph nodes, extent of the primary tumor, and size greater than 5 cm. Risk definitions now include among the low-risk group all younger patients without distant metastases, males under age 41 and females under age 51, all older patients with intrathyroid, papillary cancer or minor tumor capsular involvement of follicular cancer, and primary cancers smaller than 5 cm in diameter without distant metastases. The high-risk group comprises all patients with distant metastases, all older patients with extrathyroidal papillary cancer or major tumor capsular involvement in follicular cancer, and primary cancers 5 cm or larger, regardless of extent of disease. From 1961 to 1980, the low-risk group of 277 patients (or 89% of the total number with papillary and follicular carcinoma) seen in that time interval comprise the low-risk group having only 14 recurrences and five deaths, 5% and 1.8%, respectively. During the same interval, the high-risk group of 33 patients comprising 11% of the total experience, experienced 18 recurrences and 15 deaths, 55% and 44%, respectively. In the authors' experience, these factors were of greater prognostic significance than of any other descriptive factors.

In 1975, Byar and the European Organization for Research on Treatment of Cancer (EORTC) Thyroid Cancer Cooperative Group developed a prognostic index based on a multivariate analysis of 507 patients with thyroid cancer. In contrast to most other similar reports, medullary and anaplastic thyroid cancers were included. Age, gender, principal cell type, extrathyroidal invasion, and the presence of distant metastases were identified as important prognostic factors. Each of these variables was found to have prognostic significance when examined singly, but some were strongly correlated with others. A multivariate analysis indicated that age in years at diagnosis, sex, principal cell type, presence of anaplastic carcinoma, T category, and the number of metastatic sites were prognostically significant. The proposed EORTC prognostic index for thyroid carcinoma began with age, as follows:

+12 if male
+10 if medullary or if poorly differentiated follicular carcinoma
+45 if principal or associated cell type is anaplastic
+10 if T category is T_3
+15 if there is at least one distant metastatic site
+15 if, in addition to the above, there are multiple distant metastatic sites.

If the total score was less than 50, the patient was assigned to risk group 1 with an observed 5-year survival of 95%. A total score of 50 to 65 assigned the patient to risk group 2, with an observed 5-year survival of 80%. Risk group 3 represented a total score of 66 to 83, with an observed 5-year survival of 51%. Risk-group 4 represented a total score of 84 to 108, with a 5-year survival of 33%; when total score exceeded 109, the patient was assigned to risk-group 5 with an observed 5-year survival of 5%. Ninety-four percent of patients in risk group 5 had anaplastic tumors. Age was the single most important feature of thyroid cancer revealed in this analysis, but there was a close correlation with cell type. The status of regional lymph nodes did not add to the prediction of survival. Therapy was ignored in the analyses.

Tennvall et al. (61) in 1986, using the same EORTC prognostic index, studied 226 patients with differentiated thyroid cancer and confirmed the validity of age at diagnosis, extent of local tumor, and the presence of distant metastases as being prognostically significant. They also noted that extracapsular spread outside the thyroid gland and marked cellular atypia were equally prognostically significant. When local extent and anaplasia were taken into consideration, age alone lost its prognostic significance. The authors indicated that the biologic behavior of the papillary, follicular, and medullary carcinomas were significantly different, and that microscopic features specific for each category should be separately analyzed and separate prognostic indices be constructed.

Ito et al. (75) studied 763 patients in Japan with well-differentiated thyroid cancer and concluded that age, tumor size, sex, and degree of histologic differentiation were prognostically significant. The extent of surgical resection of the primary and the presence or absence of regional lymph node metastases did not prove to be significant. In this study, papillary and follicular carcinomas had similar survival rates. The authors questioned whether such differences from the Caucasian experience resulted from geographic and racial differences. In this series, patients with follicular carcinoma tended to be significantly younger than in a similar series of Caucasian patients. Differences in prognosis were more apparent in the older aged patients, confirming the experience of Cady et al. (72,73).

Samaan et al. (38) in 1983 reported the results of different modalities of treatment of well-differentiated thyroid cancer, retrospectively reviewing 1599 patients treated at M. D. Anderson Hospital and Tumor Institute. The median follow-up for all patients was 11 years, with a maximum follow-up of 43 years. Overall recurrence rate was 23%, and 11% had died of their disease. Eighty-one percent were papillary carcinomas. The extent of disease was defined in one of four ways:

1. Intrathyroidal, subdivided into:
   G1—encapsulated, but with microscopic evidence of capsular and/or vascular invasion
   G2—no true encapsulation, but well delineated
   G3—with marked tissue or vascular invasion
2. Adjacent cervical lymph nodes
3. Adjacent soft-tissue invasion
4. Remote metastases.

Papillary carcinoma made up 81% of the total group. Intrathyroidal carcinomas comprised 42% of the series. Of the whole patient group, 66% underwent total thyroidectomy, 7% received external radiotherapy, and 46% had radioactive iodine as part of the treatment of the original disease. Children had the best overall survival, but of the adult patients, women who had intrathyroidal papillary disease treated with total thyroidectomy and radioiodine iodine therapy, and whose disease was diagnosed between the ages of 20 and 59 of age, had the best prognosis. Those patients undergoing total thyroidectomy had significantly fewer recurrences than those treated with unilateral surgery. In those patients undergoing thyroid ablation with radioiodine, there was no statistically significant advantage between subtotal and total thyroidectomy. The larger the intrathyroidal tumor, the greater the likelihood of local recurrence. Recurrence rates for unifocal and multifocal tumor were similar. Multivariate analysis revealed the single most important prognostic factor was radioiodine treatment, which significantly increased the disease-free interval. The presence of intrathyroidal disease was the next most significant factor, and disease-free interval in these patients was significantly higher than in those with more extensive disease. Pathology was the next most significant factor: those patients with papillary carcinoma survived significantly longer than those with follicular carcinoma, who in turn had a longer disease-free survival than those with Hürthle cell carcinoma. No other factors had significant impact on disease-free survival.

Of the patients who died of thyroid cancer, the cause of death in 140 patients was documented as local recurrence in 38%, lung metastases in 31%, bone metastases in 24%, brain metastases in 4%, and liver metastases in 2%. Those patients with papillary carcinoma were much more likely to die of local disease in the neck, patients with follicular disease were much more likely to die of bone metastases, and those with Hürthle cell tumors died of local disease and lung and bone metastases in approximately equal distributions. Multiple primary tumors and regional lymph node metastases had no significant impact on survival. No benefit was seen to be derived from external radiotherapy when patients were matched for extent of disease. All patients with positive radioiodine scans after surgery did benefit from radioiodine therapy. The single most important factor influencing length of survival in this study was age at diagnosis. In those patients not treated with radioiodine, total thyroidectomy was the surgical resection of choice. Even those patients categorized as low-risk had significantly lower recurrence and death rates if they received radioiodine.

In another study from Scandinavia looking at prognostic factors of papillary, follicular, and medullary thyroid carcinoma, Tennvall et al. (76) performed a multivariate analysis of 262 patients. Age at diagnosis was an important predictor for both papillary and follicular cancers. When deaths from intercurrent disease were eliminated, marked cellular atypia and tumor invasion beyond the thyroid capsule were important prognosticators. The only significant predictor of survival in medullary cancer was tumor invasion beyond the thyroid capsule. Treatment factors were not included in the study.

In another multivariate analysis of 375 patients with well-differentiated thyroid cancer, Bacourt et al. (77) confirmed the importance of age, sex, localized disease, well-differentiated histology, and distant metastases as valid prognostic factors on univariate analysis. On multivariate analysis, the interdependence of many of these factors was confirmed, and the most important prognostic variable was the stage of the disease at the time of treatment. Of equal importance was the presence of distant metastases upon admission, with histology, age, and sex less significant.

Simpson et al. (35), in a retrospective analysis of well-differentiated thyroid cancers from multiple radiation centers in Canada, indicated that on univariate analysis of 1578 patients with papillary and follicular carcinoma, postoperative status (adequacy of removal of all gross tumor), age, extrathyroidal invasion, the presence of distant metastasis, nodal involvement, differentiation, sex, tumor size, and pathologic type were of statistically significant prognostic importance, in descending order. On multivariate analysis, using cause-specific survival rates, independently important prognostic factors for papillary carcinoma were age at the time of initial treatment, extrathyroidal invasion, and histologic differentiation. For follicular carcinomas, extrathyroidal invasion, distant metastases, primary tumor size, nodal involvement, age at diagnosis and postoperative status were important prognostic factors.

A subsequent report reviewed the treatment and outcome results (78). Surgical resection was carried out in almost all patients, with no correlation between the type of operation and recurrence or survival. Postoperative irradiation in 201 patients, radioiodine in 214 patients, or both in 107 patients were used more often in patients with a poor prognosis, and were effective in reducing local recurrences and improving survival, especially in those with microscopic postoperative residual disease. Adjuvant therapy in patients considered to have no residual disease after being operated on for both papillary and follicular carcinomas, made no significant improvement in local control or long-term survival. The control of gross residual disease was much less satisfactory; one third of patients treated by external radiation therapy or radioiodine achieved a complete remission, and an additional 43% achieved partial remission. Patients treated by both radiotherapy and radioiodine responded more often and more fully than those treated by only one of the radiation modalities.

The authors concluded that thyroid hormone was a relatively weak form of adjuvant therapy and should not be used alone when adjuvant therapy is clearly indicated. The importance of gross complete tumor removal was emphasized. In their experience, radioiodine alone was often unsuccessful in permanently eradicating gross disease, whether local or metastatic, and the addition of external radiation therapy improved the results, although ultimate survival was influenced little, if at all.

In 1986, McConahey et al. (54) reported the experience of the Mayo Clinic from 1946 through 1970 with 859 patients with papillary thyroid cancer. All but two patients underwent thyroid surgery; 319 (37%) had metastatic cervical lymph nodes. Of those 800 patients without distant metastases on initial examination who underwent a potentially curative surgical procedure, 7% postoperatively had nodal metastases, 6% had a local tumor recurrence, and 5% developed distant metastases. Of those patients having intrathyroidal tumors initially, postoperative local recurrence or distant metastases resulted in a 10-year mortality of 17% and 41%, respectively. Of those patients with extrathyroidal tumors, postoperative recurrences were associated with significantly higher death rates. Death from thyroid cancer was highly associated with age over 50 years, male sex, tumor size, tumor grade, initial extent of disease, and absence of Hashimoto's thyroiditis.

In 1987, Hay et al. (79), using the same clinical experience, proposed a prognostic scoring system and gave it the acronym AGES, for the patient's *a*ge, the histologic *g*rade of the tumor, and the *e*xtent and *s*ize of the tumor. A prognostic score was generated by regression analysis assessing the four prognostic factors. The total score was derived from 0.05 times the age in years (if age 40 or more), or +0 if less than 40 years of age, +1 if grade II, or +3 if grade III or IV, and +1 if tumor was extrathyroid and +3 if distant spread was present, and 0.2 times the tumor size in maximum dimensions. The median AGES score was 2.50, with a range of 0.00 to 11.65. Those patients having an AGES score of 3.99 or less enjoyed a cancer mortality at 25 years of 1% after ipsilateral lobectomy and 2% after bilateral resection, whether subtotal or total. In contrast, those patients with an AGES score of 4 or more who underwent lobectomy alone had a mortality from papillary thyroid carcinoma at 25 years of 65%, whereas those undergoing bilateral resection had a lower rate of 35%. In neither the minimal nor the higher risk group was the overall survival significantly improved by the performance of total thyroidectomy. Permanent unilateral vocal cord paralysis occurred in 2% and permanent hypoparathyroidism in 5% of the 859 patients who survived surgery. The extent of resection was not apparently associated with vocal cord paralysis, but it was highly associated with hypocalcemia. The authors concluded that the AGES scoring system could identify patients having papillary carcinoma who were at increased risk of mortality from the disease. This system is almost identical to the AMES system proposed by Cady and Ross; it is based primarily on simple, easily determinable clinical parameters, and it separates patients into low- and high-risk groups.

Hay (45), studying an enlarged patient sample from the Mayo Clinic with a total of 1500 patients with papillary carcinoma, confirmed the validity of the AGES scoring system. Patients in group 1 with a score of 3.99 or less represented 86% of the total 1500, with a 20-year cause-specific mortality of only 1%. The comparable mortality rates for groups 2 through 4, with scores of 4 to 4.99, 5 to 5.99, and over 6, were 20%, 67%, and 87%, respectively.

Pasieka et al. (80) in 1992 proposed the addition of nuclear DNA content to add prognostic value to existing risk factors in patients with papillary thyroid cancer. Nuclear DNA content was measured both on FNAB material and the surgical specimen in 73% of patients with primary or recurrent papillary thyroid carcinoma. The AMES risk group classification was modified to include DNA ploidy, thus creating the DAMES classification. Patients with euploid tumors that were AMES low-risk were considered to be DAMES low-risk, patients with euploid tumors that were AMES high-risk became intermediate risk, and patients with aneuploid tumors that were AMES high-risk became DAMES high-risk. Forty-eight patients were in the DAMES low-risk group. Recurrence and/or distant metastases developed in only 8% of these patients. Twenty-two patients were in the intermediate risk-group, and of these 55% had residual recurrent or distant metastatic disease, with one death from cancer at the 10-year follow-up. Three patients were in the DAMES high-risk group, and all of them developed distant metastases and died within 24 months from thyroid cancer. Thus, a statistically significant difference existed in the development of recurrence/metastasis or death from cancer in the DAMES high-risk group compared with the other risk groups combined. The authors concluded that the addition of nuclear DNA content added prognostic value to the existing AMES risk group classification.

Different conclusions were reached after the study of nuclear DNA in patients with differentiated thyroid cancer. Backdahl et al. (81) concluded that "nuclear DNA content has a predictive power significantly greater than that of all other prognostic factors combined." By contrast, in a flow cytometric study of 125 patients with differentiated thyroid carcinoma, of which 68 were papillary, Joensuu et al. (82) found that although DNA aneuploidy was a powerful adverse prognostic factor when used alone, it was not an independently significant factor in Cox's stepwise proportional hazard analysis.

In 1990, Hay (45) described the relationship of DNA-ploidy status to mortality from papillary thyroid cancer in 209 patients treated at the Mayo Clinic from 1946 through 1975 and followed for an average of 16.5 years after treatment. The highest mortality rate was found with the DNA-aneuploid tumors; the tetraploid polyploid profile was found to be intermediate between aneuploid and diploid. The differences were highly significant ($p < .001$). When the 209 patients were reanalyzed according to the EORTC score, TNM stage, AGES score, and AIMS risk group, and when they were divided into minimal and high-risk categories within each of the eight subsets, the presence of nondiploid DNA defined a group of patients with a significantly increased cancer-related death rate. When separate Cox models were constructed to adjust for each of the four schemes in each analysis, nondiploid DNA was independently associated with increased cause-specific mortality. Further experience will be required to assess the validity of DNA analysis as a vital component to the staging schema.

In a subsequent report from the Mayo Clinic, Hay et al. (83) added another variable to the prognostic scoring system for papillary thyroid carcinoma, which included completeness of the primary tumor resection but excluded histologic grade and DNA ploidy. Based on analysis of 1779 patients, the final model included five variables, including *m*etastasis, *a*ge, *c*ompleteness of resection, *i*nvasion, and *s*ize (MACIS). The final prognostic score was defined as MACIS = 3.1 if age is under 39 years, or 0.08 × age if age is over 40 years; 0.3 × tumor size in centimeters; +1 if incompletely resected; +1 if locally invasive; and +3 if distant metastasis is present. Twenty-year cause-specific survival rates for patients with MACIS less than 6, 6 to 6.99, 7 to 7.99, and 8 and over were 99%, 89%, 56%, and 24%, respectively ($p < .001$). The authors excluded histologic grade because "few surgical pathologists recognize higher grade papillary thyroid carcinoma tumors," and "ploidy, because cytometric technology is expensive and time consuming." The lowest group was defined as those having a MACIS score below 6, comprising 84% of the subjects in the group; in the 8+ MACIS group, 34% had distant metastasis, 84% had extrathyroidal invasion, and 54% underwent incomplete operation with a median age of 69.5 years and median tumor size of 4.5 cm. The authors concluded that the five variables needed for the MACIS scoring system were readily available after primary operation, and such a prognostic system could have widespread applicability in the assessment of papillary thyroid carcinoma.

DeGroot et al. (36) analyzed the University of Chicago experience with papillary carcinoma numbering 269 patients with an average 12-year follow-up. Patients were categorized into four clinical classes:

Class I—Intrathyroidal disease
Class II—With cervical nodal metastases
Class III—With extrathyroidal invasion
Class IV—With distant metastases.

Tumors averaged 2.4 cm in diameter, 21.6% had tumor capsule invasion, and 46% had multifocal tumors. Sixty-six percent of the patients had near-total or total thyroidectomy, with an overall postoperative incidence of hypoparathyroidism of 8.4%. Twenty-five percent of the patients had continuing or recurrent disease, and 8.2% died from cancer. Deaths occurred largely in patients with class III or IV disease. Cervical lymph node metastases were associated with increased recurrence but not increased mortality. Extrathyroid invasion carried an increased risk of 5.8 times for death, and distant metastases increased this risk 47-fold. Age over 45 years at diagnosis increased the risk of death 32-fold, and tumor size over 3 cm increased the risk of death 5.8-fold. Surgical resection combining lobectomy with at least contralateral subtotal thyroidectomy was associated with decreased risk of death in patients with tumors larger than 1 cm and decreased risk of recurrence among all patients. Ablation of residual thyroid tissue after surgery with radioiodine was associated with statistically significant decreased risk of recurrence of tumors larger than 1 cm and decreased risk of death in patients in classes I and II, with tumors more than 1 cm in diameter. The authors concluded that more extensive initial surgery in class I and II patients with tumors larger than 1 cm, as well as postoperative radioiodine-131 ablation of remaining thyroid tissue would improve overall results.

In a report from Memorial Sloan-Kettering Cancer Center (24) describing a consecutive series of 931 previously untreated patients with differentiated thyroid carcinoma, univariate analysis revealed female gender, multifocal primary tumors, and regional lymph node metastases to be favorable prognostic factors. Unfavorable factors included age over 45 years, follicular histology, extrathyroidal extension, tumor size greater than 4 cm, and the presence of distant metastases. On multivariate analysis, the only factors affecting prognosis were patient age, histology, tumor size, extrathyroidal extension, and distant metastases. Although histology was significant, it was a somewhat weaker predictor. Gender, nodal stage, and multifocality of the primary tumor had no prognostic significance. In this series, patients in the sixth decade of life had a 270% greater risk of death from thyroid cancer than younger patients; those in the seventh decade, a 240% increased risk; and those older than 70 years, a 710% increased risk of cancer-related mortality. Patients with tumor sizes between 3 and 5 cm had a 40% greater risk of death than patients with tumor sizes less than 3 cm, and for those whose tumors were larger than 5 cm in diameter, the mortality risk was increased by 170% compared to those whose primary tumor sizes were less than 3 cm. Men had a 10% greater risk of death from thyroid cancers than women, and patients with follicular carcinoma had an 80% increased risk compared with those with papillary carcinoma. Extrathyroidal extension increased the risk of mortality 250%, and positive nodes predicted a 40% increased mortality. Distant metastases at presentation carried a 300% increased risk of mortality from thyroid cancer. Uncensored survival for the entire study population was 78% at 10 years, and determinant survival for all patients was 87% at 10 years. In the total population, 78.5% were papillary carcinomas, 15.5% were follicular cancers, and 6% were Hürthle cell cancers. Forty-eight percent of the population had positive nodes, of which 56% of the papillary tumors and 20% of the follicular tumors were classified as N+. Tumor grade and DNA content were not systematically studied in this patient population.

The described reports document that multiple factors are of prognostic significance in assessing the risk of treatment failure of well-differentiated thyroid cancer. Most authors agree that age is a primary determinant. The older patients are much more likely to have larger tumors, more extracapsular spread, more anaplastic histology, a higher risk of distant metastases, and higher DNA content, all of which are of ominous prognostic significance.

Follicular cancers have a poorer prognosis than do papillary cancers. Well-localized intrathyroidal tumors without significant anaplasia may be successfully managed by conservative surgery with excellent long-term results. Those large tumors, usually with extracapsular spread, often more poorly differentiated histologically (with a tendency toward aneuploid DNA nuclear content), and with a higher likelihood of distant metastases, require more aggressive local/regional and systemic therapy in hopes of achieving better local control. Whereas some factors may be amenable to surgical and radiation management, the intrinsic biology of the tumor, particularly as reflected in its biologic aggressiveness implied by DNA content, may very well frustrate the most rigorous and well-directed attempts at cure.

SURGICAL TREATMENT

Few diseases have engendered more controversy than the management of thyroid cancer. There is general agreement that surgery, wherever feasible, is the primary treatment of choice, and the overall success of such treatment may well depend on the adequacy of the surgical resection. The spectrum of surgery ranges from local excision/lobectomy alone to total thyroidectomy, modified neck dissection, and even more radical resection of adjacent tissues in those patients with massive extrathyroidal cancer, up to and including laryngectomy and esophagectomy. The reports cited above outlining the prognosis of thyroid cancer help us to evaluate the overall prognosis and to reach legitimate conclusions devoid of emotionalism and tradition. Thyroid cancer is not a single disease (84). Not only are there very significant differences in the natural history and response to treatment among the different subdivisions of thyroid cancer, but also there are very significant differences depending on the extent of that disease, local/regional and distant. All of these factors impact decisions concerning the appropriateness and extent of surgery and the need for adjunctive treatment, including radioiodine, external irradiation, and chemotherapy.

Factors determining the extent of surgery include the histology and extent of the primary tumor, previous treatment, if any, overall general health of the patient, and the patient's wishes. In general, the surgical goal should be the complete removal of all gross tumor from the primary site and its local/regional extensions, including adjacent soft tissue and regional lymph nodes, without sacrifice of uninvolved adjacent structures. Less than complete removal of all tumor will require further treatment, the efficacy of which is uncertain, thus jeopardizing the ultimate outcome. Local recurrence indicates a significant risk of subsequent tumor-related mortality (22,24,35,36,40,54,70,78).

The extent of surgery should be precisely defined. Local excision is less than total removal of one thyroid lobe, usually either by enucleation or by removal of the pathological entity with little surrounding uninvolved thyroid parenchyma. Lobectomy implies the total extracapsular removal of one lobe, with or without resection of the thyroid isthmus. Subtotal thyroidectomy implies the removal of parts of both lobes of the gland, leaving a remnant of residual thyroid tissue on one or both sides. Near-total thyroidectomy implies the total extracapsular lobectomy and isthmectomy on the side of major involvement, with near-total lobectomy on the contralateral side, usually leaving a small rim of the posterior portion of that lobe to preserve parathyroid glands and their blood supply. Total thyroidectomy indicates the removal of all thyroid tissue from the neck, including a meticulous extracapsular dissection of both lobes in their entirety, including the isthmus and pyramidal lobe, while preserving recurrent laryngeal nerve and the parathyroid glands and their blood supply whenever possible. The completeness of such surgery can be documented only by subsequent radioisotopic scanning of the neck postoperatively, which studies will frequently document residual isotope uptake in the thyroid bed indicative of failure of complete removal of all microscopic evidence of radioiodine-concentrating thyroid tissue (50,51,85). Most of the radioiodine uptake will be concentrated at the superior poles of the thyroid gland and along the embryonic tract of descent and adjacent to Berry's ligament (85). Thus, the concept of total resection of all thyroid tissue may be somewhat nebulous in the absence of radioisotopic confirmation of the absence of that tissue.

There is no evidence, based on prospective randomized studies, for the superiority of total thyroidectomy for *survival* of patients with well-differentiated thyroid cancer (86). The theoretical advantages of total resection of the thyroid gland are not matched by comparable improvement in results and are accompanied by significantly increased morbidity, particularly in the hands of less-experienced surgeons (86). The risk may simply not be worth the price (48).

There appears to be no role for any surgery less than total extracapsular removal of the entire thyroid lobe at risk, for any suspicious lesions requiring thyroid resection (i.e., total thyroid lobectomy plus isthmectomy). The specimen should be submitted for frozen section examination to ascertain the histopathologic diagnosis and extent of the pathological lesion within the gland, particularly as it relates to the capsule, to whether or not there are multiple foci within the resected specimen, and to the proximity of such foci to the cut edge of the isthmus. There is general agreement that small lesions (generally less than 1 cm in diameter), totally confined to one lobe without extracapsular extension and unaccompanied by multiple other foci, are almost always cured by total lobectomy and isthmectomy, preserving the recurrent laryngeal nerve, the external branch of the superior laryngeal nerve, and the parathyroid glands with their blood supply. Any palpable abnormality in the contralateral lobe, however, must be considered suspect and appropriately sampled either by needle biopsy, complete excision, or completion total thyroidectomy for both diagnosis and treatment, particularly in the face of a malignant diagnosis.

If the pathologist reports microscopic evidence of multifocal cancer in the resected specimen, particularly if it approaches the cut edge of the isthmus, then contralateral lobectomy should be performed. This should be done conservatively, meticulously preserving associated nerves and parathyroid glands. If, for technical reasons, this is not safely possible, then subtotal lobectomy should be performed, taking care to limit one's dissection, particularly posteriorly, to within the thyroid capsule.

Upon receipt of the report of carcinoma, a careful assessment of the regional lymph nodes should be made. It seems appropriate to dissect the pericapsular, pretracheal, delphian, paratracheal, and tracheoesophageal lymph nodes on the ipsilateral side for both staging and treatment. It is apparent that clinical assessment of these lymph nodes is fraught with considerable error, even in experienced hands (65). It seems obvious that meticulous dissection of this area, including those lymph nodes lying between the recurrent laryngeal nerve and the trachea, is best accomplished in the previously undissected field rather than deferring it until the time the patient might subsequently develop clinical evidence of recurrence/metastases. Of necessity, the surgery must extensively dissect the ipsilateral recurrent laryngeal nerve, placing that nerve at significant risk of temporary paresis secondary to manipulation/devascularization in order to adequately clear the tracheoesophageal groove of metastatic disease. The other advantage of performing the surgery at this point is for the removal of potential tumor from an area in which the diagnosis of recurrence is often delayed and when the initial manifestation may frequently be the appearance of ipsilateral vocal cord paralysis secondary to invasion of the recurrent laryngeal nerve, a significantly morbid occurrence. Attention should then be directed to the jugular lymph nodes, where careful assessment of those nodes lying anterior and lateral to the internal jugular vein should be carried out by inspection and careful palpation. One or more appropriate lymph nodes should be pathologically sampled; if results are negative and no further suspicious jugular lymph nodes are apparent, then further lymph adenectomy is unnecessary.

Lore (87) has documented important anatomic and technical considerations in thyroid surgery. Total thyroidectomy may be required, with improvement in local control rates but no definite advantage to overall survival. The experience at the Lahey Clinic reported by Cady and Rossi was typical of most studies. A small but definitely increased risk of local recurrence following lobectomy occurred when compared to bilateral resection. No difference in cumulative risk of local recurrence 30 years after surgery was noted between subtotal or near-total thyroidectomy and total thyroidectomy, either in the low- or high-risk groups. Again, it was tumor that occurred outside the thyroid bed in the presence of extracapsular extension in elderly patients that ultimately proved to be fatal. Thus, unilateral resection, provided it is complete and thorough, may be adequate for the overwhelming majority of patients with papillary carcinoma.

Patients with obvious or histologically confirmed bilateral papillary carcinoma, those previously exposed to ionizing irradiation, and those in whom the surgery will be followed by radioiodine therapy are best served by total thyroidectomy. The same may be true for follicular cancer, but with less complete documentation (58,59). Relative contraindications to total thyroidectomy include questions of patient compliance with lifelong thyroid replacement or remaining under competent regular follow-up observation, or when at least one parathyroid gland cannot be safely retained with its blood supply intact, or cannot be autotransplanted into a suitable bed. The complication rate must be kept below 2% (43). When frozen section examination fails to document the true nature of the lesion, and thyroid cancer remains after unilateral lobectomy, completion total thyroidectomy may be indicated, recognizing the increased risks (42). If the original resection is considered adequate when all information is in hand, then no further surgery is indicated and the patient is closely followed.

The presence of extrathyroidal extension (ETE) is an adverse prognostic finding. In a review of the Memorial Sloan-Kettering series (88), a total of 79 patients of the overall 1012 patients (8%) had documented ETE. Those patients were more likely to fail treatment and to die of their disease than those without ETE, 77% versus 34% and 71% versus 13%, respectively ($p < .0001$). Local, regional, and distant failures were more prominent among patients with ETE than among those without it, 48% versus 9%, 41% versus 16%, and 37% versus 11%, respectively. Survival of patients with ETE in this series was adversely affected by nonpapillary histology, distant metastasis, age over 45, tumor size in excess of 4 cm, and incomplete excision. Those patients with ETE younger than 45 with negative surgical margins had survivals similar to those of patients without ETE. Survival in older patients was not affected by incomplete excision, but it was in younger patients. The presence of distant metastases did not affect survival in younger patients. If the primary tumor was completely resected, the presence of ETE did not adversely impact survival in this series. Extrathyroidal extension was defined as extension of the primary tumor outside the capsule of the thyroid gland, with invasion into adjacent surrounding structures such as trachea, larynx, strap muscles, and recurrent laryngeal nerve. Treatment of these 79 patients was exclusively surgical in 56%, with individualization in the use of postoperative radioiodine and thyroid hormone suppression. Nine percent underwent total laryngectomy and 24% required partial or segmental trachiectomy; only one patient required cervical esophagectomy and total laryngectomy. The recurrent laryngeal nerve was sacrificed in 50%, in 80% of whom the nerve was nonfunctional preoperatively; in the additional 9 (or 20%), it was sacrificed when invasion by tumor was discovered intraoperatively. A total of 55 patients underwent neck dissection as part of their initial treatment: 82% of these were therapeutic. Thirty-year disease-specific survival was reduced from 87% in the entire series of 1012 patients to 29% for the affected 79 ETE patients. Local failure rate increased from 9% overall to 48%, and the regional failure rate increased from 15% to 41%. Local and regional failure rates were adversely affected by the presence of positive surgical margins only.

Breaux and Guillamondegui (89) reported a 46.8% survival among 47 patients with ETE followed from 5 to 15 years. McCaffrey et al. (90) found a 54% survival rate in 262 patients with ETE studied at the Mayo Clinic over 15 years. The importance of clear surgical margins has been repeatedly emphasized. Resection of adjacent strap muscles, and occasionally of the recurrent laryngeal nerve, is relatively common. Resection of a normally functioning recurrent laryngeal nerve not completely surrounded or otherwise involved with well-differentiated thyroid cancer is rarely justified. The nerve can usually be spared by sharp meticulous dissection with admittedly narrow margins. Rarely is the uninvolved nerve actually invaded by well-differentiated thyroid cancer. The tumor displacing or compressing the trachea can usually be removed by sharp dissection in the appropriate plane on the thyroid and/or tracheal cartilages, but again with narrow margins. In the McCaffrey series (90), 262 patients with invasive papillary thyroid cancer were evaluated retrospectively. The sites of invasion were muscle in 53%, recurrent laryngeal nerve in 47%, trachea in 37%, esophagus in 21%, larynx in 12%, and other sites in 30%. Complete surgical removal was accomplished in 56% of the patients. When Cox's proportional hazard models were applied to the survival data, the fact most significantly impacting on survival was invasion of the trachea and esophagus. Completeness of resection approached statistical significance. Although the technique of shaving tumor from the trachea and esophagus to avoid the morbidity of resection has been successful in producing some long-term control, it is probably only effective in the absence of gross residual tumor. With frank infiltration of the airway by direct invasion of the larynx and/or trachea, the involved portions of the airway should be resected *en bloc,* with the thyroid gland and the airway and/or esophagus reconstructed by one of several appropriate measures (91–93). In rare instances, laryngotrachiectomy with establishment of a permanent tracheal stoma may be required to adequately remove massive, deeply infiltrating tumor. It is not surprising that the Mayo Clinic series documented no significant unfavorable impact on survival when ETE and invasion were minimal with no gross tumor present after resection. In those patients with tracheal and/or esophageal invasion, significant effect on survival was noted and the type of excision approached significance (90). Clearly, whether resection can be performed with an acceptable morbidity in the presence of extensive invasive thyroid carcinoma is an important consideration. Only if conservative resection would leave gross tumor behind, or if intraluminal extension is present, should major resection of critical functional components of the upper aerodigestive tract be seriously considered. Most of the current studies do not adequately include assessment of adjuvant therapy in these clinical settings (88,90). Intraluminal invasion of the larynx, trachea, or esophagus appears to carry a much graver prognostic significance than extraluminal cartilage or muscular invasion (94).

In the Mayo Clinic series of 48 patients with well-differentiated thyroid cancer invading the upper aerodigestive tract, who were treated with radical surgery and adjuvant therapy, there was no improvement in survival over those patients treated by near-total skeletonizing excisions combined with adjuvant treatment. The mean age at diagnosis of thyroid cancer in the whole series was 55.6 years with a range of 15 to 85 years. The mean age of patients with massive laryngotracheal invasion was 60.6 years, with a range of 20 to 85 years. Patients with anaplastic and medullary cancer and those considered surgically unresectable were excluded from the study. Excess mortalities from extrathyroidal invasion after treatment by total or near-total excision were 9.3%, 25.1%, and 38.5% at 5, 10, and 20 years, respectively. All patients who underwent partial debulking procedures with or without tracheostomy died of thyroid cancer with a mean survival of 3.8 years postsurgery (93).

When the final pathology report documents extension beyond the surgical margins or the presence of foci of more anaplastic carcinoma, the therapeutic decisions are more difficult. Local invasion may be controlled by adjunctive therapy, but frequently anaplastic carcinoma relentlessly recurs, leading to the patient's death. The use of combined chemotherapy and radiation has been employed in high-risk patients with poorly differentiated thyroid cancers and certain anaplastic cancers with some response and extension of disease-free survival, but with few long-term cures (95).

As noted previously, the impact on survival of the presence of regional lymph node metastases in well-differentiated thyroid cancer has been a subject of considerable debate and controversy. Frankenthaler et al. (96), in their retrospective review of 117 patients at the M. D. Anderson Hospital under the age of 20 presenting with papillary and/or follicular thyroid cancer, noted that regional lymph node metastasis was the most common presenting symptom. Sixty percent of the patients presented with clinical evidence of lymph node involvement, and of these, 13 had bilateral palpable disease. Twenty-six percent of those with initially negative necks contained pathologically confirmed nodal lymph nodes. Recurrence was highest in regional lymph nodes at 24%, with only 4% recurrence at the primary site and 3% as distant metastases. There were no deaths resulting from thyroid cancer in the entire series during the period of follow-up, certainly reflecting the young age of the patients. The current policy in these patients is to subject them to near-total or total thyroidectomy with a modified neck dissection, followed frequently by radioactive iodine therapy. Thus, the impact of nodal metastasis in this selected series of patients was insignificant.

In a retrospective review of 2282 patients with papillary and/or follicular carcinoma from the state of Illinois, with a minimum 10-year follow-up, the lymph node status had no statistically significant impact on overall survival (64). Sellars et al. (97), describing the experience in Alabama with differentiated thyroid cancer over a 34-year interval, indicated that lymph node metastases at initial presentation were prognostically significant, but older patients appeared to be the defining feature of this subgroup. In this study, older patients with cervical lymph node metastases at initial presentation were more likely to die of differentiated thyroid cancer than similar-age patients without such metastases. These data were not analyzed by multivariate analysis.

In a similar retrospective review, Coburn and Wanebo (98) found that recurrence and survival rates in thyroid cancer patients were not significantly influenced by nodal status. However, node-positive patients with the additional risk factors of age over 45, extrathyroidal invasion, and positive mediastinal nodes had more aggressive disease with comparably reduced prognosis.

In a recent report describing a matched-pair analysis of previously untreated patients with differentiated thyroid cancer with and without ipsilateral neck node metastases, Hughes et al. (99) examined the significance of nodal spread in patients with otherwise equivalent prognostic factors. Previous studies had documented that the most frequently observed adverse factors on prognosis were age above 45 years, presence of distant metastases, extrathyroidal extension from the primary lesion, increasing tumor size, and follicular histology. Hughes et al. (99) concluded that cervical lymph node involvement in older patients with thyroid cancer increased the risk of recurrence but did not statistically significantly impact survival in this age-matched series. Recurrence rates were 17% in those with positive cervical lymph nodes versus 11% in those with histologically negative nodes, the difference being not statistically significant. Five of 5 failures in the N1 neck and 5 of 8 failures in the N0 necks were subsequently successfully treated. In the older age group, disease recurred in 31% of the N+ patients, compared with only 8% of the N0 patients, and only one third of the treatment failures in those patients 45 years or older could be salvaged regardless of the original nodal status. All 13 patients who died of thyroid cancer developed distant metastases, and 3 of 5 of those occurring in the N0 patients had associated recurrence in the neck, compared with 2 of 8 in the N+ group. All in all, cervical lymph node metastases did not represent a significant prognostic factor. Extrathyroidal extension and distant metastasis at presentation were deliberately excluded from this study. Much more potent adverse factors than lymph node metastasis have been implicated in treatment failure in the overall series of patients from which this matched-pair series were derived. Thus, it is apparent that lymph node metastases should be appropriately treated when present, largely by surgical removal, and that failure to do so will result in an increased incidence of local and regional recurrence with continued follow-up. The presence of such nodal metastases in the absence of other adverse factors will not unfavorably impact overall prognosis.

This is in contrast to the conclusions reached by Mazzaferri and Jhiang (37), who, in their long-term series studied by Cox's regression analysis, concluded that the likelihood of cancer deaths was increased by the presence of regional lymph node metastases.

The role of postoperative radiation therapy in the management of well-differentiated thyroid cancer remains to be defined. This is more fully addressed in Chapter 31.

Tubiana et al. (100) summarized their experience with external radiotherapy. Surgery was the preferred treatment, with external beam irradiation indicated in those patients in whom microscopic or residual tumor remains after surgery. In the group of patients treated with external irradiation, the local recurrence at 15 years was lower than in those treated by surgery alone (11% versus 23%), even though the irradiated patients had more advanced disease and presumably were at higher risk of local failure. The study was a retrospective, nonrandomized review. The importance of adequate dose, at least 50 gray (Gy), was emphasized. Radiation therapy was more effective in the authors' hands in reducing local recurrence than was radioiodine, for well-differentiated and medullary thyroid cancers. In those patients with gross residual unresectable cancer postoperatively, external radiation was less effective, confirming the impression that the efficacy of external irradiation is inversely related to the tumor burden. When satisfactory tumor excision had been accomplished, surgery and radioiodine treatment were followed by local recurrence in 20%, compared to a rate of 39% in those patients whose excision was incomplete.

No well-controlled study documenting the efficacy of external irradiation in the adjunctive treatment of well-differentiated thyroid cancer exists. Benken et al. (101), in a study of 932 patients with papillary and follicular carcinomas, compared 346 patients treated with conventional external irradiation with 586 patients who did not receive radiotherapy. When survival rates for patients with more advanced disease were calculated on the basis of patient age, there was no obvious effect of radiotherapy in the younger-than-40 group, whereas improvement in survival by radiation just failed to reach statistical significance in the older patients ($p < .09$). The authors concluded that the retrospective analysis failed to prove that survival was prolonged in patients with differentiated thyroid carcinoma by the administration of conventional external radiotherapy.

In a recent study from Germany (102) describing the results of total thyroidectomy, ablative radioiodine therapy, and thyroid hormone therapy, patients treated with and without external irradiation were compared. There was a significant advantage for the irradiated patients with papillary carcinoma, but no beneficial effect of external radiotherapy in the follicular carcinoma patients. This beneficial effect was significantly present only in patients with papillary carcinoma and lymph node involvement, whereas those without lymph node metastases did not benefit from additional adjuvant radiotherapy. None of the patients younger than 40 died of cancer or had progressive disease during follow-up. The beneficial effect of external radiotherapy could be confirmed in the subgroup of patients older than 40 and those with positive lymph node metastases and invasive papillary thyroid cancer. The overall rate of recurrence was significantly reduced in the irradiated group compared with the nonirradiated group. It seems appropriate to consider external radiotherapy in those patients in whom there is high suspicion or histologic confirmation of residual tumor in the local/regional area, and in whom no radioisotopic concentration can be detected postoperatively. Positron emission tomography (PET) scanning may identify this residual tumor in the absence of I-131 uptake.

The alternative to resection and/or radiotherapy of extrathyroidal tumor is the use of radioactive iodine. The goal of the surgeon should be to remove as much gross tumor as possible, even in those patients with extensive invasion of the upper aerodigestive tract. These patients are frequently older, they tend to have larger, more often histologically undifferentiated tumors, and they carry a significantly poorer prognosis than those without airway invasion. In the series reported by Tsumori et al. (103), patients having resection of tumor invading the airway did significant better than patients whose smaller tumors were not resected. The use of radioactive iodine postoperatively is indicated in these patients wherever feasible.

Varma et al. (104) documented a decrease in death rate when surgery was followed by postoperative radioiodine therapy, over that of surgery alone. Similar conclusions were reached by Mazzaferri and Jhiang (37), Samaan et al. (38), and Beierwaltes (50) based on nonrandomized retrospective reviews. There is no conclusive evidence of benefit of radioiodine therapy in all patients with well-differentiated thyroid cancer. Tubiana et al. (100) and Simpson et al. (78) found radioiodine to be less effective than external irradiation in the control of local recurrence. Both groups, however, favored the use of both radioiodine and external radiotherapy wherever feasible, the former to detect distant metastases and to ablate remaining thyroid tissue in the appropriately prepared patient, and the latter to secure better local/regional control in the primary site and neck.

Factors influencing the uptake of radioiodine within metastatic thyroid tumors include the amount of residual normal thyroid tissue, serum TSH level, ambient serum iodine concentration, tumor type and differentiation, and patient age (22). Schlumberger and colleagues (105) have documented that, in approximately two thirds of patients with thyroid cancer, the metastatic thyroid cancer takes up sufficient radioiodine to be amenable to ablative therapy with I-131. Four variables had independent prognostic significance for survival: extensive metastases, older age at discovery of the metastases, absence of radioactive iodine uptake by the metastases, and moderately differentiated follicular cell type. The site of metastasis (lung or bone) was not a prognostic factor for survival after treatment of metastatic disease. Remission was achieved in only 79 of the 283 patients (28%) after metastases were found. The only predictor for 5-year disease-free survival after treatment of metastases was the original extent of disease. The authors concluded that metastases should be treated as early in the course of disease as possible. Radioactive iodine is more effective at eradicating small foci of neoplastic tissue than ablating macrometastases.

FOLLICULAR CARCINOMA

Follicular cancer represents a small proportion of the total cancer spectrum. These tumors are often solitary and are discovered in association with benign thyroid nodules or multinodular goiters. They tend to occur in areas of iodine deficiency. They often invade blood vessels and metastasize via hematogenous routes, with a smaller likelihood of regional nodal metastases.

The importance of differentiating between the follicular variant of papillary carcinoma and true follicular carcinoma cannot be overemphasized, because the behavior of the former is much more like that of papillary than follicular carcinoma. The overall treatment of follicular carcinoma is similar to that of papillary carcinoma, recognizing the significantly lower risk of regional/nodal metastasis and the higher risk of distant metastasis with follicular carcinomas. The expected survival of those patients over the age of 40 with follicular carcinoma is low, with greater disease-related mortality. Incomplete surgical excision significantly worsens the prognosis. Although most reports have not discussed treatment factors or estimation of prognosis, 30-year cancer mortality rates are likely to be higher in follicular cancers than papillary cancers because of the increased likelihood of adverse prognostic factors, including older age, larger tumors, and more mediastinal and distant involvement. In the Mazzaferri report (37), exclusion of distant metastases on admission resulted in similar papillary and follicular carcinoma mortality rates. When the patients were lumped together, the likelihood of cancer death increased with the factors of age over 40, tumor size greater than 1.5 cm, extracapsular invasion, regional/nodal metastases, and a delay in therapy over 12 months. The overall mortality rate was unaffected by tumor histologic type. The cumulative cancer mortality rate after radioiodine therapy in this series, regardless of the reason for its use, was one third that of patients not so treated.

Review of all patients who received their primary treatment for follicular thyroid cancer at the Mayo Clinic from 1946 to 1970 identified 57 female and 43 male patients with a mean of 17.4 years, and a maximum 32-year follow-up. All were treated surgically and only two of the 88 patients without distant metastases at the time of initial diagnosis underwent subsequent thyroid remnant ablation with radioiodine. Multivariate analysis of the data revealed that only age over 50 years, marked vascular invasion, and metastatic disease at the time of initial diagnosis were independent predictors of follicular cancer–related mortality. Patients with two or more of these factors were classified as high-risk. The survival percentages for the low-risk group were 99% at 5 years and 86% at 20 years, compared with the survival percentages for the high-risk group of 47% and 8%, respectively. There were no significant differences discovered between the various treatment regimens in this retrospective study. The presence of either extrathyroidal tumor extension or distant metastatic disease at the time of initial diagnosis carried a more ominous prognosis. Six of the 100 patients presented initially with regional lymph node metastases and only five were noted subsequently to have such metastases. Cervical nodal metastases did not adversely influence the overall survival. Local recurrence occurred in 5.1% at 10 years and 7.6% at 20 years in those 86 patients considered free of disease after the initial surgical procedure.

Thus, it is apparent that local/regional failure in adequately treated follicular carcinoma is much less frequent than in papillary cancer, and that the overall prognostic factors were similar to those with papillary carcinoma. The small follicular carcinoma, less than 1 cm in diameter with minimal invasion and without clinical evidence of regional or distant disease, is adequately treated by total thyroid lobectomy and isthmectomy. The rationale for total thyroidectomy in follicular carcinoma is essentially the same as in papillary carcinoma, and follicular carcinoma will require additional therapy in a higher proportion of patients (22).

HÜRTHLE CELL CARCINOMA

Hürthle cells are generally assumed to be variants of follicular cells but with distinctive cytoplasmic membranes; round, hyperchromatic, eccentrically placed nuclei with irregular chromatin; and finely granular cytoplasm with abundant mitochondria. Nodules of unencapsulated hyperplastic Hürthle cells may normally be found in the presence of benign disease including nodular goiter, Graves' disease, and Hashimoto's thyroiditis, and they represent metaplasia but not neoplasia. There are no characteristic cytologic differences between benign and malignant Hürthle cells, the diagnosis of carcinoma being made upon documentation of angioinvasion, capsular invasion, or metastatic disease. Most Hürthle cell and follicular neoplasms produce thyroglobulin. Hürthle cell tumors rarely take up radioiodine; they are commonly accompanied by regional lymph node metastases, and they are accompanied in 10% of patients by distant metastases. In 70% of patients, the disease is confined to the thyroid gland.

In a review of the Mayo Clinic experience with 1161 patients with well-differentiated thyroid cancer treated primarily at that institution, Hürthle cell carcinoma comprised 3.8% of the population. The female-to-male ratio in this series was 2:1, and the mean age was 55.5 years (108). Based on their experience with Hürthle cell neoplasms, McLeod and associates (109) concluded that all should be treated as malignant tumors, but more recent studies have suggested that both benign and malignant counterparts exist. Capsular invasion, lymph node involvement, and distant metastases clearly characterize malignant tumors. The presence of an aneuploid DNA nuclear content is frequently associated with increased risk of recurrence, distant metastases, and death.

In a review by McCloud and Thompson (109), approximately 30% of patients with Hürthle cell carcinoma were found to have coexisting or subsequent benign thyroid disease; from 7% to 39% had a history of previous head and neck irradiation; 70% to 80% present with disease confined to the thyroid gland; 11% present with lymph node metastases; and approximately 15% present with distant metastases. At one time, the authors regarded all Hürthle cell lesions larger than 2 cm as probably malignant, but a more recent review did not demonstrate a statistically significant correlation between tumor size and malignant behavior. Bilateral lesions are seen in 7% to 10% of patients with benign Hürthle cell neoplasms, but an incidence of bilateral disease as high as 40% has been reported for Hürthle cell carcinoma. Multifocal disease has been elsewhere noted in 18%, with an incidence of recurrent disease after subtotal thyroidectomy of approximately 3%.

Surgical treatment of any Hürthle cell thyroid lesion should include total lobectomy and isthmectomy with immediate frozen section analysis. In the presence of benign disease and no demonstrable contralateral thyroid abnormalities, the operative procedure is terminated at that point. A malignant diagnosis on frozen section analysis should stimulate critical assessment of the contralateral lobe, multiple frozen sections to assess the extent of disease within the resected specimen, and elective central compartment lymph adenectomy. If the patient had had previous head and neck irradiation exposure or has palpable disease in the contralateral lobe, or if the primary tumor is larger than 5 cm in diameter or is accompanied by regional lymph nodal metastases, then total thyroidectomy is recommended. In addition to removal of the central compartment lymph nodes, any suspicious nodes in the lateral neck should be resected via modified neck dissection. The adequacy of surgical resection of Hürthle cell carcinoma is paramount, because the disease frequently fails to respond to external irradiation or radioiodine therapy. If immunohistochemical studies show thyroglobulin within the tumor cells, and if serum thyroglobulin levels are elevated after total thyroidectomy, then radioiodine scintiscan should be performed after thyroid hormone administration is discontinued.

Unfortunately, this clinical setting is rare. Nuclear DNA ploidy in Hürthle cell carcinoma does not alone distinguish benign from malignant Hürthle cell tumors, but aneuploid carcinomas do behave more aggressively than did diploid tumors. In the M. D. Anderson Hospital experience documented by ElNaggar et al. (110), all patients with aneuploid carcinoma died of their disease or were alive with persistent tumors. In this limited series, none of the diploid carcinomas recurred or metastasized.

RESULTS OF TREATMENT

Most patients afflicted with well-differentiated thyroid carcinoma do well with conventional and conservative management. Most patients can be divided into low-risk and high-risk categories related to age, extrathyroidal extension, histology, adequacy of surgical treatment, and the presence or absence of distant metastases. In the Lahey Clinic series (73), the low-risk group comprised the overwhelming majority of the total series and had a death rate of only 1%, compared to the high-risk group comprising 11% of the patients who had a 46% mortality. In the Mayo Clinic series reported by Hay et al. (79), almost identical death rates in the low- and high-risk groups of papillary carcinomas were reported, at 2% and 46%, respectively.

Similarly, significant differences in overall results between the low- and high-risk groups can be identified in relation to response to treatment with surgery, radiation, and radioiodine. In those patients at high risk of local/regional failure, adequate surgical resection is paramount, up to and including total thyroidectomy and neck dissection (unilateral or bilateral), combined with mediastinal dissection and, in highly selected patients, resections of those portions of the upper aerodigestive tract significantly invaded by cancer. The extent of surgical resection is less prognostically significant in those patients with low risk of local regional failure, provided all gross tumor is adequately resected. No significant difference in overall long-term survival is noted between those patients treated by surgery alone and those treated by surgery plus adjunctive therapy, including radiation and radioiodine (78,104). External irradiation in appropriate dosage delivered to sufficiently large portals may be more effective in the control of local disease, whereas radioiodine is more effective in the detection of residual or metastatic disease and its eradication by intratumoral radiation.

The proportion of tumors that concentrate radioiodine is dependent on many factors, including patient age, proper preparation, the degree of differentiation, and other unknown factors. The efficacy of radioiodine is adversely affected by increasing tumor burden. In the cooperative Canadian study reported by Simpson et al. (78), 20-year survival varied widely in those patients in whom there was microscopic residual disease, depending on whether the patient had surgery alone or surgery plus radioiodine, with or without external irradiation. Survival varied from 35% in those patients treated surgically only, to over 80% in those patients having surgery plus additional radiation and/or radioiodine. Those patients with unresectable or incompletely resected disease leaving gross residual tumor did very poorly, with outcome much worse than for those whose surgery apparently resected gross tumor. In the same study, there appeared to be no significant difference with the addition of thyroid suppressive therapy on the specific survival of those patients with no residual or microscopic residual disease who are not treated with radioiodine or radiation therapy postoperatively. Less than half of the papillary cancers concentrated radioiodine, whereas two thirds of the follicular cancers did so.

When the final pathology report documents extension beyond the surgical margins, or the presence of foci of anaplastic carcinoma, the therapeutic decisions are difficult. Local invasions may be controlled by adjuvant therapy, but frequently anaplastic carcinoma relentlessly recurs, leading to the patient's death. The use of combined chemotherapy and radiation has been employed in high-risk patients in poorly differentiated papillary thyroid cancers and certain anaplastic cancers, with some improvement in response and extension of disease-free survival but few long-term cures (95). The value of chemotherapy for differentiated thyroid cancer is uncertain and largely disappointing, with very low response rates (78,111,112). Doxorubicin is the only antineoplastic agent with established activity in thyroid cancer, with a response rate of 30% to 45% reported, but with few complete remissions (113). The current role of chemotherapy may be as a chemosensitizer for radiation therapy in patients with poorly differentiated and anaplastic carcinomas. Much more work remains to be done to establish the role of systemic chemotherapy in the treatment of well-differentiated thyroid cancer. (See also Chapter 33.)

A rapidly increasing literature is accumulating that describes the role of molecular biology in neoplastic disease. TSH released by the pituitary gland is the predominant stimulator of thyroid growth, but there are multiple other thyroid growth stimulators and some inhibitors. Some of these growth factors, such as TSH, thyroid-stimulating immunoglobulin, and vasoactive intestinal polypeptide, work via the adenylate cyclase protein kinase, a signal transduction system. Others work via the phosphoinositide–protein kinase system, and still others work via a tyrosine kinase system. In addition, four growth-stimulatory proteins (GSP, RET, and TRK) and one inhibitory protein p53 have been identified as primary targets for mutations in human thyroid tumors. The tumor-suppressor gene, p53, has an incidence of 42% in anaplastic thyroid cancer but is rarely found in well-differentiated cancer. Further studies will be necessary to document the role and significance of these growth, inhibitory, and genetic product factors (22). (See Chapters 10, 13, and 28.)

SUMMARY

Neoplastic disease of the thyroid gland represents a varied, complex, and fascinating spectrum. Patients can be categorized into low- and high-risk categories, and treatment results can be predicted based on simple clinical parameters. Most patients respond well to adequate surgical resection, with a small segment of high-risk patients requiring more radical surgery and adjunctive irradiation and/or radioiodine treatment. There is no documentation that more radical surgery in low-risk patients will add significantly to the overall prognosis, but it will add to the potential for morbid complications. Patients with advanced tumors do significantly worse, probably unrelated to surgical management, and require more additional adjuvant and aggressive treatment, including radiation and/or radioiodine, in attempts to control this high-risk disease. Early diagnosis and effective surgical management in most patients result in excellent local/regional control and survival, especially in low-risk patients.

REFERENCES

1. Rojeski MT, Gharib H. Nodular thyroid disease. Evaluation and management. *N Engl J Med* 1985;313:428–436.
2. Maxon HR, Thomas SR, Saenger EL, et al. Ionizing irradiation and the induction of clinically significant disease in the human thyroid gland. *Am J Med* 1977;63:967–978.
3. Hauson GA, Komorowski RA, Cerletty JM, et al. Thyroid gland morphology in young adults: normal subjects versus those with prior low-dose neck irradiation in childhood. *Surgery* 1983;94:984–988.
4. Mortensen JD, Wollner LB, Bennett WA. Gross and microscopic findings in clinically normal thyroid glands. *J Clin Endocrinol Metab* 1955;15:1270–1280.
5. Clark OH, Duh QY. Thyroid cancer. *Med Clin North Am* 1991;75:211–234.
6. Fukunaga FH, Yatani R. Geographic pathology of occult thyroid carcinomas. *Cancer* 1975;36:1095–1099.
7. Komorowski RA, Hanson GA. Morphologic changes in the thyroid following low dose childhood irradiation. *Arch Pathol Lab Med* 1977;101:36–39.
8. Spitalnik PF, Straus FH. Patterns of human thyroid parenchymal reaction following low dose childhood irradiation. *Cancer* 1978;41:1098–1105.
9. Wilson SD, Komorowski R, Cerletty J, et al. Radiation associated thyroid tumors: extent of operation and pathologic technique influence the apparent incidence of carcinoma. *Surgery* 1983;94:663–669.
10. Hedinger C, Williams ED, Sobin LH. The WHO histological classification of thyroid tumors: a commentary on the second edition. *Cancer* 1989;63:908–911.
11. Harach HR, Franssila KO, Wasenius VM. Occult papillary carcinoma of the thyroid. A "normal" finding in Finland. A systematic autopsy study. *Cancer* 1985;56:531–538.
12. Sampson RJ, Oka H, Key CR, Buncher CR, Iijima S. Metastases from occult thyroid carcinoma: an autopsy study from Hiroshima and Nagasaki, Japan. *Cancer* 1970;25:803–811.
13. Allo MD, Christianson W, Koivunen D. Not all "occult" papillary carcinomas are "minimal." *Surgery* 1988;104:971–976.
14. Rosen IB, Azadian A, Walfish PG. Adverse aspects of small thyroid cancer and need for treatment. *Head Neck* 1995;17:373–376.
15. Hay ID, Grant CS, van Heerden JA, et al. Papillary thyroid microcarcinoma: a study of 535 cases observed in a 50-year period. *Surgery* 1992;112:1139–1147.
16. Parker SL, Tong T, Bolden S, et al. Cancer statistics, 1996. *CA Cancer J Clin* 1996;65:5–27.
17. Waterhouse J, Muir C, Shanmugaratnam K, Powell J, eds. Cancer incidence in five countries, vol IV. IARC Scientific Publications no. 42. Lyon: International Agency for Research on Cancer, 1982.
18. Weiss W. Changing incidence of thyroid cancer. *J Natl Cancer Inst* 1979;62:1137–1142.
19. Carroll RE, Hadden W Jr, Handy VH, Wieben EE Sr. Thyroid cancer: cohort analysis of increasing incidence in New York State, 1941–1962. *J Natl Cancer Inst* 1964;33:277–283.
20. Komorowski RA, Hanson GA. Occult thyroid pathology in the young adult: an autopsy study of 138 patients without clinical thyroid disease. *Hum Pathol* 1988;19:689–696.
21. Goodman MT, Yoshizawa CN, Kolonel LN. Descriptive epidemiology of thyroid cancer in Hawaii. *Cancer* 1988;61:1272–1281.
22. Jossart GH, Clark OH. Well-differentiated thyroid cancer. *Curr Probl Surg* 1994;31:935–1012.
23. Shah JP. Personal communication.
24. Shah JP, Loree TR, Dharker D, et al. Prognostic factors in differentiated carcinoma of the thyroid gland. *Am J Surg* 1992;164:658–661.
25. LiVolsi VA. Papillary neoplasms of the thyroid, pathologic and prognostic features. *Am J Clin Pathol* 1992;3:426–434.
26. Hutter RVP, Tollefsen HR, DeCosse JJ, Foote FW Jr, Frazell EL. Spindle and giant cell metaplasia in papillary carcinoma of the thyroid. *Am J Surg* 1965;110:660–668.
27. Reinhoff WF. The lymphatic vessels of the thyroid gland in the dog and in man. *Arch Surg* 1931;23:783–804.
28. Russell WO, Ibanez ML, Clark RL, White EC. Thyroid carcinoma—classification, intraglandular dissemination, and clinicopathological study based upon whole organ sections of 80 glands. *Cancer* 1963;16:1425–1460.
29. Sloan LW. Of origin, characteristics, and behavior of thyroid cancer. *J Clin Endocrinol* 1954;14:1309–1335.
30. Frazell EL, Foote FW Jr. Papillary cancer of the thyroid. A review of 25 years of experience. *Cancer* 1958;11:895–992.
31. Tollefsen HR, Shah JP, Huvos AG. Papillary carcinoma of the thyroid. *Am J Surg* 1972;124:468–472.
32. Buckwalter JA, Thomas CC Jr. Selection of surgical treatment for well differentiated thyroid carcinomas. *Ann Surg* 1972;176:565–578.
33. Mazzaferri EL, Young RL, Oertel JE, et al. Papillary carcinoma of the thyroid: the impact of therapy in 576 patients. *Medicine* 1977;56:171–196.
34. Rose RG, Kelsey MP, Russell WO, et al. Follow-up study of thyroid cancer treated by unilateral lobectomy. *Am J Surg* 1963;106:494–500.
35. Simpson WJ, McKinney SE, Carruthers JS, et al. Papillary and follicular thyroid cancer. Prognostic factors in 1578 patients. *Am J Med* 1987;83:479–488.
36. DeGroot LJ, Kaplan EL, McCormick M, et al. Natural history, treatment and course of papillary thyroid carcinoma. *J Clin Endocrinol Metab* 1990;71:414–424.

37. Mazzaferri EL, Jhiang SM. Long term impact of initial surgical and medical therapy on papillary and follicular thyroid cancer. *Am J Med* 1994;97:418–428.
38. Samaan NA, Schultz PN, Hickey RC, et al. The results of various modalities of treatment of well differentiated thyroid carcinoma. A retrospective review of 1599 patients. *J Clin Endocrinol Metab* 1992;75:714–720.
39. Thompson NW, Nishiyama RH, Harness JK. Thyroid carcinoma: current controversies. *Curr Probl Surg* 1978;15:1–67.
40. Grant CS, Hay ID, Gough IR, Bergstralh EJ, et al. Local recurrence in papillary thyroid carcinoma: is extent of surgical resection important? *Surgery* 1988;104:954–962.
41. Silverberg SG, Hutter RVP, Foote FW. Fatal carcinoma of the thyroid: histology, metastasis and causes of death. *Cancer* 1970;25:792–802.
42. Beahrs OH, Vandertoll DJ. Complications of secondary thyroidectomy. *Surg Gynecol Obstet* 1963;117:535–539.
43. Clark OH. Total thyroidectomy. The treatment of choice for patients with differentiated thyroid cancer. *Ann Surg* 1982;196:361–370.
44. Harness JK, Fung L, Thompson NW, et al. Total thyroidectomy: complications and technique. *World J Surg* 1986;10:781–786.
45. Hay ID. Papillary thyroid cancer. *Endocrinol Metab Clin North Am* 1990;19:545–576.
46. Foster RS. Morbidity and mortality after thyroidectomy. *Surg Gynecol Obstet* 1978;146:423–429.
47. Wingert DJ, Friesen SR, Iliopoulos J, et al. Post thyroidectomy hypocalcemia. Incidence and risk factors. *Am J Surg* 1986;152:606–610.
48. Schroder DM, Chambors A, France CJ. Operative strategy for thyroid cancer. Is total thyroidectomy worth the price? *Cancer* 1986;58:2320–2328.
49. VanHeerden JA, Groh MA, Grant CS. Early postoperative morbidity after surgical treatment of thyroid carcinoma. *Surgery* 1987;161:224–227.
50. Beierwaltes WH. The treatment of thyroid carcinoma with radioiodine. *Semin Nucl Med* 1978;8:79–94.
51. Attie JN, Moskowitz GW, Margouleff D, et al. Feasibility of total thyroidectomy in the treatment of thyroid carcinoma. Postoperative radioiodine evaluation of 140 cases. *Am J Surg* 1979;138:555–560.
52. Beierwaltes WH, Rabboni R, Durachowski C, et al. An analysis of "ablation of thyroid remnants" with I131 in 511 patients from 1947–1984: experience at the University of Michigan. *J Nucl Med* 1984;25:1287–1293.
53. Cady B, Sedgewick CE, Meissneer WA, et al. Changing clinical, pathologic therapeutic and survival patterns in differentiated thyroid carcinoma. *Ann Surg* 1976;184:541–553.
54. McConahey WM, Hay ID, Woolner LB, et al. Papillary thyroid cancer treated at the Mayo Clinic, 1946 through 1970: initial manifestations, pathologic findings, therapy and outcome. *Mayo Clinic Proc* 1986;61:976–996.
55. Brooks JR, Starnes F, Brooks DC, et al. Surgical therapy for thyroid carcinoma: a review of 1249 solitary thyroid nodules. *Surgery* 1988;104:940–946.
56. Hughes CJ, Shaha AR, Shah JP, et al. Impact of lymph node metastases in differentiated carcinoma of the thyroid: a matched pair analysis. *Head Neck* 1996;18:127–132.
57. Harwood J, Clark OH, Dunphy JE. Significance of lymph node metastases in differentiated thyroid cancer. *Am J Surg* 1978;136:107–112.
58. Young RL, Mazzaferri EL, Rahea J, Dorfman SG. Pure follicular thyroid cancer: impact of therapy in 214 patients. *J Nucl Med* 1980;21:733–737.
59. Tollefsen HR, Shah JP, Huvos AG. Follicular carcinoma of the thyroid. *Am J Surg* 1973;126:523–528.
60. Franssila KO. Is the differentiation between papillary and follicular carcinoma valid? *Cancer* 1973;32:853–864.
61. Tennvall J, Biorklund A, Moller T, et al. Is the EORTC prognostic index of thyroid cancer valid in differentiated thyroid carcinoma? Retrospective multivariate analysis of differentiated thyroid carcinoma with long follow up. *Cancer* 1986;57:1405–1414.
62. Farrar WB, Cooperman M, James AG. Surgical management of papillary and follicular carcinoma of the thyroid. *Ann Surg* 1980;192:701–704.
63. Shaha AR, Lore TR, Shah JP. Prognostic factors and risk group analysis in follicular carcinoma of the thyroid. *Surgery* 1995;118:1131–1138.
64. Cunningham MP, Duda RB, Recant W, et al. Survival discriminants for differentiated thyroid cancer. *Am J Surg* 1990;160:344–347.
65. Noguchi S, Murakami N. The value of lymph node dissection in patients with differentiated thyroid cancer. *Surg Clin North Am* 1987;67:251–261.
66. Frazell EL, Foote FW Jr. Papillary thyroid carcinoma: pathological findings in cases with and without clinical evidence of cervical node involvement. *Cancer* 1955;8:1164–1166.
67. Frable WJ. The treatment of thyroid cancer. The role of fine needle aspiration cytology. *Arch Otolaryngol Head Neck Surg* 1986;112:1200–1203.
68. Ramacciotti CE, Pretorius HT, Chu EW, et al. Diagnostic accuracy and use of aspiration biopsy in the management of thyroid nodules. *Arch Intern Med* 1984;144:1169–1173.
69. McDermott W, Morgan S, Hamlin EJ. Cancer of the thyroid. *J Clin Endocrinol Metab* 1954;14:1336–1354.
70. Tollefsen HR, DeCosse JJ, Hutter RVP. Papillary carcinoma of the thyroid. A clinical and pathological study of 70 fatal cases. *Cancer* 1964;17:1035–1044.
71. Halnan KE. Influence of age and sex on incidence and prognosis of thyroid cancer. Three hundred and forty-four cases followed for 10 years. *Cancer* 1966;11:1534–1536.
72. Cady B, Sedgewick CE, Meissner WA, et al. Risk factor analysis in differentiated thyroid cancer. *Cancer* 1979;43:810–820.
73. Cady B, Rossi R. An expanded view of risk group definition in differentiated thyroid cancer. *Surgery* 1988;104:947–953.
74. Byar DP, Green SB, Dor P, et al. A prognostic index for thyroid carcinoma. A study of the E.O.R.T.C. Thyroid Cancer Cooperative Group. *Eur J Cancer* 1979;15:1033–1041.
75. Ito I, Noguchi S, Murakami N, Noguchi I. Factors affecting the prognosis of patients with carcinoma of the thyroid. *Surg Gynec Obstet* 1980;150:535–544.
76. Tennvall J, Biorklund A, Moller T, et al. Prognostic factors of papillary, follicular and medullary carcinomas of the thyroid gland. *Acta Radiol Oncol* 1985;24:17–24.
77. Bacourt F, Asselain B, Savoie JC, et al. Multifactorial study of prognostic factors in differentiated thyroid carcinoma and a reevaluation of the importance of age. *Br J Surg* 1986;73:274–277.
78. Simpson WJ, Panyarella T, Carruthers JS, et al. Papillary and follicular thyroid cancer: impact of treatment in 1578 patients. *Int J Radiat Oncol Biol Phys* 1988;14:1063–1075.
79. Hay ID, Grant CS, Taylor WF, et al. Ipsilateral lobectomy vs. bilateral lobar resection in papillary thyroid carcinoma: a retrospective analysis of surgical outcome using a novel prognostic scoring system. *Surgery* 1987 102:1088–1095.
80. Pasieka JL, Zedenius J, Auer G, et al. Addition of nuclear DNA content to the AMES risk-group classification for papillary thyroid cancer. *Surgery* 1992;112:1154–1160.
81. Backdahl M, Carstensen J, Auer G, et al. Statistical evaluation of the prognostic value of nuclear DNA content in papillary, follicular and medullary thyroid tumors. *World J Surg* 1986;10:974–980.
82. Joensuu H, Klemi P, Eerola E, et al. Influence of cellular DNA content on survival in differentiated thyroid carcinoma. *Cancer* 1986;58:2462–2467.
83. Hay I, Bergstralh E, Goellner J, et al. Predicting outcome in papillary thyroid carcinoma: development of a reliable prognostic scoring system in a cohort of 1779 patients surgically treated at one institution during 1940 through 1989. *Surgery* 1993;114:1050–1058.
84. Block MA. Management of carcinoma of the thyroid. *Ann Surg* 1977;185:133–144.
85. Fratkin MJ, Newsome HH Jr, Sharpe AR, Tatum JL. Cervical distribution of iodine[131] following total thyroidectomy for thyroid cancer. *Arch Surg* 1983;118:864–867.
86. Harness JK, Fung L, Thompson ND, et al. Total thyroidectomy: complications and technique. *World J Surg* 1986;10:781–786.
87. Lore JM. Practical anatomical considerations in thyroid tumor surgery. *Arch Otolaryngol* 1983;109:568–574.
88. Andersen PE, Kinsella J, Loree TR, et al. Differentiated carcinoma of the thyroid with extrathyroidal extension. *Am J Surg* 1995;170:467–470.
89. Breaux EP, Guillamondegui DM. Treatment of locally invasive carcinoma of the thyroid: how radical? *Am J Surg* 1980;140:514–517.
90. McCaffrey TV, Bergstralh EJ, Hay ID. Locally invasive papillary thyroid carcinoma: 1940–1990. *Head Neck* 1994;16:165–172.

91. Lawson VG. The management of airway involvement in thyroid tumors. *Arch Otolaryngol* 1983;109:86–90.
92. Grillo HC, Zannini P. Resectional management of airway invasion by thyroid carcinoma. *Ann Thorac Surg* 1986;42:287–298.
93. Lipton RJ, McCaffrey TV, van Heerden JA. Surgical treatment of invasion of the upper aerodigestive tract by well differentiated thyroid carcinoma. *Am J Surg* 1987;154:363–367.
94. Tovi F, Goldstein J. Locally aggressive differentiated thyroid carcinoma. *J Surg Oncol* 1985;29:99–104.
95. Kim JH, Leeper RD. Treatment of locally advanced thyroid carcinoma with combination of doxorubicin and radiation therapy. *Cancer* 1987;60:2372–2375.
96. Frankenthaler RA, Sellin RV, Conger A, et al. Lymph node metastases from papillary-follicular thyroid carcinoma in young patients. *Am J Surg* 1990;160:341–343.
97. Sellers M, Beenken S, Blankenship A, et al. Prognostic significance of cervical lymph node metastases in differentiated thyroid cancer. *Am J Surg* 1992;164:578–581.
98. Coburn MC, Wanebo HJ. Prognostic factors and management considerations in patients with cervical metastases of thyroid cancer. *Am J Surg* 1992;164:671–675.
99. Hughes CJ, Shaha AR, Shah JP, et al. Impact of lymph node metastasis in differentiated carcinoma of the thyroid: a matched pair analysis. *Head Neck* 1996;18:127–132.
100. Tubiana M, Haddad E, Schlumberger M, et al. External radiotherapy in thyroid cancer. *Cancer* 1985;55:2062–2071.
101. Benken G, Olbricht T, Reinwein D, et al. Survival rates in patients with differentiated thyroid carcinoma. Influence of postoperative external radiotherapy. *Cancer* 1990;65:1517–1520.
102. Farahati J, Reiners C, Stuschke M, et al. Differentiated thyroid cancer. Impact of adjuvant external radiotherapy in patients with perithyroidal tumor infiltration (stage pT4). *Cancer* 1996;77:172–180.
103. Tsumori T, Nakao K, Miyata M, et al. Clinicopathologic study of thyroid carcinoma infiltrating the trachea. *Cancer* 1985;56:2843–2848.
104. Varma VM, Beierwaltes WH, Nofal MM. Treatment of thyroid cancer. Death rates after surgery and after surgery followed by sodium iodide I-131. *JAMA* 1970;214:1437–1448.
105. Schlumberger M, Tubiana M, deVathaire F, et al. Long term results of treatment of 283 patients with lung and bone metastases from differentiated thyroid carcinoma. *J Clin Endocrinol Metab* 1986;63:960–967.
106. Crile G Jr. The endocrine dependency of certain thyroid cancers and the danger that hypothyroidism may stimulate their growth. *Cancer* 1957;10:1119–1137.
107. Brennan MD, Bergstralh EJ, VanHeerden JA, et al. Follicular thyroid cancer treated at the Mayo Clinic 1946–1970: initial manifestations, pathologic findings therapy and outcome. *Mayo Clin Proc* 1991;66:11–22.
108. Watson RG, Brennan MD, Goellner JR, et al. Invasive Hürthle cell carcinoma of the thyroid: natural history and management. *Mayo Clin Proc* 1984;59:851–855.
109. McLeod MK, Thompson NW. Hürthle cell neoplasms of the thyroid gland. *Otolaryngol Clin North Am* 1990;23:441–452.
110. ElNaggar AK, Batsakis JG, Luna MA, et al. Hürthle cell tumors of the thyroid. A flow cytometric DNA analysis. *Arch Otolaryngol Head Neck Surg* 1988;114:520–521.
111. Shimaoka K, Schoenfeld DA, deWys WD, et al. A randomized trial of doxorubicin versus doxorubicin plus cisplatin in patients with advanced thyroid cancer. *Cancer* 1985;56:2155–2160.
112. Williams SD, Birch R, Einhorn LH. Phase II evaluation of doxorubicin plus cisplatin in advanced thyroid cancer. *Cancer Treat Rep* 1986;70:405–407.
113. Shimaoka K. There is benefit from chemotherapy for thyroid cancer. *Prog Surg* 1988;19:163–169.

CHAPTER 30

Thyroglobulin in Benign and Malignant Thyroid Disease

Andre J. Van Herle and Katja Anna Van Herle

Many publications have been devoted to the study of the thyroglobulin (Tg) molecule, a 660,000-dalton glycoprotein, produced exclusively by the thyroid gland. In recent years, major advances have expanded our knowledge of its structure, function, immunogenicity, and presence in the circulation in various physiologic and pathologic conditions. The increased knowledge about its appearance in the circulation, its regulation, and its dysregulation has added a new page to thyroidology, which we discuss in this chapter. Extensive reviews of the topic form the basis for the present discussion (1–4).

METHODOLOGY OF TG MEASUREMENTS, AND ITS LIMITATIONS

Various assay systems have been used to measure Tg in the serum, but it was not until the practical, clinically applicable radioimmunoassay (RIA) system was developed (5) that the knowledge in this field expanded rapidly. Most measurements of Tg in the serum are based on a double RIA system, although enzyme-linked immunosorbent assays (ELISA) and immunoradiometric assays (IRMA) are also extensively used. Monoclonal antibodies have also been used to develop assay systems, but in general they do not provide the same sensitivity as RIA and IRMA (<1.0 ng/mL). The specificity of these assays has been extensively tested, and thyronines that normally circulate abundantly in plasma do not cross-react in these assays. Anti-Tg autoantibodies (ATA) (5–7) interfere with the assays, but cross-reaction with other circulating substances is not clearly documented.

A. J. Van Herle, K. A. Van Herle: Department of Medicine, Division of Endocrinology, UCLA School of Medicine, Los Angeles, California 90024.

It became apparent that the normal ranges for serum Tg concentrations in humans as determined by various laboratories were vastly different. Two large international studies involving many laboratories across the United States (8) and Europe (9) clearly make this point. Both studies were conducted by blind submission of identical human sera with known concentrations of Tg to a number of laboratories. The conclusions reached by both studies were twofold. They demonstrated that the serum Tg levels obtained by different laboratories for a given thyroid disorder (e.g., thyroid cancer) cannot be compared unless every component of the RIA (or whatever assay system is being used) is identical in all the laboratories. The variations among laboratories involve all components of the assay: the Tg standards, the antibodies (first and second antibody for RIAs), and the characteristic of the label. All of these elements can play a critical role in the definition of the normal range, and consequently, the abnormal range. In general, the sensitivity of many assays varies from 1.0 to 3.0 ng/mL, and the normal range varies from 0 to 30 ng/mL, although wider ranges are frequently reported (10,11). Serum Tg levels in normal subjects and in patients with various thyroid disorders measured by our RIA system appear in Table 1. An International thyroglobulin standard has been recently made available (CRM 457) by the European Commission (12).

SERUM TG LEVELS IN NEONATES AND ADOLESCENTS

Several studies, including our own, have indicated that cord blood Tg levels are higher than those observed in the corresponding pregnant mother (5) (Fig. 1). This difference in serum Tg levels between the mother and the newborn has been used as an argument for the lack of

TABLE 1. Serum Tg levels in normal subjects and patients with various pathologic conditions of the thyroid gland

Condition (ref.)	Mean±SEM (ng/mL)	No. of subjects
Control subjects (blood donors) (5)	5.1±0.49	95
Cord blood (5)	29.3±4.7	23
Pregnancy (delivery) (5)	10.1±1.3	23
Active Graves' disease (40)	176.0±30.0	33
Euthyroid Graves' disease (40)	6.8±1.25	10
Non-Graves' disease thyrotoxicosis (40)	145.0±27.0	7
Subacute thyroiditis (acute phase) (5)	136.8±74.5	12
Differentiated thyroid carcinoma (all histologic types) (124)	103.4±125.6	32
Metastatic thyroid carcinoma (differentiated type) (51)	464.9±155.6	6
Medullary thyroid carcinoma (51)	4.9±1.6	6
Thyroid adenoma (125)	424.6±189.4	27
Endemic goiter (34)	208.1±19.8	77

From ref. 126, with permission.

transplacental transport of Tg from the fetus to the mother. Earlier studies performed in rats with radiolabeled Tg indicated that transplacental transport of Tg does not occur in either direction. The mechanisms of elevated serum Tg levels in cord blood have not been elucidated.

A recent study indicated that no correlation exists between the cord blood Tg concentration and thyroid stimulating hormone (TSH) concentration (13). Roti et al. (14) found that, after the administration of thyrotropin-releasing hormone (TRH) to mothers, cord blood TSH levels were markedly increased, yet no rise in cord serum Tg was observed. Black et al. (15) found that in a euthyroid group of "well" full-term infants, an increase in Tg occurred postnatally, which was not seen in "ill" full-term, or pre-term neonates. However, thyroid hormone levels were lower and TSH levels were higher in the "ill" and pre-term groups. This implies that there is a decreased thyroidal secretion of Tg in the latter group. In a study by Pacini et al. (16), however, cord Tg levels correlated positively with cord TSH levels in 200 newborns. This study is in agreement with levels obtained in children (17) and adults, and it suggests that Tg secretion is influenced by TSH (18,19).

The cause of the Tg surge that occurs in the infant during the first weeks of life is subject to controversy. Indeed, besides the intense release of Tg after the burst of endogenously released TSH in the first 12 hr after delivery (19), the elevated Tg may also reflect a decreased metabolic clearance rate of Tg by the immature liver of the newborn. Because Tg release has also been reported to correlate with the ratio of the weight of the thyroid gland to body weight [Torrigiani et al. (20)], it stands to reason that Tg levels are increased in cord blood, because this ratio is also increased in the newborn (21). Finally, because the perinatal thyroid gland produces hypoiodinated Tg (22), as in simple goiter, and because Tg hypoiodination leads to increased intraglandular Tg turnover and Tg hypersecretion, this mechanism could also account for the increased Tg level in the newborn. The role, if any, of the increased Tg in the neonate is unclear. Because the level of Tg in the newborn is controlled by multiple factors, it follows that various conditions of the newborn can affect the Tg level.

Although an undetectable serum Tg level in a newborn does not exclude the presence of a normal or hypofunctional gland, the athyreotic state should be accompanied by an undetectable level, and this is demonstrated by Ket et al. (13), Black et al. (15), Osotimehin et al. (23), and Czernichow et al. (24). In hypothyroid children discovered by the neonatal screening program, serum Tg can be used for the diagnosis of athyroidism if one can exclude the rare cases of congenital goiter with Tg synthesis defect described in humans (25) and goats (26). Czernichow et al. (24) showed that neonates with ectopic or eutopic hypoplastic glands all had detectable serum Tg levels, and the levels exceeded the mean concentration in normal controls.

Other factors, such as prematurity, can influence the absolute Tg levels in the newborn. Indeed, Ket et al. (13) have shown that the cord serum median Tg of premature neonates [102.0 ng/mL (27 to 38 weeks of gestation, n = 45)] was significantly higher than the median Tg level of 73.0 ng/mL of mature newborns (38 to 43 weeks of gestation, n = 158). In the premature group, a significant negative correlation was found between gestational age and the cord serum Tg level. No difference was found in cord Tg level between normal and sick full-term infants, or between normal and sick premature infants. The mean serum TSH level in sera with higher Tg levels (150 to 251 ng/mL) did not differ statistically from those with lower

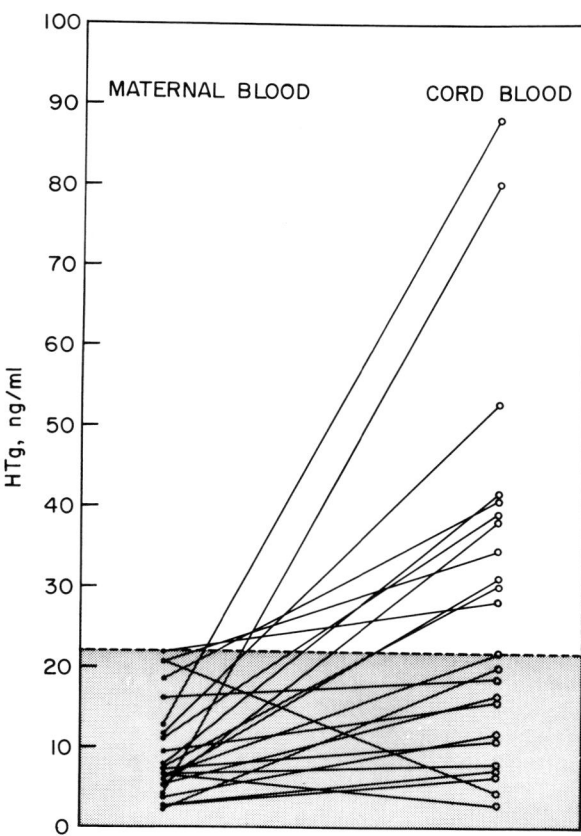

FIG. 1. Thyroglobulin concentrations in 23 maternal and cord blood sera obtained at delivery. Serum Tg levels in the mother are connected with the level in their respective infants. The *shaded area* represents the range for normal adult women. (From ref. 5, with permission.)

Tg levels (10 to 30 ng/mL). These data contrast with those from Penny et al. (27), who found a positive correlation between serum Tg and the log of the TSH levels in at least the female newborns. They also found that a difference existed in cord serum Tg levels of female infants with a low birth weight, as compared to males with a higher birth weight, which was attributed to differences in body composition rather than sex. Pacini et al. (16) showed increased cord blood Tg levels in small-for-gestational-age newborns, when compared to normal newborns. Ericsson and coworkers (28), in contrast, have found no correlation between the median cord Tg concentration, gestational age at delivery, birth rate, sex of the child, or the median cord TSH concentration. The median cord Tg, however, was significantly higher in children born by cesarean section than in those delivered by vacuum extraction. The median cord Tg concentration in children of smoking mothers was also significantly higher than in children of nonsmoking mothers (130 ng/mL versus 100 ng/mL, $p < .001$) (28). Sava and coworkers (29) have found that in an iodine-deficient area of Sicily, the newborn serum Tg levels are higher than in areas not iodine deficient, and they propose that the degree of Tg iodination partially determines Tg levels at birth.

Thus, a large variability of the Tg level in the newborn exists. A number of mechanisms have been proposed for the elevated serum Tg levels in the newborn. Rather unanimous findings are the higher Tg levels at birth, the increment in serum Tg levels in normal neonates after birth, and the subsequent decline of these levels. The absence of Tg in the serum of athyreotic infants is also supported by several studies, so that thyroid agenesis becomes a very likely diagnosis in the absence of detectable serum Tg levels. The serum Tg levels decline in the first 10 months after birth and reach the steady levels prevalent during the first decade of life (13). This decline in serum Tg levels has also been shown in individual cases (13). A similar age-related decrease of Tg in infants was reported by Pacini et al. (16), and in adolescents by Penny et al. (17). In the latter study, there were no significant differences in mean chronological age and serum Tg levels between boys and girls, and serum TSH correlated negatively with chronological age. The authors speculated that the progressive decline of serum Tg levels may represent a continuous process that is initiated *in utero* (17). The observation that TSH declines with age argues in favor of the stimulatory contribution of TSH to the observed Tg levels.

SERUM TG LEVELS IN NORMAL ADULTS

Serum Tg levels are usually steady in an individual from day to day; no major excursions seem to occur (5). Diurnal variation of serum Tg levels has not been observed in rodents (30) and was not studied in humans. No substantial rise of serum Tg levels occurs after manual, external palpation of the thyroid gland; however, the rise of serum Tg levels after open manipulation of the thyroid gland has been reported (31). Percutaneous fine-needle aspiration (FNA) biopsy of the thyroid gland leads to a rise in serum Tg levels in certain subjects, and consequently serum samples for Tg measurement should be obtained prior to FNA (31).

A recent study performed in Sweden has found a higher level of serum Tg (>30 ng/mL) in smokers (37% of smokers had elevated levels with this criterion, versus 18% of nonsmokers) (32). The authors concluded that cigarette smoking may promote goiter formation and thus increase the release of Tg. Smoking has not been considered in establishing the normal range in most laboratories. The differences in normal ranges in the various laboratories could be related to the incidental predominant selection of smokers versus nonsmokers.

The mechanism by which Tg molecules enter the circulation is still largely unknown and subject to debate, although studies in animals and humans suggest that Tg reaches the circulation via the lymphatics. It is likely that there are multiple factors that control the secretion. Studies have shown convincingly that administration of exogenous TSH, intramuscularly (33) or intravenously (34), leads to an increment in Tg release. The rise of Tg after TRH administration confirms these data (33,35).

Additional evidence supporting a stimulatory role of TSH is derived from the positive correlation observed between serum Tg concentration and the log of serum TSH levels in endemic goiter patients (36). Another stimulator that could induce elevated Tg levels is the presence of thyroid-stimulating antibodies (TSAb) (30), and the increased serum Tg levels observed in pregnancy could be related to the weak thyroid stimulatory effect of human chorionic gonadotropin (HCG). Other regulatory factors could affect serum levels, such as a change in the metabolic clearance rate of Tg. Because Tg is a glycoprotein and is cleared by the liver, a profound liver insufficiency may, for example, contribute to elevated Tg levels, as seen in liver cirrhosis (37). Finally, reduced iodination of Tg, seen in patients with goiters and the newborn, renders Tg more susceptible to *in vitro* hydrolysis and causes Tg to be more readily released from the thyroid gland. This mechanism may be responsible for the increased Tg levels in goitrous patients as well as in the newborn (29).

In adults, an age dependence was described by one group of investigators, but in this study Tg levels increased significantly with age only in women (38). Several studies have indicated the presence of higher Tg levels in women than in men. Also, Tg levels of estrogen-treated women were higher than in a control group (39). This study suggests the possibility that estrogens are involved in the physiologic regulation of Tg release. Estrogens, however, cannot explain the age-related increase in Tg levels reported by Feldt-Rasmussen et al. (38), because estrogen levels decline with advancing age in women, and it is not stated in these studies that the patients were treated with estrogens (38). The higher incidence of elevated serum Tg levels in smokers could, for example, account for the observed differences in the normal population; also, the inclusion of subjects with hepatic disease may play a role in the differences (37). The increased Tg concentration during pregnancy may also be estrogen related; however, the presence of HCG and its mild thyroid stimulatory effect is more likely responsible.

HYPERTHYROIDISM IN GRAVES' DISEASE

Graves' disease is an autoimmune disorder that usually leads to diffuse thyroid enlargement and hyperthyroxinemia. In nearly all patients with active Graves' disease, serum Tg levels have been found to be elevated (3,40–42). In contrast, in subjects with euthyroid Graves' disease, levels have been found to be normal (see Table 1). Thyroid-stimulating immunoglobulins (TSI) present in the serum of patients with Graves' disease play a causative role in the increased serum Tg and hormone levels observed in man. Indeed, serum Tg levels increase in rats after the injection of TSIs (30). A number of studies have indicated that serum Tg levels can be predictive of the outcome of Graves' disease following antithyroid drug therapy (40–42). These findings are not surprising, because TSI levels decline in certain patients following antithyroid drug therapy, and consequently the stimulatory effect on the thyroid gland and the ensuing Tg synthesis and secretion also decrease. Uller and Van Herle (40) and Gardner and coworkers (41) found that the remission rate was higher in patients with relatively low serum Tg levels who were on antithyroid drug therapy. These data were later confirmed by Kawamura et al. (42). In general, a tendency for serum Tg levels to normalize occurs in patients who go into remission on propylthiouracil (PTU) or methimazole (Tapazole) therapy (40–42). In contrast, no change in the mean serum Tg levels was seen in subjects whose condition worsened after discontinuation of therapy.

These studies could not be confirmed by others (43,44) for reasons that are not clear but may include different RIA methodology or patient population selection. Two limiting factors for the use of Tg as a predictive test in Graves' disease must be kept in mind. First, Tg levels cannot be measured accurately in patients with positive ATA titers, and second, Tg levels have no predictive value in patients who are overtreated with antithyroid drugs, because of the thyroid stimulatory role of TSH on Tg release. Therefore, it is mandatory to measure ATA titers as well as TSH levels in all patients. Normal Tg levels are frequently noted in those patients in whom a long-term remission occurs. If a recurrence develops in patients with relatively low Tg levels, a rise of Tg may be the first signal of future exacerbation, even prior to the rise in T_3 and T_4 levels (42). In patients who were treated with subtotal thyroidectomy for Graves' disease, a rapid decline in serum Tg levels occurred after an initial postoperative surge. In those patients treated with radioactive iodine, however, a gradual and sustained increase in Tg levels is observed, followed by a decline when hypothyroidism or euthyroidism occurs (40).

Sequential evaluation of serum Tg levels provides information on the status of thyroid activity in Graves' disease and helps in determining if the antithyroid medication should be discontinued and if the disease will relapse after discontinuation of therapy. The combination of serum Tg measurement together with other parameters, such as TSI levels, T_3 suppression tests, and goiter size reduction, provides the clinician with additional important information regarding the possible outcome of therapy. In patients with toxic adenomas or toxic multinodular goiter, serum Tg levels are also invariably increased (see Table 1).

SUBACUTE THYROIDITIS AND CHRONIC LYMPHOCYTIC THYROIDITIS

Subacute thyroiditis is characterized by a rapid release of Tg and thyronines into the circulation as a result of an inflammatory destruction of the thyroid gland. The elevated serum Tg levels normalize in a few weeks following steroid therapy, according to some authors (45,46). Occasionally, the serum Tg level stays elevated after apparent clinical resolution and normalization of thyroid function (47). Recently, Yamamoto and coworkers (48) found that normalization of serum Tg levels occurred in subjects with subacute thyroiditis depending on which form of therapy was used. In patients treated with prednisone therapy, serum Tg levels fell during the early phase of the disease and normalized at the end of the early phase. In contrast, in patients treated with salicylates, the decline of Tg was delayed and Tg levels remained elevated at the end of the early phase, when the thyronine levels and erythrocyte sedimentation rate (ESR) had normalized. This study suggested that prednisone led to a rapid decrease of serum Tg as a result of its inhibitory action on intrathyroidal hydrolysis.

The discovery of an elevated serum Tg level in subjects with a low iodine-123 (^{123}I) uptake is important in the differential diagnosis between subacute thyroiditis and factitial thyrotoxicosis. In the latter, the gland is suppressed and serum Tg levels are low or undetectable (49). This diagnostic application of Tg in factitial thyrotoxicosis should not, however, be used in subjects who have a history of a preexisting thyroid disorder, which in itself can lead to raised and unsuppressible Tg levels.

The study of serum Tg in chronic thyroiditis or silent thyroiditis has been only sporadically explored, because of the high incidence of Tg antibodies in the sera of these patients and the known interference of these antibodies in the RIA (5,6). Smallridge et al. (50) studied Tg levels in sera of patients with subacute thyroiditis and negative Tg antibody titers. Serum Tg levels were still moderately elevated after 4 to 6 months, and raised levels persisted up to 44 months. In patients with painless thyroiditis, the elevation of the serum Tg level was similar to that seen in subacute thyroiditis. Anti-Tg antibodies, seen with the RIA technique, were frequently present in the sera of these patients, and thus precise Tg values are not available. The serum Tg levels have been studied in a few patients with chronic thyroiditis who had no anti-Tg antibodies in their sera, and serum Tg levels appeared to be elevated (20).

ENDEMIC GOITER

Studies performed in New Guinea, an area of endemic goiter, showed a close correlation between the serum concentration of Tg and the log of serum TSH (36). The study provides us with additional evidence that chronic stimulation by TSH leads to increased serum Tg levels. In certain areas of Sicily where goiter development is endemic and iodine deficiency is also present, patients with goiters have higher serum Tg levels. In the coastal area of Sicily, however, where the iodine intake is certainly higher and sporadic goiter is demonstrable, elevated serum Tg levels are still present. Yet patients from this area experience different iodine intakes. Their increased serum Tg levels are not a result of the relative amounts of iodine present in the diet, and, therefore, it is more likely that other factors are involved. Pezzino and coworkers (18) proposed the hypothesis that the single factor that determines the Tg release is the iodination of the Tg molecule, and, according to this hypothesis, the elevated serum Tg levels may reflect an increased intraglandular turnover of Tg.

THYROID CANCER

In 1973, a suitable assay for the measurement of Tg in human sera was established in our laboratory (5). Because the assay was specific for Tg and this complex protein was known not to be produced by any other organ in the body, we felt it was reasonable to hypothesize that the serum Tg levels should be low or undetectable in patients with thyroid cancer who underwent total thyroidectomy and radioablation. Confirmation of this hypothesis came when our investigating team reported the first data in 1975 (51). It was clearly established that serum Tg as a marker could not be used to diagnose the presence of differentiated thyroid tumors, but preoperative serum Tg levels were nevertheless correlated with the histologic type of tumor present. Patients with pure papillary tumors had lower serum Tg levels than patients with mixed papillary–follicular tumors, who in turn had lower serum Tg levels than patients with pure follicular tumors (Fig. 2).

With numerous studies subsequently confirming these data, the Tg measurement has proven to be a marker for recurrent or metastatic thyroid cancer (51–75). Serum Tg has become a valuable adjunct to iodine-131 (^{131}I) total-body scanning in the evaluation of patients with differentiated thyroid tumors. However, the debate continues as to whether Tg measurements should be used as a single marker in the follow-up of these patients or be used in conjunction with ^{131}I total-body scans.

Several caveats need to be discussed. Both tests, Tg measurements and total-body scans, present false positives and false negatives. Also, the sensitivity and specificity of the Tg assay is crucial. Indeed, when various samples are tested with different assays, different results are frequently obtained. The first international standardization study (8), in which identical samples containing known amounts of Tg were submitted to a large number

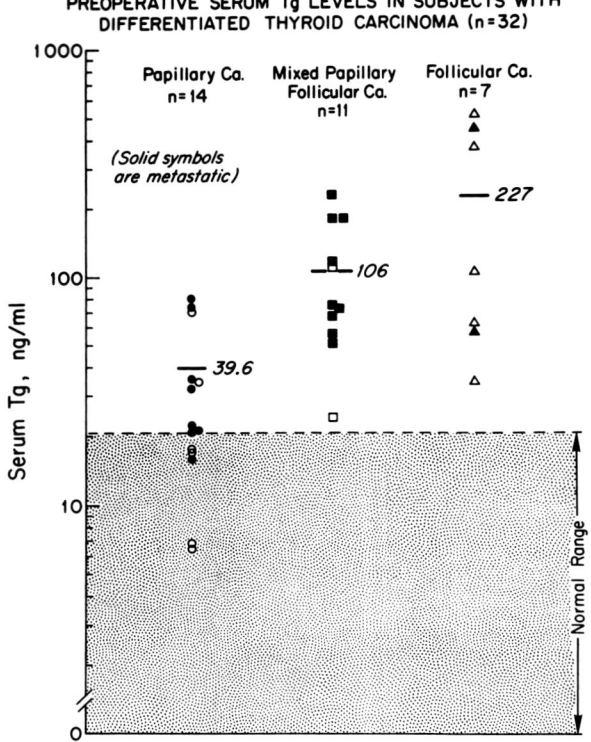

FIG. 2. Preoperative serum thyroglobulin levels in patients with differentiated thyroid carcinoma. (From ref. 126, with permission.)

of laboratories, yielded data indicating that a given laboratory was unable to detect a Tg level of 30.6 ng/mL. These findings are of concern, because the insensitive assays may lead the clinician to the false interpretation that the Tg levels are undetectable (false negative) in patients whose total-body scans are positive. Sensitive assays, however, could detect the presence of Tg in the same sera (8). Another disturbing finding came from a second international comparative study conducted by European investigators (9), in which serum Tg levels were determined for a given standard by 11 laboratories with one commercial kit (CIS-SORIN kit), yielding a mean serum Tg level of 39 ng/mL [coefficient of variation (CV), 16%], and by eight other laboratories that used another commercial kit (Henning), which found a mean Tg level of only 8.0 ng/mL (CV, 49%) in the same samples. The high Tg reading by one kit would make one suspicious of tumor recurrence or metastatic development, whereas the lower Tg reading by the other kit on the same specimen would not raise this suspicion. Thus, intercomparison of serum Tg levels using different assays from different laboratories or manufacturers is nearly impossible.

Certain studies in the literature, which compare the utility of serum Tg levels with the utility of total-body scan in patients with differentiated carcinoma who underwent thyroid ablation with ^{131}I, indicate the necessity for the ^{131}I scan as a screening method in addition to Tg (10,11,58,60,62,64,66,67,71,73–93). Other studies have proposed that only Tg levels be used as follow-up (93). Additional factors are important in this evaluation. Indeed, ATAs have been shown to interfere with the measurement of Tg (5,6). A recent study by Schaadt et al. (7) indicates that an IRMA assay for Tg is less sensitive to the presence of ATAs but is still affected by them. Thus in most if not all instances, the value of serum Tg obtained in the presence of autoantibodies is useless. The administration of a ^{131}I scanning dose to patients before obtaining samples for Tg measurement is also a source of unreliable Tg determinations. The possibility exists that Tg levels are undetectable in certain sera because the tumor and/or metastases no longer produce Tg (dedifferentiation). It is also conceivable that Tg, which is synthesized in tumor tissue, is not released, or the Tg may be immunologically altered and consequently not recognized by the anti-Tg antibody used in a given assay system. The status of suppression of endogenous TSH with T_4 or T_3 certainly affects some serum Tg values, because it is well known that the Tg released by tumors is at least in part controlled by TSH. Because most differentiated tumors have TSH receptors, they will respond to endogenous TSH with Tg release.

On the issue of false-positive scans in patients with thyroid cancer, Echenique et al. (71) reported a patient with papillary carcinoma with an equivocal uptake in the lung, who proved subsequently to have a fungus infection. Sometimes, small amounts of the patient's saliva on the scanning table, on the pillow, or on the patient's clothes can be a cause of false positive scans. The residual ^{131}I in a patient with Zenker's diverticulum can mimic areas of ^{131}I uptake in chest and neck and thus create false-positive scans. False-negative scans can also be observed in patients who are contaminated with stable iodine (e.g., x-ray contrast agents, cough syrups, vitamins containing iodine, and drugs containing iodine such as amiodarone). Therefore, a careful history of each patient should be obtained prior to the initiation of a scan. This is quite important because a false-positive scan could lead to unnecessary exposure to therapeutic doses of radioactive iodine, and a false-negative scan can lead to false security. To avoid false-positive scans, it is important to repeat the scan after repositioning of the patient on the scan table, or, in the case of Zenker's diverticulum, after the patient drinks water to flush the isotope from the diverticulum. When contamination with stable iodine is suspected, the stable iodine concentration in the urine could be used to indicate such contamination.

Serum Tg Measurement as an Indicator of the Presence of Thyroid Tumors

Because Tg is elevated in a number of thyroid conditions, the measurement of Tg in serum can be of significance only under special circumstances. Schneider et al. (94) reported that patients who have been exposed to external irradiation should be monitored with serum Tg levels, as well as clinically, because a rise in the Tg level can select individuals at higher risk for the development of thyroid nodules. In contrast, Morimoto et al. (95) performed a retrospective study in subjects exposed to radiation by atomic bomb explosions in Nagasaki and Hiroshima and concluded that serum Tg levels were not affected by atomic bomb fallout exposure when compared to a control group. Although there is agreement that Tg levels are not useful in the preoperative diagnosis of thyroid cancer *per se,* they may help to delineate higher risk groups for the development of nodules. A recent population study in Norway reported that extremely elevated serum Tg levels were observed in patients several years before clinically evident malignant thyroid tumors were found (96). The two patients with anaplastic cancer in this study had very high Tg levels, and this contrasted with the data of Pacini et al. (63) who found low levels in such patients. Extremely high serum Tg levels have been seen in patients with metastatic disease of unknown etiology. A high serum Tg level in a patient with a primary tumor of unknown type immediately points to the thyroid gland as the location of the tumor, and this could result in life-saving therapy even in the presence of metastases (87) (Fig. 3).

Scans and Serum Tg, On or Off Thyroid Hormone Therapy

Several studies have introduced various criteria to determine the need for further scanning doses based on the concentration of serum Tg and on whether these values are obtained with or without thyroid hormone therapy. Most data indicate that serum Tg levels of less than 10 ng/mL for patients on T_4 suppressive therapy are indicative of remission of the disease. In contrast, values of greater than 10 ng/mL, either with or without suppressive therapy, are suspicious for recurrence, and in such cases, total-body scans with 10 mCi of ^{131}I are called for. A clinical strategy used in our clinics is presented in Figure 4. If under these circumstances the total-body scan is negative, additional studies are done. They include ultrasound of the neck, computed tomographic (CT) scan or magnetic resonance imaging (MRI) of the neck/chest, positron emission tomographic (PET) scanning (97), thallium-201 scan, and therapeutic doses of ^{131}I with subsequent scanning, which has been advocated by several groups (10,88,98,99).

Serum Tg levels, as well as total-body scans, are difficult to interpret when the patient has undergone a partial resection of the gland and has not undergone thyroid ablation. In fact, the lack of total ablation makes the use of serum Tg and scans in the follow-up of such patients

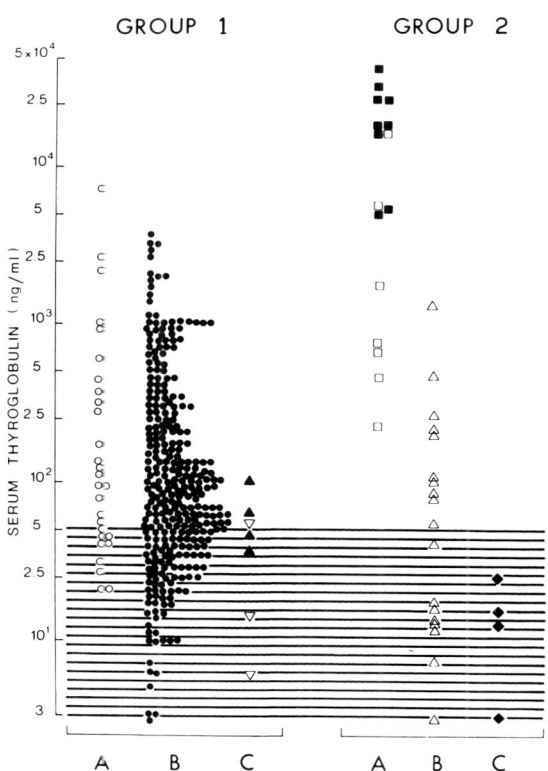

FIG. 3. Serum thyroglobulin levels in patients without (Group 1) and with (Group 2) clinical signs of malignancy. In Group 1: (A) Patients with an early (○) differentiated thyroid carcinoma (papillary, follicular, mixed); (B) patients with a benign thyroid cold nodule (●); (C) patients with a medullary (▽) and undifferentiated (▲) thyroid carcinoma. In Group 2: (A) Patients with an advanced disseminated thyroid carcinoma without (□) and with (■) bone metastases; (B) patients with a benign thyroid cold nodule with metastases from nonthyroid tumors (△) (C) patients with thyroid metastases from nonthyroid tumors (◆). *Shaded area* (fine parallel lines) represents the range of serum Tg measurements in 70 controls. (From ref. 87, with permission.)

problematic. Certain authors have indicated that Tg levels are relevant even if total thyroidectomy did not take place. Harvey et al. (100) reported that despite the presence of residual thyroid tissue, the measurement of serum Tg levels can exclude the presence of metastases in most patients after lobectomy for thyroid carcinoma. Tourniaire et al. (101) also reported that serum Tg levels are a sensitive marker after lobectomy, because a rise during the follow-up of thyroid cancer patients suggests a recurrence. In addition, Baskin (102) showed that serum Tg levels are useful in the detection of recurrences of thyroid cancer in patients who have undergone subtotal thyroidectomy and were treated with only low doses of ^{131}I (30 mCi).

It is unknown how much residual tissue or metastatic tumor tissue has to be present to elevate the serum Tg lev-

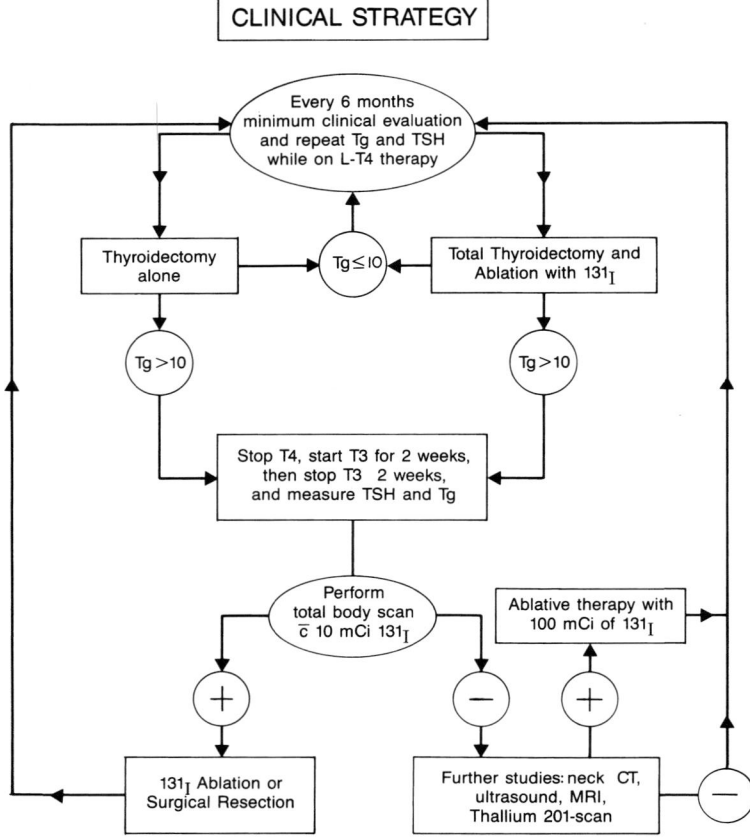

FIG. 4. Clinical strategy for follow-up study of patients with treated well-differentiated thyroid cancer, antithyroglobulin-antibody negative. Thyroglobulin (Tg) values are expressed in ng/mL.

els above set criteria, because the serum Tg levels are also dependent on other factors, such as endogenous TSH levels, the clearance rate of protein, and the histologic type of the tumor. Tg levels in general correlate well with tumor mass, and the highest levels of Tg are seen in patients with metastatic disease to the bones and the lungs (see Fig. 3).

Now that we have set forth our own strategy of using thyroid body scans and Tg in a complementary fashion, we can survey the literature of the last 10 years to see what most thyroid cancer specialists have used as follow-up criteria in their patients. The demonstration by Schlumberger et al. (65) that the production and release of Tg by thyroid tumor tissue is TSH-dependent, focused attention on whether Tg levels should be measured while "on" or "off" T_4 substitution therapy. Several groups of investigators have found that serum Tg as a marker of metastasis or tumor recurrence is most sensitive after thyroid hormone withdrawal (1,6,38,41,67,69,83,103–105). In certain patients with distant metastases, serum Tg was quite suppressed when TSH was in the normal range and became detectable only after the rise of TSH to above 50 μU/mL (58,65,75,106). However, Black and coworkers (93) have advocated the use of Tg while on replacement therapy. Others have suggested studying Tg levels on and off T_4 replacement therapy (75,76,85). Various cut-off points for serum Tg values have been proposed, but none of these can be used universally for all laboratories because of the variation in the measurement. Our own experience coincides with that of Black et al. (93), that serum Tg levels are usually obtained while the patient is on T_4 therapy. If the patient, however, has suspicious lesions for metastasis or recurrence clinically, Tg levels off T_4 therapy will also be obtained, as well as total-body scans.

Can the Serum Tg Measurement be Used as an Alternate Technique in the Follow-up of Patients with Thyroid Cancer?

There are two clinical situations in which Tg cannot be used as a sole indicator of recurrence of thyroid cancer. The first is in patients who have detectable serum Tg autoantibodies. Indeed, most authors, with a few exceptions (104,107), agree that the Tg autoantibodies affect the assay system for the measurement of Tg so profoundly that no predictive value can be attached to the measurements. However, Tg autoantibodies can fluctuate during the disease process and can disappear, which makes the Tg measurement valuable again in such patients. One could also argue that the presence of Tg autoantibodies in the patient's serum is an indicator that the corresponding antigen is still present in sufficient quantity to trigger an antibody response, and the presence of these antibodies may have significant implications for the outcome of treatment. More studies are needed to prove the significance of positive ATA titers in these patients.

The Tg measurement, nevertheless, remains an attractive testing technique in patients with thyroid cancer because of its simplicity, low cost, precision, ready availability, easy reproducibility, and utilization without necessitating withdrawal of thyroid hormone. It also allows the monitoring of patients with tumors that have lost the ability to trap radioactive iodine. The total-body scan, however, has the advantage of indicating the size, site, and functionality of the tumor. Based on cumulative data from 1323 cases of well-differentiated thyroid cancer reported in the literature (67), in which total-body scans were compared with serum Tg levels, 284 subjects had documented metastases. Of these, 37 cases (13%) were not detected by total-body scan but were suggested by abnormal Tg levels or additional clinical findings, or both. In contrast, only 12 out of the 284 cases (4.2%) had a positive scan for metastases and undetectable Tg levels by the investigator's criteria. Nine of these 12 patients were limited to two studies, with Tg values greatly discordant with most of those reported in the literature, thereby again emphasizing the need for an international reference standard. The superiority of one technique over the others has been discussed extensively in the literature. Most of the studies in the last 5 years reporting on both tests indicate that both should be used together, and this will yield the highest degree of diagnostic accuracy in patients with surgically treated cancer (71,76,82,83). Total thyroidectomy followed by ablation with ^{131}I of residual tissue is the most common modality of therapy used in patients with differentiated cancer (10,76,77,82, 108–115), and this is logical because neither Tg levels nor ^{131}I scans are interpretable in the presence of a large normal thyroid remnant.

The addition of Tg measurements to the armamentarium of the clinician has uncovered a group of patients who, if evaluated by total-body scans alone, would have to be considered cured, and yet they have tumor tissue shown with methods other than the ^{131}I scan. These tumors came to the attention of the investigators because of elevated serum Tg levels. This finding has led several groups to treat such patients with therapeutic doses of ^{131}I, despite the absence of isotopic uptake with conventional doses of ^{131}I used for scanning purposes (10,88, 103,106,116,117). The Tg level can be misleading in certain instances in which levels are low in the presence of metastasis. However, these metastases are frequently discovered clinically. The addition of Tg to the testing scheme may also have led to a reduction in the frequency of performing total-body scans (102).

What Is the Mechanism of Tg Release by Tumor Tissue?

Although the mechanism by which Tg is released in the circulation by the tumor is unknown, two mechanisms are proposed:

1. The presence of a putative abnormal stimulator could cause the release of Tg. Such a stimulator has been described (118), but these data were later retracted (119). Most thyroid tumors and metastases, however, do respond to TSH, as evidenced by the increase in Tg levels after withdrawal of thyroid hormone (65).

2. The tumor itself can release Tg into the circulation. Indeed, the fact that Tg levels are elevated in patients with no thyroid gland and Tg-producing metastases is sufficient evidence that the tumor cells produce and release Tg directly. Support for this mechanism was recently provided by in vitro studies in which perfused follicular tumor cells released Tg into the medium in a pulsatile pattern (120). Further support for the notion that Tg is released by the tumor itself comes from a study by Schneider et al. (121) who reported that the iodine content of serum Tg (TgI) from patients with thyroid cancer is low and is most likely the result of the release of newly synthesized molecules by the tumor cell, rather than from the invaded surrounding normal thyroid tissues.

The possibility, however, that serum Tg levels rise as a result of direct invasion of normal tissue is illustrated by the high Tg levels in the serum of a patient with non-Hodgkin's lymphoma involving the thyroid gland, and by the recent demonstration that medullary carcinoma of patients can present with elevated Tg levels in rare instances (87) (see Fig. 3).

Tg levels in other body fluids, such as pleural fluid (52), saliva (54), and thyroid cyst fluid (122), have been analyzed. Elevated Tg levels in pleural effusions indicate the suspicion for the presence of metastases of a differentiated thyroid carcinoma. The increase of the Tg level in pleural fluid is an important finding, especially if the primary is not known. A low Tg level in pleural fluid in a patient with an unknown primary practically excludes a differentiated thyroid tumor as the cause of the pleural effusion. This indicates that Tg measurement in pleural fluid of patients with unknown primary may be a valuable adjunct in certain clinical situations. Salivary Tg levels are elevated in patients with metastatic thyroid cancer (54), but this adds little to the diagnostic information because the serum Tg levels are always elevated in such cases (123).

Absent or low serum Tg levels in thyroid cyst fluid indicate that the cyst is nonthyroidal in origin (i.e., the cyst represents a parathyroid cyst or branchial cleft cyst). In contrast, the fluid obtained from metastatic, cystic, degenerated lymph nodes (i.e., from a papillary carcinoma) is associated with extremely high Tg levels and indicates its thyroidal origin.

CONCLUSIONS

The study of circulating Tg has created a new chapter in thyroidology. Its measurement method, although highly sensitive in most cases, is in urgent need of standardization. This becomes very clear when one analyzes the data of international cooperative studies reported in the last 5 years (8,9). Its use in clinical medicine is confined to several disorders:

1. Tg measurement can assist the pediatrician in the diagnosis of agenesis of the thyroid gland. The controversy continues over whether or not thyroid scans should be deleted. This represents a rather moot argument, because with the advent of ^{123}I and its short half-life, the risk for using this isotope in children is negligible. It is fair to state that the Tg measurement is an excellent complement for the thyroid scan in the newborn if there is suspicion for thyroid "agenesis."

2. Tg measurement can aid the physician in the diagnosis of factitial thyrotoxicosis.

3. Tg measurements are unquestionably useful in the prediction of the outcome of Graves' disease patients treated with antithyroid drugs. Obviously, only patients with serum Tg antibody–negative sera can be considered.

4. Tg measurements have made a great impact in the follow-up of patients with differentiated thyroid cancer. Although the test is not perfect, the follow-up of patients has been greatly facilitated. In certain patients, the presence of Tg in the serum may have been simply lifesaving, because it represented the only method by which metastatic disease was detected and treated.

Future developments in this field will be directed at developing an assay system in which Tg autoantibodies do not interfere with Tg measurements. Precise studies of the Tg-TSH interrelationship using the recently developed "ultrasensitive" TSH assay also need to be addressed, especially now that recombinant TSH may become available.

REFERENCES

1. Van Herle AJ, Vassart G, Dumont JE. Control of thyroglobulin synthesis and secretion (first of two parts). *N Engl J Med* 1979;301:239–249.
2. Van Herle AJ, Vassart G, Dumont JE. Control of thyroglobulin synthesis and secretion (second of two parts). *N Engl J Med* 1979;301:307–314.
3. Van Herle AJ. Measurement and clinical significance of thyroglobulin in serum and body fluids. In: Ingbar SH, Braverman LE, eds. *Werner's, the thyroid,* 5th ed. Philadelphia: JB Lippincott, 1986;534–545.
4. Refetoff S, Lever EG. The value of serum thyroglobulin measurement in clinical practice. *JAMA* 1983;250:2352–2357.
5. Van Herle AJ, Uller RP, Matthews NL, Brown J. Radioimmunoassay for measurement of thyroglobulin in human serum. *J Clin Invest* 1973;52:1320–1327.
6. Schneider AB, Pervos R. Radioimmunoassay human of thyroglobulin: effect of antithyroglobulin antibodies. *J Clin Endocrinol Metab* 1978;47:126–137.
7. Schaadt B, Feldt-Rasmussen U, Rasmusson B, et al. Assessment of the influence of thyroglobulin (Tg) autoantibodies and other interfering factors on the use of serum Tg as tumor marker in differentiated thyroid carcinoma. *Thyroid* 1995;5:165–170.
8. Van Herle AJ, Van Herle IS, Greipel MA. An international cooperative study evaluating serum thyroglobulin standards. *J Clin Endocrinol Metab* 1985;60:338–343.
9. Feldt-Rasmussen U, Schlumberger M. European interlaboratory comparison of serum thyroglobulin measurement. *J Endocrinol Invest* 1988;11:175–181.
10. Bolk JH, Bussemaker JK, Nieuwenhuijzen Kruseman AC, De Vijlder JJM, Goslings BM. Thyroglobulin measurements in the follow-up of patients with differentiated thyroid carcinoma: comparison with quantitative radioactive iodine uptake measurements and total body scans. *Neth J Med* 1985;28:340–346.
11. Valimaki M, Lamberg B-A. How to deal with undetectable and low measurable serum thyroglobulin levels in the follow-up of patients with differentiated thyroid carcinoma? *Acta Endocrinol (Copenh)* 1985;110:487–492.
12. Feldt-Rasmussen U, Profilis C, Colinet E. *Purification and certification of human thyroglobulin. Reference material: CRM 457.* Report Eur 15611 EN 1994;1–78.
13. Ket JL, De Vijlder JM, Bikker H, Gons MH, Tegelaers WHH. Serum thyroglobulin levels: the physiological decrease in infancy and the absence in athyroidism. *J Clin Endocrinol Metab* 1981;53:1301–1303.
14. Roti E, Gnudi A, Braverman LE, et al. Human cord blood concentrations of thyrotropin, thyroglobulin and iodothyronines after maternal administration of thyrotropin releasing hormone. *J Clin Endocrinol Metab* 1981;53:813–817.
15. Black EG, Bodden SJ, Hulse JA, Hoffenberg R. Serum thyroglobulin in normal and hypothyroid neonates. *Clin Endocrinol (Oxf)* 1982;16:267–274.
16. Pacini F, Lari R, La Ricca P, et al. Serum thyroglobulin in newborns' cord blood, in childhood and adolescence: a physiological indicator of thyroidal status. *J Endocrinol Invest* 1984;7:467–471.
17. Penny R, Spencer CA, Frasier SD, Nicoloff JT. Thyroid-stimulating hormone and thyroglobulin levels decrease with chronological age in children and adolescents. *J Clin Endocrinol Metab* 1983;56:177–180.
18. Pezzino V, Vigneri R, Squatrito S, Filetti S, Camus M, Polosa P. Increased serum thyroglobulin levels in patients with nontoxic goiter. *J Clin Endocrinol Metab* 1978;46:653–657.
19. Pezzino V, Filetti S, Belfiore A, Proto S, Donzelli G, Vigneri R. Serum thyroglobulin levels in the newborn. *J Clin Endocrinol Metab* 1981;52:364–366.
20. Torrigiani G, Doniach D, Roitt IM. Serum thyroglobulin levels in healthy subjects and in patients with thyroid disease. *J Clin Endocrinol Metab* 1969;29:305–314.
21. Fisher DA, Oddie TH, Burroughs JC. Thyroidal radioiodine uptake rate measurement in infants. *Am J Dis Child* 1962;103:738–749.
22. Ermans AM, Van Humskerke A, Ketelbant-Balasse P, Bordoux P, DeLange F. *Alterations of intrathyroidal iodine metabolism and increased risk of hypothyroidism in preterm infants.* Proceedings of the VIII International Thyroid Congress (abstract 4). Sydney, Australia, 1980.
23. Osotimehin B, Black EG, Hoffenberg R. Thyroglobulin concentration in neonatal blood: a possible test for neonatal hypothyroidism. *Br Med J* 1978;2:1467–1468.
24. Czernichow P, Schlumberger M, Pomarede R, Fragu P. Plasma thyroglobulin measurements help determine the type of thyroid defect in congenital hypothyroidism. *J Clin Endocrinol Metab* 1983;56:242–245.
25. Lissitzky S, Bismuth J, Jacquet P, et al. Congenital goiter with impaired thyroglobulin synthesis. *J Clin Endocrinol Metab* 1973;36:17–29.
26. De Vijlder JJM, Van Voorthuizen WF, Van Dijk JE, Rijnberk A, Tegelaers WHH. Hereditary congenital goiter with thyroglobulin deficiency in a breed of goats. *Endocrinology* 1978;102:1214–1222.
27. Penny R, Spencer CA, Frasier SD, Nicoloff JT. Cord serum thyroid-stimulating hormone and thyroglobulin levels decline with increasing birth weight in newborns. *J Clin Endocrinol Metab* 1984;59:979–985.

28. Ericsson UB, Ivarsson SA, Persson PH. Thyroglobulin in cord blood. The influence of the mode of delivery and the smoking habits of the mother. *Eur J Pediatr* 1987;146:44–47.
29. Sava L, Tomaselli L, Runello F, Belfiore A, Vigneri R. Serum thyroglobulin levels are elevated in newborns from iodine-deficient areas. *J Clin Endocrinol Metab* 1986;62:429–432.
30. Van Herle AJ, Klandorf H, Uller RP. A radioimmunoassay for serum rat thyroglobulin, physiologic and pharmacological studies. *J Clin Invest* 1975;56:1073–1081.
31. Lever EG, Refetoff S, Scherberg NH, Carr K. The influence of percutaneous fine needle aspiration on serum thyroglobulin. *J Clin Endocrinol Metab* 1983;56:26–29.
32. Christensen SB, Ericsson U-B, Janzon L, Tibblin S, Melander A. Influence of cigarette smoking on goiter formation, thyroglobulin, and thyroid hormone levels in women. *J Clin Endocrinol Metab* 1984;58:615–618.
33. Uller RP, Van Herle AJ, Chopra IJ. Thyroidal response to graded doses of bovine thyrotropin. *J Clin Endocrinol Metab* 1977;45:312–318.
34. Unger J, Van Heuverswijn B, Decoster C, Cantraine F, Mockel J, Van Herle AJ. Thyroglobulin and thyroid hormone release after intravenous administration of bovine thyrotropin in man. *J Clin Endocrinol Metab* 1980;51:590–594.
35. Belfiori A, Runello F, Sava L, La Rosa G, Vigneri R. Thyroglobulin release after graded endogenous thyrotropin stimulation in man: lack of correlation with thyroid hormone response. *J Clin Endocrinol Metab* 1984;59:974–978.
36. Van Herle AJ, Chopra IJ, Hershman JM, Hornabrook RW. Serum thyroglobulin in inhabitants of an endemic goiter region of New Guinea. *J Clin Endocrinol Metab* 1976;43:512–516.
37. Hegedus L, Kastrup J, Feldt-Rasmussen U, Peterson PH. Serum thyroglobulin in acute and chronic liver disease. *Clin Endocrinol (Oxf)* 1983;19:231–237.
38. Feldt-Rasmussen U, Petersen PH, Date J. Sex and age correlated reference values of serum thyroglobulin measured by a modified radioimmunoassay. *Acta Endocrinol (Copenh)* 1979;90:440–450.
39. Roti E, Robuschi G, Emanuele R, Bandini P, Gnudi A. Radioimmunoassay of thyroglobulin in human serum: concentrations in normal subjects and in patients with thyroid disease. *J Nucl Med Allied Sci* 1981;25:57–63.
40. Uller RP, Van Herle AJ. Effect of therapy on serum thyroglobulin levels in patients with Graves' disease. *J Clin Endocrinol Metab* 1978;46:747–755.
41. Gardner DF, Rothman J, Utiger RD. Serum thyroglobulin in normal subjects and patients with hyperthyroidism due to Graves' disease: effects of T3, iodide, ^{131}I and antithyroid drugs. *Clin Endocrinol (Oxf)* 1979;11:585–594.
42. Kawamura S, Kishino B, Tajima K, Mashita K, Tarui S. Serum thyroglobulin changes in patients with Graves' disease treated with long term antithyroid drug therapy. *J Clin Endocrinol Metab* 1983;56:507–512.
43. Feldt-Rasmussen U, Bech K, Date J, Hyltoft-Peterson P, Johansen K. A prospective study of the differential changes in serum thyroglobulin and its autoantibodies during propylthiouracil or radioiodine therapy of patients with Graves' disease. *Acta Endocrinol (Copenh)* 1982;99:379–385.
44. Ericsson UB, Tegler L, Dymling JF, Thorell JI. Effect of therapy on the serum thyroglobulin concentration in patients with toxic diffuse goitre, toxic nodular goitre and toxic adenoma. In: *Thyroglobulin and thyroglobulin autoantibodies: methodological and clinical studies [doctoral dissertation]*. Sweden: University of Lund, Malmo, 1984;99–103.
45. Glinoer D, Puttemans N, Van Herle AJ, Camus M, Ermans AM. Sequential study of the impairment of thyroid function in the early stage of subacute thyroiditis. *Acta Endocrinol (Copenh)* 1974;77:26–34.
46. Madeddu G, Casu AR, Constanza C, et al. Serum thyroglobulin levels in the diagnosis and follow up of subacute "painful" thyroiditis. *Arch Intern Med* 1985;145:243–247.
47. Izumi M, Larsen RP. Correlation of sequential changes in serum thyroglobulin, triiodothyronine, and thyroxine in patients with Graves' disease and subacute thyroiditis. *Metabolism* 1978;27:449–460.
48. Yamamoto M, Saito S, Sakurada T, et al. Effect of prednisolone and salicylate on serum thyroglobulin level in patients with subacute thyroiditis. *Clin Endocrinol (Oxf)* 1987;27:339–344.
49. Mariotti S, Martino E, Cupini C, et al. Low serum thyroglobulin as a clue to the diagnosis of thyrotoxicosis factitia. *N Engl J Med* 1982;307:410–412.
50. Smallridge RC, De Keyser RM, Van Herle AJ, Butkus NE, Wartofsky L. Thyroid iodine content and serum thyroglobulin: cues to the natural history of destruction-induced thyroiditis. *J Clin Endocrinol Metab* 1986;62:1213–1219.
51. Van Herle AJ, Uller RP. Elevated serum thyroglobulin: a marker of metastases in differentiated thyroid carcinomas. *J Clin Invest* 1975;56:272–277.
52. Lo Gerfo P, Stillman T, Colaccio D, Feind C. Serum thyroglobulin and recurrent thyroid cancer. *Lancet* 1977;1:881–882.
53. Pezzino V, Cozanni P, Filetti S, et al. A radioimmunoassay for human thyroglobulin: methodology and clinical applications. *Eur J Clin Invest* 1977;7:503–508.
54. Shah D, Dandekar S, Ganatra RD. Thyroglobulin levels in serum and saliva of patients with differentiated thyroid carcinoma. *Proc Indian Acad Sci* 1978;87B:169–175.
55. Botsch H, Schulz E, Lochner B. Serum-thyreoglobulin bestimmung zur verlaufskontrolle bei schilddrüsen karzinom patienten. *Dtsch Med Wochenschr* 1979;104:1072–1074.
56. Hay ID, Gorman CA. Serum thyroglobulin in differentiated thyroid cancer. *Br Med J* 1979;2:1076.
57. Shlossberg AH, Jacobson JC, Ibbertson HK. Serum thyroglobulin in the diagnosis and management of thyroid carcinoma. *Clin Endocrinol (Oxf)* 1979;10 17–27.
58. Tang Fui SCN, Hoffenberg R, Maisey MN, Black EG. Serum thyroglobulin concentrations and whole-body radioiodine scan in follow-up of differentiated thyroid cancer after thyroid ablation. *Br Med J* 1979;2:298–300.
59. Warwick A, Martin C. The development of a thyroglobulin radioimmunoassay in the diagnosis and management of recurrent thyroid cancer. *Aust NZ J Med* 1979;9:628A.
60. Charles MA, Dodson LE Jr, Waldeck N, et al. Serum thyroglobulin levels predict total body iodine scan findings in patients with treated well differentiated thyroid carcinoma. *Am J Med* 1980;69:401–407.
61. Hufner M, Pollmann H, Grussendorf M, Schenk P. Die Bedeutung der thyreoglobulin bestimmung im serum bei der nachsorge von patienten mit differenziertem schilddrüsen karzinom. *Schweiz Med Wochenschr* 1980;110:159–162.
62. McDougall IR, Bayer MF. Follow-up of patients with differentiated thyroid cancer using serum thyroglobulin measured by an immunoradiometric assay. Comparison with I-131 total body scans. *J Nucl Med* 1980;21:741–744.
63. Pacini F, Pinchera A, Giani C, Grasso L, Doveri F, Baschieri L. Serum thyroglobulin in thyroid carcinoma and other thyroid disorders. *J Endocrinol Invest* 1980;3:283–292.
64. Pacini F, Pinchera A, Giani C, Grasso L, Baschieri L. Serum thyroglobulin concentrations and ^{131}I whole body scans in the diagnosis of metastases from differentiated thyroid carcinoma (after thyroidectomy). *Clin Endocrinol (Oxf)* 1980;13:107–110.
65. Schlumberger M, Charbord P, Fragu P, Lumbroso J, Parmentier C, Tubiana M. Circulating thyroglobulin and thyroid hormones in patients with metastases of differentiated thyroid carcinoma: relationship to serum thyrotropin levels. *J Clin Endocrinol Metab* 1980;51:513–519.
66. Weissel VM, Bergmann H, Hofer R. Klinische wertigkeit von Serum thyroglobulin und 131I Ganzkorper retentions messungen bei der metastasensuche von differnzierten schilddrüsen karzinomen. *Acta Med Austriaca* 1980;7:114–119.
67. Ashcraft MW, Van Herle AJ. The comparative value of serum thyroglobulin measurements and iodine 131 total body scans in the follow-up study of patients with treated differentiated thyroid cancer. *Am J Med* 1981;71:806–814.
68. Schneider AB, Line BR, Goldman JM, Robbins J. Sequential serum thyroglobulin determinations, ^{131}I scans, and ^{131}I uptakes after triiodothyronine withdrawal in patients with thyroid cancer. *J Clin Endocrinol Metab* 1981;53:1199–1206.
69. Black EG, Cassoni A, Gimlette TMD, et al. Serum thyroglobulin in thyroid cancer. *Lancet* 1981;2:443–445.
70. Black EG, Hoffenberg R. Thyroglobulin and thyroid cancer. *Lancet* 1982;1:914.
71. Echenique RL, Kasi L, Haynie TP, Glenn HJ, Samaan NA, Hill CS. Critical evaluation of serum thyroglobulin levels and ^{131}I scans in post-therapy patients with differentiated thyroid carcinoma: concise communication. *J Nucl Med* 1982;23:235–240.

72. Estour B, Bornet H, Bernard MH, Fleury MC, Tourniaire J. Valeur semiologique du dosage de la thyroglobuline plasmatique dans la surveillance des cancers thyroidiens differencies. *Rev Fr Endocrinol Clin* 1982;23:490–496.
73. Roti E, Robuschi G, Emanuele R, et al. The value of serum thyroglobulin measurement as a marker of cancer recurrence in the follow-up of patients previously treated for differentiated thyroid tumor. *J Endocrinol Invest* 1982;5:43–46.
74. Holt G, Galligan J, Winship J, Roeser P, Mortimer R. Serum thyroglobulin after mantle irradiation for Hodgkin's disease. *Clin Endocrinol (Oxf)* 1983;18:605–611.
75. Panza N, De Rosa M, Lombardi G, Salvatore M. Serum thyroglobulin in patients with early thyroid cancer who have residual thyroid tissue after total thyroidectomy. *Lancet* 1984;1:398.
76. Panza N, Lombardi G, Minozzi M, et al. ^{131}I total body scan and serum thyroglobulin assay in the follow-up of surgically treated patients affected by differentiated thyroid carcinoma. *J Nucl Med Allied Sci* 1984;28:9–12.
77. Grant S, Luttrell B, Reeve T, et al. Thyroglobulin may be undetectable in the serum of patients with metastatic disease secondary to differentiated thyroid carcinoma. *Cancer* 1984;54:1625–1628.
78. Dralle H, Schwarzrock R, Lange W, et al. Comparison of histology and immunohistochemistry with thyroglobulin serum levels and radioiodine uptake in recurrence and metastases of differentiated thyroid carcinomas. *Acta Endocrinol (Copenh)* 1985;108:504–510.
79. Piekarski JD, Schlumberger M, Leclere J, Couanet D, Masselot J, Parmentier C. Chest computed tomography (CT) in patients with micronodular lung metastases of differentiated thyroid carcinoma. *Int J Radiat Oncol Biol Phys* 1985;11:1023–1027.
80. Ramanna L, Waxman AD, Brachman MB, et al. Correlation of thyroglobulin measurements and radioiodine scans in the follow-up of patients with differentiated thyroid cancer. *Cancer* 1985;55: 1525–1529.
81. Girelli ME, Busnardo B, Amerio R, et al. Serum thyroglobulin levels in patients with well-differentiated thyroid cancer during suppression therapy study on 429 patients. *Eur J Nucl Med* 1985;10:252–254.
82. Pacini F, Lari R, Mazzeo S, Grasso L, Taddei D, Pinchera A. Diagnostic value of a single serum thyroglobulin determination on and off thyroid suppressive therapy in the follow-up of patients with differentiated thyroid cancer. *Clin Endocrinol (Oxf)* 1985;23:405–411.
83. Ronga G, Fiorentino A, Fragasso G, Fringuelli FM, Todino V. Complementary role of whole body scan and serum thyroglobulin determination in the follow-up of differentiated thyroid carcinoma. *Ital J Surg Sci* 1986;16:11–15.
84. Lombardi G, Panza N, Lupoli G, D'Aiello M, Zarrilli L. Serum thyroglobulin in differentiated thyroid carcinoma: a review. *J Exp Clin Cancer Res* 1986;5(4):415–420.
85. Girelli ME, Busnardo B, Amerio R, Casara D, Betterle C, Piccolo M. Critical evaluation of serum thyroglobulin (Tg) levels during thyroid hormone suppression therapy versus Tg levels after hormone withdrawal and total body scan: results in 291 patients with thyroid cancer. *Eur J Nucl Med* 1986;11:333–335.
86. Socolov C, Pop A, Simionescu L. The value of thyroglobulin (TgL) assay in following the post-therapeutic course of differentiated thyroid cancer. *Endocrinologie* 1986;24:39–43.
87. Panza N, Lombardi G, De Rosa M, Pacilio G, Lapenta L, Salvatore M. High serum thyroglobulin levels, diagnostic indicators in patients with metastases from unknown primary sites. *Cancer* 1987;60:2233–2236.
88. Pacini F, Lippi F, Formica N, et al. Therapeutic doses of iodine-131 reveal undiagnosed metastases in thyroid cancer patients with detectable serum thyroglobulin levels. *J Nucl Med* 1987;28:1888–1891.
89. Muller-Gartner HW, Schneider C. Clinical evaluation of tumor characteristics predisposing serum thyroglobulin to be undetectable in patients with differentiated thyroid cancer. *Cancer* 1988;61:976–981.
90. Edmonds CJ, Willis CL. Serum thyroglobulin in the investigation of patients presenting with metastases. *Br J Radiol* 1988;61:317–319.
91. Harley EH, Daly RG, Hodge JW. Thyroglobulin assays in the postoperative management of differentiated thyroid cancer. *Arch Otolaryngol Head Neck Surg* 1988;114:333–335.
92. Lindegaard MW, Paus E, Hoie J, Kullman G, Stenwig AE. Thyroglobulin radioimmunoassay and ^{131}I scintigraphy in patients with differentiated thyroid carcinoma. *Acta Chir Scand* 1988;154:141–145.
93. Black EG, Sheppard MC, Hoffenberg R. Serial serum thyroglobulin measurements in the management of differentiated thyroid carcinoma. *Clin Endocrinol (Oxf)* 1987;27:115–120.
94. Schneider AB, Shore-Freedman E, Ryo UY, Bekerman C, Pinsky SM. Prospective serum thyroglobulin measurements in assessing the risk of developing thyroid nodules in patients exposed to childhood neck irradiation. *J Clin Endocrinol Metab* 1985;61:547–550.
95. Morimoto I, Yoshimoto Y, Sato K, et al. Serum TSH, thyroglobulin and thyroidal disorders in atomic bomb survivors exposed in youth: 30-year follow-up study. *J Nucl Med* 1987;28:1115–1122.
96. Thoresen SO, Myking O, Glattre E, Rootwelt K, Andersen A, Foss OP. Serum thyroglobulin as a preclinical tumour marker in subgroups of thyroid cancer. *Br J Cancer* 1988;57:105–108.
97. Adler LP, Bloom AD. Positron emission tomography of thyroid masses. *Thyroid* 1993;3:195–199.
98. Galligan JP, Winship J, Van Doorn T, et al. A comparison of serum thyroglobulin measurements and whole body ^{131}I scanning in the management of treated differentiated thyroid carcinoma. *Aust NZ J Med* 1982;12(4):248–254.
99. Schlumberger M, Tubiana M, De Vathaire F, et al. Long-term results of treatment of 283 patients with lung and bone metastases from differentiated thyroid carcinoma. *J Clin Endocrinol Metab* 1986;63: 960–967.
100. Harvey RD, Matheson NA, Grabowski PS, Rodger AB. Measurement of serum thyroglobulin is of value in detecting tumour recurrence following treatment of differentiated thyroid carcinoma by lobectomy. *Br J Surg* 1990;77:324–326.
101. Tourniaire J, Bernard MH, Ayzac L, Nicolas MH, Bornet H. Serum thyroglobulin assay after total unilateral lobectomy for differentiated thyroid carcinoma. *Presse Med* 1990;19:1309–1312.
102. Baskin HJ. Effect of postoperative ^{131}I treatment on thyroglobulin measurements in the follow-up of patients with thyroid cancer. *Thyroid* 1994;4:239–242.
103. Reiners C. Serum thyroglobulin as a substitution of ^{131}I scan in follow-up of differentiated thyroid cancer. *Acta Endocrinol Suppl (Copenh)* 1983;102(252):66–67.
104. Mariotti S, Cupini C, Giani C, et al. Evaluation of a solid-phase immunoradiometric assay (IRMA) for serum thyroglobulin: effect of anti-thyroglobulin antibody. *Clin Chim Acta* 1982;123:347–355.
105. Ozata M, Suzuki S, Miyamoto T, Liu RT, Fierro-Renoy F, Degroot LJ. Serum thyroglobulin in the follow-up of patients with treated differentiated thyroid cancer. *J Clin Endocrinol Metab* 1994;79:98–105.
106. Panza N, De Rosa M, Lombardi G, Salvatore M. Usefulness of serum thyroglobulin at replacement withdrawal after thyroidectomy for differentiated thyroid cancer. *J Nucl Med* 1985;26:316–317.
107. Black EG, Hoffenberg R. Should one measure serum thyroglobulin in the presence of anti-thyroglobulin antibodies? *Clin Endocrinol (Oxf)* 1983;19:597–601.
108. Crile G Jr. Endocrine dependence of papillary carcinoma of the thyroid. *JAMA* 1966;195:721–724.
109. Varman VM, Beierwaltes WH, Nofal NM, Nishiyama RH, Copp JE. Treatment of thyroid cancer. Death rates after surgery and after surgery followed by sodium iodide I-131. *JAMA* 1970;214:1437–1442.
110. Mazzaferri EL, Young RL, Oertel JE, Kemmerer WT, Page CP. Papillary thyroid carcinoma: the impact of therapy on 576 patients. *Medicine (Baltimore)* 1977;56:171–196.
111. Leeper RD, Shimaoka K. Treatment of metastatic thyroid cancer. In: Abe K, ed. *Endocrinology and cancer.* Philadelphia: WB Saunders, 1980;384–404.
112. Young RL, Mazzaferri EL, Rahe AJ, Dorfman SG. Pure follicular thyroid carcinoma: impact of therapy in 214 patients. *J Nucl Med* 1980; 21:733–737.
113. Christensen SB, Ljungberg O, Tibblin S. Surgical treatment of thyroid carcinoma in a defined population: 1960–1977. Evaluation of the results after a conservative surgical approach. *Am J Surg* 1983;146: 349–354.
114. Baumgartner WA. Serum thyroglobulin, a monitor of differentiated thyroid carcinoma in patients receiving thyroid hormone suppression therapy; concise communication. *J Nucl Med* 1984;25:673–676.
115. Goolden AWG. The indications for ablating normal thyroid tissue with ^{131}I in differentiated thyroid cancer. *Clin Endocrinol (Oxf)* 1985; 23:81–86.
116. Pineda JD, Lee T, Ain K, Reynolds JC, Robbins J. Iodine 131 therapy for thyroid cancer patients with elevated thyroglobulin and negative diagnostic scan. *J Clin Endocrinol Metab* 1995;80:1488–1492.
117. Clark OH, Hoelting T. Management of patients with differentiated thyroid cancer who have positive serum thyroglobulin levels and negative radioiodine scans. *Thyroid* 1994;4:501–505.

118. Greenspan FS, Lowenstein JM, West MN, Okerlund MD. Immunoreactive material to bovine TSH in plasma from patients with thyroid cancer. *J Clin Endocrinol Metab* 1972;35:795–798.
119. Greenspan FS, Lew W, Okerlund MD, Lowenstein JM. Falsely positive bovine TSH radioimmunoassay responses in sera from patients with thyroid cancer. *J Clin Endocrinol Metab* 1974;38:1121–1122.
120. Estour B, Van Herle AJ, Juillard GJF, et al. Characterization of a human follicular thyroid carcinoma cell line (UCLA RO 82 W-1). *Virchows Arch [B]* 1989;57:167–174.
121. Schneider AB, Ikekubo K, Kuma K. Iodine content of serum thyroglobulin in normal individuals and patients with thyroid tumors. *J Clin Endocrinol Metab* 1983;57:1251–1256.
122. Clark OH, Okerlund MD, Cavalieri RR, Greenspan FS. Diagnosis and treatment of thyroid, parathyroid, and thyroglossal duct cysts. *J Clin Endocrinol Metab* 1979;48:983–988.
123. Van Herle AJ, Rosenblitt PD, Van Herle TL, Van Herle P, Greipel M, Kellett K. Immunoreactive thyroglobulin in sera and saliva of patients with various thyroid disorders: role of autoantibodies. *J Endocrinol Invest* 1989;12:171–182.
124. Van Herle AJ (unpublished data).
125. Van Herle AJ. Serum thyroglobulin assay. In: DeGroot LJ, ed. *Radiation-associated thyroid carcinoma*. New York: Grune & Stratton, 1977;329–337.
126. Van Herle AJ. Serum thyroglobulin measurement in the diagnosis and management of thyroid disease. In: Oppenheimer JH, ed. *Thyroid today*, vol 4(2). Deerfield, IL: Flint Laboratories, 1981.

CHAPTER 31

Iodine-131 and External Radiation in the Treatment of Local and Metastatic Thyroid Cancer

Martin Schlumberger, Claude Parmentier, Florent de Vathaire, and Maurice Tubiana

The majority of patients with differentiated thyroid carcinoma present with localized disease, and overall long-term survival is among the best when compared with other human neoplasias. Nevertheless, mortality and morbidity rates for thyroid cancer remain a cause for concern. They are modulated by several prognostic factors (1–17). Adequate initial surgery offers the most useful contribution to both overall survival and relapse-free survival. The completeness of surgical resection, together with a knowledge of prognostic factors, will determine the subsequent choice of complementary treatment modalities, which may include additional surgery, radioiodine, and external beam irradiation.

This chapter reviews the role of radioiodine and external radiotherapy (RT) in the management of differentiated thyroid carcinoma, based on the experience obtained at the Institut Gustave-Roussy, Villejuif, where more than 2500 patients are currently followed. In patients with differentiated thyroid carcinoma, radioiodine is both a diagnostic and a therapeutic tool. Four main situations may be encountered: patients without evidence of disease, where iodine-131 (^{131}I) can be used to ablate normal thyroid remnants; patients with disease confined to the neck after incomplete surgery or relapse; patients with metastatic disease; and patients with elevated thyroglobulin (Tg) levels without other evidence of disease. RT is given to some patients with disease confined to the neck or with bone metastases. Techniques and indications for these two therapeutic tools are discussed for each of these situations.

METHODS OF TREATMENT

Radioactive Iodine

^{131}I has an 8.02-day half-life and emits β rays (mean energy, 191 keV) and γ rays (main energy, 364 keV). Its physical characteristics are remarkably well suited for therapy (18–31). The main advantage of radioiodine irradiation is that it is well tolerated. It does not induce local sequelae because the surrounding normal tissues receive only small doses. For this reason, radioiodine does not interfere with subsequent surgery.

The radiation dose is related to both tissue concentration and biologic half-life. In normal thyroid tissue, the concentration is about 1% of the administered activity per gram of thyroid tissue, and the effective half-life is about 8 days. In thyroid cancer tissue, the concentration ranges usually from 0.5% per gram to less than 0.001%. The half-life is often short, ranging from several hours to 3 days in most tumors. Therefore, the dose delivered by ^{131}I is often relatively low.

Considering an average concentration per gram in functional well-differentiated tumors of 0.1% of the activity of ^{131}I administered to the patient, the administration of 100 mCi will result in an absorbed dose of approximately 30 Grays (Gy) (when the half-life is equal to 3 days) and 15 Gy (for a half-life of 1.5 days). The dose is related to the tumor concentration and not to the tumor uptake. Considering a half-life equal to 3 days, a tumor with a mass of 5 g and an uptake of 0.5% receives a higher dose (approximately 30 Gy) than a tumor of 100 g with an uptake of 10% (approximately 3 Gy). In practice, only two thirds of the patients take up sufficient amounts of iodine in their metastases and are amenable to therapy with ^{131}I (26–29).

M. Schlumberger, C. Parmentier, F. de Vathaire, M. Tubiana: Institut Gustave-Roussy, 94805 Villejuif Cedex, France.

Dosimetric aspects of radioiodine therapy are often overlooked. These have been thoroughly discussed in many papers (28–31), and we shall only underscore a few points. The heterogeneity of the dose distribution in neoplastic tissues is caused by the spotty distribution of radioiodine (which is well visualized on autoradiographs) and by the characteristics of the radiation emitted by ^{131}I. The radiation dose is mostly delivered by the beta particles whose mean path is short, about 1 mm. This has two consequences: (a) a tumor mass that has a low concentration and that is more than 1 mm in diameter receives only a small radiation dose even if it is surrounded by normal thyroid tissue with a high radioiodine concentration; and (b) the dose received by a small mass of iodine-concentrating tissue is smaller than the dose calculated with the equations generally used for assessing the dose received by the thyroid, which assume that the size of the mass is much larger than the mean path of the particles. When the mass is small, the energy taken out by the particles leaving the iodine-concentrating tissue is not balanced by energy brought in by particles coming in from surrounding tissues. Table 1 indicates the mean dose received by tumors with the same concentration of radioiodine but of different sizes. One can see how difficult it is to deliver a sufficient dose to small micrometastases (< 1 mm), even when their concentrating ability is relatively high. However, no dosimetric evaluation can be performed in patients with small nonmeasurable metastases.

All these factors explain why the dose delivered by radioiodine is often relatively low. For a concentration of less than 0.01% per gram, it is unlikely that radioiodine alone will achieve any therapeutic benefit. In fact, recommended doses are 300 Gy for ablation of thyroid remnants and 100 Gy for treatment of metastases (28,29). In patients with distant metastases, a positive relationship has been shown between the outcome of radioiodine therapy and the effective radiation dose (29). Initial radiation doses of at least 80 Gy to metastatic foci are associated with a significant response rate to therapy, and if radiation doses to tumor are less than 35 Gy, there will be little chance for success. The range of concentration should be assessed *in vivo* by quantitative scintigraphy. Radioiodine uptake is more frequently seen and is often higher in well-differentiated carcinomas, in younger patients, and in those with small metastases. This suggests an accumulation of metabolic defects with both age and tumor progression (27). Radioiodine can eradicate small foci of neoplastic tissue, but it can seldom permanently eradicate large tumor deposits (19,26–29); therefore the addition of surgery or external irradiation is justified.

Another important dosimetric problem concerns the dose received by organs other than the thyroid tissue, including the blood, the bone marrow, and the gonads. It varies from less than 0.1 cGy to 1 cGy per mCi of iodine. Because of the short mean path of the ^{131}I beta particles, the dose delivered to tissues surrounding any functional thyroid tissue is limited.

Patients are hypothyroid at the time of the administration of radioiodine. This hypothyroid status decreases the renal clearance of ^{131}I and therefore increases the whole-body retention of ^{131}I and the radiation dose delivered to the whole body. Doses to many organs will depend on whole-body retention, which is variable among patients. On the average, the whole-body dose is double that estimated in euthyroid subjects, as shown by biologic dosimetry based on cytogenetic studies (personal data).

Several biologic studies have been undertaken with the aim of increasing radioiodine concentration. A low trapping of radioiodine and a low stable iodine concentration are observed in all differentiated thyroid cancers. The radioiodine uptake is weakly correlated with stable iodine concentration, and, more interestingly, response to thyroid stimulating hormone (TSH) stimulation is greatest in tumors with the highest iodine content.

A large number of biochemical defects have been described, and in them the iodine transport mechanism is always impaired. This may be a result of a defect in the transport mechanism of iodine itself or the result of a variety of defects. The rate of organification is generally very low, particularly in the less differentiated tumors. This may be because of defects in the enzymatic systems, such as peroxidase associated with oxidation and organification of iodine. Tg concentration is always reduced in tumors, and in many of them it can be detected only by immunochemistry. Production of Tg in the blood by neoplastic tissue can, however, be detected in almost all thyroid cancer patients (32–48). Because of the low Tg concentration, the proportion of low-molecular-weight iodoproteins is high. The hormonosynthesis yield is very low in these proteins. However, the lack of Tg is not sufficient to account for the deficiency in iodine concentration.

Hormonosynthesis requires both complex enzymatic systems and a strict structural organization. It is not surprising that several defects can impair this delicate process. The number and the variety of defects observed in malignant cells leave little hope of improving radioiodine concentration by simple means.

Most differentiated thyroid tumors possess TSH receptors on their cell membrane. Their number varies with the histologic type: most are found in follicular well-differentiated (FWD) tumors and the fewest in the less differentiated ones. Moreover, response to TSH stimulation, as

TABLE 1. *Relationship between absorbed dose and the diameter of radioiodine sphere (concentration being kept constant)*

Diameter (mm)	10	5	1	0.5	0.1
Relative absorbed dose (%)	100	90	50	33	7.5

assessed by the adenyl cyclase level and the increase in radioiodine uptake, varies widely among tumors with a given number of TSH receptors.

Stimulation by TSH increases radioiodine uptake by all thyroid tissues that are able to pick up ^{131}I. It also increases Tg release into the blood, even by tumors that cannot concentrate ^{131}I. This shows that all tumors are TSH dependent (44). TSH also plays a major role in the control of thyroid cell proliferation, as shown in the *in vitro* culture of normal human thyroid cells; suppressive therapy with T$_4$ has a favorable effect on tumor growth rate, recurrence rate, tumor progression, and death rate from thyroid cancer (23). Stimulation by supranormal levels of TSH for 2 weeks is necessary before any administration of ^{131}I for diagnostic or therapeutic purposes (44,45), but this does not induce significant tumor growth during this short period of time.

In summary, although prolonged stimulation by supranormal levels of TSH can induce the ability to concentrate iodine in a sizable proportion of thyroid tumors, there is currently no satisfactory way to predict which particular tumors will do so. Histologic type, age of the patient, size and extent of metastases, stable iodine concentration, and initial thyroid uptake remain the only valid indicators.

External Radiotherapy

The importance of combining radioiodine and external irradiation is often underestimated. With little additional toxic effect, external radiotherapy can efficiently complement radioiodine (21,25). However, external radiotherapy is not without morbidity, and its use in initial treatment of localized tumors should be restricted to patients with a high risk for local recurrence and a high likelihood of prolonged survival.

Tumor control can be achieved only if all the tumor stem cells have lost their ability to proliferate. Morphologically intact cells may not be able to proliferate. The proportion of cells surviving is inversely related to the dose delivered. At a low dose (40 Gy), there is insufficient cell kill to cause tumor control. As the dose is raised, the probability of control increases, but a small underdosage in parts of the tumor (dose less than 20% of the tumor control dose in one tenth of the tumor mass) would practically eliminate the likelihood of tumor control. There is a relationship between tumor volume and the tumor control dose: bulky tumors require higher radiation doses for control than do smaller ones. For example, the number of cells in a tumor of 6 cm in diameter is approximately 30 times greater than in a tumor of 2 cm in diameter. Thus, the tumor control dose should theoretically be increased by about 10 to 12 Gy, but in fact larger dose increments are often necessary. The volume of the largest occult metastatic foci (diameter, 4 mm) is 1000-fold smaller than that of a tumor of 4 cm in diameter; thus the tumor control dose should be 15 to 20 Gy less than the dose that controls a tumor of 4 cm. In effect, in clinical practice, a dose of 45 to 50 Gy appears to be sufficient. This dose is generally well tolerated by normal tissues, whereas the high doses required for the control of gross tumors may induce sequelae.

For a given dose, the tissue reactions are more severe when the field size is larger. Late complications of RT manifest themselves months or years after completion of irradiation. They are not reversible. Their incidence is related to the size of the irradiated volume, the total dose, and the dose per fraction. Late complications are observed mainly in tissues with a slow cell turnover, such as subcutaneous tissue. They can be particularly severe after radical irradiation to bilateral cervical regions.

Radiotherapy and surgery are complementary: surgery can excise the gross masses, and then irradiation can eradicate subclinical disease. A few decades ago, postoperative RT was used infrequently, because the prevailing view was that one should wait for recurrence in order to have something tangible to irradiate. When it was recognized that higher doses are required to eradicate gross masses than subclinical disease, prophylactic irradiation of clinically uninvolved areas at risk of containing occult deposits was advocated. This method is now widely used, with favorable clinical results. Moreover, treatment with radioiodine is still possible after beam therapy, because the decrease in the radioiodine uptake following beam therapy is generally relatively small for many months as a result of the slow cell turnover in differentiated cancers (21).

PROGNOSTIC FACTORS AND NATURAL HISTORY

Most differentiated thyroid carcinomas are extremely slow-growing, with doubling times exceeding 1 year and time courses extending over several decades. Some of the misconceptions concerning the course of thyroid cancer arose from studies with a mean follow-up of only 5 to 10 years.

In patients without distant metastases at initial treatment, total survival is significantly lower than in a reference population. These data, among others, indicate the fallacy of the idea that patients with differentiated thyroid carcinoma may die with, but not from, their thyroid cancer (1–17). Recurrent disease is frequently seen and is associated with higher mortality rates (2).

Prognostic factors have been identified by univariate analysis. Because all factors are closely interrelated, only multivariate analyses can assess the independent prognostic significance of each of them. In most reports that considered as a group patients with papillary and follicular cancer (1–6,10,12), age was found to be the most important variable. Older patients have a higher cancer-related mortality. The aggressiveness of the disease continuously increases with age, escalating sharply at 45 years of age (2) or later (9). In older patients, the probability of relapse is greater and the interval between initial treatment and relapse is shorter. Similarly, the delay between relapse and death is shorter, suggesting a more rapid growth rate (see also Chapter 28).

In children, the long-term prognosis is favorable. However, the excess mortality caused by thyroid cancer is highly significant, and the frequency of distant metastases and the relapse rate are higher than in adults. Younger children have a more aggressive course (Table 2) (8). These data clearly show that extensive treatment should be performed in children, including total thyroidectomy with lymph node dissection followed by ^{131}I treatment. Thereafter, the same protocol of follow-up should be used in both children and adults.

Histology provides highly significant prognostic information. Patients with papillary and follicular well-differentiated tumors have a similar favorable prognosis, but those with less-differentiated cancer fare worse (2,7,9–13,15,16). Some prognostic studies have considered papillary and follicular cancer separately (7,10) (see also Chapter 6).

Papillary carcinoma has a prolonged course in most patients. However, high mortality rates may be seen in some subsets of patients. Using a multivariate analysis, four variables were found to be independently predictive of survival: age, histologic grade, tumor extent, and tumor size (7). Older patients and those with less differentiated papillary carcinoma had an increased mortality rate. Prognosis is worse when the primary tumor directly invades the surrounding neck structures. In recent years, large inoperable tumor masses have virtually disappeared in developed countries. However, a small papillary carcinoma can extend through the thyroid capsule. The risk of death increases with the size of the tumor. Patients with a small tumor of less than 1 cm in diameter have an excellent prognosis. The discovery of such a tumor in a gland removed for other clinical reasons warrants long-term follow-up and suppressive treatment with L-thyroxine (LT$_4$), but it does not justify aggressive initial treatment. These four prognostic factors (age, histologic grade, tumor extent, and tumor size) have permitted classification into risk groups. Eighty-six percent of the patients were found to be in the low risk group, with a 20-year mortality rate of only 1% from papillary carcinoma (7). These data were confirmed by multivariate analyses performed on other series of patients (10,13).

In a further multivariate analysis, the same group described a scoring system based on five variables (MACIS): metastases, age, completeness of resection, invasion, and size (14). All the five variables are readily available after primary operation. Tumor cell DNA content may provide additional information because nondiploid tumors have been associated with an increased risk of mortality (17).

TABLE 2. *Younger age is associated with a more aggressive course of thyroid carcinoma in 98 children treated at Institut Gustave-Roussy*

	Age at initial treatment (yrs)		
	< 7	8–12	13–16
Patients (n)	12	48	38
Distant metastases (n)	8	19	9
Cancer deaths (n)	1	5	0

From ref. 8.

The disease-related mortality from follicular carcinoma is higher than in patients with papillary carcinoma (9–16). Multivariate analyses have determined the prognostic importance of several variables. Age, although significant, did not appear to be the most important variable. A highly significant difference in survival was observed between follicular less-differentiated tumors (FLD) and other histologic subtypes (2,12,13,15,16). Furthermore, the treatment-to-relapse and relapse-to-death intervals were shorter for FLD than for other tumors (2). These data show that these two follicular subtypes (less- and well-differentiated) should be distinguished (2,15,16). Mortality and recurrence rates are increased significantly in patients presenting with lesions with wide capsular and vascular invasion (15). Invasiveness is closely related to the grade of differentiation. Mortality from the large primary tumors is significantly higher than from small cancers, but a substantial number of patients with small follicular carcinoma die of their disease. In the Hürthle cell type, death seems to be restricted to patients with DNA aneuploid tumors (17).

The treatment approach should be based on risk groups and on extent of disease (1,2,7,10,13,14). At the time of initial treatment, prognostic factors and scoring systems enable the assessment of the patient's risk of dying from cancer (Fig. 1). The low risk group includes young patients with favorable prognostic indicators. In this group, most recurrences are curable and long-term prognosis is excellent. The high risk group includes all patients above the age of 45 and younger patients with a large thyroid tumor, with capsular invasion, or with less-differentiated histologic type. In this group, the incidence of recurrence and death from cancer is high, and treatment of the recurrence is often unsuccessful.

POSTOPERATIVE RADIOIODINE THERAPY

In all patients with thyroid carcinoma, surgery is the main primary treatment. Its extent should be based on the knowledge of prognostic factors and on the extent of the disease. Postoperatively, the use of an ablative dose of radioiodine and external radiotherapy will also depend on

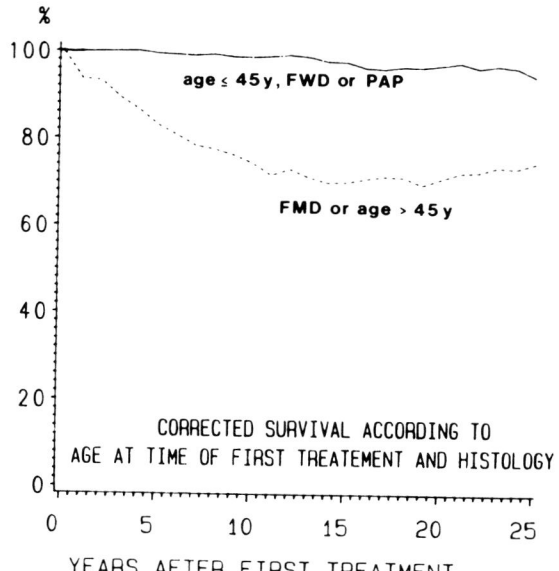

FIG. 1. Corrected survival of thyroid cancer patients without initial distant metastases according to high or low risk group (2). Only the two main prognostic factors, age at first treatment and histology, were taken into account. The low risk group includes patients aged less that 45 years with papillary (PAP) or follicular well-differentiated (FWD) carcinoma; 25 years after initial treatment, the excess of mortality is 2%. The high risk group includes patients aged more than 45 years at initial treatment or with follicular less-differentiated (FLD) carcinoma. Excess of mortality at 25 years is 30%. Corrected survival was obtained by comparison with a reference French population of the same age and sex.

the prognostic factors and the completeness of surgical excision of the neoplastic tissue. Two postoperative conditions may be encountered: complete or incomplete surgical excision.

Routine postoperative administration of ^{131}I after total surgical removal of the neoplastic tissue may have two advantages. First, total ablation of thyroid tissue increases the specificity of Tg measurement and the sensitivity of total-body ^{131}I scan during the follow-up (see later). Second, irradiation by radioiodine can destroy residual neoplastic tissue. Two issues are important relative to remnant ablation: its effectiveness in ablating ^{131}I uptake in the neck and its effect on tumor recurrence.

In some series, such as ours (2,21), the recurrence rate was similar (about 20%) whether the surgery was followed by the administration of 100 mCi or not (Table 3). It must be noted, however, that the two groups were not randomized and it is likely that the group treated by postoperative ^{131}I included patients with larger and more infiltrating tumors. On the other hand, in some series, relapse rates were lower in patients routinely treated postoperatively with ^{131}I (9,18–20,25). Two recent studies (22,23) have clearly shown that postoperative ^{131}I ablation decreases the recurrence rate and the mortality rate in patients with no residual disease and with thyroid tumor larger than 1.5 cm, with or without local invasion or regional metastases.

The reasons usually given for the nonroutine use of ^{131}I are not entirely convincing. After a single ablative dose of ^{131}I, the risks of leukemia, genetic defect, miscarriage, or infertility remain unproven (see later).

The present data do not justify the routine administration of ^{131}I to all patients, particularly young adult patients with small tumors (<1.5 cm) confined to the thyroid bed. In those patients with favorable prognostic indicators, the long-term survival is so favorable after surgery alone, that it can hardly be improved by routine ablation with ^{131}I (1–15). An ablative dose of ^{131}I is justified in patients with poor prognostic indicators, with tumors larger than 1.5 cm, with local invasion, or with regional metastases. In these patients, it will decrease the relapse and mortality rates and will facilitate the early discovery of relapses. It is also justified in patients in whom the serum Tg level remains elevated a few months after surgery (46–48). In these patients, the post-therapy total body scan can determine if surgical resection has been complete and it may indicate, in cases of ectopic uptake, further treatments.

Total ablation is easier to produce when the size of the thyroid remnant is small. Therefore, total or subtotal thyroidectomy is advocated in patients who are to be given an ablative dose of ^{131}I. Radioiodine is given after adequate TSH stimulation (see later). The use of 30 mCi of ^{131}I has been proposed because thyroid ablation (as defined by subsequent diagnostic scans that use a 2- to 5-mCi dose of ^{131}I) is achieved in 80% of patients with 30 mCi or larger doses. However, many authors still advocate the routine use of 100 mCi (24). Others recommended that ablation should be based on radiation dose delivered rather than empirical administration of a standard amount of ^{131}I (28).

In patients with incomplete surgical excision of neoplastic tissue, most authors advocate the administration of 100 mCi, and this will decrease the recurrence rate (18–23,25). In addition to its therapeutic effects, a total-body ^{131}I scan has to be performed 5 to 7 days later to delineate residual neoplastic tissue. Further surgery is warranted when foci of uptake are found in the neck, particularly behind the sternoclavicular joint or in the mediastinum. After repeat surgery, the remaining activity of radioiodine will again help to verify the completeness of excision.

Administration of several therapeutic doses of ^{131}I may be necessary to ablate uptake in metastatic lymph node. Neoplastic cells have been found in lymph nodes removed after treatment with ^{131}I, even when uptake was no longer detectable. This clearly explains the occurrence of late relapses after treatment with radioiodine alone (2,21). Therefore, surgery has been advocated to remove lymph node metastases with or without ^{131}I uptake. Similarly, radioiodine is often unsuccessful in permanently

TABLE 3. Relapse-free survival rate and overall survival rate of patients with differentiated thyroid carcinoma treated by surgery alone, or combined with postoperative radiotherapy by radioiodine or external beam

	Patients at risk	Relapse-free survival (%)				Total survival (%)			
		5 yr	10 yr	15 yr	20 yr	5 yr	10 yr	15 yr	20 yr
Surgery alone	275	80	74	66	54	93	87	81	74
Prophylactic post-op ^{131}I after surgery	61	73	64	50	43	90	81	72	72
Prophylactic post-op external RT ± ^{131}I	66	78	65	56	46	81	71	62	58
RT after incomplete surgery[a]	97	71	55	41	34	75	65	53	51
Inoperable patients	23	60	22	7	—	52	27	14	—

From refs. 2,21.
[a]Incomplete surgery means macroscopically incomplete.
Post-op, postoperative; RT, external radiotherapy.

eradicating gross local disease, and the addition of external radiation improves the results.

EXTERNAL RADIOTHERAPY TO THE NECK

The role of external radiotherapy in the treatment of thyroid cancer remains controversial. However, several series, including the 180 patients irradiated at Institut Gustave-Roussy between 1943 and 1976, have clearly shown its effectiveness in the local control of differentiated thyroid cancer (21) (see Table 3). This is documented by the low incidence of local recurrences in patients who have been irradiated. Local recurrences occurred in 9% of the 66 patients irradiated after complete surgery, and in 16% of the 97 irradiated after macroscopically incomplete surgery. This compares favorably with the 19% incidence of local recurrences in the 275 patients treated by surgery alone, 17% where surgery was complete, and 43% where the excision was questionable or incomplete. The difference is statistically significant, and it is higher when only the recurrences in the irradiated field are taken into account ($p < .001$).

It should be recalled that the irradiated patients were those who had the largest tumors, which were particularly difficult to resect and often had extension into neighboring tissues, or whose prognosis appeared to be less favorable. This is evidenced by a higher incidence of distant metastases among patients treated with external radiotherapy (27%), compared with 8% in patients treated by surgery alone.

The relapse-free survival of 23 inoperable patients treated by external beam radiotherapy was 60% at 5 years and 22% at 10 years. In the 97 patients who underwent macroscopically incomplete surgery, the relapse-free survival was 71% at 5 years and 41% at 15 years.

The data also emphasize the importance of an adequate dose. In the 95 patients (with or without residual microscopic disease) treated by cobalt 60 or megavoltage who received an average dose of 50 Gy, ten locoregional recurrences were observed (five within and five outside the irradiated field). In the 48 patients treated with conventional x-rays (average dose, 28 Gy), seven local recurrences were observed (six within the irradiated field and one outside). In the 37 patients treated with a radium mold, eight recurrences were observed (six within the irradiated field and two outside). The difference in the number of recurrences within the irradiated field between high-energy and conventional x-ray groups is significant ($p < 0.04$). The average time interval between initial treatment and local recurrence was 8.5 years.

The relapse-free survival rate was lower in irradiated patients than in those treated by surgery alone, which is not surprising because the irradiated patients had the worst prognostic factors to begin with. Nevertheless, the survival rates support the use of external radiotherapy, because a long-term cure may be achieved even in patients in whom the excision of the tumor was incomplete or impossible. The total survival rate of patients irradiated after macroscopically incomplete surgery was 75% at 5 years and 53% at 15 years, and that of the 23 patients irradiated for inoperable tumor was 52% at 5 years and 27% at 10 years. In the 66 patients irradiated after complete surgery, the survival rate was 81% at 5 years and 62% at 15 years.

These data are in keeping with those of another series of patients (25). In this series, in patients with no postoperative residual disease, adjuvant treatment using radioiodine or radiotherapy did not provide any significant improvement in local control and in survival. In contrast, in patients with microscopic residual disease, both radioiodine and radiotherapy improved local control markedly, from about one third of the patients to three quarters, for all histologic types. Patients with papillary carcinoma had a similar survival, either where microscopic residual disease was present and treated with radiotherapy, or after complete excision by surgery alone or with radioiodine. The control of gross residual disease was less satisfactory, and local control was achieved in only half of the patients treated postoperatively with radiotherapy. These data again emphasize the paramount importance of surgical excision, which should be as complete as possible. If surgery has been macroscopically incomplete, the importance of combining radioiodine and radiotherapy is shown by the fact that patients treated by both modalities responded more often and more fully than those treated by only one of those radiation modalities. However, with a longer follow-up, many authors have observed, as we have, some late recurrences.

The fall in serum Tg levels after irradiation and the low serum Tg levels in patients who had been irradiated for residual neoplastic tissue further illustrate the effectiveness of external irradiation.

In conclusion, postoperative irradiation after incomplete surgery is effective when sufficient doses are delivered. However, this should be performed only after an experienced surgeon believes that everything possible has been done, because external radiotherapy may hamper subsequent surgery for local recurrence. Conversely, after satisfactory tumor excision, external irradiation is not warranted (21,25).

Patients are irradiated with high energy radiation. The target volume should include the thyroid bed, the neck lymph nodes, and the upper part of the mediastinum. The average tumor dose is 50 Gy in 25 fractions over 5 weeks; a boost of 5 to 10 Gy is often delivered to any palpable residual tumor. Patients are irradiated with a direct anterior field shaped by lead blocks to protect the lungs and the larynx, and with a posterior field limited to the upper mediastinum. The respective dose contributions of these two fields should be adapted according to the anteroposterior diameter of the upper thorax. The choice is based on a study of the dose distribution carried out in a sagittal plane or in several transverse planes. Another technique uses a single anterior electron field of appropriate energy. Whatever the technique, assiduous attention must be paid to avoid doses greater than 42 Gy to the spinal cord, because higher doses can induce nonrecoverable transverse myelitis.

In our series of 180 irradiated patients, eight severe late complications were observed among patients irradiated with high energy radiation: two cases of brachial plexus neuropathy, two tracheal constrictions, and one laryngotracheal necrosis, necessitating a laryngectomy; two obstructions of the carotid artery; and one osteochondrosarcoma at the border of the irradiated field, 26 years after external radiotherapy was performed.

FOLLOW-UP

Long-term results in patients with metastatic thyroid carcinoma have shown that prognosis is strongly related to the size of the metastases at the time of their discovery (19,26,27,53,54). This emphasizes that the main goal of the follow-up should be the early detection of metastases, at a stage when x-rays are still normal, by the combined use of serum Tg measurement and total-body ^{131}I scan. In view of the importance of these two techniques, we shall briefly discuss them before reviewing the follow-up strategy.

Thyroglobulin

Thyroglobulin is a reliable marker for differentiated thyroid carcinoma during follow-up (32–48) (see also Chapter 30). Divergent results reported in some series appear to have been caused by poor sensitivity or accuracy of the assay. In view of the paramount prognostic importance of the size of the metastases at their discovery, Tg measurement must be sufficiently sensitive to reliably detect low Tg levels. In most commercial kits, 3 to 5 ng/mL used to be the least detectable concentration. With the availability of immunoradiometric assays based on monoclonal antibodies, the least detectable concentration, which was 1 ng/mL, is now less than 1 ng/mL. Endogenous anti-Tg antibodies are found in about 15% of cancer patients. However, interferences are found in less than 5% of sera and prevent the determination of the actual Tg level (32,33). Interferences should therefore be systematically sought, preferably by a recovery test.

When valid methods are used, an elevated serum Tg level is found during T_4 treatment in most patients with distant metastases. Among 155 patients with distant metastases, we observed only three false-negative results. However, the Tg level was below 10 ng/mL in 25 patients (27). Similar results were reported by other groups (34–37,42,43) (Table 4).

The existence of a relationship between the body tumor burden and the serum Tg level has been shown in rats grafted with transplantable thyroid cancer and in patients with lung metastases without iodine uptake, who therefore could not be treated (39) (Figs. 2,3). However, the exact amount of neoplastic tissue required to increase serum Tg level is unknown and probably varies with the biologic characteristics of the tumor. During T_4 treatment, the Tg level is elevated in patients with large metastases, frequently remains relatively low when metastases are not visible on x-rays, and is low or even undetectable in patients with small lymph node metastases. This suggests that there is a slight correlation between the level of serum Tg and the tumor burden. Indeed, among 20 patients with isolated metastatic neck lymph nodes and no other evidence of disease, serum Tg level during T_4 treatment was above 10 ng/mL in only six patients, ranged from 3 to 10 ng/mL in seven patients, was below 3 ng/mL in four, and undetectable in three patients (41). These results underscore the need for lymph node dissection at initial treatment, and if lymph node metastases are found, for routine postoperative total-body ^{131}I scan to confirm the absence of any ectopic uptake in the neck (2).

TABLE 4. *Thyroglobulin (Tg) level during T4 treatment as a function of clinical status*

Clinical status	Tg level (ng/mL)		
	<1	1–5	>5
No evidence of disease without thyroid remnants (n = 349)	99%	1%	0%
No evidence of disease after total thyroidectomy (n = 88)	93%	7%	0%
No evidence of disease after lobectomy (n = 126)	56%	20%	24%
Lymph node metastases only (n = 20)	15%	40%	45%
Distant metastases (n = 155)	2%	7%	91%

From refs. 27, 41.

Serum Tg increases after TSH stimulation in most patients with metastases, even in those whose metastases do not pick up radioiodine (44,45). Table 5 provides an example of this situation, where Tg level was above 5 ng/mL in all the 181 patients with distant metastases in whom it was measured. It was above 10 ng/mL in 175, above 40 ng/mL in 154, and above 100 ng/mL in 118 patients (27).

In patients with no evidence of disease after total thyroid ablation, Tg was undetectable in 99% during T_4 treatment and in 88% after thyroid hormone withdrawal (41). Indeed, falsely positive results have been reported even recently (42) in this situation, and may be caused by interferences in Tg measurement or by the lack of sensitivity of the assay. Therefore, an elevated Tg level is an indication for a complete workup, which may include a total-body scan carried out after the administration of 100 mCi ^{131}I, when the conventional total-body scan (2 to 5 mCi) is negative (46–48). Among 22 patients with serum Tg level above 40 ng/mL after thyroid hormone withdrawal, and no other evidence of disease, a total-body scan with 100 mCi ^{131}I discovered a relapse in 12 and thyroid remnants in eight. Total-body scan with 100 mCi ^{131}I was negative in only two patients, and in these two, lung metastases unable to pick up radioiodine were later discovered.

When interpreting results of Tg measurement, it should be remembered that thyroid cancer has a slow growth rate. Therefore, an increased Tg level may be detected long before metastases become detectable, especially when they do not pick up radioiodine.

In our initial series (35), no relapse was observed, with a follow-up now equal to or longer than 15 years, in 50 patients whose initial Tg level was undetectable during T_4 treatment and after T_4 withdrawal. It is likely, though not yet certain, that these patients are cured.

The main problem is those patients with an undetectable Tg level during T_4 treatment, but with a relatively low increase in Tg level (<10 ng/mL) after T_4 withdrawal. Among 35 patients who were in this situation, we observed four relapses during a follow-up of 15 years: two with cancer in the neck and two with it in the lungs. However, by the time the relapse was discovered, Tg level was

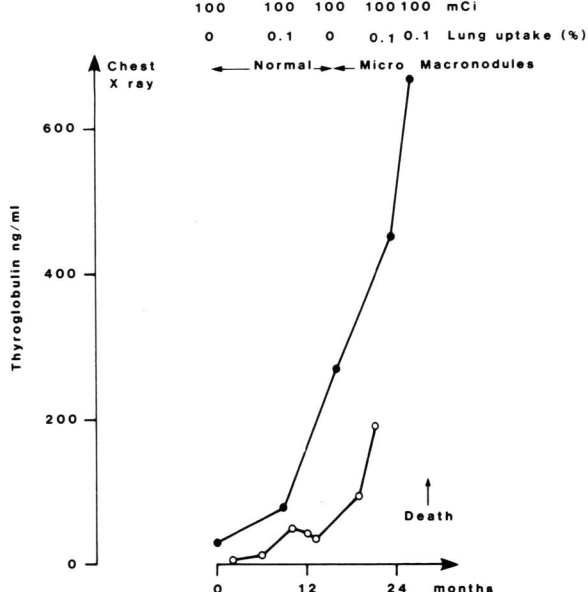

FIG. 3. Thyroglobulin level in a patient with lung metastases during T_4 treatment (○—○) and after T_4 withdrawal (●—●). There is a significant relationship between serum Tg level and the size of the metastases.

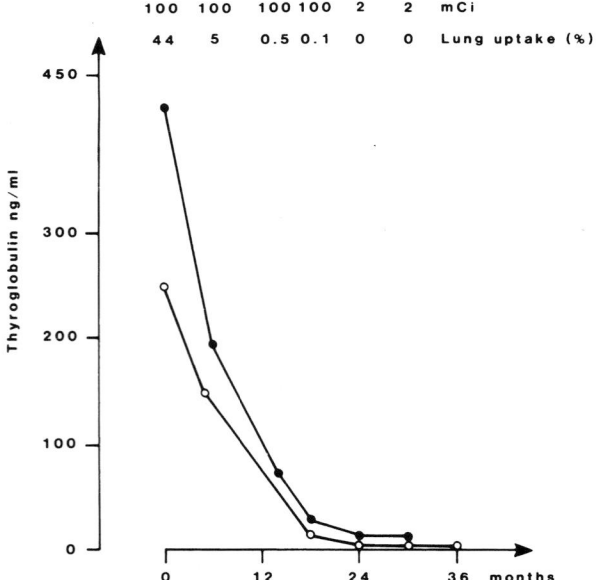

FIG. 2. Thyroglobulin (Tg) level in a patient with lung metastases during T_4 treatment (○—○) and after T_4 withdrawal (●—●). Tg level decreased with radioiodine treatments and remained low 12 years after the last treatment (not shown). Despite detectable Tg levels, no relapse occurred.

TABLE 5. *Thyroglobulin (Tg) level after thyroid hormone withdrawal*

Clinical status	Tg level (ng/mL)			
	<1	1–5	5–10	>10
No evidence of disease without thyroid remnants (n = 95)	88%	9%	3%	0%
No evidence of disease after total thyroidectomy (n = 34)	79%	9%	3%	9%
Distant metastases (n = 181)	0%	0%	4%	96%

From refs. 27,41.

TABLE 6. *Thyroglobulin (Tg) level during T_4 treatment in 192 thyroid cancer patients with thyroid remnants. Log rank test shows that the risk of relapse increases when Tg level is above 10 ng/mL*

Tg (ng/mL)	n	Observed (O)	Expected (E)	O/E
<5	62	3	7.7	0.39
6–10	39	1	5.1	0.2
11–20	37	4	4.2	0.95
21–30	24	2	3.0	0.67
31–40	8	2	0.8	2.46
>41	22	11	2.2	4.9

From ref. 38.

detectable during T_4 treatment. Patients in this situation should therefore be followed with Tg measurements both on and off T_4, and with total-body ^{131}I scans.

In patients with no evidence of disease after surgery only, serum Tg during T_4 treatment was undetectable in 93% after total thyroidectomy, but this was less specific after lobectomy only, being undetectable in this situation in only 56% (41) (see Table 4). In these latter patients, a detectable Tg level may be related to incomplete TSH suppression. However, 29% of the patients with totally suppressed TSH secretion had detectable Tg levels. This suggests the existence of infra-clinical abnormalities in the remaining lobe, as shown by ultrasonography (41). Indeed, the probability of relapse increases in those patients with high Tg levels during T_4 treatment (38) (Table 6). This shows that total thyroidectomy increases the specificity of Tg measurement during T_4 treatment for detecting relapses and should be performed in all patients with a high risk of relapse.

After thyroid hormone withdrawal, in patients after surgery only, Tg can be released either by normal thyroid remnants or by neoplastic foci. After total thyroidectomy, Tg remained undetectable in 79% of patients after thyroid hormone withdrawal, despite uptake in normal thyroid remnants in a large proportion of them (41) (see Table 5). As stated above, Tg was undetectable in 88% of these patients after total thyroid ablation but was detectable in almost all patients after lobectomy only, and in this condition Tg cannot be used as a tumor marker.

^{131}I TOTAL-BODY SCAN

As the efficacy of total-body scan depends upon the ability of malignant tissue to take up radioiodine, iodine overload should be avoided and stimulation by TSH is of critical importance. In practice, patients are taken off T_4 therapy and receive T_3 for 3 weeks. Thereafter, T_3 is withdrawn for 14 days. T_3 withdrawal for more than 2 weeks is unnecessary and may be harmful (49,50). Serum TSH level is measured before the scan is performed, because in some patients TSH fails to reach an adequate level (44,50).

In the past, bovine TSH was found to be an effective exogenous TSH preparation and was used to stimulate radioiodine uptake for the ^{131}I total-body scan. The adverse hypersensitivity reactions following its repeated use have made this approach obsolete, and the product has been removed from the market. In the future, recombinant human TSH will be available to provide exogenous TSH stimulation necessary for a ^{131}I total-body scan and a Tg test can be done while patients remain clinically euthyroid on LT_4 treatment, thereby avoiding the effects of hypothyroidism associated with thyroid hormone withdrawal (51).

The ^{131}I dose generally used in testing is 2 to 5 mCi. Higher diagnostic doses are not recommended because they may decrease the uptake of a subsequent therapeutic dose. Usually, the optimal scanning time is 72 hr after the dose of ^{131}I, when the background activity is lower and the uptake or secretion in organs such as the nasopharynx, salivary glands, stomach, breast, bladder, and colon have diminished. A diffuse liver uptake at this time is a result of the concentration of labeled iodoproteins. False-positive images are rare and may be caused by pathological transudates and inflammation, such as pulmonary edema, chronic bronchitis, skin burn, or tooth granuloma. Uptake of radioiodine has also been observed in pleuropericardial cysts and in scrotal hydroceles. Also, artifacts from nasal secretions, saliva, or urine should be avoided (see also Chapter 8).

The apparatus (rectilinear scanner with dual probes or gamma camera) should detect photons emitted by ^{131}I (main energy, 364 keV) with a high sensitivity and a high energy resolution. The apparatus is connected with computers for data acquisition and processing (Figs. 4,5). In the rectilinear scanner with two opposed probes, each probe is equipped with a thick (101-mm) crystal that provides a high sensitivity (99%) for photons emitted by ^{131}I; the collimator is adapted to the energy of these photons to provide a good spatial resolution; the simultaneous acquisition of anterior and posterior views facilitates

FIG. 4. Total-body scan performed 5 days after the administration of 100 mCi ^{131}I in a patient with a normal chest x-ray. Uptake of ^{131}I in lungs is clear. There is also some accumulation of ^{131}I in the stomach and in the colon.

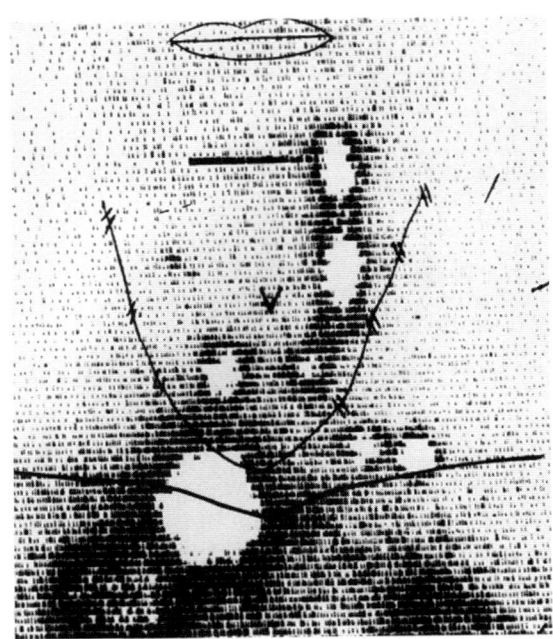

FIG. 5. Neck scintigraphy performed 5 days after the administration of 100 mCi. There is a clear uptake of ^{131}I in lymph node metastases, behind the right sternoclavicular joint. There are also two foci of uptake in the left supraclavicular area and in the left jugulocarotid chain. The total-body scan performed simultaneously allowed the discovery of lung metastases.

computerization and makes the response independent of the source depth (27). In the gamma camera, the head is equipped with a large crystal, the field of view measuring up to 500 mm in diameter; because its thickness is only 12.5 mm, its sensitivity for photons emitted by ^{131}I is low (40%); the collimator should be adapted to the energy of ^{131}I gamma rays. Gamma cameras cannot be used when high activities are present, because of counting errors at high counting rates.

When using a digitalized dual probe rectilinear scanner, uptake in the lungs as low as 1 µCi, and uptake as low as 0.1 µCi could be detected in lymph nodes (27). On a single scintigram, it is difficult to obtain a precise image of the areas with high iodine uptake and to visualize the lesions that pick up only small amounts of radioiodine. Thus, in patients with thyroid remnants, one should accept a blurred overexposed image of the thyroid remnants in order to detect uptakes in small foci of neoplastic tissue. In fact, previous ablation of thyroid remnants increases the sensitivity of total-body scan by facilitating the discovery of these small foci.

In 1963, we introduced scintigraphies performed after the administration of 100 mCi, because this technique enabled us to detect metastases that are far too small to be seen even at the present time on ultrasound images or even on computerized tomography (CT) scan, and with uptake of radioiodine too small to be detected by conventional scintigrams (2 to 5 mCi) (52). This technique proved useful and is currently used by several groups (46–48). Hence, a total-body scan is warranted 4 to 7 days after each administration of 30 or 100 mCi ^{131}I, as it may detect occult neoplastic disease not shown after a diagnostic dose (46–48). It is sometimes argued that this increase in sensitivity is without practical interest, because if the activity taken up by the neoplastic tissue is not high enough to be detectable on routine total-body scan performed with 2 to 5 mCi ^{131}I, it has no therapeutic value. This is debatable for two reasons. First, radioiodine is not the only form of treatment. For instance, an involved mediastinal node can be resected by surgery. Second, the total iodine uptake can be misleading, because tumor concentration of radioiodine is the only relevant parameter for therapy. A low uptake in a very small metastasis results in a higher concentration than a higher uptake in a bulky metastasis. Indeed, experience has shown that small tumors that are barely detectable on routine total-body scan because the uptakes are low are more easily cured by radioiodine than larger tumors with a higher uptake but with a lower tumor concentration (26,27,46–48,53,54).

Finally digitalized scanning is mandatory for measuring the iodine uptake in metastases and for assessing the effect of treatment on this uptake (26–29). With current methods, it is possible to measure uptakes with a precision of less than 20%.

Strategy of Follow-Up

Relapses are discovered usually during the first years of follow-up, but they may also emerge clinically after decades of apparently complete remission (2). Therefore, follow-up ought to be intensive during the first 2 to 3 years but should also be pursued throughout the patient's life.

L-Thyroxine treatment is advocated for all patients with differentiated thyroid carcinoma, with the aim of suppressing TSH secretion without inducing thyrotoxicosis (43). This is achieved by obtaining an undetectable TSH level and an FT_3 level within the normal range, if possible. This may avoid thyrotoxicosis and its long-term effects such as osteoporosis and cardiac complications. The mean daily dose of LT_4 is 2.4 µg/kg body weight. TSH and FT_3 levels are checked 3 months after initiation of LT_4 treatment. When necessary, the LT_4 daily dose is modified by 25 µg. In patients without any evidence of disease, including an undetectable Tg level after LT_4 withdrawal, the TSH level may remain detectable, at the lower limit of the normal range (see also Chapters 4 and 27).

A strategy has been developed for the follow-up of patients in which Tg assays have a prominent role (Fig. 6). The ablation of thyroid remnants increases the sensitivity of both Tg measurement and total-body ^{131}I scan and is advocated in patients at high risk of developing relapses (note the ^{131}I ablative dose in Figure 6). Of note, serum Tg level may decline slowly during the first months after initial therapy.

A total-body ^{131}I scan is performed each year for 2 years after initial therapy, with the first scan performed after an initial ablative dose of ^{131}I. Thereafter, in patients with negative total-body scan and undetectable or low Tg levels after thyroid hormone withdrawal, follow-up is resumed with clinical evaluation, FT_3, TSH, and Tg measurements, once a year, while on T_4 therapy. Diagnostic ^{131}I total-body scan is performed 5 years after initial treatment.

When Tg level is detectable, and especially if it increases with time during T_4 treatment in patients without thyroid remnants, a total-body ^{131}I scan and a chest x-ray are performed and Tg is measured again after thyroid hormone withdrawal. Patients with positive total-body scans are treated with 100 mCi ^{131}I. In those patients with a negative total-body ^{131}I scan, in whom Tg levels increased significantly after thyroid hormone withdrawal, additional attempts to localize thyroid tissue are made (neck ultrasound, neck and thorax CT scan). Administration of 100 mCi ^{131}I with a total-body scan 5 days later permits the detection of unknown normal or neoplastic thyroid tissue in a large proportion of these patients, who can subsequently be cured (46–48). If this post-therapy total-body scan is negative, venous sampling catheterization did not reveal any Tg concentration gradient, and scanning with ^{131}I labeled anti-Tg monoclonal antibody or with thallium-201 (55) has not proved to be useful. We have recently studied these patients using scintigraphy with an analog of somatostatin labeled with indium-111 for the localization of neoplastic foci (56).

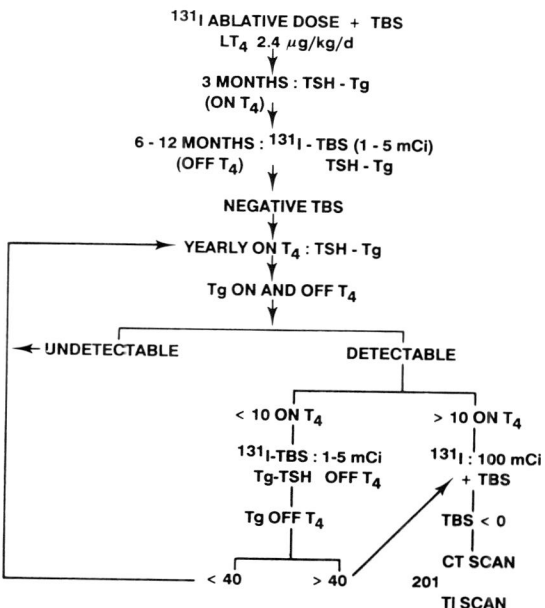

FIG. 6. Strategy of follow-up in patients without thyroid remnants and in the absence of serum interference in the method of Tg measurement. Follow-up is based on the combined use of thyroglobulin (Tg) measurement and total-body ^{131}I scan (TBS). An IRMA method (Dynotest Tg) was used.

Patients with thyroid remnants after total thyroidectomy, whose Tg levels are elevated during T_4 treatment, are given 100 mCi of radioiodine to ablate the thyroid remnant with a total-body scan 5 days later. This may be an indication for further surgery.

Patients with large thyroid remnants, for instance after lobectomy only, whose Tg levels are elevated during T_4 treatment, should first undergo further surgery.

Since the routine use of the Tg assay, the number of total-body ^{131}I scans performed has been reduced, but they are more effective because their indications are better defined. This allows an earlier discovery of relapse that should improve long-term treatment results.

LOCAL RECURRENCE

Recurrent disease may be associated with a higher mortality rate. However, treatment of local recurrence is often curative. A local recurrence often precedes or is associated with the emergence of distant metastases. Therefore, patients with recurrent disease should be assessed with a view to further treatment by all modalities (2,25).

The treatment of local recurrence should include the administration of 100 mCi of ^{131}I with a scan 5 days later, which allows for a better delineation of known neoplastic tissue and sometimes the discovery of unsuspected neoplastic foci. A neck or chest CT scan may be helpful to localize lymph node metastases, particularly in the mediastinum. Tracheal and esophageal extension can be assessed by CT scan and endoscopic examination. When feasible, further surgery is then undertaken. The use of an intraoperative probe may help the localization of functioning neoplastic foci (57). With the remaining ^{131}I activity, the patient is scanned again after surgery to ensure the completeness of surgical excision. Recurrences only rarely require extensive resection. At Institut Gustave-Roussy, however, three patients with a massive neck recurrence underwent tracheal resection and laryngectomy, and two of them also underwent a total esophagectomy. Neoplastic tissue was totally removed, two of these patients lived 11 and 12 years after surgery, and none of the three experienced a neck relapse. Extensive surgical procedures allow a good quality of life, avoid death from local growth and suffocation, and, even if small distant metastases are present, the life expectancy of the patients is several years or even decades.

In our series, survival after neck recurrences was 62% ± 10% at 10 years (2). It was significantly shorter among older patients, in those with FLD tumors, and in the absence of radioiodine uptake. For recurrent tumor with radioiodine uptake, survival after treatment of recurrence was 91% at 5 years, 86% at 10 years, and 50% at 15 years. In these patients, when a complete surgical resection of the recurrent mass has been performed, no complementary treatment is warranted. For recurrent tumor without ^{131}I uptake or with uptake too low for significant radiation dose to be delivered, survival was only 53% at 5 years, 32% at 10 years, and 30% at 15 years after recurrence. In these patients, external radiotherapy to the neck is indicated after radical surgery (2,21,25). Its usefulness has been demonstrated in a series of 16 patients who were irradiated for local recurrence (21). Irradiation was given after incomplete surgical excision of the local recurrence in 11 patients. Only two of them experienced a local recurrence, 2 and 3 years after irradiation. Irradiation was performed in another five patients for inoperable local recurrence, three of whom experienced a local relapse 1, 2, and 4 years after irradiation. Of the 11 patients without further local recurrence, five are alive without evidence of disease and six are dead; in five of these, deaths were caused by distant metastases.

DISTANT METASTASES

Incidence

Metastases outside the neck occur in 10% to 15% of patients with differentiated thyroid cancer (20,22,26,27, 53,54,58–61). Almost half of them are present initially, but in recent years, in industrialized countries, large neck masses and synchronous distant metastases have almost disappeared as presenting signs.

Pre-Treatment Evaluation

Patients with metastatic disease need a complete workup. The extent of disease is first appreciated by total-body scan performed after the administration of 100 mCi, after as complete a thyroidectomy as possible.

In patients with lung metastases, a chest CT scan is performed to search for mediastinal involvement. In patients with macronodular metastases, it often reveals micronodular lung metastases not visible on plain x-rays. Even when the chest x-ray is normal, a lung CT scan may show peripheral micronodular lung metastases in cases with diffuse uptake of ^{131}I in the lungs (Table 7).

In patients with bone metastases, x-rays are performed on painful bones and where radioiodine uptake has been demonstrated. A CT scan or magnetic resonance imaging (MRI) helps to delineate the extent of these metastases. MRI is particularly useful for the workup of metastases localized in the spine and the skull. Most bone metastases are hypervascularized, and if surgery is to be performed, arteriography and presurgical embolization may be warranted.

Strategy of Treatment

Surgery

Surgery should be considered for bone metastases in patients with orthopedic or neurologic complications, or in those at high risk of such complications. Surgery

TABLE 7. *Findings in 67 patients with lung metastases and normal chest x-rays. Experience at Gustave-Roussy Institute*

	Negative	Positive
Chest x-ray	67	0
Lung tomograms	25	1
Lung CT scan	15	8
Tg level during T$_4$ treatment	3	43 (2–85 ng/mL)
Total-body ^{131}I scan		
1–2 mCi	15	52
100 mCi	0	67

From ref. 27.

should also be considered with a curative intent in patients with a single or a few bone metastases, where remarkable results have been produced (62), and in those with a single or a few cerebral metastases. Lung metastases are often multiple and surgery on lungs is rarely beneficial.

Radioiodine

^{131}I is the most frequently employed form of treatment of metastatic cancer. However, only two thirds of the patients take up sufficient amount of iodine in their metastases to be amenable to therapy with ^{131}I (26,27). Radioiodine can eradicate small foci of neoplastic tissue but can seldom permanently eradicate large tumor deposits (26,27,53,54,60); therefore the addition of surgery or external irradiation may be warranted. For this reason, in patients with large mediastinal lymph node metastases and lung metastases not visible on plain x-rays, mediastinal dissection is performed whenever possible and lung metastases are thereafter treated with ^{131}I.

The treatment dose is 100 to 150 mCi in adults and approximately 1 mCi/kg body weight in young children. High treatment doses (200 mCi) have been advocated by several authors, but the effectiveness of these higher doses remains to be established. The dose is given after TSH stimulation. A post-therapy scan is performed 5 to 7 days later, and T$_4$ treatment is resumed. Successive treatments with ^{131}I are given 3 to 6 months later until total ablation of residual uptake or adverse reactions are seen. There is no upper limit for the cumulative ^{131}I dose administered. However, cumulative doses of ^{131}I higher than 600 mCi appeared of limited benefit (27). The early discovery of metastases, at a stage when they are not visible on plain x-rays, will permit a reduction in the total dose of ^{131}I necessary for cure and hence in body irradiation (26,27) (see Figs. 3,4).

Response to ^{131}I therapy is monitored with x-rays, radioiodine uptake, and Tg levels on and off T$_4$ (26,27,46–48).

External Radiotherapy

External radiotherapy is mandatory for bone metastases not amenable to surgery, especially when they are located in the vertebral column, near the base of skull, or in sites where a pathological fracture would result in a serious disability. Generally, it induces rapid relief of bone pain and recalcification of bone metastases (21,63).

External radiotherapy can efficiently complement radioiodine, delivering 40 to 45 Gy to large volumes, or larger doses to smaller volumes, with little additional toxic effect. Moreover, treatment with radioiodine is still possible after beam therapy (63).

Chemotherapy

Of the drugs administered to patients with metastatic differentiated thyroid carcinoma, the only one that appeared effective was doxorubicin, with a response rate ranging from 0% to 33% in various series (64). Responses were partial and lasted only a few months. In two reports (64,65), doxorubicin was combined with cisplatin, and similar response rates were found to that of doxorubicin alone, but with major toxicity. Also, the combination of doxorubicin and external radiotherapy appeared to be effective in patients with large tumor masses in the neck (66).

Treatment with interferon-α or interleukin 2, either alone or in combination with doxorubicin, did not result in any tumor response.

Therefore, chemotherapy should be given only in pilot studies to patients with progressing metastases, unable to pick up radioiodine. Even in these patients, the indication for chemotherapy should always be balanced with possible long survivals without treatment (see also Chapter 33).

Treatment Results and Prognostic Factors

After treatment of metastases, 122 of 263 patients (46%) with demonstrable radioiodine uptake, had a complete response, as demonstrated by x-rays and total-body ^{131}I scans (27). Seven relapses were observed in those patients in complete remission after treatment of distant metastases, with follow-up periods of up to 30 years (27). This agrees with other large series of patients with metastatic disease (53,54,58–60).

Overall survival rates from the time of detection of metastases were 55% at 5 years, 40% at 10 years, and 33% at 15 years (27). This is in agreement with other series in which overall 10-year survival rates were 25% (60), 29% (58), 27% (59), and, in patients with pulmonary metastases, 14% (20) and 44% (53).

Favorable responses to treatment are marked by parallel decreases in tumor volume, ^{131}I uptake, and Tg levels. In contrast, a decrease in ^{131}I uptake without a parallel decrease or with an increase in tumor volume announces histologic progression (see Figs. 2,3). In these cases, other treatment modalities, including chemotherapy, should be considered as alternatives.

In keeping with the low cell turnover rate in differentiated thyroid cancer, 66% of these remissions occurred within 5 years after initiation of treatment of metastases. In our series, logistic regression analysis showed that young age at the time of discovery of the metastases, presence of ^{131}I uptake, and small extent of metastases had a significantly favorable prognostic impact on remission when all variables had been taken into account (27). Complete remission occurred in 83% of the patients with a normal x-ray examination at discovery of the metastases, and in only 15% of patients with metastases visible on initial x-ray ($p < .001$) (Table 8). In a high proportion of patients in complete remission, the Tg level remained detectable but at a low level during T_4 treatment or after LT_4 withdrawal. In the majority of these patients, the Tg level remained stable with time (27). This shows the persistence of neoplastic thyroid cells in a large proportion of patients considered in complete remission, but these cells are unable to grow because of previous irradiation.

Univariate analysis has shown the prognostic influence of several variables on survival. They are strongly interrelated: radioiodine uptake is more frequently seen in younger patients, in those with papillary or well-differentiated carcinoma, and in those with small metastases (26,27).

A multivariate analysis showed that histology of the thyroid tumor, age at the time of discovery of the metastases, ^{131}I uptake, and extent of the metastases have a significant prognostic impact on survival (27). In this analysis, the site (bone or lung) had no independent prognostic value. However, bone metastases were associated with a poor prognosis when they were visible on x-rays, and such is the case in general. In most cases, they cannot be eradicated with radioiodine treatment alone, which underscores the need to combine it with surgery and external radiotherapy. Patients with metastases at the sternum or at the base of the skull were more frequently cured than patients with skeletal metastases in other locations, and this curability may be a result of their relatively early detection (63).

The better survival observed in patients with ^{131}I uptake in their metastases who consequently were treated with radioiodine cannot be explained by differences in growth rate, despite the rare possibility of long-term survival without treatment (26,27). The effectiveness of radioiodine is clear in some patients, and survival at 10 years was 93% in patients in remission after therapy for distant metastases and 14% in those who do not enter remission (27). In fact, thyroid hormone therapy alone is insufficient for lung metastases, even when they are not visible on chest x-rays. In these patients, despite relatively low uptake, favorable results were obtained with radioiodine (26,27,46–48).

As already reported (60,61), two factors (age and extent of tumor) establish three discrete groups of patients in whom the risk of death from thyroid cancer differs considerably. ^{131}I uptake or its absence in metastases was not taken into consideration in this analysis. It has been claimed that ^{131}I treatment does not affect survival (60,61) and that the better survival rates found in patients with small metastases may be linked only to earlier detection of distant spread. However, caution must prevail because the prognostic factors are closely interrelated, and in such subgrouping over 95% of younger patients with limited disease exhibited ^{131}I uptake and invariably responded to ^{131}I therapy, whereas 56% of patients aged over 40 years had ^{131}I uptake and only 19% responded to therapy. Further evidence of the impact of treatment is the increase in survival with the year of discovery of the metastases (27).

In conclusion, disseminated thyroid cancer can be cured in a significant proportion of patients. In others, durable palliation was achieved, and the presence of metastases was compatible with decades of survival. Furthermore, these treatments provided in most patients a good quality of life. Even patients who had lung macronodules or who had been paraplegic may return to a normal quality of life.

Complications of Treatment with ^{131}I

Acute Side Effects

Therapeutic doses of ^{131}I cause few acute side effects. Occasionally, patients complain of nausea. Transient sialadenitis is frequently observed but has rarely led to long-term xerostomia. This will diminish with high salivary flow and sufficient hydration. However, long-term xerostomia is frequently observed after treatment with external irradiation and radioiodine.

Radiation thyroiditis usually starts 3 or 4 days after the therapeutic dose has been given. The symptoms (pain while swallowing) are usually trivial if small amounts of thyroid tissue are being destroyed, but they may be severe if one lobe or more is being destroyed, sometimes requiring corticosteroids for a few days.

Patients with brain or spinal cord metastases can develop edema or sudden hemorrhage into the tumor, which can cause serious central nervous system compression symptoms.

Genetic Defects and Infertility

Estimated absorbed doses from an oral administration of ^{131}I to an euthyroid adult are approximately 0.14 cGy/mCi (0.038 mGy/MBq) to the ovaries, and 0.085 cGy/mCi (0.023 mGy/MBq) to the testes (67).

Particular attention must be given to avoid the use of ^{131}I in pregnant women. It is noteworthy that pregnancy does not appear to enhance tumor aggressiveness.

In men, a dose-related depression of spermatogenesis accompanied by an elevation of serum FSH has been observed after ^{131}I treatment for thyroid carcinoma. These deleterious effects were reversible but may be permanent after repeated treatments with ^{131}I (68,69).

In approximately 30% of nonmenopausal women, a transient ovarian failure has been observed during the first year after radioiodine therapy, with amenorrhea and increased serum gonadotropin concentrations, with older women being the most affected (70).

Genetic damage induced by exposure to ^{131}I was sought in three recent studies (71–73). The incidence of

TABLE 8. *Distant metastases from differentiated thyroid carcinoma: remission rate as a function of the size of the metastases*

	Patients (n)	Remission (%)
Lung metastases		
Normal chest x-ray	73	83
Micronodules	64	53
Macronodules	77	14
Total	214	50
Bone metastases		
Single	37	22
Multiple	71	3
Total	108	9
Lung and bone metastases	72	7

From ref. 27.

miscarriages increased slightly after surgery for thyroid cancer, both before and after ^{131}I, but did not vary with the cumulative ^{131}I dose. Miscarriages were more frequent in women treated with ^{131}I during the year preceding the conception. Stillbirth, pre-term birth, low birth weight, congenital malformation, and death during the first year of life were not different before and after ^{131}I.

The incidences of thyroid disease or nonthyroidal malignancy were similar in children born before and those born after ^{131}I exposure of their mother. Therefore, it is recommended to postpone conception for 1 year after the administration of a therapeutic dose of ^{131}I, and until the control of thyroid hormonal status has been achieved. In case of pregnancy, TSH level should be checked every 3 months, because LT$_4$ requirement may increase during pregnancy.

Carcinogenesis and Leukemogenesis

Mild pancytopenia may occur in patients with bone metastases after extended-field external radiotherapy and repeated treatments with ^{131}I. The risk of cancer and leukemia after the administration of tens of mCi for benign conditions has not been detected (74). The overall relative risk of secondary carcinoma was found to be increased only in patients treated with high cumulative dose of ^{131}I (72,75,76). For a cumulative dose below 400 mCi, no excess risk was found. Similarly, the risk of leukemia appeared to be significantly increased only in patients treated with high cumulative doses of ^{131}I, or in association with external radiotherapy (72,75–77). A site-by-site study has shown that only the risk of colon cancer was increased after ^{131}I treatments (76). This may be related to the hypothyroid status of these patients at the time of ^{131}I treatment. This status decreases the intestinal motility and is responsible of an accumulation of radioiodine in the colonic lumen. This fact underscores the need for laxative treatment after each therapeutic dose of ^{131}I.

Pulmonary Fibrosis

Radiation fibrosis may develop in patients with diffuse lung metastases, and eventually prove fatal, when excessive doses (> 150 mCi) are administered at short intervals (< 3 months) (78).

REFERENCES

1. Byar DP, Green SB, Dor P, et al. A prognostic index for thyroid carcinoma. A study of the EORTC thyroid cancer cooperative group. *Eur J Cancer* 1979;15 1033–1041.
2. Tubiana M, Schlumberger M, Rougier P, et al. Long term results and prognostic factors in patients with differentiated thyroid carcinoma. *Cancer* 1985;55 794–804.
3. Bacourt F, Asselain B, Savoie JC, et al. Multifactorial study of prognostic factors in differentiated thyroid carcinoma and a re-evaluation of the importance of age. *Br J Surg* 1986;73:274–277.
4. Hannequin P, Liehn JC, Delisle MJ. Multifactorial analysis of survival in thyroid cancer: pitfalls of applying the results of published studies to another population. *Cancer* 1986;58:1749–1755.
5. Kerr DJ, Burt AD, Boyle P, et al. Prognostic factors in thyroid tumours. *Br J Cancer* 1986;54:475–482.
6. Tennvall J, Björklund A, Möller T, Ranstam J, Åkerman M. Is the EORTC prognostic index of thyroid cancer valid in differentiated thyroid carcinoma? Retrospective multivariate analysis of differentiated thyroid carcinoma with long follow-up. *Cancer* 1986;57:1405–1414.
7. Hay ID, Grant CS, Taylor WF, McConahey WM. Ipsilateral lobectomy versus bilateral lobar resection in papillary thyroid carcinoma: a retrospective analysis of surgical outcome using a novel prognostic scoring system. *Surgery* 1987;103:1088–1095.
8. Schlumberger M, De Vathaire F, Travagli JP, et al. Differentiated thyroid carcinoma in childhood: long term follow-up of 72 patients. *J Clin Endocrinol Metab* 1987;65:1088–1094.
9. Simpson WJ, McKinney SE, Carruthers JS, et al. Papillary and follicular thyroid cancer. Prognostic factors in 1578 patients. *Am J Med* 1987;83:479–488.
10. Cady B, Rossi R An expanded view of risk-group definition in differentiated thyroid carcinoma. *Surgery* 1988;104:947–953.
11. Schelfhout LJDM, Creutzberg CL, Hamming JF, et al. Multivariate analysis of survival in differentiated thyroid cancer: the prognostic significance of the age factor. *Eur J Cancer* 1988;24:331–337.
12. Thoresen SO, Akslen LA, Glattre E, et al. Survival and prognostic factors in differentiated thyroid cancer. A multivariate analysis of 1055 cases. *Br J Cancer* 1989;59:231–235.
13. Shah JP, Loree TR, Dharker D, Strong EW, Begg C, Vlamis V. Prognostic factors in differentiated carcinoma of the thyroid gland. *Am J Med* 1992;164:658–661.
14. Hay ID, Bergstrah EJ, Goellner JR, Ebersold JR, Grant CS. Predicting outcome in papillary thyroid carcinoma: development of a reliable prognostic scoring system in a cohort of 1779 patients surgically treated at one institution during 1940 through 1989. *Surgery* 1993;114:1050–1058.
15. Lang W, Choritz H, Hundeshagen H. Risk factors in follicular thyroid carcinomas: a retrospective follow-up study covering a 14-year period with emphasis on morphological findings. *Am J Surg Pathol* 1986;10:246–265.
16. Sakamoto A, Kasai N, Sugano H. Poorly differentiated carcinoma of the thyroid. A clinico-pathologic entity for a high risk group of papillary and follicular carcinomas. *Cancer* 1983;52:1846–1853.
17. Ryan JJ, Hay ID, Grant CS, et al. Flow cytometric DNA measurements in benign and malignant Hürthle cell tumors of the thyroid. *World J Surg* 1988;12:482–487.
18. Beierwaltes WH. Carcinoma of the thyroid. Radionuclide diagnosis, therapy and follow-up. *Clin Oncol* 1986;5:23–27.
19. Maheshwari YK, Hill CS, Haynie TP, Hickey RC, Samaan NA. ^{131}I therapy in differentiated thyroid carcinoma: M.D. Anderson Hospital experience. *Cancer* 1981;47:664–671.
20. Massin JP, Savoie JC, Garnier H, Guiraudon G, Leger FA, Bacourt F. Pulmonary metastases in differentiated thyroid carcinoma. Study of 58

cases with implications for the primary tumor treatment. *Cancer* 1984; 53:982–992.
21. Tubiana M, Haddad E, Schlumberger M, Hill C, Rougier P, Sarrazin D. External radiotherapy in thyroid cancers. *Cancer* 1985;55:2062–2071.
22. Samaan NA, Schultz PN, Hickey RC, Goepfert H, Haynie TP, Johnson DA, Ordonez NG. The results of various modalities of treatment of well differentiated thyroid carcinoma: a retrospective review of 1599 patients. *J Clin Endocrinol Metab* 1992;75:714–720.
23. Mazzaferri EL, Jhiang SM. Long term impact of initial surgical and medical therapy on papillary and follicular thyroid cancer. *Am J Med* 1994;97:418–428.
24. Kuni CC, Klingensmith WC. Failure of low doses of ^{131}I to ablate residual thyroid tissue following surgery for thyroid cancer. *Radiology* 1980;137:773–774.
25. Simpson WJ, Panzarella T, Carruthers JS, Gospodarowicz MK, Sutcliffe SB. Papillary and follicular thyroid cancer: impact of treatment in 1578 patients. *Int J Radiat Oncol Biol Phys* 1988;14:1063–1075.
26. Schlumberger M, Tubiana M, De Vathaire F, et al. Long-term results of treatment of 283 patients with lung and bone metastases from differentiated thyroid carcinoma. *J Clin Endocrinol Metab* 1986;63:960–967.
27. Schlumberger M, Challeton C, De Vathaire F, et al. Radioactive iodine treatment and external radiotherapy for lung and bone metastases from thyroid carcinoma. *J Nucl Med* 1996;37:598–605.
28. Maxon HR, Smith HS. Radioiodine-131 in the diagnosis and treatment of metastatic well differentiated thyroid cancer. *Endocrinol Metab Clin North Am* 1990;19:685–718.
29. Maxon HR, Thomas SR, Hertzberg VS, et al. Relation between effective radiation dose and outcome of radioiodine therapy for thyroid cancer. *N Engl J Med* 1983;309:937–941.
30. Coliez R, Tubiana M, Dutreix J. Problèmes de dosimétrie posés par le traitement du cancer de la thyroïde par l'iode radioactif. *J Radiol Electrol (Paris)* 1954;35:22–27.
31. Pochin EE. Radioiodine therapy of thyroid cancer. *Semin Nucl Med* 1971;1:503–515.
32. Van Herle AJ, Uller RP, Matthews NL, Brown J. Radioimmunoassay for measurement of thyroglobulin in human subjects. *J Clin Invest* 1973;52:1320–1327.
33. Mariotti S, Barbesino P, Caturegli P, et al. Assay of thyroglobulin in serum with thyroblogulin autoantibodies: an unobtainable goal? *J Clin Endocrinol Metab* 1995;80:468–472.
34. Ashcraft MW, Van Herle AJ. The comparative value of serum thyroglobulin measurements and iodine 131 total body scans in the follow-up study of patients with treated differentiated thyroid cancer. *Am J Med* 1981;71:806–814.
35. Schlumberger M, Fragu P, Parmentier C, Tubiana M. Thyroglobulin assay in the follow-up of patients with differentiated thyroid carcinomas: comparison of its value in patients with or without normal residual tissue. *Acta Endocrinol (Copenh)* 1981;98:215–221.
36. Pacini F, Lari R, Mazzeo S, Grasso L, Taddei D, Pinchera A. Diagnostic value of a single serum thyroglobulin determination on and off thyroid suppressive therapy in the follow-up of patients with differentiated thyroid cancer. *Clin Endocrinol* 1985;23:405–411.
37. Girelli ME, Busnardo B, Amerio R, Casara D, Betterle C, Piccolo M. Critical evaluation of serum thyroglobulin (Tg) levels during thyroid hormone suppression therapy versus Tg levels after hormone withdrawal and total body scan: results in 291 patients with thyroid cancer. *Eur J Nucl Med* 1986;11:333–335.
38. De Vathaire F, Blanchon S, Schlumberger M. Thyroglobulin level helps to predict recurrence after lobo-isthmectomy in patients with differentiated thyroid carcinoma. *Lancet* 1988;i:52–53.
39. Schlumberger M, Tubiana M. Serum Tg measurements and total body ^{131}I scans in the follow-up of thyroid cancer patients. In: Hamburger JI, ed. *Diagnostic methods in clinical thyroidology*. New York: Springer-Verlag, 1989;147–157.
40. Schlumberger M, Fragu P, Gardet P, Lumbroso J, Violot D, Parmentier C. A new immunoradiometric assay (IRMA) system for thyroglobulin measurement in the follow-up of thyroid cancer patients. *Eur J Nucl Med* 1991;18:153–157.
41. Schlumberger M. Follow-up of patients with differentiated thyroid carcinoma. In: Johnson JT, Didolkar MS, eds. *Head and neck cancer,* vol. III. New York: Elsevier Science Publishers, 1993;903–910.
42. Ozata M, Suzuki S, Miyamoto T, Liu RT, Fierro-Renoy F, De Groot LJ. Serum thyroglobulin in the follow-up of patients with treated differentiated thyroid cancer. *J Clin Endocrinol Metab* 1994;79:98–105.
43. Dulgeroff AJ, Hershman JM. Medical therapy for differentiated thyroid carcinoma. *Endocr Rev* 1994;15:500–515.
44. Schlumberger M, Charbord P, Fragu P, Lumbroso J, Parmentier C, Tubiana M. Circulating thyroglobulin and thyroid hormones in patients with metastases of differentiated thyroid carcinoma: relationship to serum thyrotropin levels. *J Clin Endocrinol Metab* 1980;51:513–519.
45. Schneider AB, Line BR, Goldman JM, Robbins J. Sequential serum thyroglobulin determination ^{131}I scans and ^{131}I uptakes after triiodothyronine withdrawal in patients with thyroid cancer. *J Clin Endocrinol Metab* 1981;53:1199–1206.
46. Pacini F, Lippi F, Formica N, Elisei R, Anelli S, Ceccarelli C, Pinchera A. Therapeutic doses of iodine-131 reveal undiagnosed metastases in thyroid cancer patients with detectable serum thyroglobulin levels. *J Nucl Med* 1987;28:1888–1891.
47. Schlumberger M, Arcangioli O, Piekarski JD, Tubiana M, Parmentier C. Detection and treatment of lung metastases of differentiated thyroid carcinoma in patients with normal chest x-ray. *J Nucl Med* 1988;29:1790–1794.
48. Pineda JD, Lee T, Ain K, Reynolds JC, Robbins J. Iodine-131 therapy for thyroid cancer patients with elevated thyroglobulin and negative diagnostic scans. *J Clin Endocrinol Metab* 1995;80:1488–1492.
49. Goldman JM, Line BR, Aamodt RL, Robbins J. Influence of triiodothyronin withdrawal time on ^{131}I uptake post-thyroidectomy for thyroid cancer. *J Clin Endocrinol Metab* 1980;50:734–739.
50. Schlumberger M, Charbord P, Fragu P, et al. Relationship between thyrotropin stimulation and radioiodine uptake in lung metastases of differentiated thyroid carcinoma. *J Clin Endocrinol Metab* 1983;57:148–151.
51. Meier CA, Braverman LE, Ebner S, et al. Diagnostic use of recombinant human thyrotropin in patients with thyroid carcinoma (phase I/II study). *J Clin Endocrinol Metab* 1994;78:188–196.
52. Tubiana M, Mabille JP. L'iode radioactif et le cancer de la thyroïde. Problèmes diagnostiques. *J Radiol Electrol (Paris)* 1963;44:179–186.
53. Samaan NA, Schultz PN, Haynie TP, Ordonez NG. Pulmonary metastasis of differentiated thyroid carcinoma: treatment results in 101 patients. *J Clin Endocrinol Metab* 1985;60:376–380.
54. Casara D, Rubello D, Saladini G, et al. Different features of pulmonary metastases in differentiated thyroid cancer: natural history and multivariate statistical analysis of prognostic variables. *J Nucl Med* 1993;34:1626–1631.
55. Hoefnagel CA, Delprat CC, Marcuse HR, De Vijlder JJM. Role of thallium-201 total body scintigraphy in follow-up of thyroid carcinoma. *J Nucl Med* 1986;27:1854–1857.
56. Tenenbaum F, Lumbroso J, Schlumberger M, Caillou B, Fragu P, Parmentier C. Radiolabeled somatostatin analog scintigraphy in differentiated thyroid carcinoma. *J Nucl Med* 1995;36:807–810.
57. Ricard M, Tenenbaum F, Schlumberger M, Travagli JP, Lumbroso J, Revillon Y, Parmentier C. Intra-operative detection of pheochromocytoma with iodine-123 labelled meta-iodobenzylguanidine: a feasibility study. *Eur J Nucl Med* 1993;20:426–430.
58. Høie J, Stenwig AE, Kullmann G, Lindegaard M. Distant metastases in papillary thyroid cancer. A review of 91 patients. *Cancer* 1988;61:1–6.
59. Brown AP, Greening WP, McCready VR, Shaw HJ, Harmer CL. Radioiodine treatment of metastatic thyroid carcinoma: the Royal Marsden Hospital experience. *Br J Radiol* 1984;57:323–327.
60. Ruegemer JJ, Hay ID, Bergstralh EJ, Ryan JJ, Offord KP, Gorman CA. Distant metastases in differentiated thyroid carcinoma: a multivariate analysis of prognostic variables. *J Clin Endocrinol Metab* 1988;67:501–508.
61. Dinneen SF, Valimaki MJ, Bergstralh EI, Goellner JR, Gorman CA, Hay ID. Distant metastases in papillary thyroid carcinoma: 100 cases observed at one institution during 5 decades. *J Clin Endocrinol Metab* 1995;80:2041–2045.
62. Roy-Camille R, Leger FA, Merland JJ, Saillant G, Savoie JC, Riche MC. Perspectives actuelles dans le traitement des métastases osseuses des cancers thyroïdiens. *Chirurgie (Paris)* 1980;106:32–36.
63. Tubiana M, Lacour J, Monnier JP, et al. External radiotherapy and radioiodine in the treatment of 359 thyroid cancers. *Br J Radiol* 1975;48:894–907.
64. Shimaoka K, Schoenfeld DA, De Wys WD, Creech RH, De Conti R. A randomized trial of doxorubicin versus doxorubicin plus cisplatin in patients with advanced thyroid carcinoma. *Cancer* 1985;56:2155–2160.
65. Williams SD, Birch R, Einhorn LH. Phase II evaluation of doxorubicin

plus cisplatin in advanced thyroid cancer: a Southeastern Cancer Study Group Trial. *Cancer Treat Rep* 1986;70:405–407.
65. Kim JH, Leeper RD. Treatment of locally advanced thyroid carcinoma with combination doxorubicin and radiation therapy. *Cancer* 1987;60: 2372–2375.
67. MIRD. *MIRD primer for absorbed dose calculations.* New York: The Society of Nuclear Medicine, 1988.
68. Handelsman DJ, Turtle JR. Testicular damage after radioiodine (I-131) therapy for thyroid cancer. *Clin Endocrinol* 1983;118:465–472.
69. Pacini F, Gasperi M, Fugazzola L, et al. Testicular function in patients with differentiated thyroid carcinoma treated with radioiodine. *J Nucl Med* 1994;35:1418–1422.
70. Raymond JP, Izembart M, Marliac V, et al. Temporary ovarian failure in thyroid cancer patients after thyroid remnant ablation with radioactive iodine. *J Clin Endocrinol Metab* 1989;69:186–190.
71. Casara D, Rubello D, Saladini G, et al. Pregnancy after high therapeutic doses of iodine-131 in differentiated thyroid cancer: potential risks and recommendations. *Eur J Nucl Med* 1993;20:192–194.
72. Dottorini ME, Lomuscio G, Mazzucchelli L, Vignati A, Colombo L. Assessment of female fertility and carcinogenesis after iodine-131 therapy for differentiated thyroid carcinoma. *J Nucl Med* 1995;36:21–27.
73. Schlumberger M, De Vathaire F, Ceccarelli C, et al. Exposure to radioactive iodine (131-I) for scintigraphy or therapy does not preclude pregnancy in thyroid cancer patients. *J Nucl Med* 1996;37: 606–612.
74. Holm LE, Hall P, Wiklund K, et al. Cancer risk after iodine-131 therapy for hyperthyroidism. *J Natl Cancer Inst* 1991;83:1072–1077.
75. Hall P, Holm LE, Lundell G, et al. Cancer risks in thyroid cancer patients. *Br J Cancer* 1991;64:159–163.
76. De Vathaire F, Schlumberger M, Delisle, et al. Leukemias and cancers following ^{131}I administration for thyroid cancer. *Br J Cancer* 1997 *(in press)*.
77. Brincker H, Hansen HS, Andersen AP. Induction of leukemia by ^{131}I treatment of thyroid carcinoma. *Br J Cancer* 1973;28:232–237.
78. Rall JE, Alpers JB, Lewallen CG, Sonenberg M, Berman M, Rawson RW. Radiation pneumonitis and fibrosis: a complication of radioiodine treatment of pulmonary metastases from cancer of the thyroid. *J Clin Endocrinol Metab* 1957;17:1263–1276.

CHAPTER 32

Medullary Thyroid Carcinoma and the Multiple Endocrine Neoplasia Syndromes

Donald T. Donovan and Robert F. Gagel

Malignancy of the thyroid parafollicular or calcitonin-producing cells (C cell) comprises 5 to 10% of all thyroid neoplasms (1). This neoplasm has distinct characteristics that separate it from malignancies of the follicular epithelium and make it necessary to discuss this tumor as a separate entity. In this chapter, we focus on the basic and clinical aspects, with special emphasis on the integrated medical and surgical management, of this tumor, both in its sporadic and in its two familial forms, multiple endocrine neoplasia (MEN) types IIA and IIB.

THE NORMAL C CELL

Anatomy and Histology of the Normal C Cell

The parafollicular or C cell of the thyroid is a characteristic cell type that is located adjacent to but outside of the thyroid follicle in humans and other mammals (Fig. 1). It has several features that differentiate it from follicular epithelium, including calcitonin production (2), a biogenic amine uptake mechanism, and secretion of other small polypeptide hormones (3). Elegant studies performed by Le Douarin and Le Lievre (4) demonstrated migration of the C cells from the neural crest during embryonic life. Although the C cell is located within the thyroid gland, there is little evidence to indicate either hormonal or cellular interactions between the follicular epithelium and the C cell. In avian or teleost species, the C cell exists as a separate structure (the ultimobranchial body), unassociated with the thyroid gland (5).

The C cells are distributed in a characteristic pattern within the mammalian thyroid gland. The greatest concentration of C cells is located in the upper portion of each lobe of the thyroid gland, at the juncture of the upper one third and lower two thirds of the lobe along a hypothetical central vertical axis (Fig. 2) (6). The normal distribution of C cells is significant because it explains the characteristic location of hereditary medullary thyroid carcinoma (see Fig. 2).

FUNCTION OF THE C CELL

Secretory Products

The primary secretory product of the C cell is a polypeptide hormone called calcitonin. This small peptide (32 amino acids) was first characterized approximately 35 years ago (7,8). Within the last 15 years, the gene encoding calcitonin has been cloned (9) (Fig. 3) and subsequently shown to contain the coding sequence for a second peptide called calcitonin gene-related peptide (10). By a molecular mechanism called alternative RNA processing, the C cell splices and cleaves the primary transcript of the calcitonin gene to calcitonin messenger RNA, whereas neural cells process the same transcript to produce the messenger RNA for the calcitonin gene-related peptide. The specific factors in the C cell or neural tissue responsible for alternative processing of the calcitonin gene primary transcript have not been elucidated.

D. T. Donovan: Department of Otorhinolaryngology and Communicative Sciences, Baylor College of Medicine, Houston, Texas 77030.

R. F. Gagel: Department of Endocrine Neoplasia and Hormonal Disorders, University of Texas M. D. Anderson Cancer Center, Houston, Texas 77030.

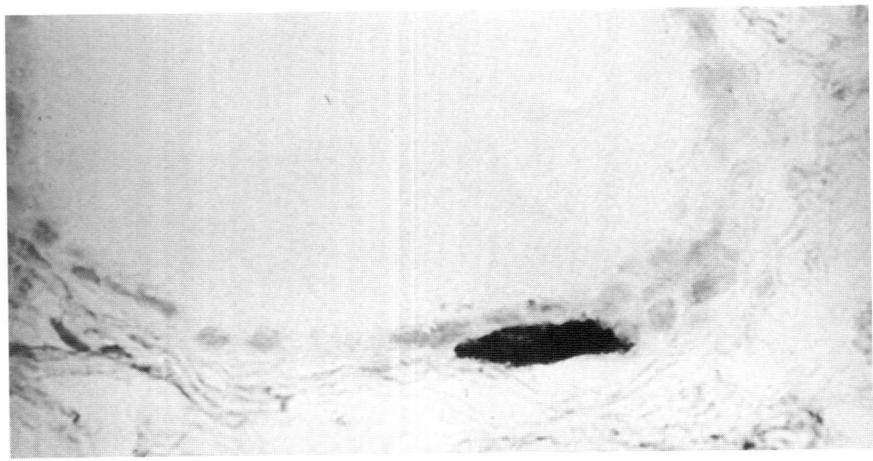

FIG. 1. Histologic section of normal thyroid tissue demonstrating positive immunohistochemical staining for calcitonin in a parafollicular or C cell. In the normal thyroid gland one observes no more than one or two C cells per high-powered field.

Regulation of Production

Calcitonin production by the C cell can be regulated at two different levels. Transcription of the calcitonin gene can be positively enhanced by adenosine 3',5'-cyclic monophosphate (cyclic AMP) and phorbol esters (11,12), and by glucocorticoids (11,13), or negatively by 1,25-dihydroxyvitamin D_3 (14). Release or secretion of calcitonin by the C cell is primarily regulated by the extracellular calcium concentration (15). Other substances, such as pentagastrin (16–18), β-adrenergic agonists (19,20), growth hormone–releasing hormone (21), and other gastrointestinal peptides (20–24), can stimulate calcitonin release from the C cell. Identification of individuals who have an exaggerated calcitonin release in response to either calcium (25–27) or pentagastrin (16,17,28) has formed the basis for screening techniques for medullary thyroid carcinoma.

Calcitonin Function

Once secreted into the plasma, calcitonin binds to specific receptors on the osteoclast, where it acts to inhibit bone resorption (29). The precise physiologic role for calcitonin in the regulation of bone cell metabolism is still debated. There are also specific calcitonin receptors in kidney and brain whose function is less clearly understood, although some evidence exists that calcitonin receptors in the brain may play a role in pain perception.

Expression of Calcitonin Gene Products Outside the Thyroid Gland

Calcitonin gene-related peptide, the peptide produced as a result of alternative RNA processing of the primary calcitonin gene transcript, is expressed primarily in neural tissue. It has been shown to have a number of biologic effects, including vasodilation (30), effects on pancreatic secretion (31), and regulation of acetylcholine receptor synthesis and function (32,33), and it is likely to be of fundamental importance in the regulation of neural function.

Cells outside the thyroid gland that produce primarily calcitonin include the Kulchitsky cells of the lung (34), the pituitary gland (35,36), and isolated cells within the thymus gland. The function of the calcitonin produced by these cell types is not known. In addition, calcitonin can be produced by cell types that do not normally produce calcitonin. Examples include hepatoma, lung carcinoma (37,38), and benign liver disease. In most of these diseases, the primary calcitonin gene product appears to be a partially processed form of calcitonin (procalcitonin) that can be identified in serum on the basis of its immunochemical heterogeneity (39,40), or by specific radioassays for procalcitonin (41). In many cases, release of calcitonin does not appear to be regulated by the same factors that stimulate calcitonin release in the normal C cell and, therefore, calcitonin secretion from these tumor cell types may not be increased by either calcium or pentagastrin (42).

PATHOLOGY OF MEDULLARY THYROID CARCINOMA

Medullary thyroid carcinoma (see also Chapter 6) is usually hard and firm in consistency and either chalky white or red in color on cross-section. On histologic examination, there are frequently sheets of spindle-shaped or rounded cells divided by fibrous septa, in a nested pattern characteristic of endocrine tumors (Fig. 4). The nuclei are usually uniform in shape with infrequent mitoses. The cytoplasm is eosinophilic with a finely granular appearance. Amyloid, which is thought to consist, in part, of calcitonin gene products, is frequently seen deposited between tumor cells (43).

Medullary thyroid carcinoma may be confused with anaplastic carcinoma, Hürthle cell tumor, or papillary thyroid carcinoma, especially if the medullary thyroid carcinoma contains pseudopapillary elements or giant

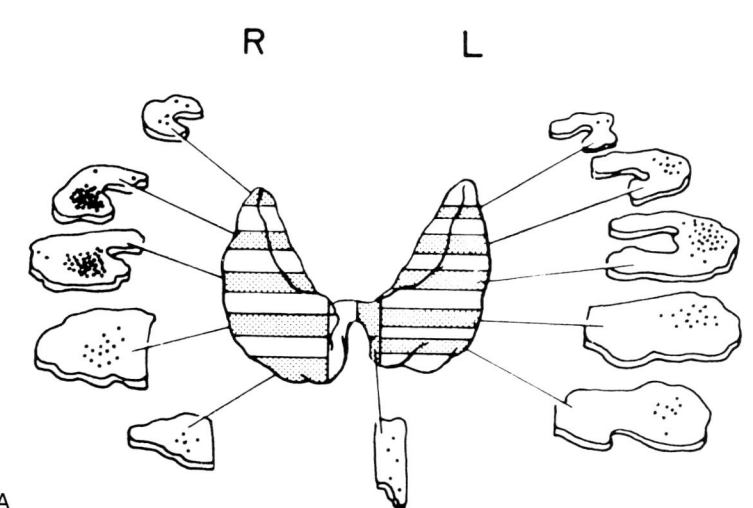
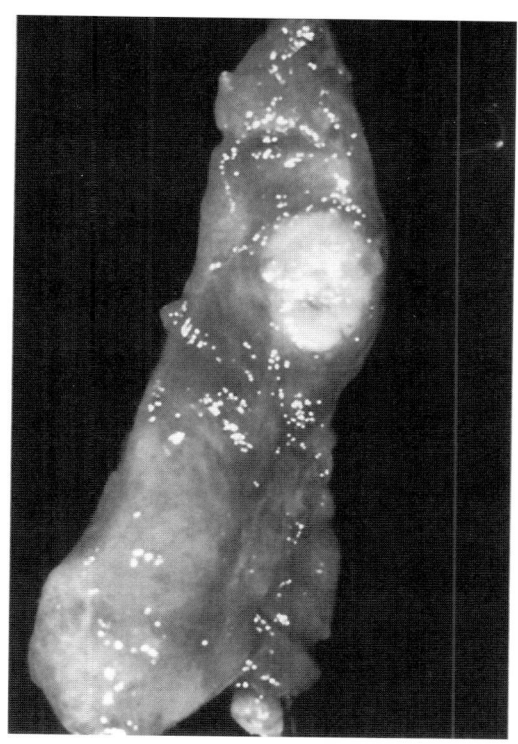

FIG. 2. Distribution of C cells in the thyroid gland. **A:** Figurative reconstruction of C-cell distribution in alternate sections of a thyroid gland. The *points* on the surface of each section represent a single stained C cell observed microscopically at 10× magnification and projected onto a surface for marking of immunoperoxidase-reactive sites. Note the predominance of C cells in the middle third of the lateral lobes, and that they are in the central region of each lobe. (Reproduced from ref. 6, with permission.) **B:** The distribution of C cells explains the characteristic location of hereditary medullary thyroid carcinoma in a thyroid gland from a patient with MEN type IIA. The tumor is located at the junction of the upper one third and lower two thirds of the thyroid gland. The contralateral lobe in this patient showed only microscopic medullary thyroid carcinoma, demonstrating that this disease may present asymmetrically.

cells. In such cases, a positive diagnosis can be made by positive immunohistochemical staining for calcitonin or by special stains for amyloid. The tumor characteristically metastasizes to paratracheal and cervical lymph nodes; it may spread hematogenously to liver, lung, and bone in later stages of the disease.

Medullary thyroid carcinoma may express a number of genes usually not expressed, or expressed at low levels, in the normal C cell. The protein products of these genes include carcinoembryonic antigen (44–47), somatostatin (48,49), pro-opiomelanocortin (50,51), vasoactive intestinal peptide, and neurotensin (52). Genes normally expressed in the C cell that may be expressed at higher levels in medullary thyroid carcinoma include histaminase (53), calcitonin, and chromogranin A (54). Little is known about the mechanism by which ectopic or altered expression of these proteins occurs, although one might hypothesize the production of one or more transcriptional activators by the transformed C cell. Ectopic production of several of these hormones can produce clinical syndromes, including corticosteroid excess and diarrheal syndromes (50,51,55,56).

Features That Can Be Used to Separate Hereditary from Sporadic Medullary Thyroid Carcinoma

The characteristic histologic findings associated with hereditary medullary thyroid carcinoma are bilateral and multicentric neoplasia (57). Sporadic medullary thyroid carcinoma generally presents with a large single focus in one lobe of the thyroid gland. Hereditary medullary thyroid carcinoma arises in the areas of the thyroid gland where the distribution of C cells is greatest (see Fig. 2). The first histologic abnormality observed in hereditary medullary thyroid carcinoma is C cell hyperplasia (Fig. 5). Each of these hyperplastic foci is thought to arise from a single clonal population of cells (58). As this clonal cell population expands, there are a series of histologic stages (59) that have been characterized as hyperplasia, nodular hyperplasia, microscopic carcinoma (see Fig. 5), and finally grossly detectable tumor (see Figs. 2,4). In the earliest stages of the disease, these foci may be detected only by microscopic examination of the area of the thyroid containing the greatest C cell concentration (see Fig. 2). Later, visible lesions (pin-

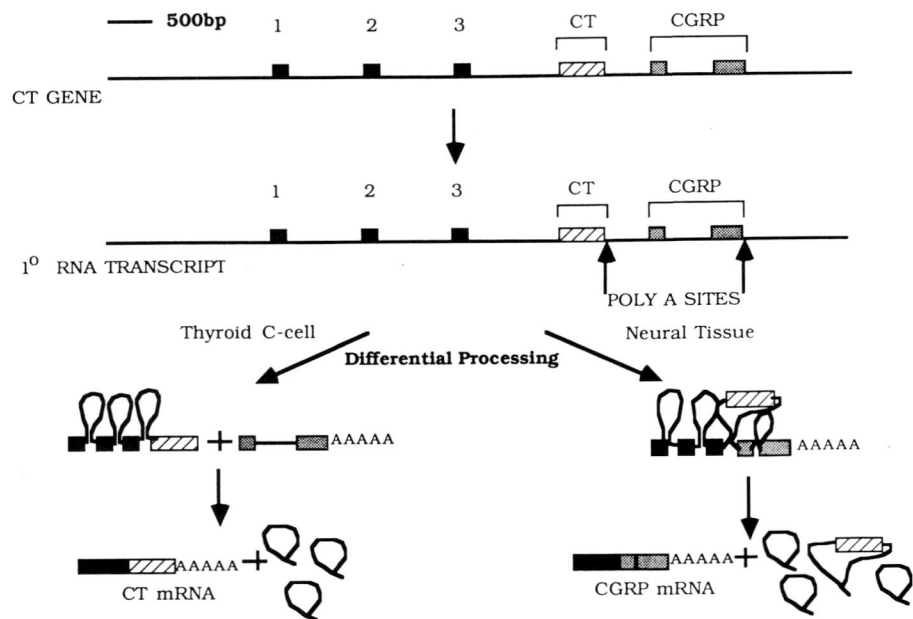

FIG. 3. Alternative RNA processing of the calcitonin gene produces either calcitonin or calcitonin gene-related peptide. The primary RNA transcript of the calcitonin gene includes exon (designated by a *box*) and intron (designated by *thin line*) sequence, which can be processed to produce calcitonin mRNA by cleavage and polyadenylation at the polyadenylation site following the calcitonin exon or calcitonin gene-related peptide mRNA by alternatively splicing out the calcitonin exon and flanking introns. Calcitonin is the primary product in the C cell, whereas calcitonin gene-related peptide is the preferred product in neural tissue. CT, calcitonin; CGRP, calcitonin gene-related peptide; bp, base pairs; mRNA, messenger RNA; AAAAA, poly A tail.

point, white and chalky) will be found in these same locations. Identification of these small lesions requires systematic 1- to 5-mm sectioning and histologic examination of the thyroid gland. Tumor formation may be an asymmetric process in hereditary medullary thyroid carcinoma, but the incidence of bilaterality approaches 100%. There may be a large tumor in one lobe (see Fig. 2) and only histologic evidence of carcinoma or C cell hyperplasia in the contralateral lobe of the thyroid gland.

Little is known about the evolution of the C cell abnormality in sporadic medullary thyroid carcinoma. Although C cell hyperplasia has been found with sporadic medullary

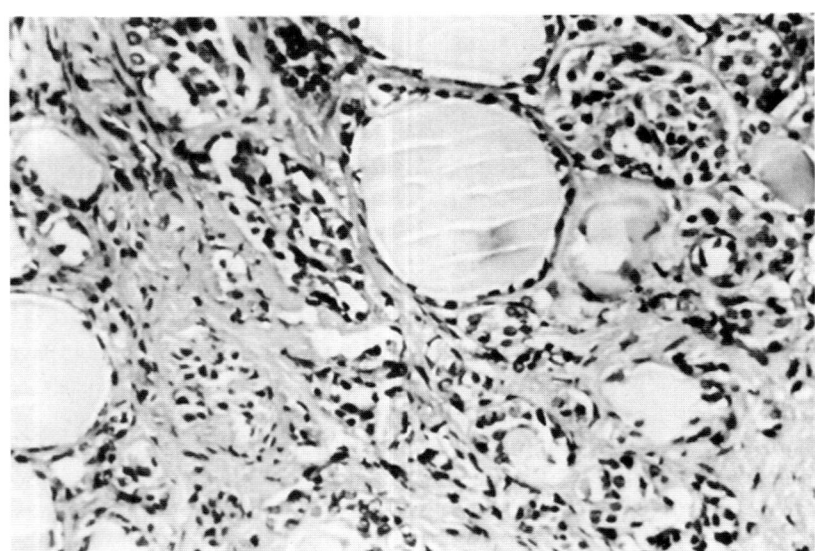

FIG. 4. Characteristic hereditary medullary thyroid carcinoma demonstrating the "nested" appearance of the tumor and deposition of amyloid. Note that the tumor cells appear to be infiltrating into the thyroid follicle.

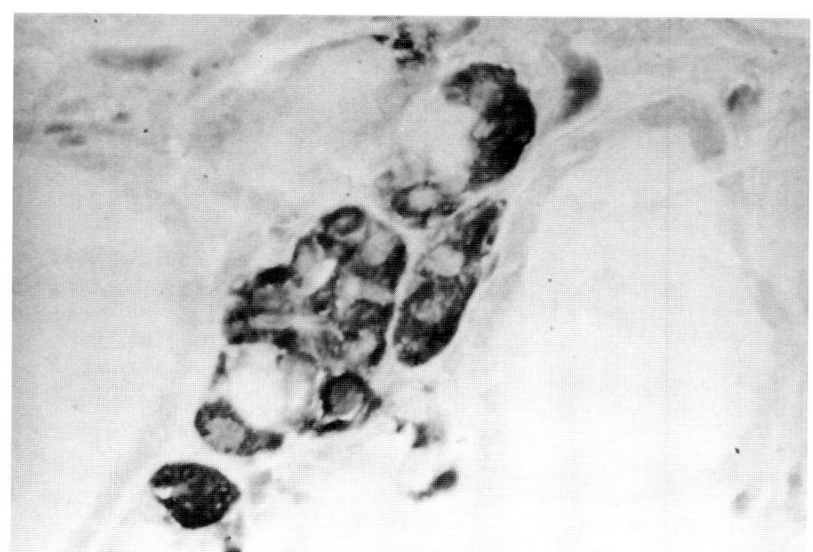

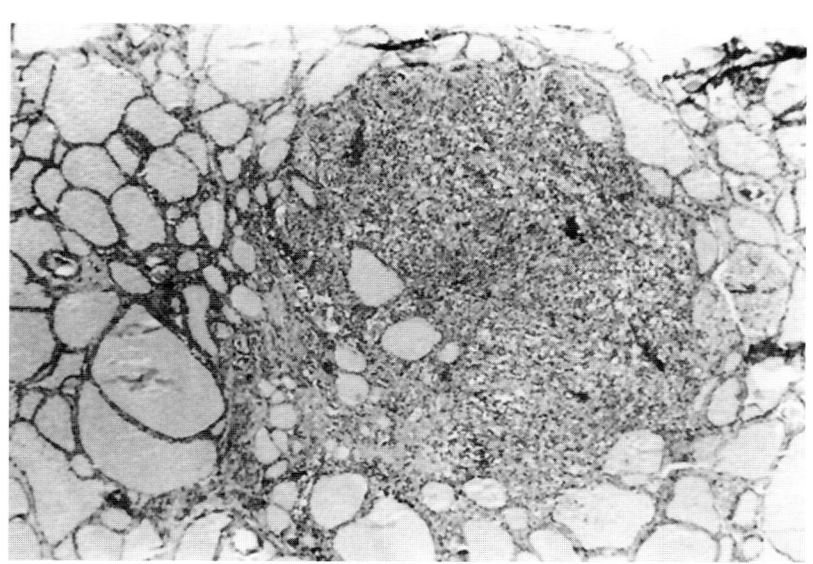

FIG. 5. Stages in the development of hereditary medullary thyroid carcinoma. **A:** C cell hyperplasia. The first stage in the development of hereditary medullary thyroid carcinoma is a hyperplastic expansion of the C cell population. These cells have been positively identified by positive immunohistochemical staining for calcitonin. **B:** Microscopic medullary thyroid carcinoma. A microscopic focus of hereditary medullary thyroid carcinoma in which one or more foci of hyperplastic C cells have expanded into surrounding thyroid tissue. This lesion may be visible only as a small white pinpoint lesion on gross examination of sections of the thyroid gland.

thyroid carcinoma in a few cases (60), it is far less common. Whether C cell hyperplasia in cases of apparent sporadic medullary thyroid carcinoma represents a new mutation causing hereditary medullary thyroid carcinoma or is indicative of a factor stimulating diffuse C cell hyperplasia is not known with certainty (61).

Fine-Needle Biopsy Diagnosis of Medullary Thyroid Carcinoma

Increased application of fine-needle aspiration (FNA) biopsy as a diagnostic procedure for thyroid nodule evaluation has made it possible to diagnose medullary thyroid carcinoma prior to surgery (62,63). Several different cell types may be seen, including oval to round cells with eccentrically located nuclei, large polygonal or spindle-shaped cells, and small round cells with scanty cytoplasm. Variable amounts of cytoplasm are observed, and there may be acidophilic granulation observed with certain stains. Nuclei are usually pleomorphic and may contain vacuoles. Amyloid may be observed as clumps of amorphous material. The diagnosis is confirmed by the demonstration of amyloid and positive immunohistochemical staining for calcitonin (Fig. 6). A preoperative diagnosis of medullary thyroid carcinoma is helpful because it alerts the surgeon to the necessity for total thyroidectomy and the possibility of parathyroid or adrenal medullary disease.

THE CLINICAL SYNDROMES ASSOCIATED WITH MEDULLARY THYROID CARCINOMA

There are three major types of clinical presentations for medullary thyroid carcinoma. More than 50% of medullary thyroid carcinoma will be diagnosed as a re-

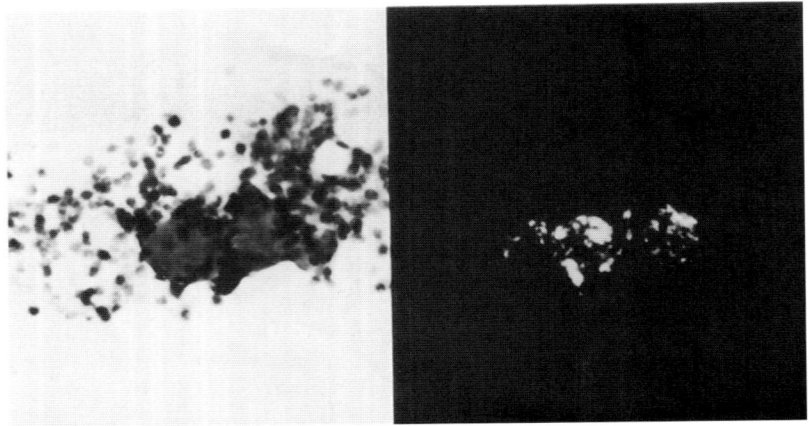

FIG. 6. Fine-needle biopsy of medullary thyroid carcinoma. **Left:** Cytologic examination demonstrates small, uniform cells with surrounding amyloid. **Right:** The diagnosis was proven by the demonstration of positive immunohistochemical staining for calcitonin (courtesy of Dr. Thomas Wheeler).

sult of evaluation for a thyroid nodule or metastatic carcinoma with an unknown primary source. A smaller percentage will be identified as a result of family screening for MEN IIA. The least common but most distinctive presentation is the clinical syndrome of medullary thyroid carcinoma, mucosal neuromata, and marfanoid body habitus classified as MEN type IIB.

Sporadic Medullary Thyroid Carcinoma

Evaluation of a cold thyroid nodule is the most common clinical presentation leading to the diagnosis of medullary thyroid carcinoma. The only clinical features that may lead the clinician to suspect medullary thyroid carcinoma are the presence of a diarrheal syndrome (64) or radiographic evidence of a calcified thyroid nodule. The diagnosis is usually suspected during the surgical procedure as a result of frozen-section analysis of tumor tissue or less commonly as a result of a preoperative FNA. A patient with advanced medullary thyroid carcinoma may present with hepatic, pulmonary, or bony metastasis.

Multiple Endocrine Neoplasia Type IIA

Multiple endocrine neoplasia type IIA is a syndrome composed of medullary thyroid carcinoma, pheochromocytoma, and parathyroid neoplasia genetically transmitted as an autosomal dominant trait. The clinical disorder was first described clearly by Sipple in 1961 (65), and it was classified as a separate syndrome by Steiner et al. in 1968 (66) to differentiate it from MEN type I (primary hyperparathyroidism, pituitary adenoma, islet-cell tumor). Williams (67) was the first to classify the thyroid tumor in this syndrome as the medullary type of thyroid carcinoma. He postulated it to be a neoplastic process of the C cells and, therefore, likely to produce the then newly discovered peptide calcitonin (7,8). Subsequent work by several investigators demonstrated production of this peptide by the tumor (26).

In 1971, Melvin and his coworkers (26,68) demonstrated the usefulness of provocative testing for the identification of hereditary medullary thyroid carcinoma. They found 12 members of an MEN IIA kindred, 11 of whom had no clinical evidence of thyroid disease, with consistent elevations of the serum calcitonin after a calcium infusion. Each of these individuals was found to have medullary thyroid carcinoma at surgery. These studies led to the concept that it might be possible to identify medullary thyroid carcinoma in its early stages, perhaps prior to the development of metastatic disease, by prospective screening techniques. Shortly thereafter, several patients with C cell hyperplasia without evidence of metastatic disease were identified by application of these techniques (69). In this same kindred, annual prospective screening of all family members has resulted in the identification of an additional 28 family members with either C cell hyperplasia or microscopic medullary thyroid carcinoma and no evidence of metastases (17,18,70).

Studies in this and other MEN IIA kindreds (28,71–74) form the basis for our current understanding of the hereditary disease process. There is a histologic progression of the thyroidal C cell disease process from the earliest detectable lesion of C cell hyperplasia to frank medullary thyroid carcinoma. It is now possible to consistently detect these abnormalities by prospective screening of potentially affected family members. The result has been a decrease in the mean age of diagnosis from 33 years prior to prospective screening to a mean age of 13 in the early 1980s (75).

The recent identification of germline mutations of the *ret* proto-oncogene in hereditary medullary thyroid carcinoma and MEN IIA offers the prospect of simplified DNA-based screening strategies and will make it possible to determine gene carrier status at birth. The use of these techniques will be discussed in a subsequent section.

Adrenal Medullary Disease

Pheochromocytoma occurs in approximately 50% of MEN IIA gene carriers. In prospectively screened families, diagnosis of clinically significant adrenal medullary disease invariably follows diagnosis of C cell disease, although there are a few examples of pheochromocytoma preceding C cell disease (18,76). The pheochromocytomas are almost always located in an intra-adrenal location, although exceptions have been described (77). The earliest clinical manifestations include intermittent jitteriness, headaches, palpitations, and a sense of anxiety. It is frequently difficult to separate these symptoms from

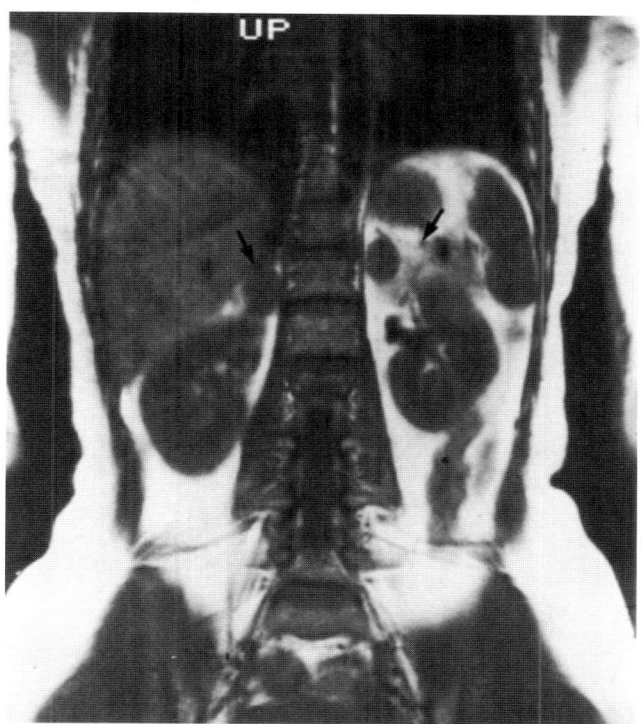

FIG. 8. Magnetic resonance image demonstrating bilateral pheochromocytoma in a patient with MEN type IIA.

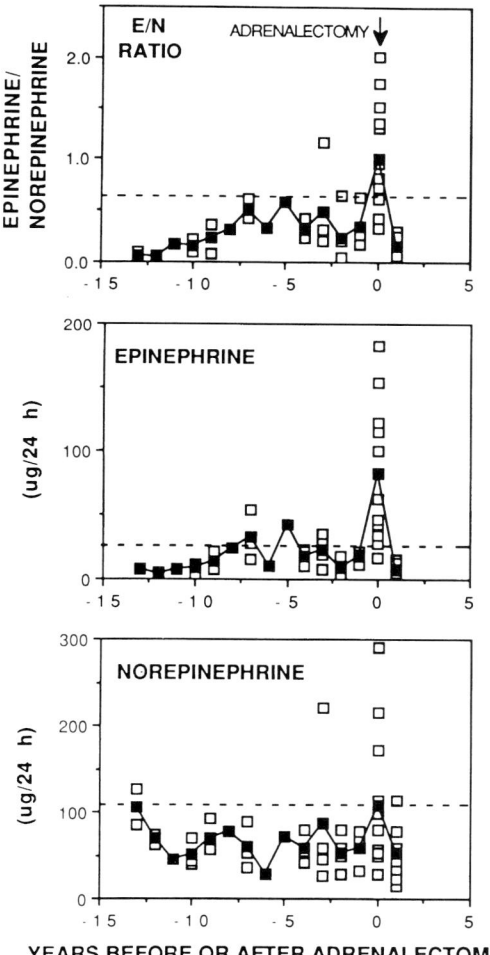

FIG. 7. The 24-hr urinary norepinephrine excretion, epinephrine excretion, and ratio of epinephrine to norepinephrine in 11 prospectively screened patients proved to have pheochromocytoma. Each *open square* indicates a value or the mean of two or more values in a patient, and each *solid square*, the mean for all the subjects in a particular year; the latter symbols are connected by a *solid line*. The *dashed line* shows the upper limit of normal. (From ref. 18, with permission.)

those that could be caused by anxiety. Hypertension is almost never observed at this stage. The earliest biochemical abnormality observed during prospective screening is an elevation of the 24-hr urine epinephrine excretion and an elevated epinephrine-to-norepinephrine ratio (Fig. 7) (18,70,78,79). Excretion of norepinephrine does not usually increase until later in the course of the disease, and even with large tumors there is a greater relative increase of epinephrine production as characterized by an increased epinephrine-to-norepinephrine ratio in a 24-hr urine collection (18). Hypertension may or may not be present with large pheochromocytomas. It is likely that the relative increase of epinephrine production, with its predominant β-adrenergic-like effects, explains the lack of hypertension early in the course of this disease. There is also a progression of histologic abnormalities from adrenal medullary hyperplasia to multicentric pheochromocytoma (80,81). Although invasion of the adrenal medullary capsule is commonly seen in advanced pheochromocytomas, clinical evidence of metastasis is rare.

Diagnosis of an advanced pheochromocytoma is made by the demonstration of abnormal catecholamine production and an intra-adrenal mass by computerized tomography (CT) or magnetic resonance imaging (MRI) (Fig. 8). In cases where an extra-adrenal pheochromocytoma is suspected, ^{131}I-meta-iodobenzylguanidine, a catecholamine analog concentrated in chromaffin tissue, can be used to localize the tumor (82). The diagnosis of early adrenal medullary disease may be more difficult. Intermittent symptoms suggestive of pheochromocytoma may not always be associated with abnormal urine catecholamine excretion, and there may be no demonstrable adrenal mass by CT or MRI scanning. In this situation, ^{131}I-meta-iodobenzylguanidine scanning may demonstrate abnormal uptake in one or both adrenal glands (83). Surgical exploration may be the only way to prove the diagnosis.

Hyperparathyroidism

Hyperparathyroidism is the least common of the three clinical manifestations of MEN IIA. This contrasts with the findings in MEN type I, where almost 100% of affected family members will develop hypercalcemia by

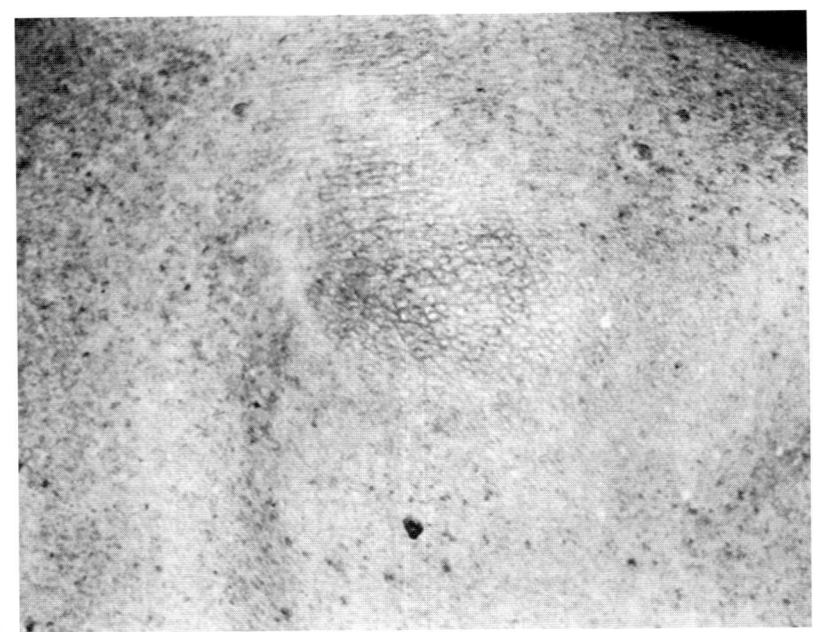
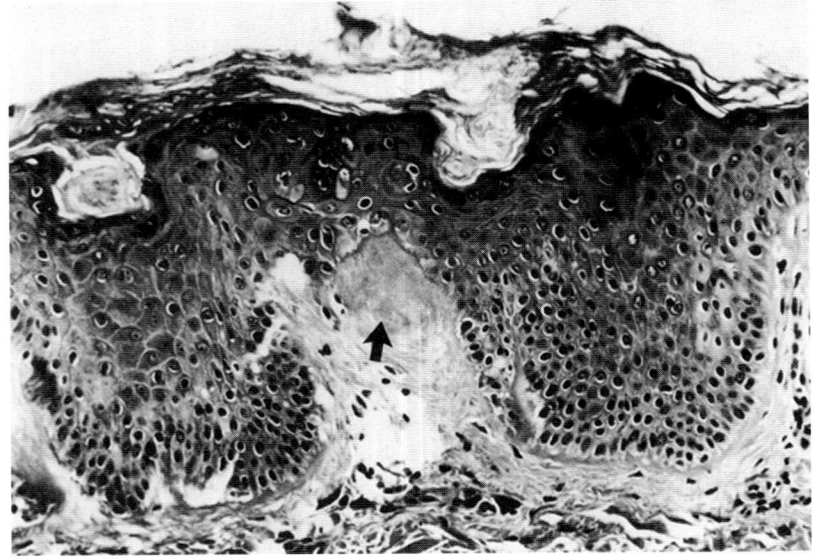

FIG. 9. Cutaneous lichen amyloidosis and MEN type IIA. **A:** The characteristic appearance and location over the upper back of cutaneous lichen amyloidosis in one family with multiple endocrine neoplasia type IIA. **B:** Histologic section through the cutaneous lesion demonstrating the amyloid deposition *(arrow)* at the basement membrane (×400).

the age of 40 (84,85). Ten percent to 25% of known MEN IIA gene carriers will develop hyperparathyroidism, usually after the third decade (26,66,72,86). The clinical features do not differ from those seen with sporadic hyperparathyroidism and include hypercalcemia, hypercalciuria, urolithiasis, and parathyroid hormone–induced bone disease. Multiglandular parathyroid hyperplasia (26,87) is most commonly seen, although in older patients with advanced disease there is superimposition of multiglandular adenoma formation (72,86). The earliest functional abnormalities detected are incomplete suppression of parathyroid hormone secretion by a calcium infusion (88).

Clinical evidence of hyperparathyroidism is almost never seen in young, prospectively screened family members, although hyperplasia of parathyroid glandular tissue may be observed (18,89). The most likely explanation for the failure to find evidence for hyperparathyroidism in affected young patients is the late onset of the disease and partial treatment by the potential removal of one or two parathyroid glands during the thyroidectomy for C cell disease (18). It seems likely that some of these patients will develop hyperparathyroidism at a later date, and measurement of the serum calcium concentration once or twice a decade throughout life is an important part of continued follow-up in kindred members.

Variant Forms of MEN IIA

Hereditary medullary thyroid carcinoma is usually associated with other components of the MEN IIA syndrome, but there have been a number of families described in which hereditary medullary thyroid carcinoma (known as familial MTC or FMTC) was the only observed manifestation of MEN IIA (90). The clinical course of the medullary thyroid carcinoma in these families is indolent when compared with that of other families with MEN IIA. Whether this represents a separate syndrome or merely a variant of MEN IIA, in which the genetic component is modified to delay the onset of all manifestations of the MEN IIA syndrome, is not clear.

There are now reports of several MEN IIA families with cutaneous skin lesions (91,92). In two of these families, a pruritic and pigmented papular skin lesion occurred in the periscapular area of the back (Fig. 9). In one of these reports (91), the investigators have characterized this lesion as a form of cutaneous lichen amyloidosis (see Fig. 9), a disease which, like medullary thyroid carcinoma, is transmitted as an autosomal dominant trait. The characteristic features of this lesion in these geographically diverse families lead to the conclusion they likely represent the same condition. In one of these families, the skin lesion preceded the development of C cell hyperplasia, making the skin lesion potentially useful as a predictor of gene carrier status (92).

Multiple Endocrine Neoplasia Type IIB

The clinical syndrome of medullary thyroid carcinoma, pheochromocytoma, and ganglioneuromatosis has been called MEN type IIB (or MEN III). The clinical features of the syndrome were first convincingly assembled by Williams and Pollock in 1966 (93); they include mucosal neuromas that are located on the distal tongue, in subconjunctival areas, and ganglioneuromatosis throughout the gastrointestinal tract. Patients with this syndrome are identified by the characteristic mucosal neuromas located on the distal portion of the tongue, thickened lips, and marfanoid features (Fig. 10). Hyperparathyroidism is almost never observed in MEN IIB (94).

The most common presentation in early childhood may be gastrointestinal disorders, including colic, cramping, obstructive symptoms, and diarrhea, which are related to the presence of neuromas throughout the gastrointestinal tract (93,95,96). Marfanoid features include long, thin extremities, an altered upper-to-lower-body ratio, slipped femoral epiphysis, and pectus excavatum (93,95,96). The clinical spectrum of the mucosal neuroma syndrome may vary considerably, with some patients demonstrating prominent neuromas and other patients presenting with more subtle manifestations (see Fig. 10).

Medullary thyroid carcinoma associated with MEN IIB is generally more aggressive than that found in MEN IIA. Metastatic disease generally occurs early (28,97), and spread of tumor beyond the neck at the time of primary surgery is now uncommon (93,94). The bilateral and multicentric histologic changes associated with medullary thyroid carcinoma in MEN IIA are also found in MEN IIB; in rapidly growing tumors, there may be less amyloid deposited within the tumor.

Pheochromocytomas are eventually identified in about one half of individuals with this syndrome. The pheochromocytomas are bilateral, multicentric, and have many of the same characteristics found in MEN IIA. Malignant pheochromocytoma in MEN IIB is uncommon, and management of pheochromocytoma should not differ from that described for MEN IIA.

MEN type IIB is transmitted as an autosomal dominant trait. Families with the syndrome have been described (98–100), but these families represent a minority of the patients described in the literature. The virulence of the medullary thyroid carcinoma is the most likely reason for the relative rarity of large kindreds (28,101), although survival into middle or old age has been described (94,102).

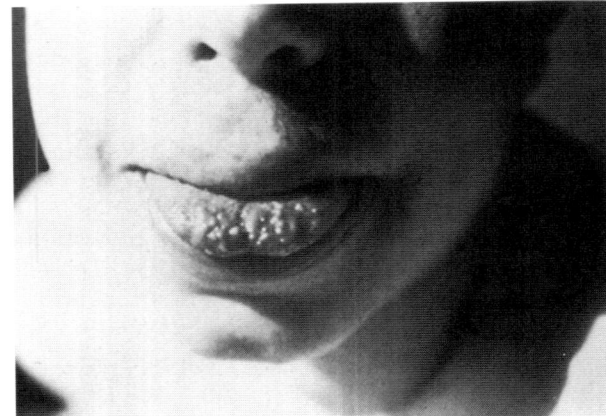
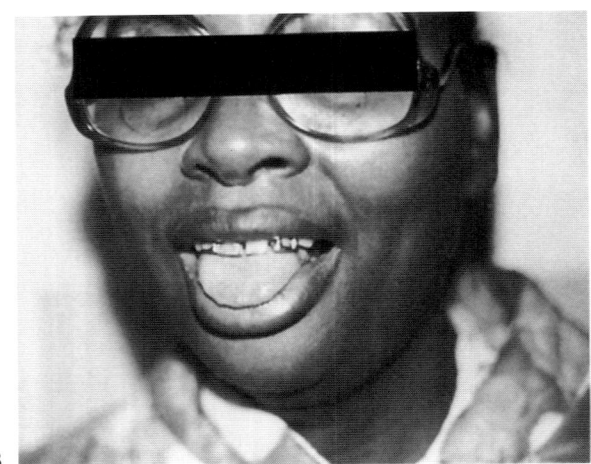
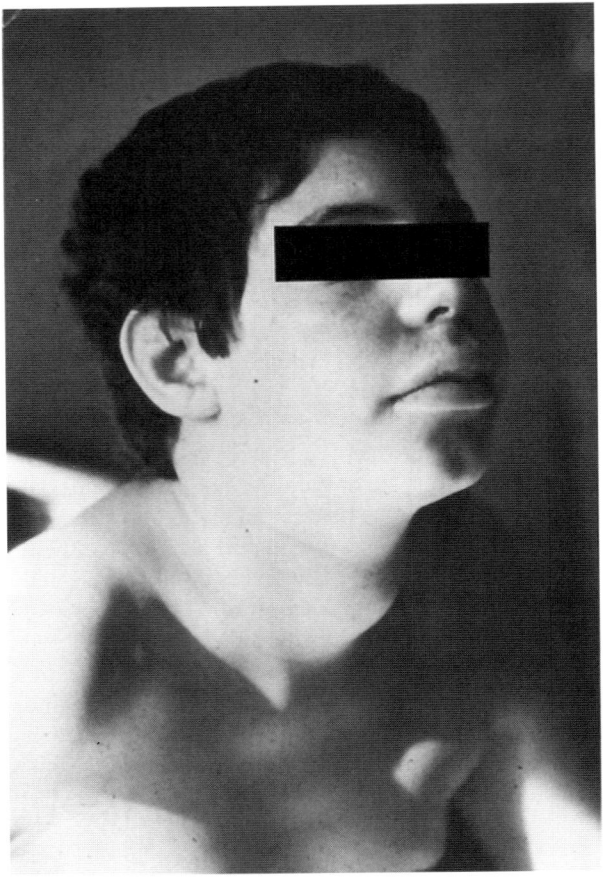

FIG. 10. Clinical features of MEN type IIB. The characteristic mucosal neuromas may be obvious **(A)** or more subtle **(B)**. Other clinical features include thick lips and thickened eyelids **(C)**. A thyroid area mass is shown (C), which was subsequently found to be a medullary thyroid carcinoma.

GENETIC ABNORMALITIES IN HEREDITARY AND SPORADIC MEDULLARY THYROID CARCINOMA

Multiple Endocrine Neoplasia Type IIA and Familial Medullary Thyroid Carcinoma

Genetic linkage analysis led, in 1987, to the localization of the MEN II gene to centromeric chromosome 10 (103,104). The chromosomal region containing the causative gene was progressively narrowed over the next several years, leading to the identification of mutations of the *ret* proto-oncogene in 1993 (105,106). This gene encodes a tyrosine kinase receptor, and mutations causing MEN IIA affect an extracellular domain, each converting a cysteine to another amino acid at codon 609, 611, 618, 620, or 634 (Fig. 11) (Table 1). The most common mutation, accounting for over 80% of all mutations associated with MEN IIA, affects codon 634 (107). A single mutation, a codon 634 cysteine to arginine (TGC to CGC) substitution, accounts for 50% of all MEN II mutations. All examples of the MEN IIA/cutaneous lichen amyloidosis syndrome have been found to have a codon 634 mutation (107). The handful of families with the MEN IIA and Hirschsprung variant of MEN IIA have a codon 609, 618, or 620 mutation (108).

Mutations of codons 609, 611, 618, and 620 most commonly cause FMTC (without pheochromocytoma or parathyroid neoplasia), although some have classic MEN IIA. Pheochromocytoma has not been reported with a codon 609 mutation (108). A few families with hereditary MTC have been found to have codon 768 and 804 mutations (107).

Ninety-three percent to 95% of kindreds with MEN IIA or FMTC have a mutation of one of these seven codons (107). In the remaining 5% of families with proven germline transmission of MTC, mutations of the *ret* proto-oncogene have not been identified.

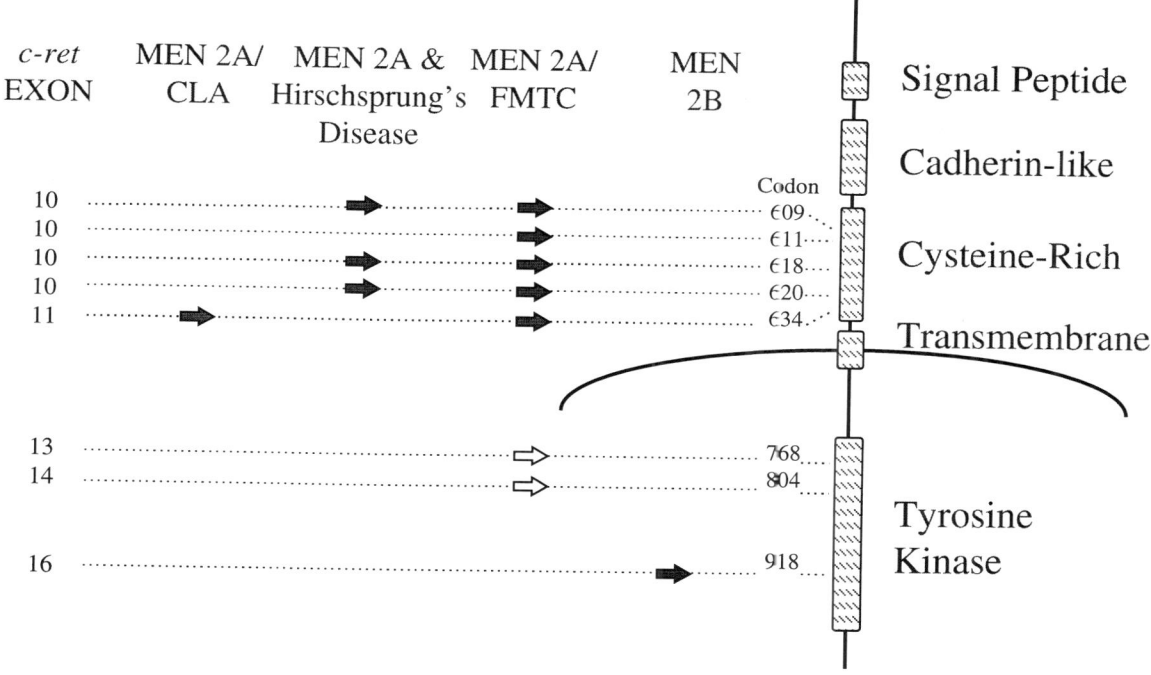

FIG. 11. Mutations of the *ret* proto-oncogene associated with MEN type II. This figure shows a schematic description of the *ret* proto-oncogene. Mutations of eight codons have been identified as germline (codons 609, 611, 618, 620, 634, 768, 804, 918) and two as sporadic (codons 768 and 804) mutations in medullary thyroid carcinoma. The net effect of these mutations is to activate the receptor, thereby causing transformation. On the left side of the figure is shown the genomic exon that contains the affected codon. CLA, cutaneous lichen amyloidosis; FMTC, familial medullary thyroid carcinoma.

Multiple Endocrine Neoplasia Type IIB

A single mutation converting a methionine to a threonine at codon 918 has been identified in MEN IIB (109,110). Approximately 92% to 94% of individuals with MEN IIB have a germline mutation at this codon (see Fig. 11 and Table 1). No mutation of the *ret* proto-oncogene has been identified in the other 6% to 8%.

Sporadic Medullary Thyroid Carcinoma

Somatic mutations (those that occur only in the tumor) of codon 918 of the *ret* proto-oncogene have been identified in approximately 25% of sporadic medullary thyroid carcinomas (111–113). The mutation in these patients is identical to that identified in MEN IIB and converts a methionine to threonine. Codon 768 and 804 mutations have been identified in a few tumors (see Fig. 11 and Table 1).

The Mechanism of Transformation

The point mutations of the *ret* proto-oncogene result in unregulated activation of the tyrosine kinase receptor. Detailed studies have shown the extracellular cysteine (codon 634) and the intracellular tyrosine kinase (codon 918) mutations transform NIH 3T3 cells (114–116). The codon 634 mutation results in receptor dimerization in the absence of a ligand, increased autophosphorylation of the receptor, and phosphorylation of downstream substrate proteins. The codon 918 mutation causes autophosphorylation and phosphorylation of a different set of substrate proteins, but it does not cause receptor dimerization. Cells transformed by expression of mutant receptors develop tumors when injected into mice (114,115).

SCREENING FOR MEDULLARY THYROID CARCINOMA

Multiple Endocrine Neoplasia Type IIA

Current recommendations for prospective screening are based on almost two decades of experience (108, 117). The introduction of DNA-based diagnostic studies, however, has had a profound effect on the management of hereditary medullary thyroid carcinoma. The first step in the management of a kindred with MEN IIA or FMTC is to perform a *ret* proto-oncogene analysis on all mem-

TABLE 1. Mutations of the RET proto-oncogene associated with hereditary medullary thyroid carcinoma

Affected codon	Amino acid change (normal → mutant)	Nucleotide change (normal → mutant)	Clinical syndrome	Percentage of MEN II mutations
609	cys → arg	TGC → CGC[b]	MEN IIA/ FMTC[a]	0–1
	cys → tyr	TGC → TAC		
611	cys → tyr	TGC → TAC	MEN IIA/ FMTC[a]	2–3
	cys → trp	TGC → TGG		
618	cys → ser	TGC → AGC	MEN IIA/ FMTC[a]	3–5
	cys → gly	TGC → GGC		
	cys → arg	TGC → CGC		
	cys → phe	TGC → TTC		
	cys → ser	TGC → TCC		
	cys → end	TGC → TGA		
620	cys → arg	TGC → CGC	MEN IIA/ FMTC[a]	6–8
	cys → tyr	TGC → TAC		
	cys → phe	TGC → TTC		
	cys → ser	TGC → TCC		
634	cys → ser	TGC → AGC	MEN IIA	80–90
	cys → gly	TGC → GGC[b]		
	cys → arg	TGC → CGC[b]	*MEN IIA/ Cutaneous lichen amyloidosis	
	cys → tyr	TGC → TAC[b]		
	cys → phe	TGC → TTC[b]		
	cys → ser	TGC → TCC		
	cys → trp	TGC → TGG[b]		
768	glu → asp	GAG → GAC	FMTC	0–1
804	val → leu	GTG → TTG	FMTC	0–1
918	met → tyr	ATG → ACG	MEN IIB	10–20

[a]Mutations of exon 10 codons 609, 611, 618, and 620 are most commonly associated with FMTC, although overlap with MEN IIA exists.
[b]FMTC, familial medullary thyroid carcinoma; MEN II, multiple endocrine neoplasia type II.

bers of the family to determine which individuals are gene carriers. In most cases, this analysis should be repeated twice on separate blood draws to exclude the possibility of a sample mix-up or laboratory error (108, 118). This is an important point because a sample mix-up within a family could result in an unaffected individual being designated as a gene carrier and an affected individual as normal. Once a specific mutation has been identified, two approaches have been utilized to guide further management.

The first is based on two decades of experience with pentagastrin testing. This approach advocates annual pentagastrin testing starting at age 4 or 5 years, only in children who are gene carriers (119). The pentagastrin test is performed by intravenous injection of 0.5 µg pentagastrin per kg body weight, diluted into 1 mL normal saline, over a 10-second period with measurement of serum calcitonin prior to injection and then 2, 5, and 10 minutes after. In most subjects, the peak calcitonin value will be observed at 2 or 5 minutes. Each gene carrier should also have a yearly 12- or 24-hr measurement of catecholamines and/or metanephrines, and a serum calcium measurement every other year (18,70,78,120). Thyroidectomy should be performed when the pentagastrin test result becomes abnormal, on average around the age of 10 to 13 (Fig. 12). Studies of children who were managed using this approach indicate that approximately 90% have evidence of long-term (15 to 20 years) cure, although recurrences have been noted in a few (18). Why a few children have recurrent disease is not clear. Approximately 50% of these children had evidence of microscopic medullary thyroid carcinoma at the time of pentagastrin test conversion from normal to abnormal. It is therefore possible that metastasis to local lymph nodes was present at the time of primary surgery and was undetected in the children who have developed recurrent disease 15 to 20 years later. An alternative explanation is the possibility that the thyroidectomy was less than complete, resulting in a few residual normal C cells being subsequently transformed by continued expression of the mutant *ret* proto-oncogene.

An alternative approach to management of MEN IIA, which is gaining favor, is to make a decision regarding thyroidectomy based solely on the genetic test results (108,117,118,121). A positive genetic test result, confirmed in a second independent blood draw, indicates that the affected child has a 90% probability of developing medullary thyroid carcinoma at some point during life (122). The earliest age at which medullary thyroid carcinoma has been diagnosed is 3 years, and a single child with metastatic disease at age 6 has been described (123). A thyroidectomy performed at the age of 5 years would be ex-

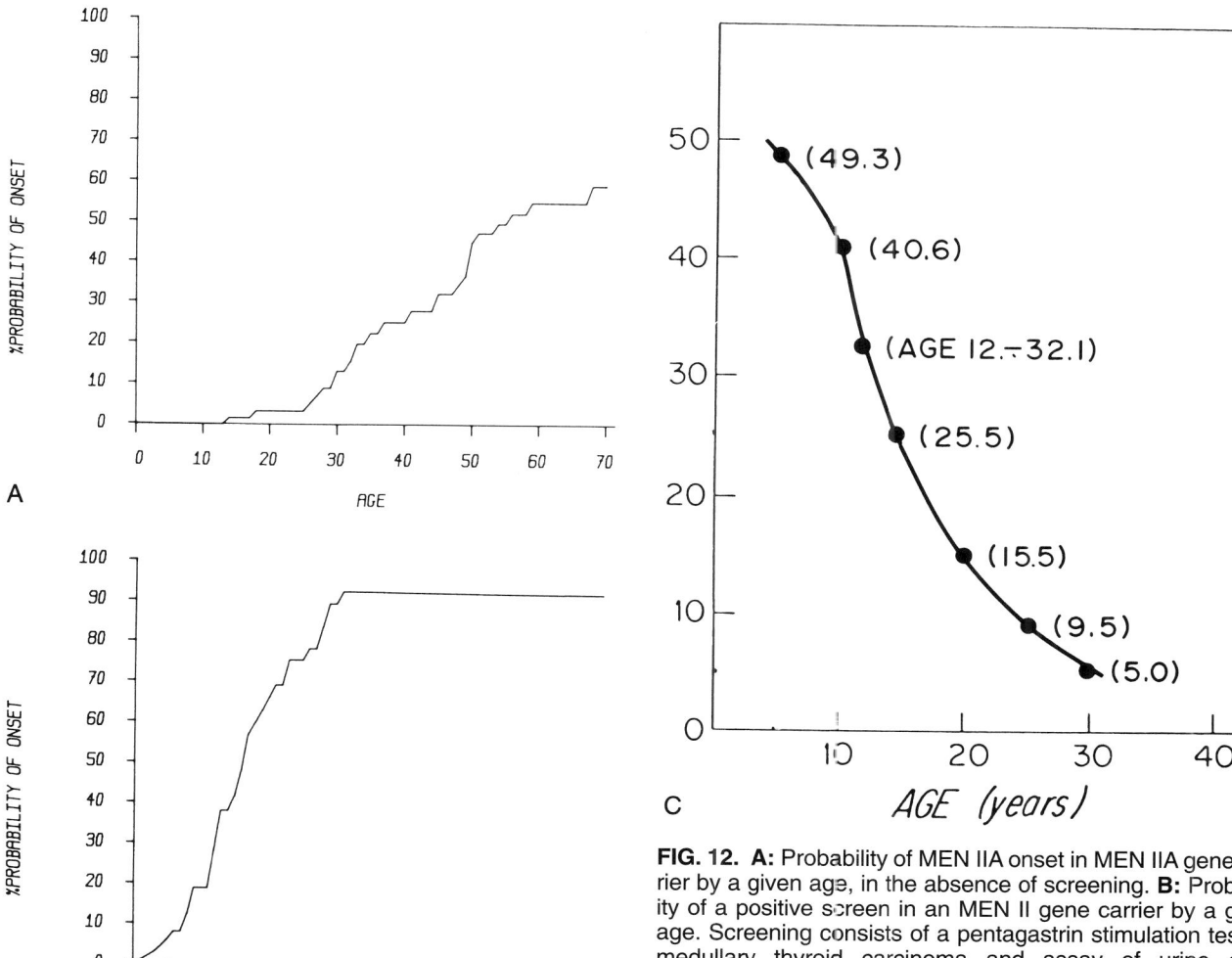

FIG. 12. **A:** Probability of MEN IIA onset in MEN IIA gene carrier by a given age, in the absence of screening. **B:** Probability of a positive screen in an MEN II gene carrier by a given age. Screening consists of a pentagastrin stimulation test for medullary thyroid carcinoma and assay of urine catecholamines for pheochromocytoma. **C:** Probability of subsequent conversion (development of disease) for an individual at 50% risk who had a negative provocative test result at a given age. [Reproduced with permission from ref. 122 (A and B) and ref. 75 (C).]

pected to remove normal or malignant C cells prior to the development of metastasis. The advantages of this approach include the simplicity of the decision process, avoidance of preoperative pentagastrin screening, and the highest probability that any transformed C cells can be removed prior to the development of metastatic disease. Although concerns have been expressed about the potential for a higher incidence of complications such as hypoparathyroidism or recurrent laryngeal nerve damage in young children, the available experience suggests that the risks are no greater in children than adults (118,121,124). Whether long-term studies of children who are thyroidectomized at an earlier age based solely on genetic testing will result in a cure rate greater than the 90% found in children in whom the decision was based on pentagastrin testing is not clear at this time. At present, either of the approaches described is acceptable.

Multiple Endocrine Neoplasia Type IIB

The identification of the mucosal neuronal phenotype in a child should alert the physician to the diagnosis of medullary thyroid carcinoma. Although it is important to confirm the diagnosis by a *ret* proto-oncogene analysis or pentagastrin test, the overwhelming likelihood of medullary thyroid carcinoma in such an individual will, in almost every case, lead to the decision for thyroidectomy during the first year of life or at the time of diagnosis. Because experience with early thyroidectomy in this syndrome is limited (28), it is not possible to determine at this time if such treatment will be curative. Parents, siblings, and children of an affected individual should also be examined by genetic testing because the penetrance of the mucosal neuroma phenotype may be less than 100%. A mother and one child were found to have mucosal neuromas and medullary thyroid carcinoma, and a second child had medullary thyroid carcinoma but no evidence of the mucosal neuroma syndrome (125). Other routine screening tests do not differ from the recommendations for MEN IIA, except that hyperparathyroidism is rare in MEN IIB (98).

Other Screening Studies

The key to screening for pheochromocytoma in known families is the application of simple screening procedures over an extended period of time. Prospective annual screening for pheochromocytoma by measurement of 12- or 24-hr urinary catecholamines permits detection of early pheochromocytoma. Experience indicates that it is difficult to identify more than 5% to 10% of these tumors at the stage of adrenal medullary hyperplasia, but small pheochromocytomas can be identified before they become significant clinical problems (18,70,77,126). Measurement of the urinary vanillylmandelic acid is not useful for diagnosis of early pheochromocytoma (70). A combination of urine catecholamine and metanephrine measurements enhances the probability of detecting early disease.

Interpretation of Test Results

The pentagastrin test (127,128) and the combined calcium/pentagastrin test (16) have been used in prospective screening efforts. The relative merits of each test have been debated (129). The choice now seems less important than the measurement of the calcitonin samples in an assay that is capable of measuring the normal basal serum calcitonin concentration. Definition of the normal basal calcitonin concentration and the response to pentagastrin or calcium/pentagastrin in a normal subject permits greater precision in determining the significance of an abnormal result in a potentially affected kindred member. There are several excellent commercial assays or kits that are based on previously developed research assays (27,130,131), so sensitive assays should be available to most physicians for screening purposes.

It is useful to have normative data in a particular kindred to determine the significance of a particular result. In an individual MEN IIA gene carrier, there will inevitably be a period of conversion from a normal to an abnormal test result, during which results may fluctuate (17). The decision to perform a total thyroidectomy should be based on a combination of an abnormal pentagastrin test and a positive genetic test.

Interpretation of test results can be difficult in certain situations. An elevated basal serum calcitonin with no further increase after pentagastrin injection may be indicative of assay artifact (131), another tumor ectopically producing calcitonin (42), renal failure (132), or abnormal calcitonin release associated with exercise or thyroiditis. Uncommonly, a patient with medullary thyroid carcinoma may have a basal elevation of the serum calcitonin concentration without further stimulation by calcium or pentagastrin.

Clarification of the cause of the calcitonin elevation may be difficult. An elevation of the serum calcitonin concentration caused by assay artifact can usually be identified by measurement of the sample in another calcitonin radioimmunoassay (where a normal result would be observed), or by utilizing a technique that is specific for monomeric calcitonin, such as a concentrating technique (133) or a two-site immunoradiometric assay (134,135). Renal failure as a cause of an elevated serum calcitonin can be confirmed by measurement of the serum creatinine (132). Exercise-induced elevations of the serum calcitonin (136) or thyroiditis can usually be identified by careful history-taking and repeat testing.

Should Families of Patients with Sporadic Medullary Thyroid Carcinoma Be Screened?

Recent studies have demonstrated that approximately 5% to 7% of patients with apparent sporadic medullary thyroid carcinoma have germline mutations of the *ret* proto-oncogene, indicating that they have hereditary medullary thyroid carcinoma (137–139). The discovered cases include several *de novo* germline mutations that can be passed to subsequent generations or members of previously unidentified kindreds (111,113). A consensus is developing that all patients with apparent sporadic medullary thyroid carcinoma should have a peripheral blood *ret* proto-oncogene analysis performed to detect germline mutations (113). If the test is negative, the probability that this individual could be a member of a kindred with hereditary medullary thyroid carcinoma without a *ret* proto-oncogene mutation is 5% to 7%. Application of the Bayes theorem indicates that first-degree relatives of an individual with medullary thyroid carcinoma and a negative *ret* proto-oncogene analysis would have less than a 0.5% probability of developing medullary thyroid carcinoma (113). In most cases, families of an affected individual will find this risk level acceptable and no further testing is required unless there is a family history. In situations where a family finds a probability of 0.5% to be unacceptable, all first-degree relatives should have a pentagastrin test performed. If pentagastrin test results are normal, the probability of hereditary medullary thyroid carcinoma falls to an insignificant level.

Application of these screening approaches to index cases with apparent sporadic medullary thyroid carcinoma has resulted in the identification of at least 15 new kindreds (111,113,137–139). Most importantly, it has been possible to identify gene carrier status in children within these kindreds at a stage in the development of medullary thyroid carcinoma when they can be cured.

Sporadic Medullary Thyroid Carcinoma

Several recent reports have identified medullary thyroid carcinoma in a high percentage of patients with multinodular goiter and elevation of the basal serum calcitonin (140,141). In one report, 41% of multinodular goiter patients with an elevated basal serum calcitonin, determined by two-site immunoradiometric assay, had a microscopic or macroscopic focus of medullary thyroid carcinoma (142). In more than one half of these patients, the basal calcitonin concentration was below 200 pg/mL. These results provide a compelling argument for inclusion of calcitonin measurement in the routine evaluation of a multinodular goiter or thyroid nodule, because there are few other screening studies for detection of medullary thyroid carcinoma at a potentially curable stage. Routine preoperative use of FNA of thyroid nodules is likely to increase the yield of preoperative diagnosis of medullary thyroid carcinoma and result in the appropriate operation during the first surgical procedure.

TREATMENT OF MEDULLARY THYROID CARCINOMA

The definitive treatment of medullary thyroid carcinoma is surgical removal of the entire thyroid gland and its primary lymphatic drainage. This is accomplished by total thyroidectomy and a meticulous central compartment node dissection. The extent of additional surgical dissection and other management considerations are dependent on several factors: the stage of the disease at the time of diagnosis, the presence or absence of associated endocrine abnormalities, and the risk of cervical or distant metastasis. We believe the primary operation provides the greatest chance for cure and, therefore, the appropriate procedure should be performed at that time.

Total thyroidectomy is indicated in both the hereditary and sporadic forms of medullary carcinoma of the thyroid for several reasons. First, the C cells, from which the tumor originates, have a diffuse and bilateral anatomic distribution (6), frequently resulting in multifocal and bilobar tumor. In the sporadic form of medullary thyroid carcinoma, bilateral disease may be seen in 30% of the cases (143), and in hereditary cases, the incidence approaches 100% (18,57,143). Second, in hereditary medullary thyroid carcinoma, a high incidence of C cell hyperplasia exists in the contralateral thyroid lobe, even in early medullary thyroid carcinoma. This pathological change is a precursor of the development of frank carcinoma (95, 144). Third, 5% to 7% of patients presumed to have sporadic medullary thyroid carcinoma prove to be index cases for MEN IIA with germline mutations of the *ret* proto-oncogene, assuring they will have bilateral disease (111,113,137–139,145).

Central node dissection is indicated during the initial operation because of the high incidence of regional lymphatic involvement in medullary thyroid carcinoma. In several large series, cervical metastases at the time of presentation have been observed in 50% to 63% of cases (146–148). In a smaller selected series, metastases to regional lymph nodes were found in 33%, 81%, and 70.6% of MEN IIA, MEN IIB, and sporadic disease cases, respectively (101). Metastases may be seen even with primary lesions less than 1.0 cm in diameter. Performing central node dissection at the initial procedure also obviates the need to reexplore this area of the neck at a future date should calcitonin levels remain elevated after the initial procedure. This significantly decreases the risk of hypoparathyroidism and recurrent laryngeal nerve injury if a patient requires further surgery for persistent disease.

In patients detected by prospective family screening who have no overt thyroid lesion, total thyroidectomy and central compartment node dissection may be curative for this disease. Surgery in this group of patients has resulted in normalization of calcitonin levels and rendered patients free of any apparent clinical disease in over 90% of the cases (18,28,149).

Technique of Total Thyroidectomy

The technique of total thyroidectomy is described in greater detail elsewhere in this text (see Chapter 36), but in the treatment of this particular disease several points should be highlighted. First, every effort should be made to remove all thyroid tissue in the neck. This requires complete dissection of the inferior and superior poles of the gland. The arteries and veins should be isolated individually and ligated proximal to the gland. Placing a single surgical clamp on the entire superior pole should be avoided, because it increases the possibility of leaving thyroid tissue in the neck, and it enhances the risk of injuring the external branch of the superior laryngeal nerve. Second, identification and dissection of the right and left recurrent laryngeal nerves as they course through the neck is strongly recommended. The nerve should be isolated inferiorly in the tracheoesophageal groove and traced superiorly, and the thyroid gland should be dissected free. The nerve should be followed into the posterior aspect of the cricothyroid membrane. This allows thorough dissection of the gland and removal of surrounding soft-tissue lymphatics while minimizing inadvertent injury to the nerve. Third, precise identification and examination of all four of the parathyroid glands is mandatory in this disease, because of the associated incidence of parathyroid hyperplasia and adenomas. Preservation of the blood supply is critical for each parathyroid gland left in the paratracheal region. Reimplantation of parathyroid tissue into the patient's nondominant forearm should be performed in cases in which a partial parathyroidectomy is indicated.

Technique of Central Compartment Node Dissection

A central node dissection (dissection of level VI lymphatic compartment) is defined as the removal of lymph nodes and soft tissue from the hyoid bone superiorly, to the sternal notch inferiorly, and to the internal jugular veins bilaterally (Fig. 13). The anterior limit of the dissection is the superficial layer of the deep cervical fascia as it invests infrahyoid and sternocleidomastoid musculature. The posterior limit of the dissection is the visceral prevertebral fascia overlying the deep neck musculature. In the midline region, the fascial dissection is carried down to the visceral compartment with preservation of the larynx, trachea, esophagus, and recurrent laryngeal nerves. Laterally, the dissection is extended to the carotid sheath. All of the soft tissue contained within the superficial layer of the deep fascia to the deep layer of the deep cervical fascia from the sternal notch to the hyoid bone is removed. The sternohyoid, thyrohyoid, sternothyroid, omohyoid, and sternocleidomastoid muscles and the contents of the visceral compartment and carotid sheath are preserved. Meticulous dissection and removal of the lymphatic compartments of the paratracheal node region overlying the prevertebral fascia are critical. Dissection should be carried down inferiorly to the sternal notch and, some authors advocate (150), to the superior aspect of the great vessels.

Management of Lateral Cervical Lymphatics

In familial MEN IIA or IIB patients with a palpable thyroid mass or cervical adenopathy at presentation, and in all sporadic cases of medullary thyroid carcinoma, a total thyroidectomy and central compartment node dissection as described previously should be carried out. In addition, if palpable disease is present in the thyroid and the central compartment lymph nodes, the surgeon

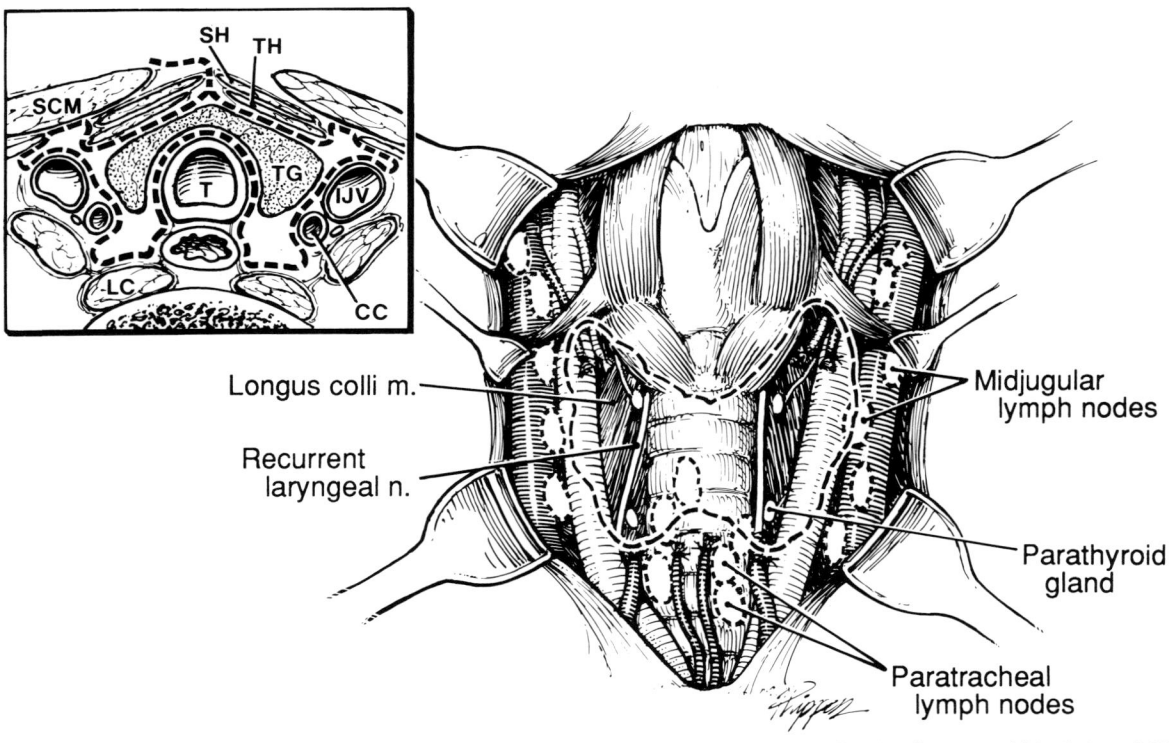

FIG. 13. The extent of initial surgical dissection in the treatment of medullary carcinoma of the thyroid includes removal of the thyroid gland and its primary lymphatic drainage. The location of resected thyroid gland and the middle jugular, lower jugular, and paratracheal node-bearing areas *(dotted lines)* included in a central node dissection are outlined. **Inset:** Transverse depiction of the deep cervical fascial envelope *(dashed line)* that encompasses the central node compartment and the thyroid gland. IJV, internal jugular vein; CC, common carotid artery; SH, sternohyoid muscle; TH, thyrohyoid muscle; SCM, sternocleidomastoid muscle; LC, longus colli muscle; T, trachea; TG, thyroid gland.

should explore both lateral cervical lymphatics. This includes careful systematic evaluation of the lower, mid, and upper jugular regions, as well as anterior aspects of the posterior triangles and jugulodigastric regions not encompassed in central neck dissections (see Fig. 13). All soft tissue should be carefully examined, and enlarged lymph nodes should be sampled for the presence of metastases. If metastases are found, then a definitive modified neck dissection originally described by Bocca (151) and modified by Tisell et al. (150) should be performed. This entails complete dissection from the clavicle inferiorly, to the trapezius posteriorly, to the mandible and infratemporal fossa superiorly. The soft tissue and lymphatic drainage contained within the deep cervical fascia (from the superficial to deep layer of the deep cervical fascia) should be removed, with preservation of the sternocleidomastoid muscle, contents of the carotid sheath, spinal accessory, and hypoglossal nerves.

The rationale for this recommendation is the observation that patients with a palpable thyroid mass have clinical or pathologic evidence of metastasis in a significant number of cases (147,148). In patients with hereditary disease, there is a 50% incidence of micrometastasis, as evidenced by elevated pentagastrin-stimulated calcitonin after initial surgery (26,57). In sporadic medullary thyroid carcinoma, control of disease is achieved in only 45% of cases (57). Most of these series do not define their compartment dissection technique, but support for an aggressive surgical approach in the neck was first provided by the studies of Tisell et al. (150), who demonstrated a surgical cure achieved with reoperation in approximately 30% of patients with local metastasis; these authors employed a meticulous modified neck dissection for hereditary medullary thyroid carcinoma. These latter results suggest that surgical cure is potentially attainable and adequate dissection at the primary operation will offer the greatest chance for cure.

MANAGEMENT OF PERSISTENT CALCITONIN ELEVATION

After definitive surgical treatment for medullary thyroid carcinoma, a pentagastrin test should be performed. Patients with normal or nondetectable calcitonin levels on two follow-up evaluations are likely to be free of disease (18).

Even with aggressive surgical intervention, however, a small group of patients will have persistent elevation of either basal or pentagastrin-stimulated calcitonin levels after their initial surgery. This is likely to represent persistent metastatic disease. In this clinical situation, the challenge is establishing the location of the residual disease. If tumor is localized to the neck and a definitive node dissection was not performed initially, then reoperation is indicated. If disease has metastasized outside the neck, it is unlikely that surgical reintervention will result in cure. Techniques for localizing tumor include conventional CT or MRI techniques to image the neck, chest, and liver, and radionuclide scan to detect the uptake of thallium, indium-labeled octreotide, or radioiodinated meta-iodobenzylguanidine by tumor tissue (152,153). Each of these techniques is dependent on the presence of a sizable tumor and is not likely to detect micrometastasis.

A technique we and others (154–156) have used to localize occult metastatic disease is the application of selective venous catheterization. In our studies, we have placed several indwelling catheters (right and left neck, hepatic vein, and peripheral venous) through the femoral veins and injected pentagastrin (dose identical to the standard pentagastrin test), with withdrawal of blood samples at 0, 1, 2, and 5 min after injection from each of the catheters. This technique has enabled us to localize disease to the neck and determine laterality in several cases. A step-up in the calcitonin concentration gradient from the hepatic vein would suggest distant metastatic disease. Experience with these diagnostic techniques and reoperation based on the results are not likely to improve the cure rate by more than 5% to 30% (149,150,157,158), but identification of diffuse disease outside the neck may prevent reoperation in a patient with distant metastatic disease.

The best results with reoperation in this disease were originally reported by Tisell et al. (150), who described normalization of the serum calcitonin concentration in 4 of 11 patients reoperated for persistent elevations of the serum calcitonin concentration after the primary surgical procedure. In each of their 11 patients, there was evidence of central and lateral node micrometastasis, which was detectable as a mass in only one case preoperatively. All patients underwent extensive modified neck dissection involving microdissection with the aid of magnification, and meticulous dissection of all the node-bearing compartments from the clavicle to the base of the skull. Four patients had normalization of their pentagastrin-stimulated calcitonin levels postoperatively. The remaining seven patients had persistent elevation of calcitonin levels. Subsequent studies have corroborated Tisell's initial experience (159,160). Dralle et al. (159) demonstrated normalization of pentagastrin-stimulated serum calcitonin after systematic compartment lymphadenectomy in 29.2% of 82 patients, versus 8.5% of patients who underwent a selective neck dissection. Reoperation with microdissection compartment lymphadenectomy resulted in normalization of calcitonin in 28% of 32 patients reported by Moley et al. and a 40% decrease in calcitonin in 42% of the remaining patients in the study (160). The data from the latter study suggested that patients whose medullary thyroid carcinoma at the time of presentation penetrated beyond the thyroid gland capsule or had extracapsular lymph node extension were much less likely to benefit from reoperation. Taken cumulatively, this broader experience indicates that 15% to 25% of carefully selected patients will have normalization of their serum calcitonin values after reoperation with systematic compartment lymphadenectomy (150,159–161). It is important to select carefully patients who are most likely to benefit from this type of procedure by exclusion of distant metastatic disease before consideration of reoperation. Detailed imaging studies of the neck, chest, and abdomen should be performed to exclude distant metastatic disease.

We conclude that an adequate primary operation provides the best chance for surgical cure in patients with palpable or occult locally metastatic tumor. Appropriate subsequent surgical procedures may result in cure or delay progression of disease, and therefore they can be justified. The clinician should not, however, raise false expectation of a surgical cure for patients who have persistent elevation of pentagastrin-stimulated calcitonin levels after definitive therapy.

PARATHYROID GLAND CONSIDERATIONS

Management of the parathyroid glands during a surgical procedure for medullary thyroid carcinoma falls into three general categories: sporadic medullary thyroid carcinoma and a normal serum calcium concentration; hereditary medullary thyroid carcinoma and associated primary hyperparathyroidism; and prospectively screened patients with early hereditary medullary thyroid carcinoma and a normal serum calcium concentration.

In patients with apparent sporadic medullary thyroid carcinoma and a normal serum calcium concentration, all four parathyroid glands should be identified and care taken to preserve the respective blood supply of each gland. If it is necessary to resect parathyroid tissue to perform adequate surgical removal of tumor and lymph nodes, the parathyroid tissue should be implanted in the sternocleidomastoid muscle or forearm after frozen-section histologic documentation of parathyroid tissue (150,162). Overly aggressive management of normal glands is associated with high incidence of hypoparathyroidism and should be avoided (158).

In patients with hereditary medullary thyroid carcinoma and clinical evidence of primary hyperparathyroidism, it is likely there will be multiple parathyroid gland involvement with either hyperplasia or adenomatous changes (18,86,87,163). The correct management in patients with hyperparathyroidism requires that all four parathyroid glands be identified. If an enlarged gland is found and an adenoma is clearly present, the gland should be removed. The remaining glands should then be transplanted to either the sternocleidomastoid muscle (150) or the nondominant forearm (164–166). The location of transplanted glands needs to be clearly marked, as some patients may continue to have persistently elevated calcium requiring reexploration and further removal of glandular tissue. If diffuse hyperplasia of each of the glands is found, then removal of three and one-half glands is appropriate with autotransplantation of only a portion of one remaining gland to the nondominant forearm (164–166). If no abnormalities are found in the hypercalcemic patient, careful dissection during the removal of the central node compartment is advisable to ensure that the patient does not have additional parathyroid glands in the paratracheal or upper mediastinal region. If no other glands are found, removal of three glands with autotransplantation of the remaining tissue is indicated. In the event of persistent or recurrent hypercalcemia, further glandular excision can more easily be accomplished.

The latter approach, routine transplantation of parathyroid tissue to the nondominant forearm, has been used extensively for management of hyperparathyroidism in MEN type I, where hyperparathyroidism is inevitably the primary manifestation and recurrent disease is common (165–167). The major advantages of this approach include the ability to monitor graft function by measurement of parathyroid hormone in the venous effluent, and management of recurrent hyperparathyroidism by local resection of parathyroid tissue. This technique has been applied in some families with MEN IIA in whom recurrent hyperparathyroidism has been a problem (72,121). An additional advantage of this approach is that it will permit neck reoperation without risk for development of hypoparathyroidism.

The correct management of the third category, prospectively screened patients with early hereditary medullary thyroid carcinoma and a normal serum calcium concentration, is not clear. In several recent series, no parathyroid abnormalities have been found in prospectively screened patients (18,28), and a 10-year follow-up in one series (18) demonstrated no subsequent hyperparathyroidism. It is possible that the inevitable removal of some parathyroid tissue as a result of a total thyroidectomy (162) has prevented or delayed the development of parathyroid disease (18). It is unclear if these patients will eventually develop clinical evidence of parathyroid disease. At this point, a reasonable approach would suggest preservation of parathyroid glandular tissue in these patients.

The application of genetic screening to kindreds with hereditary disease has led to early operation of gene carriers. One concern has been that any residual C cells may undergo transformation in the decades after the initial surgery. Recognizing that it is difficult to perform a total thyroidectomy and preserve parathyroid function, Wells and colleagues (121) have advocated a total thyroidectomy and removal of all parathyroid tissue from the neck in these children, with transplantation of parathyroid tissue to the nondominant forearm. This approach makes it possible to remove the posterior capsule of the thyroid gland without concern for parathyroid vascularity and function. The initial report from these investigators described no permanent hypoparathyroidism in these children (121). Whether cure rates in these children will be better than those obtained using a more conservative approach will require long-term follow-up studies (108).

These studies point out the concern about the possibility of hypoparathyroidism in young patients. The necessity to take calcium and vitamin D supplementation for a lifetime is a significant issue, with the attendant problems of hypercalciuria and renal calcification. Where possible, parathyroid tissue removed should be cryopreserved if not transplanted. Postoperatively, calcium levels should be monitored closely. Appropriate calcium and vitamin D supplements should be implemented. After the surgical procedure, the serum calcium should be monitored on a regular basis until it is stabilized in the normal range.

ADRENAL GLAND CONSIDERATIONS

Management in Sporadic Medullary Thyroid Carcinoma

The risk of pheochromocytoma in a nonfamilial case of medullary thyroid carcinoma would, indeed, be low; however, a patient may be an index case of medullary thyroid carcinoma and the surgeon should be prepared for that eventuality. In patients in whom a diagnosis of medullary thyroid carcinoma is made by FNA, preoperative screening for pheochromocytoma (see preceding) should be conducted.

Management in Hereditary Medullary Thyroid Carcinoma

All patients with hereditary or familial medullary thyroid carcinoma are at risk for development of a pheochromocytoma. Familial cases of medullary thyroid carcinoma should be screened preoperatively with 24-hr urine epinephrine and norepinephrine levels, as well as appropriate imaging studies of the adrenal glands. If all these studies are normal, the risk of a hypertensive crisis during the induction of anesthesia is extremely low. If catecholamine abnormalities are detected or there is a clinical suspicion of pheochromocytoma, additional studies should be performed to determine the presence or absence of adrenal medullary abnormalities. The anesthesiologist should always be alerted in advance to the familial history of these patients, so that in the event of a crisis, appropriate hypotensive medications are readily available.

In the event of an undiagnosed pheochromocytoma being present at the time of anesthetic induction, a hypertensive crisis may ensue. Appropriate management would include β-adrenergic blockade with intravenous phentolamine (given in 5-mg increments until the blood pressure is controlled) or a nitroprusside infusion (168,169). In addition β-adrenergic blockage (propranolol, 1 mg given intravenously in incremental doses) is indicated to treat tachyarrhythmias.

In patients with proven adrenal medullary disease, the abnormal adrenal medullary tissue should be surgically removed in a separate operation prior to thyroidectomy. How much adrenal tissue to remove is more controversial. All clinicians would agree that removal of both adrenal glands is mandatory in the rare families with proven adrenal medullary malignancy, preferably as soon as the diagnosis of gene carrier status is made (82). There are different approaches to the management of adrenal medullary disease in other families with MEN II. Some surgeons remove only those adrenal glands in which there are demonstrable pheochromocytomas (18,170,171). Other physicians, concerned about the rare possibility of adrenal medullary malignancy (82) and the 50% likelihood of development of a pheochromocytoma in the contralateral adrenal gland, recommend bilateral adrenalectomy at the time of primary operation (77,82,126,172). The latter approach eliminates the need for a second, later operation, but it exposes patients who would not have developed a clinically significant pheochromocytoma to the risks associated with adrenal corticosteroid deficiency. Two deaths secondary to adrenal insufficiency in this setting have been described. Our approach has been to remove only affected adrenal glands (18). The adrenal gland(s) should be removed through an anterior abdominal or flank approach (77). All patients should receive preoperative treatment with pharmacologic α- and β-adrenergic antagonists (18,173,174).

CLINICAL COURSE OF MEDULLARY THYROID CARCINOMA

The clinical course of untreated medullary thyroid carcinoma is likely to include progressive growth of the thyroid tumor, eventual local, regional, and distant (pulmonary, hepatic, and bone) metastases, and, in a large percentage of cases, death related to either metastatic thyroid tumor or pheochromocytoma. There is general agreement that surgical management has favorably influenced the clinical course of the disease. The main factors that influence survival include the size of the tumor, the presence or absence of extracapsular spread, the extent of cervical or distant metastasis, and the type of tumor syndrome. The impact of tumor size and extent of metastatic disease on the course of the disease is shown most clearly by the work of Samaan et al. (175) (Fig. 14). In their studies, patients with intraglandular disease were much less likely to die from their disease than patients with nodal or distant metastases. The impact of the type of tumor syndrome will be discussed in the following sections.

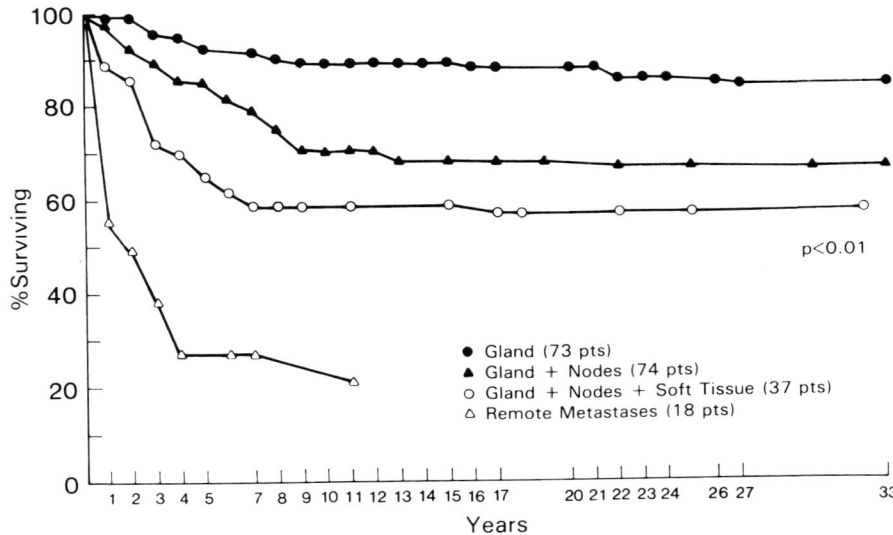

FIG. 14. Survival rates of patients with familial (50 patients) and sporadic (152 patients) medullary thyroid carcinoma, according to extent of disease. (Reproduced with permission from ref. 175.)

It is important to note that over the past decade there has been a reevaluation of some of the factors affecting survival, and more information has been gathered about the impact of early surgical intervention on the course of the disease.

Sporadic Medullary Thyroid Carcinoma

It had long been felt that patients with sporadic medullary thyroid carcinoma have a much worse prognosis than those with the hereditary form of the disease. This was supported by studies demonstrating a poorer survival in patients with sporadic than hereditary disease. Kakuda et al. (101) found 5-, 10-, and 20-year survival in 18 patients with hereditary medullary thyroid carcinoma detected by family screening to be 100%, 90%, and 90%, respectively (Fig. 15). This is contrasted with only 82.4%, 64.7%, and 43.1% survival, respectively, for 17 cases of sporadic medullary thyroid carcinoma (see Fig. 15). The fundamental differences in these comparisons were the age of the patients and the extent of tumor metastasis at the time of diagnosis. Samaan and coworkers (175) had earlier reached similar conclusions, but in a more recent analysis of their survival data in 152 patients with sporadic and 50 patients with hereditary (MEN IIA) disease, they have shown that there are no statistically significant differences in survival rates when the groups were matched for age and extent of involvement. The latter results are important because they suggest that the biologic behavior of the primary tumor is not different; rather, it is the greater size and extent of tumor metastasis associated with sporadic medullary thyroid carcinoma that is the determining factor in survival.

Hereditary Medullary Thyroid Carcinoma and Multiple Endocrine Neoplasia Type IIA

Improved survival in patients with MEN can be attributed not only to earlier detection of the thyroid tumor, but also to appropriate management of adrenal medullary disease. Although specific data were difficult to obtain prior to the development of techniques for prospective screening for this syndrome, the average life expectancy in patients with hereditary MEN IIA was approximately 50 years of age (26,86). Death was caused by spread of the thyroid tumor, or it occurred suddenly as a result of the pheochromocytoma.

The early 1970s brought a dramatic change in the approach to this disease. Work by several groups demonstrated that surgical cure of medullary thyroid carcinoma is possible even in the presence of local nodal metastasis. In the initial work described by Melvin et al. (26,68), 7 of 12 patients with local metastases were rendered disease free, and an 18-year follow-up of this same group demonstrated 6 of 12 remain disease free, with three deaths (18). Experience in other groups has resulted in cure rates in patients with palpable disease ranging from 15% to 50% (71,72,74,101,158,172–174).

The application of prospective screening techniques has further improved the cure rate. In patients with MEN IIA discovered by prospective family screening and treated by total thyroidectomy and central node dissection, normalization of the serum calcitonin concentration can be attained in a high percentage of cases. Jackson et al. (149) achieved this in 26 out of 26 patients who had no palpable disease. In the series of Telander et al. (28), 14 of 14 children with no palpable disease, prospectively

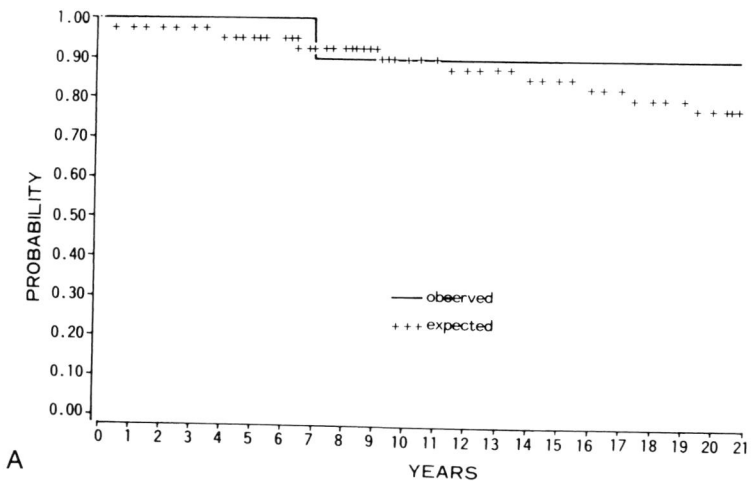

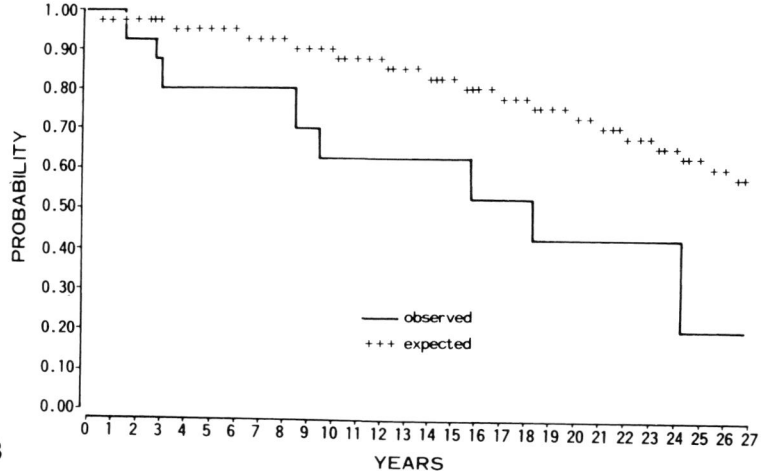

FIG. 15. Survival in hereditary or familial medullary thyroid carcinoma. Cumulative survival curve of 18 MEN IIA patients (A) and 17 sporadic medullary thyroid carcinoma (B) patients from the Mayo Clinic experience. (Reprinted with permission from ref. 101.)

screened between 1975 and 1985, had normal pentagastrin-stimulated calcitonin levels after their surgery. In an 18-year follow-up on the effect of prospective screening, Gagel et al. (18) reported long-term follow-up in 35 family members who had undergone thyroidectomy for hereditary medullary carcinoma of the thyroid since 1968. After the initiation of their prospective screening in 1972, 23 patients underwent thyroidectomy as soon as abnormal serum calcitonin levels developed. More than 90% remain disease free, with follow-up periods of 10 to 23 years. Patients detected by family screening with an elevated serum calcitonin level and no palpable disease have an excellent long-term prognosis and can most probably be considered cured of their disease.

Multiple Endocrine Neoplasia Type IIB

Separate survival statistics for MEN IIB patients are difficult to obtain because of the relative rarity of the syndrome. In a report by Kakudo et al. (101), 11 cases of

MEN IIB had cumulative survivals of 90.9%, 81.8%, and 40.9% at 5, 10, and 20 years, respectively (compare to Fig. 15), which is considerably lower than the survival for either MEN IIA or sporadic tumors. Isolated experience with individual cases would generally support this clinical experience. A number of three-generation families exist, and the diagnosis of MEN IIB does not necessarily mean the clinical course will be dismal (94,102,149).

ADJUNCTIVE FORMS OF THERAPY

Although the experience in eliminating all the metastatic disease by reoperation of the neck for metastatic disease has been disappointing, it is hoped that newer techniques in localization of the disease and more meticulous surgical dissections may be of benefit. Management of distant metastatic disease is at the present time directed by symptomatic relief. Although some authors have advocated the addition of radiation therapy, with favorable response (148,179,180), the general consensus is that medullary thyroid carcinoma responds poorly to radiotherapy (146,175). In a recent report by Samaan et al. (175), a relatively large number of patients with medullary thyroid carcinoma, matched for age, extent of disease, and surgical intervention, had a much shorter survival than those who had received no radiation therapy. Similarly, treatment of patients with radioactive iodine has not been shown to be effective in clinical settings (181–183). From a theoretical standpoint, radioactive iodine should not affect C cells directly, as they do not have any function in thyroid hormone production and, therefore, do not take up circulating iodine. However, radioactive iodine covalently linked to meta-iodobenzylguanidine may prove to be more effective (153).

Experience with chemotherapeutic agents has likewise been disappointing. Doxorubicin, streptozocin, etoposide, and bleomycin have been used as single agents in patients, without significant response. Agents used in combination have included cis-platinum and 5-fluorouracil, and cyclophosphamide and methotrexate, but these agents have likewise not been effective in inducing any significant tumor regression. Recent small series suggest the response rate may be greater in combinations containing dimethyltriazenoimidazole carboxamide (DTIC). No chemotherapeutic regimens reported to date have been found to be particularly effective, and response rate has been generally poor. In various series, the response rate to chemotherapy has not exceeded 15% (146,148,184) (see also Chapter 33).

THE FUTURE

A ligand for the *ret* tyrosine kinase receptor has recently been identified (185,186). Several lines of evidence support a role for glial cell line–derived neurotrophic factor (GDNF), a transforming growth factor-β–like factor (187), as an endogenous ligand for the *ret* receptor, including specific interaction, support of biologic functions mediated by *ret* (185,186), and expression in tissues where *ret* is expressed at an appropriate time in development (185). There is no current information regarding mutations of GDNF in MEN II, medullary thyroid carcinoma, or Hirschsprung's disease, although this gene becomes an obvious candidate for mutational analysis in Hirschsprung's disease and in the 5% to 7% of families with hereditary medullary thyroid carcinoma in whom no *ret* mutation has been identified.

The identification of a ligand will also foster research on the ligand–receptor interaction and potentially lead to the development of analogs that modify receptor function, strategies which may alter the therapeutic approach to treatment of medullary thyroid carcinoma in the future.

REFERENCES

1. Woolner LB, Beahrs OH, Black BM, McConahey WM, Keating FR Jr. Classification and prognosis of thyroid carcinoma. *Am J Surg* 1961;102:354–394.
2. Bussolati G, Pearse AGE. Immunofluorescent localization of calcitonin in the "C" cells of pig and dog thyroid. *J Endocrinol* 1967;37:205–209.
3. Pearse AGE. Common cytochemical and ultrastructural characteristics of cells producing polypeptide hormones (the APUD series) and their relevance to thyroid and ultimobranchial C cells and calcitonin. *Proc R Soc Lond (Biol)* 1968;170:71–80.
4. Le Douarin N, Le Lievre C. Demonstration de l'origine neurales des cellules a calcitonine du corps ultimobranchial chez l'embryon de poulet. *C R Soc Biol (Paris)* 1970;270:2857–2860.
5. Pearse AGE. Morphology and cytochemistry of thyroid and ultimobranchial C cells. In: Greep and Astwood, eds. *Handbook of physiology, section 7: endocrinology*. Washington, DC: American Physiological Society, 1976;411–421.
6. Wolfe HJ, Voelkel EF, Tashjian AH Jr. Distribution of calcitonin-containing cells in the normal adult human thyroid gland: a correlation of morphology with peptide content. *J Clin Endocrinol Metab* 1974;38:688–694.
7. Copp DH, Cameron EC, Cheney BA, Davidson AGF, Henze KG. Evidence for calcitonin—a new hormone from the parathyroid that lowers blood calcium. *Endocrinology* 1962;70:638–649.
8. Hirsch PF, Gauthier GF, Munson PL. Thyroid hypocalcemic principle and recurrent laryngeal nerve injury as factors affecting the response to parathyroidectomy in rats. *Endocrinology* 1963;73:244–252.
9. Jacobs JW, Goodman RH, Chin WW, et al. Calcitonin messenger RNA encodes multiple polypeptides in a single precursor. *Science* 1981;213:457–459.
10. Rosenfeld MG, Mermod JJ, Amara SG, et al. Production of a novel neuropeptide encoded by the calcitonin gene via tissue-specific RNA processing. *Nature* 1983;304:129–135.
11. Cote GJ, Gould JA, Huang SC, Gagel RF. Studies of short-term secretion of peptides produced by alternative RNA processing. *Mol Cell Endocrinol* 1987;53:211–219.
12. de Bustros A, Baylin SB, Berger CL, Roos BA, Leong SS, Nelkin BD. Phorbol esters increase calcitonin gene transcription and decrease c-myc mRNA levels in cultured human medullary thyroid carcinoma. *J Biol Chem* 1985;260:98–104.
13. Muszynski M, Birnbaum RS, Roos BA. Glucocorticoids stimulate the production of preprocalcitonin-derived secretory peptides by a rat medullary thyroid carcinoma cell line. *J Biol Chem* 1983;258:11678–11683.
14. Cote GJ, Rogers DG, Huang ES, Gagel RF. The effect of 1,25-dihydroxyvitamin D_3 treatment on calcitonin and calcitonin gene-related

peptide mRNA levels in cultured human thyroid C-cells. *Biochem Biophys Res Commun* 1987;149:239–243.
15. Cooper CW, Deftos LJ, Potts JT Jr. Direct measurement of in vivo secretion of pig thyrocalcitonin by radioimmunoassay. *Endocrinology* 1971;88:747–754.
16. Wells SA Jr, Baylin SB, Linehan WM, et al. Provocative agents and the diagnosis of medullary carcinoma of the thyroid gland. *Ann Surg* 1978;188:139–141.
17. Graze K, Spiler IJ, Tashjian AH Jr, et al. Natural history of familial medullary thyroid carcinoma: effect of a program for early diagnosis. *N Engl J Med* 1978;299:980–985.
18. Gagel RF, Tashjian AH Jr, Cummings T, et al. The clinical outcome of prospective screening for multiple endocrine neoplasia type 2a. An 18-year experience. *N Engl J Med* 1988;318:478–484.
19. Zeytinoglu FN, Gagel RF, Tashjian AH Jr, Hammer RA, Leeman SE. Regulation of neurotensin release by a continuous line of mammalian C-cells: the role of biogenic amines. *Endocrinology* 1983;112:1240–1246.
20. Gagel RF, Zeytinoglu FN, Voelkel EF, Tashjian AH Jr. Establishment of a calcitonin-producing rat medullary thyroid carcinoma cell line. II. Secretory studies of the tumor and cells in culture. *Endocrinology* 1980;107:516–523.
21. Zeytin FN, Rusk SF, Baird A, et al. Induction of c-fos, calcitonin gene expression, and acidic fibroblast growth factor production in a multipeptide-secreting neuroendocrine cell line. *Endocrinology* 1988;122:1114–1120.
22. Roos BA, Bundy LL, Bailey R, Deftos LJ. Calcitonin secretion in vitro. I. Preparation of monolayer C-cell cultures. *Endocrinology* 1974;95:1142–1149.
23. Roos BA, Deftos LJ, Rorabaugh P. Calcitonin secretion in vitro. II. Regulatory effects of enteric mammalian polypeptide hormones on trout C-cell cultures. *Endocrinology* 1976;98:1284–1288.
24. Zeytinoglu FN, DeLellis RA, Gagel RF, Wolfe HJ, Tashjian AH Jr. Establishment of a calcitonin-producing rat medullary thyroid carcinoma cell line. I. Morphological studies of the tumor and cells in culture. *Endocrinology* 1980;107:509–515.
25. Parthemore JG, Bronzert D, Roberts G, Deftos LJ. A short calcium infusion in the diagnosis of medullary thyroid carcinoma. *J Clin Endocrinol Metab* 1974;39:108–111.
26. Melvin KEW, Tashjian AH Jr, Miller HH. Studies in familial (medullary) thyroid carcinoma. *Recent Prog Horm Res* 1972;28:399–470.
27. Heath H III, Body JJ, Fox J. Radioimmunoassay of calcitonin in normal human plasma: problems, perspectives and prospects. *Biomed Pharmacother* 1984;38:241–245.
28. Telander RL, Zimmerman D, van Heerden JA, Sizemore GW. Results of early thyroidectomy for medullary thyroid carcinoma in children with multiple endocrine neoplasia type 2. *J Pediatr Surg* 1986;21:1190–1194.
29. Lin HY, Harris TL, Flannery MS, et al. Expression cloning of an adenylate cyclase-coupled calcitonin receptor. *Science* 1991;254:1022–1024.
30. Fischer JA, Born W. Novel peptides from the calcitonin gene: expression, receptors and biological function. *Peptides* 1985;6(suppl 3):265–271.
31. Beglinger C, Koehler E, Born W, et al. Effect of calcitonin and calcitonin gene-related peptide on pancreatic functions in man. *Gut* 1988;29:243–248.
32. New HV, Mudge AW. Calcitonin gene-related peptide regulates muscle acetylcholine receptor synthesis. *Nature* 1986;323:809–811.
33. Fontaine B, Klarsfeld A, Changeux JP. Calcitonin gene-related peptide and muscle activity regulate acetylcholine receptor alpha-subunit mRNA levels by distinct intracellular pathways. *J Cell Biol* 1987;105:1337–1342.
34. Linnoila RI, Becker KL, Silva OL, Snider RH, Moore CF. Calcitonin as a marker for diethylnitrosamine-induced pulmonary endocrine cell hyperplasia in hamsters. *Lab Invest* 1984;51:39–45.
35. Catherwood BD, Deftos LJ. Presence by radioimmunoassay of a calcitonin-like substance in porcine pituitary glands. *Endocrinology* 1980;106:1886–1891.
36. Gagel RF, O'Brian DS, Voelkel EF, et al. Pituitary immunoreactive calcitonin-like material: lack of evidence for cross-reactivity with pro-opiomelanocortin. *Metabolism* 1983;32:686–696.
37. Gazdar AF, Carney DN, Becker KL, Deftos LJ, Liang V, Go W, Marangos PJ, Moody TW, Wolfsen AR, Zweig MH. Expression of peptide and other markers in lung cancer cell lines. *Recent Results Cancer Res* 1985;99:167–174.
38. Becker KL, Silva OL, Snider RH, et al. The surgical implications of hypercalcitonemia. *Surg Gynecol Obstet* 1982;154:897–908.
39. Deftos LJ, Roos BA, Bronzert D, Parthemore JG. Immunochemical heterogeneity of calcitonin in plasma. *J Clin Endocrinol Metab* 1975;40:409–412.
40. Roos BA, Parthemore JG, Lee JC, Deftos LJ. Calcitonin heterogeneity: in vivo and in vitro studies. *Calcif Tissue Res* 1977;22(suppl):298–302.
41. Ghillani P, Motte P, Bohuon C, Bellet D. Monoclonal antipeptide antibodies as tools to dissect closely related gene products. A model using peptides encoded by the calcitonin gene. *J Immunol* 1988;141:3156–3163.
42. Samaan NA, Castillo S, Schultz PN, Khalil KG, Johnston DA. Serum calcitonin after pentagastrin stimulation in patients with bronchogenic and breast cancer compared to that in patients with medullary thyroid carcinoma. *J Clin Endocrinol Metab* 1980;51:237–241.
43. Sletten K, Westermark P, Natvig JB. Characterization of amyloid fibril proteins from medullary carcinoma of the thyroid. *J Exp Med* 1976;143:993.
44. Raue F, Schmidt GH, Ziegler R. Tumor markers in C-cell cancer. *Deutsche Med Wochenschr* 1983;108:283–287.
45. DeLellis RA, Rule AH, Spiler I, et al. Calcitonin and carcinoembryonic antigen as tumor markers in medullary thyroid carcinoma. *Am J Clin Pathol* 1978;70:587–594.
46. Kodama T. Identification of carcinoembryonic antigen in the C-cell of the normal thyroid. *Cancer* 1980;45:98.
47. Jackson CE, Norum RA, Talpos GB, Feldkamp CS, Tashjian AH Jr. Clinical value of calcitonin and carcinoembryonic antigen doubling times in medullary thyroid carcinoma. *Henry Ford Hosp Med J* 1987;35:120–121.
48. Cote GJ, Palmer WN, Leonhart K, Leong SS, Gagel RF. The regulation of somatostatin production in human medullary thyroid carcinoma cells by dexamethasone. *J Biol Chem* 1986;261:12930–12935.
49. Gagel RF, Palmer WN, Leonhart K, Chan L, Leong SS. Somatostatin production by a human medullary thyroid carcinoma cell line. *Endocrinology* 1986;118:1643–1651.
50. Rosenberg EM, Hahn TJ, Orth DN, Deftos LJ, Tanaka K. ACTH-secreting medullary carcinoma of the thyroid presenting a severe idiopathic osteoporosis and senile purpura: report of a case and review of the literature. *J Clin Endocrinol Metab* 1978;47:255–262.
51. Steenberg PH, Hoppener JW, Zandberg J, Roos BA, Jansz HS, Lips CJ. Expression of the proopiomelanocortin gene in human medullary thyroid carcinoma. *J Clin Endocrinol Metab* 1984;58:904–908.
52. Zeytinoglu FN, Gagel RF, Tashjian AH Jr, Hammer RA, Leeman SE. Characterization of neurotensin production by a line of rat medullary thyroid carcinoma cells. *Proc Natl Acad Sci USA* 1980;77:3741–3745.
53. Baylin SB, Beaven MA, Keiser HR, et al. Serum histaminase and calcitonin levels in medullary carcinoma of the thyroid. *Lancet* 1972;1:455–458.
54. Deftos LJ, Woloszczuk W, Krisch I, et al. Medullary thyroid carcinomas express chromogranin A and a novel neuroendocrine protein recognized by monoclonal antibody HISL-19. *Am J Med* 1988;85:780–784.
55. Bernier JJ, Rambaud JC, Cattan D, et al. Diarrhoea associated with medullary carcinoma of the thyroid. *Gut* 1969;10:980–985.
56. Melvin KEW, Tashjian AH Jr, Cassidy CE, et al. Cushing's syndrome caused by ACTH- and calcitonin-secreting medullary carcinoma of the thyroid. *Metabolism* 1970;19:831–838.
57. Block MA, Jackson CE, Greenawald KA, et al. Clinical characteristics distinguishing hereditary from sporadic medullary thyroid carcinoma. *Arch Surg* 1980;115:142–148.
58. Baylin SB, Gann DS, Hsu SH. Clonal origin of inherited medullary thyroid carcinoma and pheochromocytoma. *Science* 1976;193:321–323.
59. Wolfe HJ, DeLellis RA. Familial medullary thyroid carcinoma and C-cell hyperplasia. *Baillieres Clin Endocrinol Metab* 1981;10:351–365.
60. Ekblom M, Valimaki M, Pelkonen R, Jansson R, Sivula A, Franssila K. Familial and sporadic medullary thyroid carcinoma: clinical and immunohistological findings. *Q J Med* 1987;65:899–910.
61. Ponder BA, Ponder MA, Coffey R, et al. Risk estimation and screening in families of patients with medullary thyroid carcinoma. *Lancet* 1988;1:397–401.

62. Soderstrom N, Telenius-Berg M, Akerman M. Diagnosis of medullary thyroid carcinoma of the thyroid by fine needle aspiration biopsy. *Acta Med Scand* 1975;197:71–76.
63. Lew W, Orel S, Henderson DW. Intranuclear vacuoles in nonpapillary carcinoma of the thyroid. *Acta Cytol* 1984;28:581–586.
64. Cox TM, Fagan EA, Hillyard CJ, et al. Role of calcitonin in diarrhoea associated with medullary carcinoma of the thyroid. *Gut* 1979;20:629.
65. Sipple JH. The association of pheochromocytoma with carcinoma of the thyroid gland. *Am J Med* 1961;31:163–166.
66. Steiner AL, Goodman AD, Powers SR. Study of a kindred with pheochromocytoma, medullary carcinoma, hyperparathyroidism and Cushing's disease: multiple endocrine neoplasia, type 2. *Medicine (Baltimore)* 1968;47:371–409.
67. Williams ED. A review of 17 cases of carcinoma of the thyroid and pheochromocytoma. *J Clin Pathol* 1965;18:288–292.
68. Melvin KEW, Miller HH, Tashjian AH Jr. Early diagnosis of medullary carcinoma of the thyroid gland by means of calcitonin assay. *N Engl J Med* 1971;285:1115–1120.
69. Wolfe HJ, Melvin KEW, Cervi-Skinner SJ, et al. C-cell hyperplasia preceding medullary thyroid carcinoma. *N Engl J Med* 1973;289:437–441.
70. Gagel RF, Melvin KE, Tashjian AH Jr, et al. Natural history of the familial medullary thyroid carcinoma-pheochromocytoma syndrome and the identification of preneoplastic stages by screening studies: a five-year report. *Trans Assoc Am Physicians* 1975;88:177–191.
71. Wells SA Jr, Ontjes DA, Cooper CW, et al. The early diagnosis of medullary carcinoma of the thyroid gland in patients with multiple endocrine neoplasia type II. *Ann Surg* 1975;182:362–370.
72. Cance WG, Wells SA Jr. Multiple endocrine neoplasia Type IIa. *Curr Probl Surg* 1985;22:1–56.
73. Brouwers Smalbraak GJ, Vasen HF, Struyvenberg A, Nieuwenhuijzen Kruseman AC, Helsloot MH, Lips CJ. Multiple endocrine neoplasia type 2A (MEN-2A): natural history, screening, and central registration. *Neth J Med* 1986;29:111–117.
74. Telenius-Berg M, Berg B, Hamberger B, et al. Impact of screening on prognosis in the multiple endocrine neoplasia type 2 syndromes: natural history and treatment results in 105 patients. *Henry Ford Hosp Med J* 1984;32:225–231.
75. Gagel RF, Jackson CE, Block MA, et al. Age-related probability of development of hereditary medullary thyroid carcinoma. *J Pediatr* 1982;101:941–946.
76. Jadoul M, Leo JR, Berends HH, et al. Pheochromocytoma-induced hypertensive encephalopathy revealing MEN IIa syndrome in a 13-year-old boy. *Horm Metab Res* 1989;21(suppl):46–49.
77. Lips KJ, Van der Sluys Veer J, Struyvenberg A, et al. Bilateral occurrence of pheochromocytoma in patients with the multiple endocrine neoplasia syndrome type 2A (Sipple's syndrome). *Am J Med* 1981;70:1051–1060.
78. Hamilton BP, Landsberg L, Levine RJ. Measurement of urinary epinephrine in screening for pheochromocytoma in multiple endocrine neoplasia type II. *Am J Med* 1978;65:1027–1032.
79. Miyauchi A, Masuo K, Ogihara T, et al. Urinary epinephrine and norepinephrine excretion in patients with medullary thyroid carcinoma and their relatives. *Nippon Naibunpi Gakkai Zasshi* 1982;58:1505–1516.
80. De Lellis RA, Wolfe HJ, Gagel RF, et al. Adrenal medullary hyperplasia. A morphometric analysis in patients with familial medullary thyroid carcinoma. *Am J Pathol* 1976;83:177–196.
81. Carney JA, Sizemore GW, Tyce GM. Bilateral adrenal medullary hyperplasia in multiple endocrine neoplasia, type 2: the precursor of bilateral pheochromocytoma. *Mayo Clin Proc* 1975;50:3–10.
82. Sisson JC, Shapiro B, Beierwaltes WH. Scintigraphy with I-131 MIBG as an aid to the treatment of pheochromocytomas in patients with the multiple endocrine neoplasia type 2 syndromes. *Henry Ford Hosp Med J* 1984;32:254–261.
83. Yobbagy JJ, Levatter R, Sisson JC, Shulkin BL, Polley T. Scintigraphic portrayal of the syndrome of multiple endocrine neoplasia type-2B. *Clin Nucl Med* 1988;13:433–437.
84. Marx SJ, Vinik AI, Santen RJ, Floyd JC Jr, Mills JL, Green J III. Multiple endocrine neoplasia type I: assessment of laboratory tests to screen for the gene in a large kindred. *Medicine (Baltimore)* 1986;65:226–241.
85. Rizzoli R, Green J III, Marx SJ. Primary hyperparathyroidism in familial multiple endocrine neoplasia type I. Long-term follow-up of serum calcium levels after parathyroidectomy. *Am J Med* 1985;78:467–474.
86. Keiser HR, Beaven MA, Doppman J, et al. Sipple's syndrome: medullary thyroid carcinoma, pheochromocytoma, and hyperparathyroidism. *Ann Intern Med* 1973;78:561–579.
87. Carney JA, Roth SI, Heath H III, Sizemore GW, Hayles AB. The parathyroid glands in multiple endocrine neoplasia type 2b. *Am J Pathol* 1980;99:387–398.
88. Heath H III, Sizemore GW, Carney JA. Preoperative diagnosis of occult parathyroid hyperplasia by calcium infusion in patients with multiple endocrine neoplasia, type 2a. *J Clin Endocrinol Metab* 1976;43:428–435.
89. Gagel RF, Tashjian AH Jr, Cummings T, Papathanasopoulos N, Reichlin S. Impact of prospective screening for multiple endocrine neoplasia type 2. *Henry Ford Hosp Med J* 1987;35:94–98.
90. Farndon JR, Leight GS, Dilley WG, et al. Familial medullary thyroid carcinoma without associated endocrinopathies: a distinct clinical entity. *Br J Surg* 1986;73:278–281.
91. Gagel RF, Levy ML, Donovan DT, Alford BR, Wheeler T, Tschen JA. The association of multiple endocrine neoplasia, type 2a and cutaneous lichen amyloidosis. *Ann Intern Med* 1990:112(7):551–552.
92. Nunziata V, Giannattasio R, di Giovanni G, D'Armiento MR, Mancini M. Hereditary localized pruritus in affected members of a kindred with multiple endocrine neoplasia type 2A (Sipple's syndrome). *Clin Endocrinol (Oxf)* 1989;30:57–63.
93. Williams ED, Pollock DJ. Multiple mucosal neuromata with endocrine tumours: a syndrome allied to Von Recklinghausen's disease. *J Pathol Bacteriol* 1966;91:71–80.
94. Carney JA, Sizemore GW, Hayles AB. Multiple endocrine neoplasia, type 2b. *Pathol Annu* 1978;8:105–153.
95. Carney JA, Sizemore GW, Hayles AV. C-cell disease of the thyroid gland in multiple endocrine neoplasia, type 2b. *Cancer* 1979;44:2173–2183.
96. Rashid M, Khairi MR, Dexter RN, Burzynski NJ, Johnston CC Jr. Mucosal neuroma, pheochromocytoma and medullary thyroid carcinoma: multiple endocrine neoplasia type 3. *Medicine (Baltimore)* 1975;54:89–112.
97. Stjernholm MR, Freudenbourg JC, Mooney HS, Kinney FJ, Deftos LJ. Medullary carcinoma of the thyroid before age 2 years. *J Clin Endocrinol Metab* 1980;51:252–253.
98. Dyck PJ, Carney JA, Sizemore GW, Okazaki H, Brimijoin WS, Lambert EH. Multiple endocrine neoplasia, type 2b: phenotype recognition; neurological features and their pathological basis. *Ann Neurol* 1979;6:302–314.
99. Hubner A, Holschneider AM. Multiple endocrine neoplasias in 3 generations. *Langenbecks Arch Chir* 1987;372:747–750.
100. Aine E, Aine L, Huupponen T, Salmi J, Miettinen P. Visible corneal nerve fibers and neuromas of the conjunctiva—a syndrome of type-3 multiple endocrine adenomatosis in two generations. *Graefes Arch Clin Exp Ophthalmol* 1987;225:213–216.
101. Kakudo K, Carney JA, Sizemore GW. Medullary carcinoma of thyroid. Biologic behavior of the sporadic and familial neoplasm. *Cancer* 1985;55:2818–2821.
102. O'Neal L. Multiple endocrine neoplasia, type IIb: medullary carcinoma of the thyroid, pheochromocytomas, neuromas, and ganglioneuromatosis. *Proc Annu Conf Res Med Educ* 1983;1:7–16.
103. Simpson NE, Kidd KK, Goodfellow PJ, et al. Assignment of multiple endocrine neoplasia type 2A to chromosome 10 by linkage. *Nature* 1987;328:528–530.
104. Mathew CG, Chin KS, Easton DF, et al. A linked genetic marker for multiple endocrine neoplasia type 2A on chromosome 10. *Nature* 1987;328:527–528.
105. Mulligan LM, Kwok JBJ, Healey CS, et al. Germline mutations of the RET proto-oncogene in multiple endocrine neoplasia type 2A (MEN 2A). *Nature* 1993;363:458–460.
106. Donis-Keller H, Shenshen D, Chi D, et al. Mutations in the RET proto-oncogene are associated with MEN 2A and FMTC. *Hum Molec Genet* 1993;2:851–856.
107. Mulligan LM, Marsh DJ, Robinson BG, et al. Genotype-phenotype correlation in multiple endocrine neoplasia type 2: report of the international RET mutation consortium. *J Intern Med* 1995;238:343–346.
108. Wohllk N, Cote GJ, Evans D, et al. Application of genetic screening information to the management of medullary thyroid carcinoma and multiple endocrine neoplasia. *Endocr Metab Clin North Am* 1996;25:1–25.
109. Carlson KM, Dou S, Chi D, et al. Single missense mutation in the tyrosine kinase catalytic domain of the RET proto-oncogene is associ-

ated with multiple endocrine neoplasia type 2B. *Proc Natl Acad Sci U S A* 1994;91:1579–1583.
110. Hofstra RM, Landsvater RM, Ceccherini I, et al. A mutation in the RET proto-oncogene associated with multiple endocrine neoplasia type 2B and sporadic medullary thyroid carcinoma. *Nature* 1994;367:375–376.
111. Zedenius J, Wallin G, Hamberger B, et al. Somatic and MEN 2A de novo mutations identified in the RET proto-oncogene by screening of sporadic MTCs. *Hum Molec Genet* 1994;3:1259–1262.
112. Hofstra RMW, Landsvater RM, Ceccherini I, et al. A mutation in the RET proto-oncogene associated with multiple endocrine neoplasia type 2B and sporadic medullary thyroid carcinoma. *Nature* 1994;367:376–376.
113. Wohllk N, Cote GJ, Bugalho MMJ, et al. Relevance of ret proto-oncogene mutations in sporadic medullary thyroid carcinoma. *J Clin Endocrinol Metab* 1996;81:3740–3745.
114. Xing S, Smanik PA, Oglesbee MJ, Trosko JE, Mazzaferri EL, Jhiang SM. Characterization of ret oncogenic activation in MEN2 inherited cancer syndromes. *Endocrinology* 1996;137:1512–1519.
115. Asai N, Iwashita T, Matsuyama M, Takahashi M. Mechansims of activation of the ret proto-oncogene by multiple endocrine neoplasia 2A mutations. *Molec Cell Biol* 1995;15:1613–1619.
116. Santoro M, Carlomagno F, Romano A, et al. Activation of ret as a dominant transforming gene by germline mutations of MEN 2A and MEN 2B. *Science* 1995;267:381–383.
117. Wells SA Jr, Donis-Keller H. Current perspectives on the diagnosis and management of patients with multiple endocrine neoplasia type 2 syndromes. *Endocrinol Metab Clin North Am* 1994;23:215–228.
118. Gagel RF, Cote GJ, Martins Bugalho MJG, et al. Clinical use of molecular information in the management of multiple endocrine neoplasia type 2A. *J Intern Med* 1995;238:333–341.
119. Lips CJ, Landsvater RM, Hoppener JW, et al. Clinical screening as compared with DNA analysis in families with multiple endocrine neoplasia type 2A. *N Engl J Med* 1994;331:828–835.
120. Takai S, Miyauchi A, Matsumoto H, et al. Multiple endocrine neoplasia type 2 syndromes in Japan. *Henry Ford Hosp Med J* 1984;32:246–250.
121. Wells SA, Chi DD, Toshima K, et al. Predictive DNA testing and prophylactic thyroidectomy in patients at risk for multiple endocrine neoplasia type 2A. *Ann Surg* 1994;220:237–250.
122. Easton DF, Ponder MA, Cummings T, et al. The clinical and screening age-at-onset distribution for the MEN-2 syndrome. *Am J Hum Genet* 1989;44:208–215.
123. Graham SM, Genel M, Touloukian RJ, Barwick KW, Gertner JM, Torony C. Provocative testing for occult medullary carcinoma of the thyroid: findings in seven children with multiple endocrine neoplasia type IIa. *J Pediatr Surg* 1987;22:501–503.
124. Leape LL, Miller HH, Graze K, et al. Total thyroidectomy for occult familial medullary carcinoma of the thyroid in children. *J Pediatr Surg* 1976;11:831–837.
125. Sciubba JJ, DAmico E, Attie JN. The occurrence of multiple endocrine neoplasia type IIb, in two children of an affected mother. *J Oral Pathol Med* 1987;16:310–316.
126. van Heerden JA, Sizemore GW, Carney JA, Grant CS, ReMine WH, Sheps SG. Surgical management of the adrenal glands in the multiple endocrine neoplasia type II syndrome. *World J Surg* 1984;8:612–621.
127. Hennessey JF, Gray TK, Cooper CW, Ontjes DA. Stimulation of thyrocalcitonin secretion by pentagastrin and calcium in 2 patients with medullary carcinoma of the thyroid. *J Clin Endocrinol Metab* 1973;36:200–203.
128. Hennessy JF, Wells SA, Ontjes DA, Cooper CW. A comparison of pentagastrin injections and calcium infusion as provocative agents for the detection of medullary carcinoma of the thyroid. *J Clin Endocrinol Metab* 1974;39:487.
129. McLean GW, Rabin D, Moore L, Deftos LJ, Lorber D, McKenna TJ. Evaluation of provocative tests in suspected medullary carcinoma of the thyroid: heterogeneity of calcitonin responses to calcium and pentagastrin. *Metabolism* 1984;33:790–796.
130. Catherwood BD, Deftos LJ. General principles, problems and interpretation in the radioimmunoassay of calcitonin. *Biomed Pharmacother* 1984;38:235–241.
131. Body JJ, Heath H III. Nonspecific increases in plasma immunoreactive calcitonin in healthy individuals: discrimination from medullary thyroid carcinoma by a new extraction technique. *Clin Chem* 1984;30:511–514.
132. Lee JC, Parthemore JG, Deftos LJ. Immunochemical heterogeneity of calcitonin in renal failure. *J Clin Endocrinol Metab* 1977;45:528–533.
133. Body JJ, Heath H III. "Nonspecific" increases in plasma immunoreactive calcitonin in healthy individuals: discrimination from medullary thyroid carcinoma by a new extraction technique. *Clin Chem* 1984;30:511–514.
134. Seth R, Motte P, Kehely A, et al. A sensitive and specific two-site enzyme-immunoassay for human calcitonin using monoclonal antibodies. *J Endocrinol* 1988;119:351–357.
135. Motte P, Ait-Abdellah M, Vauzelle P, Gardet P, Bohuon C, Bellet D. A two-site immunoradiometric assay for serum calcitonin using monoclonal anti-peptide antibodies. *Henry Ford Hosp Med J* 1987;35:129–132.
136. Aloia JF, Rasulo P, Deftos LJ, Vaswani A, Yeh JK. Exercise-induced hypercalcemia and the calciotropic hormones. *J Lab Clin Med* 1985;106:229–232.
137. Eng C, Mulligan L, Smith D, et al. Mutation of the ret proto-oncogene in sporadic medullary thyroid carcinoma. *Genes Chromosom Cancer* 1995;12:209–212.
138. Decker RA, Peacock ML, Borst MJ, Sweet JD, Thompson NW. Progress in genetic screening of multiple endocrine neoplasia type 2A: is calcitonin testing obsolete? *Surgery* 1995;118:257–264.
139. Komminoth P, Kunz EK, Matias-Guiu X, et al. Analysis of ret proto-oncogene point mutations distinguishes heritable from nonheritable medullary thyroid carcinomas. *Cancer* 1995;76:479–489.
140. Pacini F, Fontanelli M, Fugazzola L, et al. Routine measurement of serum calcitonin in nodular thyroid diseases allows the preoperative diagnosis of unsuspected sporadic medullary thyroid carcinoma. *Clin Endocrinol* 1994;78:826–829.
141. Rieu M, Lame MC, Richard A, et al. Prevalence of sporadic medullary thyroid carcinoma: the importance of routine measurement of serum calcitonin in the diagnostic evaluation of thyroid nodules. *Clin Endocrinol* 1995;42:453–460.
142. Niccoli P, Wion-Barbot N, Caron P, et al. Routine measurement of serum calcitonin in multinodular goiter. *J Clin Endocrinol Metab* 1997;82(2).
143. Graham SM, Genel M, Touloukian RJ, Barwick KW, Gertner JM, Torony C. Provocative testing for occult medullary carcinoma of the thyroid: findings in seven children with multiple endocrine neoplasia type IIa. *J Pediatr Surg* 1987;22:501–503.
144. Wolfe HJ, DeLellis RA. Familial medullary thyroid carcinoma and C-cell hyperplasia. *Baillieres Clin Endocrinol Metab* 1981;10:351–365.
145. Sizemore GW, Carney JA, Heath H III. Epidemiology of medullary carcinoma of the thyroid gland: a 5-year experience (1971–1976). *Surg Clin North Am* 1977;57:633–645.
146. Saad MF, Ordonez NG, Rashid RK, et al. Medullary carcinoma of the thyroid: a study of the clinical features and prognostic factors in 161 patients. *Medicine (Baltimore)* 1984;63:319–342.
147. Chong GC, Beahrs OH, Sizemore GW, Woolner LH. Medullary carcinoma of the thyroid gland. *Cancer* 1975;35:695–704.
148. Rougier P, Parmentier C, Laplanche A, et al. Medullary thyroid carcinoma: prognostic factors and treatment. *Int J Radiat Oncol Biol Phys* 1983;9:161–169.
149. Jackson CE, Talpos GB, Kambouris A, Yott JB, Tashjian AH Jr, Block MA. The clinical course after definitive operation for medullary thyroid carcinoma. *Surgery* 1983;94:995–1001.
150. Tisell L, Hansson G, Jansson S, Salander H. Reoperation in the treatment of asymptomatic metastasizing medullary thyroid carcinoma. *Surgery* 1986;99 60–66.
151. Bocca S. A conservative technique in radical neck dissection. *Ann Otol Rhinol Laryngol* 1967;76:975–987.
152. Talpos GB, Jackson CE, Froelich JW, Kambouris AA, Block MA, Tashjian AH Jr. Localization of residual medullary thyroid cancer by thallium/technetium scintigraphy. *Surgery* 1985;98:1189–1196.
153. Keeling CA, Basso LV. Iodine-131 MIBG uptake in metastatic medullary carcinoma of the thyroid. A patient treated with somatostatin. *Clin Nucl Med* 1988;13:260–263.
154. Sizemore GW, Sheedy PF, George JM, et al. Localization of residual medullary thyroid carcinoma (MTC) by transfemoral venous catheterization and measurement of immunoreactive plasma calcitonin (iCT). In: *Program of the Annual Meeting of the Endocrine Society.* 1974;56:A-303.

155. Wells SA Jr, Baylin SB, Johnsrude IS, et al. Thyroid venous catheterization in the early diagnosis of familial medullary thyroid carcinoma. *Ann Surg* 1982;196:505–511.
156. Raue F, Boden M, Girgis S, Rix E, Ziegler R. Katacalcin—a new tumor marker in C-cell cancer of the thyroid gland. *Klin Wochenschr* 1987;65:82–86.
157. Block MA, Jackson CE, Tashjian AH Jr. Management of occult medullary thyroid carcinoma of thyroid: evidenced only by serum calcitonin elevations after apparently adequate neck operation. *Arch Surg* 1978;113:368–372.
158. Sizemore GW, Carney JA, Heath H III. Epidemiology of medullary carcinoma of the thyroid gland: a 5-year experience. *Surg Clin North Am* 1977;57:633–645.
159. Dralle H, Damm I, Scheumann GF, et al. Compartment-oriented microdissection of regional lymph nodes in medullary thyroid carcinoma. *Surgery Today* 1994;4(2):112–121.
160. Moley JF, Wells SA, Dilley WG, Tisell LE. Reoperation for recurrent or persistent medullary thyroid cancer. *Surgery* 1993;114(6):1090–1095.
161. Dralle H, Scheumann G, Proye C, et al. The value of lymph node dissection in hereditary medullary thyroid carcinoma: a retrospective, European, multicentre study. *J Intern Med* 1995;238:357–361.
162. Miller HH, Melvin KEW, Gibson JM, Tashjian AH Jr. Surgical approach to early familial medullary carcinoma of the thyroid gland. *Am J Surg* 1972;123:438–443.
163. Block MA, Jackson CE, Tashjian AH Jr. Management of parathyroid glands in surgery for medullary thyroid carcinoma. *Arch Surg* 1975; 110:617–624.
164. Niederle B, Roka R, Brennan MF. The transplantation of parathyroid tissue in man: development, indications, techniques and results. *Endocr Rev* 1982;3:245–279.
165. Mallette LE, Blevins T, Jordan PH, Noon GP. Autogenous parathyroid grafts for generalized primary parathyroid hyperplasia: contrasting outcome in sporadic hyperplasia versus multiple endocrine neoplasia type I. *Surgery* 1987;101:738–745.
166. Wells SA Jr, Ellis GJ, Gunnells JC, Schneider AB, Sherwood LM. Parathyroid autotransplantation in primary parathyroid hyperplasia. *N Engl J Med* 1976;195:57–62.
167. Nakamura Y, Leppert M, Lathrop GM, et al. A primary genetic linkage map of chromosome 10. Human Gene Mapping 9: Ninth International Workshop on Human Gene Mapping. *Cytogenet Cell Genet* 1987;46:667.
168. Flacke WE, Bloor BC, Flacke JW. Adrenal medulla. *Semin Anesth* 1984;3:194–206.
169. Desmonts JM, Marty J. Anaesthetic management of patients with phaeochromocytoma. *Br J Anaesth* 1984;56:781–789.
170. Tibblin S, Dymling JF, Ingemansson S, Telenius-Berg M. Unilateral versus bilateral adrenalectomy in multiple endocrine neoplasia IIA. *World J Surg* 1983;7:201–208.
171. Jansson S, Tisell LE, Fjalling M, Lindberg S, Jacobsson L, Zachrisson BF. Early diagnosis of and surgical strategy for adrenal medullary disease in MEN II gene carriers. *Surgery* 1988;103:11–18.
172. Lips CJ, Minder WH, Leo JR, Alleman A, Hackeng WH. Evidence of multicentric origin of the multiple endocrine neoplasia syndrome type 2a (Sipple's syndrome) in a large family in the Netherlands. Diagnostic and therapeutic implications. *Am J Med* 1978;64: 569–578.
173. Nicholson JP Jr, Vaughn ED, Pickering TG, et al. Pheochromocytoma and prazosin. *Ann Intern Med* 1983;99:477–479.
174. Cubeddu LX, Zarate NA, Rosales CB, Zschaek DW. Prazosin and propranolol in preoperative management of pheochromocytoma. *Clin Pharmacol Ther* 1982;32:156.
175. Samaan NA, Schultz PN, Hickey RC. Medullary thyroid carcinoma: prognosis of familial versus sporadic disease and the role of radiotherapy. *J Clin Endocrinol Metab* 1988;67:801–805.
176. Lips CJ, Vasen HF, Lamers CB. Multiple endocrine neoplasia syndromes. *CRC Crit Rev Oncol Hematol* 1984;2:117–184.
177. Sizemore GW, Heath H III, Carney JA. Multiple endocrine neoplasia type 2. *Baillieres Clin Endocrinol Metab* 1980;9:299–315.
178. Jackson CE, Talpos GB, Kambouris A, Yott JB, Tashjian AH Jr, Block MA. The clinical course after definitive operation for medullary thyroid carcinoma. *Surgery* 1983;94:995–1001.
179. Steinfield AD. The role of radiation therapy in medullary carcinoma of the thyroid. *Radiology* 1977;123:745.
180. Halman KE. The nonsurgical treatment of thyroid cancer. *Br J Surg* 1975;62:769.
181. Hellman DW, Kartchner M, Van Antwerp JD, et al. Radioiodine in the treatment of medullary carcinoma of the thyroid. *J Clin Endocrinol Metab* 1979;48:451–455.
182. Deftos LJ, Stein MF. Radioiodine as an adjunct to the surgical treatment of medullary thyroid carcinoma. *J Clin Endocrinol Metab* 1980: 50:967–968.
183. Gagel RS. The pathogenesis and clinical course of multiple endocrine neoplasia, type 2a. In: Kleerkoper and Krane, eds. *Clinical disorders of bone and mineral metabolism.* New York: Mary Ann Liebert, 1989; 563–571.
184. Gottlieb JA, Hill CS Jr. Chemotherapy of thyroid cancer with adriamycin: experience with 30 patients. *N Engl J Med* 1974;290: 193–107.
185. Trupp M, Arenas E, Falnzilber M, et al. Functional receptor for GDNF encoded by the c-ret proto-oncogene. *Nature* 1996;381:785–788.
186. Durbec P, Marcos-Gutierrez CV, Kilkenny C, et al. GDNF signaling through the ret receptor tyrosine kinase. *Nature* 1996;381: 789–793.
187. Lin LF, Dohtery DH, Lile JD, Bektesh S, Colline F. GDNF: a glial cell line-derived neurotrophic factor for midbrain dopaminergic neurons. *Science* 1993;260:1130–1132.

CHAPTER 33

Anaplastic Carcinoma, Lymphoma, Unusual Malignancies, and Chemotherapy for Thyroid Cancer

M. William Audeh, Leslie Memsic, and Allan Silberman

The thyroid gland is unique in the large number of primary tumors that may arise within its parenchyma. Malignancies of epithelial, mesothelial, and endothelial origin have all been described, perhaps reflecting the complex embryology of the thyroid, derived in part from ectoderm, mesoderm, and endoderm (1). At least 14 pathologically distinct primary thyroid malignancies are recognized (1,2), and numerous case reports of secondary metastases to this relatively small organ may be found in the medical literature (3,4). Approximately 90% of all thyroid malignancies, however, are well-differentiated tumors arising from papillary, follicular, or parafollicular C cells, and these are adequately managed with surgery and/or radiotherapy. The remainder are the subject of this chapter; they include anaplastic carcinoma (which also arises from the papillary/follicular compartment), primary thyroid lymphoma, and other rare malignancies. It is their distinct biologic behavior and the use of chemotherapy in their management, rather than their rarity, that warrants a separate analysis of these unusual diseases.

ANAPLASTIC CARCINOMA AND PRIMARY THYROID LYMPHOMA

Epidemiology

Anaplastic carcinoma has been declining in incidence in the past few decades (5) and now represents less than 5% of all thyroid malignancies, whereas thyroid lymphoma has been increasing to 3% to 5% of all thyroid malignancies. Anaplastic carcinoma often arises in a setting of multinodular, endemic goiter (6), or a prior history of well-differentiated thyroid cancer (7,8). A prior history of radioiodine therapy for thyrotoxicosis has been implicated in some cases (9,10). The decreasing incidence observed may be the result of dietary improvements or more widespread use of thyroidectomy for these conditions. Primary thyroid lymphoma has been strongly associated with autoimmune (Hashimoto's) thyroiditis (11), and prior to the use of immunohistochemistry it was erroneously identified as the "small cell" variant of anaplastic carcinoma. The increasing incidence of thyroid lymphoma may therefore be the result of improved case-finding, rather than a true epidemiologic trend.

Clinical Presentation

Anaplastic carcinoma and thyroid lymphoma are both rapidly growing malignancies presenting in the thyroid. The survival rate of anaplastic carcinoma differs markedly from that of primary thyroid lymphoma, with 5-year survivals of under 1% for the former and 70%, for the latter (2,12). However, early diagnosis and intensive therapy of anaplastic carcinoma may yield long-term survival in some patients with tumors smaller than 4 cm, limited to the thyroid (13,14). Therefore, there is an urgent need to distinguish between these diseases immediately, a goal that is complicated by the striking similarities in their clinical presentation (Table 1).

Both occur most commonly in the elderly population, with a median age of 63 to 70 years (13,15), and they typically present as rapidly enlarging neck masses. They may

M. W. Audeh, L. Memsic, and A. Silberman: Cedars-Sinai Cancer Center, Los Angeles, California 90033.

TABLE 1. *Clinical presentation*

	Anaplastic carcinoma	Thyroid lymphoma
Incidence	<5% (? decreasing)	3%–5% (? increasing)
Median age	63–70 years	63–70 years
Male:female ratio	1:1.5	1:3
Prior history	Multinodular goiter, well-differentiated thyroid carcinoma	Autoimune thyroiditis
Presenting symptoms	Dysphagia, dyspnea, hoarseness, pain	Dysphagia, dyspnea, hoarseness, pain
Presenting signs	Rapidly enlarging neck mass	Rapidly enlarging neck mass
	Fever, leukocytosis	Fever, ±leukocytosis
Noninvasive diagnostics	Nonspecific	? Gallium-67
Median survival	8 months	>2 years

produce obstructive symptoms of dysphagia and dyspnea with stridor, as well as hoarseness and pain. Both have been associated with fever, which in anaplastic carcinoma has recently been attributed to ectopic secretion of granulocyte-colony stimulating factor (G-CSF) (16–18), with attendant leukocytosis (thus adding the question of an infectious process to the differential diagnosis).

Distinguishing clinical features include a female predominance for thyroid lymphoma (approximately 3:1) and past medical history. A rapidly developing neck mass with a prior history of autoimmune thyroiditis suggests lymphoma, whereas a longstanding goiter or prior diagnosis of well-differentiated thyroid carcinoma suggests anaplastic carcinoma.

Noninvasive diagnostic tests are of little value in distinguishing these entities. Radioiodine scanning is likely to be negative in both, whereas newer scanning agents such as technetium-99 and methoxy-isobutyl-isonitrile (MIBI) have shown uptake in both (19). Gallium-67 citrate may be preferentially accumulated by thyroid lymphoma but is not definitive. Other diagnostic tests, such as ultrasound, computed tomography (CT), and magnetic resonance imaging (MRI) scans, are unable to reliably distinguish lymphoma from carcinoma in all cases. Tissue biopsy with immunohistochemistry remains the only reliable method of diagnosis.

ANAPLASTIC CARCINOMA OF THYROID

The Biology of Anaplastic Carcinoma

The observation that anaplastic carcinoma often arises within a thyroid gland containing a multinodular goiter or well-differentiated papillary or follicular carcinoma led to the assumption that the anaplastic carcinoma cell evolves from these less malignant processes. This has been difficult to prove, although the coexistence of anaplastic and well-differentiated carcinoma within the same gland has supported this view (20). Molecular biology has provided further support for the fundamental difference between well-differentiated and anaplastic carcinoma, in keeping with clinical observations.

DNA Ploidy

Aneuploidy appears to be typical of anaplastic carcinoma. Aneuploidy was detected in 68% in a series of 19 cases of anaplastic large cell or spindle cell carcinoma, and a DNA index (DI) of less than 1.3 was associated with improved survival (21). In a Swedish study of 36 cases of anaplastic giant cell carcinoma, however, all tumors were aneuploid (22). In a follow-up study of 126 cases from the same institution, 17 (13.5%) were found to contain adjacent foci of well-differentiated carcinoma, primarily papillary. In this subset, all anaplastic areas were aneuploid, whereas nearly half of the differentiated foci showed an aneuploid DNA content (23). In a separate study of 15 cases, including eight with coexistent differentiated components, all anaplastic areas showed aneuploid DNA content, as did all differentiated areas (24). It is possible that aneuploidy within a well-differentiated carcinoma may be a feature suggestive of transformation to anaplastic carcinoma. The rare cases of diploid anaplastic carcinoma may have an improved prognosis.

Cancer Genes

Loss of tumor suppressor genes and oncogene activation may also be markers of anaplastic transformation. The p53 tumor suppressor gene appears mutated in anaplastic carcinoma, but not in papillary carcinoma (25). H-*ras* may also be activated in anaplastic carcinoma, as shown by transfection experiments with thyroid malignancies in which only anaplastic carcinoma tumors contained this oncogene (26). This is in contrast to DNA histochemical data that show H-*ras* activation in a variety of thyroid neoplasms (27). As with other more common malignancies such as colon and breast cancer, it is apparent that a combination of suppressor gene loss and oncogene activation is required for neoplastic transformation and progression.

Cell Biology

The biology of anaplastic carcinoma has been further characterized by the availability of cell lines that may be studied *in vitro* or transplanted into animal models. The results of these studies have provided biologic data that may be applied to clinical observations. Anaplastic carcinoma is one of the most rapidly progressive malignancies known, with a tumor doubling time measured in days, rivaling Burkitt's lymphoma and acute myelogenous leukemia. The cause of this phenomenon appears to be an extremely short cell cycle time of 23.5 hours, rather than an unusually high growth fraction (28), which may have implications for the design of chemotherapy regimens in the treatment of this disease.

The extremely poor prognosis and low response rate to chemotherapy is likely a result of the inherent drug resistance of anaplastic carcinoma to available agents. The multidrug resistance gene, *mdr*-1, and its protein product, p-glycoprotein (p-gp) were overexpressed in only 30% of cases studied, and they showed no correlation with clinical outcome (29). Drug resistance may be mediated by another factor, multidrug resistance-associated protein (mrp), which was found overexpressed in 100% of cell lines and 60% of patient samples (30).

The frequent presence of fever and leukocytosis in patients with anaplastic carcinoma has recently been attributed to ectopic production of G-CSF by the malignant cells (16–18,31). Serum levels of G-CSF have been measured in patients with these findings and are elevated. White blood cell counts may be as high as 40,000 to 50,000/mm^3, with the majority being mature granulocytes (17). Tumor cells stain positively for G-CSF by immunohistochemical techniques (16,18), and cell lines derived from these tumors produce high levels of G-CSF *in vitro* (18,31). It is not known whether the ectopic production of G-CSF defines a subset of patients with a different prognosis, or a response to therapy.

Clinical Spectrum of Anaplastic Carcinoma

Histologic Subtypes

A variety of histologic subtypes of anaplastic carcinoma have been reported, including spindle cell, giant cell, and squamoid (32), although at least 30% display a total lack of differentiation by morphology or marker studies (33). It is unclear whether these subtypes carry prognostic significance. Anaplastic giant cell carcinoma is sometimes described as having sarcomatoid features (5), with osteoclast-like giant cells or divergent differentiation displaying osseous, vascular, and myogenic elements (34–37). No differences in clinical behavior have been clearly established for these histologic subtypes. The occasional presence of features resembling sarcoma may cause diagnostic confusion, particularly because primary sarcoma of the thyroid and sarcoma metastatic to the thyroid have been reported (3,38–40) (see later). Angiomatoid features may mimic angiosarcoma (37), but yet they are are compatible with anaplastic carcinoma, a view supported by the observation that endothelial cell growth factors are actively secreted by anaplastic carcinoma cell lines in animal models (34). Awareness of these histologic variants is important, primarily to avoid misdiagnosis.

A separate entity with clinical behavior intermediate between well-differentiated and anaplastic carcinoma has been proposed, the so-called insular carcinoma (32,41), which appears histologically similar to anaplastic carcinoma yet retains the ability to concentrate iodine. This may be a transitional form of well-differentiated carcinoma in the process of transformation to anaplastic carcinoma, and other clinical patterns suggestive of on-going transformation have been described. Most significant of these is the finding of anaplastic transformation within metastatic lesions, such as lymph nodes or lung nodules in patients with well-differentiated papillary and follicular carcinoma within the thyroid (42,43). It is clear that anaplastic transformation is not limited to the primary tumor, and it may instead present as rapidly progressive metastatic disease in a patient after thyroidectomy for well-differentiated carcinoma.

Local and Metastatic Behavior

Anaplastic carcinoma is frequently lethal without metastasizing, so significant is the problem of local invasion into the structures of the neck and upper airway. A German series of 170 cases of locally invasive anaplastic carcinoma reported the use of tracheostomy in 40% of patients, half for active bleeding and half for prophylaxis against asphyxiation (44). As might be expected, the need for tracheostomy was associated with the poorest prognosis. The local tumor progression may be so rapid as to cause symptomatic destruction of the functional thyroid, with destructive thyrotoxicosis followed by hypothyroidism (45). This aggressive behavior has led to the current designation of all cases of anaplastic carcinoma as stage IV, regardless of anatomic extent of disease (46).

Distant metastases also occur frequently, primarily to lung and bone (1). In the lung they may present as nodular masses, diffuse infiltration, or hemorrhagic pleural effusion (47). Solitary bone metastases may be mistaken for primary sarcoma of bone (48), particularly in view of the occasional presence of osteosarcomatoid features in giant cell anaplastic carcinoma. Many unusual sites of metastatic involvement have been reported, including metastases to the tonsil (49), small bowel (50), and right ventricle (51).

The Role of Chemotherapy in Malignancies of the Thyroid—Overview

The role of chemotherapy in the management of malignancies of the thyroid has evolved over the past 20 to

25 years, as the distinct clinical entities of anaplastic carcinoma and primary thyroid lymphoma have become better defined and addressed separately from the majority of thyroid malignancies. It is now clear that chemotherapy is an integral part of the therapy of these uncommon malignancies, although this has not always been the case. Much of the uncertainty regarding the value of systemic chemotherapy in thyroid malignancies resulted from the inclusion in early clinical trials of these biologically different entities along with differentiated thyroid cancer, yielding survival rates ranging from a few months to several years within the study population.

At the time of the first edition of *Thyroid Disease* in 1990, a major advance in the management of unusual malignancies of the thyroid was the use of immunohistochemistry to identify lymphoid malignancies, which have an average 5-year survival of 70% for localized disease (1). When cases of previously diagnosed anaplastic carcinoma were restudied using these techniques, as many as 20% were reclassified, many as lymphomas (52). The entity of small cell anaplastic carcinoma was then identified as primary thyroid lymphoma, and it was separated from the better-defined non-small cell or true anaplastic carcinoma, with a median survival of 8 months and rare long-term survivors. Indeed, some still contend that any long-term survivors of anaplastic carcinoma are more likely to have been misdiagnosed rather to have been true responders to therapy (53).

At the time of this second edition, significant new information regarding the cellular biology and molecular genetics of anaplastic carcinoma and thyroid lymphoma has become available, and the therapeutic approaches to these diseases have been further refined. Clinically distinct subtypes within these entities may now be defined, allowing more appropriate application of therapy. Unfortunately, in view of the extremely poor prognosis associated with anaplastic carcinoma, it is clear that this disease requires further study in the form of clinical trials with new chemotherapeutic agents in combination with surgery and radiotherapy.

Multimodality Therapy of Anaplastic Carcinoma

The therapy of anaplastic carcinoma has evolved from primarily local therapy to the addition of systemic therapy during or following local therapy. The preferred initial therapy for small, localized disease remains surgical resection, although few patients present at this stage. There appears to be little benefit to radical neck dissection (54). Frequently, surgical resection is incomplete or technically unfeasible, and radiation therapy as primary or adjuvant therapy has been used palliatively to obtain local control, in an attempt to avoid death resulting from local tumor invasion. A retrospective analysis of 51 patients treated in this manner from 1970 to 1986 illustrates the results of this approach (55). At the conclusion of primary radiotherapy, patients without residual local disease or evidence of metastases had a median survival of 8 months, generally due to the subsequent development of metastases. Patients with lung metastases at presentation who were locally free of tumor after radiotherapy to the neck had a median survival of 7.5 months. However, those patients with residual local disease after therapy had a median survival of 1.6 months, regardless of the presence or absence of distant metastases. These observations confirmed the importance of local control as the primary aim of therapy, because of the extremely poor survival if local control is not achieved. However, despite local control, distant metastases are common and contribute to mortality.

Further improvement in local control rates has resulted from intensification of local therapy when definitive surgery is not possible. Early studies suggested that hyperfractionation of radiotherapy was more effective than conventional dose therapy, particularly with the addition of low dose doxorubicin as a radiosensitizer, although toxicity was high (56,57). Kim and Leeper (57) initially reported nine patients treated at Memorial Sloan-Kettering Cancer Center with hyperfractionated external beam radiotherapy at a dose of 160 cGy twice daily, three times per week, to a total of 5760 cGy. Doxorubicin 10 mg/m^2 was given once weekly, 90 minutes prior to radiotherapy for 6 weeks. Toxicity consisted of reversible pharyngoesophagitis, tracheitis, and local erythema. Eight of 9 patients achieved a complete response, although two developed marginal recurrences after 4 months. Despite excellent local control, 5 of 8 developed distant metastases within 3 to 10 months. This same group expanded their initial report, with 16 of 19 patients (84%) achieving complete local control, and 68% maintaining local control up to the time of death from metastatic disease, with a median survival of less than 1 year. This experience clearly illustrates that local control may be successful with intensive radiotherapy therapy, but that chemotherapy with low dose doxorubicin is inadequate to prevent distant metastases.

Tennval et al. (58) further refined this approach by employing preoperative or neoadjuvant therapy, followed by surgical resection if possible. Preoperative radiotherapy by twice daily fractions of 100 to 130 cGy was delivered to a dose of 3000 cGy, and postoperatively to a total dose of 4600 cGy. Doxorubicin 20 mg was administered weekly throughout radiotherapy. Of 33 patients treated from 1984 to 1992, debulking surgery was possible in 23 (70%). Forty-eight percent had no evidence of local recurrence, and eight (24%) died as a result of local failure. Four patients (12%) survived beyond 2 years without evidence of disease. It is unclear whether surgical resection contributed to local control beyond that obtained by intensive radiotherapy with radiosensitization. Experience with other radiosensitizing drugs, such as methotrexate, or a combination of bleomycin, cyclophosphamide, and 5-fluorouracil has been unpromising, with significant toxicity (54).

Modern therapy of anaplastic carcinoma has led to the addition of full dose systemic chemotherapy, in combination with intensive local therapy, to reduce the incidence of distant metastases. The following section describes the development of chemotherapy in advanced thyroid cancer.

Chemotherapy in Thyroid Malignancies—Initial Studies

Early clinical trials involving chemotherapy in the treatment of thyroid malignancies are of limited value because of the heterogeneity of histologic entities included in these studies. However, the observations made during these trials have formed the basis of our current therapy and as such warrant review.

Single Agents

The most active single chemotherapeutic agent in thyroid cancer is doxorubicin, with a response rate of 37% in an initial series of 30 patients with various histologies, including recurrent differentiated thyroid cancer, medullary carcinoma, and anaplastic carcinoma (59). Median survival of responding patients was 11 months, compared with 4 months for nonresponders. Responders were seen in all cell types (including anaplastic carcinoma), and a meta-analysis of 248 patients yielded overall response rates of 22% to 42%, depending on histology (60). The recommended single agent dose for systemic therapy with doxorubicin is 60 to 75 mg/m^2 every 3 weeks, not to exceed a total cumulative dose of 550 mg/m^2.

A note of caution is appropriate regarding the use of doxorubicin in this patient population. Some authors limit the use of this agent to euthyroid patients (61), as it is uncertain whether either hypo- or hyperthyroidism may predispose the myocardium to doxorubicin-induced cardiotoxicity. Predictors of subsequent development of cardiotoxicity are a lowering of QRS voltage on the electrocardiogram (62), and a decrease in ejection fraction by radionuclide ventriculography or two-dimensional echocardiogram (63). Therefore, prior to initiating therapy with doxorubicin, it is recommended that thyroid hormone levels be measured and baseline measurements of cardiac function be obtained.

Other single agents have been studied less extensively. Activities ranging from 0% to 20% have been reported with bleomycin (64), cisplatin, etoposide (64,65), and mitoxantrone (58).

Combination Chemotherapy

A number of studies combining chemotherapeutic agents with single-agent activity have been reported, although the majority has been nonrandomized trials with small numbers of patients. All combination therapies have included doxorubicin, the most extensively studied combination being doxorubicin with cisplatinum (66–68).

The first randomized trial comparing single-agent to combination therapy was reported by the Eastern Cooperative Oncology Group (ECOG) (66), with patients randomized to receive doxorubicin 60 mg/m^2, with or without cisplatinum 40 mg/m^2 on day 1. Therapy was repeated every 21 days. The group evaluated 84 patients, including 39 with anaplastic carcinoma, 35 with differentiated carcinoma, and 10 with medullary carcinoma. Twelve had nodal metastases, 27 had bone metastases, and 47 had visceral metastases, primarily pulmonary. Seven of 41 (17%) treated with doxorubicin alone responded, versus 11 of 43 (26%) in the combination arm, but this difference was not statistically significant. Of note is the fact that five complete responses were seen in the combination arm, whereas none was seen in the doxorubicin arm.

When stratified by histology, subset analysis suggested a benefit of combination therapy for anaplastic carcinoma, with 6 of 18 (33%) responding in the combination arm, including three complete responses, versus 1 of 21 (4.7%) in the single-agent arm. Predictors of poor response were weight loss greater than 10%, nonambulatory status, and presence of pulmonary metastases. Toxicity consisted mainly of myelosuppression, which was similar in both arms. The single-agent response rate of 17% is significantly lower than earlier reports with doxorubicin, and may represent the rigorous histologic criteria employed in this trial to rule out cases of lymphoma. The ECOG trial was the first to suggest a superiority of combination therapy in thyroid cancer, although the benefits were limited to anaplastic carcinoma.

A criticism of the ECOG trial was that a relatively low dose of cisplatinum was employed. Surprisingly, a smaller single-arm phase II trial failed to confirm the ECOG study, despite utilizing escalating doses of cisplatinum (68). Twenty-two patients received doxorubicin 60 mg/m^2 and cisplatinum 60 mg/m^2 every 4 weeks, with escalation to 75 mg/m^2 in the absence of hematologic or renal toxicity. This series included seven anaplastic carcinomas and 15 patients with other histologies. Only two partial responses were seen (9%). Regimens combining doxorubicin with other agents have also been reported, with results similar to doxorubicin alone. A Milan study described 23 patients with thyroid cancer treated with doxorubicin and vincristine, with an overall response rate of 26% (69). Bukowski et al. (70) reported a 36% response rate utilizing doxorubicin, vincristine, bleomycin, and oral melphalan. However, rigorous methods to exclude lymphoma from the anaplastic category were not employed. Overall, response rates with chemotherapy for anaplastic carcinoma have been similar to those seen in refractory well-differentiated carcinoma (60,66).

The chemotherapy of choice for anaplastic carcinoma remains doxorubicin, either alone or in combination with cisplatinum. The rarity of anaplastic carcinoma precludes large clinical trials, but several new therapeutic agents have become available in the past few years, including carboplatinum, ifosphamide, taxol, and, most recently, the camptothecins, irinotecan and topotecan. Their unique mechanisms of action, and the poor response rates documented in anaplastic carcinoma with "standard" therapy, argue for the evaluation of these agents in the management of anaplastic carcinoma.

Therapy of Anaplastic Carcinoma—Summary

Despite the frequently poor prognosis of this locally aggressive and rapidly metastasizing tumor, a subset of patients with good prognostic features may achieve long-term survival. Favorable features include unilateral tumors, size less than 4 cm, and absence of invasion of local structures (54). Surgery followed by local radiotherapy and systemic chemotherapy may lead to long-term survival. For unresectable tumors, intensive local therapy with hyperfractionated radiotherapy and low-dose doxorubicin may render some tumors operable, and it may produce long-term local control without surgery in some patients, thereby avoiding the significant morbidity of locally advanced disease. However, despite the adequacy of local control, systemic therapy appears to be essential to achieving long-term survival, as distant metastases are frequent. The current standard chemotherapy of doxorubicin with or without cisplatinum offers a modest response rate of approximately 20% to 30%, with some long-term survivors. Future studies with new chemotherapeutic agents may substantially improve the current survival rates with anaplastic carcinoma.

PRIMARY LYMPHOMA OF THE THYROID

Primary lymphoma of the thyroid is a relatively rare disorder, representing approximately 5% of thyroid neoplasms and 2% of extranodal lymphomas (71,72). The incidence of this disease has increased in recent years with the standard use of immunohistochemistry to distinguish lymphoid tumors from anaplastic carcinoma. Approximately 15% of thyroid malignancies were formerly described as small cell anaplastic carcinoma, and many have subsequently been reclassified as lymphomas (73). One such study reevaluated 53 patients originally classified as small cell anaplastic, applying common leukocyte antigen (CLA) staining to the specimens. This antigen, a membrane protein common to all hematolymphoid cells, was present in 33 (62% of cases), whereas epithelial markers for carcinoma were present in only 6 (11%), and 14 (26%) stained with neither and remained undefined. No cases displayed dual expression of CLA and epithelial markers. The pathologic distinction between lymphoma and carcinoma is much clearer in the case of anaplastic giant cell or spindle-cell variants, or in those cases where coexisting papillary and follicular elements suggest evolution from differentiated to undifferentiated carcinoma (73). Other identifying markers are the presence of B-cell (and, rarely, T-cell) antigens, and surface or cytoplasmic immunoglobulin.

Within the category of thyroid lymphoma, however, further advances in immunohistochemistry have led to improved definition of at least two main subsets with differing biology and clinical behavior (72,74). As will be discussed later, stage and clinicopathologic subtype are of the greatest importance in determining prognosis and guiding therapy.

Diagnosis

The clinical presentation of thyroid lymphoma is similar to that of anaplastic carcinoma and has been discussed previously in this chapter. As for diagnostic testing, ultrasound and nuclear isotope scanning are helpful, but there is no noninvasive diagnostic test that will reliably distinguish between these two entities, and biopsy is always recommended for definitive diagnosis. Although fine-needle aspiration may yield sufficient tissue to provide a diagnosis of lymphoma (75), the importance of observing the cellular pattern of growth and the use of multiple immunohistochemical markers to fully define subsets of lymphoma argues for a subsequent biopsy by core needle or an open procedure (76). A Japanese study analyzing 119 cases of biopsy-proven thyroid lymphoma arising in the setting of Hashimoto's thyroiditis reported that only 78% were correctly identified as lymphoma by fine-needle aspiration (76). Ultrasound showed an asymmetrical pseudocystic or nodular pattern in most cases, although other studies have indicated similar findings in adenomatous goiter, chronic thyroiditis, and thyroid carcinoma (77). Open biopsy or core needle biopsy yielded a definitive diagnosis in 100% of cases.

Staging

A diagnosis of primary lymphoma of the thyroid can be made with certainty only in the setting of localized disease at presentation. Patients presenting with widespread lymphoma who also display involvement of the thyroid may have primary lymphoma of the thyroid, or of another site, with secondary spread to the thyroid. As a result, the majority of cases of primary thyroid lymphoma reported in the medical literature has presented with localized disease and are stage IE or IIE by the Ann Arbor classification of lymphoma staging (78). The numerical stage refers to involvement of the thyroid and local soft tissue (I), or local lymph node groups (II) as well. The *E* is applied to any extranodal presentation of lymphoma, which is the case, by definition, with thyroid lymphoma.

Staging for any patient with thyroid lymphoma should include chest x-ray, CT or MRI of the thyroid and neck, CT of the chest to evaluate for mediastinal adenopathy, and CT of the abdomen. Bone marrow biopsy should be included, although it is rarely positive when all other studies have been negative. Although the need for gastrointestinal imaging is not firmly established, there is an increased risk of gastrointestinal involvement with thyroid lymphoma (79). Thyroid lymphoma is often considered similar to other extranodal lymphomas arising in mucosa-associated lymphoid tissue, or MALT lymphomas (72,79). MALT lymphomas include those presenting in breast, lung, parotid, thyroid, or gastrointestinal tract, and they have a predilection for recurrence in any of these sites. Because of the potential for Waldeyer's ring involvement, a thorough head and neck exam is mandatory.

Histopathology and the Etiology of Thyroid Lymphoma

The majority of thyroid lymphomas are non-Hodgkin's B-cell type, although T-cell lymphoma and Hodgkin's disease of the thyroid have been reported (80,81). The classification of malignant lymphomas has developed over the past 40 years, with the 1982 Working Formulation (82) being the most comprehensive system to date to effectively combine histopathologic subsets with relevance to clinical and biologic behavior (83). According to this system, the majority of thyroid lymphomas, at least 60% to 75%, are diffuse, large cell type (DLC), and are of intermediate grade (71,72,84,85). As many as 10% are high grade, aggressive lymphomas of immunoblastic type, and the remainder are of low grade, less aggressive histologies such as plasmacytoid lymphoma or intermediate lymphocytic lymphoma (ILL) (86). The latter group has been associated most frequently with Hashimoto's thyroiditis and may represent 20% to 30% of all thyroid lymphoma.

The Working Formulation designates low, intermediate, and high grade lymphoma as separate categories on the basis of the many differences in their clinical behavior. As all grades may present within the thyroid, it is apparent that full definition of the nature of the malignant lymphoid infiltrate is essential. Some authors have concluded that all lymphomas presenting within the thyroid should be considered MALT-type by anatomic definition (72). However, a new classification system for lymphoid neoplasms from the International Lymphoma Study Group would restrict this definition to a subset of thyroid lymphomas, based on histology, immunohistochemistry, and possible etiology (74).

Attempting to more accurately define lymphomas according to their cell of origin in the normal immune system, the Revised European-American Lymphoma, or REAL, classification identifies a specific entity known as marginal zone B-cell lymphoma, which in the normal counterpart is a nodal or extranodal lymphocyte with the capacity to respond to antigen and "home" to certain tissues. The extranodal malignant form corresponds to the MALT lymphoma histology, or low grade lymphoma in the Working Formulation. This category combines all lymphomas that are thought to arise from chronic antigen stimulation, and therefore it includes lymphomas developing in the setting of Sjögren's syndrome in the parotid, *Helicobacter* gastritis in the stomach, and Hashimoto's thyroiditis, for example. Studies of the lymphocytic infiltrates in chronic Hashimoto's thyroiditis revealed a monoclonal B-cell proliferation by immunoglobulin gene rearrangement in nearly half the cases (87). Epstein-Barr virus (EBV) has been implicated as a possible factor in the transformation of Hashimoto's thyroiditis to malignant lymphoma, with EBV-related RNA detected in some lymphomas, but not in Hashimoto's thyroiditis (88).

Low grade MALT lymphomas often remain limited to the site of antigenic stimulation, and these may be adequately treated with local therapy or removal of the antigenic stimulus, as is the case with *Helicobacter* gastritis-related lymphomas in early stages. These cells lack surface immunoglobulin (Ig), but 40% stain for cytoplasmic Ig. They possess general B-cell markers of CD 19, 20, 22, and they are CD5 and CD10 negative, thereby excluding chronic lymphocytic leukemia, mantle, and follicular-center cell lymphomas. Cytogenetics show no *bcl*-1 or *bcl*-2 translocations, although trisomy 3 and t(11,18) have been reported. As is the case with all low grade lymphomas, transformation to a higher grade, usually DLC lymphoma, often occurs, and this may explain the high frequency of this histology in thyroid lymphomas.

Diffuse large cell lymphoma of the thyroid may therefore arise *de novo* or as a result of the transformation of a subclinical low grade MALT lymphoma. Unlike MALT lymphomas, *bcl*-2 rearrangement is seen in 30% to 40% of large cell lymphomas, and, in addition to CD19, 20, and 22 positivity, they are often CD45 positive, in further distinction to the marginal zone MALT lymphomas. EBV has also been implicated in the transformation of low grade to intermediate grade histologies (89). Other markers of aggressive biology, such as acquisition of p53 mutations, were not found in a study of 27 thyroid lymphomas, all of which were negative for p53 mutations (90).

Therapy of Thyroid Lymphoma

The rarity of thyroid lymphoma, as with anaplastic carcinoma, has precluded the study of large series of patients treated in similar fashion at a single institution. Surgery was initially the treatment of choice, in the era when preoperative evaluation could not distinguish lymphoma from other entities, and thyroidectomy was primary therapy (72,91). Radiotherapy later became the standard therapy of localized lymphoma in other sites, and it was increasingly applied to thyroid lymphoma, either as primary therapy or in combination with surgery. Despite excellent local response rates, distant relapses occurred in as many as 50% (72,85). The risk of systemic relapse in a significant proportion of patients presenting with early-stage disease led to the use of combination chemotherapy, with dramatic improvement in overall survival and disease-free survival. Combination chemotherapy then superseded surgery or radiotherapy alone as the treatment of choice. The evolution of this therapy will be described next.

Radiotherapy With or Without Surgery

The mainstay of therapy for stage IE and IIE thyroid lymphoma has been radiotherapy, with or without surgery (70,85). Overall 5-year survival rates as high as 75% to 80% were initially reported (11), in keeping with the results in other localized lymphomas of intermediate grade treated with radiotherapy alone. An early Stanford study reported eight patients with stage I/IIE disease treated with regional radiotherapy after surgery, which consisted of total or subtotal thyroidectomy in five patients, and biopsy only in three (84). The field encompassed a full-mantle field in five patients, and neck and mediastinum in three, at a dose of 4300 to 5200 cGy. The extent of surgery did not appear to affect outcome in this small study, and an 83% 3-year survival was reported, with 75% disease free at 2 years. Further support for primary radiotherapy came from several larger studies (85,91). However, despite documented benefit for most patients, a subset was identified at high risk for failure or relapse.

The Mayo Clinic reported a series of 38 patients, 34 stage I/IIE, treated with 2400 to 6000 cGy, to the neck only in ten, and to the neck and mediastinum in the remainder (85). Disease-free survival at 5 years was 59%. Fourteen patients relapsed, 75% within 12 months of therapy. Ten of the 14 (71%) relapsed at multiple sites, and in six (43%), relapse also occurred within the radiated field. There were no relapses in the treated field in patients rendered disease free by prior surgery, and bulky residual disease appeared to predispose to relapse. Radiotherapy doses may also have been inadequate in some cases. Of those recurrences at distant sites, the most frequent sites were para-aortic nodes and the gastrointestinal tract. The authors recommended a dose of 4000 cGy to the neck, axillae, and mediastinum, and they did not recommend blocks to the larynx or spinal cord, as these may prevent complete eradication of local disease. The frequency of subdiaphragmatic recurrences indicated the probable value of systemic therapy.

A subsequent study identified subgroups at risk for recurrence and confirmed the value of regional radiotherapy for some patients with localized thyroid lymphoma. The Royal Marsden group reported a retrospective study of 46 patients, all with disease limited to the thyroid or cervical lymph nodes (stage I/IIE), but with extension into the thoracic inlet or retrosternal region in 40% (92). Of these patients, 78% had DLC histology. All patients had undergone surgery prior to radiotherapy, with definitive resection in 60%. The majority received radiotherapy to the neck and mediastinum to a dose of at least 4000 cGy. Overall survival was 40% at 5 years, and 30% at 10 years. Half of all recurrences occurred at local sites, despite full-dose radiotherapy. Adverse prognostic features included residual tumor bulk after surgery, fixation to surrounding structures, extracapsular extension, and retrosternal involvement. It was concluded that patients with these adverse factors should be considered for chemotherapy as well.

Combined Modality Therapy

An early study examining the addition of chemotherapy from the M. D. Anderson Cancer Center reported 38 patients, 12 stage IE and 26 stage IIE (93). Of these, 15 were treated with radiotherapy alone, 6 with chemotherapy alone, and 14 with both radiotherapy and chemotherapy. Radiotherapy was given initially in eight patients, to a total dose of 4000 cGy, to the neck and mediastinum, followed by chemotherapy. In six patients, chemotherapy was given first for four cycles, followed by radiotherapy. Chemotherapy consisted primarily of CHOP (cyclophosphamide, doxorubicin, vincristine, and prednisone), sometimes in combination with bleomycin. The 5-year survival for all stages was 75%, with 64% disease-free survival, regardless of type of therapy. Stage IE patients had a 5-year survival of 91%, versus 62% for stage IIE. Nine patients relapsed, only one of whom had had combined modality therapy. Five relapses were in retroperitoneal nodes or in the stomach. Small numbers precluded statistically significant subset analysis, but the results suggested that stage IIE patients with mediastinal involvement were at highest risk for relapse, and that initial chemotherapy followed by local radiotherapy appeared to be the optimal strategy for this subgroup.

A recent meta-analysis from Yale has yielded the largest number of patients for evaluation, and it has concluded that chemotherapy significantly reduces relapse rates in thyroid lymphoma (72). A total of 211 patients with stage I/IIE thyroid lymphoma, taken from a Yale series of 11 patients combined with a literature review from 1980 to 1992, were collected. Only those patients treated with adequate radiotherapy or anthracycline-containing chemotherapy were analyzed; they included 159 treated with radiotherapy alone, 13 with chemotherapy alone, and 39 with both radiation and chemotherapy. Only relapse rates were studied. The overall relapse rate was 37.1% for radiotherapy, 43% for chemotherapy, and 7.7% for combined modality therapy. Distant relapses occurred in 30.8% of patients treated with radiotherapy alone. A subset with small-volume disease limited to the neck appeared to be adequately treated by radiotherapy or chemotherapy. The authors concluded unequivocally that the addition of chemotherapy to radiotherapy lowered both distant and local relapse.

This approach was further confirmed by a large single institution study from Japan, in which 119 patients with thyroid lymphoma associated with Hashimoto's thyroiditis were treated with a combination of six cycles of CHOP chemotherapy and radiotherapy, with a resultant 100% 8-year survival (76). The histologic subtypes were not reported. It is possible that true MALT lymphomas, particularly of lower grade, will respond best to aggressive therapy while still localized, whereas transformation to DLC and subsequent dissemination is associated with the worst prognosis, regardless of the site of origin.

The overall approach to extranodal stage I and II lymphomas has been to attempt to reach the minimum therapy required for cure. The Vancouver group has reported the use of three cycles of CHOP, with radiotherapy limited to the involved field to a dose of 3000 cGy to 4400 cGy, with an overall survival of 85% at 2 years (94). This approach remains standard for localized lymphoma, and it should be considered for all cases of thyroid lymphoma.

Therapy of Thyroid Lymphoma—Summary

Surgery and radiotherapy are effective modalities for local control of early-stage thyroid lymphoma. However, the inability to predict which patients may have disseminated disease at diagnosis has led to the application of systemic chemotherapy for reduction of distant relapses and improvement in local control. Unlike anaplastic carcinoma, the chemotherapy of lymphoma is often curative, and 85% to 100% cure rates are possible with either three or six cycles of CHOP chemotherapy, combined with radiotherapy. A subset of patients with small amounts of disease limited to the neck may be adequately treated with radiotherapy alone, but all others with stage I/IIE disease should be considered for combined modality therapy, utilizing an anthracycline-containing chemotherapy regimen, and adequate radiotherapy fields encompassing likely sites of involvement.

UNUSUAL TUMORS OF THE THYROID

Much rarer than anaplastic carcinoma or thyroid lymphoma are primary squamous cell carcinoma and sarcoma of the thyroid.

Squamous carcinoma of the thyroid is the subject of case reports, and it is more often thought to be metastatic or locally invasive from another structure within the head and neck than arising as a primary thyroid tumor (95–97). However, a unique embryologic relationship exists between the thyroid and the tongue, a frequent site of squamous carcinoma, because of the thyroglossal duct. Thyroglossal duct cysts are not uncommon, and indeed case reports exist of intrathyroid thyroglossal duct cysts developing squamous carcinoma and presenting as a hard thyroid mass (96) Interestingly, lingual thyroid associated with squamous carcinoma of the base of tongue has also been reported (98). The presumed rarity of primary squamous cell carcinoma of the thyroid has been challenged by an autopsy study of 67 cases of thyroid cancer in Japan (4). A surprising 28.4% of cases harbored foci of squamous carcinoma within the thyroid, although 90% of these were coexistent with papillary or anaplastic carcinoma. Other than surgical excision, or local radiotherapy, no specific therapy may be recommended for this rare entity.

Sarcoma involving the thyroid is more frequently metastatic than primary, with malignant fibrous histiocytoma and leiomyosarcoma diagnosed as metastases by fine-needle aspirate (3). Kaposi's sarcoma metastatic to the thyroid in a patient with human immunodeficiency virus (HIV) infection has also been reported (38). It should be considered in the differential diagnosis of an enlarging neck mass with adenopathy in patients with HIV, along with lymphoma. Primary leiomyosarcoma and liposarcoma of the thyroid have been reported, the latter ascribed to prior radiation to the neck and considered to be a case of radiation-induced thyroid sarcoma (39,40).

REFERENCES

1. Hansen JT. Surgical anatomy and embryology of the lower neck and superior mediastinum. In: Falk S, ed. *Thyroid disease.* New York: Raven Press. 1990;15–27.
2. Norton JA, Levin B, Jensen RT. Cancer of the endocrine system. In: DeVita V, Hellman S, Rosenberg S, eds. *Cancer: principles and practice of oncology.* Philadelphia: JB Lippincott, 1993;1333–1435.
3. Gattuso P, Castelli J, Reyes CV. Fine needle aspiration cytology of metastatic sarcoma involving the thyroid. *South Med J* 1989;82:1158–1160.
4. Harada T, et al. Rarity of squamous cell carcinoma of the thyroid: autopsy review. *World J Surg* 1994;18:542–546.
5. Lampertico P. Anaplastic carcinoma of the thyroid gland. *Semin Diagn Pathol* 1993;10:159–168.
6. Hofstadter F. Frequency and morphology of malignant tumors of the thyroid before and after the introduction of iodine prophylaxis. *Virchows Arch* 1980;385:263.
7. Hill CS, Aldinger KA. Management of anaplastic carcinoma of the thyroid. In: Greenfield LP, ed. *Thyroid cancer.* Boca Raton, FL: CRC Press, 1978;165.
8. Willems JS, Lowhagen T, Palombini L. The cytology of of a giant cell, osteoclastoma-like thyroid neoplasm. *Acta Cytol* 1979;23:214–216.
9. Peters J, O'Reilly S, Barragry JM. Anaplastic carcinoma of the thyroid following radio-iodine therapy. *Ir J Med Sci* 1993;162:3–4.
10. Bridges AB, Davies RR, Newton RW, McNeill GP. Anaplastic carcinoma of the thyroid in a patient receiving radio-iodine therapy for amiodarone-induced thyrotoxicosis. *Scott Med J* 1989;34:471–472.

11. Hamburger J, Miller JM, Kini S. Lymphoma of the thyroid. *Ann Intern Med* 1983;99:685–693.
12. Laing RW, Hoskin P, Hudson BV, et al. The significance of MALT histology in thyroid lymphoma. *Clin Oncol* 1994;6:300–304.
13. Tan RK, et al. Anaplastic carcinoma of the thyroid: a 24 year experience. *Head Neck* 1995;17:41–47.
14. Meng G, Ma DB, Wang HS. Anaplastic carcinoma of the thyroid: an analysis of 33 cases. *Chung Hua Wai Ko Tsa Chih* 1994;32:46–48.
15. Brownlie BE, et al. Primary thyroid lymphoma. *N Z Med J* 1994;107: 301–304.
16. Yazawa S, et al. Thyroid anaplastic carcinoma producing granulocyte-colony stimulating factor. *Intern Med* 1995;34:584–588.
17. Iwasa K, et al. Anaplastic carcinoma producing the granulocyte-colony stimulating factor (G-CSF). *Surg Today* 1995;25:158–160.
18. Oka Y, et al. Establishment of a human anaplastic thyroid cancer cell line secreting granulocyte-colony stimulating factor. *In Vitro Cell Dev Biol Anim* 1993;29A:537–542.
19. Maurea S, et al. Non-Hodgkin's lymphoma in a patient with follicular thyroid cancer. *J Nucl Biol Med* 1994;38:18–21.
20. Spires JR, Schwartz MR, Miller RH. Anaplastic thyroid carcinoma. Association with differentiated thyroid cancer. *Arch Otolaryngol Head Neck Surg* 1988;114:40–44.
21. Klemi PJ, Joensuu H, Eerola E. DNA aneuploidy in anaplastic carcinoma of the thyroid gland. *Am J Clin Pathol* 1988;89:154–159.
22. Ekman ET, et al. Nuclear DNA content in anaplastic giant-cell thyroid carcinoma. *Am J Clin Oncol* 1989;12:442–446.
23. Wallin G, et al. Co-existent anaplastic and well-differentiated thyroid carcinomas: a nuclear DNA study. *Eur J Surg Oncol* 1989;15:43–48.
24. Galera-Davidson H, et al. Nuclear DNA in anaplastic thyroid carcinoma with a differentiated component. *Histopathology* 1987;11:715–722.
25. Matias-Guiu X, et al. p53 expression in anaplastic carcinomas arising from thyroid papillary carcinomas. *J Clin Pathol* 1994;47:337–339.
26. Stringer BM, et al. Detection of the H-ras oncogene in human anaplastic carcinomas. *Experientia* 1989;45:372–376.
27. Lemoine NR, et al. High frequency of ras oncogene activation in all stages of human thyroid tumorigenesis. *Oncogene* 1989;4:159.
28. Yoshido A, et al. Study of cell kinetics in anaplastic thyroid carcinoma transplanted to nude mice. *J Surg Oncol* 1989;41:1–4.
29. Yamashita T, et al. Multidrug resistance gene an P-glycoprotein expression in anaplastic carcinoma of the thyroid. *Cancer Detect Prev* 1994;18:407–413.
30. Sugawara I. Expression of multidrug resistance-associated protein (mrp) in anaplastic carcinoma of the thyroid. *Cancer Lett* 1994;82:185–188.
31. Ono I, et al. Heterotransplantability of human anaplastic thyroid carcinoma line in nude mice. *Hum Cell* 1989;2:74–79.
32. Carcangiu ML. Anaplastic thyroid carcinoma. A study of 70 cases. *Am J Clin Pathol* 1985;83:135–158.
33. LiVolsi VA, Brooks JJ, Arendish-Durand B. Anaplastic thyroid tumors. Immunohistology. *Am J Clin Pathol* 87:434–442.
34. Itoh K, et al. Human endothelial cell growth factors derived from thyroid anaplastic cell carcinoma. *Laryngoscope* 1989;99:533–537.
35. Blasius S, et al. Anaplastic thyroid carcinoma with osteosarcomatous differentiation. *Pathol Res Pract* 1994;190:507–510.
36. Pascal-Vigneron V, et al. Osteogenic anaplastic carcinoma of the thyroid. *Thyroid* 1993;3:319–323.
37. Mills SE, Stallings RG, Austin MB. Angiomatoid carcinoma of the thyroid gland. Anaplastic carcinoma with follicular and medullary features mimicking angiosarcoma. *Am J Clin Pathol* 1986;86:674–678.
38. Krauth PH, Katz JF. Kaposi's sarcoma involving the thyroid in a patient with AIDS. *Clin Nucl Med* 1987;12:848–849.
39. Griem KL, et al. Radiation-induced sarcoma of the thyroid. *Arch Otolaryngol Head Neck Surg* 1989;115:991–93.
40. Kawahara E, et al. Leiomyosarcoma of the thyroid. *Cancer* 1988;62: 2558–2563.
41. Bal C, et al. Insular carcinoma of the thyroid. *Clin Nucl Med* 1993; 18:1056–1058.
42. Kawahara E, et al. Papillary carcinoma of the thyroid gland with anaplastic transformation in the metastatic foci. *Acta Pathol Jpn* 1986; 36:921–927.
43. Moore JH, Bacharach B, Choi HY. Anaplastic transformation of metastatic follicular carcinoma of the thyroid. *J Surg Oncol* 1985;29: 216–221.
44. Holting T, Meybier H, Buhr H. Problems of tracheostomy in locally invasive anaplastic thyroid cancer. *Langenbecks Arch Chir* 1989;374:72–76.
45. Murakami T, et al. Destructive thyrotoxicosis in a patient with anaplastic thyroid cancer. *Endocrinol Jpn* 1989;36:905–907.
46. American Joint Committee on Cancer. *Manual for staging*. Philadelphia: JB Lippincott, 1988.
47. Koppl H, Scheer E, Herbst EW. Extensive pulmonary tumor embolisms of anaplastic thyroid carcinoma as a rare cause of hemorrhagic pleural effusion. *Pneumologie* 1993;47:593–596.
48. Paksoy N, et al. Metastatic follicular carcinoma of the thyroid simulating sarcoma of the limb. *Pathologica* 1994;86:314–315.
49. Hadar T, et al. Anaplastic thyroid carcinoma metastatic to the tonsil. *J Laryngol Otol* 1987;101:953–956.
50. Phillips FL, et al. Isolated metastasis to small bowel from anaplastic thyroid carcinoma. *J Clin Gastroenterol* 1987;9:563–567.
51. Lind T, Jensen F, Petri C. Anaplastic thyroid carcinoma with metastasis to the right heart ventricle. *Ugeskr Laeger* 1986;148:1684–1685.
52. Shvero J, et al. Anaplastic thyroid carcinoma. A clinical, histologic, and immunohistochemical study. *Cancer* 1988;62:319–325.
53. Cannizzaro MA, et al. Anaplastic carcinoma of the thyroid. Long term survival. *Minerva Chir* 1993;48:1293–1299.
54. Nel C, et al. Anaplastic carcinoma of the thyroid. A clinicopathologic study of 82 cases. *Mayo Clin Proc* 1985;60:51–58.
55. Levendag PC, De Porre PM, van Putten WL. Anaplastic carcinoma of the thyroid gland treated by radiation therapy. *Int J Rad Oncol Biol Phys* 1993;26:125–128.
56. Simpson W. Anaplastic carcinoma: a new approach. *Can J Surg* 1980; 23:25–27.
57. Kim J, Leeper R. Treatment of anaplastic giant and spindle cell carcinoma of the thyroid gland with combination adriamycin and radiotherapy. *Cancer* 1983;52:954–957.
58. Tennval J, et al. Combined doxorubicin, hyperfractionated radiotherapy and surgery in anaplastic thyroid carcinoma. *Cancer* 1994;74: 1348–1354.
59. J, et al. Chemotherapy of thyroid cancer. *Cancer* 1972;30:848–885.
60. Ahuja S, Ernst H. Chemotherapy of thyroid carcinoma. *J Endocrinol Invest* 1987;10:303–310.
61. Durie B, et al. High risk thyroid cancer. Prolonged survival with early multimodality therapy. *Cancer Clin Trials* 1981;4:67–73.
62. Minow R, et al. Adriamaycin cardiomyopathy-risk factors. *Cancer* 1977;39:1397–1402.
63. Schwartz R, McKenzie W, Alexander J. Congestive heart failure and left ventricular dysfunction complicating doxorubicin therapy. *Am J Med* 1987;82:1109–1118.
64. Poster D, et al. Current status of chemotherapy in the treatment of advanced carcinoma of the thyroid gland. *Cancer Clin Trials* 1981;4: 301–307.
65. Hoskin P, Harmer C. Chemotherapy for thyroid cancer. *Radiother Oncol* 1987;10:187–194.
66. Shimaoka K, et al. A randomized trial of doxorubicin versus doxorubicin plus cisplatin in patients with advanced thyroid carcinoma. *Cancer* 1985;56:2155–2160.
67. Droz JP, et al. Phase II trials of adriamycin, cisplatin, and their combination in thyroid cancer—a review of 44 cases. *Int Congr Ser* 1985;684:203–208.
68. Williams S, Birch R, Einhorn L. Phase II evaluation of doxorubicin plus cisplatin in advanced thyroid cancer: a southeastern cancer study group trial. *Cancer Treat Rev* 1986;70:405–407.
69. Luporini G, et al. *Phase II study with doxorubicin and vincristine in metastatic thyroid cancer* (abstract 10). Presented at Third European Conference on Clinical Oncology, 1985.
70. Bukowski R, et al. Combination chemotherapy of metastatic thyroid cancer. *Am J Clin Oncol* 1983;6:579–581.
71. Aozasa K, et al. Malignant lymphoma of the thyroid. *Cancer* 1986;58:100–104.
72. Doria R, Jekel J, Cooper D. Thyroid lymphoma: the case for combined modality therapy. *Cancer* 1994;73:200–206.
73. Tober A, Maurer R, Hedinger CE. Undifferentiated thyroid tumors of diffuse small cell type. *Virchows Arch [A]* 1984;404:117–126.
74. Harris NL, et al. A revised European-American classification of lymphoid neoplasms: a proposal from the International Lymphoma Study group. *Blood* 1994;84:1361–1393.
75. Das DK, et al. Fine needle aspiration cytology diagnosis of non-Hodgkin's lymphoma of the thyroid. *Diagn Cytopathol* 1993;9: 639–645.
76. Matsuzuka F, et al. Clinical aspects of primary thyroid lymphoma: di-

agnosis and treatment based on our experience of 119 cases. *Thyroid* 1993;3:93–99.
77. Komatsu M, et al. Ultrasonography in the diagnosis of malignant lymphoma of the thyroid. *Nippon Geka Gakkai Zasshi* 1994;95:187–191.
78. Jacobs CJ. Lymphomas of extranodal head and neck sites. In: Jacobs CJ, et al., eds. *Cancers of the head and neck.* Boston: Martinus Nijhoff, 1987.
79. Stone CW, et al. Thyroid lymphomas with gastrointestinal involvement. *Am J Hematol* 1986;21:357–365.
80. Oertel JE, Hefess CS. Lymphoma of the thyroid and related disorders. *Semin Oncol* 1987;14:333–342.
81. Mizukami Y, et al. Primary T-cell lymphoma of the thyroid. *Acta Pathol Jpn* 1987;37:1987–1995.
82. National Cancer Institute-sponsored study of the classification of non-Hodgkin's lymphoma. *Cancer* 1982;49:2112–2135.
83. Rosenberg S. Classification of lymphoid neoplasms. *Blood* 1994;84:1359–1360.
84. Clark LY, et al. Non-Hodgkin's lymphoma presenting as thyroid enlargement. *Cancer* 1981;48:2712–2716.
85. Blair JJ, et al. Radiotherapeutic management of primary thyroid lymphoma. *Int J Radiat Oncol Biol Phys* 1985;11:365–370.
86. Aozasa K, et al. Intermediate lymphocytic lymphoma of the thyroid. *Cancer* 1986;57:1762–1767.
87. Tiemann M, et al. Temperature gradient gel electrophoresis for analysis of clonal evolution in non-Hodgkin's lymphoma of the thyroid. *Electrophoresis* 1995;16:729–732.
88. Takahashi K, et al. Contribution of Epstein-Barr virus to development of malignant lymphoma of the thyroid. *Pathol Int* 1995;45:366–374.
89. Maehara N, et al. Malignant lymphoma of the thyroid with evidence of an Epstein-Barr viral infection concomitant with thalassemia minor. *Surg Today* 1995;25:151–154.
90. Iyota K, et al. Absence of p53 mutation in Japanese patients with malignant thyroid lymphoma. *J Endocrinol Invest* 1994;17:775–772.
91. Sirota D, Segal R. Primary lymphomas of the thyroid gland. *JAMA* 1979;242:1743–1746.
92. Tupchong MB, Hughes F, Harmer CL. Primary lymphoma of the thyroid. *Int J Radiat Oncol Biol Phys* 1986;12:1813–1821.
93. Vigliotti A, et al. Thyroid lymphomas stage I and IIE. *Int J Radiat Oncol Biol Phys* 1986;12:1807–1812.
94. Connors J, et al. Chemotherapy and involved field radiotherapy for limited stage histologically aggressive lymphoma. *Ann Intern Med* 1987;107:25–30.
95. Theander C, et al. Primary squamous cell carcinoma of the thyroid. *J Laryngol Otol* 1993;107:1155–1158.
96. Kresnik E, et al. Squamous cell carcinoma of the thyroid originating from a thyroglossal duct cyst. *Nuklearmedizin* 1995;34:76–78.
97. Almeida F, et al. Technetium-99m-mdp uptake in thyroid cartilage in invasive squamous cell laryngeal carcinoma. *J Nucl Med* 1994;35:1170–1173.
98. Bengoechoea-Beeby MP, et al. Concomitant lingual thyroid and squamous carcinoma of the base of tongue. *J Oral Maxillofac Surg* 1994;52:494–495.

CHAPTER 34

Management of Thyroid Carcinoma Invading the Upper Aerodigestive System

Judith M. Czaja and Thomas V. McCaffrey

Well-differentiated carcinoma of the thyroid gland is a predominantly curable disease with a mortality of 11% to 17%. Although invasion of local and regional structures is common with anaplastic carcinoma of the thyroid gland, invasion of regional structures by well-differentiated papillary and follicular carcinomas of the thyroid gland is less frequent. In a postmortem pathologic study, Silliphant et al. (1) found extracapsular extension in only 17 of 122 cases of well-differentiated thyroid carcinoma. Of the 859 patients treated at the Mayo Clinic for papillary thyroid carcinoma, 138 (16%) had invasion of 242 extrathyroidal sites (2). In another study, Batsakis (3) found that laryngotracheal invasion by thyroid carcinoma has a frequency of 7%, with all histologic types of thyroid carcinoma represented. This is supported by other studies of invasive thyroid carcinoma (4).

When local invasion of upper aerodigestive tract structures by well-differentiated thyroid carcinomas occurs, it is a cause of considerable morbidity and mortality. Life-threatening airway hemorrhage and suffocation can be consequences of airway invasion by thyroid malignancy. Local invasion, with its associated morbidity, is a common direct cause of death from thyroid carcinoma. In the review by McConahey et al. (2), the cause of death from papillary carcinoma was related to untreatable local disease in 36% of cases and metastatic disease in 39%. Tollefson et al. (5), in a review of postmortem examinations of patients who died from papillary thyroid carcinoma, concluded that 47% of these patients died from local disease. Others have shown that 80% to 86% of those who die from all forms of thyroid cancer have active local disease (5). The control of locally invasive thyroid carcinoma is therefore an important clinical problem. It would be expected that successful treatment of these locally invasive tumors would improve survival and reduce morbidity. Improved management of patients with invasive thyroid malignancy requires a thorough understanding of the natural history of the disease, the patterns of invasion, and the techniques of surgical resection of these tumors (see Chapters 25, 28, 29, and 36).

ANATOMIC RELATION OF THE THYROID GLAND TO UPPER AERODIGESTIVE STRUCTURES

The proximity of the thyroid gland to the larynx, laryngeal nerves, pharynx, and cervical esophagus (see Chapter 2) is the prime reason for the involvement of these structures in thyroid carcinoma when extracapsular invasion occurs. The sites of extrathyroidal invasion in 292 patients treated for papillary thyroid carcinoma at the Mayo Clinic between 1940 and 1995 is shown in Table 1. The trachea, recurrent laryngeal nerves, and esophagus have the highest incidence of invasion, after the commonly involved overlying strap muscles. Invasion of the larynx by thyroid carcinoma occurs by direct extension of the tumor, because the laryngeal cartilages do not pose a significant barrier to invasion. The route of invasion can be through the thyroid and cricoid cartilage (Fig. 1) or into the paraglottic space by extension around the posterior border of the thyroid cartilage. The pharynx is usually invaded by posterior extension of the thyroid carci-

---

J. M. Czaja: Department of Otolaryngology—Head and Neck Surgery, University of Cincinnati, Cincinnati, Ohio 45267-0528.
T. V. McCaffrey: Department of Otolaryngology, Mayo Clinic, Rochester, Minnesota 55905.

TABLE 1. *Sites of invasion from 292 invasive papillary thyroid carcinomas*

Location	Number
Muscle only	66
Muscle	143
Trachea	109
Laryngeal nerve	131
Esophagus	63
Larynx	30
Other	82
Total	624 sites from 292 tumors

noma around the thyroid cartilage and into the pyriform sinus (Fig. 2). When the carcinoma extends into the wall of the pyriform sinus, intraluminal extension is not uncommon. This results in dysphagia and hemorrhage. The esophagus can be invaded by direct extension of the primary thyroid tumor or by invasion from a metastatically involved paratracheal lymph node (Fig. 3). Tracheal invasion by thyroid carcinoma also occurs by direct extension of the primary tumor or by invasion from a paratracheal lymph node bearing metastatic tumor.

Recent histopathologic studies by Shin et al. (6) have critically evaluated the pathways of direct spread of thyroid carcinoma into the trachea. The perithyroidal fascia adjacent to the trachea is continuous with fibrous tissue between tracheal rings. Points of weakness in the intercartilaginous spaces of the tracheal wall correspond to areas where there is communication between tracheal submucosa (containing nerves, blood vessels, and scant lymphatics) and the perithyroidal adventitia (with its own nerves, blood vessels, and lymphatics). These points of weakness are considered to be the portals of entry of thyroid carcinoma into the trachea. Study of the regional lymphatics in cases of invasive thyroid carcinoma has shown a paucity of carcinoma present, suggesting that direct spread is the primary mode of invasion (Fig. 4).

Because of the proximity to the thyroid gland and the paratracheal lymph nodes, the recurrent laryngeal nerves are often involved by the extension of thyroid carcinoma from either its primary site or metastatically involved nodes (see Fig. 3). The dysphonia that results from laryngeal nerve paralysis is one of the first symptoms of extrathyroidal extension of thyroid carcinoma and may be the first indication of the presence of thyroid disease. However, invasion of the trachea, larynx, or esophagus can occur without recurrent nerve paralysis.

Perhaps the greatest morbidity of invasive thyroid carcinoma is intraluminal invasion of the larynx, pharynx, or trachea. Once intraluminal invasion occurs, the airway becomes compromised, either because of mass effect or laryngeal nerve paralysis. In addition, hemorrhage from the intraluminal tumor mass is common because of the vascularity of most thyroid tumors. Once intraluminal invasion occurs, successful treatment requires radical excision of tumor to control the symptoms of hemorrhage and airway obstruction.

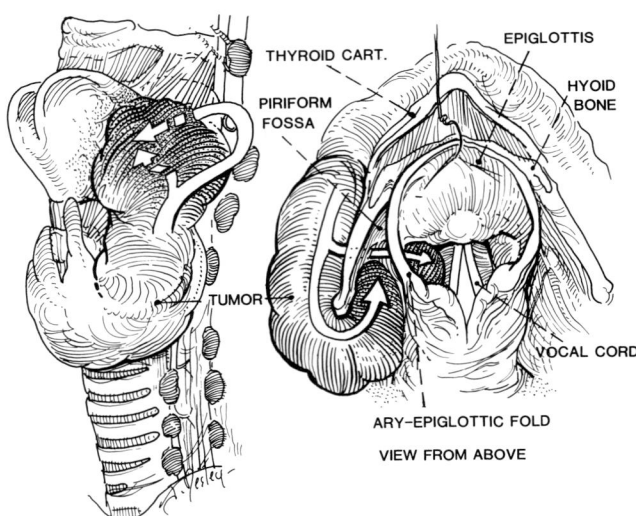

FIG. 1. Laryngeal invasion by a thyroid tumor. Direct invasion of the thyroid cartilage is shown on the *left*. Invasion of the paraglottic space by a thyroid tumor wrapping around the posterior edge of the thyroid cartilage is shown on the *right* in cross-section.

EFFECT OF INVASION ON SURVIVAL

Extracapsular spread and invasion of adjacent structures by anaplastic thyroid carcinoma cannot be successfully treated or palliated. Anecdotal reports in the literature of successful aggressive management of patients with anaplastic thyroid carcinoma imply that long-term survival is improved. However, widespread opinion regarding the management of this neoplasm is to the contrary. Such anecdotes should not be extrapolated to the population of patients with this aggressive, uniformly fatal neoplasm (7). Although extracapsular spread and invasion have been shown to have a negative prognostic significance in well-differentiated thyroid carcinoma, well-differentiated thyroid carcinoma with extracapsular extension and local invasion can be treated successfully.

In the study of papillary thyroid cancer by McConahey et al. (2), extrathyroidal invasion was highly associated ($p < .005$) with risk of development of postoperative metastatic cervical lymph nodes, risk of local recurrence, risk of development of postoperative distant metastases, and risk of death from thyroid carcinoma regardless of the patient's age or sex, or the grade or size of the primary tumor. Intraluminal invasion of the larynx, trachea, or esophagus appears to have a more grave prognostic significance than extraluminal cartilage invasion (8).

In a more recent study by Anderson et al. (4), multivariate analysis of patients with extrathyroidal extension

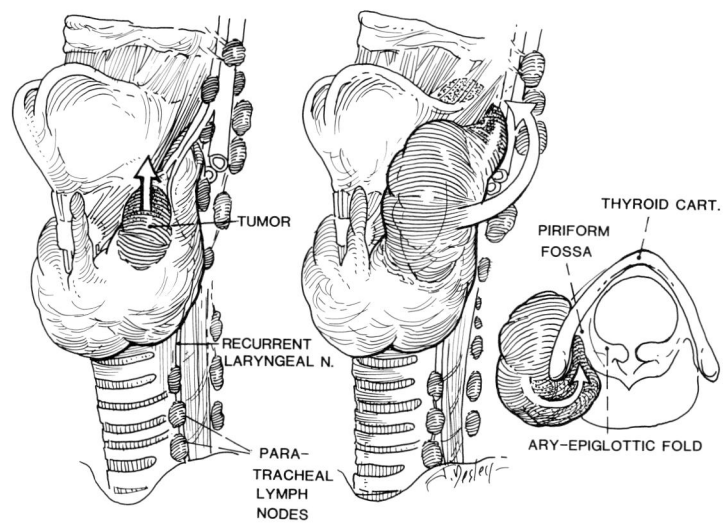

FIG. 2. Example of a large thyroid carcinoma invading the pyriform sinus and pharynx by posterior extension around the thyroid cartilage and through the substance of the thyroid cartilage.

of differentiated thyroid carcinoma demonstrated that an age greater than 45 years old, nonpapillary (Hürthle cell, follicular cell) histology, distant metastases at presentation, tumor size over 4 cm, and incomplete excision all adversely affect long-term survival. In this study, further analysis of patients aged over 45 years old showed no impact on survival when the tumor was incompletely excised. This may suggest a more aggressive course of the disease in older patients with an overall poorer prognosis.

MANAGEMENT

Diagnosis of Upper Aerodigestive Tract Invasion

Symptoms

The predominant symptoms of upper aerodigestive tract invasion are stridor, hoarseness, hemoptysis, and dysphagia. Stridor and hoarseness are most common and can arise from either obstruction of the airway lumen by tumor or paralysis of the laryngeal muscles as a result of invasion of the recurrent laryngeal nerves. Hemoptysis, often severe, is always the result of intraluminal extension of tumor (Fig. 5). Invasion of the pharynx or esophagus, or extrinsic compression of these structures, can result in dysphagia.

Endoscopy

Office endoscopy, using either the laryngeal mirror or the fiberoptic nasopharyngoscope, provides critical information in evaluating thyroid carcinoma. Vocal cord paralysis can readily be detected by laryngoscopy and provides information on invasion of the recurrent laryngeal nerves. If direct intraluminal invasion has occurred, it can be seen, and the site of hemoptysis can be determined. Of all the tests for evaluating the upper aerodigestive tract in thyroid carcinoma, the endoscopic examination is by far the most valuable and must be performed routinely before thyroid surgery so that the need for extended resection of invasive tumors can be anticipated.

Imaging

Diagnostic imaging (see Chapter 9) is helpful in predicting invasion of the upper aerodigestive tract by thyroid

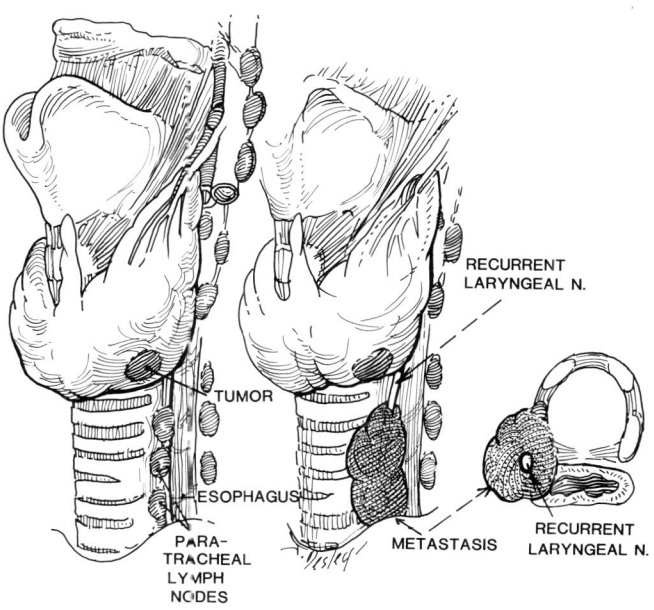

FIG. 3. Invasion of the recurrent laryngeal nerve, tracheal wall, and esophagus by extension of thyroid carcinoma from a paratracheal lymph node.

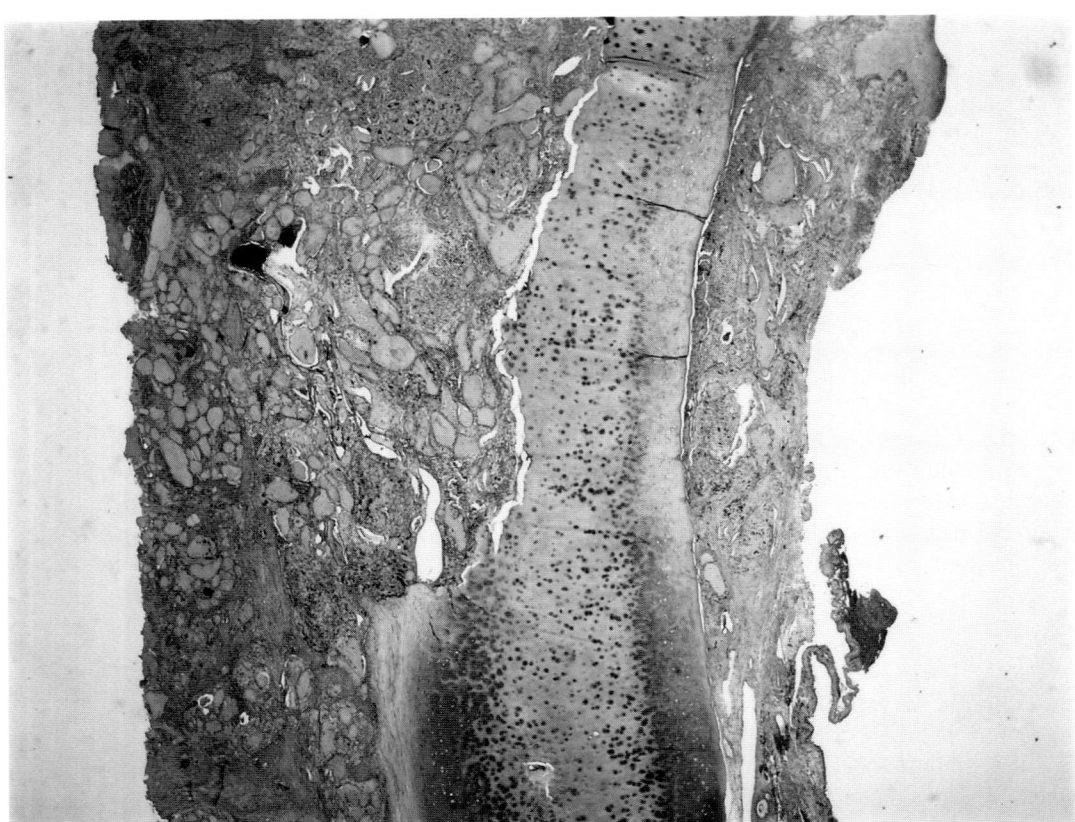

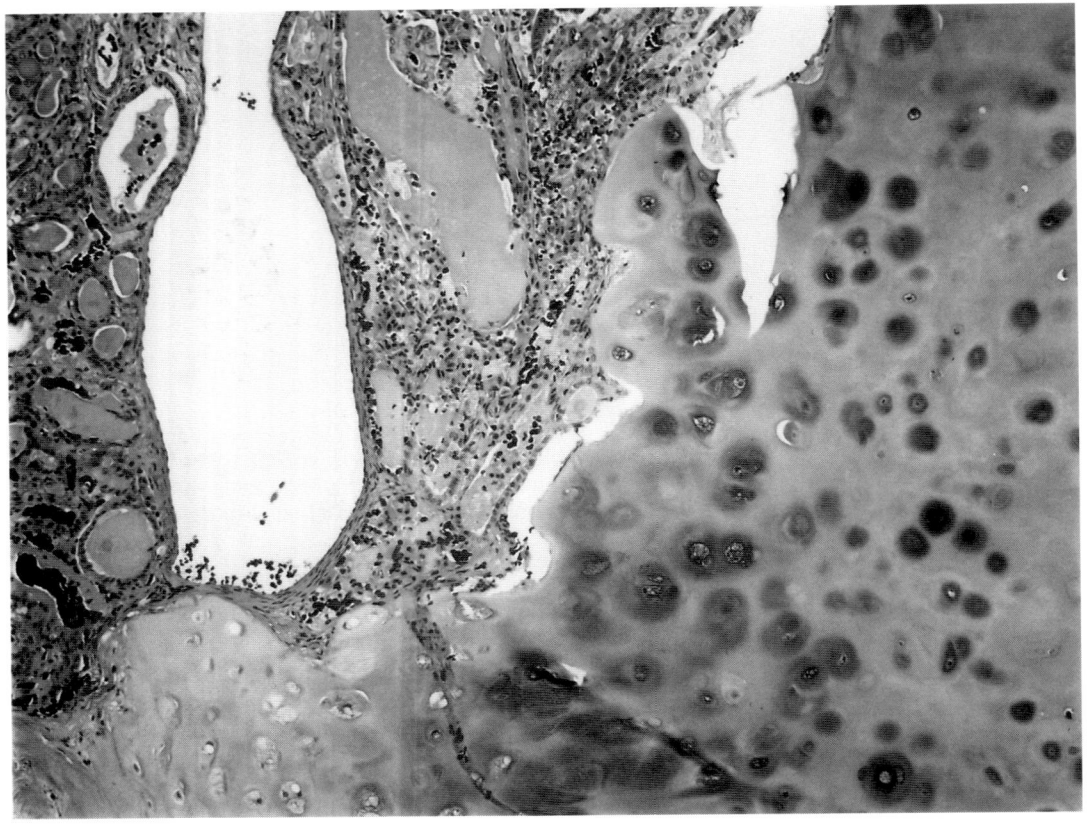

FIG. 4. A: Invasive papillary thyroid carcinoma involving the trachea. Horizontal sectioning of the tracheal wall shows tumor invading deeply into the anterior wall with submucosal extent on the intraluminal surface. (*Top: thyroid margin;* bottom: tracheal lumen.) (×12.) **B:** Higher power magnification shows direct tumor extension into tracheal cartilage. (×100.)

carcinoma. Computed tomography (CT) has been the most useful imaging technique in defining invasion of the cartilaginous framework of the larynx and trachea, which may not be apparent on endoscopic examination or palpation. With better definition of the extent of invasion and preoperative planning, techniques can be used that preserve the functional integrity of the airway while still accomplishing resection of the tumor (Fig. 6). More recently, magnetic resonance imaging (MRI) has also been valuable in evaluating aerodigestive tract invasion. In rare cases, based on CT or MRI evidence of invasion of the carotid artery, preoperative angiography with balloon occlusion of the carotid artery may be necessary to predict the safety of carotid resection. Extensive involvement of the great vessels may require resection of the carotid to remove invasive disease in the field of resection.

Although diagnostic ultrasound examination is sensitive for detecting intrathyroidal tumors and nodal metastases, it is not useful in evaluating aerodigestive tract invasion.

Treatment Planning

Treatment planning begins after the local extent and invasiveness of the tumor, as well as the location and extent of metastatic disease, are determined. The potential curability of the disease must be considered before radical resection of locally invasive disease is undertaken. Several studies have shown no significant difference in survival of patients with locally invasive well-differentiated thyroid carcinoma when treated by radical resection of aerodigestive structures, compared to those treated by near-complete conservative resection (8–11). The technique of shaving tumor from the trachea and larynx to avoid the morbidity of resection has been successful in producing long-term local control of invasive well-differentiated thyroid carcinoma, but only if no gross residual tumor is left behind (7,12). This technique removes gross disease from vital structures in the neck, but it can be assumed that microscopic foci of disease remain, leaving microscopically positive tumor margins that are later treated with adjuvant radiotherapy or radioiodine. The survival curve in Figure 7 shows the similar survivals after radical resection (group I) and conservative resection (group II) of invasive well-differentiated thyroid carcinomas. There is no statistical difference in survival between group I and group II. However, if gross tumor is left behind (group III), death from local recurrence is certain (13).

There is controversy throughout the literature regarding the shave technique for the management of superficially invasive thyroid carcinoma. Grillo et al. (14) state that procedures in which tumors are shaved off the airway and treated postoperatively with radioiodine or external beam radiotherapy are seldom successful and have a high local recurrence rate. Likewise, a study by Park et al. (15) in 1993 showed that shave resection and postoperative adjuvant therapy with radioiodine or radiotherapy failed to control the disease in 12 of 16 patients. It was their conclusion that aggressive local resection should be performed for invasive thyroid carcinoma. The benefits of surgical resection in cases of upper aerodigestive tract invasion must outweigh surgical morbidity. Sacrifice of upper aerodigestive tract function in the absence of residual gross disease to increase cure rate is not justified; conservative management of these patients with preservation of voice, airway, and swallowing results in similar survival when compared to patients undergoing more aggressive resection.

In the presence of intraluminal invasion and hemorrhage, the necessity of controlling life-threatening hemoptysis requires radical excision that may include laryngectomy, pharyngectomy, or tracheal resection (16–18).

The Question of Resectability

Unlike primary squamous cell carcinomas encountered in the upper aerodigestive tract, invasive thyroid carcinoma may often be successfully resected with little margin of normal tissue. Adjuvant therapy with iodine-131 (^{131}I) or external beam radiotherapy can be used to control close or microscopically involved margins (19). For these reasons, the criteria for resectability of invasive thyroid carcinoma are distinctly different from those of squamous cell carcinoma arising in the upper aerodigestive tract. An attempt at resection followed by adjuvant therapy is usually justified with even extensive tumors, because long-term survivals can often be achieved and the morbidity of tumor invasion minimized.

Surgical Techniques

The ability to successfully manage invasive thyroid carcinoma requires a knowledge of surgical techniques that conserve the upper aerodigestive tract. Because a thyroid tumor can invade the larynx, trachea, pharynx, or esophagus, suitable surgical procedures with the potential to preserve function must be utilized by the surgeon. Likewise, aggressive techniques may require the assistance of many disciplines, including thoracic and vascular surgery as well as otolaryngology. Preoperative planning and expertise in the surgical skills necessary for adequate tumor extirpation are critical to the successful management of these patients. Each region of the aerodigestive tract poses unique problems, so techniques will be discussed by region.

Larynx

As discussed previously, invasion of the larynx by thyroid carcinoma can occur into or around the thyroid cartilage lamina or through the cricoid cartilage or cricothy-

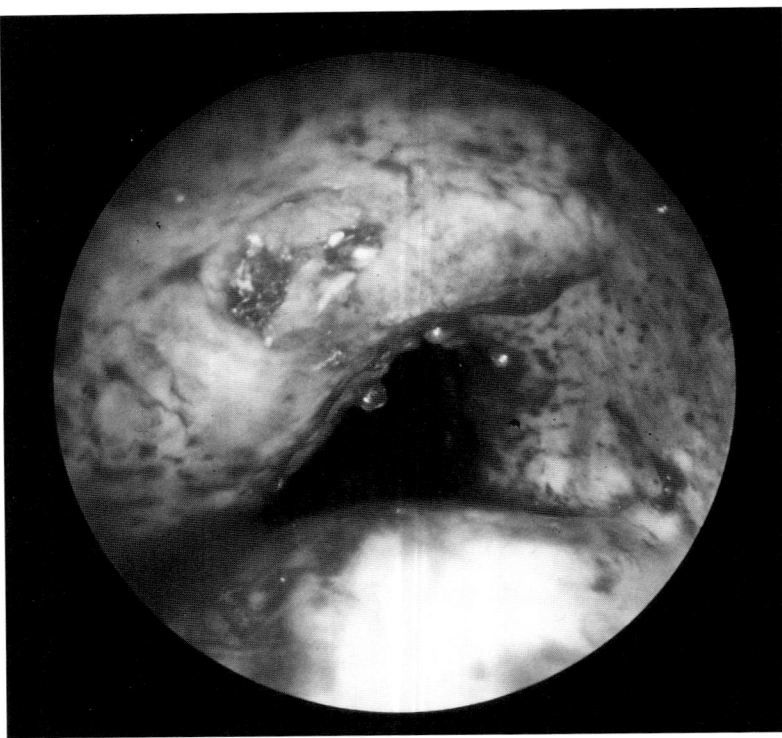

FIG. 5. Intraoperative tracheoscopy demonstrates anterior tracheal wall invasion by well-differentiated papillary thyroid carcinoma. Multiple foci of tumor nodules give the tracheal wall a cobblestone appearance. This was seen and photodocumented on office endoscopy. Patient's presenting symptom was hemoptysis for 1 year. Management included tracheal resection with primary anastomosis and postoperative ^{131}I.

roid membrane. Because invasion is often unilateral, it is possible in many cases to completely excise the carcinoma by performing a vertical hemilaryngectomy or by excision of a thyroid cartilage lamina (Fig. 8). This procedure will preserve airway and voice and permit complete excision of the invading tumor.

Anterior invasion via the cricoid or cricothyroid membrane is less common but entails careful consideration of the structural integrity of the cricoid ring. Excision of a substantial portion of the cricoid cartilage may impair airway function by producing collapse and stenosis of the subglottic airway. If more than one third of the total circumference of the cricoid cartilage is resected, a cartilage graft may be required to reconstruct the cricoid ring, as in laryngotracheoplasty. If more cricoid destruction is present, or resection includes greater than one third of the ring, then total laryngectomy is usually necessary.

Laryngeal Nerve Preservation

Thyroid tumor frequently invades the recurrent laryngeal nerve. If laryngeal paralysis has occurred as a presenting symptom, resection of the nerve with the tumor is required. If voice is subsequently impaired and no compensation occurs, voice rehabilitation by Teflon paste injection or thyroplasty can be performed later.

In some cases, when CT imaging suggests close invasion of the region of the recurrent laryngeal nerves without paralysis, an attempt to preserve laryngeal function is warranted. This is the case when both laryngeal nerves are involved, or when the involved nerve is the only functioning nerve, and resection would result in bilateral laryngeal paralysis and the need for a tracheotomy.

Although there are many techniques for locating the laryngeal nerves during thyroidectomy using well-recognized anatomic landmarks, the presence of invasive tumor or scarring from previous procedures may make precise identification difficult. In such cases, intraoperative monitoring of laryngeal muscle activity has been shown to be helpful (20). This is performed by transoral placement of wire hook electrodes into the thyroarytenoid muscles (Fig. 9). This permits accurate placement of the electrodes into the muscle even in the presence of a large thyroid tumor. Electromyographic monitoring during the dissection in the region of the laryngeal nerves will show muscle discharges as the nerves are approached. More definitive localization of the nerves can be obtained by stimulation of the tissue using a bipolar stimulator. In this way, it is possible to locate a functioning nerve in the midst of scar or encompassing tumor.

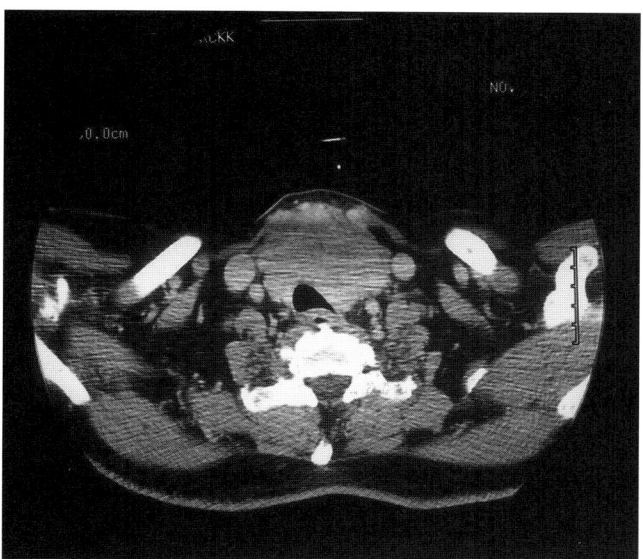

FIG. 6. CT scan of thyroid carcinoma demonstrates obvious deformation of the airway without evidence of gross intraluminal involvement. (Same patient as shown in Figure 5.)

Trachea

Tracheal invasion may occur by direct extension from the primary thyroid tumor or as a result of extension from a metastatically involved paratracheal lymph node. If the tracheal wall is not invaded, shaving the tumor off the trachea is indicated. However, if there is erosion of the tracheal wall and intraluminal extension, complete excision requires segmental resection of the trachea and reanastomosis (Fig. 10). Smaller regions of invasion, involving less than one quarter of the tracheal circumference, can be resected by cutting a window from the involved trachea, and then reconstructed by covering with adjacent fascia or muscle flap (Fig. 11) (17,21). A recent study by Ozaki et al. (22) suggests that window techniques of tracheal resection be abandoned for a circumferential resection and end-to-end anastomosis in management of tracheal involvement. This is based on a histopathologic study of patterns of tumor spread on adventitial and mucosal surfaces of the circumferential trachea. Examination of circumferential tumor spread in the trachea demonstrated invasion on the mucosal surface that exceeded the invasion on the adventitial side in 5 of 21 patients undergoing resection. These results suggest that window sectioning of the tracheal wall in the area of invasion may leave residual disease (22). In settings where control of surgical margins by frozen-section pathology is not adequate, it is speculated that this may predispose to recurrence despite adjuvant postoperative therapy.

Pharynx and Esophagus

Pharyngeal invasion can accompany laryngeal invasion. When thyroid carcinoma invades the larynx around the posterior edge of the thyroid lamina, invasion into the pyriform sinus may occur. Even with intraluminal involvement of the pyriform sinus, resection of the pyriform sinus by lateral pharyngotomy, including a portion of the thyroid lamina, can accomplish complete resection without sacrificing voice or swallowing. More extensive invasion of the larynx and pharynx with intraluminal extension and hemorrhage may require total laryngopharyngectomy to control symptoms and maintain the airway. In these cases, reconstruction can be accomplished

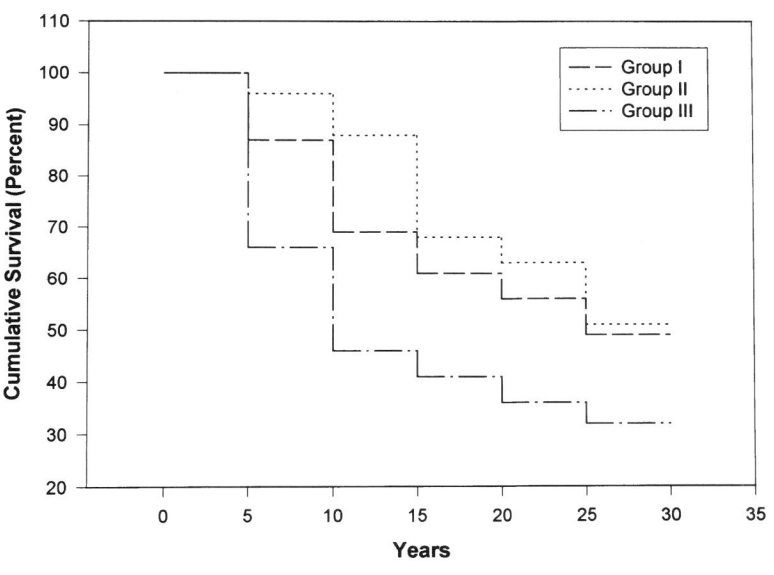

FIG. 7. Survival after aerodigestive tract invasion by well-differentiated thyroid carcinoma for three separate treatment groups. Group I: radical excision; Group II: near-complete excision with preservation of function (shaving technique); Group III: no excision, biopsy only. There is no statistical difference in survival between Groups I and II. All patients in Group III died of locally invasive thyroid disease.

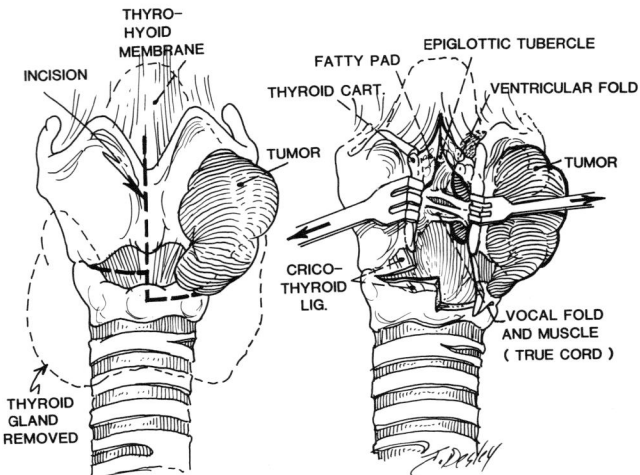

FIG. 8. Partial vertical hemilaryngectomy for removal of thyroid carcinoma invading the left hemilarynx and paraglottic space. Reconstruction is performed using a sternocleidomastoid muscle flap. This technique permits preservation of voice and laryngeal function as well as complete removal of the tumor.

by regional cutaneous or myocutaneous flaps, microvascular tissue transfer, or gastric pull-up.

Invasion of the esophagus may be difficult to manage. Esophageal involvement is often associated with tracheal extension. It is advocated by some authors that extensive removal of gross disease be performed, including the esophageal muscular layers. This leaves the underlying mucosa intact and remaining muscle may be reapproximated in certain cases. Anecdotal reports in the literature state that postoperative dysphagia is minimal and may resolve spontaneously or after dilatation (14). If the wall of the esophagus is invaded with intraluminal extension, treatment will involve resection of the esophagus. Reconstruction in these cases is best accomplished by free microvascular jejunal transfer or by gastric pull-up (23).

Mortality of Disease Versus Morbidity of Surgery

Whether resection can be performed with acceptable morbidity in cases of extensive invasive thyroid carcinoma must be considered. Determining a level of acceptable morbidity will depend on the desires of the patient, the presence of metastatic disease, and the availability of reconstructive options. In the presence of metastatic disease, resection of symptomatic local disease should still be considered. In such cases, less than total excision may be appropriate, especially if such a resection can minimize morbidity and improve the condition of the patient. Extensive resections to establish wide margins are not appropriate when resecting well-differentiated thyroid carcinoma, especially if such a resection would introduce significant morbidity itself. By choosing from the variety of conservation techniques, a locally invasive tumor can be removed while airway, voice, and swallowing function are preserved. Only if conservative resection would leave behind a gross or intraluminal tumor should functional aerodigestive tract structures be sacrificed. With a wide variety of function-preserving operations available, even invasive thyroid tumors can be resected with minimal morbidity, providing extended survival for many patients.

Use of Adjuvant Therapy (see also Chapter 31)

Adjuvant therapy is widely used in the treatment of well-differentiated thyroid carcinoma. It is agreed that the presence of aerodigestive tract invasion is an indication for aggressive use of adjuvant therapy. ^{131}I should be considered in all cases of invasive thyroid carcinoma with sufficient iodine uptake. This will significantly reduce the chance of local recurrence (19).

Less widely used in well-differentiated thyroid carcinoma is external beam radiotherapy. However, this modality has been quite effective in controlling local and regional disease, especially in cases of incomplete excision

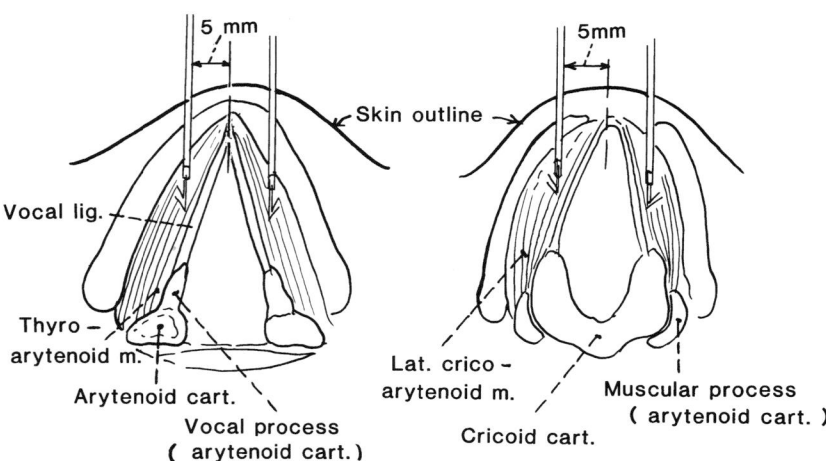

FIG. 9. Endoscopic placement of bipolar wire hook electrodes into the thyroarytenoid and lateral cricoarytenoid muscles for intraoperative monitoring of laryngeal muscle activity. Muscle stimulation indicates dissection in the proximity of the recurrent laryngeal nerve.

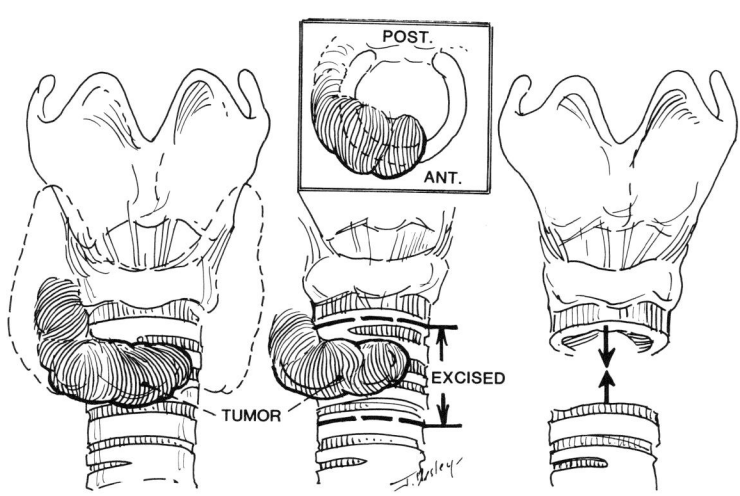

FIG. 10. Segmental tracheal resection for extensive invasion of tracheal wall by thyroid carcinoma.

or microscopic residual tumor or in tumors with minimal iodine uptake that would reduce the effectiveness of ^{131}I. The effectiveness of external beam radiotherapy in moderate doses (4000 cGy over 3.5 weeks) surpasses that of radioiodine when close or microscopically involved margins are present. Although external beam radiotherapy is effective in treating gross local residual tumors, higher doses of radiation are required and the regression of the tumor may be slow (19).

SUMMARY

Well-differentiated thyroid carcinoma infrequently invades the upper aerodigestive tract. When invasion occurs, it is the source of significant morbidity and mortality. The most common structures invaded by thyroid carcinoma are the strap muscles, trachea, recurrent laryngeal nerves, esophagus, and larynx. This may produce symptoms of airway obstruction, dysphagia, and hemoptysis.

Locally invasive thyroid carcinoma can often be successfully treated while preserving function of the upper airway. If the tumor involves only the wall of the larynx or trachea without intraluminal extension, shaving of the tumor from the trachea or larynx will produce survival rates comparable to more radical and destructive procedures. Intraluminal extension is a more serious problem that will usually require resecting a portion of the aerodigestive tract. In this situation, partial laryngeal or tracheal resection with preservation of function may be possible and should be done.

Adjuvant therapy using radioiodine or external beam radiotherapy should be considered an integral part of any treatment plan for these tumors. These modalities will

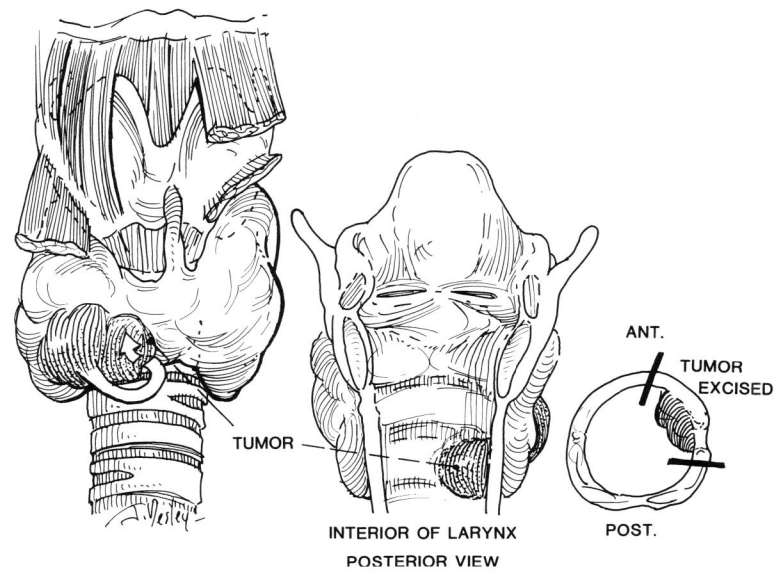

FIG. 11. Limited anterior tracheal invasion by thyroid carcinoma. **Insert:** Resection with a tracheal window. This can be performed when less than one quarter of the tracheal circumference is removed. The tracheal wall can be reconstructed using adjacent muscle or fascia.

significantly reduce the rate of local recurrence and control symptomatic local disease.

REFERENCES

1. Silliphant WM, Klink GH, Levitin MS. Thyroid carcinoma and death: a clinicopathological study of 193 autopsies. *Cancer* 1964;17:513–525.
2. McConahey WM, Hay ID, Woolner LB, van Heerden JA, Taylor WF. Papillary thyroid cancer treated at the Mayo Clinic, 1946-1970:initial manifestations, pathologic findings, therapy, and outcome. *Mayo Clinic Proc* 1986;61:978–996.
3. Batsakis J. Laryngeal involvement by thyroid disease. *Ann Otol Rhinol Laryngol* 1987;96(6):718–719.
4. Andersen PE, Kinsella J, Loree TR, Shaha AR, Shah JP. Differentiated carcinoma of the thyroid with extrathyroidal extension. *Am J Surg* 1995;170:467–470.
5. Tollefson H, DeCosse J, Hutter R. Papillary carcinoma of the thyroid: a clinical and pathological study of 70 fatal cases. *Cancer* 1964;17:1035–1044.
6. Shin DH, Mark EM, Suen HC, Grillo HC. Pathologic staging of papillary carcinoma of the thyroid with airway invasion based on the anatomic manner of extension to the trachea. *Hum Path* 1993;24(8):866–870.
7. Melliere DJM, Ben Yahia NE, Becquemin JP, Lange F, Boulahdour H. Thyroid carcinoma with tracheal or esophageal involvement: limited or maximal surgery? *Surgery* 1993;113(2):166–172.
8. Tovi F, Goldstein J. Locally aggressive differentiated thyroid carcinoma. *J Surg Oncol* 1985;29(2):99–104.
9. Lipton RJ, McCaffrey TV, van Heerden JA. Surgical treatment of invasion of the upper aerodigestive tract by well-differentiated thyroid carcinoma. *Am J Surg* 1987;154(4):363–367.
10. Breaux G, Guillamondegui O. Treatment of locally invasive carcinoma of the thyroid: how radical? *Am J Surg* 1980;140(4):514–517.
11. Segal K, Abraham A, Levy R, Schindel J. Carcinomas of the thyroid gland invading larynx and trachea. *Clin Otolaryngol* 1984;9(1):21–25.
12. Cody HS, Shah JP. Locally invasive, well-differentiated thyroid cancer. 22 years experience at Memorial Sloan-Kettering Cancer Center. *Am J Surg* 1981;142(4):480–483.
13. McCaffrey TV, Bergstralh EJ, Hay ID. Locally invasive papillary thyroid carcinoma: 1940-1990. *Head Neck* 1994;16:165–172.
14. Grillo HC, Suen HC, Mathisen DJ, Wain JC. Resectional management of thyroid carcinoma invading the airway. *Ann Thorac Surg* 1992;54:3–10.
15. Park CS, Suh KW, Min JS. Cartilage-shaving procedure for the control of tracheal cartilage invasion by thyroid carcinoma. *Head Neck* 1993;15:289–291.
16. Fujimoto Y, Obara T, Ito Y, et al. Aggressive surgical approach for locally invasive papillary carcinoma of the thyroid in patients over forty-five years of age. *Surgery* 1986;100(6):1098–1107.
17. Grillo HC, Zannini P. Resectional management of airway invasion by thyroid carcinoma. *Ann Thorac Surg* 1986;42(3):287–298.
18. Nakao K, Miyata M, Izukura M, Monden Y, Maeda M, Kawashima Y. Radical operation for thyroid carcinoma invading the trachea. *Arch Surg* 1984;119(9):1046–1049.
19. Simpson WJ, Carruthers JS. The role of external radiation in the management of papillary and follicular thyroid cancer. *Am J Surg* 1978;136:457–460.
20. Lipton RJ, McCaffrey TV, Litchy WJ. Intraoperative electrophysiologic monitoring of laryngeal muscle during thyroid surgery. *Laryngoscope* 1989;98(12):1292–1296.
21. Friedman M, Toriumi DM, Owens R, Grybauskas VT. Experience with the sternocleidomastoid myoperiosteal flap for reconstruction of subglottic and tracheal defects: modification of technique and report of long-term results. *Laryngoscope* 1988;98(9):1003–1011.
22. Ozaki O, Sugino K, Mimura T, Ito K. Surgery for patients with thyroid carcinoma invading the trachea: circumferential sleeve resection followed by end-to-end anastomosis. *Surgery* 1995;117:268–271.
23. McCaffrey TV, Fisher J. Repair of traumatic cervical esophageal stenosis using microvascular free jejunum transfer. *Ann Otol Rhinol Laryngol* 1984;93:512–516.

CHAPTER 35

General and Regional Anesthesia for Thyroid Surgery

Wen-hsien Wu, Jay Jong-il Choi, and Steven S. C. Cheng

There are two different situations in which patients with thyroid disorders may require surgery: they may need definitive surgical treatment for hyperthyroidism, or they may have underlying hyper- or hypothyroidism and need an operation unrelated to the thyroid problem (1). In either instance, profound disturbances in thyroid homeostasis can ensue during or immediately after surgery.

In this chapter, we discuss the pathophysiology of the thyroid hormones and some of their biochemical, metabolic, and pharmacologic interactions. The optimal anesthetic management of the patient with hyperthyroidism, and of the patient with thyroid storm, during the perioperative period is also discussed.

PHYSIOLOGIC EFFECTS OF THYROID HORMONES

The principal effect of the thyroid hormones is to increase the metabolic activities of most tissues of the body. In humans, the thyroid hormones [thyroxine (T_4) and triiodothyronine (T_3)] exert several functions: (a) stimulation of carbohydrate metabolism; (b) enhancement of protein anabolism and catabolism; (c) stimulation of lipid metabolism; (d) stimulation of the cardiovascular system, as reflected by increase in blood flow, cardiac output, heart rate, blood volume, and arterial pressure; and (e) enhancement of bone resorption by stimulating osteoclasts, leading to mild hypercalcemia, with concomitant suppression of serum parathyroid hormone levels, modest elevations in levels of bone alkaline phosphatase, and negative calcium balance (2,3).

INTERRELATION BETWEEN THYROID, PITUITARY, AND ADRENAL HORMONES

The control of normal thyroid function rests with thyroid stimulating hormone (TSH) of the anterior pituitary gland. In turn, the plasma concentration of thyroid hormones regulates the secretion of TSH, thus establishing a feedback mechanism (4). Cortisone administration for several weeks in euthyroid patients can cause depression of thyroid function (5). In addition, a clinically euthyroid state has been produced in some patients receiving steroid therapy for hyperthyroidism (6).

It has been suggested that the corticosteroids diminish thyroid function by suppressing secretion of TSH (7,8). The relationship between the adrenal medulla and the thyroid is a complex one (9). Hormones react with adenylate cyclase on all membranes to catalyze the formation of cyclic adenosine $3',5'$-cyclic monophosphate (AMP) from adenosine triphosphate (ATP). In turn, cyclic AMP meditates many of the hormonal effects. Catecholamines promote the activity of adenylate cyclase to form cyclic AMP. Thyroxine stimulates adenylate cyclase production by increasing protein synthesis. Thus, the formation of cyclic AMP is accelerated in hyperthyroidism (10).

There is a striking similarity in the clinical manifestation of adrenergic hyperactivity and hyperthyroidism. The influence of thyroid hormones on the serum catecholamines is controversial. It is generally believed that thyroid hormones do not alter serum catecholamine levels or tissue sensitivity to catecholamines, but there are some exceptions (11–13). Nevertheless, the clinical picture appears to present a summation effect of augmented adrenergic and thyroid responses.

W. Wu, J. Jong-il Choi, and S. S. C. Cheng: Department of Anesthesiology, University of Medicine and Dentistry of New Jersey Medical School, Newark, New Jersey 07103.

PHARMACOLOGIC INTERACTIONS

Under physiologic conditions, T_4 increases hepatic mixed-function oxidase activity and so stimulates hepatic drug metabolism in rats (14). As the dose of T_4 is increased well beyond the physiologic range, the stimulatory effect is diminished and, in some cases, inhibition of drug metabolism results. The mechanisms responsible for the dose-dependent effects of T_4 on hepatic drug metabolism in rats probably involves cytochrome P-450. T_4 treatment produces dose-dependent decreases in hepatic cytochrome P-450 activity in hypophysectomized rats of both sexes. Because the concentration of cytochrome P-450 is normally not rate-limiting for hepatic drug metabolism, the effect of the hormone to increase nicotinamide adenine dinucleotide (NADH) cytochrome C reductase activity probably accounts for the stimulation of drug metabolism. With higher doses of thyroxine and progressively diminishing amounts of hepatic cytochrome P-450, it may become rate-limiting and ultimately produce a decline in the rate of drug metabolism. Abnormalities of thyroid function can markedly influence human metabolism of some drugs, including antipyrine (15), morphine (16), and anticoagulants (17). In humans, the half-life of antipyrine is consistently prolonged in hypothyroidism, shortened in hyperthyroidism, and returns to the normal range only when patients are rendered euthyroid (15). Because antipyrine is eliminated from the body mainly by transformation (18), changes in the plasma half-life of antipyrine reflect alterations in its rate of biotransformation. Hypothyroid patients have increased sensitivity to a variety of drugs, particularly narcotics (19,20).

Influence of Anesthetics on Serum Thyroxine

The effects of various anesthetic agents on serum thyroxine levels have been reviewed (21,22). In humans, elevated serum T_4 levels (22% to 35%) were found during anesthesia using diethyl ether (23), halothane (24), and isoflurane (25) without measurable changes in serum binding or increasing the output of T_4 from the thyroid gland. The elevated T_4 levels return to the resting level usually within 2 hr of the end of anesthesia. This represents rapid mobilization of the bound T_4 from the intracellular compartment, particularly in the liver, to the extracellular compartment (23). Methoxyflurane (26) and spinal anesthesia (27) have little effect, whereas nitrous oxide-thiopental anesthesia (23) decreases serum T_3 and T_4. The antithyroid property of thiopental is related to its thiourylene nucleus. In animals, after a single large dose of thiopental (40 mg/kg), impairment of thyroid activity is virtually instantaneous and persists 6 to 7 days (28). Thiourylene, a chemical similar to thiouracil (29), inhibits peripheral deiodination of T_4 to T_3 (30).

Minimal Alveolar Concentration and Thyroid Status

The minimal alveolar concentration (MAC) is defined as the anesthetic concentration at 1 atmosphere that produces immobility in 50% of animal subjects exposed to a noxious stimulus. The MAC has been used extensively to evaluate factors that influence anesthetic requirements. The level of thyroid activity in animals has a minor effect on the MAC for halothane and cyclopropane (31,32). MAC values are temperature dependent, and thyroid-induced changes in the MAC may be attributable to the effect of thyroid-induced changes in temperature on lipid solubility (31). Cerebral metabolism is maintained independently of thyroid activity. This has been shown in brain tissues, where there is no significant change in oxygen consumption in response to T_4 administration (33). Pender et al. (34) suggested an increased sensitivity to anesthetics in the hypothyroid patient, in whom decreases in cardiac output may produce a more rapid anesthetic induction with volatile agents, and, combined with decreased circulating volume and abnormal baroreceptor function, may readily produce hypotension. Similarly, reductions in hepatic drug metabolism and renal drug excretion, as well as depression of respiratory drive, can prolong elimination of both intravenous and volatile anesthetics, leading to delayed recovery from anesthesia (35).

HYPERTHYROIDISM

Pathophysiology

Hyperthyroidism is a complex of physiologic and biochemical aberrations resulting from hypersecretion of the thyroid hormones, T_4 and/or T_3. The most common manifestation of hyperthyroidism is diffuse toxic goiter (Graves' disease). Typically, hyperthyroidism occurs approximately 4.5 times more frequently in women, with a peak incidence in the third and fourth decades of life (36). The other variants of hyperthyroidism include adenoma (Plummer's disease), toxic multinodular goiter, iodine-induced hyperthyroidism (Jod-Basedow disease), chorionic tissue of a hydatidiform mole (37) or choriocarcinoma, hyperthyroidism from thyroiditis, and others (see Chapter 14). Hyperthyroidism during pregnancy occurs in about 0.2% of patients and is most often a result of diffuse toxic goiter (38).

Signs and Symptoms

Signs and symptoms of hyperthyroidism reflect the impact of excess amounts of thyroid hormones on the speed of biochemical reactions, total body oxygen consumption, and energy production. Thyroid hormones increase the number and the activity of mitochondria, as well as their size and total membrane surface (39).

The process of oxidative phosphorylation takes place in the mitochondria. The energy liberated by oxidation is transformed into the high-energy bonds of ATP. This transformation of the energy is termed coupling. Thyroxine induces uncoupling both *in vivo* and *in vitro* (40). Hence, energy cannot be stored and heat production increases. Some of the clinical manifestations of hyperthyroidism are related to compensatory mechanisms for elimination of excess heat. These include sweating, tachycardia, and vasodilation (41).

The cardiovascular responses of Graves' disease are classified as a hyperdynamic circulatory state, characterized by cardiomegaly, pulmonary edema, peripheral edema, tachycardia, mitral valve prolapse (42), and increased cardiac output, imposed by the hypermetabolic state (43). These suggest hyperactivity of the sympathetic nervous system as well as vasodilation of the circulatory beds supplying muscle and skin. The heart responds to the low peripheral resistance with an accelerated rate and augmented stroke volume. These cardiovascular responses, including abnormal left ventricular function, are presumably direct effects of an excess in circulating thyroid hormones, independent of beta-adrenoceptor activation (44,45). Thyrotoxic patients may have electrocardiographic (ECG) changes consistent with left ventricular hypertrophy (46). Thyrotoxicosis in elderly patients, who account for 10% to 17% of the thyrotoxic population, is characterized by insidious onset ("masked" or "apathetic") or by monosystemic presentation with a cardiovascular complaint (47–50). The signs and symptoms include tachycardia, irregular heart beat, atrial fibrillation, heart failure, and occasionally papillary muscle dysfunction (51,52). Atrial fibrillation occurs in 39% of elderly thyrotoxic patients, frequently associated with a heart rate of less than 100 beats per minute (53). In the presence of atrial fibrillation without known etiology, one needs to consider the possibility of apathetic hyperthyroidism.

Thyroid myopathy is associated with weakness of skeletal muscle because of excess protein catabolism (54–56). Thyroxine inhibits the activity of creatine phosphokinase both *in vitro* and *in vivo* (57). The muscles of thyrotoxic patients perform with decreased efficiency as a result of uncoupling of oxidative phosphorylation as well as the inability of muscle to synthesize phosphocreatine (58). Experimental hyperthyroidism showed a reduction of resting membrane potential, rate of rise (dV/dt), and threshold of action potentials recorded in the extensor muscle (59).

Ocular pathology includes varying degrees of exophthalmos, some mild changes, such as upper lid retraction, lid lag, and infrequent blinking (in 50% of thyrotoxic patients), and some serious changes, such as proptosis, and extraocular muscle and corneal and optic nerve involvement (in 5%) (60). A major degree of exophthalmos occurs in about one third of the hyperthyroid patients, and the condition on rare occasions becomes severe enough that the eyeball protrusion stretches the optic nerve enough to damage vision. Exophthalmos is a result of an infiltrative process involving the retro-orbital tissues, and degenerative changes in the extraocular muscles. The etiology of exophthalmos, like that of hyperthyroidism itself, appears to be an autoimmune process. Hepatosplenomegaly occurs in about 2% of patients (36). Decreased hepatic glycogen content is presumably an etiologic factor.

Preoperative Drug Therapy and Other Treatments

It is of paramount importance that patients with hyperthyroidism be brought as close to a euthyroid condition as possible prior to operation in order to avoid perioperative thyroid storm. Thus, only patients in a life-or-death emergency situation should be taken to surgery without the benefit of being rendered euthyroid. In general, treatment for hyperthyroidism includes the use of antithyroid drugs, propylthiouracil (Propacil) or methimazole (Tapazole), beta-adrenergic blockers, radioactive iodine, or subtotal thyroidectomy (61).

Antithyroid Drugs

When time and individual tolerance permit, the patient should receive antithyroid drugs, propylthiouracil or methimazole, which decrease the synthesis of thyroxine. The average onset of action of the thiourylenes is 8 days, and 6 to 7 weeks are required to achieve the euthyroid state (62). The most serious untoward reaction from treatment with these drugs is agranulocytosis, with an incidence of 1 in 500 (63). This reaction usually occurs during the first few months of therapy. The development of sore throat or fever usually heralds the onset of this reaction.

The most common untoward reaction is a mild, sometimes pruritic, papular rash. It often subsides spontaneously without interrupting the treatment. Intraoperative bleeding resulting from drug-induced thrombocytopenia or hypoprothrombinemia has been reported in patients being treated with propylthiouracil (64,65).

Oral Iodide

Lugol's solution (or the tablet) is effective in reducing vascularity of hyperplastic glands in addition to inhibiting hormone synthesis and secretion. Iodine should be administered for 7 to 10 days prior to operation. Acute administration of excess iodine causes a transient inhibition of thyroid hormone formation, the Wolff-Chaikoff effect (66). Lithium has been shown to act similarly to iodide in preventing iodine release from the thyroid (67). If antithyroid drugs cannot be administered for any reason before surgery, adrenergic blockers, in conjunction with steroids and iodide, are used to prepare the patient for emergency surgery.

Beta-Adrenergic Blockers

Beta-adrenergic receptor blockade has been shown to control the peripheral manifestations of hyperthyroidism (68–71) in pregnant patients (72–74) and neonates (75). Thyroid storm in both adults (76) and children (77) has been managed with propranolol in conjunction with antithyroid therapy. However, seemingly adequate propranolol therapy does not invariably prevent thyroid storm (78). Cardiac output is reduced, but oxygen consumption is unchanged (79,80). Heart rate is usually slowed, although it does not decrease to normal levels, suggesting that the circulatory changes in hyperthyroidism are mediated only in part through the beta-adrenergic receptors, and that the T_4 exerts an independent action on the myocardium (44,81).

The combination of oral propranolol (80 mg every 8 hr) and potassium iodide (60 mg every 8 hr) is effective in attenuating cardiovascular manifestations of hyperthyroidism and reducing circulating plasma concentrations of T_3 and T_4 (82). However, we have reported a case in which more than 1000 mg of propranolol per day was not effective in decreasing heart rate below 95 beats per minute (83). The efficacy of propranolol is attributed to beta-adrenergic blockade and to the ability of this drug to interfere with the deiodination of T_4 to T_3 in the peripheral circulation and tissues (84). The half-life of propranolol has been shown to be 3.4 to 6 hr (85). In a patient dependent on beta-adrenergic blockade to control cardiovascular symptoms, the withdrawal of propranolol can precipitate a thyroid crisis or cardiac decompensation. Therefore, the continuation of the drug in these patients is essential. However, beta-adrenergic blocker should be used with extreme caution in managing patients with cardiac failure. Water-soluble beta-adrenergic blockers (atenolol, nadolol, sotalol) are less well absorbed than the lipid-soluble agents (propranolol, oxprenolol, metoprolol), are not metabolized in the liver, and are more slowly eliminated, primarily by the kidneys (86). Nadolol is effective in controlling sympathetic nervous system manifestations of hyperthyroidism with a single daily oral dose of 160 mg (87). Furthermore, plasma concentrations of nadolol are maintained at therapeutic concentrations in the 24-hour perioperative period.

Beta-adrenergic blockers are divided into cardioselective (beta-1 selective) and noncardioselective agents (88). The noncardioselective beta-adrenergic blockers (propranolol, oxprenolol, timolol, nadolol, and stalol) antagonize catecholamine effects at both cardiac beta-1 receptors and at noncardiac beta-2 receptors. Cardioselective beta-1 receptor blockers (atenolol, metoprolol, acebutolol) are therefore preferable in patients with chronic lung disease, asthma, peripheral vascular disease, or insulin-dependent diabetes mellitus. It is known that beta-adrenergic blockade with propranolol may potentiate the hypoglycemic action of insulin and delay the return to normoglycemia in normal subjects, perhaps by inhibition of gluconeogenesis (89). Hyperthyroid patients have diminished hepatic glycogen reserves (90) and are at even greater risk of beta-adrenergic blockade–induced hypoglycemia. As the clinical manifestations of hypoglycemia in the anesthetized beta-adrenergic-blocked patient may not be obvious and may thus go uncorrected, parenteral glucose should be given from the onset of surgery (87). Spot checks for plasma glucose levels should be carried out intraoperatively. Cardioselectivity declines or disappears at high doses. No beta-blocker is completely safe in an asthmatic patient.

One of the recently introduced beta-blockers is esmolol (Brevibloc), which is an ultra-short-acting cardioselective beta-blocker that is rapidly converted to inactive metabolites by blood esterases. After an intravenous dose of 50 to 400 µg/kg per min, full recovery occurs within 30 min in patients with a normal cardiovascular system (91). The indications for esmolol are situations where "on-off" control of beta-adrenergic blockade is desired, as in supraventricular tachycardia (92), perioperative tachycardia, or hypertension.

Definite clinical improvement is seen in patients receiving reserpine and guanethidine (93,94). This is presumably secondary to depletion of catecholamine stores. Elevated heart rate, blood pressure, cardiac output, and cardiac index of the thyrotoxic patient tend to return toward normal. Oxygen consumption is not significantly lowered (95).

Alpha-Methyldopa

Alpha-methyldopa (Aldomet) exerts a centrally mediated antihypertensive effect and interferes with the actions of biogenic catecholamine by forming a false transmitter. It slows the heart rate but does not alter cardiac output and oxygen consumption in the hyperthyroid state (96,97).

Combined Alpha- and Beta-Adrenergic Blockade

Phenoxybenzamine (Dibenzyline) and propranolol have been shown to alleviate thyrotoxic symptoms and to reduce oxygen consumption by 12%, while leaving results of laboratory tests unaltered (98). Labetalol is a combined alpha- and beta-adrenergic blocking agent that causes less bronchospasm and vasoconstriction than propranolol and lowers the blood pressure more rapidly. Labetalol is a more powerful beta-adrenergic blocker than alpha-adrenergic blocker (beta to alpha ratio 3:1 after oral and 7:1 after IV dosage) (88). Usual dosage of labetalol is 2 mg/min. The infusion should be continued until a satisfactory response is obtained. The effective intravenous dose is usually in the range of 50 to 200 mg. When there is bronchospasm in asthmatic patients, beta-adrenergic blocking agents are not advisable. Calcium channel blockers may be an alternative. Their single most important property is the selective inhibition of the slow inward calcium current in those tissues where there is a slow rising calcium-dependent upstroke of the action potential not fired by a fast sodium signal (99). Such tissues are vascular smooth muscle and nodal tissue (sinus and atrioventricular nodes). Beta-blockade tends to enhance smooth muscle contraction, but it impairs myocardial contraction.

Calcium Channel Blockers

Calcium channel blockers hinder the entry of calcium through the calcium channel in both smooth muscle and myocardium, so that less calcium is available to the contractile apparatus in both tissues. The result is vasodilation and a negative inotropic effect (99). Introduced in Europe in 1963, verapamil is the prototype of calcium channel blockers. Although originally used as an antianginal and antihypertensive agent, these properties were soon overshadowed by a dramatic effect on supraventricular arrhythmias (100,101). The usual oral dose is 80 to 120 mg, three times daily. When used for uncontrolled atrial fibrillation, verapamil is infused at a very slow dose (0.0001 mg/kg per min) and titrated against the ventricular response. When there is no myocardial depression, a bolus of 5 to 10 mg (0.1–0.15 mg/kg) can be given over 1 min and repeated 10 min later, if needed; the infusion rate after a successful bolus is 0.005 mg/kg per min for about 30 to 60 min, decreasing thereafter (99).

Corticosteroids

Corticosteroid therapy has been recommended for 1 week prior to surgery. However, it is infrequently used in the hyperthyroid patient rendered euthyroid with antithyroid drugs. Corticosteroids have been shown to diminish thyroid function by suppressing secretion of TSH (7,8). Prednisolone 25 mg, dexamethasone (Decadron) 4 mg, or hydrocortisone 100 mg may be used.

An additional 200 mg of hydrocortisone or its equivalent is administered intravenously during the operation (102).

Preoperative Assessment and Medication

Because of the potential for sudden exacerbation of cardiovascular abnormalities in hyperthyroidism, the effectiveness of antecedent therapy must be evaluated preoperatively. Principal concerns include the patient's cardiovascular status, dehydration secondary to diarrhea, pulmonary ventilatory reserve, psychologic status, the size and consistency of the thyroid gland, and the presence of deviation and obstruction of the trachea or bronchus (1). Mild anemia, thrombocytopenia, increased serum alkaline phosphatase, hypercalcemia, muscle wasting, and bone loss (3) frequently occur in hyperthyroidism. Preoperative laboratory assessment of the hyperthyroid patient includes thyroid indices (total T_4, free T_4, and total T_3), serum electrolytes, arterial blood gases, chest roentgenogram, and ECG. Laryngoscopy, bronchoscopy, computed tomographic (CT) scans of the neck, and pulmonary function tests with flow-volume loop are useful in determining the extent of airway compression. Adequate premedication is essential.

Apprehension aggravates the already elevated metabolic state and causes release of more catecholamines. Short-acting barbiturates and/or diazepam help to relieve apprehension (102). Narcotics decrease the metabolic rate. Anticholinergic drugs in excessive doses tend to aggravate the already present tachycardia and interfere with the normal heat-regulating mechanism. Chlorpromazine reduces the autonomic manifestations of thyrotoxicosis and decreases the basal metabolic rate (103). However, it may be contraindicated in the presence of deranged liver function.

Intraoperative Management

The patient with a large thyroid mass may have a compromised airway because of vocal cord paralysis and/or airway compression. This should be handled in the same way as any other upper airway compromise. Transoral or transnasal tracheal intubation in the awake patient should be used. Preanesthetic preparation must include a detailed explanation of the procedure to ensure maximal patient cooperation. Most patients will require additional sedation as well as adequate topical anesthesia of the upper airway. Topical anesthesia via an in-line nebulizer with a mask may be supplemented by superior laryngeal nerve block or transtracheal injection of 3 to 4 mL of 4% lidocaine to prevent coughing and laryngeal spasm.

A flexible fiberoptic laryngoscope will provide less traumatic and more often successful intubation in some patients. In an awake patient, the time required for intubation is not limited by apnea. Fiberoptic nasotracheal intubation in an awake patient is often easier than an orotracheal approach, because the tracheal tube via the nasopharyngeal route is more in line with the glottis. A lubricated endotracheal tube is advanced through the nostril into the oropharynx and the fiberscope is advanced through the tube for visualization of the glottis. When the vocal cords are exposed as shown in Figure 1, the tip of the fiberscope is positioned just proximally, then 2 mL of 4% lidocaine is sprayed through the working channel of the fiberscope. Thirty seconds later, the tip of the fiberscope is advanced between cords and an additional 2 mL of 4% lidocaine is sprayed into the larynx and trachea.

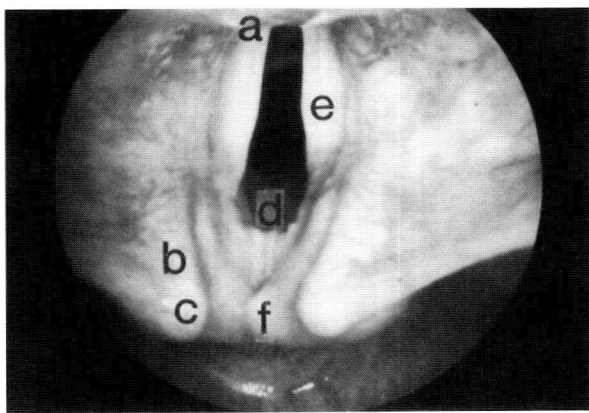

FIG. 1. View of vocal cords obtained prior to intubation. a, epiglottis; b, aryepiglottic fold; c, cuneiform tubercle; d, rima glottis; e, vocal cord; f, corniculate tubercle. (Courtesy of Dr. C. L. Tsay and Dr. W. H. Wu.)

The tip of the fiberscope is advanced to the mid trachea and the tracheal tube is advanced over the shaft of the scope into the trachea. A firm armored endotracheal tube is preferable and should be passed beyond the point of extrinsic compression.

Thiopental sodium is a reasonable choice for induction of anesthesia, as it possesses antithyroid and sympatholytic activities. During maintenance of anesthesia, the goals are to avoid administration of drugs that stimulate the sympathetic nervous system and to provide sufficient anesthetic to prevent exaggerated responses to surgical stimuli (102). Inhalation agents that stimulate the sympathoadrenal axis (e.g., diethyl ether and cyclopropane) are contraindicated. Methoxyflurane (Penthrane) possesses depressant effects on the sympathoadrenal system (104). However, methoxyflurane-induced nephrotoxicity (105, 106) and the possibility of organ toxicity caused by altered drug metabolism in hyperthyroidism do not make methoxyflurane a reasonable choice of inhalation anesthesia. Ketamine should not be used because of its sympathomimetic effect (107–109). Alarm reactions, including severe hypertension and tachycardia, to ketamine in patients taking thyroid replacement medication have been reported (110).

Increasing experimental evidence indicates that the hyperthyroid state enhances hepatotoxicity by volatile anesthetic agents in rodents (111–115). Exposure of T_3-treated rats to halothane, enflurane, or isoflurane results in hepatic centrilobular necrosis (113). The incidence of hepatic necrosis with halothane is approximately 4 times more than with either enflurane or isoflurane. In addition, drug-related hepatotoxicity occurs in patients with hyperthyroidism almost exclusively with propylthiouracil, whereas cholestatic jaundice has been typically associated with methimazole (116). However, patients with hyperthyroidism who are rendered euthyroid preoperatively are not likely to have a higher risk of postoperative hepatic dysfunction after exposure to halothane or enflurane (117). The ability of isoflurane to reduce myocardial sensitivity to catecholamines makes this agent a better choice among inhalation anesthetics (if an inhalation anesthetic is ever called for). Sevoflurane (Sevo), a new nonflammable inhalational anesthetic agent, is similar to enflurane with respect to biotransformation in humans (118). However, this agent has not undergone extensive testing in hyperthyroid patients.

Selection of muscle relaxants must be based on the impact of these drugs on the sympathetic nervous system. Succinylcholine may produce an elevation in heart rate and arterial pressure secondary to the mechanism of ganglionic stimulation (119,120), probably mediated by activation of nicotinic receptors on ganglion cells. Pancuronium causes a moderate increase in heart rate, and, to a lesser extent, in cardiac output secondary to a vagolytic action (121) produced by muscarinic receptor blockade (121–123). Also, pancuronium inhibits re-uptake of norepinephrine by adrenergic nerves (124–126). Gallamine increases heart rate by both vagolytic (127) and sympathomimetic actions (128). Likewise, histamine release after administration of d-tubocurarine, metocurine, atracurium, and succinylcholine would be undesirable. However, histamine-related cardiovascular responses may be prevented by slow injection or by prophylactic administration of antihistamines (both H_1 and H_2 blockers) (129). Vencuronium and Rocuronium are good choices for facilitating endotracheal tube intubation in hyperthyroid patients. Both drugs have hemodynamic effects even in higher doses. As skeletal muscle weakness is frequently present in hyperthyroidism, it is reasonable to reduce the dose of muscle relaxants and monitor the neuromuscular blockade, using a peripheral nerve stimulator. Reversal of nondepolarizing neuromuscular blocking agents should be done, preferably with glycopyrrolate, which causes less tachycardia than atropine. A balanced anesthetic technique using nitrous oxide, thiopental, narcotic, and a muscle relaxant may be used.

Narcotics have been shown to stimulate the sympathoadrenal axis (130,131). However, anesthetic doses of fentanyl (24 to 75 µg/kg) decrease rather than increase plasma catecholamine and cortisol concentrations in humans (132). The effect of fentanyl on plasma catecholamines may be dose dependent. Sufentanil presents a lower incidence of hypertension when used in anesthetic doses (10 to 20 µg/kg) as compared with equipotent doses of fentanyl (133,134). With the exception of meperidine, opioid analgesics usually produce a decrease in heart rate because of the stimulation of the central vagal nucleus in the medulla (135). Sufentanil tends to be more effective in blocking sympathetic activation associated with surgical stimuli, especially in patients prone to intraoperative hypertension (136). Alfentanil is another fentanyl derivative, approximately one-forth as potent as fentanyl. The small volume of distribution of alfentanil at steady state results in an elimination half-life considerably less than that of fentanyl (1.5 to 3.5 hr), and its lower hepatic clearance renders that clearance less dependent on hepatic blood flow (137,138). Because alfentanil provides rapid onset of action, short duration of analgesic effect, moment-to-moment control, protection against hemodynamic swing from surgical stimuli, and prompt recovery, it makes a better choice of analgesic than other narcotics in hyperthyroidism.

Close monitoring of drug delivery and hemodynamics is essential. Controlled animal studies have not demonstrated a clinically significant change in anesthetic requirements for halothane in hyperthyroidism (139). However, increased cardiac output and tissue blood flow in hyperthyroidism accelerate uptake of inhaled anesthetics, resulting in the need to raise the inspired anesthetic concentration to achieve cerebral anesthetic concentration, thus giving a clinical impression that hyperthyroidism leads to increased anesthetic requirements (140,141). Likewise, elevation in body temperature as a result of hyperthyroidism is expected to increase anesthetic requirements about 5% for each degree the temperature rises above 37°C (142).

In general, the induction of general anesthesia in hyperthyroid patients should be done slowly. When using sympathomimetic drugs for the treatment of hypotension, one must consider the possibility of exaggerated responsiveness of hyperthyroid patients to catecholamines. Therefore, direct-acting vasopressors, such as phenylephrine and methoxamine, are better choices than indirect-acting vasopressors, such as ephedrine, which act in part by releasing catecholamines. Laryngeal mask airway (LMA) has been used during thyroid surgery. LMA not only can avoid complications from endotracheal intubation but also can identify and preserve the recurrent laryngeal nerve (143), but further study is necessary to establish the role of LMA for thyroid surgery.

Regional anesthesia, both spinal and epidural, reduces the effects of hyperthyroidism, probably by decreasing catecholamines released by the adrenal medulla and from nerve endings. Whenever applicable, local and regional anesthesia are reasonable choices. The primary innervation of the thyroid derives from superficial branches of the cervical plexus. Thus, anesthesia for thyroid surgery can be provided with blocking bilateral deep and superficial cervical plexuses and the branches of the superior laryngeal nerves supplying the upper pole of the thyroid. One of the advantages of this technique is that the patient's phonation can be tested throughout the surgery to ensure that no nerve damage occurs. Blocking the superior laryngeal nerve and the recurrent laryngeal nerve are therefore undesirable. Only those branches of the superior laryngeal nerve that supply the superior pole of the thyroid are blocked, under direct vision, during surgery (146,147). Epinephrine-containing local anesthetic solutions should be avoided, as systemic absorption can produce exaggerated circulatory responses.

Monitoring

Monitoring during maintenance of anesthesia in hyperthyroid patients includes obtaining an electrocardiogram, the heart rate, and the blood pressure, and using a precordial or an esophageal stethoscope. Monitoring of core body temperature (by esophageal probe) is mandatory. Pulmonary arterial pressure monitoring may be necessary in a patient with congestive heart failure. In addition, transcutaneous pulse oximetry, neuromuscular blockade, and inspired and end-tidal concentrations of oxygen, carbon dioxide, nitrous oxide, and inhalational anesthetics by mass spectrometry should be continuously monitored.

The patient should be placed on a cooling blanket. Refrigerated intravenous solutions and ice should be readily accessible. Arterial blood gas analysis may be needed. Intraoperative problems include dysrhythmia (such as atrial fibrillation), cardiac decompensation, and acute pulmonary edema (148). Oxygen consumption is elevated. Both respiratory and metabolic acidosis occur more rapidly than in euthyroid patients (34). Hyperthermia is likely to occur because heat production is increased (149). Adequate intravenous fluids and electrolytes must be provided to allow copious perspiration and urine output. Serum glucose should be periodically checked. Special care must be taken to prevent drying or abrasion of the corneas of exophthalmic eyes.

Thyroid Storm

Thyroid storm is a severe exacerbation of hyperthyroidism resulting from sudden excessive release of thyroid hormones from the gland into the circulation (140) (see Chapter 40). It is a syndrome characterized by exaggerated thyrotoxic manifestations, fever, and symptoms and signs of prominent cardiovascular, gastrointestinal, and central nervous system function. The cardiovascular signs include marked sinus tachycardia, atrial fibrillation, and congestive heart failure. Gastrointestinal symptoms include diarrhea. Central nervous system signs include agitation to various degrees, mental obtundation, or coma.

The clinical presentation of thyroid storm varies from a febrile reaction after a subtotal thyroidectomy, to hypotension, coma, and ultimately death (150). Thyroid storm associated with surgery can occur intraoperatively, but is more likely to manifest in the first 6 to 18 hr after surgery and is nearly always abrupt in onset. It can mimic the onset of malignant hyperthermia (149). The similarity of these two disorders has been previously reported (149–151). Many of the clinical manifestations of both disorders are compensatory mechanisms for dissipation of excessive heat. Peters et al. (149) have reported two pediatric patients in whom thyrotoxicosis was mistaken for malignant hyperthermia. Both can lead to tachydysrhythmias, fever, and cardiac arrest.

The incidental use of dantrolene in hyperthyroidism has not been reported. Dantrolene produces a generalized muscle weakness by direct action on excitation–contraction coupling, perhaps by decreasing the amount of calcium released from the sarcoplasmic reticulum. It does not alter neuromuscular transmission, but it does produce some CNS depressant effects.

Thyrotoxicosis should be considered as part of the differential diagnosis of malignant hyperthermia in any age group. Serum creatine phosphokinase is approximately half of normal in hyperthyroidism (152), whereas it is elevated in 70% of patients susceptible to malignant hyperthermia (153). Hyperglycemia is likely, reflecting impairment of insulin secretion by thyroid hormone and increased glycogenolysis. The differential diagnosis of intraoperative tachycardia includes paroxysmal atrial tachycardia, cardiac failure, drug actions, early hypoxia, hypercarbia, hypovolemia, "light" anesthesia, fever and sepsis, malignant hyperthermia, myocardial infarction, pulmonary embolus, transfusion reaction, and thyrotoxicosis (154). Symptoms and signs of the differential diagnosis are described in Table 1.

Treatment

The objectives of treatment are to provide supportive care, to inhibit further production of thyroid hormones, and to use various agents that antagonize the effects of thyroid hormones already in the circulation (1). Intravenous infusion of cold crystalloid solutions along with glucose to provide caloric intake is necessary to replace fluid loss that accompanies hyperthermia. Sedation with adequate doses of narcotics, barbiturates, and phenothiazines is necessary. Diuretics, digitalis, vasodilator, and oxygen may be used for congestive heart failure. Drugs including propylthiouracil, sodium iodide, propranolol, and cortisol are essential. Propylthiouracil, 200 to 400 mg orally every 8 hr, inhibits thyroid hormone synthesis and the extrathyroidal conversion of T_4 to T_3 (30). Sodium iodide 500 to 1000 mg IV every 8 hr blocks release of thyroid hormones stored in the gland. It may be started an hour after the administration of an antithyroid drug.

The rationale for giving iodide after the propylthiouracil administration is to avoid any thyroidal accumulation of the iodide that may later be used to synthesize new thyroid hormones (150). Propranolol is necessary to alleviate the cardiac and psychomotor manifestations of thyrotoxicosis, which it does within 2 to 10 min when given intravenously at a rate of 1 mg per min for a total dose of 2 to 10 mg (155). The effects last for 3 to 4 hr after a single dose. Propranolol in doses of 20 to 120 mg given by mouth is effective in about 1 hr, lasting for 4 to 8 hr. Increased metabolism and use of corticosteroids during thyroid storm can result in acute primary adrenal insufficiency, requiring exogenous cortisol re-

TABLE 1. *Differential diagnosis of intraoperative tachycardia*

Diagnosis	Symptoms and signs
Paroxysmal atrial tachycardia	Electrocardiographic recognition of AV nodal reentry at a rate of 150–200 beats/min, hypotension, chest pain, and dyspnea
Cardiac failure	Decreased cardiac output, elevated left atrial pressure, pulmonary venous congestion, dyspnea, cough and orthopnea
Drug actions	Beta-adrenergic agonists, anticholinergics, ketamine, and Pavulon
Early hypoxia	Cyanosis, decreased OxyHb saturation
Hypercarbia	Elevated end-tidal PCO_2, hypertension
Hypovolemia	Hypotension, decreased urine output
Light anesthesia	Hypertension, irregular respiration, vomiting, sweating, lacrimation, increased muscle tone
Sepsis	Bacteremia, fever, early hyperdynamic signs (hypotension, decreased systemic vascular resistance, increased cardiac output), late hypovolemic signs (decreased cardiac output, lactic acidosis, oliguria)
Malignant hyperthermia	Fever, dysrhythmia, unstable blood pressure, cyanosis, diaphoresis, muscle rigidity, respiratory and metabolic acidosis, hyperkalemia, elevated levels of creatine phosphokinase, lactic dehydrogenase, and myoglobinuria
Myocardial infarction	Unexplained cardiac dysrhythmias, hypotension, congestive heart failure, and chest pain
Pulmonary embolus	Pertinent history, dyspnea, tachycardia, substernal chest pain, hypotension, increased central venous pressure, and wheezing
Transfusion reactions	Allergic reactions (pruritis, erythema, urticaria, eosinophilia, laryngobronchospasm, fever, pulmonary edema, and cough) Hemolytic reactions (substernal pain, nausea, dyspnea hypotension, skin flushing, hemoglobinuria, oliguria, and intractable hemorrhage) Delayed hemolytic reactions (jaundice, positive indirect Coomb's test)
Thyrotoxicosis	Cardiac dysrhythmias, fever, increased cardiac output, congestive heart failure, skeletal muscle weakness, diaphoresis, agitation, and coma

placement (140). The dose of cortisol is 100 to 200 mg IV every 8 hr. In addition, pharmacologic quantities of cortisol inhibit peripheral conversion of T_4 to T_3 (1). Acetaminophen is preferred over salicylates in the treatment of hyperpyrexia, because salicylates may displace thyroid hormones from serum binding proteins, leading to increased tissue availability (1).

The duration of thyroid storm varies from one to several days, averaging 3 days (156). Improvement begins within 12 hr of institution of therapy. It has been suggested that the level of consciousness and state of mentation of the patient in crisis are reliable prognostic signs.

Intraoperative Complications of Surgery

Manipulation of the carotid sinus may cause profound hypotension with marked bradycardia or asystole. Infiltration of the area around the bifurcation of the common carotid artery with a local anesthetic may successfully block the carotid sinus reflex. Intravenous administration of atropine is also useful. Venous air embolism is uncommon, but if a large vein is opened, it is possible for as much as 200 mL of air to be aspirated during a deep inspiration (157).

Postoperative Period

The aims of postoperative management are similar to those in the intraoperative period. Thyroid storm is more likely to manifest in the first 6 to 18 hr after surgery, and the treatment modalities are those described above. Other postoperative problems include injury to the phrenic or cervical sympathetic nerves, pneumomediastinum, pneumothorax, and tracheal laceration (102). Removal of a tumor that has exerted pressure on the trachea may produce tracheomalacia, and the trachea may collapse when the endotracheal tube is removed (34). Thus, the patient's airway should be checked carefully during extubation. Immediate reintubation may be lifesaving. The airway may be compromised by hematoma or laryngeal edema. Unilateral recurrent laryngeal nerve injury is usually tolerated; however, bilateral damage may necessitate tracheostomy. Injury to the superior laryngeal nerve results in loss of sensation in the larynx above the vocal cords, thus causing the risk of aspiration.

Accidental removal or injury of the parathyroid glands during thyroidectomy may lead to hypocalcemia. The intrinsic muscles of the larynx are exquisitely sensitive to calcium deficiency. Inspiratory stridor occurs long before overt tetany and results in partial or complete laryngospasm (157). The first symptoms of hypocalcemia (see also Chapter 39) include circumoral or extremity paresthesias and increased neuromuscular irritability (34). Treatment consists of elevation of plasma calcium concentration to an approximately normal range by slow intravenous administration of up to 1 g of calcium chloride, using extreme care, especially if the patient has been receiving digitalis. In the patient with exophthalmos, the cornea should be protected. It is desirable to observe the postthyroidectomy patient in an intensive care facility for 24 to 72 hr postoperatively if the surgeon and anesthesiologist anticipate significant complications.

HYPOTHYROIDISM

Although surgery is not often undertaken for the treatment of hypothyroidism, anesthesia may be necessary for a patient with the disease. *Hypothyroidism* is the generic term for exposure of the body to subnormal amounts of physiologically active thyroid hormones (see Chapter 20). Decreased function of the thyroid gland may be secondary to dysfunction of the hypothalamus or anterior pituitary, or primary as a result of destruction of the thyroid gland. The symptoms of hypothyroidism include dry skin, constipation, fatigue, cold intolerance, hoarseness, menorrhagia, and impairment of memory. Physical examination may disclose hoarseness, periorbital edema, lateral thinning of the eyebrows, brittle hair, dry skin, goiter, hypothermia, bradycardia, and prolongation of the relaxation phase of the deep tendon reflexes (158).

Subclinical hypothyroidism is diagnosed entirely by laboratory studies showing minimally elevated serum TSH with normal serum T_3 and T_4 (159). It does not present any particular anesthetic problem. Mild hypothyroidism is characterized by elevations of serum TSH and low-to-normal T_4 levels. Required surgery in patients with mild or moderate hypothyroidism need not be deferred until the hypothyroid state has been corrected (160). In patients with overt hypothyroidism, T_4 serum levels are markedly depressed, and greatly elevated levels of TSH are seen. Elective procedures are contraindicated in overt hypothyroidism because of the potential for precipitation of hypothyroid coma following general anesthesia (161). Treatment is with exogenous replacement of thyroid hormones. Thyroxine therapy requires up to 10 days to exert a physiologic effect and therefore is not effective for emergency treatment. Intravenous T_3 exerts a physiologic effect within 6 hr and reaches a peak effect within 48 to 72 hr (141). The important anesthetic considerations include profound sensitivity to narcotics (19, 162), somnolence and lethargy resulting from the depressant effect on the CNS (163), depression of myocardial function (164), anemia (165), hypertension (166), impaired free water clearance (167,168), coagulation and hemostatic abnormalities, reduced platelet adhesiveness (169), and low levels of factors VII, VIII, IX, and XI (170), hypothermia (1), and hypoglycemia owing to adrenocortical insufficiency (171). Respiratory abnormalities include impaired ventilatory regulation, alveolar hypoventilation, reduced diffusion capacity for carbon monoxide, and difficulties associated with mechanical ventilation and weaning caused by obesity and chest muscle weakness (172,173). An enlarged tongue may be present in the hypothyroid patient, often associated with amyloidosis, and may hamper tracheal intubation (174).

Hoarseness and dysarthria can indicate myxedematous infiltrations of the tongue and vocal cords (175), whereas dysphagia may be an early manifestation of goitrous esophageal compression.

Intraoperative Management

Induction of anesthesia can be accomplished with the slow intravenous administration of ketamine, a positive inotropic agent in humans (176). Barbiturates or benzodiazepines are not the first choices. Cardiac arrest temporarily related to injection of 200 mg of thiopental in overt hypothyroidism (162) may be attributable to relative overdosage in this hypovolemic state. Maintenance of anesthesia is best achieved by nitrous oxide and oxygen with controlled ventilation if indicated, with minimal doses of short-acting opioids, benzodiazepines, or ketamine (19,162,177). Potent volatile anesthetics are not recommended because of the exquisite sensitivity to drug-induced myocardial depression, particularly in the presence of hypovolemia and/or attenuated baroreceptor reflex response (140). The clinical impression of a reduced anesthetic requirement is most likely derived from a rapid induction of anesthesia, which is a result of the reduced cardiac output, thus accelerating the establishment of a steady state of anesthesia (140). Narcotics, including fentanyl or morphine, may be associated with prolonged recovery from anesthesia (19) or they may precipitate hypothyroid coma (20). Because of its mild sympathomimetic effect, pancuronium may be a useful muscle relaxant, if needed, in hypothyroid patients (140).

Monitoring

Monitoring of hypothyroid patients during anesthesia is directed toward early recognition of congestive heart failure and hypothermia. Measurement of central venous pressure as an index of central blood volume is essential during major surgery. A solution containing dextrose and saline should be utilized for intravenous fluid therapy and must be closely monitored to avoid progressive hyponatremia resulting from impaired free water excretion (178). Because of an increased incidence of adrenocortical insufficiency in hypothyroidism (171), and impaired adrenocortical response to stress in overt hypothyroidism (179), it is recommended that patients with severe overt hypothyroidism receive 300 mg of hydrocortisone daily during any acute stress (158,177). Body temperature must be continuously monitored intraoperatively, as refractory hypothermia-induced cardiac arrhythmias may occur when body temperature falls below 32°C (180). Late postoperative complications seen with overt hypothyroidism include hyponatremia, inappropriate vasopressin secretion, and adynamic ileus (162,181). Postoperative analgesia, if necessary, should be provided with minimal doses of opioids, because these patients are extremely vulnerable to the ventilatory depressant effects of opioids (140).

ACKNOWLEDGMENT

The authors thank Ms. Traci M. Monroe for her dedicated performance in typing this manuscript.

REFERENCES

1. Izenstein BZ, Dluhy RG, Willliams GH. Thyroid. In: Vandam LD, ed. *To make the patient ready for anesthesia: medical care of the surgical patient.* Menlo Park, CA: Addison Wesley, 1980;126–133.
2. Guyton AC. The thyroid metabolic hormones. In: *Textbook of medical physiology,* 7th ed. Philadelphia: WB Saunders, 1986;897–908.
3. Cooper DS. Thyroid hormone and the skeleton: a bone of contention. *JAMA* 1988;259:3175.
4. Pearson OH. Endocrine consequences of hypophysectomy. *Anesthesiology* 1963;24:563–67.
5. Frederickson DA. Effect of massive cortisone therapy on thyroid function. *J Clin Endocrinol Metab* 1951;11:760.
6. Werner SC, Platman SR. Remission of hyperthyroidism (Graves' disease) and altered pattern of serum-thyroxine binding induced by prednisone. *Lancet* 1965;2:751–755.
7. Ingbar SH, Freinkel N. ACTH, cortisone and the metabolism of iodine. *Metabolism* 1956;5:652–666.
8. Wilber JF, Tiger RD. The effect of glucocorticoids on thyrotropin secretion. *J Clin Invest* 1969;48:2096–2103.
9. Crile GW. The interdependence of the thyroid, adrenals and nervous system. *Am J Surg* 1929;6:61–620.
10. Sutherland E. On the biological role of cyclic AMP. *JAMA* 1970;214:1281–1288.
11. Goldfien A, Zileli S, Goldman D, et al. The estimation of epinephrine and norepinephrine in human plasma. *J Clin Endocrinol Metab* 1961;21:281–295.
12. Harrison TS. Adrenal medullary and thyroid relationships. *Physiol Rev* 1964;44:161–185.
13. Stoffer SS, Jiang NS, Gomam GA, Pikler GM. Plasma catecholamines in hypothyroidism and hyperthyroidism. *J Clin Endocrinol Metab* 1973;36:587–589.
14. Rumbaugh RC, Kramer RE, Colby HD. Dose-dependent actions of thyroxine on hepatic drug metabolism in male and female rats. *Biochem Pharmacol* 1978;27:2027–2031.
15. Eichelbaum M, Bodem G, Gugler R, Schneider-Deters C, Dengler HJ. Influence of thyroid status on plasma half-life of antipyrine in man. *N Engl J Med* 974;290:1040–1042.
16. Lund C, Benedict EB. The influence of the thyroid gland on the action of morphine. *N Engl J Med* 1929;201:345–353.
17. Walters MB. The relationship between thyroid function and anticoagulant therapy. *Am J Cardiol* 1963;11:112–114.
18. Brodie BB, Axelrod J. The fate of antipyrine in man. *J Pharmacol Exp Ther* 1950;98:97–104.
19. Kim JM, Hackman L. Anesthesia for untreated hypothyroidism: report of three cases. *Anesth Analg* 1977;56:299–302.
20. Nordquist P, Dhuner KG, Stenberg K, Omdahl G. Myxedema coma and CO_2 retention. *Acta Med Scand* 1960;166:189–194.
21. Halevy S. Effects of anesthesia and surgery on thyroid function. In: Brown BR, Blitt CD, Giesecke AH, eds. *Anesthesia and the patient with endocrine disease.* Philadelphia: FA Davis, 1980;55–90.
22. Oyama T. Endocrine response to anesthetic agents. *Br J Anesth* 1973;45:276–281.
23. Oyama T, Shibata S, Matsuki A. Thyroxine distribution during ether and thiopental anesthesia in man. *Anesth Analg* 1969;48:1–6.
24. Oyama T, Shibata S, Matsuki A. Thyroxine distribution during halothane anesthesia in man. *Anesth Analg* 1969;48:715–719.
25. Oyama T, Latto P, Haladay DA, Chang H. Effect of isoflurane anesthesia and surgery on thyroid function in man. *Can Anaesth Soc J* 1975;22:474–477.

26. Oyama T, Shibata S, Matsuki A, Kudo T. Effect of methoxyflurane anesthesia on thyroid function in man. *Can Anaesth Soc J* 1969;16:204–208.
27. Oyama T, Matsuki A, Kudo T. Serum level of thyroxine in man during spinal anesthesia and surgery. *Anaesthesia* 1972;27:2–8.
28. Wase AW, Foster WC. Thiopental and thyroid metabolism. *Proc Soc Exp Biol Med* 1956;91:89–91.
29. Wase AW, Greenspan J. Effect of sodium 5-allyl-5 (1-methylbutyl) 2-thiobarbiturate on uptake of I^{131} by rat thyroid. *Proc Soc Exp Biol Med* 1953;84:154–155.
30. Oppenheimer JH, Schwartz HL, Surks MI. Propylthiouracil (PTU) inhibits the conversion of L-thyroxine (T_4) to L-triiodothyronine (T_3), a possible explanation of the anti-T_4 effect of PTU and further support of the concept that T_3 is the primary thyroid hormone. *J Clin Invest* 1972;51:2493–2497.
31. Munson ES, Hoffman JC, DiFazio CA. The effects of acute hypothyroidism and hyperthyroidsm on cyclopropane requirement (MAC) in rats. *Anesthesiology* 1968;29:1094–1098.
32. Badad AA, Eger EI II. The effects of hyperthyroidism and hypothyroidism on halothane and oxygen requirements in dogs. *Anesthesiology* 1968;29:1087–1093.
33. Sokoloff L, Wechsler RL, Mangold R, Balls K, Katz SS. Cerebral blood flow and oxygen consumption in hyperthyroidism before and after treatment. *J Clin Invest* 1953;32:202–208.
34. Pender JW, Fox M, Basso LV. Diseases of the endocrine system. In: Katz J, Benunof, Kadis LB, eds. *Anesthesia and uncommon diseases.* Philadelphia: WB Saunders, 1981;155–220.
35. Murkin JM. Anesthesia and hypothyroidism: a review of thyroxine physiology, pharmacology, and anesthetic implications. *Anesth Analg* 1982;61:371–383.
36. Wemer SC. Hyperthyroidism, introduction. In: Wemer SC, Ingbar SH, eds. *The thyroid,* 3rd ed. New York: Harper and Row, 1971;501.
37. Hershman JM, Higgins HP. Hydatidiform mole—a cause of clinical hyperthyroidism. *N Engl J Med* 1971;28:573–577.
38. Burrow GN. The management of thyrotoxicosis in pregnancy. *N Engl J Med* 1985;313:562–568.
39. Peachey LD, Greif RL. Alterations of mitochondrial structure induced by thyroid hormones in vivo and in vitro. *Endocrinology* 1965;77:61–77.
40. Hoch FL. Thyrotoxicosis as a disease of mitochondria. *N Engl J Med* 1962;266:446–454.
41. Hoch FL. Biochemistry of hyperthyroidism and hypothyroidism. *Postgrad Med J* 1968;44:347–362.
42. Channick BJ, Adlin EV, Marks AD, Deneberg BS, McDonough MT, Chakko CS, Spann JF. Hyperthyroidism and mitral-valve prolapse. *N Engl J Med* 1981;305:497–500.
43. De Grook WJ, Leonard JJ. Hyperthyroidism as a high cardiac output state. *Am Heart J* 1970;79:265–275.
44. McDevitt DG, Shanks RG, Hadden DR, et al. The role of the thyroid in the control of heart rate. *Lancet* 1968;1:998–1000.
45. Forfar JC, Muir AL, Sawers SA, Toft AD. Abnormal left ventricular function in hyperthyroidism. *N Engl J Med* 1982;307:1165–1170.
46. Sandler G. The effects of thyrotoxicosis on the electrocardiogram. *Br Heart J* 1959;21:111–16.
47. Bartels EC, Kingsley JW Jr. Hyperthyroidism in patients over 60. *Geriatrics* 1949;4:333–340.
48. Iversen K. Thyrotoxicosis in aged individuals. *J Gerontol* 1953;8:65–69.
49. Seed L, Lindsay AM. Hyperthyroidism in the aged. A review of 100 cases over 60 years of age. *Geriatrics* 1949;4:136–145.
50. Lahey FH. Apathetic thyroidism. *Ann Surg* 1931;93:1026–1030.
51. Forfar JC, Miller HC, Toft AD. Occult thyrotoxicosis: a correctable cause of "idiopathic" atrial fibrillation. *Am J Cardiol* 1979;44:9–12.
52. Symons C. Thyroid heart disease. *Br Heart J* 1979;41:257–262.
53. Davis PJ, Davis FB. Hyperthyroidism in patients over the age of 60 years. Clinical features in 85 patients. *Medicine (Baltimore)* 1974;53:161–181.
54. Adams DD, Rosman NP. Hyperthyroidism: neuromuscular system. In: Werner SC, Ingbar SH, eds. *The thyroid,* 3rd ed. New York: Harper and Row, 1971;615–627.
55. Ramsay I. Thyrotoxic muscle disease. *Postgrad Med J* 1968;44:385–397.
56. Grob D. Myopathies and their relations to thyroid disease. *NY State J Med* 1963;63:218–228.
57. Askonas BA. Effect of thyroxine on creatine phosphokinase activity. *Nature* 1967;167:933–934.
58. Thom GW. Creatine studies in thyroid disorders. *Endocrinology* 1936;20:628–634.
59. McArdle JJ, Games RC, Sellin LC. Membrane electrical properties of fast- and slow-twitch muscle from rats with experimental hyperthyroidism. *Exp Neurol* 1977;56:168–178.
60. Day RM. Hyperthyroidism: clinical and pathological manifestations. In: Werner SC, Ingbar SH, eds. *The thyroid,* 3rd ed. New York: Harper and Row, 1971;535–543.
61. Waldstein SS. The assessment and management of hyperthyroidism. *Otolaryngol Clin North Am* 1980;13:13–27.
62. Solomon DH. Hyperthyroidism: antithyroid drug treatment. In: Werner SC, Ingbar SH, eds. *The thyroid,* 3rd ed. New York: Harper and Row, 1971;682–690.
63. Gilman AG, Murad F. Thyroid and antithyroid drugs. In: Goodman LS, Gilman AG, eds. The pharmacological basis of therapeutics, 5th ed. New York: Macmillan, 1975;1398–1422.
64. Gotta AW, Sullivan CA, Seaman J, Jean-Giles B. Prolonged intraoperative bleeding caused by propylthiouracil-induced hypoprothrombinemia. *Anesthesiology* 1972;37:562–563.
65. Ideda S, Schwess JF. Excessive blood loss during operation in the patient treated with propylthiouracil. *Can Anaesth Soc J* 1982;29:477–480.
66. Thomas WC. Thyroid disease. *Int Anaesthesiol Clin* 1968;6:179–187.
67. Temple R, Berman M, Robbins J. The use of lithium in the treatment of thyrotoxicosis. *J Clin Invest* 1972;51:2746–2756.
68. Shanks RG, Lowe DC, Hadden DR. Controlled trial of propranolol in thyrotoxicosis. *Lancet* 1969;1:993–998.
69. Vinik AJ, Pimstone BL, Hoffenberg R. Sympathetic nervous system blocking in hyperthyroidism. *J Clin Endocrinol Metab* 1968;28:725–727.
70. Lee TC, Coffey RJ, Mackin J. The use of propranolol in surgical treatment of thyrotoxic patients. *Ann Surg* 1973;177:643–647.
71. Michie W, Hamer-Hodges DW, Pegg CAS. Beta-blockade and partial thyroidectomy for thyrotoxicosis. *Lancet* 1974;1:1009–1011.
72. Jackson GL. Treatment of hyperthyroidism in pregnancy. *Penn Med* 1973;76:56–57.
73. Langer A, Hung CT, McAnulty JA. Adrenergic blockade: a new approach to hyperthyroidism during pregnancy. *Obstet Gynecol* 1974;44:181–186.
74. Bullock JL, Harris RE, Young R. Treatment of thyrotoxicosis during pregnancy with propranolol. *Am J Obstet Gynecol* 1975;121:242–245.
75. Pemberton PJ, McConnell B, Shanks RG. Neonatal thyrotoxicosis treated with propranolol. *Arch Dis Child* 1974;40:813–815.
76. Buckle RM. Treatment of thyroid crisis by beta-adrenergic blockade. *Acta Endocrinol (Copenh)* 1968;57:168–176.
77. Galaburda M, Rosman NP, Haddow JE. Thyroid storm in an 11-year old boy managed by propranolol. *Pediatrics* 1974;53:920–922.
78. Eriksson M, Rubenfeld S, Garber AJ, Kohler PO. Propranolol does not prevent thyroid storm. *N Engl J Med* 1977;296(5):263–264.
79. Howitt G, Rowlands DJ. Beta-sympathetic blockade in hyperthyroidism. *Lancet* 1966;1:628–631.
80. Howitt G, Rowlands DJ, Leung DY. Myocardial contractility and the effects of beta adrenergic blockade in hypothyroidism and hyperthyroidism. *Clin Sci* 1968;34:485–495.
81. Pietras RJ, Real MA, Poticha GS. Cardiovascular responses in hyperthyroidism. The influence of adrenergic receptor blockade. *Arch Intern Med* 1972;129:426–429.
82. Feek CM, Sawers SJ, Irvine WJ. Combination of potassium iodide and propranolol in preparation of patients with Graves' disease for thyroid surgery. *N Engl J Med* 1980;302:883–885.
83. Choi JJ, Rosenblum CS, Wu WH. "Surgery" as one of preoperative managements in the thyrotoxic patient. 1990 (manuscript submitted.)
84. Verhoeven RP, Visser TJ, Docter R, Hennemann G, Schalekamp MADH. Plasma thyroxine, 3,3′,5-thiiodothyronine and 3,3′,5′-triiodothyronine during beta-adrenergic blockade in hyperthyroidism. *J Clin Endocrinol Metab* 1977;44:1002–1005.
85. Faulkner L, Hopkins JT, Boerth RC. Time required for complete recovery from chronic propranolol therapy. *N Engl J Med* 1973;289:607–609.
86. Feely J, DeVane F, MacLean D. Beta-blockers and sympathomimetics. *Br Med J [Clin Res]* 1983;286:1043–1047.
87. Hamilton WFD, Forrest AL, Gunn A, Peden NR, Feely J. Beta-

adrenoceptor blockade and anesthesia for thyroidectomy. *Anaesthesia* 1984;39:335–342.
88. Opie LH, Sonnenblick EH, Kaplan NM, Thadani U. Beta-blocking agents. In: Opie LH, ed. *Drugs for the heart.* Orlando, FL: Grune & Stratton, 1987;1–18.
89. Newman RJ. Comparison of propranolol, metoprolol and acebutol in insulin-induced hypoglycaemia. *Br Med J [Clin Res]* 1976;2:447–449.
90. Kimberg, DV. Liver. In: Werner SC, Ingbar SH, eds. *The thyroid,* 3rd ed. New York: Harper and Row, 1971;569–573.
91. Gorczynski RJ, Quon CY, Krasula RW, Matier WL. Esmolol. In: Scriabine A, ed. *New drugs annual: cardiovascular drugs,* vol. 3. New York: Raven Press, 1985;99–119.
92. Byrd RC, Sung RJ, Marks J. Safety and efficacy of esmolol for control of ventricular rate in supraventricular tachycardia. *J Am Coll Cardiol* 1984;3:394–399.
93. Canary JJ, Schaaf M, Duffy BJ. Effects of oral and intramuscular administration of reserpine in thyrotoxicosis. *N Engl J Med* 1957;257:435–442.
94. Lee NW, Bronsky D, Waldstein SS. Studies of thyroid and sympathetic nervous systems interrelationships. II. Effects of guanethidine on manifestations of hyperthyroidism. *J Clin Endocrinol Metab* 1962;22:879–885.
95. Goldstein S, Killip T. Catecholamine depletion in thyrotoxicosis. Effects of guanethidine on cardiovascular dynamics. *Circulation* 1965;31:219–227.
96. Theilen EO, Wilson WR, Tutunji EJ. The acute hemodynamic effects of alphamethyldopa in thyrotoxic patients and normal subjects. *Metabolism* 1963;12:625–630.
97. Ingenito AJ, Barrch JP, Procita L. A centrally mediated peripheral hypotensive effect of methyldopa. *J Pharmacol Exp Ther* 1970;175:593–599.
98. Stout BD, Wiener L, Cox JW. Combined alpha and beta sympathetic blockade in hyperthyroidism. Clinical and metabolic effects. *Ann Intern Med* 1969;70:963–970.
99. Opie LH, Singh BN. Calcium channel antagonists. In: Opie LH, ed. *Drugs for the heart.* Orlando, FL: Grune & Stratton, 1987;34–53.
100. Schamroth L, Krikler DM, Garrett C. Immediate effects of intravenous verapamil in cardiac arrhythmias. *Br Med J [Clin Res]* 1972;1:660–662.
101. Talano JV, Tommaso C. Slow channel calcium antagonists in the treatment of supraventricular tachycardia. *Prog Cardiovasc Dis* 1982;25:141–156.
102. Stehling LC. Anesthetic management of the patient with hyperthyroidism. *Anesthesiology* 1974;41:585–595.
103. Boutros AR. Anesthesia and the thyroid gland: a review. *Can Anaesth Soc J* 1961;8:586–615.
104. Li TH, Shaul MS, Etsten BE. Decreased adrenal venous catecholamine concentrations during methoxyflurane anesthesia. *Anesthesiology* 1968;29:1145–1152.
105. Mazze RI, Cousins MJ, Kosek JC. Dose-related methoxyflurane nephrotoxicity in rats: a biochemical and pathologic correlation. *Anesthesiology* 1972;36:571–587.
106. Richley JE, Smith RB. Renal failure after methoxyflurane anesthesia. *Anaesthesia* 1972;27:9–13.
107. Traber DL, Wilson RD, Priano LL. Blockade of the hypertensive response to ketamine. *Anesth Analg* 1970;49:420–426.
108. Traber DL, Wilson RD, Priano LL. A detailed study of the cardiopulmonary response to ketainine and its blockade by atropine. *South Med J* 1970;83:1077–1081.
109. Traber DL, Wilson RD, Priano LL. Involvement of the sympathetic nervous system in the pressor response to ketamine. *Anesth Analg* 1969;48:248–252.
110. Kaplan JA, Cooperman LH. Alarming reactions to ketamine in patients taking thyroid medication—treatment with propranolol. *Anesthesiology* 1971;35:229–230.
111. Calvert DN, Brody TM. The effects of thyroid function upon carbon tetrachloride hepatotoxicity. *J Pharmacol Exp Ther* 1961;134:304–310.
112. Wood M, Berman ML, Harbison RD, Hoyle P, Phythyon JM, Wood AJJ. Halothane-induced hepatic necrosis in triiodothyronine-pretreated rats. *Anesthesiology* 1980;52:470–476.
113. Berman ML, Kuhnert L, Phythyon JM, Holaday DA. Isoflurane and enflurane induced hepatic necrosis in triiodothyronine pretreated rats. *Anesthesiology* 1983;58:1–5.
114. Holaday DA, Berman ML, England R, Abumrad N. The effect of halothane on metabolic pathways in the hyperthyroid rat *(abstract). Anesthesiology* 1984;61:A266.
115. Berman ML, Kuhnert L, Phythyon JM, Holaday DA. Lack of gender effect of triiodothyronine enhancement of halothane induced hepatotoxicity *(abstract). Anesthesiology* 1984;61:A275.
116. Smith AC, Berman ML, James RC, Harbison RD. Characterization of hyperthyroidism enhancement of halothane-induced hepatotoxicity. *Biochem Pharmacol* 1983;32:3531–3539.
117. Seino H, Dohi S, Aiyoshi Y, Mizutani T, Nakamura K, Naito H. Postoperative hepatic dysfunction after halothane or enflurane anesthesia in patients with hyperthyroidism. *Anesthesiology* 1986;64:122–125.
118. Holaday DA, Smith FR. Clinical characteristics and biotransformation of sevoflurane in healthy human volunteers. *Anesthesiology* 1981;54:100–106.
119. Galindo AHF, Davis TB. Succinylcholine and cardiac excitability. *Anesthesiology* 1962;23:32–40.
120. Goat VA, Feldman SA. The dual action of suxamethonium on the isolated rabbit heart. *Anaesthesia* 1972;27:149–153.
121. Miller RD, Eger EI II, Stevens WC, Gibbons R. Pancuronium induced tachycardia in relation to alveolar halothane, dose of pancuronium, and prior atropine. *Anesthesiology* 1975;42:353–355.
122. Hughes R, Chapple DJ. Effects of non-depolarizing neuromuscular blocking agents on autonomic mechanisms in cats. *Br J Anaesth* 1976;48:59–68.
123. Marshall IG. The ganglion blocking and vagolytic action of three short-acting neuromuscular blocking agents in the cat. *J Pharm Pharmacol* 1973;25:530–536.
124. Doherty JR, McGrath JC. Sympathomimetic effects of pancuronium bromide on the cardiovascular system of the pithed rat. *Br J Pharmacol* 1978;64:589–599.
125. Quintana A. Effect of pancuronium bromide on the adrenergic reactivity of the isolated rat vas deferens. *Eur J Pharmacol* 1977;46:275–277.
126. Ivankovich AD, Miletich DJ, Albrecht RF, Zahed B. The effect of pancuronium on myocardial contraction and catecholamine metabolism. *J Pharm Pharmacol* 1975;27:837–841.
127. Eiselle JH, Marta JA, Davis HS. Quantitative aspects of the chronotropic and neuromuscular effects of gallamine in anesthetized man. *Anesthesiology* 1971;35:630–633.
128. Brown BB Jr, Crout JR. The sympathomimetic effect of gallamine on the heart. *J Pharmacol Exp Ther* 1970;172:266–273.
129. Scott RRF, Savarese JJ, Alil H-H, Gargarian M. Atracurium: clinical strategies for preventing histamine release and attenuating the hemodynamics response. *Anesthesiology* 1984;61:A287.
130. Giesecke AH, Jenkins MT, Crout JR. Urinary epinephrine and norepinephrine during Innovar-nitrous oxide anesthesia in man. *Anesthesiology* 1967;28:701–704.
131. Zauder HL. The effect of certain analgesic drugs and adrenal cortical hormones on the brain of normal and hypophysectomized rats as measured by the thiobarbituric acid reagent. *J Pharmacol Exp Ther* 1951;101:40–46.
132. Stanley TH, Berman L, Green O, Robertson D. Plasma catecholamine and cortisol response to fentanyl-oxygen anesthesia for coronary artery operations. *Anesthesiology* 1980;53:250–253.
133. Sebel PS, Bovill JG. Cardiovascular efects of sufentanil anesthesia. *Anesth Analg* 1982;61:115–119.
134. Sebel PS, Bovill JG, Boekhorst RAA, Rog N. Cardiovascular effects of high dose fentanyl anaesthesia. *Acta Anaesthesiol Scand* 1982;26:308–315.
135. Reitan JA, Stendert KB, Wymore ML, Martucci RW. Central vagal control of fentanyl induced bradycardia during halothane anesthesia. *Anesth Analg* 1978;57:31–36.
136. Rosow CE, Philbin DM, Keegan CR, Moss J. Hemodynamics and histamine release during induction with sufentanil or fentanyl. *Anesthesiology* 1984;60:489–491.
137. Stanski DR, Hug CC Jr. Editorial: Alfentanil—a kinetically predictable narcotic analgesic. *Anesthesiology* 1982;57:435–438.
138. Hug CC Jr, Stanski DR. In reply. *Anesthesiology* 1983;59:257.
139. Babad AA, Eger EI. The effects of hyperthyroidism and hypothyroidism on halothane and oxygen requirements in dogs. *Anesthesiology* 1968;29:1087–1093.
140. Stoelting RK, Dierdorf SF, McCammon RL. Thyroid gland. In: *Anesthesia and co-existing disease,* 2nd ed. New York: Churchill Livingstone, 1988;473–486.
141. Pender JW, Fox M, Basso LV. Thyroid gland. In: Kadis J, Kadis LB, eds. *Anesthesia and uncommon diseases; pathophysiologic and clinical correlations.* Philadelphia: WB Saunders, 1973;108–115.

142. Steffey EP, Eger EI. Hyperthermia and halothane MAC in the dog. *Anesthesiology* 1974;41:392–396.
143. Greatorex RA, Denny NM. Application of the laryngeal mask airway to thyroid surgery and preservation of the recurrent laryngeal nerve. *Ann R Coll Surg Engl* 1991;7B(b):352–354.
144. Knight RT. Use of spinal anesthesia to control sympathetic overactivity in hyperthyroidism. *Anesthesiology* 1945;6:225–238.
145. Brewster WR Jr, Issacs JP, Osgood PF, King TL. The hemodynamic and metabolic interrelationships in the activity of epinephrine, norepinephrine and the thyroid hormones. *Circulation* 1956;13:1–20.
146. Bahr VV. Local anesthesia for thyroid surgery. In: Erikson E, ed. *Illustrated handbook in local anaesthesia*. Philadelphia: WB Saunders, 1980;43–45.
147. Raj PP. *Handbook of regional anesthesia*. New York: Churchill Livingstone, 1985;55–56.
148. Kadis LB, Bennett EJ, Dalal FV, Zauder HL. Anesthetic management of thyrotoxicosis. *Anesth Analg* 1966;45:415–421.
149. Peters KT, Nance P, Wingard DW. Malignant hyperthyroidism or malignant hyperthermia? *Anesth Analg* 1981;60:613–615.
150. MacKin JF, Canary JJ, Pittman CS. Thyroid storm and its management. *N Engl J Med* 1974;291:1396–1398.
151. Murray JF. Hyperpyrexia of uncertain origin. *Br J Anaesth* 1978;50:387–388.
152. Nevins MA, Madhukar S, Bright M, Lyon LF. Pitfalls in interpreting serum creatine phosphokinase activity. *JAMA* 1973;224:1382–1386.
153. Gronert GA. Malignant hyperthermia. *Anesthesiology* 1980;53:395–423.
154. Thornton HL, Knight PF. *Emergency anesthesia*. Baltimore: Williams and Wilkins, 1965;386–387.
155. Parsons V, Jewitt D. Beta-adrenergic blockade in the management of acute thyrotoxic crisis, tachycardia, and arrhythmias. *Postgrad Med J* 1967;43:756–762.
156. Waldstein SS, Slodki SJ, Kaganiec GI. A clinical study of thyroid storm. *Ann Intern Med* 1960;52:626–642.
157. Kritchman MM, Papper EM. Anesthesia in thyroid disease. In: Werner SC, Ingbar SH, eds. *The thyroid*, 3rd ed. New York: Harper and Row, 1971;481–488.
158. White VA, Kumagai LF. Preoperative endocrine and metabolic considerations. *Med Clin North Am* 1979;63:1321–1334.
159. Evered DC, Ormstron BJ, Smith PA, Hall R, Bird T. Grades of hypothyroidism. *Br Med J [Clin Res]* 1973;1:657–662.
160. Weinberg AD, Brennan MD, Gorman CA, Marsh HM, O'Fallon WM. Outcome of anesthesia and surgery in hypothyroid patients. *Arch Intern Med* 1983;143:893–897.
161. Senior RM, Birge SJ, Wessler S, Avioli SV. The recognition and management of myxedema coma. *JAMA* 1971;217:61–65.
162. Abbott TR. Anaesthesia in untreated myxoedema: report of two cases. *Br J Anaesth* 1967;39:510–514.
163. Kudrjavcev T. Neurologic complications of thyroid dysfunction. *Adv Neurol* 1978;19 619–636.
164. Bough EW, Crowley WF, Ridgway EC. Myocardial function in hypothyroidism. *Arch Intern Med* 1978;138:1476–1480.
165. Hines JD, Halsted CH, Griggs RC. Megaloblastic anemia secondary to folate deficiency associated with hypothyroidism. *Ann Intern Med* 1968;68:792–805.
166. Fuller H Jr, Spittel JA Jr, McConahey WM, Schirger A. Myxedema and hypertension. *Postgrad Med* 1966;40:425–428.
167. Goldberg M, Reivich M. Studies on the mechanism of hyponatremia and impaired water excretion in myxedema. *Ann Intern Med* 1962;56:120–130.
168. Pettinger WA, Talner L, Ferris TF. Inappropriate secretion of antidiuretic hormone due to myxedema. *N Engl J Med* 1965;272:363–364.
169. Edson JR, Fecher DR, Doe RP. Low platelet adhesiveness and other hemostatic abnormalities in hypothyroidism. *Ann Intern Med* 1975;82:342–346.
170. Simone JV, Abildgaard CF, Schulman I. Blood coagulation in thyroid dysfunction. *N Engl J Med* 1965;273:1057–1061.
171. Carpenter CCJ, Solomon N, Silverberg SG. Schmidt's syndrome (thyroid and adrenal insufficiency): a review of the literature and report of fifteen new cases including ten instances of co-existent diabetes mellitus. *Medicine (Baltimore)* 1964;43:153–180.
172. Wilson WR, Bedell GN. The pulmonary abnormalities in myxedema. *J Clin Invest* 1960;39:42–55.
173. Zwillich CW, Pierson DJ, Hofeldt FD. Ventilatory control in myxedema and hypothyroidism. *N Engl J Med* 1975;292:662–665.
174. Roizen MF. Anesthesia for the patient with endocrine disease. In: Moya F, ed. *Current reviews in clinical anesthesia. Curr Rev* 1987;8:41–48.
175. Ritter RN. The effects of hypothyroidism upon the ear, nose, and throat: a clinical and experimental study. *Laryngoscope* 1967;77:1427–1479.
176. Tweed WA, Minuck M, Myrnia D. Circulatory response to ketamine anesthesia. *Anesthesiology* 1972;37:613–619.
177. James ML. Endocrine disease and anesthesia. *Anaesthesia* 1970;25:232–252.
178. Shalev O, Naparestek Y, Brezis M, Ben Yishai D. Hyponatremia in myxedema: a suggested therapeutic approach. *Isr J Med Sci* 1979;15:913–916.
179. Ridgway EC, McCammon JA, Benotti J, Maloof F. Acute metabolic responses in myxedema to large doses of intravenous l-thyroxin. *Ann Intern Med* 1972;77:549–555.
180. Reuler JB. Hypvothermia: pathophysiology, clinical settings and management. *Ann Intern Med* 1978;89:519–527.
181. Nelson JC, Palmer FJ, Bowyer AF. The successful treatment of myxedema and coronary artery disease in patients intolerant of thyroid hormone. *Med Arts Sci* 1974;29:15–22.

CHAPTER 36

The Technique of Thyroidectomy by Cervical and Thoracic Approaches

Eric A. Birken, Stephen A. Falk, and Richard H. Feins

In describing thyroidectomy, a variety of terms are applied to similar procedures, making current nomenclature confusing. To avoid confusion, one should specify separately for each side of the thyroid gland which portions are removed (unnecessary in the case of total thyroidectomy) and the procedure performed. The surgical procedures include partial thyroid lobectomy, subtotal lobectomy, total lobectomy, bilateral subtotal thyroidectomy, near-total thyroidectomy, and total thyroidectomy.

Partial thyroid lobectomy is not advocated, because it is a nonanatomic biopsy technique. An exception to this is when a biopsy is performed of suspected anaplastic thyroid carcinoma or lymphoma. Unilateral thyroid lobectomy consists of removal of one thyroid lobe with division of the gland at the isthmus, and it is considered the minimal operation performed on the thyroid gland, often providing an anatomic biopsy technique. This is so because the thyroid gland is not violated during the course of the procedure until the end, when the isthmus is divided between clamps. This technique, therefore, offers the advantages of maintaining a bloodless field and allowing excellent visualization with identification and preservation of all important anatomic structures, as well as avoiding the possible transection of tumor and subsequent seeding of the wound with tumor cells.

Subtotal lobectomy is simply a lobectomy that spares the posterior capsule to minimize the risk of potential complications such as hypoparathyroidism. We advocate the identification of all important structures in subtotal lobectomy, with sparing of the posterior capsule and a portion of adjacent thyroid tissue in the event that the parathyroid glands are not identified. Bilateral subtotal thyroidectomy is an alternative to total thyroidectomy, performed to decrease the risk of postoperative hypocalcemia. Near-total thyroidectomy consists of total lobectomy with contralateral subtotal lobectomy, with the subtotal portion performed for the reasons stated, or simply to attempt to avoid rendering the patient hypothyroid. Total thyroidectomy is defined as the attempted removal of all thyroid tissue present, with the two lobes of the thyroid removed independently or in continuity.

The decision of which operation to perform is beyond the scope of this chapter. (For further discussion of indications and choice of procedure, see Chapters 17, 22, 23, 25, and 28 through 34. Also, Chapter 2 has a discussion of the surgical anatomy relevant to thyroidectomy.) This chapter will specifically focus on lobectomy as the basic component of any of the aforementioned procedures. A discussion concerning thoracic extension will conclude the chapter.

CERVICAL SURGICAL TECHNIQUE

Instrumentation

A general head and neck instrument tray is needed to perform thyroid surgery. In addition, we recommend the use of Green retractors for lateral retraction of the strap muscles, and the McCabe facial nerve dissector for dissecting the recurrent and superior laryngeal nerves (Fig. 1). A fiberoptic headlight is essential for adequate visualization, as dissection of the superior pole is performed under the shadow of the superior flap, and dissection of the recurrent laryngeal nerves and parathyroid tissue is frequently performed under the shadow of the thyroid lobe.

In general, we do not recommend the use of Lahey retractors or other instruments that penetrate the gland. They can cause troublesome bleeding and theoretically could

---

E. A. Birken, S. A. Falk, R. H. Feins: Department of Surgery, University of Rochester School of Medicine and Dentistry, Rochester, New York 14642.

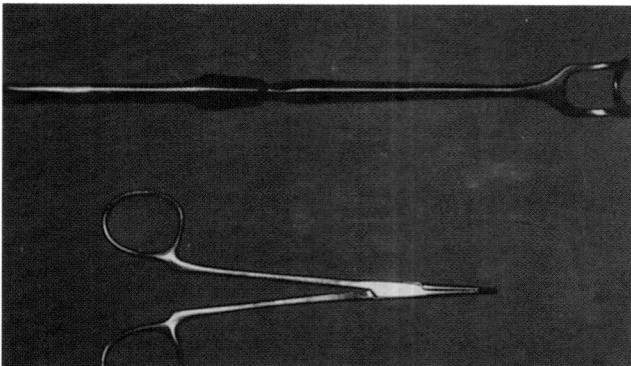

FIG. 1. The McCabe facial nerve dissector is useful for dissecting recurrent laryngeal nerve and parathyroid vessels. The Green retractor is useful for retraction of the strap musculature.

lead to seeding of the wound with tumor cells in cancer cases. It is preferable to use a gauze sponge over the fingers for retraction of the gland. A complete list of instruments necessary for thyroidectomy is listed in Table 1. It is very helpful to use a second assistant for retraction, particularly during the dissection of the superior pole.

Positioning of the Patient

The patient is placed supine on the operating table and a general anesthetic is administered. A shoulder roll is placed under the scapulae, extending the neck and throwing the shoulders back, thereby facilitating the inferior aspect of the dissection. The head is then elevated approximately 15 degrees and the knees are slightly flexed (modified reverse Trendelenburg's position) to minimize venous blood pressure in the operative site. Both arms should be tucked in so as to provide the surgeon and assistants unimpeded access to the patient (Fig. 2). The patient is then prepped in a sterile fashion (to include the margin of the mandible, both necks, and the anterior upper chest) and draped.

Marking the Incision

The anterior neck is inspected and the thyroid eminence and sternal notch are marked. If available, an appropriate relaxed skin tension line (RSTL) two finger breadths above the sternal notch is chosen. The incision will be placed as much as possible in an RSTL at this location. The proposed incision line extends from one anterior border of the sternocleidomastoid to the other, descending gently toward the midline in a curvilinear fashion. It is important that the line be gently curved and absolutely symmetrical for optimal cosmesis. Using a 2-0 silk suture, this line is then marked with firm pressure, followed by a standard surgical skin marker (Fig. 3). A

TABLE 1. *Suggested list of instruments for thyroidectomy*

1 nylon needle holder
4 short needle holders
6 large towel clips
2 straight Mayo scissors
1 baby Metzenbaum scissors
1 regular Metzenbaum scissors
1 nurses' scissors
1 fine iris scissors
4 No. 3 knife handles (1 calibrated)
1 No. 7 knife handle
6 No. 10 blades
4 No. 15 blades
1 short plain forceps
1 short multitoothed forceps
2 vascular forceps
1 fine Cushing forceps
2 regular Cushing forceps
1 Freer elevator
2 Kelly clamps
2 Ochsner clamps
36 Crile clamps
12 curved Mosquito clamps
6 straight Mosquito clamps
2 Babcock clamps
2 Senn rakes
2 pairs of double skin hooks
1 pair of single skin hooks
1 pair vein retraction
1 adenoid suction
1 pair Green retractors
1 double-ended and medium small Richardson retractor
1 McCabe nerve dissector
5 bullets (peanuts)
2 army-navy retractors
1 fiberoptic headlight
1 bipolar cautery unit

19-gauge needle is then dipped into methylene blue and puncture marks are placed on opposing sides of the incision to facilitate accurate closure (Fig. 4). It is helpful to inject the incision line with 1% Xylocaine containing 1:100,000 epinephrine 10 min prior to making the incision, to decrease skin bleeding.

Elevating the Flaps

The incision is made and carried down through the subcutaneous tissue and platysma muscle laterally. A layer of loose areolar tissue is then identified superficial to the superficial layer of the deep cervical fascia. Just deep to this fascia are the anterior jugular veins, which should be preserved as landmarks to facilitate dissection (Fig. 5). The superior flap is then elevated to the level of the thyroid notch. The inferior flap is elevated over a distance of approximately 1 cm, which may be necessary to perform the inferior portion of the dissection and will improve the appearance of the closure. By taking care to elevate the flaps in this plane of loose areolar tissue, a rel-

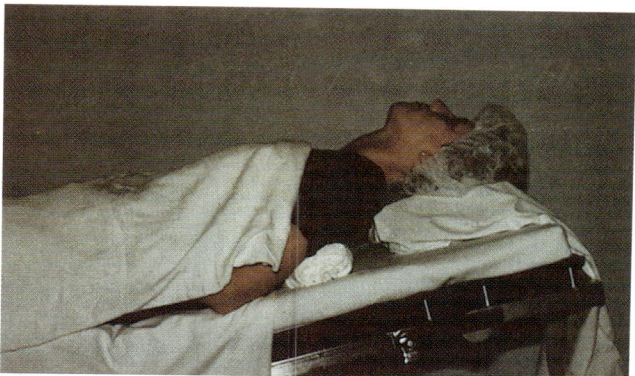

FIG. 2. Patient position for thyroidectomy. Reverse Trendelenburg decreases venous engorgement, and shoulder roll throws shoulders back and extends neck.

atively bloodless operative field is maintained. The flaps are then retracted with 2-0 silk ligatures placed subdermally and affixed to the drapes with Crile clamps.

Exposing the Thyroid Gland

The superficial layer of the deep cervical fascia is then grasped on either side of the approximate midline and opened sharply. If possible, the anterior jugular veins should be avoided, but it is likely that bridging veins will require ligation. It is often helpful to place a Crile clamp under this fascial layer and superficial to the sternohyoid muscle to assist in the opening of the fascial layer from the thyroid notch to the sternal notch. The linea alba, located between the medial borders of the sternohyoid muscles, is identified and incised sharply while the muscles are retracted laterally, thus exposing the thyroid isthmus (Fig. 6). The sternothyroid muscle, which is intimately associated with the anterior surface of the thyroid gland, is next identified. Using gentle blunt finger dissection,

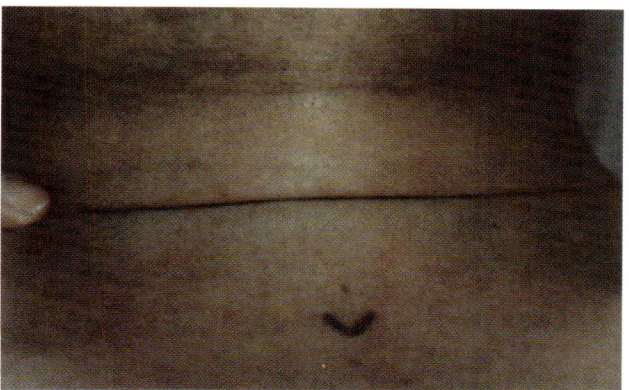

FIG. 3. Silk suture is used to mark the skin symmetrically in the proposed incision line, ideally in a relaxed skin tension line 1 to 2 cm above the suprasternal notch.

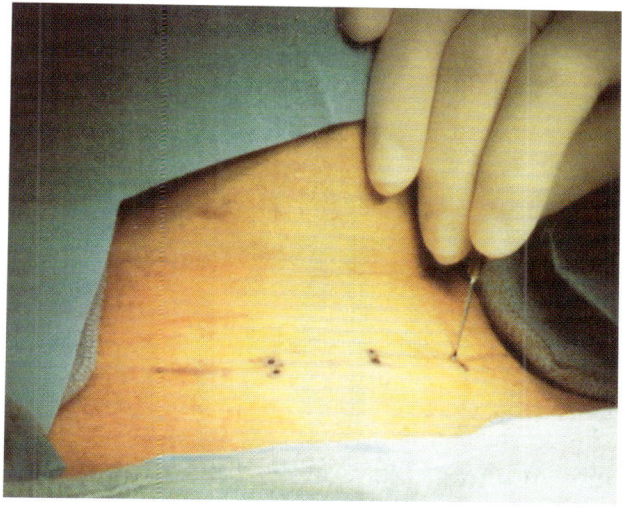

FIG. 4. Marking of the incision line with a 19-gauge needle dipped into methylene blue to aid in accurate approximation of flaps at closure.

the sternothyroid and sternohyoid muscles are swept off the surface of the thyroid gland (Fig. 7). If difficulty or bleeding is encountered in attempting to deliver the gland, it is most often a result of the fact that strap musculature is still attached to the surface of the gland. Rarely is it necessary to section the strap muscles to deliver the gland. However, a recent study demonstrated that no functional or cosmetic deformity occurs if the strap muscles are severed (1). Before publication of this recent study, traditional teaching was that, should it be necessary to cut the muscles, such as in the case of a large goiter, it is preferable to section the muscles in their upper portion as they are innervated by branches of the ansa hypoglossi entering the muscle at the inferior aspect. These strap muscles are then retracted laterally using a Green retractor. At this point, the thyroid gland should be well exposed and the field bloodless (2,3).

Mobilizing the Thyroid Gland

Using a combination of sharp and blunt dissection, the thyroid gland is dissected from the surrounding loose areolar tissue. Great care is taken to coagulate any small vessels extending to or from the gland. Bipolar electrocautery is generally used, or if necessary 4-0 silk suture is used. The authors recommend a lateral to medial approach as being safest, as the recurrent laryngeal nerve will be identified early and will less likely be injured. When the anterior and lateral surfaces of the gland are dissected free from surrounding tissue, middle thyroid vein(s) will next be identified (Fig. 8). After these vessels are clamped, divided, and ligated with 4-0 silk, the gland may be rotated medially by the first assistant. A moist

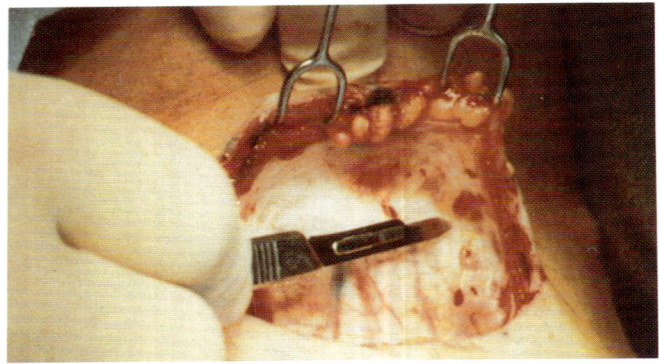
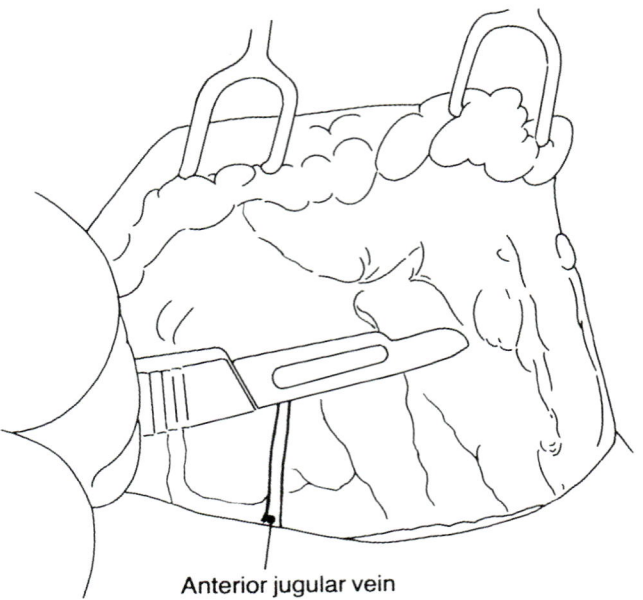

FIG. 5. A: Elevation of superior flap to the thyroid notch in a subplatysmal plane. Inferior flap is raised to clavicles (not shown). **B:** Line drawing corresponding to (A).

gauze draped over the index finger for rotating the gland is preferable to using penetrating instrument such as an Allis or Lahey clamp. These instruments can easily cause the thyroid gland to bleed, and it is paramount at this point to maintain an absolutely bloodless field.

Dissection of the Recurrent Laryngeal Nerve and Parathyroid Glands

The dissection next proceeds to the inferior aspect of the thyroid gland, initially taking great care to stay immediately on the surface of the gland. Small bridging and surface vessels that are encountered may be cauterized using a bipolar cautery, to minimize any possibility of recurrent laryngeal nerve injury. When the thyroid gland is well mobilized and rotated medially, the undersurface of the gland and tracheoesophageal space are apparent. Using a technique of gentle spreading with minimal cutting, the recurrent laryngeal nerve should next be located. The recurrent laryngeal nerve is usually found 1 to 2 cm lateral to the tracheoesophageal groove, and often deep to the inferior thyroid artery (Fig. 9). The relationship to the inferior thyroid artery is variable,

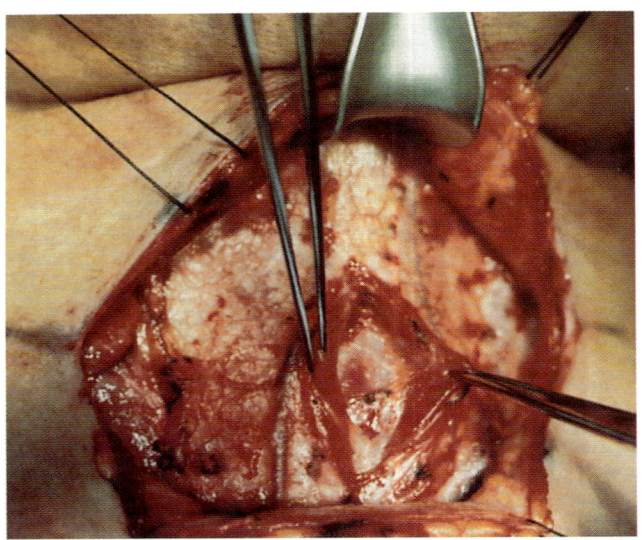
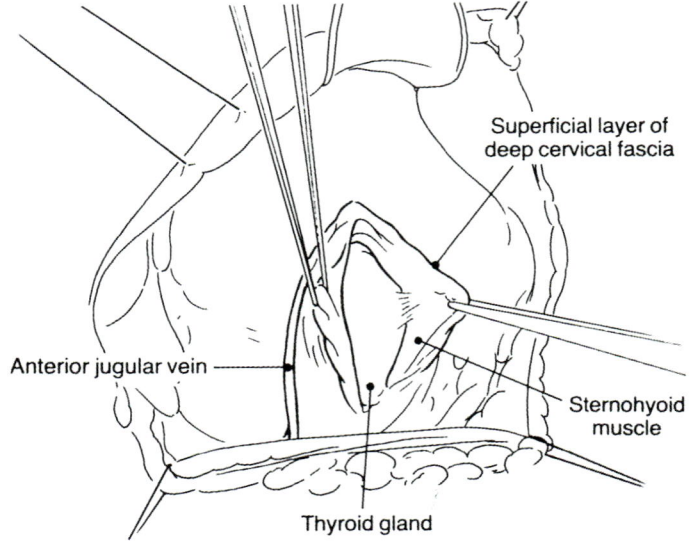

FIG. 6. A: Exposure of the thyroid gland is accomplished by incising the superficial layer of the deep cervical fascia in the midline and retracting the strap muscles laterally. **B:** Line drawing corresponding to (A).

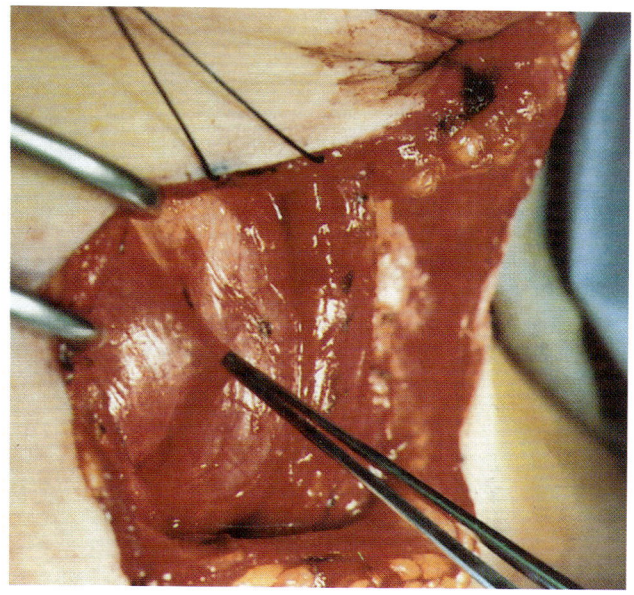
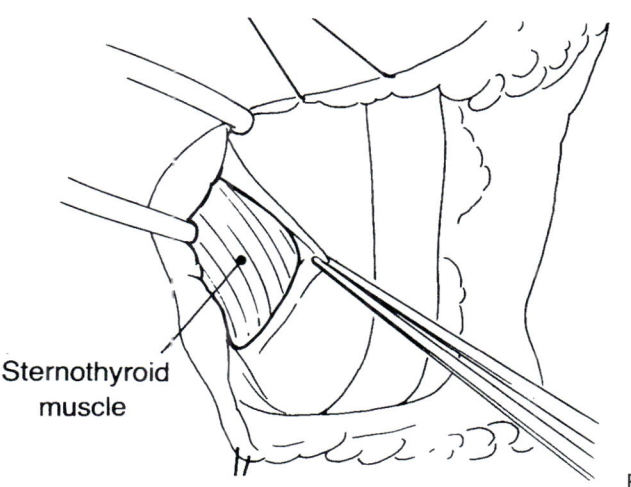

FIG. 7. A: Mobilization of the thyroid gland is facilitated by removing all fibers of the sternohyoid and sternothyroid muscles from the thyroid capsule. If a plane of dissection between the sternothyroid muscle and thyroid capsule is maintained, minimal bleeding will be encountered. **B:** Line drawing corresponding to (A).

though, and one must respect all tissue as nerve until it is identified with certainty (4,5).

From an inferior to superior direction, the recurrent laryngeal nerve courses in a slightly lateral-to-medial and deep-to-superficial fashion. The surgeon must be aware of the rare situation of a nonrecurrent laryngeal nerve, which arises directly from the cervical vagus. This anomaly occurs in 0.3% to 1.8% of patients and is found more commonly on the right side, being associated with an aberrant right subclavian artery. When this occurs on the left side, it is associated with an abnormal left-to-right aortic arch. A nonrecurrent laryngeal nerve will course in a directly lateral to medial direction. The recurrent laryngeal nerve must be identified and kept in view throughout the dissection, for this assures its preservation. The recurrent laryngeal nerve should be dissected as it courses under or

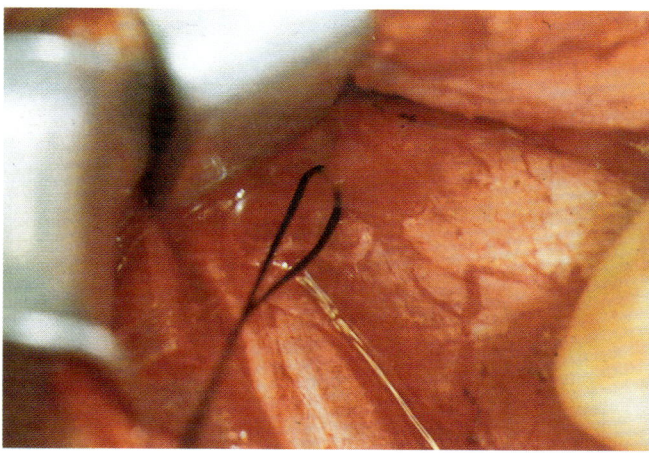
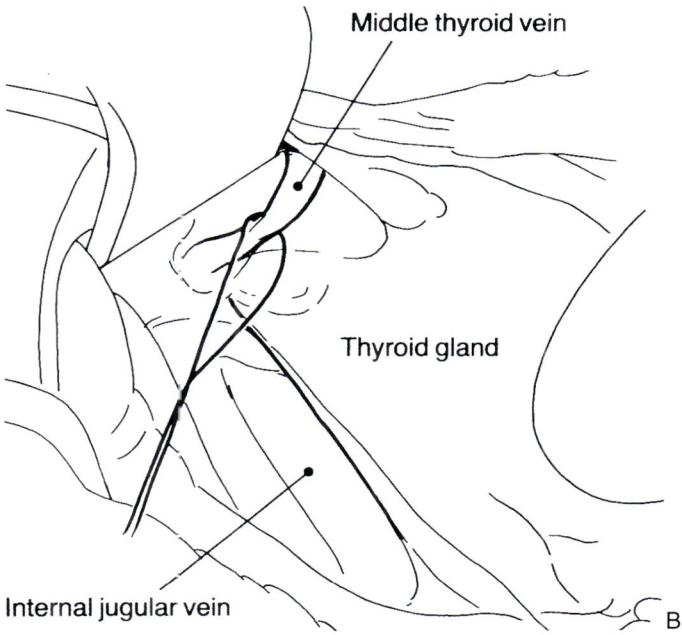

FIG. 8. A: The middle thyroid vein is identified and sacrificed, which further facilitates mobilization of the gland toward the midline. **B:** Line drawing corresponding to (A).

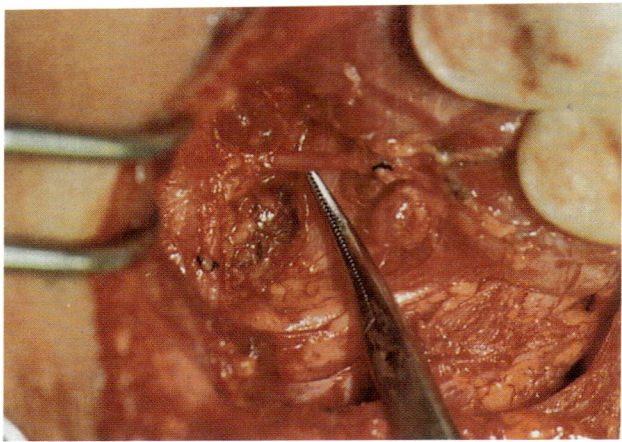
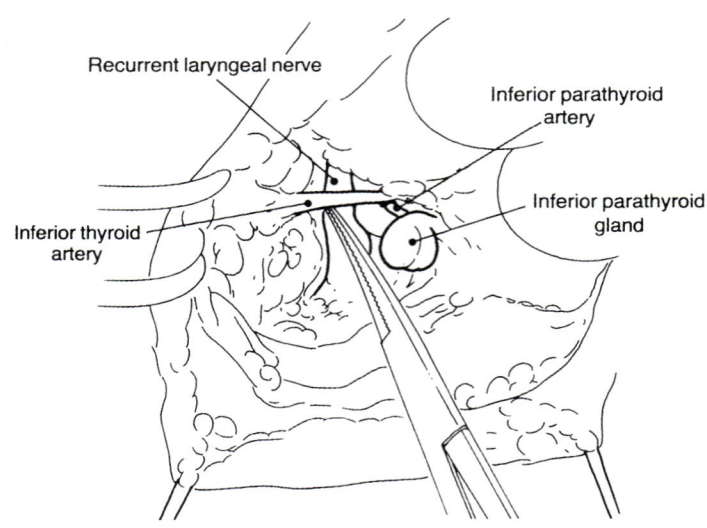

FIG. 9. A: Identification of the inferior thyroid artery, inferior parathyroid artery, recurrent laryngeal nerve, and inferior parathyroid gland (see text for detailed description). **B:** Line drawing corresponding to (A).

through Berry's (suspensory) ligament, and it should be followed to the point where it bifurcates and enters the cricothyroid joint, thereby absolutely confirming its identity (Fig. 10). Completing the superior portion of the dissection may be difficult at this point, and tracing the nerve completely into the larynx is not always possible because of overlying thyroid tissue. This may need to be completed after the superior pole dissection has been performed. Also, the nerve may actually enter the substance of the thyroid gland for a short distance in the region of the suspensory ligament in 7% to 10% of patients. If dissection of the recurrent laryngeal nerve is difficult because of previous thyroid surgery or radiated field, intraoperative nerve monitoring may be helpful (6,7).

The inferior thyroid artery, arising from the thyrocervical trunk, is identified entering the field laterally from behind the carotid artery. This vessel courses in a lateral to medial direction and enters the middle third of thyroid substance. When this vessel, the inferior parathyroid gland, and the recurrent laryngeal nerve are identified, the vessel may be taken. The inferior thyroid artery provides blood supply to the inferior and usually superior parathyroid glands, and by carefully dissecting the vessel the glands, may be identified. Most often, the parathyroid glands are identified and their vascular supply becomes apparent after their identification. The inferior thyroid artery should be taken at the thyroid capsule to preserve blood supply to the parathyroid glands (Figs. 11,12,13).

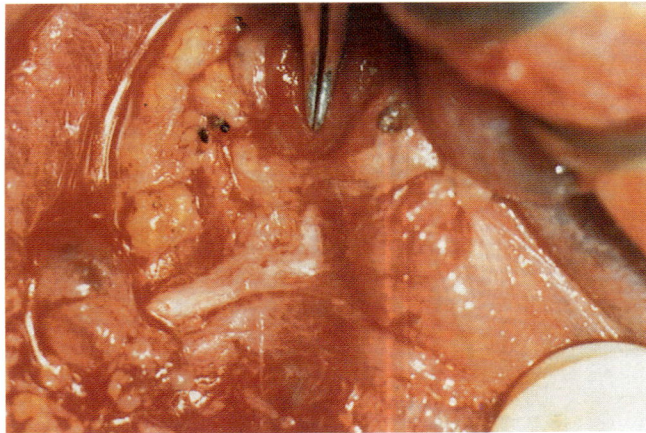
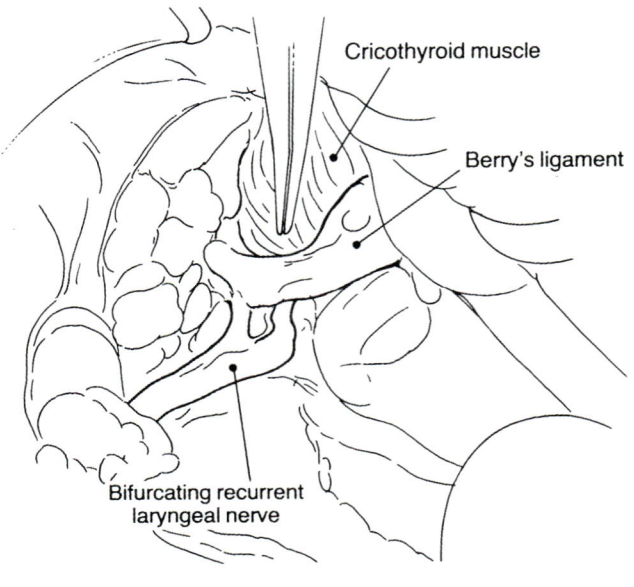

FIG. 10. A: The recurrent laryngeal nerve often bifurcates deep to Berry's ligament before entering the cricothyroid joint. **B:** Line drawing corresponding to (A).

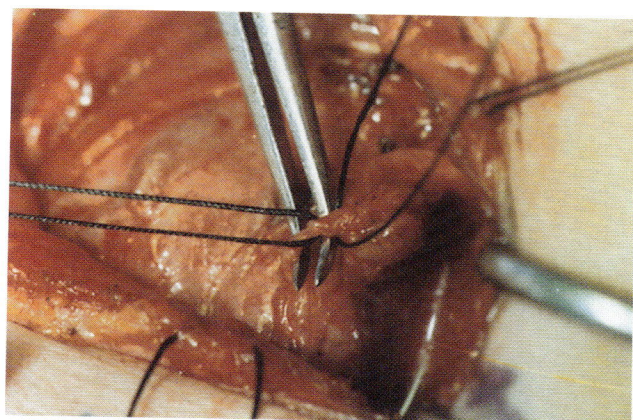
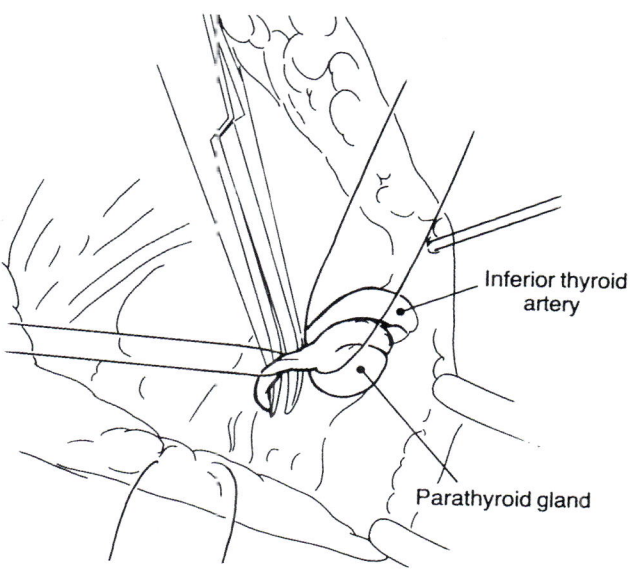

FIG. 11. A: The inferior thyroid artery is taken at the thyroid capsule (medially to the parathyroid gland) to preserve blood supply to the parathyroid glands. **B:** Line drawing corresponding to (A).

Next, the remaining inferior pole vessels should be taken individually (Fig. 14).

If parathyroid glands are not identified, the thyroid capsule should be incised over its posterior aspect and careful inspection made for parathyroid glands located in a subcapsular or intrathyroidal location. The superior parathyroid glands are often found in a subcapsular location. Should the normally tan parathyroid gland appear devitalized, suffer venous engorgement, or be accidentally or unavoidably removed, autoimplantation should be performed. The suspected parathyroid tissue should be carefully minced into 1-mm pieces and frozen-section confirmation obtained (8). The tissue is then kept in normal saline until the end of the procedure and, after confirmation is received, implanted into the sternocleidomastoid muscle or brachioradialis muscle. A small pocket is developed in the muscle, and the minced gland placed within the pocket. This area is then oversewn with nonabsorbable suture and marked with stainless steel clips.

Dissection of the Superior Pole

The dissection next proceeds to the superior pole. By carefully dissecting the thyroid gland from surrounding tissue, preferably with a second assistant providing retraction of the superior flap and the first assistant retracting the gland inferiorly, the superior pole vessels will be identified. These include the superior thyroid artery and often more than one vein. These vessels should all be carefully dissected, and individually clamped, divided,

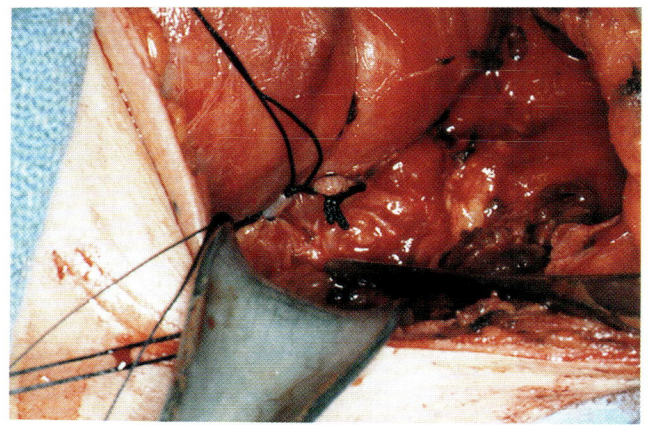
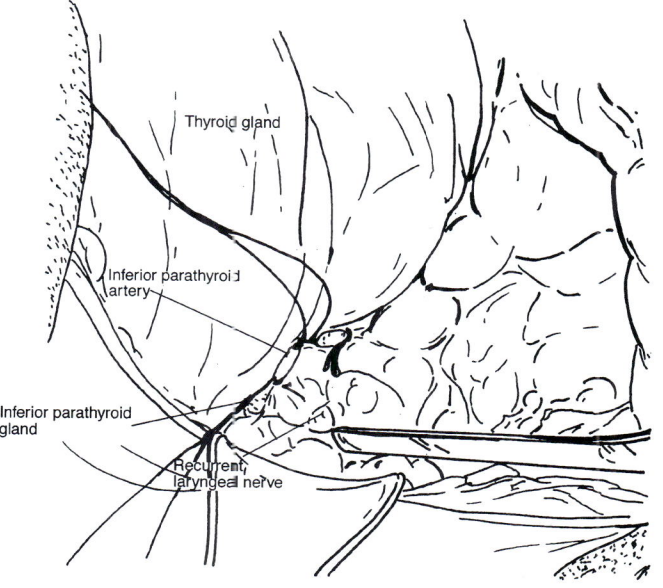

FIG. 12. A: High power magnification of inferior parathyroid artery tied at thyroid capsule, preserving the blood supply to the parathyroid gland. Note the position of the recurrent laryngeal nerve. **B:** Line drawing corresponding to (A).

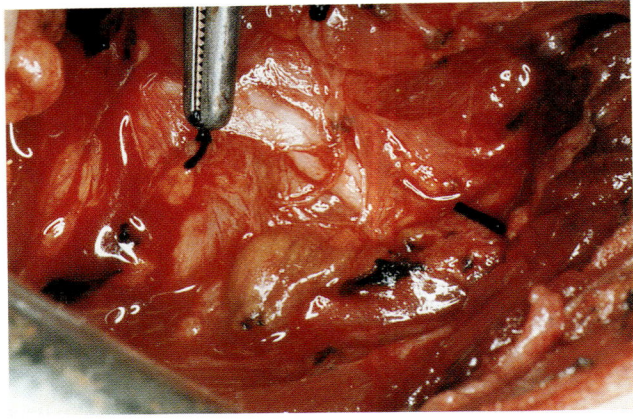
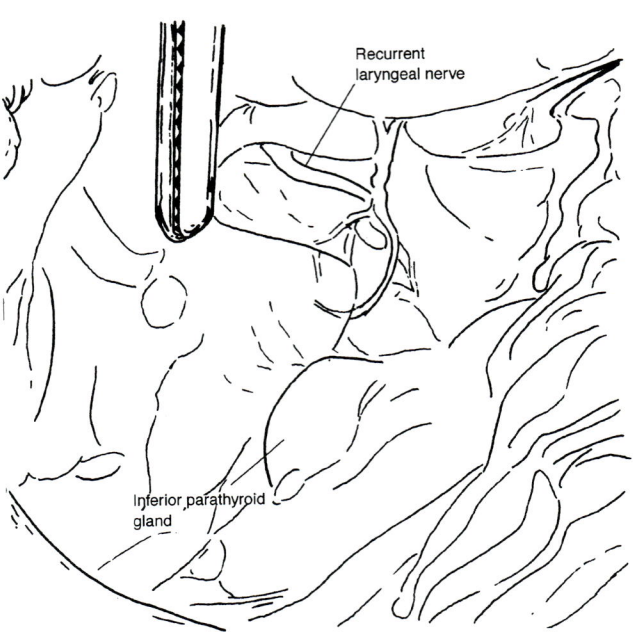

FIG. 13. A: Higher power magnification of Figure 12. Cutting the inferior parathyroid artery between the parathyroid gland and the thyroid gland enables the parathyroid gland to be preserved with its blood supply and further mobilizes the thyroid gland. **B:** Line drawing corresponding to (A).

and ligated with 4-0 silk at the surface of the gland (Fig. 15). Division of these vessels individually and close to the gland is important for two reasons. First, individual ligation provides more secure hemostasis and avoids the possibility of arteriovenous shunting. Second, this technique reduces the possibility of superior laryngeal nerve injury. The superior laryngeal nerve has a variable relationship with the superior pole vessels, often passing nearby or even between them. This often overlooked nerve is important to preserve vocal quality, particularly in those whose professions demand a high-performance voice (e.g., singers, attorneys).

In some instances, the superior pole dissection may be performed prior to identification of the recurrent laryngeal nerve and parathyroid glands to facilitate gland rotation. When this is necessary, we recommend the division of only the superior pole vessels, and we stress that there be no division of Berry's ligament (the suspensory ligament) prior to the identification of the recurrent laryngeal nerve.

With the recurrent laryngeal nerve in view, Berry's ligament may be divided, if not done so earlier in the dissection (Fig. 16). This ligament is often associated with multiple small vessels and may best be taken after hemostasis is assured with bipolar cautery. The recurrent laryngeal nerve is then identified coursing into the lateral aspect of the cricothyroid space, entering the larynx as it passes through the inferior pharyngeal constrictor muscle (see Fig. 10).

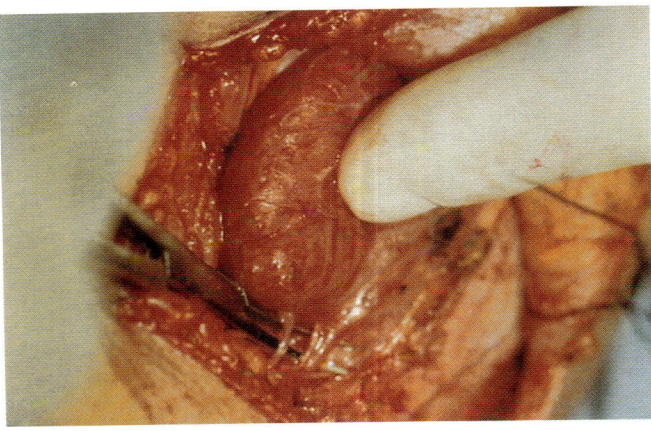
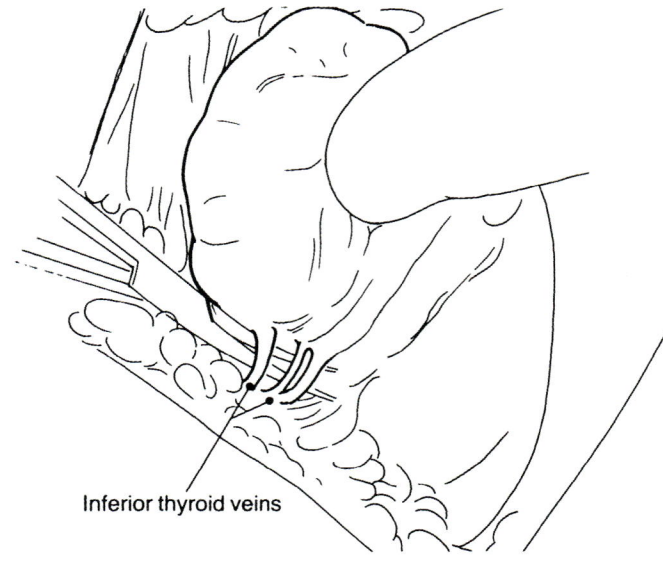

FIG. 14. A: The inferior thyroid veins are taken. **B:** Line drawing corresponding to (A).

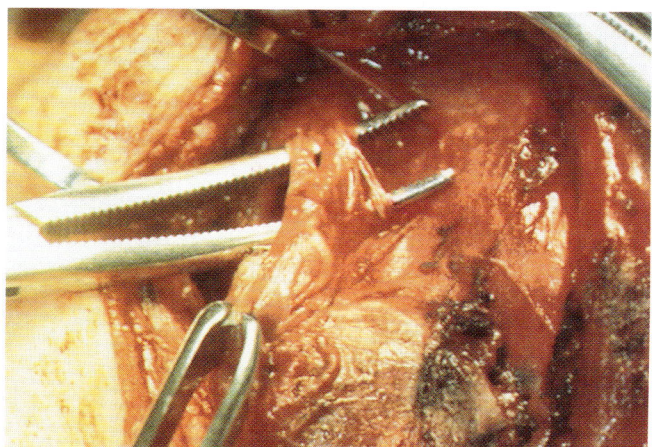
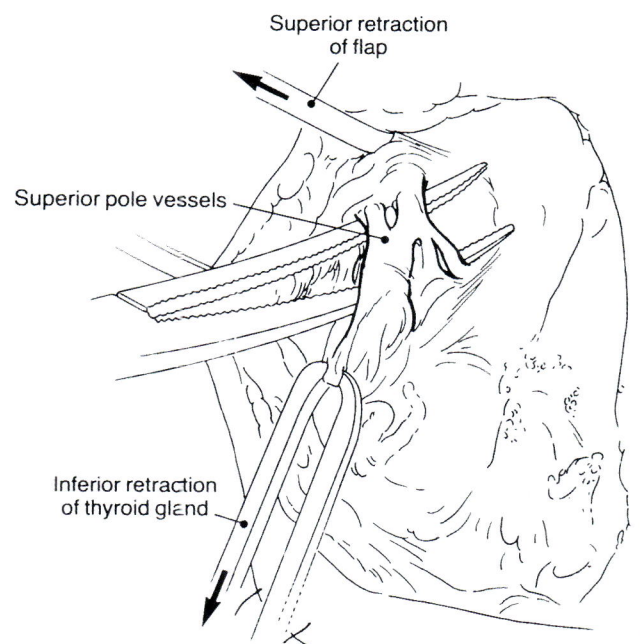

FIG. 15. A: The superior pole vessels are individually ligated close to the superior pole to assure preservation of the external branch of the superior laryngeal nerve. **B:** Line drawing corresponding to (A).

Division of the Isthmus and Removal of the Lobe

The thyroid isthmus is next divided. The space between the thyroid gland and anterior tracheal wall is carefully dissected with Crile clamps and clamped (Fig. 17). After sharp division of the isthmus, suture ligatures are placed on the remaining contralateral portion of isthmus. The portion to be removed is also ligated in a similar fashion to facilitate the remaining dissection. The remaining thyroid is removed from the anterior trachea superiorly, again with the recurrent laryngeal nerve in view at all times. The lobe is then delivered as specimen. If a pyramidal lobe is present on the side dissected or emanating from the isthmus it should be removed in continuity. As mentioned previously, if total thyroidectomy is indicated, the contralateral lobe may be removed in continuity or separately. If subtotal lobectomy is performed on either side, the dissection is identical with the exception that the thyroid gland is transected between clamps just anterior to the posterior capsule and oversewn with absorbable suture for hemostasis.

Wound Closure

After meticulous hemostasis has been achieved, closure is initiated. It is important to be certain that no oozing

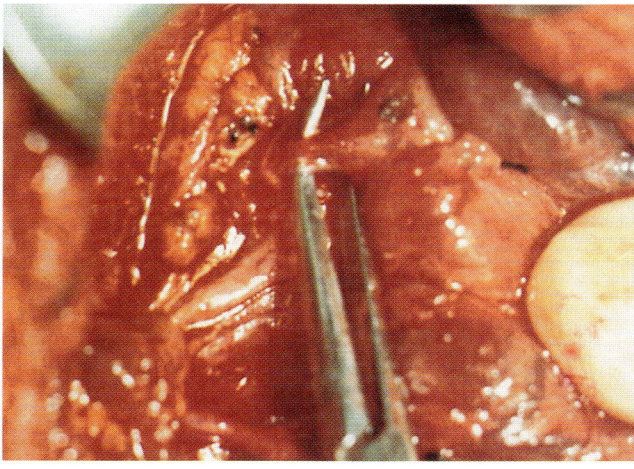
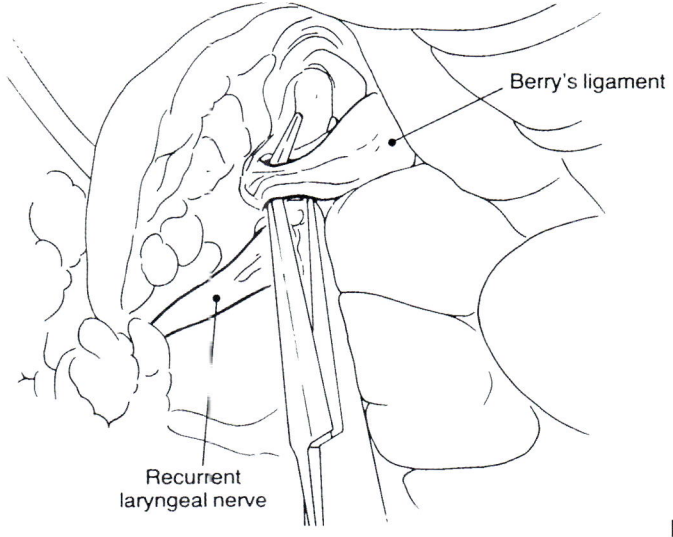

FIG. 16. A: The recurrent laryngeal nerve is completely dissected by division of the ligament of Berry. **B:** Line drawing corresponding to (A).

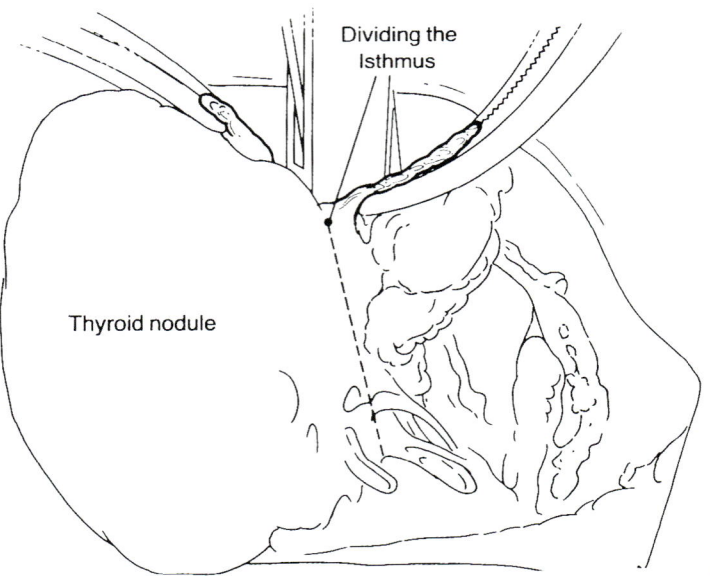

FIG. 17. A: The isthmus is divided between clamps and suture-ligated. **B:** Line drawing corresponding to (A).

exists, because any bleeding that may occur after the wound has been closed may lead to airway compromise, necessitating immediate open drainage of the surgical site. Immediately prior to closure, the patient should be given positive pressure by the anesthesiologist, while the wound is inspected for absolute hemostasis. The wound is then closed in three layers. Using absorbable suture, the strap muscles are first approximated to restore normal anterior cervical contour. This should be performed in a running fashion to facilitate rapid wound decompression in the event of hematoma and airway compromise. Perhaps a safer alternative is to approximate the strap muscles in the superior aspect of the wound, but leave a space between the two inferiorly, through which a ¼-inch Penrose drain may extend to the depth of the wound. We have found no difference in the cosmetic result and prefer the latter approach for patient safety. Although there have been several reports advocating not using postoperative drains (9), some patients have copious amounts of drainage (despite meticulous hemostasis at the conclusion of surgery).

The next layer of closure is in the deep subcutaneous and superficial subcutaneous layers. In the midline, there is no platysmal layer, but approximation should be at this level medially and at the platysmal level laterally. The superficial subcutaneous sutures preferably should be 4-0 chromic sutures that catch a portion of the deep layer of the dermis, thus resulting in eversion of the skin. The skin may be closed with either simple or running nonabsorbable suture. We prefer a skin closure of running subcuticular 4-0 Prolene. Any minor mismatched levels of skin may be corrected with intraepithelial 6-0 Prolene using loupe magnification. Finally, a "sleeper stitch" is placed in the skin at the drain site and the first throw of the knot is made (Fig. 18). When the Penrose drain is removed, this suture is tied down to minimize scarring at the drain site. Steri-strips are then placed, and a pressure dressing is applied. The "Queen Anne" pressure dressing has been shown to apply no more pressure than fluffed gauze and tape applied in a simple fashion to the anterior neck, and we therefore recommend the latter for simplicity.

Postoperative Care

During the first 2 postoperative days, serum calcium levels are checked and exogenous calcium and thyroid hormone are administered as necessary. The pressure dressing is removed approximately 24 hr after surgery. Should the drainage be minimal, the drain may be removed and the "sleeper stitch" tied. If the drainage is heavy, then the drain should be left in place and removed only when the drainage falls to minimal levels. Another light pressure dressing is applied and may be removed 1 or 2 days later. If running or simple skin sutures have been placed, they should be removed in 1 week. A running subcuticular suture may be removed 2 weeks later. We recommend the reapplication of Steri-strips after the skin is treated with benzoin, and that the Steri-strips be left in place as long as the patient tolerates them. We have found that patient tolerance is improved through the use of skin colored Steri-strips. Indirect laryngoscopy should be performed to document recurrent laryngeal nerve function. The patient is seen for routine wound checks, with further follow-up dictated by the nature of the disease state.

THORACIC SURGICAL TECHNIQUE

Although most thyroid surgery can be done through a cervical incision, there are occasions when extension into

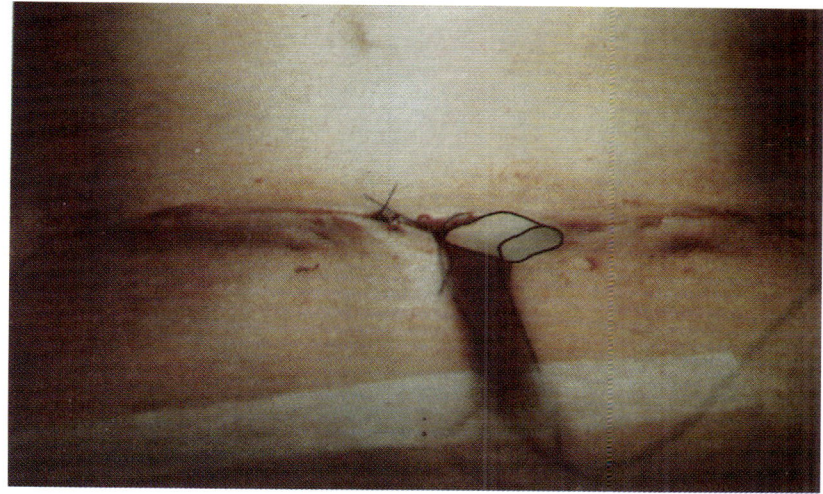

FIG. 18. Subcuticular closure over a ¼-inch Penrose drain. A "sleeper stitch" is placed to approximate the drain site after the drain is removed, improving wound cosmesis.

the thorax proper is necessary for a safe procedure. This is particularly true with reoperations. All patients undergoing surgery for substernal goiter should have the entire anterior chest prepared so that options for intrathoracic extension are kept open.

There are basically four types of incisions that may help to provide safer exposure in the rare instances when extension from the cervical approach is necessary. These are the upper partial median sternotomy, the complete median sternotomy, the anterior thoracotomy, and the standard posterolateral thoracotomy.

Most substernal goiters extend into the middle or posterior mediastinum, a position dictated by embryologic development. An anterior approach to the mediastinum therefore may not provide optimal exposure, because the goiter is behind the great vessels and sometimes even the trachea. A posterolateral incision gives excellent exposure to the posterior mediastinum, but it has the disadvantage of not being able to give ready access to the inferior thyroid vessels in the neck. The anterior thoracotomy provides improved exposure of the mediastinum and full access to the neck vessels.

Upper Partial Median Sternotomy

When substernal extension of a thyroid goiter is limited to the superior mediastinum, improved visualization can be obtained by a median sternotomy that is limited to the upper part of the sternum. The cervical collar incision is extended in a T-shaped fashion to just below the manubrium. The sternal saw is used to divide the sternum, starting superiorly, down to this level. A small Finachetto retractor is then placed and the sternal halves are distracted (Fig. 19). Care must be taken to control the internal mammary artery and vein and a small vein that usually is present at the top of the sternum. Cautery usually readily controls this latter vessel. Periosteal bleeders are also controlled by cautery. Bleeding from the upper sternal bone marrow is usually not of sufficient amount to require bone wax. Each sternal half can be elevated individually with a right-angle retractor.

Once the anterior mediastinum is opened, the mass is usually readily palpable, and since it is most often well encapsulated, it can be readily mobilized from the thymic remnant. The left innominate vein runs in this tissue in a horizontal direction and care must be taken that it not be injured. The same is true of the small thymic vein that comes off the inferior surface of the innominate vein. Other areas of concern are the right internal mammary vein and the phrenic nerves that come quite anterior, near the origins of the internal mammary arteries. The recurrent laryngeal nerves are usually not a problem at this level if one stays close to the goiter. Once fully mobilized, the goiter and appropriate contiguous thyroid tissue can be readily removed. A drain is placed in the space prior to closure.

If the upper limited sternotomy provides only marginally better exposure than that provided by the cervical incision, the incision can be carried out laterally to create a trap-door incision that usually enters the chest at the third intercostal space (Figs. 20,21). The trap-door incision is quite painful and should be done only if absolutely necessary to improve exposure.

Complete Median Sternotomy

A full median sternotomy has been proposed by some to offer good exposure to the mediastinum. Unfortunately, this is true primarily for the anterior mediastinum but it may not provide any advantage for the substernal border that extends posteriorly behind the great vessels.

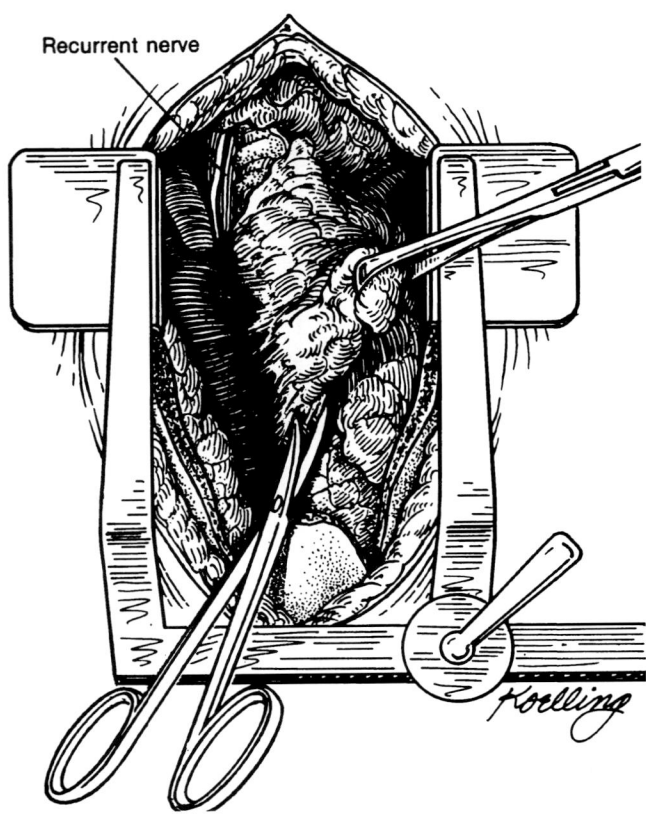

FIG. 19. Partial median sternotomy, showing removal of the thymus gland prior to removal of substernal goiter. (From ref. 10.)

The full median sternotomy does provide complete control of most blood vessels that may have grown secondarily into residual thyroid tissue left from a previous exploration (Figs. 21–23). The full median sternotomy is accomplished in much the same way as the limited upper sternotomy, with the saw being brought through the entire length of the sternum. Care must be taken to stay in the midline of the sternum. During the actual sternotomy, the breathing should be stopped in expiration by the anesthesiologist to avoid entry into either pleural space. Bleeding from the periosteum and bone marrow can be quite brisk but is readily controlled by cautery for the periosteum and bone wax for the marrow. Any of a variety of sternal retractors can be used to open the mediastinum. At the conclusion of the procedure, a substernal chest tube is placed and brought out through a small separate incision just inferior to the main incision. The sternal halves are reapproximated with No. 7 sternal wire. The fascia is closed with running absorbable suture, and the skin is closed with a subcuticular absorbable suture. The chest tube can usually be removed the morning after surgery if drainage is low.

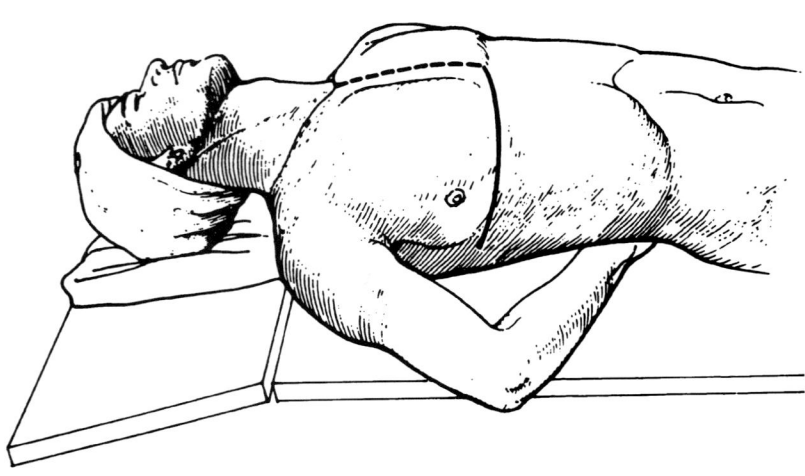

FIG 20. Incision for trap-door extension *(solid line)* of median sternotomy. The incision is submammary, but the trap-door extension enters the chest at the third intercostal space. (From ref. 11.)

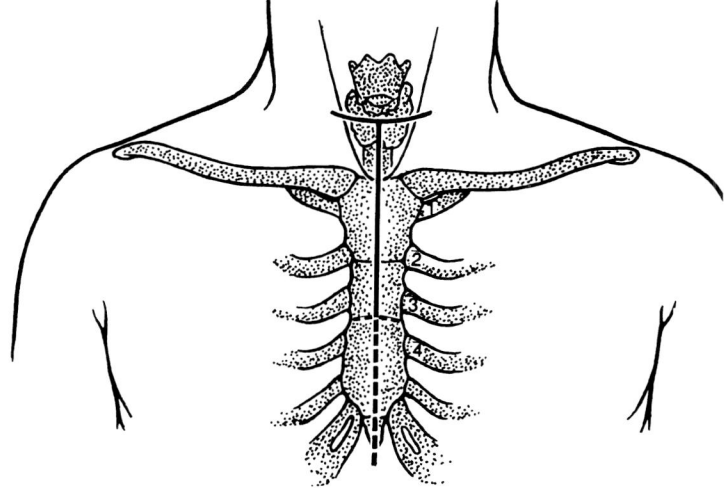

FIG 21. Incision for upper partial median and full median sternotomy with transverse collar incision. Incision for upper partial median sternotomy is the *vertical solid line.* Incision for the full median sternotomy is the *vertical solid and dashed line.* The point at the third interspace for the trap door extension is shown by the *horizontal dashed line.* (From ref. 10.)

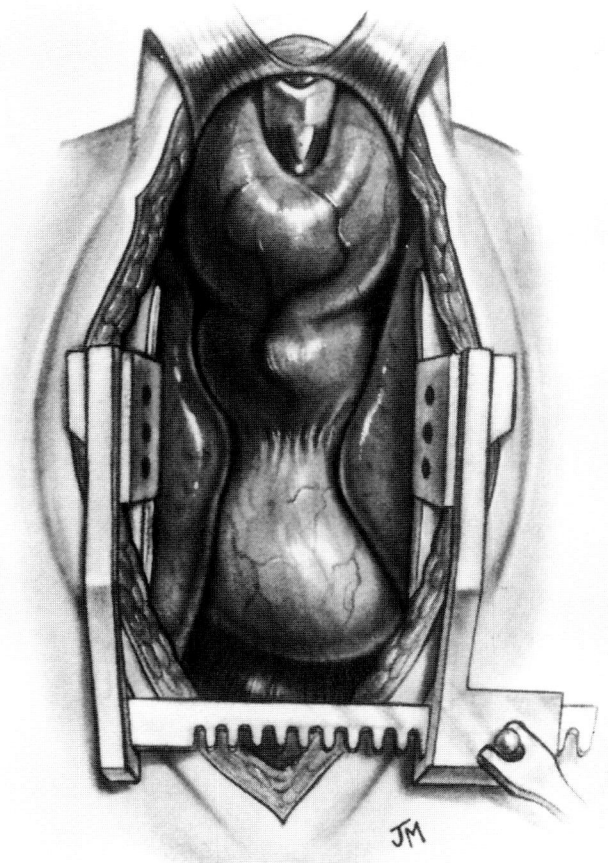

FIG 22. Anterior mediastinum after median sternotomy, with left-sided substernal goiter. (From ref. 12.)

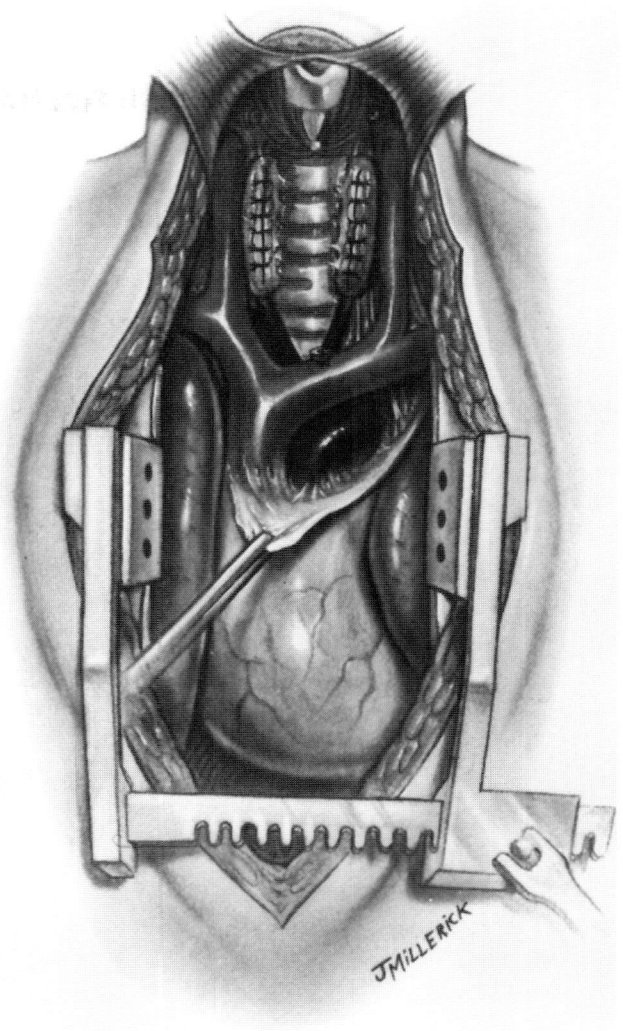

FIG 23. Goiter being removed from anterior mediastinum via anterior median sternotomy. (From ref. 12.)

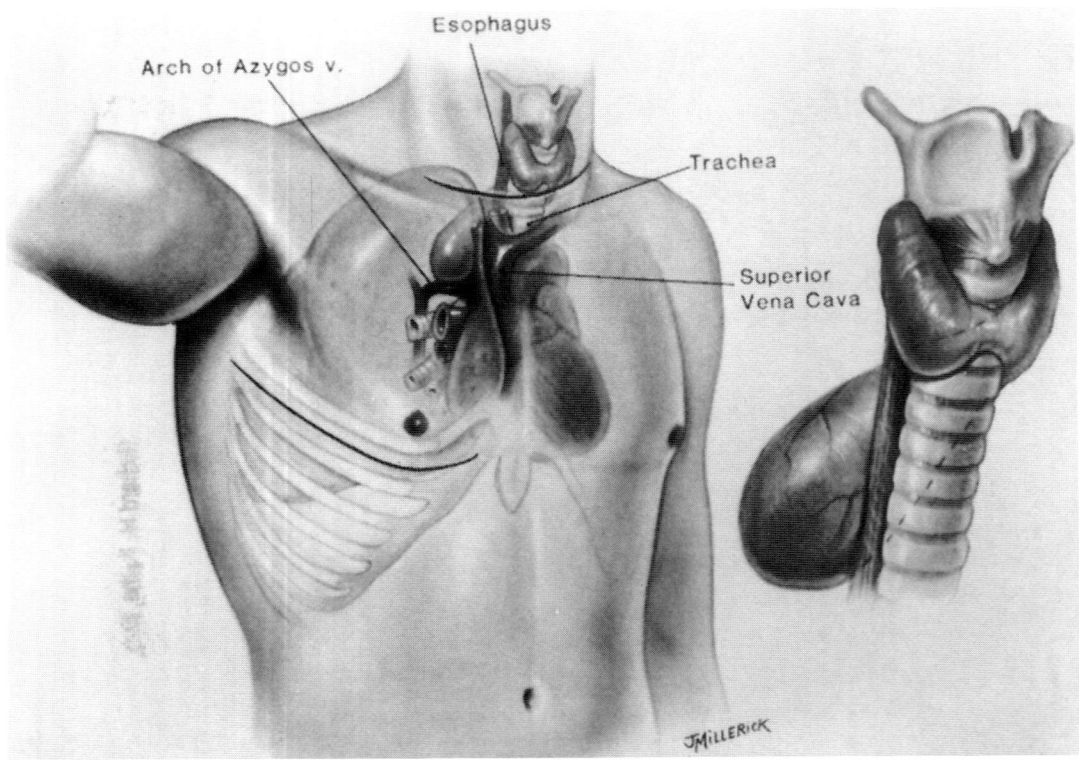

FIG 24. Combined cervical and anterior thoracotomy for posterior intrathoracic goiter. The incision is submammary, but the chest is entered in the second or third intercostal space on the right or left of the sternum. (From ref. 12.)

Anterior Thoracotomy

One of the best thoracic incisions to provide extended exposure from a cervical collar incision is the anterior thoracotomy. This incision can be placed to the right or left of the sternum and enters the chest in the second or third intercostal space (Figs. 24,25). The incision should be placed lateral enough that the internal mammary artery is preserved. With this incision, good exposure of even posterior mediastinal thyroid goiters can be obtained. The combination of this incision with the cervical collar incision provides control in the chest and control of

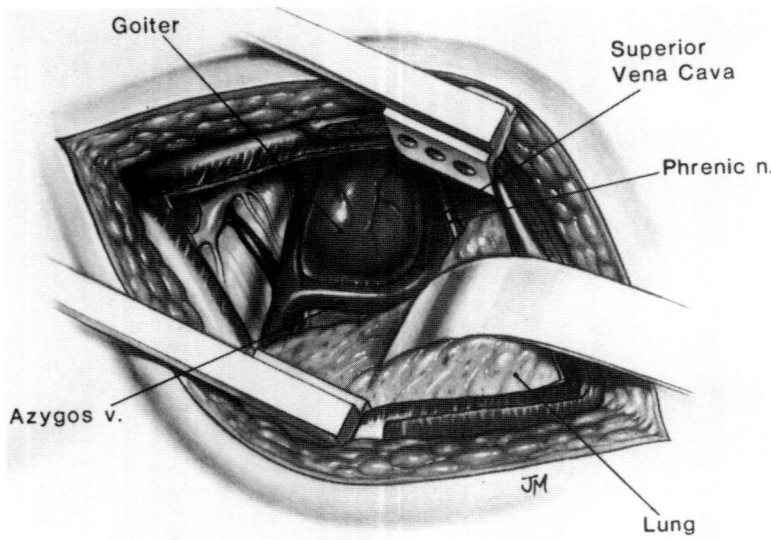

FIG 25. Exposure of posterior mediastinal goiter via anterior thoracotomy. Lung is retracted inferiorly. Mass can be readily delivered into the cervical incision. (From ref. 12.)

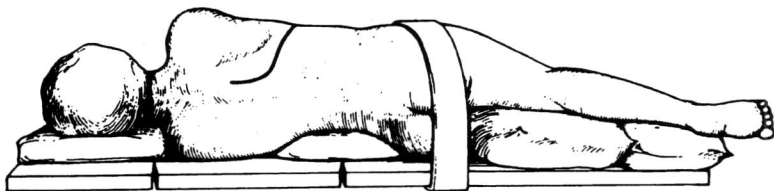

FIG 26. Standard posterolateral thoracotomy incision for true intrathoracic goiter with intrathoracic blood supply. (From ref. 11.)

/the inferior thyroid vessels. Exposure is facilitated by a double-lumen endotracheal tube, placed previously so that the lung on the thoracotomy side can be deflated.

With the chest and the neck open, the goiter can be mobilized from posterior to the anterior mediastinal structures under direct vision. In many cases, the thoracic mass is easiest to remove after separation from the thyroid, if such a connection exists.

Twenty-four-hour drainage with a chest tube is advisable. Most often the intercostal space does not need to be closed with paracostal sutures.

Posterolateral Thoracotomy

The standard posterolateral thoracotomy provides excellent exposure for the rare true ectopic thyroid tissue that resides in the thorax and derives its blood supply from intrathoracic vessels. The patient is in a full lateral thoracotomy position and the chest is entered in the fourth or fifth interspace (Fig. 26). The main disadvantage of this approach is that it gives very poor control of the inferior thyroid vessels. The exposure is again facilitated by the use of a double-lumen endotracheal tube, so that the lung can be deflated on the operated side. The gland is dissected from the mediastinum with care being taken to stay on the gland capsule. The aberrant blood supply must be identified and ligated. The chest should be drained until drainage is less than 100 cc/24 hr.

In general, it should be a very rare occasion when extension of the operative field beyond that provided by a cervical incision is necessary to remove a substernal goiter. Techniques such as the use of a suspended anterior self-retaining retractor, marsupialization, and the use of a sterile spoon to release intrathoracic suction, allow over 98% of these tumors to be delivered into the neck and removed. A knowledge of the upper partial median sternotomy, the complete median sternotomy, the anterior thoracotomy, and the standard posterolateral thoracotomy is important, however, when the mass cannot be safely delivered, when attempts at delivery result in excessive bleeding, or when extracapsular malignancy is present.

REFERENCES

1. Jaffe V, Young AE. Strap muscles in thyroid surgery: to cut or not to cut? *Ann R Coll Surg Engl* 1993;5:378–379.
2. Thompson NW, Olsen WR, Hoffman GL. The continuing development of the technique of thyroidectomy. *Surgery* 1973;73(6):913–917.
3. Falk SA, Birken EA. Surgery of the thyroid gland, a study guide for surgeons. *Official course manual, annual meeting of the American Academy of Otolaryngology, Head and Neck Surgery.* 1982–1989.
4. Karlan MS, Catz B, Dunkelman D, et al. A safe technique for thyroidectomy with complete nerve dissection and parathyroid preservation. *Head Neck Surg* 1984;6:1014–1019.
5. Attie JN, Khafif RA. Preservation of parathyroid gland during total thyroidectomy. *Am J Surg* 1975;130:399–404.
6. Rice DH, Cone-Wesson B. Intraoperative recurrent laryngeal nerve monitoring. *Otolaryngol Head Neck Surg* 1991;105:372–375.
7. Maloney RW, Murcek BW, Stoebler KW, et al. A new method for intraoperative recurrent laryngeal nerve monitoring. *ENT J* 1994;73:30–33.
8. Lore JM Jr, Pruet CW. Retrieval of the parathyroid glands during thyroidectomy. *Head Neck Surg* 1983;5:268–269.
9. Wax MK, Valiulis AP, Hurst KH. Drains in thyroid and parathyroid surgery: are they necessary? *Arch Otolaryngol Head Neck Surg* 1995;121:981–983.
10. Abele JS, Gavin LA, Greenspan FS, Miller TR, Rapoport B. Surgical treatment. In: Clark OH, ed. *Endocrine surgery of the thyroid and parathyroid glands.* St. Louis: CV Mosby, 1985;287–288.
11. Moores DM, Foster ED, McKneally MF. Incisions. In: Pearson FG, et al., eds. *Thoracic surgery.* New York: Churchill Livingstone, 1995;118–123.
12. Shahian DM. Surgical treatment of intrathoracic goiter. In: Cady B, Rossi RL. eds. *Surgery of the thyroid and parathyroid glands.* Philadelphia: WB Saunders, 1991;219–221.

CHAPTER 37

Complications of Thyroid Surgery: An Overview

Stephen A. Falk

The last four chapters of this book present complications of thyroidectomy, including pathophysiology, diagnosis, incidence, treatment, and prevention. These chapters consist of (a) an overview, (b) nonmetabolic complications (nerve injury, hemorrhage, airway obstruction, flap necrosis, and chyle leak), (c) the metabolic complications of hypocalcemia and hypoparathyroidism, hypocalcitonemia, and hypo- and hyperthyroidism, and (d) the metabolic complication of thyroid storm.

In contrast to medical storm, surgical thyroid storm is almost unheard of now because of the universal practice of adequately preparing hyperthyroid patients (with Graves' disease, toxic multinodular goiter, and toxic solitary nodule) for surgery. Such preparation achieves clinical and optimally chemical euthyroidism prior to thyroidectomy. Also, there are unavoidable circumstances when a hyperthyroid patient, who is either previously undiagnosed or under initial treatment, but not euthyroid, requires urgent surgery. Thyroid storm, surgery for hyperthyroidism, and general anesthesia are addressed in Chapters 40, 17, and 35, respectively.

There is less than a 4% incidence of all significant complications after thyroidectomy. Complications can be kept to a minimum by a thorough knowledge of the anatomy and its variations, by understanding thyroid pathology, and by meticulous hemostasis and delicate surgical technique.

Every operation has a tempo. The tempo of thyroidectomy is, at first, fast and flashy, with exposure of a large surgical field. The tempo then markedly changes. Movements slow and the field of interest becomes small, as the recurrent laryngeal nerve and parathyroid glands and their blood supply are identified and preserved. This part of the operation requires of the surgeon a different emotional input—more akin to microsurgery—of increased concentration, meticulous attention to detail, and strict hemostasis. Lighting and instrumentation should be available to meet the demands here (see Chapter 36). After this part is complete, the original tempo is resumed as the gland is removed and the operation is terminated. Surgeons having the least complications have an innate feeling for the changes in tempo; they have had intensive training and wide experience in head and neck surgery; they have an avid interest in the normal and abnormal thyroid gland, and they perform thyroid operations frequently.

COMPLICATION OR NATURAL SEQUELA?

A complication is an unexpected adverse result caused by thyroidectomy. This is to be contrasted with (a) natural sequelae of either a temporary or a permanent nature associated with thyroidectomy, and (b) changes noted after thyroidectomy but actually caused by the disease for which the surgery was performed, or caused by another disease, either related or unrelated to the primary one. It is instructional to consider complications within this frame of reference.

Hypothyroidism

Hypothyroidism is not a complication of thyroidectomy, because it is an expected result. It is a permanent, natural sequela of occasional cases of unilateral thyroid lobectomy and of almost all cases of total or near-total thyroidectomy. To treat adequately the pathology (suspicious cold nodules, small carcinomas of less than 2 cm, and toxic solitary nodules in unilateral lobectomy cases; Graves' disease, toxic multinodular goiter, compressive benign multinodular goiter, and carcinoma in total thyroidectomy cases), sufficient thyroid tissue is removed. Hypothyroidism is a natural consequence.

S. A. Falk: Department of Surgery, University of Rochester School of Medicine and Dentistry, Rochester, New York 14642.

This situation is most readily appreciated in Graves' disease. A smaller size and poorer vascular integrity of the thyroid remnant predispose to hypothyroidism. Remnant size is a key factor in determining postoperative hypothyroidism and recurrent hyperthyroidism, and the only factor under the direct control of the surgeon. Because hypothyroidism is more readily treatable (by thyroid hormone) than is hyperthyroidism [which usually requires iodine-131 (^{131}I), and this was probably avoided in the first place in favor of surgery], the surgeon tends to remove more thyroid tissue, favoring total or near-total thyroidectomy, as opposed to bilateral subtotal thyroidectomy. In so doing, the chance of recurrent hyperthyroidism is decreased but the chance of hypothyroidism is increased. Postoperative hypothyroidism is a reasonable price for the patient to pay to avoid recurrent hyperthyroidism. In this way, hypothyroidism is an unavoidable, expected, and natural sequela of the surgery and not, strictly speaking, a complication (1).

Some element of hypothyroidism occurring after thyroidectomy for Graves' disease occurs as a consequence of the disease itself. The natural history of Graves' disease is variable. The hyperthyroidism may be persistent or cyclic, with exacerbations and remissions. However, in some patients, as originally described by Graves, the hyperthyroidism spontaneously leads to hypothyroidism, as the immunoglobulins that stimulated the gland to diffuse toxic hyperplasia eventually destroy it.

But another element of the hypothyroidism appearing after thyroidectomy for Graves' disease and other diseases occurs as a consequence of another disease, sometimes related to the primary one for which surgery was performed. For example, Graves' disease is often accompanied histologically by lymphocytic infiltration. Histologic Hashimoto's thyroiditis (lymphoid follicles, Hürthle cells, fibrosis) is found in about one third of Graves' patients (2), and frequently in patients with carcinoma and benign pathologies. The lymphocytic infiltration or the Hashimoto's thyroiditis reduces the functional capacity of remnant thyroid tissue, predisposing to hypothyroidism.

Hypocalcemia and Hypoparathyroidism

Temporary

Hypocalcemia and hypoparathyroidism, adverse effects of thyroidectomy, are either natural sequelae or true complications (see Chapter 39). Temporary postthyroidectomy hypocalcemia occurs after unilateral thyroid lobectomy because of dilution of serum albumin, with a fall in total calcium and with stable levels of free (ionized) calcium and serum parathormone (3). These changes represent only adverse natural sequelae associated with the thyroidectomy. After bilateral thyroid lobectomy, in addition to the same dilutional effects that cause temporary hypocalcemia, temporary hypoparathyroidism frequently occurs despite careful and meticulous preservation of parathyroid glands and their vascular integrity. The mechanisms for such temporary hypoparathyroidism have not been fully elucidated. It is assumed that the mechanism is ischemia of parathyroid tissue, although only a few studies have measured blood flow to parathyroid glands. Ischemia is a logical explanation, but so are hypothermia of parathyroid tissue and the effects of endothelin 1, which will be discussed in Chapter 39. Changes in serum calcitonin are probably not the reason. Until the pathogenesis is determined, the question of whether temporary hypoparathyroidism is an adverse natural sequela or a true complication of thyroidectomy remains unanswered.

Permanent

The mechanisms of permanent hypoparathyroidism are clearer. The surgeon removed or devascularized the parathyroid tissue. In benign thyroid cases and in encapsulated carcinoma, permanent hypoparathyroidism is a true complication. However, in carcinomas that have penetrated the thyroid capsule or in the presence of significant cervical metastases with paratracheal disease, the surgeon's judgment may dictate complete removal of the disease at all cost. In so doing, permanent hypoparathyroidism is a natural sequela, because it is expected. It is a trade-off—the patient pays the price of permanent hypoparathyroidism in achieving complete tumor removal. My personal philosophy in cases of aggressive carcinoma is to avoid permanent hypoparathyroidism if at all possible, even if this means leaving behind small areas of carcinoma and relying on ^{131}I to eradicate residual carcinoma. This approach serves well in papillary and follicular carcinomas, which usually avidly take up ^{131}I. In medullary carcinoma, external radiation therapy could achieve eradication of small areas of residual tumor.

Conclusion

In common parlance, adverse natural sequelae from thyroid surgery and adverse changes caused by the underlying disease or other diseases are usually called complications. Accordingly, in this book we have listed them as complications. However, it is important for the surgeon to differentiate such changes from those that are true complications of thyroidectomy. Just as surgery is often erroneously blamed for all or most adverse effects in the postoperative period, in a similar manner adverse effects may be erroneously ascribed to radiation and medical therapy. The origin of adverse effects is usually known, but sometimes truly unknown, poorly known, or multiple. By keeping our thinking clear, physicians can provide patients with more complete and accurate explanations of treatment results and thereby avoid misinformation, misinterpretations, and manipulations by attorneys and an American public obsessed with lawsuits.

COMPLICATIONS OF TOTAL VERSUS BILATERAL SUBTOTAL THYROIDECTOMY

Reasons to perform total thyroidectomy (TT) versus bilateral subtotal thyroidectomy (BST) are addressed elsewhere in terms of disease control in carcinoma (see Chapters 28–34) and in terms of risks of recurrent hyperthyroidism and hypothyroidism in Graves' disease (see Chapter 17). Here, I discuss the controversy of whether or not TT increases the chance of complications as compared to BST, regardless of the benefits of each in treating thyroid disease.

The literature on the risks of TT and BST is confusing and conflicting because these terms refer to two factors—how much thyroid tissue, if any, should be left behind (the size of the remnant) and the technique used. In terms of the thyroid remnant, there is agreement that TT is an attempt to remove all thyroid tissue; *attempt*, because even when a good surgeon performs TT, small areas of thyroid tissue are left behind in about 70% of cases (4). BST means leaving behind a small thyroid remnant on each side. However, TT and BST are performed with various techniques that give rise to different rates of complications. So, when comparing studies of TT and BST, we must compare the actual techniques used and also separately consider preservation of the recurrent laryngeal nerve and parathyroid tissue. We also must specify the remnant for each lobe. BST means subtotal lobectomy on each side. TT means total lobectomy on each side. Total lobectomy on one side and contralateral subtotal lobectomy (TL and SL) should also be specified.

Proper modern technique of thyroidectomy requires identification and dissection of the recurrent laryngeal nerve from the thoracic inlet to the cricothyroid joint where it enters the larynx. Such a technique, done with proper instrumentation, lighting, and gentleness, is extremely safe and much safer than the old practice of not dissecting the nerve and assuming it is safely behind the thyroid remnant. The old practice invites nerve transection and/or contusion as the thyroid remnant is clamped, especially as the nerve courses under the ligament of Berry and then anteriorly as it enters the larynx. Mountain et al. (5) reported that the incidence of nerve paralysis is 3 to 4 times greater in cases when the nerve is not exposed than in cases when it is routinely exposed. The technique of identification and dissection of the nerve is used during TT. However, in the literature, BST is reported both with this technique and with the old technique. Therefore, it is illogical to think that nerve paralysis is more common after TT than BST.

In terms of nerve preservation, BST and TT are equally safe if the nerve is positively identified and traced throughout its course in the surgical field. Indeed, if BST refers to the old technique, then TT is a more anatomic, technically easier, and safer operation than BST. In terms of preservation of parathyroid glands and their blood supply, TT can be done safely with permanent hypoparathyroidism occurring in 0% (6–9), 0.4% (10), 0.6% (11), 0.8% (12), 1% (13), 1.3% (4), 2.0% (14), 2.7% (15), and 2.8% (16) of cases. The technique employed consists of the identification of the parathyroids (by following the inferior thyroid artery to the glands) and the preservation of their blood supply. The parathyroid glands are separated from the thyroid with intact vascularity (see Chapters 36,39). Then both lobes are removed entirely.

BST or SL can be performed using this same technique and then leaving behind a remnant. This is the preferred way to do BST or SL and the incidence of hypoparathyroidism is the same as after TT or TL. However, BST or SL is also performed as follows: If the parathyroids cannot be positively identified and/or their blood supply cannot be identified or becomes precarious, then a remnant (posterior capsule of thyroid gland) is left behind with the assumption that it contains parathyroid tissue and its blood supply. This technique is acceptable considering the uncertain status of parathyroid tissue and its blood supply.

BST or SL is also performed in a third way: No attempt is made to identify parathyroid tissue, and its blood supply and/or the main trunk of the inferior thyroid artery is divided. A thyroid remnant is left and assumed to contain viable parathyroid tissue. This technique is an outmoded one and is to be condemned and abandoned because of the increased incidence of hypoparathyroidism. When BST is done in this outmoded way, hypoparathyroidism is more common than after TT.

TT is associated with an increased risk of hypoparathyroidism if the surgeon's primary purpose is to remove all thyroid parenchyma, as in cancer cases, regardless of the consequences. Even in cancer cases, I do not adhere to this philosophy, but rely on ^{131}I to eradicate small areas of residual thyroid tissue that I leave behind if I feel their presence will aid the vascular integrity of parathyroid glands. Rigid adherence to the goal of TT will increase the incidence of hypoparathyroidism as compared with BST, as shown in some series (17).

A LOGICAL APPROACH TO TOTAL THYROIDECTOMY VERSUS BILATERAL SUBTOTAL THYROIDECTOMY

Determining which thyroid operation to do means balancing the risks and benefits of TT, BST, or TL and SL. Each surgeon must choose an approach individualized for each patient and arrived at during preoperative discussions with the patient, balancing the risks and benefits, and modified by good surgical judgment of the findings at operation. Endocrinologists who dictate to surgeons the type of operation to be performed and the surgeons who comply are doing a disservice to their patients.

My own approach is based on the following convictions. Permanent hypocalcemia is a very serious and lifelong complication and is to be avoided if at all possible and even in cancer cases. Less serious, but still representing a colossal failure of surgery, is recurrent hyperthyroidism in Graves' disease cases, for which ^{131}I is usually necessary but not desirable because it was avoided in the first place in favor of surgery. I consider hypothyroidism not even a complication of surgery, since it is an expected, natural sequela that is readily treatable. During the procedure, I try to apply these convictions.

I approach each case by attempting to perform TT, but only if I can dissect out and preserve at least two parathyroid glands and their intact arterial supply. TT can still be done with autotransplantation of vascular compromised parathyroids. However, the average success of fresh parathyroid autografts is 82% (18). So I prefer a subtotal lobectomy that will preserve parathyroid function in nearly all cases, rather than a total lobectomy and autotransplantation of parathyroids that do not readily dissect on a vascular pedicle. If a TT (or a TL) cannot be done, a flexible response is warranted. I do a subtotal lobectomy if I cannot identify at least one parathyroid on a side. With these principles in mind, I perform, preferably, a TL and SL, or a BST if I cannot do a TT.

COMPLICATIONS OF COMPLETION (REOPERATIVE) THYROID SURGERY

Over the last 10 years, a number of studies have addressed complications of completion thyroid surgery. These studies were prompted by the increasing use of total or near-total thyroidectomy, which offers a number of advantages for treatment of thyroid cancer when compared with less-than-total thyroidectomy (which includes BST; TL and SL; unilateral total, subtotal, or partial lobectomy; and nodulectomy). The advantages of total or near-total thyroidectomy include the following:

1. It removes the primary cancer and multifocal cancer in the same and opposite side (80% of cases) or in the opposite lobe (30% of cases).
2. It eliminates the small chance that residual papillary or follicular carcinoma will undergo transformation to anaplastic carcinoma.
3. It allows for preparation of the patient for ^{131}I scanning by permitting the patient to become hypothyroid.
4. By removing as much normal thyroid tissue as possible, it allows therapeutic ^{131}I, the total dose of which is limited because of the risk of leukemia, to be used specifically to eradicate metastases but not large amounts of residual normal thyroid tissue.
5. It permits using elevation of serum thyroglobulin as a tumor marker for recurrence.

These benefits of total or near-total thyroidectomy are proven; they probably translate into decreased recurrences and greater cure rates (see Chapters 28,29).

Table I summarizes a number of studies of completion thyroid surgery. A 1963 study showed that in patients receiving two or more operations for cancer, 17% had permanent vocal cord paralysis and 13.3% had permanent hypoparathyroidism (19). These high rates occurred because many operations were performed for clinical recurrence, and aggressive surgery was done with purposeful sacrifice of the recurrent laryngeal nerve. More recent studies demonstrate low rates of complications, with a range of 0% to 5% for temporary and 0% to 4% for permanent vocal cord paralysis, and 0% to 15% for temporary and 0% to 7.4% for permanent hypoparathyroidism. With varying definitions of completion thyroid surgery and inclusion of varying types of cases, the reported incidence of complications shows wide variability. Nevertheless, these studies confirm low and acceptable complication rates that are similar to those that occur after primary total or near-total thyroidectomy (see Chapters 38,39).

These studies also show a high rate of finding thyroid cancer in the ipsilateral or contralateral lobe (with a range of 25% to 92%) and in lymph nodes (with a range of 4% to 23%). Optimal time for reoperation is immediately after the primary operation, usually within 1 week, or else 3 months later. Between these times, surgery is difficult because of healing and granulating tissue.

Complications occurred more frequently when reoperation was performed on a lobe or lobes that had previously received surgery. For this reason, nodulectomy of solitary nodules is to be condemned, because pathologic evaluation to diagnose carcinoma frequently requires analysis of the tumor–capsule–thyroid interface to identify capsular invasion. Also, a frozen-section diagnosis of a nodule may be benign, but a permanent section may prove malignant. If a nodulectomy only were done, reoperation would be required to complete at least the total lobectomy. Also, a surgeon performing a nodulectomy may dispense with proper identification and preservation of the recurrent laryngeal nerve and parathyroid glands and their blood supply and increase the chance of complications. Reoperations are more difficult because of postoperative scarring, loss of normal tissue planes, and difficulty in identifying parathyroid glands and recurrent laryngeal nerves.

Techniques to help find these structures include the following:

1. Identifying the nerve either high, where it enters the larynx at the cricothyroid joint, or low in the neck in the superior mediastinum, and then tracing the nerve through the scarred area.
2. Using an approach lateral to the strap muscles to avoid at first the scarred area, while working through the standard anterior Kocher incision.

TABLE 1. Summary of studies of completion thyroidectomy

Author year (ref.)	Definition	Vocal cord paralysis (%)		Hypoparathyroidism (%)		Time from initial surgery to reoperation	Residual cancer (%)		Notes
		Temporary	Permanent	Temporary	Permanent		Thyroid	Lymph nodes	
Beahrs 1963 (19)	2,3,5	6.7	17	7.4	13.3	variable	100	—	Includes only cancer cases; all cases reoperated for clinically recurrent cancer
Thompson 1970 (20)	all	—	3.7	—	7.4	—	—	—	
Rao 1987 (21)	1,1&4	0	2.7	5.4	0	>3 months	58	0	A
Calabro 1988 (22)	1,1&4	1.5	0	12.1	0	immediate or >3 months	42	12	A B
Auguste 1990 (23)	1,4	2.5	0	12.5	0	1 to 280 days	38	16	A B
DeGroot 1991 (24)	1,4	0	0	0	0	<6 months	31	—	A
deJong 1992 (25)	1	2	0	3	0	10 weeks to 9 months	43	4	A B
Wax 1992 (26)	1	3	0	15	3	<4 months	25	—	A
Levin 1992 (27)	1,2,3,4	0.8	0.8	3.4	0	1 day to 45 years	64	23	B C Includes surgery for benign and malignant disease
Pasieka 1992 (28)	1,2,3,5	5	—	8	1.7	<7 days or >3 months	43* 92**	11*	
Wagner 1994 (29)	all	—	4	—	0.5	—	—	—	D
Summary ranges#		0–5	0–4	0–15	0–7.4		25–92	4–23	

The table contains: Author, year of publication, and reference. Definition of completion thyroid surgery varies. This term refers to:
1. Contralateral lobectomy performed shortly after an initial unilateral total or subtotal lobectomy for cancer when preoperative needle biopsy or frozen section failed to diagnose the cancer. In these cases, the contralateral lobe is clinically normal and on pathologic examination may be normal or contain microscopic or small cancers.
2. Contralateral lobectomy for clinical recurrence of cancer in a patient who had previously received lobectomy for cancer.
3. Repeat surgery on the same side for clinical recurrence or persistence.
4. Repeat surgery on the same side without clinical recurrence.
5. Repeat surgery on both sides for clinical recurrence.
6. Combinations of 1 and 3, 1 and 4, 2 and 3, 2 and 4.
Some studies include patients who also received neck dissections.
Frequency (%) of temporary and permanent vocal cord paralysis and temporary and permanent hypoparathyroidism, time from initial surgery to reoperation, frequency (%) of finding cancer in thyroid (ipsilateral or contralateral lobe) and cervical lymph nodes during completion thyroid surgery, and other important points. A dash indicates that information was not available.
A, No patients had reoperation for clinical recurrence.
B, Some cases with lymph node dissection are included.
C, No hypoparathyroidism or vocal cord paralysis occurred in any patient with a prior total lobectomy.
D, 2% rate of vocal cord paralysis for primary cases versus 4% for reoperative cases.
*, For completion thyroid surgery with definition 1.
**, For completion thyroid surgery with definitions 2, 3, 5.
#, Study of Beahrs not included because all cases reoperated for clinically recurrent cancer.

Therefore, the minimal initial thyroid operation for any lesion suspected of being cancer is a total or subtotal lobectomy. During that procedure, the opposite lobe should be palpated, but its parathyroid glands and recurrent laryngeal nerve should not be dissected. This limits the postoperative scarring that would increase the risk of complications if reoperation of that lobe became necessary in the future.

CHANGING TRENDS IN THYROID SURGERY

Over the last half-century, significant changes in thyroid surgery have occurred. In the 1950s, a palpable nodule was often an indication for surgery without any preoperative investigation as to the nature of the nodule. The development of serum tests of thyroid function, radionuclide scanning, ultrasonography, and, less often, computed tomographic (CT) and magnetic resonance image (MRI) scanning, help in the selection of surgery in patients who may have a malignancy. Although none of these tests individually can reliably distinguish benign from malignant disease, the use of several of them can help select patients for surgery. The use of thyroid stimulating hormone (TSH) suppression by administering exogenous thyroxine (T_4) also can aid in the selection of patients for surgery and increase the proportion of operated nodules that contain cancer. Fine-needle aspiration (FNA) also reduced the number of thyroidectomies yet increased the proportion of cancer found in operative cases. With advances in all of these modalities (with FNA providing the greatest benefit), the percentage of thyroidectomies in which cancer was found increased from 6% in the early 1950s to 47% in the late 1980s (30). FNA has caused an increase in the percentage of preoperative malignant diagnoses. With the use of preoperative FNA, thyroid surgery is used less for diagnosis (e.g., lobectomy for possible malignant nodule) and more for therapy (31). Along with FNA, total thyroidectomy has been more frequently performed.

Complications have decreased even though total thyroidectomies are more commonly done. This decrease has been noted when comparing separate studies over the last half century that were reported from the experiences of individual institutions (30,31). Recent reports of complications from thyroid surgery usually show lower rates.

MORTALITY: PAST AND PRESENT

Today we perform thyroid surgery with a mortality rate very close to zero. Prior to the 1870s, mortality was 40%. Only by looking from a historical perspective can we really appreciate the significance of these statistics, which represent the tremendous developments that have taken place in those brief 130 years. These developments constitute our surgical inheritance to which our patients are the fortunate heirs.

Unremitting hemorrhage, sepsis, tetany, and thyroid storm frequently resulted in a fatal outcome of thyroid surgery prior to the 1870s. As each of these complications became understood and therefore largely preventable, the mortality rate of thyroidectomy gradually declined.

Hemorrhage

Prior to the 1870s, ligature, cautery, and extended periods of manual pressure did not adequately control the hemorrhage associated with surgery on the thyroid, a highly vascular and delicate organ especially in cases of exophthalmic goiter (Graves' disease). The situation has been glibly described (32): "Can the thyroid gland when in the stage of enlargement be removed with a reasonable hope of saving the patient? Experience emphatically answers, no! If a surgeon should be so foolhardy as to undertake it . . . every step he takes will be followed by a torrent of blood and lucky will it be for him if his victim lives long enough to enable him to finish his hard butchery. No honest and sensible surgeon would ever engage in it."

The discovery and use of the hemostatic forceps in European clinics during the 1870s enabled the operation to be conducted with reasonable control of bleeding. To help further, Kocher and Mayo (33) staged thyroidectomy. At successive operations they ligated inferior and superior thyroid arteries and then removed first one lobe and then the other. Staging was done as late as the 1940s by Lahey (34) for selected patients with advanced cardiac complications (congestive heart failure, atrial fibrillation) of Graves' disease.

Sepsis

Joseph Lister's discovery of antisepsis in 1867, based on an understanding of the microbiology of infection as established by Pasteur, completely revolutionized surgery. The operative death rate before Lister was 25% to 40% under the best conditions, and 75% to 90% in military hospitals and during the American Civil War, little different since the days of Ambroïse Paré (1517 to 1590). St. Clair Thomson, Lister's house surgeon, wrote: "No wonder that the public dreaded the mention of an operation and shrank and shuddered at the suggestion of entering a hospital. Admission to a surgical ward was looked upon as the entrance to the valley of the shadow of death. . . . Lister, this genius, created anew the ancient art of healing. He did more for surgery and mankind in his lifetime than all the surgeons of all the ages had been able to effect since the days of Hippocrates... the history of Medicine and Surgery... will always be divided into the times before and after Lister" (35).

With hemorrhage and infection under reasonable control, Emil Theodur Kocher, the father of thyroid surgery, was able to achieve a mortality rate of 2.4% in 250 patients in 1889 (36), with deaths still resulting from tetany and thyroid storm.

Tetany

The parathyroid glands were recognized in 1891. In 1896, myxedema after thyroidectomy was distinguished as a separate entity from tetany. In 1898, tetany was shown to result from removal of the parathyroids and not the thyroid (37). Hypocalcemia following parathyroidectomy was demonstrated in 1909 (38).

These discoveries led the way for thyroidectomy with preservation of the parathyroids and a marked reduction in the incidence of tetany (36). In 1908, Mayo (33) reported on 979 thyroidectomies with an overall mortality rate of 2.3%. The mortality for simple, or colloid, goiter or adenoma was 0.7%, with deaths resulting from hemorrhage. However, surgery for Graves' disease was accompanied by a mortality of 25% early in Mayo's series. Surgical treatment often consisted only of ligation of the superior thyroid arteries and veins for mild cases. In more advanced cases, a unilateral lobectomy was done, with or without a contralateral partial lobectomy. In cases where part of the gland was removed, mortality was 6%. Combined mortality for actual thyroidectomy cases and ligation cases was 4.7%, with deaths resulting mainly from thyroid storm.

Thyroid Storm

Thyroid storm remained a significant problem, and it was not until 1915 that Kendall (39) isolated thyroxine, leading to an early understanding of storm. Crile, believing that anxiety caused storm after observing spontaneous storm in nonoperated patients, developed the concept of "stealing" the gland in 1912 (40). After preoperative medication with scopolamine and morphine calmed the patient's mind, the operation was conducted under general and local anesthesia (procaine) with gentle dissection and followed by further local anesthesia (quinine and urea), often without the patient's actual consent and knowledge (a remarkable contrast with the present emphasis on informed consent). This system of anesthesia minimized the effect of surgical shock and decreased storm (41). When Plummer (42) in 1923 introduced Lugol's iodine to suppress the toxic gland, the incidence of storm was significantly reduced (43). This enabled Crile to report on 22,000 thyroidectomies in 1932, half for Graves' disease, with only a 1% mortality. The risk of storm essentially ended in 1945 when Astwood and Vanderlaan (44) reported on the use of antithyroid drugs. All of these improvements enabled Lahey (34) to perform, throughout his career, 18,000 thyroidectomies including 5000 for Graves' disease, with an overall 0.7% mortality.

THE PRESENT

A review of 24,000 thyroidectomies, representing one third of all thyroidectomies performed in the United States during 1971 in both teaching and community hospitals, showed an overall mortality rate of 0.3%. Mortality increased with age, being less than 0.1% in patients younger than 50 years of age, and 2% in those older than 70 (45). Of 1300 thyroidectomies (total, subtotal, and lobectomy) performed between 1974 and 1987 for varied pathologies, the overall mortality rate was 0.13% (46). Over the following decades, refinements in anesthesia, airway and pulmonary management, intensive medical treatment, antibiotics, and surgical training, and dozens of other advances have combined with control of hemorrhage, sepsis, tetany, and storm to produce today's mortality of close to zero.

Reports of 4690 patients undergoing bilateral subtotal thyroidectomy for hyperthyroidism (Graves' disease, toxic multinodular goiter) revealed a zero mortality (47–55). Similarly, surgery for cold nodules, suspicion of carcinoma, and toxic solitary nodules almost always consisting of unilateral lobectomy, can be accomplished with a similar mortality of zero. Recent large series of total thyroidectomy for papillary, follicular, and medullary carcinoma, Graves' disease, and toxic and nontoxic multinodular goiter also show a zero mortality (6,15,16,56). A rising mortality would be expected with total removal, which is very difficult in cases of advanced medullary cancer. For this reason among others, if anaplastic carcinoma, which is often deeply invasive, extends beyond the immediate confines of the thyroid capsule, resection is not attempted. Generally, mortality increases in elderly and medically fragile patients, in patients with substernal goiter, and especially in those with tracheal compression, who require thyroidectomy on an emergency basis (tracheotomy will not relieve airway obstruction that is located inferior to the tracheotomy site). However, a recent report showed no mortality in 12 patients over 80 years of age undergoing thyroidectomy for tracheal compression and malignancy (57). Operative mortality of substernal goiter is low but still significant. Recent reports of thyroidectomy for substernal goiter show mortality rates of 0.8% (58), 3% (59), 3.5% (60), and 7% (61).

ACKNOWLEDGMENTS

The author wishes to thank Lee Reussner, M.D., and Ronald Pulli, M.D., for their helpful suggestions during the preparation of this manuscript.

REFERENCES

1. Falk SA. The management of hyperthyroidism. A surgeon's perspective. *Otolaryngol Clin North Am* 1990;23:361–80.
2. Falk SA, Birken EA, Ronquillo A. Graves' disease associated with histologic Hashimoto's thyroiditis. *Otolaryngol Head Neck Surg* 1985;93:86–91.
3. Falk SA, Birken EA, Baran DT. Temporary postthyroidectomy hypocalcemia. *Arch Otolaryngol Head Neck Surg* 1988;114:168–174.
4. Attie JN, Khaf f RA. Preservation of parathyroid glands during total thyroidectomy. *Am J Surg* 1975;130:399–404.
5. Mountain JC, Stewart GR, Colcock BP. The recurrent laryngeal nerve in thyroid operations. *Surg Gynecol Obstet* 1971;133:978–980.
6. Reeve TS, Delbridge L, Cohen A, Crummer P. Total thyroidectomy: the preferred option for multinodular goiter. *Am J Surg* 1987;206:782–786.
7. Demeester-Mirkine N, Hooghe L, Van Geertruyden J, et al. Hypocalcemia after thyroidectomy. *Arch Surg* 1992;127:854–848.
8. Winsa B, Rastad J, Akerstrom, et al. Retrospective evaluation of subtotal and total thyroidectomy in Graves' disease with and without endocrine ophthalmopathy. *Eur J Endocrinol* 1995;132:406–412.
9. Rao RS, Jog VB, Baluja CA, et al. Risk of hypoparathyroidism after surgery for carcinoma of the thyroid. *Head Neck* 1990;12:321–325.
10. Karlan MS, Catz B, Dunkelman D, et al. A safe technique for thyroidectomy with complete nerve dissection and parathyroid preservation. *Head Neck Surg* 1984;6:1014–1019.
11. Khadra M, Delbridge L, Reeve TS, et al. Total thyroidectomy: its role in the management of thyroid disease. *Aust N Z J Surg* 1992;62:91–95.
12. Perzik SL. The place of total thyroidectomy in the management of 909 patients with thyroid disease. *Am J Surg* 1976;132:480–483.
13. Clark OH. Total thyroidectomy: the treatment of choice for patients with differentiated thyroid cancer. *Ann Surg* 1982;196:361–370.
14. Thompson NG, Olsen WR, Hoffman GL. The continuing development of the technique of thyroidectomy. *Surgery* 1973;73:913–927.
15. Harness JK, Fung L, Thompson NW, Burney RE, McLeod MK. Total thyroidectomy: complications and technique. *World J Surg* 1986;10:781–786.
16. Jacobs JK, Alard JW, Ballinger JF. Total thyroidectomy. *Ann Surg* 1983;197:542–548.

17. Chonkich GD, Petti GH, Goral W. Total thyroidectomy in the treatment of thyroid disease. *Laryngoscope* 1987;97:897–900.
18. Saxe AW, Spiegel AM, Marx SJ, Brennan MF. Deferred parathyroid autografts with cryopreserved tissue after reoperative surgery. *Arch Surg* 1982;117:538–543.
19. Beahrs OH, Vandertoll DJ. Complications of secondary thyroidectomy. *Surg Gynecol Obstet* 1963;117:535–539.
20. Thompson NW, Harness JK. Complications of total thyroidectomy for carcinoma. *Surg Gynec Obstet* 1970;131:861–868.
21. Rao RS, Fakih AR, Mehta AR, et al. Completion thyroidectomy for thyroid carcinoma. *Head Neck Surg* 1987;9:284–288.
22. Calabro S, Auguste L, Attie JN. Morbidity of completion thyroidectomy for initially misdiagnosed thyroid carcinoma. *Head Neck Surg* 1988;10:235–238.
23. Auguste L, Attie JN. Completion thyroidectomy for initially misdiagnosed thyroid cancer. *Otolaryngol Clin North Am* 1990;23:429–439.
24. DeGroot LJ, Kaplan EL. Second operations for "completion" of thyroidectomy in treatment of differentiated thyroid cancer. *Surgery* 1991;110:936–940.
25. De Jong SA, Demeter JG, Lawrence AM, et al. Necessity and safety of completion thyroidectomy for differentiated thyroid carcinoma. *Surgery* 1992;112:734–739.
26. Wax MK, Briant TDR. Completion thyroidectomy in the management of well-differentiated thyroid carcinoma. *Otolaryngol Head Neck Surg* 1992;107:63–68.
27. Levin KE, Clark AH, Duh Q, et al. Reoperative thyroid surgery. *Surgery* 1992;111:604–609.
28. Pasieka JL, Thompson NW, McLeod MK, et al. The incidence of bilateral well-differentiated thyroid cancer found at completion thyroidectomy. *World J Surg* 1992;16:711–717.
29. Wagner HE, Seiler CA. Indications for and results of recurrent surgery of the thyroid gland. *J Suisse Med* 1994;124:1222–1226.
30. Galloway JW, Sardi A, DeConti RW, et al. Changing trends in thyroid surgery. *Am J Surg* 1991;57:18–20.
31. Puls T. The changing aspect of thyroid surgery: a review of 130 consecutive cases. *Acta Otorhinolaryngol Belg* 1993;47:351–354.
32. Gross SD. *A system of surgery,* vol 2, 4th ed. Philadelphia: HC Lea, 1886;394.
33. Mayo CH. A consideration of the mortality in one thousand operations for goitre. *Trans South Surg Gynecol Assoc* 1908;21:225–287.
34. Lahey FH. Aids in avoiding serious complications in thyroidectomy. *Trans South Surg Assoc* 1940;53:89–105.
35. Thomson S. Lister: a house surgeon's memories. *King's College Hospital Gazette,* 1937, Oct.
36. Halsted W. The operative story of goitre. *Johns Hopkins Hosp Rev* 1920;19:71–257.
37. Welsh DA. On the parathyroid glands of the cat. A preliminary study in experimental pathology. *J Pathol* 1898;5:202.
38. McCallum WC, Voegtlin C. On the relation of tetany to the parathyroid glands and to calcium metabolism. *J Exp Med* 1909;11:118.
39. Kendall EC. The isolation in crystalline form of the compound containing iodine which occurs in the thyroid: its chemical nature and physiological activity. *Trans Assoc Am Physicians* 1915;70:420.
40. Crile GW. The identity of cause of aseptic wound, fever, and post-operative hypothyroidism and their prevention. *Trans South Surg Assoc* 1912;25:417–421.
41. Colcock BP. Lest we forget: a story of five surgeons. *Surgery* 1968;64:1162–1172.
42. Plummer HS. Results of administering iodine to patients having exophthalmic goiter. *JAMA* 1923;80:1955.
43. Sistruck WE. The part which iodine played in the treatment of patients with exophthalmic goitre. *Trans South Surg Assoc* 1928;41:112–119.
44. Astwood EB, Vanderlaan WP. Thiouracil derivations of greater activity for the treatment of hyperthyroidism. *J Clin Endocrinol Metab* 1945;5:424–430.
45. Foster RS. Morbidity and mortality after thyroidectomy. *Surg Gynecol Obstet* 1978;146:423–429.
46. Carditello A. Nodular thyropathies. *J Chirurgie* 1990;127:330–333.
47. Osoux JP, DeCalan L, Portier G, et al. Surgical treatment of Graves' disease. *Am J Surg* 1988;156:177–181.
48. Califano G, Abate S, Ferulano GP, Danzi M. Surgery of toxic goiter: indications and long-term results. *Ital J Surg Sci* 1985;15:233–237.
49. Simms JM, Talbot CH. Surgery for thyrotoxicosis. *Br J Surg* 1983;70:581–583.
50. Cusick EL, Krukowski ZH, Matheson NA. Outcome of surgery for Graves' disease re-examined. *Br J Surg* 1987;74:780–783.
51. Melliere F, Etienne G, Becquemin JP. Operations for hyperthyroidism. *Am J Surg* 1988;155:395–399.
52. Sugrue DD, Drury MI, McEvoy M, Heffernan SJ, O'Malley E. Long term follow up of hyperthyroid patients treated by subtotal thyroidectomy. *Br J Surg* 1983;70:408–411.
53. Blondeau P. Surgical treatment of hyperthyroidism from a personal experience of 2395 cases. *Bull Acad Natl Med* 1991;175:1065–1073.
54. Patwardhan NA, Moront M, Rao S, et al. Surgery still has a role in Graves' hyperthyroidism. *Surgery* 1993;114:1108–1113.
55. Menegaux F, Ruprecht T, Chigot J. The surgical treatment of Graves' disease. *Surg Gynecol Obstet* 1992;176:277–282.
56. Winsa B, Rastad J, Larsson E, et al. Total thyroidectomy in therapy-resistant Graves' disease. *Surgery* 1994;116:1068–1075.
57. Miccoli P, Iacconi P, Cecchini GM, et al. Thyroid surgery in patients aged over 80 years. *Acta Chirurg Belg* 1994;94:222–223.
58. DeAndrade MA. A review of 128 cases of posterior mediastinal goiter. *World J Surg* 1977;1:789–797.
59. Georgiadis N, Katsas A, Leoutsakos B. Substernal goiter. *Int Surg* 1970;54:116–121.
60. Watt-Boolsen S, Blichert-Toft M, Folke K, et al. Surgical treatment of benign nontoxic intrathoracic goiter: a long term observation. *Am J Surg* 1981;141:721–722.
61. Lamke LO, Bergdahl L, Lamke B. Intrathoracic goiter: a review of 29 cases. *Acta Chir Scand* 1979;145:83–86.

CHAPTER 38

Nonmetabolic Complications of Thyroid Surgery

David D. Caldarelli and Andrew J. Lerrick

Essential to the successful surgical management of thyroid disease are recognition of variations in regional neurovascular anatomy, knowledge of diverse surgical approaches, and an understanding of current intraoperative monitoring techniques. Despite significant advances in surgical technique and postoperative management, complications following thyroid surgery continue to produce significant morbidity. Recurrent laryngeal nerve trauma and hypoparathyroidism cause temporary or permanent injury, often requiring aggressive medical or surgical management. Although less frequent, postoperative bleeding and upper airway obstruction may be life-threatening and require emergency intervention. This chapter discusses methods used to identify the recurrent and superior laryngeal nerves; variations of neurovascular anatomy in the viscerovertebral angle; common neurovascular and upper airway complications attendant to thyroid surgery; newly developed intraoperative nerve monitoring methods; immediate and long-term management of common nonmetabolic complications; and recent research in vocal fold rehabilitation after laryngeal nerve injury.

ANATOMY (See also Chapter 2)

Thyroid Gland

The thyroid gland consists of a left and a right lobe, which extend superolaterally to the thyroid cartilage from a connecting isthmus, which usually overlies the second and third tracheal rings (1). The thyroid gland derives its blood supply bilaterally from the inferior thyroid artery, a branch of the thyrocervical trunk, and the superior thyroid artery, the first branch of the external carotid artery (2). An embryologic remnant may persist, the thyroidea ima artery, which arises from the aorta, inominate, or carotid artery and travels on the anterior surface of the trachea to supply the isthmus (3). Blood from the gland drains into the superior, middle, and inferior thyroid veins. Fifty percent of glands have a pyramidal lobe. Occasionally, the isthmus is absent and the gland is in two parts (1). Autonomously functioning accessory thyroid tissue can be found anywhere between the suprahyoid tissue and the aortic arch. Sympathetic nerve fibers arising from the cervical ganglion innervate the gland. Parasympathetic fibers are derived from the vagus nerve via laryngeal nerve branches.

Recurrent Laryngeal Nerve

The right recurrent laryngeal nerve arises from the main vagal trunk at the first part of the subclavian artery and loops posteriorly around the undersurface of the artery before ascending superiorly and medially in the upper mediastinum to the tracheoesophageal groove in the lower cervical region. The nerve then travels superiorly in a vertical direction for almost the entire length of the thyroid gland, passing deep to the inferior constrictor muscle and medially behind the posterior suspensory ligament of Berry to enter the larynx posteriorly at the cricothyroid junction, at a site known as Killian's space. The end branch of the recurrent laryngeal nerve, known as the inferior laryngeal nerve, accompanies the inferior laryngeal artery into the larynx. The left recurrent laryngeal nerve courses around the arch of the aorta in a posterior direction before ascending in the tracheoesophageal groove to follow a course similar to the right recurrent laryngeal nerve.

The recurrent laryngeal nerve carries motor, sensory, and parasympathetic fibers. The nerve divides into an internal branch, which supplies sensation to the vocal cords and subglottic region, and an external branch, which provides motor function to four of the five intrinsic laryngeal

---

D. D. Caldarelli and A. J. Lerrick: Department of Otolaryngology/Bronchoesophagology, Rush-Presbyterian-St. Luke's Medical Center, Chicago, Illinois 60612.

muscles (4). These five muscles are the thyroarytenoid (vocalis), the posterior cricoarytenoid, the lateral cricoarytenoid, the transverse and oblique arytenoid, and the cricothyroid. Prior to entering the larynx, the nerve sends branches to the inferior constrictor and cricopharyngeus muscles.

It has been hypothesized that the recurrent laryngeal nerve divides into selective motor fibers before entering the larynx. In fact, were extralaryngeal divisions of the recurrent laryngeal nerve present, selective injury to abductor and adductor fibers would occur (5). In anatomic studies, Rustad (6) found 43% of recurrent laryngeal nerves divided externally into one or more branches. The anterior division passed either anteriorly or posteriorly to the cricothyroid articulation and then coursed along the cricoarytenoid muscle to innervate all intrinsic laryngeal muscles, whereas the posterior branch usually innervated only the posterior cricoarytenoid and arytenoideus muscles.

Alternatively, most current anatomic, physiologic, and surgical evidence supports Galen's original concept of internal division (7). Using microscopic evaluation, staining techniques, and radioactive tracers to determine neural pathways, other investigators support the concept of intralaryngeal ramification. Kratz (8) used the operating microscope to identify the recurrent laryngeal nerves, noting that the nerve divides internally almost 100% of the time. Dedo (9) mapped recurrent laryngeal nerve ramifications, demonstrating that intrinsic nerve fibers branch after entering the larynx, suggesting that extralaryngeal trauma, injury, or disease affect the entire recurrent laryngeal nerve and are not site specific. The course of the recurrent laryngeal nerve frequently varies despite normal anatomy, or as a consequence of congenital vascular anomalies, maldevelopment of adjacent structures, and/or distortion of regional anatomy by neoplasms, trauma, or inflammation (Fig. 1).

Hunt et al. (10) noted that the recurrent laryngeal nerve was located in the tracheoesophageal groove on the right 65% of the time and on the left 77% of the time. The recurrent laryngeal nerve was lateral to the trachea on the right 33% of the time, as opposed to 22% on the left. In six instances on the right and four on the left of 151 cases, the nerve was anterolateral to the trachea and highly vulnerable to iatrogenic injury.

Numerous neural pathway variations occur in the vicinity of the thyroid, especially when glandular disease is present. At the level of the inferior pole, the inferior thyroid artery may traverse the recurrent laryngeal nerve anteriorly or posteriorly; alternatively, the nerve may pass between arterial ramifications. Hunt et al. (10) noted that the recurrent laryngeal nerve is embedded in the posterior suspensory ligament of Berry in 50% of cases.

One significant anatomic variation altering the pathway of the recurrent laryngeal nerve is an aberrant right subclavian artery. When this anomaly occurs, the recurrent laryngeal nerve emanates directly from the vagus nerve and traverses medially toward the adjacent thyroid gland without recurring around the subclavian artery. Similarly, when only a right aortic arch is present, the left recurrent laryngeal nerve is nonrecurrent. When a double aortic arch is present, each nerve is recurrent around its respective aorta.

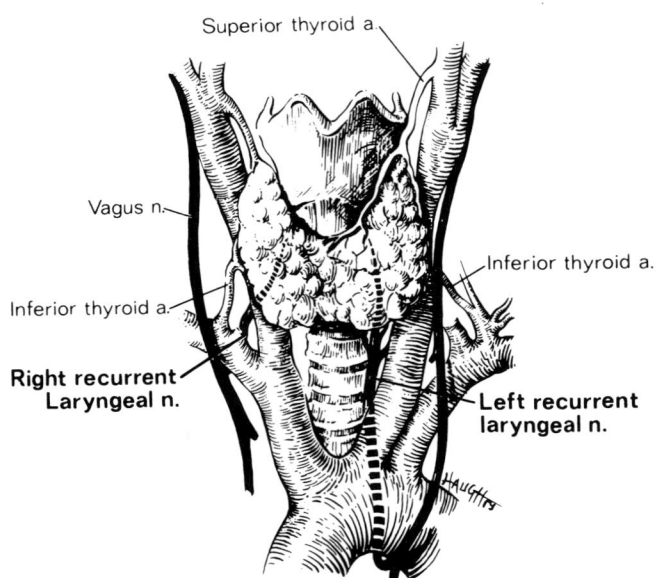

FIG. 1. Usual relationships of recurrent laryngeal nerve to thyroid parenchyma and vasculature.

Superior Laryngeal Nerve

The superior laryngeal nerve is a branch of the vagus nerve arising from the lower ganglion that travels inferomedially between the internal and external carotid arteries. At the level of the hyoid bone, the superior laryngeal nerve divides into a large medial internal branch that penetrates the thyrohyoid membrane to provide sensory and secretory fibers to the supraglottic larynx, and a small lateral external branch that carries motor fibers to the cricothyroid muscle and inferior constrictor (1). The cricothyroid muscle is innervated by the motor division of the superior laryngeal nerve; it is the only intrinsic laryngeal muscle not innervated by the recurrent laryngeal nerve. The external branch of the superior laryngeal nerve travels medially to the superior thyroid artery and continues its descent superficial to the investing fascia of the inferior pharyngeal constrictor muscle (Fig. 2). The branch is separated from the superior pole of the thyroid gland and the superior thyroid vasculature by loose connective tissue. The nerve and artery pass beneath the sternothyroid muscle. Sun and Chang's study (11) of superior laryngeal nerve pathways in 120 cadavers found that 118 had an anatomic variant consisting of a neural loop con-

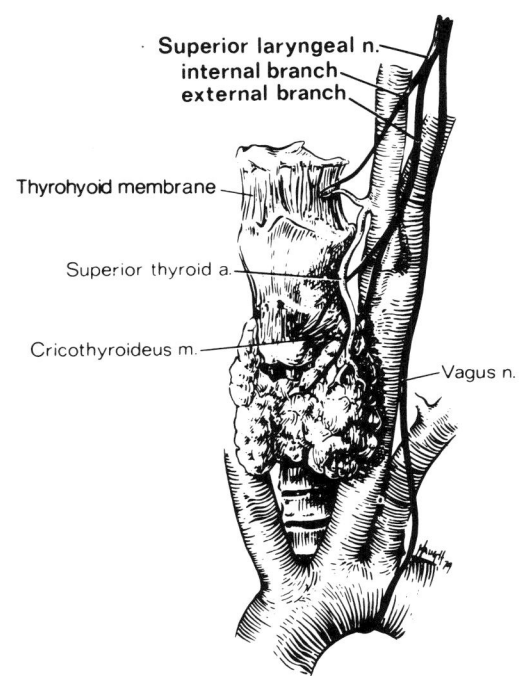

FIG. 2. Usual relationships of superior laryngeal nerve to thyroid parenchyma and vasculature.

necting the cervical sympathetic chain with the superior laryngeal nerve and its external and internal branches.

METHODS OF IDENTIFICATION

Recurrent Laryngeal Nerve

Most surgeons advise identifying rather than avoiding the recurrent laryngeal nerve when performing thyroid surgery. Nerve preservation is best accomplished through careful surgical technique that uses important anatomic landmarks to identify the nerve. Initial steps are elevation of subplatysmal flaps, lateral retraction of the sternocleidomastoid muscles, incision of the midline raphe, retraction of the strap muscles for exposure, and release of the surrounding soft tissue by gentle dissection. Identification of the recurrent laryngeal nerve is crucial after exposure and gross examination of the gland.

Loré et al. (12) proposed that the nerve be identified following the principles of parotid gland excision, in which the main trunk of the facial nerve is identified prior to gland mobilization and removal. The inferior thyroid artery is a reliable anatomic landmark for identifying the recurrent laryngeal nerve. Beahrs (13) described a triangle formed by the common carotid artery posteriorly, the inferior thyroid artery superiorly, and the recurrent laryngeal nerve anteroinferiorly. However, identification of the artery does not assure subsequent detection of the nerve, because of numerous variations in their neurovascular relationship. Dissection has generally shown the left inferior thyroid artery to be situated anteriorly to the recurrent laryngeal nerve in 60% of cases, whereas the right inferior thyroid artery is anterior to the nerve in 40%. In 10%, the nerve is so interlaced with branches of the artery that the relationship is uncertain. Loré et al. (12) and Sedgwick (14) believe that the nerve should be identified in the tracheoesophageal groove if not found after isolating the inferior thyroid artery. Using this approach, the recurrent laryngeal nerve is exposed in a triangle formed by the trachea and esophagus medially, the common carotid artery laterally, and the thyroid lobe superiorly. Wang (15) proposed a more constant anatomic relationship between the recurrent laryngeal nerve and the inferior cornu of the thyroid cartilage. Once identified, the nerve can be followed superiorly, where it may nonetheless become trapped in gland parenchyma. During particularly difficult dissections, magnification and electrical nerve monitoring may be needed.

The posterior suspensory ligament of Berry is another important landmark used to identify the recurrent laryngeal nerve. This ligament originates from the cricoid cartilage and upper tracheal rings and attaches to the posteromedial aspect of each thyroid lobe. The recurrent laryngeal nerve passes deep to the ligament. The nerve is at increased risk in this area, particularly if there is glandular enlargement or fibrosis caused by carcinoma, Graves' disease, or Hashimoto's thyroiditis. During glandular traction, embedded nerve fibers may be pulled forward and are thus vulnerable to injury. At times, a portion of the thyroid gland enveloped within the suspensory ligament may be mistaken for tumor invasion of the recurrent laryngeal nerve, leading to unnecessary sacrifice of the nerve. Alternatively, a posteromedial extension of the thyroid lobe lying medial to Berry's ligament may be overlooked during total thyroidectomy. Examination of the anterior neck from foramen cecum to the suprasternal notch is essential to prevent overlooking residual disease; there have been numerous instances of carcinoma arising in a thyroglossal remnant (16).

Gross tumor invasion by malignant disease is an indication for nerve sacrifice. Nerve preservation is possible if a plane of dissection can be established between the tumor and the epineurium.

Superior Laryngeal Nerve

A lateral approach to expose the superior pole of the thyroid gland, with division and ligation of the superior thyroid vessels, is one of the final steps during thyroidectomy. A medial approach to the superior thyroid artery provides limited exposure and risks nerve injury. Anatomic distortion, adherence of the nerve to a chronically inflamed thyroid gland, and displacement of the neurovascular pedicle may cause technical problems.

Mooseman and DeWeese (17) noted that the course of the superior laryngeal nerve varied 21% of the time; in 15%, the nerve adhered to the superior thyroid artery or its branches, and in 6% it was entrapped while looping around or through the arterial branches.

Beahrs (13) described a method for superior laryngeal nerve identification in the sternothyrolaryngeal triangle. Within this triangle, the nerve is usually medial to the superior thyroid vasculature and adjacent to the inferior pharyngeal constrictor. If there is unusual enlargement of the superior pole, transection of the sternothyroid muscle below its attachment to the thyroid cartilage allows easier access, and, consequently, better exposure of the neurovascular structures. Another technical maneuver to facilitate exposure of the superior thyroid vessels is to superiorly retract or divide the sternothyroid muscle and inferiorly retract the upper pole of the thyroid. Gentle retraction of the vascular pedicle permits identification of the external branch as it courses along the surface or enters the body of the cricothyroid muscle. To minimize the risk of nerve damage, indiscriminate use of electrocautery should be avoided in the area of the superior pole, and caution should be exercised when cross-clamping the superior pedicle.

INTRAOPERATIVE NERVE MONITORING

Several electrophysiologic methods of assessing nerve function by monitoring laryngeal musculature contraction have recently been developed to help detect the recurrent laryngeal nerve during dissection (18,19). Electromyographic and nerve action potentials can be recorded using an endotracheal tube with electrical sensors (20) or by placing a recording electrode endoscopically in the thyroarytenoid muscle (19). The simplest technique employs a disposable nerve stimulator similar to the one used to identify the facial nerve during parotid surgery. Alternatively, the recurrent laryngeal nerve can be stimulated while an assistant palpates the arytenoid cartilage and posterior cricoarytenoid muscle, noting the presence or absence of motion in these structures (21).

NEURAL INJURY

Vocal cord function should be evaluated and documented preoperatively because of the multiple risks for neurologic injury during thyroid surgery. To prevent recurrent laryngeal nerve injury, the surgeon must anticipate anatomic variations in the course of the nerve and recognize that its course may be altered by pathologic conditions of the thyroid gland or adjacent lymph nodes. A review of the literature reveals that when the recurrent laryngeal nerve is identified, there is a statistically significant lower rate of temporary and permanent paralysis than that for procedures performed without obligatory nerve identification ($p < .01$) (22). Risk factors for transient and permanent recurrent laryngeal nerve paralysis include underlying thyroid disease, the extent of resection, and failure to expose the nerve (23).

Inadvertent recurrent laryngeal nerve trauma during thyroid surgery has decreased over the past two decades, especially during secondary or extensive thyroid procedures, as a result of increased awareness of the intrinsic relationship between the recurrent laryngeal nerve and the thyroid gland, use of magnification (e.g., loupes, operating microscope), and advances in intraoperative electrical methods to identify the nerve. After detection, injury is usually caused by stretching, crushing, suturing, or severing the main nerve trunk. Indiscriminate attempts at hemostasis may result in injury to the recurrent laryngeal nerve at any level. Delicate dissection and meticulous hemostasis are essential.

Should nerve transection occur, immediate microsurgical anastomosis is advisable. Repair of the severed nerve may prevent vocal cord atrophy (24,25). Epineural anastomosis is superior to perineural repair. Suggested suture size is 7-0 or 8-0 nylon or polypropylene. Unfortunately, neural anastomosis rarely restores normal function. Recovery is greater in the event of partial transection.

Acute denervation leads either to nerve regeneration (complete reinnervation with synkinesis, partial reinnervation with synkinesis, or mixed recurrent laryngeal nerve injuries) or to chronic denervation (complete paralysis) (4).

Unilateral Recurrent Laryngeal Nerve Injury

Unilateral recurrent laryngeal nerve injury is the most common traumatic neurolaryngologic lesion (4). The glottis alteration after recurrent laryngeal nerve injury is complex. Acute effects range from vocal fold flaccidity with loss of abduction and adduction causing dysphonia, to complete paralytic aphonia with periodic aspiration and an ineffective cough (4). Long-term effects include paralysis of the vocal fold in a median or paramedian position; a shortened membranous segment of the paralyzed vocal fold; and hyperadduction of the normal vocal fold during phonation in an attempt to close the posterior gap (26). Clinically, inadequate glottic closure causes weak phonation and a breathy voice. Representative studies report an incidence of recurrent and superior laryngeal nerve injury of 1% to 17.5% for all types of thyroid and concomitant surgery (27).

Wagner and Seiler (23) found that recurrent laryngeal nerve palsy occurred in 5.9% of 1026 patients, of which 59% were transient and 2.4% were permanent. The incidence of nerve injury was as follows: euthyroid goiter (1.7%), recurrent goiter (3.8%), Graves' disease (4%), chronic lymphocytic thyroiditis (5%), and thyroid carcinoma (8%). The incidence of permanent recurrent laryngeal nerve palsy was 1.1% for subtotal lobectomy and

4.0% for total lobectomy. Risk of recurrent laryngeal nerve paralysis greatly increases to as high as 17.5% in retrosternal goiters (28).

Recent studies (6,12) show recurrent laryngeal nerve injury has decreased. In 488 instances of nerve dissection, Loré (24) reported permanent laryngeal nerve paralysis of under 0.5%; temporary paralysis was 2.6%. One study reported a 2% incidence of nerve damage in patients who underwent primary surgery for thyroid carcinoma (29). Concomitant regional or radical neck dissection increased the incidence of nerve injury to 13% in 39 patients. Mediastinal exploration puts the nerve at greater risk.

Beahrs (13) noted that nerve injury increases markedly during secondary thyroid surgery, to 9.5% for benign disease and 17% for secondary and tertiary procedures for carcinoma. Despite inherent risk, reoperation for recurrent or persistent thyroid carcinoma should be performed to permit effective radioactive iodine treatment and scanning for metastatic disease (30).

Loré (24) advocates intraoperative and postoperative steroids for difficult dissections. Nerve identification and preservation is particularly challenging if the patient has a thyroid malignancy or a history of chronic thyroiditis, thyroid surgery, or radiotherapy. Early exploration is advocated when unilateral vocal cord paralysis occurs in the immediate postoperative period if the cause is entrapment. Removal of a constricting ligature usually results in neural recovery (31). Surgically related temporary neuropraxia is far more common, in which case exploration is unwarranted.

Preoperative vocal cord paralysis is not always caused by thyroid malignancy. One study of 2453 patients, 29 of whom had preoperative vocal cord palsy, found that 75% had benign disease; function returned postoperatively in 89% (32). Approximately 1% to 2% of preoperative paralysis is caused by a benign thyroid mass compressing the nerve against the cervical spine or trachea. Nerve preservation makes postoperative recovery possible (33). Imaging studies of the brainstem, skull base, neck, and chest are warranted to rule out other etiologies in the absence of thyroid disease.

Bilateral Recurrent Laryngeal Nerve Injury

Bilateral vocal cord paralysis remains one of the most severe complications of thyroid surgery and a challenging problem in laryngology. In a review of 389 cases of bilateral abductor vocal cord paralysis, 58% were secondary to thyroid surgery (34). The condition is marked by varying degrees of inspiratory stridor, dyspnea, and minimal dysphonia. It is often manifest upon extubation immediately after thyroidectomy if neuropraxia and/or neural transection have occurred. Patients developing severe respiratory stridor require immediate rigid or flexible fiberoptic laryngoscopy to assess cord mobility; emergency endotracheal intubation is warranted. Tracheotomy may be required to maintain a patent airway until definitive treatment is undertaken.

Bilateral recurrent laryngeal nerve paralysis may remain clinically undetected for long periods of time. Many patients tolerate a minimal airway for years until a severe respiratory infection compromises it. To rule out asymptomatic bilateral vocal cord paralysis, all patients should undergo laryngoscopic examination after thyroidectomy. Postthyroidectomy hypothyroidism precipitates airway distress in over 50% of patients with bilateral vocal cord paralysis. This condition is usually associated with myxedema infiltration of the paralyzed cords, causing further closure of a previously narrowed airway (35). Laryngospasm, associated with hypocalcemic tetany of hypoparathyroidism, may produce sudden airway obstruction (36).

Superior Laryngeal Nerve Injury

Thyroid surgery is the most common cause of injury to the external branch of the superior laryngeal nerve; the internal branch is rarely involved (37). Unilateral and bilateral superior laryngeal nerve paralysis is frequently overlooked. Electromyography of the cricothyroid muscle reveals a fairly high incidence of unilateral and bilateral, transient and permanent, paralysis (38). In 325 patients evaluated for voice preservation after thyroidectomy, permanent changes were noted in 11% after lobectomy and 25% after subtotal thyroidectomy. When the superior laryngeal nerve was identified and preserved, voice changes occurred in only 5% of patients (39).

Symptoms of unilateral superior laryngeal nerve injury include frequent throat clearing, a breathy voice, loss of upper vocal registers, fatigue while vocalizing, huskiness, and difficulty maintaining or changing vocal pitch (27,40). On indirect laryngeal examination, the paralyzed vocal cord appears shorter, hyperemic, and at a lower level than the contralateral cord. The glottic chink may appear oblique, because of rotation of the posterior commissure toward the paralyzed side. Contraction of the intact cricothyroid muscle causes the epiglottis and anterior larynx to shift toward the nonparalyzed side.

After bilateral superior laryngeal nerve injury, the larynx appears symmetric because both cricothyroid muscles are paralyzed. Signs of bilateral paralysis are subtle: the absence of vertical tilt of the thyroid on the cricoid cartilage and failure of the vocal cords to lengthen and tense during phonation. Visualization of the vocal cords may be obscured by the epiglottis, which may overhang the anterior glottis. The cords appear bowed, flaccid, and hyperemic, and they allow excess escape of air during phonation, producing a weak, poorly controlled, breathy, low-pitched voice. Stroboscopic evaluation and laryngeal electromyography aid in evaluating subtle vocal cord pathology (41).

Combined Superior and Recurrent Laryngeal Nerve Injury

Combinations of superior and recurrent laryngeal nerve paralysis produce symptoms of varying degree and severity. Unilateral paralysis of both the superior and recurrent nerves, with preservation of the internal branch of the superior laryngeal nerve, is the most common injury resulting from thyroid surgery. The voice is weak and breathy. The paralyzed cord is bowed and may appear erythematous. During respiration, the affected cord is immobile and remains in a lateral position, providing a better airway than that of isolated recurrent nerve paralysis (37). With phonation, the normal cord is slightly superior to the flaccid, paralyzed cord, the epiglottis and anterior larynx shift toward the intact contracting cricothyroid muscle, and the posterior larynx moves toward the paralyzed cord (37).

LARYNGEAL REHABILITATION

The goals of treatment after nerve injury are restoration of normal phonation, elimination of aspiration, and preservation of airway (42). If a traumatized nerve has not recovered spontaneous function within 6 months and glottic incompetence persists, phonosurgery can achieve permanent glottic competence. Many surgeons prefer to wait 1 year before intervention. Indications for phonosurgery are a breathy voice, chronic aspiration, and poor pulmonary clearance from a diminished cough. Treatment includes voice therapy alone or in combination with vocal fold augmentation, laryngoplastic phonosurgery (medialization thyroplasty, arytenoid adduction), or laryngeal reinnervation (nerve–nerve anastomosis, nerve–muscle transfer) (4,42).

Analysis of Vocal Quality

Historically, the evaluation of patients with vocal fold paralysis has included subjective assessment, self-evaluation, objective measures, and perceptual judgment of voice recordings (43,44). Currently, acoustic signal analysis, aerodynamic flow, videostroboscopic, and perceptual patient self-evaluation are used for analysis of the voice pre- and posttreatment (26,45). Aerodynamic measures include subglottal pressure, airflow, and laryngeal resistance (42,43,46,47). Speech therapists look for improvement in voice quality, jitter, shimmer, and maximum intensity (47). Electromyography is used to record laryngeal muscle function during phonation and respiration, and at rest. It can distinguish between paralysis and mechanical fixation of the vocal cord (41). Laryngeal electromyography can detect recurrent and superior laryngeal nerve damage and can predict the potential for recovery of a paralyzed vocal cord in 90% of cases (4).

TREATMENT OF UNILATERAL RECURRENT LARYNGEAL NERVE INJURY

Management of unilateral vocal fold paralysis is controversial (48). Currently, vocal fold injection, thyroplasty, and reinnervation techniques are employed to surgically rehabilitate the paralyzed larynx (49). Teflon injection is the quickest and least expensive procedure, although many prefer newer techniques that provide superior phonatory quality and are fully reversible.

Endoscopic Techniques

Intrafold injection into the paralyzed thyroarytenoid muscle of allogenic or xenogenic substances augments the vocal fold medially to provide competent glottic closure. Increasing the bulk of the vocalis muscle permits apposition with the functioning cord during phonation, coughing, and swallowing (45). Injection is performed under topical and local anesthesia by suspension laryngoscopy or transorally, using a curved laryngeal needle. Ward et al. (50) recommended percutaneous injection for patients with trismus or who cannot tolerate laryngoscopy, in which case a 16-gauge spinal needle is introduced into the subglottic lumen via the cricothyroid membrane and directed to the undersurface of the cord. Vocal cord visualization for transoral or percutaneous injection is provided by a televised fiberoptic laryngoscope. McCaffrey et al. (51) safely performed 62 transcutaneous injections in the office without anesthesia.

Patients may be injected under general anesthesia using the operating microscope, which permits better exposure and more accurate injection (52). The drawback is the inability to assess the voice or airway prior to extubation.

Resorbable Agents

In acute situations, temporary augmentation is achieved with glyceride, which is resorbed in 2 to 3 days. Repeated injections are required until the nerve recovers or a permanent rehabilitative procedure is performed. Gelfoam paste can be injected to achieve an effect of 6 to 10 weeks' duration (53).

Teflon Injection

Teflon (polytef, polytetrafluoroethylene) paste injection remains the easiest method of achieving permanent vocal fold augmentation after unilateral vocal cord paralysis. Teflon injection has been the mainstay of treatment for three decades for glottic insufficiency, despite the drawback of being essentially irreversible (45). Improvement is greater for controlling aspiration than correcting dysphonia (54). The major defect of unilateral vocal cord paralysis, a soft and breathy voice, can be diminished by injecting Teflon into the paralyzed cord to move the immobile edge to the midline, eliminating the air leak and permitting the mobile cord to vibrate firmly against the edge of the paralyzed cord during phonation (55). Teflon causes vocal fold stiffness with loss of the mucosal wave (56). Teflon injection should not be performed for 6 months after traumatic nerve dissection but should be offered to patients with terminal disease in spite of their poor prognosis (57).

Complications of Teflon Injection

Poor voice quality following Teflon injection is usually the result of inaccurate placement on either the undersurface or in the phonating edge of the cord. The poorest results were seen in patients with scarring and atrophy. Late vocal cord recovery or injection into mobile vocal folds that did not warrant Teflon is disastrous and requires Teflon excision (45,58). Overinjection and granulomatous foreign body reaction are the two most common problems associated with Teflon injection. Overfilling may result in acute respiratory distress. Excess Teflon should be immediately removed by microlaryngoscopy, by incising the vocal cord and extracting the compound with an aspirator or cupped forceps, which causes considerable scarring. An alternative approach for managing convex vocal folds and granulomas is cordectomy (59). Complications of granulomatosis include arytenoid fixation necessitating arytenoidectomy, replacement of the thyroarytenoid muscle, and endotracheal migration (60,61). One patient presented with a cold thyroid nodule 3 years after intracordal injection (62). Airway obstruction occurring as a late consequence of granuloma formation may require tracheotomy (60,63,64). Teflon histology reveals intracellular refractile material of irregular shape with epithelioid histiocytes and giant cells (61). In many instances, adequate coverage with microflaps cannot be achieved (64). A prospective analysis of lung function using spirometric and flow-volume loop studies demonstrated an increase in airway resistance after Teflon injection that was not evident clinically (58).

Autologous Lipoinjection

Limitations of Teflon prompted use of other materials to augment the vocal fold. Autologous fat has been used as an alternative to alloplastic substances (65). Fat imparts soft bulk, allows the cord to retain vibratory qualities, and does not migrate (65,66). Histologic studies confirm the preservation of viable fat 6 months after injection. Drawbacks of lipoinjection include unsatisfactory voice quality, and respiratory compromise from overinjection. Fat is an autologous material that can be retrieved successfully if overinjected (66).

Collagen Injection

Soluble bovine collagen has been an alternative agent to restore glottic competence for more than 10 years (44). Collagen is structurally similar to host connective tissue and rarely causes a hypersensitivity reaction. It provides better vocal cord vibration and better phonation than Teflon (67). Collagen possesses unique advantages as a bioimplant, making it well suited to treat vocal fold atrophy, vocal cord defects, minimal glottic insufficiency, and scarred vocal cords that are not optimally managed with Teflon (44,47). If the injected collagen is improperly distributed, the implant can be removed with little damage. Another agent that has been injected into the paralyzed vocal cord is a hydrophilic gel; this material assumes an elastic property similar to the surrounding tissue, improves voice quality, and reduces vocal fatigue (68).

Laryngeal Framework Surgery

Laryngeal framework surgery is one type of phoniatric surgery (69). Patients who require laryngeal framework surgery generally fall into two categories: those with paralytic dysphonias (arytenoid rotation technique, Isshiki's type I thyroplasty) and those seeking adjustments in vocal fold tension to produce changes in vocal pitch (cricothyroid approximation, Isshiki's type III thyroplasty, and LeJeune's anterior commissure laryngoplasty) (69). This discussion will address only the former. Laryngoplastic procedures are best performed using local anesthesia to permit fine-tuning of the voice intraoperatively.

Medialization laryngoplasty (Isshiki's type I thyroplasty) achieves vocal cord medialization by placing an implant below the inner perichondrium of the thyroid cartilage (70–72). Proper size, shape, and placement of the implant can achieve medialization of the anterior, middle, and posterior vocal fold, as well as the functionally important interarytenoid area. Thyroplasty preserves the mucosal wave, it is reversible, and it can be utilized early in vocal cord paralysis. Postoperatively, patients have been able to vocalize more than two octaves with good volume (56,70).

Thyroplasty has gained acceptance slowly despite offering many advantages over Teflon. Comparison between Teflon injection and thyroplasty found that the thyroplasty group had significantly better voice quality, quantitative aerodynamic findings, and laryngeal function. As a result of violation of the true vocal fold, particularly by increasing its mass and stiffness, the Teflon group was more likely to have an irregular vocal fold edge and an abnormal glottal closure pattern (46).

Reinnervation Techniques

Medialization improves the strength, loudness, durability, and projectability of the voice, but only reinnervation improves vocal quality. Nerve–nerve anastomoses and nerve–muscle pedicles are used to reinnervate paralyzed vocal cords. Crumley (49) proposed that nerve transfer offers the best opportunity to achieve a normal phonatory voice. Reinnervation leaves the vocal cord undisturbed and is reversible, which is important if either vocal fold injection or thyroplasty becomes necessary (49,73). Nerve–muscle pedicles have been used to reinnervate the posterior cricoarytenoideus (opening), cricothyroideus (elongation), and the thyroarytenoideus (closure), permitting coordinated stimulation of each of the principal intrinsic laryngeal muscles by perineural electrodes (74).

Patients who underwent anastomosis of the ansa cervicalis to the recurrent laryngeal nerve achieved normal to excellent phonatory quality by videostroboscopic and glottographic analysis (73). The technique's success is best explained by excellent vocal fold medialization, correction of thyroarytenoid muscle atrophy, and arytenoid repositioning, because the reinnervated cord rarely abducts or adducts (73). Tucker (75) achieved glottic closure for unilateral vocal cord paralysis using the ansa hypoglossi with a segment of strap muscle as a nerve–muscle pedicle to reinnervate the thyroarytenoideus. Because nerve transfer achieves better phonatory quality, this is the procedure of choice in younger patients and those who use their voices professionally.

A physician skilled in laryngeal framework or reinnervation surgery should consider these techniques prior to Teflon injection (48). Although the proponents of each procedure often exclude the other, optimal repair may require a combination of two or more approaches, with refinements made as needed. Tucker (76) considerably improved voice quality by combining thyroplasty with nerve–muscle pedicle reinnervation.

TREATMENT OF BILATERAL RECURRENT LARYNGEAL NERVE INJURY

Permanent rehabilitative laryngeal surgery is usually not performed for 6 to 12 months after injury, because recovery of vocal cord motion may occur in either or both paralyzed cords. Laryngeal electromyography can distinguish between mechanical fixation of the vocal cord and nerve injury, identify the presence or absence of nerve damage, quantify the extent of injury, predict recovery in over 90% of patients, and provide a predictive value for patients who might require corrective laryngeal surgery (18,41). When it is apparent that spontaneous nerve function will not return, various rehabilitative options are available.

Nonendoscopic Techniques in the Treatment of Bilateral Vocal Cord Paralysis

Permanent use of a valved tracheotomy tube eliminates the need for further surgery and provides a reasonably normal voice. However, the patient must be willing to tolerate the inconvenience and care of a tracheotomy.

In 1946, Woodman (77) described extralaryngeal arytenoidectomy and suture lateralization of the vocal cord. Most open laryngeal procedures in the treatment of bilateral vocal cord paralysis are modifications of his technique. Following thyrotomy, arytenoidectomy and cordectomy are performed (78). To achieve an adequate airway, a temporary laryngeal stent is placed, but it must be removed before decannulation. Using a thyrotomy approach, Singer et al. (79) described arytenoidectomy without cordectomy or laryngeal stent. This method has the additional advantage of allowing excellent phonation by not disturbing vocal cord apposition and by providing a posterior glottic airway that permits decannulation.

In a nerve–muscle pedicle reinnervation technique, Tucker (80) transposed the anterior belly of the omohyoid muscle with a branch of the ansa hypoglossi nerve to the posterior cricoarytenoid muscle. Successful reinnervation achieved adequate abductor function.

Endoscopic Techniques in the Treatment of Bilateral Vocal Cord Paralysis

Developments in endolaryngeal surgery have permitted patients with bilateral vocal cord paralysis to be decannulated, while maintaining an adequate airway and a near-normal voice. Lateral fixation of the vocal cord is a simple procedure that often obviates the need for a tracheotomy. If unsuccessful, this procedure does not compromise more complicated endoscopic or open laryngeal procedures (81).

In 1949, Thornell (82) provided the first description of an endolaryngeal arytenoidectomy; most current procedures are based on his concept. The carbon dioxide laser is currently used to perform endoscopic arytenoidectomy and cordectomy, successfully treating bilateral vocal cord paralysis by securing an open airway and maintaining adequate phonation (83,84). Endoscopic arytenoidectomy may be combined with partial resection of the thyroarytenoid muscle and false cord, along with suture lateralization of the vocal cord into an abducted position (85).

TREATMENT OF SUPERIOR LARYNGEAL NERVE INJURY

Patients with isolated unilateral and bilateral superior laryngeal nerve injury usually compensate adequately and do not require treatment. Training exercises by a speech pathologist can assist patients in techniques to compensate for their deficit. Patients who persistently aspirate and fail to develop adequate speech usually have recurrent laryngeal nerve involvement.

TREATMENT OF COMBINED LARYNGEAL NERVE INJURY

In the case of unilateral recurrent and superior laryngeal nerve injury, the posterior glottic chink may be too wide to achieve adequate closure by manipulation of the vocal cord. By closing the posterior gap, arytenoid adduction addresses the problem and improves glottic competence (26). Arytenoid adduction is particularly effective in acute cases. Failure to achieve vocal fold lengthening in cases of long-term paralysis, presumably because of soft-tissue contracture, leads to poor functional results. Tucker (74,86) achieved excellent pitch control and vocal quality using a nerve–muscle pedicle to reinnervate the thyroarytenoideus muscle, the primary laryngeal adductor.

NONNEURAL COMPLICATIONS OF THYROID SURGERY

Postoperative Hemorrhage

Ordinary discharge after thyroidectomy is adequately managed with the use of closed suction drainage and pressure dressings. Although relatively uncommon, postthyroidectomy hemorrhage may be early or delayed, usually occurring within the first 12 hours. Immediate hemorrhage often presents in the operating room after extubation, especially if the patient coughs repeatedly or vomits (87). Delayed hemorrhage, occurring hours later, is characterized by excessive bloody discharge, swelling in the anterior neck, cervical venous distention, and/or dyspnea secondary to tracheal compression. Acute airway obstruction from tracheal compression or laryngeal edema may develop. Emergency treatment requires immediate removal of neck sutures or surgical clips, evacuation of the hematoma, and securing the airway by reintubation, prior to exploration and establishing hemostasis. In rare instances, an emergency cricothyrotomy or tracheotomy is required. The larynx should be examined prior to extubation; if significant edema is present, a tracheotomy or prolonged intubation is necessary. Intravenous steroids and head elevation may resolve the condition (87).

In a review of 1800 thyroid procedures, Spinelli et al. (87) reported nine early and ten late hemorrhages, the source usually being strap muscles and the inferior pole, but rarely the superior pole. All 19 required reoperation and general anesthesia. Unsuspected hematologic or vascular abnormalities may cause untoward postoperative bleeding. According to Hunt (10), the inferior thyroid artery is absent on the left in 5% of cases and on the right in 2% of cases. Large branches from the left subclavian artery enter the gland at a level lower than normal, appearing to replace the inferior thyroid arteries. Retrosternal bleeding from these aberrant vessels may go unnoticed. Inadvertent injury of the thyroidea ima artery may result in a mediastinal hematoma.

Airway Obstruction

Postoperative airway obstruction is one of the major causes of morbidity and mortality following thyroid surgery. The airway may be partially or totally obstructed by a hematoma, laryngeal edema, or bilateral vocal cord paralysis. Tracheal compression by a longstanding benign mass or invasion by a malignant neoplasm may compromise the airway (16). Bilateral vocal cord paralysis can even be caused by endotracheal cuff compression of peripheral branches of the recurrent laryngeal nerve (88,89). One case report of upper airway obstruction was caused by ectopic intratracheal thyroid tissue (16).

Swelling, neck pain, and stridor caused by hematoma usually precede complete airway obstruction. Some surgeons forego dressings to permit visualization of the anterior neck. Management of tracheal compression has been discussed in the section on postoperative hemorrhage. Airway obstruction consequent to laryngeal edema may occur more insidiously than from tracheal compression caused by an expanding hematoma, bilateral vocal cord paralysis, laryngospasm, or tracheal obstruction. Flexible fiberoptic laryngoscopy can assess the degree of airway obstruction without precipitating further swelling; laryngeal edema may be managed satisfactorily with high doses of intravenous steroids over 24 to 48 hours.

Sudden postoperative airway obstruction may occur secondary to bilateral vocal cord paralysis. Obstruction may be safely documented using the flexible fiberoptic laryngoscope at bedside. Depending on the severity of the symptoms, emergent reintubation may be necessary, followed by a tracheotomy.

Arytenoid Dislocation

Bilateral arytenoid dislocation causing vocal cord fixation as a result of traumatic intubation rarely occurs (90,91). When odynophagia accompanies a weak and breathy voice, arytenoid dislocation consequent to endotracheal intubation must be considered. Cricoarytenoid joint disarticulation is relatively uncommon, with only 57 cases of dislocation or subluxation having been reported through 1994 (91). On laryngoscopic examination, the arytenoid cartilage is usually dislocated posterolaterally, whereas the vocal cord is fixed in abduction and may quiver during phonation. A forced duction test should be conducted prior to performing a tracheotomy for presumed bilateral vocal cord paralysis. The dislocated arytenoid should be reduced to its normal position within 1 week of surgery; surgery can effectively achieve good voice quality even when the diagnosis has been delayed (90,91).

Sympathetic Nerve Injury

Horner's syndrome, which results from cervical sympathetic chain injury, is an unusual complication of thyroid surgery (92). The vulnerability of the sympathetic chain results from its proximity to the place where the inferior thyroid artery arches medially from the thyrocervical trunk. When the carotid sheath is laterally retracted to expose the artery, the sympathetic chain may be stretched, causing injury. The sympathetic chain can also be injured by a retractor compressing it against the vertebral column.

Chylous Fistula

Chylous fistula is rare following thyroidectomy. It is manifested by milky-white discharge that increases with resumption of oral intake, despite pressure dressings and suction drainage. Injury to the thoracic duct may occur during excision of a markedly enlarged gland, dissection of an invasive thyroid tumor, or while performing a concurrent neck dissection. If the thoracic duct is interrupted during surgery, it should be ligated. Use of the operating microscope may aid in identification and repair. Continuous closed suction drainage is the initial treatment of a chylous fistula, because most lymphatic vessels will seal off during the first 48 to 72 hours. Inadvertent injury to the thoracic duct in the left lower neck or, more rarely, on the right, may result in profuse and continuous chylous drainage. A persistent chylous fistula over 3 to 5 days usually warrants exploration and ligature.

Skin Flap Necrosis

Partial or total skin flap necrosis following thyroidectomy is rare because the standard skin incision causes minimal interruption of the blood supply to the anterior neck, and flaps are elevated in the subplatysmal plane. Extended incisions for a radical neck dissection or mediastinal dissection increases the risk, especially at trifurcation sites. Prior radiotherapy compromises flap viability. Flap infection and necrosis can be minimized by careful planning of the skin incisions for extended procedures, use of prophylactic antibiotics, closure of wounds without tension, and use of closed suction drainage.

Tracheoesophageal Blood Supply

The blood supply to the anterior cervical esophagus and posterior tracheal wall originate mainly from branches of the inferior thyroid artery (93). Ligation of these vessels along with surgical separation of the tracheoesophageal tissue plane during dissection can compromise the blood supply in patients with poor collateral blood flow.

Minor Complications

Seromas occur infrequently and are best managed by pressure dressings and repeated aspiration. Occasionally, an open drainage procedure is necessary. Tracheomalacia caused by gland compression may compromise the airway, requiring a tracheotomy below the involved segment. Severe cases may require tracheal resection and complex reconstruction with flaps and/or prosthetic materials (16).

Hypertrophic scarring and keloid formation are best managed by serial injection of steroids for several weeks. Scar revision should be performed judiciously, as keloids often recur. Inadequate closure of the strap muscles occasionally causes tethering of the cervical skin to the anterior tracheal wall. Patients may complain of neck discomfort while swallowing. Release of the fibrous adhesions and placement of an intervening layer of soft-tissue corrects the problem.

Laryngeal Pacing Research

Recovery of nerve function is a primary goal of research to rehabilitate the paralyzed larynx. Using microprocessor technology, implantable devices capable of electrical neurostimulation have been designed to stimulate various functions of the denervated larynx (94). Selective electrical stimulation of the posterior cricoarytenoid muscle preserves the airway, permits adequate phonation, diminishes aspiration, and can be reversed (95).

One method of controlling vocal cord position has used transcutaneous electrical stimulation of the recurrent laryngeal nerve. Cord position was directly related to the frequency of applied current: 30 Hz resulted in maximal vocal cord abduction, whereas stimulation from 10 to 30 Hz resulted in graded vocal cord abduction. Stimulation above 30 Hz produced progressive adduction (96). Frequency-dependent movement of the vocal cords was attributed to the difference between contraction times of the abductor and adductor muscles (97). Vocal cord abduction has been achieved by direct electrical stimulation of the posterior cricoarytenoid muscles (98). A laryngeal pacemaker system has been used to stimulate the lateral cricothyroid and thyroarytenoid muscles on the paralyzed side of the larynx based on the activity of the normal, nonparalyzed side (99).

Proposed methods of nerve–muscle pedicle pacing of the laryngeal dilators, synchronous with respiration, use electrical stimulation modulated by rhythmic information derived from the chest wall, diaphragm, phrenic nerve, or accessory muscles of respiration (100). Using a linear strain gauge secured to the tracheal rings, one unique device determines mechanical lengthening of the trachea during inspiration to send an efferent impulse to a monopolar electrode that stimulates a crossover nerve–muscle pedicle (100). An implanted pressure transducer has been developed to detect negative intrathoracic pressure to trigger vocal cord abduction in synchrony with respiration (101).

A sensor that detects thermal changes in the pharynx during respiration has been used to stimulate the recurrent laryngeal nerve (102). Successful abduction of a paralyzed vocal cord has been achieved through radiofrequency electrical stimulation of the posterior cricoarytenoid muscle using a chest wall expansion transducer (103).

ACKNOWLEDGMENTS

The authors wish to acknowledge the assistance of Patricia Howard in the preparation of this chapter.

REFERENCES

1. Anderson JE. *Grant's atlas of anatomy,* 7th ed. Baltimore: Williams & Wilkins, 1978;30–35.
2. Dozois RR, Beahrs OH. Surgical anatomy and technique of thyroid and parathyroid surgery. *Surg Clin North Am* 1977;57:(4)647–661.
3. Pick TP, Howden R. *Gray's anatomy,* 30th ed. Philadelphia: Lea & Febiger, 1985;666.
4. Crumley RL. Unilateral recurrent laryngeal nerve paralysis. *J Voice* 1994;8(1):79–83.
5. Hawe P, Lothian KR. Recurrent laryngeal nerve injury during thyroidectomy. *Surg Gynecol Obstet* 1960;110:488–494.
6. Rustad WH. Revised anatomy of recurrent laryngeal nerves: surgical importance based on the dissection of 100 cadavers. *J Clin Endocrinol Metab* 1954;14:87–96.
7. Galen C. *On anatomical procedures: the later books* (translated by WLN Duckworth). Cambridge: Cambridge University Press, 1962.
8. Kratz RC. The identification and protection of the laryngeal motor nerves during thyroid and laryngeal surgery: a new microsurgical technique. *Laryngoscope* 1973;83:59–78.
9. Dedo HH. The paralyzed larynx: an electromyographic study in dogs and humans. *Laryngoscope* 1970;80:1455–1517.
10. Hunt PS, Poole M, Reeve TS. A reappraisal of the surgical anatomy of the thyroid and parathyroid glands. *Br J Surg* 1968;55:63–66.
11. Sun SQ, Chang RW. The superior laryngeal nerve loop and its surgical implications. *Surg Radiol Anat* 1991;13(3):175–180.
12. Loré JM, Duck JK, Elias S. Preservation of the laryngeal nerves during total thyroid lobectomy. *Ann Otol* 1977;86:7–8.
13. Beahrs OH. Complications of surgery of the head and neck. *Surg Clin North Am* 1977;57(4):823–829.
14. Sedgwick C. *Major problems in clinical surgery,* vol 15. Philadelphia: WB Saunders, 1974;1–4.
15. Wang D. The use of the inferior cornu of the thyroid cartilage in identifying the recurrent laryngeal nerve. *Surg Gynecol Obstet* 1975;140:91–94.
16. Ogden CW, Goldstraw P. Intratracheal thyroid tissue presenting with stridor. A case report. *Eur J Cardiothorac Surg* 1991;5(2):108–109.
17. Mooseman DA, DeWeese MS. The external laryngeal nerve as related to thyroidectomy. *Surg Gynecol Obstet* 1968;126:1011–1016.
18. Miller RH, Rosenfield DB. The role of electromyography in clinical laryngology. *Otolaryngol Head Neck Surg* 1984;92(3):287–291.
19. Lipton RJ, McCaffrey TV, Litchy WJ. Intraoperative electrophysiologic monitoring of laryngeal muscle during thyroid surgery. *Laryngoscope* 1988;98:129–196.
20. Maloney RW, Murcek BW, Steehler KW, Sibley D, Maloney RE. A new method for intraoperative recurrent laryngeal nerve monitoring. *Ear Nose Throat J* 1994;73(1):30–33.
21. Gavilan J, Gavilan C. Recurrent laryngeal nerve: identification during thyroid and parathyroid surgery. *Arch Otolaryngol Head Neck Surg* 1986;112:1286–1288.
22. Jatzko GR, Lisborg PH, Muller MG, Wette VM. Recurrent nerve palsy after thyroid operations—principal nerve identification and a literature review. *Surgery* 1994;115(2):139–144.
23. Wagner HE, Seiler C. Recurrent laryngeal nerve palsy after thyroid gland surgery. *Br J Surg* 1994;812(2):226–228.
24. Loré JM. The thyroid gland. In: Loré JM, ed. *An atlas of head and neck surgery,* 3rd ed. Philadelphia: WB Saunders, 1988;728–807.
25. Ezaki H, Ushio H, Harada Y, Takeichi N. Recurrent laryngeal nerve anastomosis following thyroid surgery. *World J Surg* 1982;6:342–346.
26. Woodson GE, Murray T. Glottic configuration after arytenoid adduction. *Laryngoscope* 1994;104(8):965–969.
27. Balanzoni S, Altini R, Pasi L, Fussi F. Prevention of laryngeal nerve lesions in thyroid surgery. *Minerva Chir* 1994;49(4):299–302.
28. Sinclair IS. The risk to the recurrent laryngeal nerves in thyroid and parathyroid surgery. *J R Coll Surg Edinb* 1994;39(4):253–257.
29. van Heerden JA, Groh MA, Grand CS. Early post operative morbidity after surgical treatment of thyroid carcinoma. *J Surg* 1987;101(2):224–227.
30. Levin KE, Clark AH, Duh QY, Demeure M, Siperstein AE, Clark OH. Reoperative thyroid surgery. *Surgery* 1992;111(6):604–609.
31. Holl-Allen RTJ. A new look at recurrent nerve paralysis associated with thyroid disease. *Proc R Soc Med* 1973;66:753–754.
32. Rowe-Jones JM, Rosswick RP, Leighton SE. Benign thyroid disease and vocal cord palsy. *Ann R Coll Surg Engl* 1993;75(4):241–244.
33. Rueger RG. Benign disease of the thyroid gland and vocal cord paralysis. *Laryngoscope* 1974;84:897–907.
34. Holinger LD, Holinger PC, Holinger PH. Etiology of bilateral abductor vocal cord paralysis. *Ann Otol* 1976;85:428–437.
35. Holinger PC, Holinger LD, Seibel MS, Holinger PH. Psychiatric manifestations of the post-thyroidectomy bilateral abductor vocal cord paralysis syndrome. *J Nerv Ment Dis* 1980;168:46–49.
36. Young HA, Ferguson IT. Laryngeal tetany: an unusual presentation of chronic renal failure. *J Laryngol Otol* 1977;91:373–377.
37. Ward PH, Berci G, Calcaterra TC. Superior laryngeal nerve paralysis: an often overlooked entity. *Trans Am Acad Ophthalmol Otolaryngol* 1977;84:78–89.
38. Zerilli M, Scarpini M, Bisogno ML, Di Giorgio A, Chiavellati L, Flammia M. Superior laryngeal nerve in thyroid surgery. *Ann Ital Chir* 1994;65(2):193–197; discussion, 197–198.
39. Kark AE, Kissin MW, Auerbach R, Meikle M. Voice changes after thyroidectomy: role of the external laryngeal nerve. *Br Med J [Clin Res]* 1984;289:1412–1415.
40. Blaugrund SM, Carroll LM. Technique and perioperative quantitative analysis of thyroplasty type I. *Op Tech Head Neck Surg* 1993;4:186–190.
41. Parnes SM, Satya-Murti S. Predictive value of laryngeal electromyography in patients with vocal cord paralysis of neurogenic origin. *Laryngoscope* 1985;95:1323–1326.
42. Benninger MS, Crumley RL, Ford CN, Gould WJ, Hanson DG, Ossoff RH, Sataloff RT. Evaluation and treatment of the unilateral paralyzed vocal fold. *Otolaryngol Head Neck Surg* 1994;111(4):497–508.
43. Ford CN, Unger JM, Zundel RS, Bless DM. Magnetic resonance imaging (MRI) of vocal fold medialization surgery. *Laryngoscope* 1995;105(5):498–504.
44. Ford CN, Bless DM, Loftus JM. Role of injectable collagen in the treatment of glottic insufficiency: a study of 119 patients. *Ann Otol Rhinol Laryngol* 1992;101(3):237–247.
45. Nakayama M, Ford CN, Bless DM. Teflon vocal fold augmentation: failures and management in 28 cases. *Otolaryngol Head Neck Surg* 1993;109(3):493–498.
46. D'Antonio LL, Wigley TL, Zimmerman GJ. Quantitative measures of laryngeal function following Teflon injection or thyroplasty type I. *Laryngoscope* 1995;105(3):256–262.
47. Ford CN, Bless DM. Selected problems treated by vocal fold injection of collagen. *Am J Otolaryngol* 1993;14(4)257–261.
48. Odland RM, Wigley T, Rice R. Management of unilateral vocal fold paralysis. *Am Surg* 1995;61(5):438–443.
49. Crumley RL. Teflon versus thyroplasty versus nerve transfer: a comparison. *Ann Otol Rhinol Laryngol* 1990;99(10):759–763.
50. Ward PH, Hanson DG, Abemayor E. Transcutaneous teflon injection of the paralyzed vocal cord: a new technique. *Laryngoscope* 1985;95:644–649.
51. McCaffrey TV. Transcutaneous Teflon injection for vocal cord paralysis. *Otolaryngol Head Neck Surg* 1993;09(1):54–59.
52. Sadek SAA. Teflon injection of the vocal cords under general anesthesia. *J Laryngol Otol* 1987;101:695–705.
53. Schramm VL Jr, May M, Lavorato AS. Gelfoam paste injection for vocal cord paralysis: temporary rehabilitation of glottic incompetence. *Laryngoscope* 1978;88:1268–1273.
54. Woo JK, van Hasselt CA, Chan HS. Teflon injection for unilateral vo-

cal cord paralysis and its effect on lung function. *Clin Otolaryngol* 1992;17(6):497–500.
55. Dedo HH. Injection and removal of Teflon for unilateral cord paralysis. *Ann Otol Rhinol Laryngol* 1992;101(1):81–86.
56. Desrosiers M, Ahmarani C, Bettez M. Precise vocal cord medialization using an adjustable laryngeal implant: a preliminary study. *Otolaryngol Head Neck Surg* 1993;109(6):1014–1019.
57. Paaske PB, Illum P, Tranberg H. Treatment of vocal cord paresis with Teflon injections. *Ugeskr Laeger* 1992;154(12):780–783.
58. Habashi S, Croft CB. Intracordal Teflon injection: a question of timing. *J Laryngol Otol* 1992;105(2):128–129.
59. Russell JD, Perry A, Cheesman AD. Cordectomy: a solution to Teflon granuloma of the vocal fold. *J Laryngol Otol* 1995;109(1):53–55.
60. Ossoff RH, Koriwchak MJ, Netterville JL, Duncavage JA. Difficulties in endoscopic removal of Teflon granulomas of the vocal fold. *Ann Otol Rhinol Laryngol* 1993;102(6):405–412.
61. McCarthy MP, Gideon JK, Schnadig VJ. A Teflon granuloma presenting as an endotracheal nodule. *Chest* 1993;104(1):311–313.
62. Wassef M, Achouche J, Guichard JP, Tran Ba Huy P. A delayed teflonoma of the neck simulating a thyroid neoplasm. *ORL J Otorhinolaryngol Relat Spec* 1994;56(6):352–356.
63. Goff WF. Intracordal polytef (Teflon) injection: a histologic study of two cases. *Arch Otolaryngol* 1973;97:371–372.
64. Rontal E, Rontal M. The immobile cord. In: Cummings CW, Fredrickson JM, Harker LA, Krause CJ, Schuller DE, eds. *Otolaryngology—head and neck surgery*, no. 3. St. Louis: CV Mosby, 1986;2055–2071.
65. Zaretzky LS, Shindo ML, deTar M, Rice DH. Autologous fat injection for vocal fold paralysis: long-term histologic evaluation. *Ann Otol Rhinol Laryngol* 1995;104(1):1–4.
66. Mikaelian DO, Lowry LD, Sataloff RT. Lipoinjection for unilateral vocal cord paralysis. *Laryngoscope* 1991;101(5):465–468.
67. Ford CN, Bless DM. A preliminary study of injectible collagen in human vocal fold augmentation. *Otolaryngol Head Neck Surg* 1986;94(1):104–112.
68. Kresa Z, Rems J, Wichterle O. Hydrogen gel implants in the vocal cords. *Otolaryngol Head Neck Surg* 1988;98(3):242–246.
69. New surgical techniques for voice improvement. *Arch Otolaryngol* 1989;246(5):397–402.
70. Rothman W. Laryngoplasty for the treatment of vocal cord paralysis in an amateur singer. *Arch Otolaryngol Head Neck Surg* 1992;118(2):209–210.
71. Isshiki N, Okamura H, Ishikawa T. Thyroplasty type I (lateral compression) for dysphonia due to vocal cord paralysis or atrophy. *Acta Otolaryngol (Stockh)* 1975;80:465–473.
72. Koufman JA. Laryngoplasty for vocal cord medialization: an alternative to Teflon. *Laryngoscope* 1986;96:726–731.
73. Crumley RL. Update: ansa cervicalis to recurrent laryngeal nerve anastomosis for unilateral laryngeal paralysis. *Laryngoscope* 1991;101(4):384–387; discussion, 388.
74. A canine model for global control of the reimplanted larynx. A potential avenue for human laryngeal transplantation. *ASAIO Trans* 1991;35(3):487–489.
75. Tucker HM. Reinnervation of the unilaterally paralyzed larynx. *Ann Otol Rhinol Laryngol* 1977;86:789–791.
76. Tucker HM. Combined laryngeal framework medialization and reinnervation for unilateral vocal fold paralysis. *Ann Otol Rhinol Laryngol* 1990;99:778–780.
77. Woodman G. A modification of the extralaryngeal approach to arytenoidectomy for bilateral abductor paralysis. *Arch Otol* 1946;43:63–65.
78. Helmus C. Microsurgical thyrotomy and arytenoidectomy for bilateral recurrent laryngeal nerve paralysis. *Laryngoscope* 1969;79:491–503.
79. Singer SL, Hamaker RC, Miller SM. Restoration of the airway following bilateral recurrent laryngeal nerve paralysis. *Laryngoscope* 1985;95:1204–1207.
80. Tucker HM. Nerve-muscle pedicle reinnervation of the larynx: avoiding pitfalls and complications. *Ann Otol Rhinol Laryngol* 1982;91:440–444.
81. Ejnell H, Mansson I, Hallen O, Bake B, Stenborg R. A simple operation for bilateral vocal cord paralysis. *Laryngoscope* 1984;94:954–958.
82. Thornell WC. New intralaryngeal approach for bilateral abductor paralysis of vocal cords. *Trans Am Acad Ophthalmol Otolaryngol* 1949;53:631.
83. Remsen K, Lawson W, Patel N, Biller HF. Lateralization for bilateral vocal cord abductor paralysis. *Otolaryngol Head Neck Surg* 1985;93(5):645–649.
84. Ossoff RH, Sisson GA, Duncavage JA, Moselle HI, Andrews PE, McMillan WG. Endoscopic laser arytenoidectomy for the treatment of bilateral vocal cord paralysis. *Laryngoscope* 1984;94:1293–1297.
85. Kirchner F. Endoscopic lateralization of the vocal cord in abductor paralysis of the larnyx. *Laryngoscope* 1979;89:1179.
86. Rusnov M, Tucker HM. Laryngeal reinnervation for unilateral vocal cord paralysis: long-term results. *Ann Otol Rhinol Laryngol* 1981;90:1–5.
87. Spinelli C, Berti P, Miccoli P. The postoperative hemorrhagic complication in thyroid surgery. *Minerva Chir* 1994;49(12):1245–1247.
88. Hahn FW Jr, Martin JT, Lilly JC. Vocal cord paralysis with endotracheal intubation. *Arch Otolaryngol* 1970;92:226–229.
89. Brandwein M. Bilateral vocal cord paralysis following endotracheal intubation. *Arch Otolaryngol Head Neck Surg* 1986;112:887–892.
90. Quick CA, Merwin GC. Arytenoid dislocation. *Arch Otolaryngol* 1978;104:267–270.
91. Sataloff RT, Bough ID Jr, Spiegel JR. Arytenoid dislocation: diagnosis and treatment. *Laryngoscope* 1994;104(11):1353–1361.
92. Caldarelli DD, Holinger LD. Complications and sequelae of thyroid surgery. *Otolaryngol Clin North Am* 1980;13(1):85–97.
93. Burger D, Piehlsinger E. The blood supply of the cervical esophagus. *Acta Anat (Basal)* 1991;142(3):204–207.
94. Broniatowski M, Tucker HM, Nose Y. The future of electronic pacing in laryngeal rehabilitation. *Am J Otolaryngol* 1990;11(1):51–62.
95. Opert PM, Young KA, Tobey DN. Use of direct posterior cricoarytenoid stimulation in laryngeal paralysis. *Arch Otolaryngol* 110(1):88–92.
96. Sanders I, Aviv J, Kraus WM, Racenstein MM, Biller HF. Transcutaneous electrical stimulation of the recurrent laryngeal nerve in monkeys. *Ann Otol Rhinol Laryngol* 1987;96(1):38–42.
97. Sanders I, Aviv J, Biller HF. Transcutaneous electrical stimulation of the recurrent laryngeal nerve: a method of controlling vocal cord position. *Otolaryngol Head Neck Surg* 1986;95(2):152–157.
98. Zrunek M, Bigenzahn W, Mayr W, Unger E, Feldner-Busztin H. A laryngeal pacemaker for inspiration-controlled, direct electrical stimulation of the denervated posterior cricoarytenoid muscle in sheep. *Eur Arch Otorhinolaryngol* 1991;248(8):445–448.
99. Goldfarb D, Keane WM, Lowry LD. Laryngeal pacing as a treatment for vocal fold paralysis. *J Voice* 1994;8(2):179–185.
100. Broniatowski M, Tucker HM, Kaneko S, Jacobs G, Nose Y. Laryngeal pacemaker. Part I. Electronic pacing of reinnervated strap muscles in the dog. *Otolaryngol Head Neck Surg* 1986;94(1):41–44.
101. Otto RA, Davis W. Functional electrical stimulation for the treatment of bilateral recurrent laryngeal nerve paralysis. *Otolaryngol Head Neck Surg* 1986;95(1):47–51.
102. Kim KM, Choi HS, Kim GR, Hong WP, Chun YM, Park YJ. Laryngeal pacemaker using a temperature sensor in the canine. *Laryngoscope* 1987;97(10):1207–1210.
103. Bergmann K, Warzel H, Eckhardt HU, Hopstock U, Hermann V, Gerhardt HJ. Long-term implantation of a system of electrical stimulation of paralyzed laryngeal muscles in dogs. *Laryngoscope* 1988;98(4):455–459.

CHAPTER 39

Metabolic Complications of Thyroid Surgery: Hypocalcemia and Hypoparathyroidism; Hypocalcitonemia; and Hypothyroidism and Hyperthyroidism

Stephen A. Falk

HYPOCALCEMIA AND HYPOPARATHYROIDISM

The first part of this chapter addresses the influence of thyroid surgery on calcium metabolism. (Parathyroid function and calcium homeostasis are discussed in Chapter 5.) Hypocalcemia after thyroidectomy can be either temporary or permanent. Temporary hypocalcemia, although not a serious complication of thyroidectomy, has several undesirable results. Whether or not the patient requires treatment with calcium, frequent monitoring and blood tests are required. The hypocalcemia is considered temporary only when calcium levels return to normal. Until then, the prospect of permanent hypocalcemia is real. Also, the occurrence of temporary hypocalcemia may convince the surgeon to perform less than a complete lobectomy or less than a total or near-total thyroidectomy. Such incomplete thyroid surgery may compromise or change management in several ways. For example, patients with thyroid cancer will usually require higher doses of radioactive iodine to ablate residual thyroid tissue before radioiodine scanning and serum thyroglobulin levels can detect recurrent metastatic disease. Also, patients with Graves' disease experience an increased incidence of recurrent hyperthyroidism.

S. A. Falk: Department of Surgery, University of Rochester School of Medicine and Dentistry, Rochester, New York 14642.

Pathophysiology of Temporary Hypocalcemia

An understanding of temporary hypocalcemia provides an understanding of permanent hypocalcemia, because the pathogenesis of the former is more complicated. There are many causes of temporary hypocalcemia, as listed in Table 1. Some have been proven and others are controversial. The table emphasizes that hypocalcemia may be a result of hypoparathyroidism or independent of parathyroid function. The evidence for and the pathophysiology of each cause will be discussed separately.

Ischemia

Ischemia of parathyroid glands is the most commonly accepted cause of hypoparathyroidism. If the parathyroid glands became dusky at surgery or their blood supply was compromised, then ischemia is likely to be the cause. In cases of temporary hypoparathyroidism, even though the blood supply is not obviously compromised, ischemia is often still assumed to be the cause. However, this logical assumption is unproven. This chapter will describe many other causes of temporary hypocalcemia besides ischemia.

Ischemia may arise from the temporary vascular spasm of parathyroid vessels that results from surgical trauma, or from permanent impairment of blood flow through parathyroid vessels, also resulting from surgical trauma. Parathyroid function returns as neovascularization is established after surgery. One must consider embarrassment of arterial supply and/or venous drainage. An understanding of the blood supply to the parathyroids, and

TABLE 1. *Causes of hypocalcemia associated with thyroidectomy*

Temporary hypoparathyroidism
   Ischemia of parathyroid glands
   Release of endothelin 1
   Hypothermia of parathyroid glands
   Parathyroid suppression
Temporary hypocalcemia without hypoparathyroidism
   Calcitonin release
   Hungry bone syndrome
   Reduced renal reabsorption of calcium
Permanent hypoparathyroidism
   Removal or vascular necrosis of parathyroids
Spurious—lowered total calcium with normal ionized calcium

proper surgical technique for the preservation of the parathyroids with their intact vascularity, will decrease ischemia (and the necrosis that causes permanent hypoparathyroidism).

Traditionally, it has been taught that the inferior parathyroid artery that supplies the inferior parathyroid glands usually (in 90% to 95% of cases) arises from the inferior thyroid artery. In the remaining cases (5% to 10%), it comes from the superior thyroid artery. The superior parathyroid artery that supplies the superior parathyroid glands usually (in 80% to 86% of cases) arises from the inferior thyroid artery. In the remaining cases (14% to 20%), it arises from the superior thyroid artery. The parathyroid glands receive nearly all their blood supply from the superior and inferior parathyroid arteries, which are considered terminal or end arteries (as are the central retinal, renal, and cochlear arteries). The glands are nearly completely dependent on the integrity of the parathyroid arteries for their viability and are very vulnerable to a decreased blood flow in these vessels (1). This traditional understanding of parathyroid vascular anatomy was determined by cadaver injection studies.

Figure 1 depicts the blood supply to the parathyroid glands. Small vessels are often found between the thyroid gland and the parathyroid glands (silk loops in Fig. 1). If the parathyroid artery is interrupted, the parathyroid glands will not receive sufficient blood supply from the adjacent thyroid gland through these small vessels, and the parathyroid glands will undergo vascular necrosis (2). Furthermore, these small bridging vessels can be divided without affecting the viability of the parathyroids, as long as the parathyroid arteries are preserved.

However, a recent *in vivo* study using laser Doppler flowmetry during thyroid and parathyroid surgery demonstrated that parathyroid blood supply is not mainly dependent on the inferior thyroid artery (3). Temporary selective occlusion was carried out on the inferior or superior thyroid artery, or on vessels from the thyroid capsule and thymus region, and flow was measured in parathyroid glands. Occlusion of either the inferior or superior thyroid artery reduced the flow to both superior and inferior parathyroid glands by only one third. Therefore, blood supply came equally from the inferior thyroid artery, the superior thyroid artery, and the thyroid capsule/thymus vessels.

At thyroidectomy, an attempt is made to identify all parathyroid glands and preserve them with an intact blood supply. The inferior thyroid artery is identified on each side, and its branches to the parathyroid glands, the superior and inferior parathyroid arteries, usually can be dissected and preserved. The parathyroid glands are separated from the thyroid gland by tying the small vessels between them, thus allowing the parathyroids to separate from the thyroid in a lateral direction. The parathyroids are usually preserved *in situ* on a pedicle supplied by branches of the inferior thyroid artery. Branches of the inferior thyroid artery supplying the thyroid gland (silk knots in Fig. 1) are ligated only if they are located medially to the parathyroid glands (4–7).

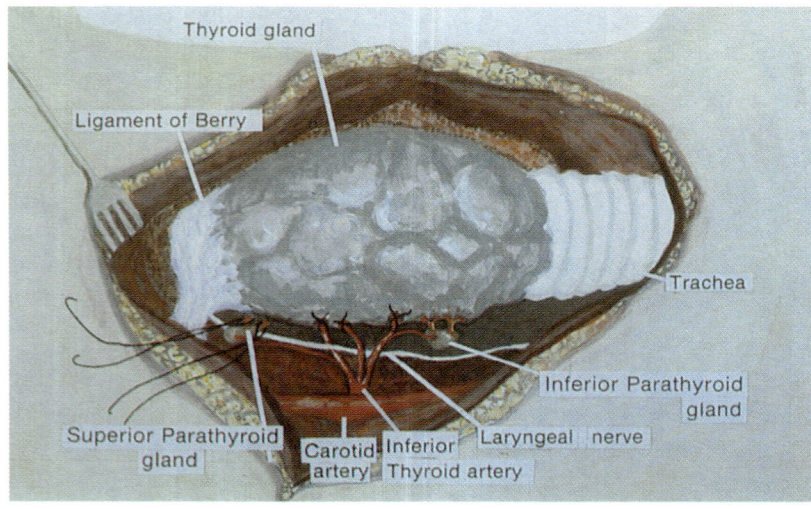

FIG. 1. Blood supply to the parathyroid glands.

In a minority of cases, the blood supply of the superior parathyroid glands arises from the superior thyroid artery. For this reason, identification and preservation of the parathyroid glands are always attempted before ligation of the superior pole of the thyroid gland, so that branches of the superior thyroid artery supplying the superior parathyroid glands can be identified and preserved if needed.

The optimal technique for preservation of parathyroid function is the dissection, identification, and isolation of the glands and their blood supply, followed by small vessel ligation at the level of the thyroid capsule, as described. This method decreases the incidence of postthyroidectomy hypocalcemia (5–8). In cases where one or more parathyroids cannot be so managed, a posterior cuff of thyroid tissue should be preserved, although this technique is not as reliable. There are several explanations for not finding the parathyroids. Possibly, "unidentified" parathyroid glands do not really exist and the patient has only three glands (5% incidence) or two glands (0.6% incidence) (4,9), not four.

Identification of parathyroid glands is often most easily accomplished by following branches of the inferior thyroid arteries to them. The glands may be located between the lobules of the thyroid gland in a subcapsular location (especially the superior parathyroids), or in an intrathyroidal location (4% of parathyroids). It is helpful to nick with a No. 15 blade the capsule of the superior pole in several places to find the superior parathyroid glands that are often present in the subcapsular location. Also, with increasing fat deposition in the parathyroids, as occurs with age, they are more easily confused with the fatty areolar tissue located adjacent to the thyroid gland, or with small nodules of thyroid tissue at the thyroid capsule. For these reasons, some parathyroid glands may not be identified because they are not supplied by a dissectible branch of the inferior thyroid artery. These glands may have a tenuous blood supply that becomes impaired by the operation.

Just when most thyroid surgeons agree that lateral (truncal) ligation of the main inferior thyroid artery should be avoided, two recent studies support this method. Cakmakli et al. (10) compared two groups of patients undergoing bilateral subtotal thyroidectomy. One group received truncal ligation of the inferior thyroid artery; the other group received small vessel ligation at the thyroid capsule. No difference in total calcium levels were found between the groups on postoperative days 1, 2, or 3. Although ionized calcium was not measured, total calcium was corrected for changes in albumin. However, parathormone (PTH), the main concern, was not measured. Nies et al. (11), in a similar study of two identical groups of patients, found no difference in serum levels of ionized calcium and PTH. Both studies concluded that bilateral truncal ligation of the inferior thyroid arteries during bilateral subtotal thyroidectomy does not cause hypoparathyroidism or hypocalcemia. However, Reyes et al. (12) found a decrease in hypoparathyroidism from 17.6% to 0% when the inferior thyroid artery was not ligated.

There are thus two viewpoints concerning the cause of hypoparathyroidism. According to one, truncal ligation is to be condemned and abandoned because of the loss of blood supply to the parathyroids and the increased incidence of hypoparathyroidism. All parathyroid vessels should be preserved and vessels to the thyroid can be ligated only at the thyroid capsule. This technique is supported by the concept that the inferior thyroid artery is the main source of blood supply to the parathyroids, and by the terminal nature of the parathyroid arteries which mostly arise from the inferior thyroid artery. According to the other viewpoint, the main inferior thyroid arteries can be routinely ligated laterally in the neck (truncal ligation), as done in some major centers reporting large series of thyroidectomies (13–16) with no increased incidence of hypoparathyroidism. This technique is supported by studies showing that the inferior thyroid artery is only one source (along with the superior thyroid artery, thyroid capsule, and thymus vessels) of blood supply to parathyroids and not more important than the others.

How do we reconcile these viewpoints? Even if only one third of the blood supply to the parathyroids comes from the inferior thyroid artery, why remove that supply by truncal ligation? Because it is safe to assume that hypoparathyroidism can be kept to a minimum by preserving as much blood supply as possible, surgeons should avoid truncal ligation and preserve all parathyroid vessels.

Release of Endothelin 1

Endothelin 1 (ET-1) is a vasoconstricting peptide (17) produced as an acute phase reactant. Plasma ET-1 levels are transiently elevated after major physical stress, such as acute myocardial infarction, subarachnoid hemorrhage, and abdominal surgery. In 20 patients with carcinoma who received hemithyroidectomy with preservation of parathyroid glands and lymph node dissection, 13 (65%) showed transient hypoparathyroidism and hypocalcemia. In 12 of these 13 patients, plasma ET-1 levels rose, and the peak level coincided with the onset of the transient hypoparathyroidism and hypocalcemia. Plasma ET-1 levels obtained during surgery from the internal jugular vein on either the operated or unoperated side were higher than levels from the antecubital vein. This finding was in keeping with known high concentrations of ET-1 in parathyroid and thyroid tissue and in endothelial cells. Also, ET-1 has a direct inhibitory effect on PTH secretion, as shown by the finding that infusion of ET-1 into the arterial supply of the parathyroid glands of the rat produces hypoparathyroidism and hypocalcemia. Therefore, ET-1 may be involved in the development of transient hypoparathyroidism after thyroidectomy. A transient increase in plasma ET-1 from injured thyroid, parathyroid, and endothelial tissue after surgical manipulation may cause transient hypoparathyroidism and hypocalcemia, either indirectly through its vasoconstrictive effect on the superior and inferior parathyroid arteries or directly by its inhibitory effect on PTH secretion (or both) (18).

Hypothermia

Ischemia is often assumed to be the cause of temporary hypoparathyroidism after thyroidectomy, even in cases in which the parathyroid glands and their blood supply were thought to be preserved. Therefore, direct impairment of blood supply by the surgeon and consequent ischemia were not the mechanisms for the hypoparathyroidism. Also, in the literature, proof of impaired blood flow to the parathyroids is almost always lacking, except for the study of Johansson et al. (3) in which blood flow to the parathyroids was measured. By assuming that ischemia is the mechanism of hypoparathyroidism, the responsibility for causing hypoparathyroidism is unjustly placed squarely on the surgeon; without foundation, it is assumed that the surgeon must have interfered with the delicate parathyroid blood supply during surgery. However, physiologic changes causing hypoparathyroidism can occur during surgery; some changes are under the control of the surgeon and some are not. One such physiologic change is hypothermia. Evidence for hypothermia as a cause of hypoparathyroidism is presented based on an index case, animal studies, *in vitro* studies, and observations during thyroid surgery.

Index Case

A 38-year-old woman with Graves' disease elected surgery as treatment. For several years she was unable to become pregnant, most likely because of longstanding Graves' disease. As she desired to have a child as soon as possible, and she did not want to wait the 6 to 12 months after treatment with iodine-131 (^{131}I) before trying to become pregnant, and she was not interested in thionamide treatment because of the high relapse rate.

Six parathyroid glands were found during thyroidectomy. The right and left inferior parathyroids located near the junction of the inferior thyroid artery and recurrent laryngeal nerve were preserved on a vascular pedicle and appeared completely viable at the conclusion of surgery. The right superior parathyroid gland was preserved on a vascular pedicle but appeared dusky. The left superior parathyroid gland could not be preserved with its blood supply and was autotransplanted. Of great interest were two parathyroid glands located 2 cm inferior to the lower thyroid poles and superficially on the fatty areolar tissue. These two parathyroid glands and their vascularity were completely and readily preserved without dissection or any manipulation because of their superficial location far from the thyroid gland. Nevertheless, this patient developed temporary hypoparathyroidism lasting 6 weeks.

Ischemia could be invoked as the cause of the hypoparathyroidism only if we postulate differential function for the parathyroids [i.e., before surgery the superior parathyroids (which were dusky and autotransplanted) were more active in PTH synthesis and secretion than the other four]. Differential function occurs with parathyroid adenoma and hyperplasia, which the patient did not have because the superior parathyroids were normal in size and appearance, as were the other four glands. Differential function of normal-appearing parathyroids has not been described. Ischemia cannot be the cause because four parathyroid glands and their blood supply were preserved; most workers state that two parathyroids are sufficient for calcium homeostasis (some state that one is sufficient). In this case, the rare occurrence of six parathyroid glands, with two found without dissection in a superficial location, together with the surprising finding of temporary hypoparathyroidism, pointed to hypothermia as a possible explanation.

Animal studies

White rabbits, whose thyroid and parathyroid glands are physiologically similar to humans, were divided into three groups. After exposure under general anesthesia, taking care to avoid disturbing their blood supply, the thyroid and parathyroid glands of each group were irrigated with body temperature saline (group A, control), room temperature saline (21°C) to cool them as they would be cooled in an operating room environment by ambient air (group B), or iced saline (group C). The temperatures of the parathyroid glands were taken every 5 minutes while the neck was left open for 90 minutes. The neck was closed and the animals recovered. As baseline parathyroid hormone levels can vary widely among animals, the levels were expressed as a percentage of the preoperative level, which was given a value of 100%. On the first postoperative day, PTH levels were 90% for group A, 65% for B, and 53% for C. The difference between the groups approached significance despite a small sample size. The decrease in PTH levels correlated with the decrease in temperature of the irrigating solution (19).

In Vitro Studies

In vitro studies of bovine parathyroid cell preparations have shown a 75% reduction of PTH after 30 to 60 minutes of incubation at 20°C. Recovery was rapidly reversible after warming to 37°C (E. Brown, M.D., Harvard Medical School, *unpublished observations*). The reduction represented decreased secretion of stored hormone. Such reduction in protein secretion is in keeping with its known sensitivity to decreased temperatures. It is possible that reduction in PTH secretion reverses slowly after several hours of cooling of human tissue (as in the operating room), in conjunction with minor degrees of ischemia from vasospasm.

Observations During Thyroid Surgery

During thyroid surgery, temperature measurements of exposed parathyroid glands with intact vascularity show hypothermia to 90°F, which can last for several hours. Hypothermia results from exposure in the operating room to an ambient temperature (65° to 70°F) that is well below body temperature. Lowered temperatures are observed in parathyroid glands that are exposed for a longer time (19).

Conclusions

During thyroid surgery, hypothermia of parathyroid glands frequently occurs because of exposure in the operating room to an ambient temperature below body temperature. Animal and *in vitro* studies show that hypothermia causes a reduction of PTH secretion. Temporary hypoparathyroidism is often observed after thyroid surgery in which the parathyroid glands and their blood supply were preserved. Therefore, direct impairment of blood supply by the surgeon and consequent ischemia were not the mechanisms for the hypoparathyroidism.

Hypothermia of parathyroids can cause or, in combination with other mechanisms, contribute to temporary hypoparathyroidism. Return of PTH secretion can be expected after restoration of normal temperature. Figure 2 presents an overview of the mechanisms of temporary hypocalcemia after thyroid surgery. Surgery can result in hypothermia of parathyroids with and without (as in the index case) manipulation of thyroid and parathyroid glands. Hypothermia decreases PTH secretion by a direct effect, and it may also do so indirectly by causing ischemia of the parathyroid glands. Ischemia, a central mechanism, also results from thyroid and parathyroid gland manipulation, which causes vasoconstriction of parathyroid vessels. Hypothermia also results from ischemia of parathyroid glands. By taking appropriate precautions to maintain parathyroid tissue substantially at body temperature, surgeons can prevent hypothermia-induced temporary hypoparathyroidism.

Parathyroid Suppression

Hyperthyroidism causes an increase in both bone resorption (osteoclastic activity) and bone formation (osteoblastic activity). Resorption is greater than formation, resulting is a negative calcium balance, mild hypercalcemia in 50% of patients, hypercalciuria, and skeletal decalcification (20). Hyperthyroid patients with hypercalcemia have secondary hypoparathyroidism. This parathyroid suppression is expected based on the mechanism of feedback inhibition of calcium levels on PTH synthesis and secretion. After thyroidectomy, the stimulus for hypercalcemia, which is elevated serum thyroxine (T_4) and triiodothyronine (T_3), disappears. However, suppression of parathyroid tissue persists temporarily, with con-

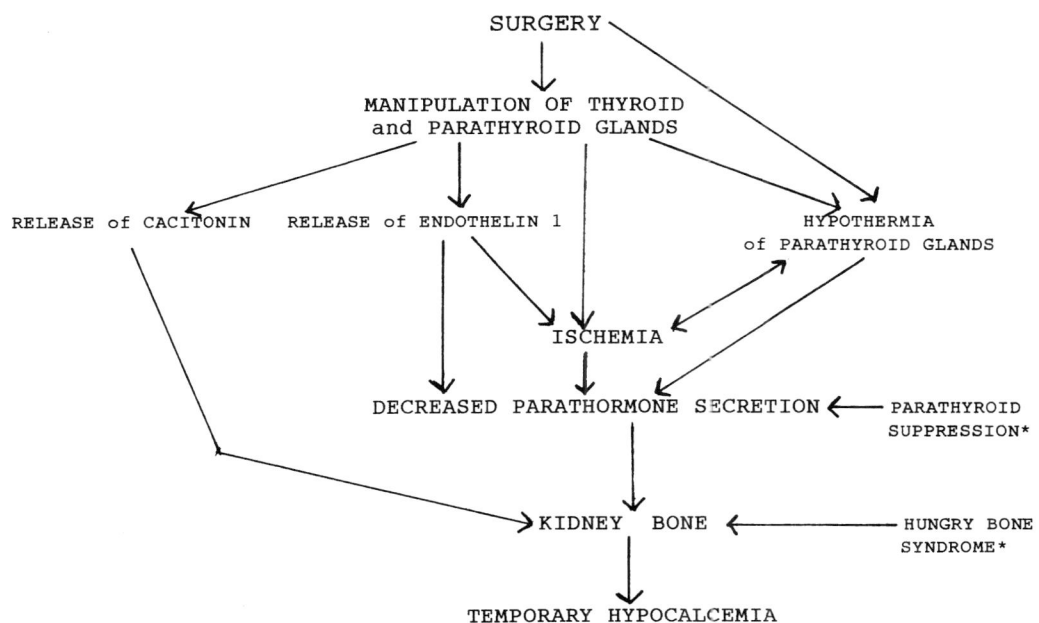

FIG. 2. Pathogenesis of temporary hypocalcemia after thyroid surgery.

*Can occur only in surgery for hyperthyroidism.

sequent hypocalcemia, until the lowering serum calcium levels stimulate parathyroid tissue (21,22).

The explanation of temporary parathyroid suppression could occur in Graves' patients prepared for thyroidectomy with only propranolol, in whom serum T_4 and T_3 become normal 3 to 4 days after thyroidectomy (23,24). However, temporary parathyroid suppression probably does not account for hypocalcemia for the great majority of patients with Graves' disease who are prepared with antithyroid drugs. Their hyperthyroidism, the consequent hypercalcemia, and the consequent parathyroid suppression were corrected for many weeks before thyroidectomy. Also, parathyroid suppression cannot explain the temporary hypocalcemia associated with thyroidectomy for non-Graves' cases.

Calcitonin Release

Calcitonin reduces serum calcium by inhibiting osteoclastic activity (osteoclastic activity raises serum calcium) and by decreasing renal reabsorption of calcium (thereby increasing renal excretion). Calcitonin release associated with thyroid surgery could theoretically cause transient hypocalcemia. Such calcitonin release could occur in two ways—as a leak of calcitonin from the thyroid remnant, or as a release from the gland during the manipulation of surgery. The parafollicular cells (C cells) responsible for calcitonin synthesis and secretion are located predominantly in the central region of the middle third of the thyroid lobe (25) (an area removed at thyroidectomy) and not in the posterior part of the gland (the area that becomes the thyroid remnant and contains very little calcitonin). Therefore, if calcitonin produces temporary hypocalcemia, it would be released at the time of surgery and not leaked from the damaged thyroid remnant (26).

The preponderance of evidence favors no significant role for calcitonin in producing temporary postthyroidectomy hypocalcemia. Three studies demonstrated a rise in serum calcitonin that was closely correlated with a fall in serum calcium for several days after thyroidectomy (27–29). However, Franz et al. (26) demonstrated a marginal increase in calcitonin that followed but did not precede the fall in calcium. They concluded that calcitonin release was not important. Similarly, Falk et al. (8) demonstrated completely unchanged serum calcitonin levels after unilateral lobectomy and bilateral subtotal and total thyroidectomy. Six other studies (30–35) also could not show any significant rise in calcitonin in patients with transient postthyroidectomy hypocalcemia.

Proponents of the mechanism of calcitonin release assume that manipulation of the thyroid gland during surgery releases calcitonin. This simple explanation seems logical and is consistent with the known release of catecholamines and development of hypertensive crisis from surgery for pheochromocytomas. This explanation also is consistent with the widely held, yet erroneous, assumption that thyroid surgery for hyperthyroidism stimulates the intraoperative release of T_4 and T_3 into the circulation. Hermann et al. (36) studied patients undergoing thyroidectomy for hyperthyroidism, who were prepared only with propanolol and not with antithyroid medications. Free T_4 and T_3 levels were at least 3 times normal. Intraoperative levels of free T_4 and T_3 in the thyroid venous effluent (middle thyroid vein) did not exceed those in peripheral blood (cubital vein). Because thyroidectomy for hyperthyroidism does not release thyroid hormones, it is illogical to assume that thyroidectomy will cause calcitonin release, especially when parafollicular cells (the source of calcitonin) comprise 0.1% of the mass of the normal thyroid gland and a much smaller amount in cases of hyperthyroidism where thyroid follicles have hypertrophied.

Calcitonin is a calcium-lowering hormone but only in patients with hypercalcemia, in whom its effect is transient. Acute administration of even large doses of calcitonin to normal subjects does not produce hypocalcemia; patients with medullary thyroid carcinoma and markedly elevated levels of calcitonin on a chronic basis have normal levels of serum calcium. In patients with medullary carcinoma, the often-described escape or resistance to calcitonin could also explain normocalcemia. Based on the consensus of these studies and our knowledge of calcitonin physiology, calcitonin release is a very unlikely cause of hypocalcemia.

Hungry-Bone Syndrome

Because bone resorption (osteoclastic activity) is greater than its formation (osteoblastic activity) in hyperthyroidism, the result is a net negative calcium balance, mild hypercalcemia in 50% of patients, hypercalciuria (yet rare renal stones), skeletal decalcification, and generalized bone disease (20,21). The bone disease has been called thyrotoxic osteodystrophy and consists of osteoporosis (decalcification), osteitis fibrosa (increased osteoclastic activity with tissue proliferation in the marrow), and osteomalacia (impaired mineralization of newly formed bone osteoid) (37). Elevation of serum alkaline phosphatase (with normal 5′-nucleotidase, bilirubin, and transaminases to eliminate the possibility of liver disease sometimes caused by the hyperthyroidism itself), or, more accurately, elevation of the bone fraction of alkaline phosphatase, can be used as a biochemical marker of bone formation. Elevation of urinary hydroxyproline that largely derives from the catabolism of the collagenous matrix of bone can be used as a biochemical marker of bone resorption (21,30). Wartofsky (38) has provided an excellent review of calcium metabolism in hyperthyroidism.

After thyroidectomy for Graves' disease, acute reversal of osteodystrophy can occur as thyroid hormone levels normalize. Such normalization abolishes the excess stimulation of osteoclasts secondary to hyperthyroidism. Osteoblasts continue to remineralize bones, resulting in avid retention of calcium and phosphorus by bone (thus, *hungry-bone* syndrome) and temporary hypocalcemia and hypophosphatemia. Hungry-bone syndrome has been suggested on the basis of one positive-balance study in which a large intake of calcium was needed to maintain a stable serum calcium level with little fecal and urinary loss (37). Laitinen (39) compared hypocalcemia after thyroidectomy in patients with hyperthyroidism, versus nontoxic nodular goiter. Urinary hydroxyproline, a derivative of the collagenous matrix of bone, served as an indicator of bone resorption. The hyperthyroid patients had elevated hydroxyproline; patients with nontoxic nodular goiter had normal hydroxyproline. After thyroidectomy, hypocalcemia was demonstrated in the hyperthyroid patients but not in the nontoxic goiter patients. It was interpreted that thyrotoxic bone disease was responsible for the hypocalcemia. Because direct or indirect measurements of calcium flux into the skeleton were not made, the only possible conclusion was an association between thyrotoxic bone disease and hypocalcemia, but not necessarily a causal relationship.

Wilkin et al. (40) performed a similar study but used serum alkaline phosphatase as an indicator of bone disease. In contrast to Laitinen's study (39), the frequency of hypocalcemia after thyroidectomy was similar in Graves' disease patients with bone disease (elevated alkaline phosphatase), Graves' disease patients without bone disease (normal alkaline phosphatase), and patients with nontoxic goiter. They concluded that hypocalcemia was not related to thyrotoxic osteodystrophy. Percival et al. (30) found transient hypocalcemia (with a maximal fall at 12 hr and lasting 5 days) in 30% of patients after thyroidectomy. Their study of patients before and after thyroidectomy is the most thorough of the investigations to date. Serum alkaline phosphatase, a biochemical marker of bone formation, did not change after thyroidectomy, nor did urinary hydroxyproline, a biochemical marker of bone resorption. Therefore, the hypocalcemia was not the result of a change in calcium turnover in the skeleton, in which case an increase in bone formation and/or a decrease in bone resorption would be expected. The fasting calcium-to-creatinine ratio in the urine provides an index of net calcium flux (the major source of calcium for excretion is bone, once intestinal absorption is not a factor because of fasting). The fasting calcium-to-creatinine ratio in urine did not change. If the hypocalcemia were the result of an increase in calcium deposition in the skeleton, a decrease in this ratio is expected. Thus, hungry-bone syndrome (reversal of thyrotoxic osteodystrophy) did not occur.

Hungry-bone syndrome as a cause of hypocalcemia is known to occur after parathyroidectomy for primary hyperparathyroidism in 12.6% of cases (41). Evidence of this syndrome as a cause of hypocalcemia after thyroidectomy for Graves' disease is circumstantial (37,39); indeed, the evidence that it is not causal is more convincing (30). In addition, hungry-bone syndrome as an explanation for hypocalcemia after thyroidectomy for Graves' disease can be seriously questioned on other accounts. We need to know why hypocalcemia begins immediately after thyroidectomy (within 24 hr). The normalization of elevated serum T_4 and T_3 levels after thyroidectomy would at first seem a likely reason for reversal of osteodystrophy. However, serum T_4 and T_3 become normal 3 to 4 days after thyroidectomy in patients prepared with propranolol only (23,24). Because the hypocalcemia occurs before normalization of serum T_4 and T_3, normalization of T_4 and T_3 cannot be an explanation. Also, most patients with hyperthyroidism who undergo thyroidectomy have been rendered euthyroid with antithyroid drugs for many weeks preoperatively, and the osteodystrophy has largely been corrected before surgery (28,40). Therefore, the lack of some reasonable explanation of why the hypocalcemia begins immediately after thyroidectomy, and the available data, make the hungry-bone syndrome a very unlikely cause of hypocalcemia after thyroidectomy for Graves' disease. Hungry-bone syndrome also cannot explain hypocalcemia after thyroidectomy for non-Graves' disease cases.

Reduced Renal Reabsorption of Calcium

Percival et al. (30) found transient hypocalcemia in 30% of patients after thyroidectomy. They demonstrated a decrease in renal tubular reabsorption of calcium. Both calcitonin and PTH affect reabsorption of calcium: calcitonin decreases reabsorption, causing hypocalcemia, and parathyroid hormone increases reabsorption, causing hypercalcemia. Therefore, the decrease in reabsorption of calcium could result from either an increased secretion of calcitonin or a decreased secretion of PTH. However, both hormones failed to change after thyroidectomy. Thus, the explanation for the reduced renal reabsorption of calcium remains to be elucidated.

Summary of Pathophysiology of Temporary Hypocalcemia

Figure 2 presents an overview of mechanisms of temporary hypocalcemia after thyroid surgery. Some mechanisms are well proven, but others are less so. Hypocalcemia is a multifactorial phenomenon. All mechanisms are not involved in every case; one, several, or all mechanisms can be involved in a particular case. The figure emphasizes that some of the mechanisms result from hypoparathyroidism (those that cause decreased parathormone secretion). Other mechanisms (release of calcitonin and hungry-bone syndrome) are independent of parathyroid function and directly affect kidney and bone. Some mechanisms are under the control of the surgeon but some are not.

Endothelin 1 decreases PTH secretion by a direct effect, and also indirectly by causing ischemia of parathyroid glands. Hypothermia acts similarly by a direct effect on PTH secretion and indirectly via ischemia. Ischemia, a central mechanism, also results from thyroid and parathyroid gland manipulation, which causes vasoconstriction of parathyroid vessels. Hypothermia results from surgery with or without manipulation of the glands during exposure to the ambient temperature in the operating room, below body temperature. Hypothermia also results from ischemia of parathyroid glands. Effects of decreased PTH secretion, hungry-bone syndrome, and calcitonin on the function of kidney and bone can cause hypocalcemia.

Pathophysiology of Permanent Hypoparathyroidism

Permanent hypoparathyroidism may occur as a result of vascular necrosis or removal of the parathyroid glands. Techniques for identifying and preserving parathyroids and their blood supply to prevent vascular necrosis have been described.

Removal of parathyroids with the thyroid specimen, and their microscopic identification by the pathologist, should occur in only a small number of cases. In 4% of cases, parathyroid glands are present in an intrathyroid location. Actually, they may be present between lobules of thyroid tissue and not in a true intrathyroid location, but nevertheless they cannot be seen by inspecting the thyroid capsule. These glands can be salvaged by slicing and inspecting the specimen under sterile conditions and, if found, they can be autotransplanted into a suitable muscle bed (see later).

Spurious Hypoparathyroidism (Lowered Total Calcium, with Normal Ionized Calcium)

Calcium exists in three forms in the blood and body fluids: (a) ionized or free calcium, (b) calcium complexed with organic acids, and (c) protein-bound calcium (Table 2). The free and complexed calciums are referred to as the nonprotein-bound or ultrafilterable fraction, and they comprise 50% of the total calcium. The other 50% is protein bound. Ninety-five percent of the ultrafilterable fraction is free calcium, and only 5% is the complexed calcium. For practical purposes, therefore, measurement of the ultrafilterable fraction represents free calcium. The physiologic properties of calcium are all functions of the free or ionized calcium. Of the calcium that is protein bound, the majority (80%) is bound to albumin and the rest (20%) to globulins.

During the first 2 postoperative days, patients who have undergone nonthyroid surgery (parotidectomy, hemilaryngectomy, cholecystectomy) exhibit a decrease in total serum calcium, albumin, and hematocrit, whereas free calcium, PTH, and calcitonin remain stable (8). The decrease in total calcium is caused by the decrease in albumin. Another study of patients undergoing nonthyroid surgery (cholecystectomy, vagotomy, herniorraphy, varicose vein stripping) showed a similar fall of total calcium and albumin and also a fall of serum sodium, chloride, potassium, magnesium, phosphorus, and osmolarity (34). The decrease in albumin, total calcium, hematocrit, and electrolytes is caused by the nonspecific release of antidiuretic hormone (ADH) from the general stress of surgery, with consequent water retention by the kidneys and hemodilution (42). The lowering of the serum albumin level cannot be explained by decreased synthesis associated with fasting and increased degradation associated with surgery, anesthesia, or other factors over such a short period (43). The half-life of serum albumin is 21 days under normal conditions, and 12 days under stress conditions (43). In addition to this hemodilutional effect, major surgery changes the permeability of vessel walls, causing a large transcapillary leak of albumin into the extravascular space (26,44) with consequent lowering of serum albumin. These very same changes (lowered total calcium and lowered albumin, but unchanged ionized calcium, PTH, and calcitonin) are observed after unilateral lobectomy (UL) (8). The transient hypocalcemia after UL as measured by total calcium reflects a fall in albumin-bound calcium and has little physiologic importance. Anatomic studies of the parathyroid glands have shown a zero incidence of one parathyroid gland, a 0.2% (45) and 0.6% (4,9) incidence of two glands, a 6% (45) and 5% (4,9) incidence of three glands, a 91% (4,9) incidence of four glands, a 4% (4,9) incidence of five glands, a 0.5% (28) incidence of six glands, and an extremely rare occurrence of more than six glands. Therefore, it is rare for a patient to have fewer than three glands. For this reason, it is our practice not to measure calcium level routinely after UL.

Nevertheless, it is important to preserve all parathyroid tissue even during UL, because a contralateral lobectomy, which will place the remaining parathyroids at risk of necrosis, removal, and ischemia, could become necessary. The contralateral lobectomy may be performed immediately or delayed if a solid nodule proves to be carcinoma on frozen or permanent sections, respectively. Also, a patient found to have a benign lesion at UL has an increased chance of ultimately developing other nodules in the remaining thyroid lobe (benign multinodular goiter). These nodules may require lobectomy for diagnosis. Therefore, it is important for the surgeon to make every attempt to preserve all parathyroid tissue during UL just as during bilateral lobectomy.

TABLE 2. *Components of total calcium*

Ultrafilterable (nonprotein-bound) fraction: 50%
Free, ionized—physiologically active (95%)
Complexed to organic acids (5%)
Protein-bound fraction: 50%
Bound to albumin (80%)
Bound to globulins (20%)

Incidence

The reported incidence of hypocalcemia after thyroidectomy is highly variable in the literature and depends on many factors such as the following:

1. The extent and type of thyroid disease. Incidence of hypocalcemia is higher after surgery for large benign multinodular goiters and for cancer, especially large cancers with extracapsular spread, invasion of adjacent structures (recurrent laryngeal nerve, trachea, larynx, esophagus), and paratracheal or lateral cervical metastases.
2. Type of thyroidectomy performed. In general, a decreasing incidence of hypocalcemia occurs after total thyroidectomy, total lobectomy and subtotal lobectomy, bilateral subtotal thyroidectomy, and hemithyroidectomy.
3. The technique of thyroidectomy, especially that used to preserve parathyroid tissue and its blood supply, and the use of autotransplantation.
4. Neck dissection performed with thyroidectomy. In cases of advanced cancer where central or lateral neck dissection is performed, the incidence of hypocalcemia is higher.
5. Primary versus completion (reoperative) thyroid surgery.
6. Expertise of the surgeon.
7. Reporting of symptomatic or asymptomatic (laboratory) hypocalcemia.
8. Reporting of temporary or permanent hypocalcemia.
9. Diligence in looking for hypocalcemia in the postoperative period.
10. Interval between operation and postoperative assessment.
11. Variation in the proportion of original cohort of patients available for study. Such variation will produce a selection bias in the results.

Permanent Hypocalcemia

Some studies support and others refute thyroidectomy as an extremely safe procedure with very infrequent occurrence of hypocalcemia. Based on the consensus of the studies, permanent hypocalcemia is more frequently reported after total thyroidectomy (TT) than after bilateral subtotal thyroidectomy (BST) (34,46–48). However, in some series, TT produces permanent hypocalcemia at just as low an incidence as does BST. One study (49) reported a higher incidence of permanent hypocalcemia after BST (1.3%) than after TT (0%). This finding depended on the surgeon performing the surgery: senior endocrine surgeons performed TT, whereas a larger number of surgeons (and presumably less skilled ones) performed BST. Permanent hypocalcemia after TT has been reported to occur in 13.8% (46), 13.5% (50), 5% to 10% (47), 9% (51), 8.4% (52), 6.2% (53), 5.4% (6), 3% (7), 2% (5,6), 0.4% (48), and 0% (34,49,54,55) of cases, and after BST in 1.9% (56), 1.3% (49), 0.2% (48), and 0% (34,51,57) of cases.

Temporary Hypocalcemia

Temporary hypocalcemia after thyroidectomy occurs more often than does the permanent variety and is usually more commonly observed after TT [51% (51), 26% (49), 25% (7), 22% (34), 10% (48), 8.4% (52), 7% (54), 6.9% (46)] than after BST [39% (51), 30% (30), 22.2% (49), 12% (34,57), 9.1% (55), 2% (48), 1.6% (46)].

In a study of hypocalcemia after thyroidectomy, in which serum total and ionized calcium, PTH, and calcitonin were determined every 6 hours after surgery, Falk et al. (8) showed that BST and TT produced asymptomatic, temporary chemical hypoparathyroidism in the majority of patients. In other words, if one searches diligently for hypoparathyroidism, it can frequently be found. Most of these patients had asymptomatic, chemical hypocalcemia. Only 9% of patients developed temporary hypocalcemia that required treatment, and none developed permanent hypoparathyroidism. Similarly, Demeester-Mirkine et al. (34) also showed a high incidence of temporary hypocalcemia (12% after BST, 22% after TT) and temporary hypoparathyroidism (8% after BST, 22% after TT). Only 2% of patients developed temporary hypocalcemia that required treatment, and none developed permanent hypocalcemia. Likewise, Flynn et al. (51) showed a high incidence of temporary hypoparathyroidism (39% after BST, 51% after TT).

Temporary Hypoparathyroidism After Hemithyroidectomy

The incidence of hypoparathyroidism and consequent hypocalcemia after hemithyroidectomy is small. Because this is an unusual problem, only a few studies have addressed it. The incidence is 1% (34), 4% (35), and 0% (8,58). All cases were temporary, none were permanent, and none required treatment for symptomatic hypocalcemia. These incidences approximate the chance of a patient having only three parathyroid glands (5% incidence) or two glands (0.6% incidence) (4,9) on one or both sides of the neck. The chance that a patient has three or two parathyroid glands on only one side of the neck is less than 5% or 0.6%, respectively. The chance occurrence that a patient has only three or two glands on one side of the neck *and* undergoes lobectomy on that side *and* the surgeon did not preserve the glands can explain the low incidence of hypoparathyroidism after hemithyroidectomy.

Hemithyroidectomy causes a significant temporary decrease (39%) in PTH level measured intraoperatively (59). In 20 patients with thyroid carcinoma receiving hemithyroidectomy with preservation of parathyroid glands and lymph node dissection, 13 (65%) showed temporary hypoparathyroidism and hypocalcemia (18). Such a high incidence is surprising and secondary to node dissection in combination with hemithyroidectomy. One patient required treatment for symptomatic hypocalcemia.

Conclusion

Despite careful preservation of the parathyroids and their blood supply by experienced thyroid surgeons, the glands are sensitive to surgical manipulation, and BST and TT are associated with a high propensity for temporary hypocalcemia. The hypocalcemia is inversely related to the number of parathyroid glands preserved with their vascular integrity intact.

In the hands of experienced thyroid surgeons who are well trained in major head and neck surgery, who perform frequent thyroid operations, and who preserve parathyroid tissue and its vascularity as described earlier, the incidence of temporary hypocalcemia (chemical, asymptomatic) is high, that of temporary hypocalcemia (symptomatic and/or requiring treatment) is moderate (about 10%), and that of permanent hypoparathyroidism is small (under 2%).

Diagnosis

Clinical Symptoms and Signs

The clinical features of hypocalcemia are secondary to increased neuromuscular excitability and include extremity and circumoral paresthesias, anxiety, tetany, carpopedal spasm, laryngospasm, and convulsions. Serum calcium levels should be determined daily and when necessary twice daily during the early postoperative period, and at longer intervals thereafter. Bedside clinical maneuvers to demonstrate the increased neuromuscular excitability include Chvostek's sign (tapping of facial nerve trunk and observing facial twitch), Trousseau's sign (occlusion of brachial artery causing carpal spasm), and deliberate hyperventilation. Hyperventilation produces a respiratory alkalosis; alkalosis increases binding of calcium to albumin, causing a decrease in free calcium (see later). Hypocalcemia may first present as tetany, convulsions (60), or psychiatric symptoms, years after thyroidectomy. This is called latent or borderline hypoparathyroidism. Here, parathyroid damage was partial and normocalcemia was maintained unless there are increasing demands on calcium homeostasis resulting in hypocalcemia, which can occur years after thyroidectomy. High calcium requirements, which accompany periods of rapid growth, pregnancy, and lactation (61), predispose to postoperative and latent hypocalcemia. Chronic diseases such as bone disease, which decreases calcium reserves, and renal disease, which decreases serum calcium levels, can predispose to hypocalcemia. Reduced intestinal absorption of calcium (caused by corticosteroids or a low calcium, high phosphate diet) and increased urinary calcium excretion (caused by diuretic therapy) can also lead to hypocalcemia.

Temporary Versus Permanent Hypocalcemia

Hypocalcemia after thyroidectomy usually prompts the question whether it will be temporary or permanent. This question carries great import for the future care of the patient. Although it requires frequent blood tests and doctor visits, patients will accept temporary hypocalcemia as a mere temporary inconvenience. However, patients have more difficulty accepting permanent hypocalcemia with the necessary lifelong testing and care. Unfortunately, on occasion, some patients erroneously consider permanent hypocalcemia as malpractice even though they were well informed of its possible occurrence and accepted it as a known risk of thyroidectomy and the surgeon took all necessary precautions to prevent its occurrence. If the parathyroids were preserved *in situ* or autotransplanted, the surgeon can often reassure the patient that hypocalcemia will probably be temporary. The presence of two or more parathyroid glands in the surgical specimen likely portends future permanent hypocalcemia. During the postoperative period, increasing serum levels of PTH and less dependency on calcium and vitamin D to maintain normocalcemia are also reassuring findings that the hypocalcemia will probably be temporary. Murakami et al. (62) predicted the outcome of postoperative hypocalcemia: patients with permanent hypocalcemia had lower concentrations of urinary inorganic phosphate than patients with temporary hypocalcemia or controls.

Hypoparathyroidism lasting 3 to 6 months after thyroidectomy will usually be permanent. Rarely, parathyroid function can return late. A case of delayed recovery of parathyroid function occurred 6 months after thyroidectomy. During the eleventh week of gestation, a pregnant patient received BST for Graves' disease. Postoperative PTH was undetectable. Six months after thyroidectomy, she delivered a normal baby; 1 month later, calcium levels rose and PTH eventually normalized. Although increased requirements for calcium associated with pregnancy worsened her hypocalcemia, such delayed recovery of PTH levels is rare (63).

Interaction of Calcium and Magnesium

On occasion, a patient will be found to have symptoms and clinical findings compatible with hypocalcemia, although the total and even the ionized calcium levels are normal. In this circumstance, magnesium levels should be determined because hypomagnesemia can reduce end-organ (kidney, bone) responses to PTH and suppress PTH secretion (64). On rare occasions, tetany can develop with normal serum levels of total and ionized calcium and magnesium (64). This situation results from a precipitous fall in serum calcium from high levels (e.g., 13 mg/dL) into the normal range, and it has been seen after parathyroidectomy for primary hyperparathyroidism but not after thyroid surgery (where such high levels are rare). The neuromuscular system had adapted to the elevated calcium levels. When these levels returned to normal, neuromuscular irritability resulted.

Laboratory Evaluation

Laboratory findings include low levels of serum calcium (total or ionized). Parathormone and phosphate levels may or may not be low, depending on the pathophysiology of the hypocalcemia. The electrocardiogram shows a prolonged QT interval and T-wave abnormalities, and it can reveal arrhythmias including torsade de pointes (65).

Total calcium as measured routinely in a clinical setting may often fail to reflect ionized (free) calcium levels, especially in patients with changing albumin concentrations, alkalosis, or acidosis. A knowledge of these effects is of practical significance clinically.

For example, if the albumin level decreases, as in cirrhosis, in nephrotic syndrome, or in the postoperative patient because of the dilutional effects of ADH, the total calcium level will be low but the free calcium level will remain normal. If globulins increase, as in sarcoidosis and myeloma, the total calcium level will be high but the free calcium level will remain normal. (Free calcium may be increased in these two diseases for various reasons.)

The normal protein affinity for calcium is such that 1 g of albumin binds approximately 0.7 mg of calcium. The binding of calcium to albumin increases with alkalosis, so alkalosis causes a decrease in free calcium and an increase in bound calcium, but no change in total calcium level. The opposite effects occur under the influence of acidosis. After bilateral lobectomy, free calcium should be measured, as this is becoming increasingly available. However, if only the total calcium level is available, the albumin level should be determined, and for every decrease in the albumin level of 10 g/L (1 g/dL), 0.17 mmol/L (0.7 mg/dL) of bound calcium should be subtracted from the total calcium value to arrive at an estimate of free calcium (i.e., serum calcium should be corrected to a normal albumin concentration).

Index Case

As shown in Table 3, a patient has a preoperative total calcium level of 2.37 mmol/L (9.50 mg/dL) and an albumin level of 40 g/L (4 g/dL). On the first day after thyroidectomy, the total calcium level is 2.12 mmol/L (8.50 mg/dL) and the albumin level is 30 g/L (3 g/dL). Although the patient's total calcium level is below the normal limits of 2.25 to 2.74 mmol/L (9 to 11 mg/dL), an estimate of free calcium is a more reliable indicator of calcium status. The total calcium level of 2.37 mmol/L (9.50 mg/dL) consists of half bound and half free, or 1.19 mmol/L (4.75 mg/dL) each. Because 1 g of albumin binds 0.7 mg calcium, the fall in albumin level by 10 g/L (1 g/dL) causes the bound calcium to decrease from 1.19 to 1.01 mmol/L (4.75 to 4.05 mg/dL). The drop of 0.25 mmol/L (1 mg/dL) in total calcium value is explained by a decrease in 0.17 mmol/L (0.7 mg/dL) bound and 0.07 mmol/L (0.3 mg/dL) free. So the free calcium level decreased from 1.19 to 1.11 mmol/L (4.75 to 4.45 mg/dL) and is still within the normal limits of 0.92 to 1.33 mmol/L (3.76 to 5.32 mg/dL). The patient is not hypocalcemic, although the total calcium level of 2.12 mmol/L (8.50 mg/dL) is below normal.

On the second postoperative day (POD), the total calcium level is 1.87 mmol/L (7.50 mg/dL) and the albumin value is still 30 g/L (3 g/dL). The bound calcium value fell by 0.17 mmol/L (0.7 mg/dL), as on POD 1, and is still 1.01 mmol/L (4.05 mg/dL). However, the fall in total calcium level of 0.50 mmol/L (2 mg/dL) is explained by a decrease in 0.17 mmol/L (0.7 mg/dL) bound and 0.32 mmol/L (1.3 mg/dL) free. So the free calcium value fell to 0.86 mmol/L (3.45 mg/dL), and the patient can be considered truly hypocalcemic. If the surgeon considered only the total calcium level of 2.12 mmol/L (8.50 mg/dL) on POD 1, he would consider the patient hypocalcemic, when in reality the patient is not (free calcium value is normal). If the surgeon considered only the total calcium value, he would be very concerned about 1.87 mmol/L (7.50 mg/dL) on POD 2. However, in terms of free calcium, the patient is only mildly hypocalcemic at 0.86 mmol/L (3.45 mg/dL).

In most clinical situations after thyroidectomy, calculating the free calcium level as in the preceding example suffices for an estimate. However, measured free calcium level is higher than the calculated value (8). This discrepancy is caused by changes in calcium binding associated with changes in the acid–base balance, varying affinities

TABLE 3. *Total calcium, bound calcium, free calcium, and albumin levels before and after total thyroidectomy in a representative patient*

	Normal	Before	After (day 1)	After (day 2)
Calcium levels mmole/L (mg/dL)				
Total	2.24–2.74 (9–11)	2.37 (9.50)	2.12 (8.50)[b]	1.87 (7.50)[b]
Bound[a]	1.32–1.42 (5.24–5.68)	1.19 (4.75)	1.01 (4.05)[b]	1.01 (4.05)[b]
Free[a]	0.92–1.32 (3.76–5.32)	1.19 (4.75)	1.11 (4.45)	0.86 (3.45)[b]
Albumin levels g/L (g/dL)				
	35–50 (3.5–5.0)	40 (4.0)	30 (3.0)[b]	30 (3.0)[b]

[a]Bound and free calcium levels are calculated values.
[b]Below normal.

of albumin for calcium, and other variables. For these reasons, measuring free calcium after thyroidectomy is sometimes necessary to assess the patient's calcium status accurately.

Evaluation of Postthyroidectomy Hypocalcemia

The evaluation of the patient with hypocalcemia after thyroidectomy should include serum levels of total and ionized calcium, albumin, phosphate, magnesium, and PTH. Hypocalcemia and hypophosphatemia suggest the hungry-bone syndrome, which usually requires treatment with large infusions of vitamin D, calcium, and often magnesium. Hypocalcemia and hyperphosphatemia suggest hypoparathyroidism, which can be confirmed with reduced serum PTH level. Table 1 lists causes of hypocalcemia after thyroidectomy. Regardless of these causes, no specific therapy is required other than calcium and vitamin D replacement. However, other causes of hypocalcemia (i.e., hypomagnesemia, alkalosis, renal failure, pancreatitis, blood transfusions) could also occur in the postoperative thyroid patient, and these would require specific therapy (see Chapter 5).

Prevention

Prevention of hypoparathyroidism requires a thorough understanding of parathyroid embryology and anatomy, and it is best accomplished by meticulous dissection and preservation of parathyroid glands and their vessels with proper instrumentation, lighting, and magnification (see previous section on ischemia, and also Chapter 36).

In both unilateral and bilateral thyroid surgery, our goal is to remove as much normal and abnormal thyroid tissue as possible and thus perform total lobectomy, or total or near-total thyroidectomy. We favor such complete surgery because removal of less than all thyroid tissue can compromise patient management, such as in the patient receiving less than unilateral lobectomy for a solitary nodule that proves to be carcinoma. Also, in the patient receiving less than total thyroidectomy for thyroid carcinoma, the effectiveness of postoperative ^{131}I scanning, and the reliability of serum thyroglobulin levels for detecting recurrences and following treatment with ^{131}I will be compromised. Furthermore, in the patient electing to have surgery for Graves' disease, we prefer to perform total lobectomy on one side and total lobectomy or near-total lobectomy on the other side to reduce the incidence of recurrent hyperthyroidism to as close to zero as possible. A small thyroid remnant is a key factor and the only factor under the direct control of the surgeon in achieving a low incidence of recurrent hyperthyroidism or carcinoma.

However, in each case, we temper our goal of total lobectomy or total thyroidectomy with our judgment of parathyroid status. When a parathyroid gland cannot be identified, we often preserve a small posterior cuff of thyroid tissue with adjacent areolar tissue under the assumption that the unidentified parathyroid gland is located in or around this tissue. In addition, after its removal, we slice and inspect the thyroid gland under sterile conditions for any parathyroid glands located in a subcapsular or intraglandular location. If found, they would be autotransplanted into a suitable muscle bed. At the conclusion of the procedure, we regularly inspect the parathyroid glands preserved *in situ* for signs of vascular compromise such as hemorrhage or duskiness. If found, they also would be autotransplanted. Intact vascularized nonpathologic parathyroid glands are left *in situ*.

Over 85 years ago, Halsted (66) demonstrated that autotransplanted parathyroid tissue can function. Parathyroid autotransplantation has been used during thyroid and parathyroid surgery. The thyroid surgery has included total and subtotal thyroidectomy and a second lobectomy to complete the thyroidectomy for carcinoma (67–73), lobectomy for cold nodules, and thyroidectomy for Graves' disease (72,74). Funahashi et al. (75) aggressively treated papillary thyroid carcinoma with total thyroidectomy and bilateral lymph node dissections, which placed the parathyroids at high risk for damage if left *in situ*. They, therefore, deliberately removed all parathyroid glands before the node dissections and then autotransplanted them into the pectoralis major muscle. This recipient site is chosen because it is accessible through the neck incision, and because the sternomastoid muscle, although preserved during the node dissection, is so mobilized that its compromised blood supply would decrease the success of the grafts. Parathyroid autotransplantation has been used during total and subtotal parathyroidectomy for primary hyperparathyroidism [caused by adenoma, hyperplasia (76) (sporadic, familial, or associated with the multiple endocrine neoplasia syndromes), or carcinoma], for secondary hyperparathyroidism caused by chronic renal failure (77), and during reoperation for persistent and recurrent hyperparathyroidism (78). The success of parathyroid autografts is generally high. A combined success rate of 82% has been reported from numerous studies after both thyroid and parathyroid surgery (79). However, the success is very variable. After total thyroidectomy, reported success rates are 31% (73), 78% (9), 94% (69), 98% (71), and 100% (67,70). After parathyroidectomy, reported success rates are 77% (78), 81% (80), 95% (77), 94% (81), and 100% (82). Despite the high success rate of autografted parathyroid tissue, latent hypoparathyroidism can be a significant problem under conditions of increased demands for calcium (periods of rapid growth, pregnancy, and lactation), increased urinary excretion (use of diuretics), or decreased intestinal absorption (low calcium, high phosphate diet; steroids) (70).

Devascularized and unavoidably or inadvertently removed parathyroid glands are placed in saline. These glands can be confirmed histologically by frozen section if there is any doubt as to their identity, especially in cases of thyroid or parathyroid cancer. They are minced into pieces so they have the consistency of a gel and inserted into a well-vascularized muscle bed. Minced tissue probably has a greater chance of success as a graft than small pieces of solid tissue have, as there is greater surface area for contact between the minced tissue and muscle. A suitable muscle bed includes the sternomastoid muscle or the brachioradialis exposed through a longitudinal incision in the lateral aspect of the flexor surface of the nondominant forearm. Parathyroid tissue is placed in a muscle pocket that is identified with a metal clip and closed with nonabsorbable suture. Autografting to the forearm has an advantage over autografting to the sternomastoid muscle: Confirmation of graft function can be made using the former, by measuring an efferent (e.g., antecubital vein) venous PTH gradient of 2:1 or greater between grafted and nongrafted forearms (76). However, such function does not indicate the absolute need for the autograft, because viable parathyroid tissue could be remaining *in situ* in the neck. For this reason, postoperative normocalcemia and normal PTH levels do not prove graft function. The only way to prove that an autograft is needed is to defer it, observe postoperative hypoparathyroidism, treat with calcium and vitamin D, and then autograft cryopreserved (as opposed to "fresh") tissue (79,81). In cases of thyroid carcinoma where the graft would not need to be removed (as opposed to surgery for hyperparathyroidism, where recurrent hypercalcemia may occur) transplanting into the neck and avoiding a second incision is preferable than into the forearm.

Treatment

Surgical

Although the standard treatment for permanent hypoparathyroidism is medical (see later), even large doses of calcium and 1,25-dihydroxyvitamin D_3 and careful monitoring of the patient may not prevent recurrent bouts of dangerous hypocalcemia often associated with pregnancy, intercurrent illnesses, and trauma. Hypocalcemia can be dangerous and frequent, especially in the noncompliant patient. Preliminary attempts at allotransplantation of parathyroid tissue hold promise as a cure for permanent hypoparathyroidism (83,84). A successful parathyroid isograft from an identical twin cured permanent postoperative hypoparathyroidism. Although hypoparathyroidism and the availability of an identical twin are a rare occurrence, in this situation parathyroid isografting can be curative (85).

Medical

The goal of medical treatment is to stabilize serum calcium levels in the low-normal or mildly subnormal range, because hypocalcemia is a stimulus of PTH secretion and may hasten recovery of parathyroid function. In addition to monitoring serum levels of total or ionized calcium, determination and correction of any abnormalities in serum albumin, phosphate, and magnesium are often necessary for proper calcium homeostasis. Because hypothyroidism has manifold effects on calcium metabolism, including decreasing calcium absorption from the gut, treatment of postthyroidectomy hypothyroidism with thyroxine is necessary. Euthyroidism is basic for the resumption of normal calcium homeostasis (86).

An approach to the treatment of temporary hypocalcemia after bilateral thyroid surgery, recently mentioned at conferences and in one report (55), is the routine placing of all patients on oral calcium that is then discontinued 1 to 2 weeks after surgery. Although this approach allows easy follow-up of patients during the treatment period, eventually they must be weaned from calcium to find those with permanent hypocalcemia (or at least lasting more than the treatment period).

Objections to this approach include the following:

1. Treating all patients, although only some have hypocalcemia, strikes me as unsound practice; such "shot gun" medicine violates a fundamental principle of establishing a diagnosis before instituting treatment.
2. Monitoring the need for calcium and, just as importantly, educating the patient (regarding the importance of taking calcium and having its level frequently monitored) is often more easily, safely, and successfully done with the patient in the hospital than in an outpatient setting.
3. If calcium levels are not monitored during the treatment period to keep them in the low-normal or mildly subnormal range, this approach could delay or prevent return of parathyroid function, because hypocalcemia is a stimulus for PTH secretion and may hasten recovery of parathyroid function.
4. This approach prevents the surgeon from knowing and monitoring the incidence of temporary hypocalcemia in his patients and making modifications of surgical technique to reduce the incidence. Such modifications include better preservation of blood supply to parathyroid glands and avoidance of hypothermia.

Medical Treatment, by Daniel T. Baran and Jessica C. Rockwell

Treatment of hypocalcemia (Table 4) depends on the severity and rate of onset. Patients with a serum calcium of less than 3 mg/dL, seizures, or tetany must be treated emergently with intravenous calcium. Calcium gluconate (10%) is supplied in 10-mL vials containing 93 mg elemental calcium. Calcium chloride is supplied in 10-mL vials and contains 272 mg elemental calcium. One or two ampules of calcium gluconate (93 to 186 mg) can be diluted in 50 to 100 mL dextrose and infused

TABLE 4. Drugs for acute and chronic management of hypocalcemia[a]

Drug	Treatment of choice	Alternate treatment	Assessment	Comments
Acute (patient with tetany, seizures)				
Calcium parenteral	Calcium-gluconate 10%,[b] 2 ampules in 100 ml, D5W over 10–15 min	Calcium chloride 10%,[c] 1/2 ampule (5 mL) over 10–15 min	Monitor SCa, SP, I SMg, ECG; S albumin, ionized calcium, PTH if appropriate	If SMg low, replace (see below)
Stable patient				
Calcium parenteral	Calcium gluconate 10%, 1–2 mg/kg per hr over 6–12 hr		Monitor SCa q 4 hr; stop infusion or reduce to maintenance when SCa≥8.0 mg/dL; check for Chvostek and Trousseau signs	
Maintenance				
Calcium parenteral	Calcium gluconate 10%, 0.3–0.5 mg/kg per hr			
Chronic				
Calcium oral	Calcium carbonate: Os-Cal 500 (500 mg),[d] Tums (200 mg), Extra Strength Tums (400 mg)	Calcium lactate 625 mg (80 mg),[d] calcium gluconate 1 g (90 mg)[d]		Dosage: 1.0–2.5 g elemental calcium/d; calcium carbonate preferred because concentration of elemental calcium per tablet is greatest requiring ingestion of fewer tablets
Vitamin D	Ergocalciferol (Drisdol) 50–100,000 U/d	Dihydrotachysterol (DHT) 250–1000 μg/d; 1,25(OH)$_2$D (Rolcaltrol) 0.25–1.00 μg/d	With all vitamin D preparations, monitor for hypercalcemia	Ergocalciferol: inexpensive; must be 25- and 1α-hydroxylated; slow onset of action; long half-life DHT: less potent than 1,25(OH)$_2$D; does not require 1α-hydroxylation 1,25(OH)$_2$D; does not require 25- or 1α-hydroxylation; very potent; short half-life; expensive
Magnesium parenteral	Magnesium sulfate 10%,[e] day 1: 1 mEq/kg per 24 hr, 16 mEq IM q 4–6 hr or 3–4 mEq/hr IV; days 2–5: 0.5 mEq/kg per 24 hr, 8 mEq IM q 6 hr or 1–2 mEq/hr IV		With all magnesium preparations, rule out renal insufficiency; if present, monitor levels closely	
Magnesium oral	Magnesium gluconate 500 mg (2.2 mEq)[d]; magnesium oxide 400 mg (20 mEq)[d] 1–2 tabs qd			May cause diarrhea

[a] Abbreviations: D5W, 5% dextrose in water; S, serum; Ca, calcium; Pi, inorganic phosphate; Mg, magnesium; ECG, electrocardiogram; PTH, parathyroid hormone; 1,25(OH)$_2$D, 1α,25-dihydroxyvitamin D; IM, intramuscular: IV, intravenous.
[b] 1 g in 10 mL ampule provides 90 mg elemental calcium.
[c] 1 g in 10 mL ampule provides 272 mg elemental calcium.
[d] Numbers in parentheses are amount of the element per tablet.
[e] 1 g in 10 mL ampule provides 98 mg or 8.13 mEq elemental magnesium. (Magnesium sulfate 50% = 49.3 mg/mL) Prepared by Jessica Rockwell, M.D., and Daniel Baran, M.D.

over 10 to 15 minutes (to avoid venous irritation). After the initial bolus for severe hypocalcemia, or in the stable patient requiring intravenous replacement, an infusion of 1 to 2 mg/kg per hour (10 ampules calcium gluconate in 1 liter = 930 mg), should be initiated with improvement of hypocalcemia expected in 6 to 12 hours (resolution of symptoms and serum calcium greater than 7 mg/mL). If the patient is unable to take oral calcium supplements, a maintenance infusion of 0.3 to 0.5 mg/kg per hour can be given.

Dietary or oral supplements should provide 1.5 to 2.5 g of calcium per day. Calcium preparations vary in the content of elemental calcium per tablet. Calcium carbonate contains more elemental calcium per dose than calcium gluconate or lactate, thus requiring the ingestion of fewer tablets.

Vitamin D replacement may be required to treat hypocalcemia. Vitamin D preparations vary in price, potency, rate of onset of action, and half-life. All of these factors are important in monitoring therapy, which may be lifelong. With all preparations, the therapeutic-to-toxic ratio is small, and thus the risk of inducing hypercalcemia is significant. Serum calcium should be monitored regularly and maintained in the low-normal range. Ergocalciferol is the most frequently administered preparation because of its availability and low cost. The dose is 50,000 to 100,000 U/day. This preparation has a slow onset of action because it must be 25- and 1-alpha-hydroxylated, and it has a long half-life because it is stored in fat. Calcitriol [$1,25(OH)_2D_3$] and dihydrotachysterol (DHT), a synthetic analog of $1,25(OH)_2D_3$, have more rapid onset of action and shorter half-lives, but they are more potent and more expensive for long-term management of hypocalcemia. The dose of calcitriol is 0.25–1.0 μg/day, and the dose of DHT is 0.25–1.0 mg/day.

If magnesium deficiency is present, this must be corrected as well. Parenteral replacement of magnesium can be given intravenously or intramuscularly. Magnesium sulfate is provided in 10% or 50% solutions, which contain 0.5 g/5 mL or 0.5 g/mL of magnesium, respectively (0.5 g = 4 mEq). The total replacement dose of magnesium is 2–4 mEq/kg, which is administered over 3 to 5 days by giving 1 mEq/kg in the first 24 hours, followed by 0.5 mEq/kg over the next 3 to 4 days. For intramuscular replacement, a schedule of 16 mEq every 4 to 6 hours for the first 24 hours, followed by 8 mEq every 6 hours for 3 to 4 days, is recommended. For intravenous replacement, 40 mEq per liter (5 ampules of 10% or 1 ampule of 50% $MgSO_4$/L saline) giving 2 liters over the first 24 hours followed by 1 liter over 24 hours for 3 to 4 days. Oral magnesium supplementation is limited by diarrhea, but it can be provided by magnesium oxide (400 mg) at 1 or 2 tablets per day (20–40 mEq).

When replacing calcium and magnesium in the acute setting, it is important to monitor blood levels frequently, to monitor the electrocardiogram [particularly in patients on digoxin (as calcium potentiates the toxic effects of digoxin)], and to be certain of the patient's renal status to assure adequate clearance of magnesium and phosphate. The long-term management of the patient with hypocalcemia requires regular monitoring of therapy. The goal should be to maintain calcium levels in the low-normal range. The patient should wear a medical alert bracelet.

HYPOCALCITONEMIA

Of the three hormones (thyroid hormones, PTH, calcitonin) produced by the thyroid and parathyroid glands, the consequences of a deficiency of calcitonin (CT) are the least understood. After thyroidectomy, patients have permanent hypocalcitonemia (below-normal serum levels). We must carefully evaluate the consequences, if any, of chronic hypocalcitonemia, both as an isolated event and in conjunction with other endocrine and nonendocrine abnormalities. With the availability of a convenient way to administer CT by nasal spray, is it necessary to provide CT replacement after thyroidectomy for hypocalcitonemia, just as we provide thyroid hormone replacement for hypothyroidism and calcium for hypoparathyroidism?

Calcitonin: Discovery, Sources, Physiology, and Pharmacology

Copp et al. (87) perfused with calcium-rich blood the dog from which the thyroid and parathyroid glands had been removed. He expected the blood calcium to fall, because the parathyroid glands were absent; this would support the concept that hypercalcemia was controlled by suppressing secretion of PTH. Instead, the calcium level rose, indicating that the thyroid and parathyroid glands contained a calcium-lowering hormone, which he named calcitonin (87,88). CT is a 32-amino-acid peptide synthesized predominantly by the parafollicular cells (C cells, which arise from neural crest) in the thyroid gland, and also by thymus, lung, gastrointestinal tract, and central nervous system.

Calcitonin is found in fish in the ultimobranchial bodies, the embryologic equivalent of parafollicular cells in humans. Salmon CT is extremely potent (4000 U/mg) compared with human CT (120 U/mg) and pig CT (200 U/mg). CT can be administered by nasal spray. This convenient way of administering CT has renewed interest in this hormone among clinicians, because previously it was effective only when given by intramuscular injection, which lowered compliance during chronic treatment (88).

The exact role of calcitonin in normal physiology is not known. It may preserve calcium in bones during periods when large amounts of calcium are mobilized from the skeleton, such as during pregnancy, lactation, and growth (89). Because release of gastrin, pancreozymin, and glucagon increases the secretion rate of CT, CT may prevent hypercalcemia after eating a meal high in calcium (90).

In pharmacologic doses, the main action of CT is to reduce plasma calcium and phosphate by inhibiting osteoclastic activity (bone resorption, osteolysis). CT is the only hormone that directly inhibits osteoclasts. Prolonged administration of CT results in a loss of responsiveness to CT. This is called resistance or the escape phenomenon, and it can be seen in two clinical situations. CT can be used only acutely to treat hypercalcemia, and patients with medullary carcinoma with extremely high levels of CT are normocalcemic. Reasons for resistance include formation of antibodies, secondary hyperparathyroidism, and down-regulation of CT receptors on osteoclasts (91,92). In addition to its inhibitory effects on osteolysis, CT enhances osteoblastic bone formation (93). CT also has several extraosseous effects. It has natriuretic, diuretic, and calciuric effects, the latter mediated by decreasing renal reabsorption of calcium. CT is also a potent analgesic, 30 to 50 times more potent than morphine.

Through its inhibition of osteolysis and its calciuric effect, CT is effective in treating hypercalcemia. Through its inhibition of osteolysis, CT is effective in treating bone diseases characterized by excessive osteolysis, such as Paget's disease, multiple myeloma, hyperparathyroidism, osseous metastases, osteoporosis (92), osteogenesis imperfecta, familial hyperphosphatemia, and chronic steroid therapy.

Hypocalcitonemia Caused by Surgery, ^{131}I Treatment, and Disease of the Thyroid

The parafollicular cells responsible for calcitonin production are located predominantly in the central region of the middle third of the thyroid lobe (25), which is an area removed by subtotal and total thyroidectomy. Therefore, it is not surprising that after thyroidectomy, patients have lower basal calcitonin levels than controls and less increase in calcitonin after calcium and pentagastrin infusion (94–98). [However, one study found that serum CT was not reduced after total thyroidectomy (99).]

Hypocalcitonemia, like hypothyroidism, is a natural sequela of thyroidectomy, because it is an expected outcome. Neither should be considered a complication.

Lower basal calcitonin levels than controls and less increase in calcitonin after calcium and pentagastrin infusion are also observed after treatment of hyperthyroidism with ^{131}I, which also affects parafollicular cell function (95,100,101). Because calcitonin is produced at several extrathyroid locations, basal calcitonin levels are reduced (to about 50% of controls) but not absent (95). Patients with autoimmune primary hypothyroidism (102) and agenesis and ectopic thyroid glands (103) also have low CT levels.

The Role of Hypocalcitonemia in Osteoporosis

Osteoporosis is a huge public health problem affecting 1 in 3 women over age 60; $10 to $12 billion is spent annually as a result of fractures in the spine, hip, and wrist, and vertebral compression with associated pain, loss of height, and kyphosis. The etiology of involutional osteoporosis is multifactorial; it includes female sex; postsurgical and natural menopause (estrogen deficiency); advancing age; inadequate dietary intake of calcium, vitamin D, or protein; impaired absorption of calcium; Caucasian or Asian race; smoking; excessive caffeine and alcohol intake; inactivity; small body build with low body weight; nulliparity; and genetic factors. CT deficiency may play a role. Secondary osteoporosis can be caused by hyperparathyroidism, hyperthyroidism, immobilization, malabsorption, chronic hepatic and renal disease, alcoholism, and therapy with corticosteroids and other medications.

The role of calcitonin deficiency in the pathogenesis of osteoporosis, in the general population but especially in postmenopausal women, is a complex and controversial topic. Wartofsky (38) and Mundy (104) have provided excellent reviews. The facts that women have a lower capacity to secrete CT than men and that CT levels are lower with increasing age, have led to the theory that CT is related to osteoporosis, which is highest in older women. Similarly, blacks have less osteoporosis and higher CT levels than whites. However, more recent studies (with an improved extraction method and newer immunometric assays that permit more sensitive and specific measurement of monomeric CT, the biologically active form of CT) have confirmed decreased CT levels in women, but they showed no change in adults with increasing age (105). However, CT levels have been reported as low, normal, or high (105) in women with osteoporosis. High CT levels associated with osteoporosis were caused by excess skeletal release of calcium, which stimulated CT secretion (105). Therefore, changes in CT levels are likely secondary to osteoporosis and do not cause it.

Hyperthyroidism and Thyroid Hormone Overreplacement and Osteoporosis

Because hyperthyroidism is known to cause negative calcium balance, hypercalcemia, hypercalciuria, and osteoporosis, it is not surprising that suppressive doses of thyroid hormone also can be associated with osteoporosis (106–110) in patients who have subclinical hyperthyroidism (suppressed TSH with normal T_4 and T_3). However, other studies have failed to show osteoporosis after T_4 therapy. To resolve this discrepancy, an extensive review of the literature was performed, and it concluded that women (especially postmenopausal women) who have subclinical hyperthyroidism and receive T_4 have reduced bone density (111). Also, a meta-analysis of the available studies did not find any significant reduction in bone mass (0.31% annual loss) in premenopausal women during prolonged T_4 treatment (164 µg/day for 8.5 years) resulting in reduced serum thyroid stimulating hormone (TSH). However, a significant reduction in bone mass (0.91% annual loss) was found in postmenopausal women during T_4 treatment (171 µg/day for 9.9 years) (112). Burman (113) recently provided an excellent review of the risks of hyperthyroidism and thyroid hormone overreplacement.

Combination of Hyperthyroidism and Hypocalcitonemia on Osteoporosis

After thyroidectomy, it is difficult to separate the effects of administration of excess exogenous thyroid hormone from those of CT deficiency. CT deficiency could make the skeleton more sensitive to subclinical hyperthyroidism (105). Simultaneous CT deficiency in patients who underwent thyroidectomy or ^{131}I treatment (for cancer or Graves' disease) and suppressive T_4 therapy may cause or exacerbate osteoporosis. Data in this area are conflicting (114), with some studies showing (96,115) and some not showing (95) a reduced bone-mineral density in CT-deficient (thyroidectomized or ^{131}I-treated) patients. Osteoporosis could be worsened in patients with known risk factors for its development.

Further research is needed to define the role of CT deficiency in patients with subclinical hyperthyroidism. For now, judicious use of thyroxine is warranted to decrease the risk of osteoporosis (21), especially in post menopausal women (see Chapters 4 and 27). For replacement therapy, T_4 should be given to keep TSH in a normal range. For suppressive therapy, T_4 should be given to titrate TSH into a low-normal or below-normal level, but suppressing TSH below 0.1 µU/mL provides no further advantage in terms of preventing cancer growth yet increases osteoporosis (116).

The question posed at the beginning of this section was whether it is necessary to provide CT replacement after thyroidectomy for hypocalcitonemia, just as we provide thyroid hormone replacement for hypothyroidism and calcium for hypoparathyroidism. We don't have the answer yet, but stay posted.

HYPOTHYROIDISM AND HYPERTHYROIDISM

Pathophysiology and Diagnosis

Hypothyroidism

Hypothyroidism is not a complication but a natural sequela of thyroidectomy (see Chapter 37), in which sufficient abnormal and normal thyroid tissue is removed as part of the surgery to result in hypothyroidism as a natural consequence. In addition, hypothyroidism can occur as a consequence of a disease such as Hashimoto's thyroiditis, found frequently in patients with carcinoma and in one third of Graves' disease patients. Hashimoto's thyroiditis reduces the functional capacity of remnant thyroid tissue predisposing to hypothyroidism (117). Also, some part of hypothyroidism occurring after thyroidectomy for Graves' disease occurs as a consequence of the Graves' disease itself. Without treatment, as originally described by Graves, or after medical treatment only (i.e., without ablative treatment), hypothyroidism ensues. Hypothyroidism is a readily treatable and expected natural sequela of thyroidectomy and concomitant thyroid disease. Viewed in this light, hypothyroidism is not a complication of thyroid surgery.

The protean clinical manifestations of hypothyroidism and hyperthyroidism are detailed in Chapters 14 and 20. The laboratory diagnosis is presented in Chapter 4. Measurements of pituitary function are the most sensitive ways to detect hypo- and hyperthyroidism and are far more sensitive than measurements of thyroid function. Regarding hypothyroidism, the pituitary is exquisitely sensitive to tiny decreases in the optimal level of circulatory thyroid hormones, and it adapts appropriately by increasing secretion of TSH. Despite serum levels of T_4 and T_3 within the normal range, increases in basal TSH secretion can be detected by measurements of serum TSH (by radioimmunoassay or by the sensitive techniques) or by an exaggerated response of TSH to thyrotropin-releasing hormone (TRH). Depending on the laboratory criteria used, various degrees of primary hypothyroidism (i.e., the disease in the thyroid gland, as opposed to central hypothyroidism caused by pituitary or hypothalamic disease) can be detected. They include the following:

1. Clinical (overt) hypothyroidism. Low serum T_4 and/or T_3 and elevated serum TSH. Patients have clear clinical symptoms and signs of hypothyroidism.

2. Mild hypothyroidism. Normal or low-normal serum T_4 and/or T_3, elevated serum TSH, and exaggerated response of TSH to TRH. Patients have mild and nonspecific symptoms associated with hypothyroidism and usually do not show classic signs on physical examination.

3. Subclinical, compensated, or preclinical hypothyroidism. Normal serum T_4 and/or T_3, mild elevation of serum TSH, and exaggerated response of TSH to TRH. (Note that some physicians refer to patients in group 2 as having subclinical hypothyroidism.) These patients have the earliest laboratory findings of thyroid failure, with few or no symptoms and physical signs.

Temporary Hypothyroidism

Pathogenesis

In addition to the preceding degrees of hypothyroidism, several studies have confirmed and elucidated the nature of temporary hypothyroidism after thyroidectomy for hyperthyroidism [occurring with Graves' disease (118–121), toxic solitary nodule, and toxic multinodular goiter (122)] and after ^{131}I treatment of Graves' disease (123). The hypothalamic–pituitary–thyroid axis is suppressed in patients who have had chronic high levels of thyroid hormones. Recovery of suppressed pituitary function requires several months after treatment of hyperthyroidism with surgery or ^{131}I (124) and after withdrawal of thionamide therapy (125). This situation is similar to the suppression of the pituitary–adrenal axis seen in patients treated chronically with glucocorticoids. Suppression of pituitary function is evidenced by the failure of TSH to increase in response to low serum T_4 and T_3, and by a flat or subnormal response by TSH to TRH. The latter indicates continued pituitary suppression caused by postoperative subclinical hyperthyroidism (see later) if T_4 and T_3 were in the elevated or high normal range. The pituitary suppression lasts for several months in some patients after thyroidectomy for hyperthyroidism.

Recovery of pituitary function can be assessed by observing the appropriate rise in serum TSH level in response to persistently low T_4 and/or T_3. Under the influence of elevated TSH levels, the thyroid remnant can be stimulated to undergo enough hyperplasia so that serum T_4 and T_3 become normal, followed by normalization of serum TSH. Such a sequence of events could explain temporary hypothyroidism lasting several months after thyroidectomy. In addition, increase in iodine intake, increase in thyroid stimulating antibodies, and autonomy of the remnant could also cause an inadequately functioning remnant to increase secretion of thyroid hormones, with conversion of thyroid status from hypothyroidism to euthyroidism. Such change in thyroid status can occur years after thyroidectomy.

Incidence and Management

Temporary hypothyroidism after surgery for hyperthyroidism occurs often and over a long period of time, as shown in the following studies:

1. Toft et al. (119) observed that 20% of their patients after bilateral subtotal thyroidectomy for hyperthyroidism developed temporary hypothyroidism at 2 and 3 months after surgery, but at 6 months they were euthyroid.
2. Of patients who were hypothyroid 4 months after thyroidectomy, Cusick et al. (120) found that 37% had temporary hypothyroidism—they became euthyroid at 1 year after thyroidectomy without treatment.
3. After bilateral subtotal thyroidectomy, Kuma et al. (118) observed that temporary subclinical hypothyroidism occurred often (46% of patients) and throughout a long period of follow-up (12 years).

Of patients with subclinical hypothyroidism at 1 year after surgery, 34.5% spontaneously became euthyroid by the 6th year after surgery. Of patients with clinical hypothyroidism at 1 year after surgery, 25% spontaneously became euthyroid by the 6th year after surgery. Of patients with subclinical hypothyroidism at 6 years after surgery, a surprisingly large number (48%) spontaneously became euthyroid by the 12th year after surgery.

Recognition of temporary hypothyroidism is important to prevent thyroid replacement therapy from being started or continued unnecessarily. Patients found to have subclinical hypothyroidism during the first year after surgery can be followed without treatment, because 34.5% will become euthyroid spontaneously. Patients who require T_4 treatment for clinical hypothyroidism during the first postoperative year should be evaluated to determine whether they continue to need T_4. Two convenient ways to assess their need for T_4, and to prevent overt hypothyroid symptoms from developing if they are still hypothyroid, are as follows:

1. Decrease the dose of T_4 to one half. After several weeks, a rise in serum TSH and a fall in free T_4 indicate continued need for T_4 replacement, and the original dose can be resumed. If TSH and free T_4 remain normal, the hypothyroidism was probably temporary. Then, all T_4 can be stopped, but thyroid status should be checked several months later.
2. The second method takes advantage of the occurrence of physiologic nonsuppressible thyroid secretion. Exogenous T_3 (100 μg/day for 6 weeks) suppresses serum T_4 to only about one third of the basal level (average of 2.7 μg/dL, range 1.4 to 5.0 μg/dL) in patients with normal hypothalamic–pituitary–thyroid axis, but to levels less than 0.6 μg/dL in patients with hypothyroidism (primary or secondary). To assess whether a patient with previous hypothyroidism still requires T_4 replacement, substitute T_3 for T_4. After 6 weeks of T_3, if serum T_4 level is below 0.6 μg/mL, the patient is still hypothyroid; T_4 can be resumed and T_3 discontinued. If the serum T_4 level is higher than 1.4 μg/mL, the patient is euthyroid, because he shows nonsuppressible thyroid secretion; all thyroid hormones can be stopped, but thyroid status should be checked several months later (125,126) (see Chapter 27).

Hyperthyroidism

The pituitary is also exquisitely sensitive to tiny increases in the optimal level of thyroid hormones, and it adapts appropriately by decreasing TSH secretion. Despite serum levels of T_4 and T_3 within the normal range, decreases in basal TSH secretion can be detected by measurements of serum TSH by the newer sensitive techniques, but not by the older radioimmunoassays, which cannot distinguish euthyroid from hyperthyroid patients. Pituitary suppression by thyroid hormone levels that are slightly raised from steady state but still "normal" can also be detected by a flat or blunted response of TSH to

TRH. As with hypothyroidism, depending on the laboratory criteria used, various degrees of hyperthyroidism can be detected, as follows:

1. Clinical hyperthyroidism. High serum T_4 and/or T_3 and low TSH by sensitive assay. Patients have clear clinical symptoms and signs of hyperthyroidism.
2. Subclinical hyperthyroidism. Normal or high normal T_4 and/or T_3, low TSH by sensitive assay, and flat or blunted response of TSH to TRH. These patients have the earliest laboratory findings of thyroid hyperfunction, with mild and nonspecific symptoms and physical signs of hyperthyroidism.

Incidence

The reported incidences of hypothyroidism and hyperthyroidism after thyroidectomy are highly variable, because they depend on many factors such as the extent and type of thyroid disease, type of thyroidectomy performed (total, subtotal, lobectomy), the technique of thyroidectomy, the expertise of the surgeon in preserving blood supply to the thyroid remnant, the definition of hypothyroidism (clinical, mild, subclinical) and hyperthyroidism (clinical, subclinical), the reporting of temporary and permanent hypothyroidism, and the varying intervals between operation and postoperative assessment. Unless these factors are specified, incidence figures of hypothyroidism and hyperthyroidism reported after thyroidectomy are fairly meaningless. Permanent hypothyroidism occurs frequently after surgery; reports span a wide range: 4% (127), 9.6% (128), 19% (129), 21% (130–132), 22% (133), 30% (134–136), 33% (118), 40% (57), 51% (137), 58% (138), 59% (55), and 70% (139). Reports of a large series of thyroidectomies for Graves' disease show incidences of recurrent hyperthyroidism of 11.5% (137), 4% (138), 3.2% (134,140), and 1.2% (55).

Changing Thyroid Function After Thyroidectomy

Thyroid function after bilateral subtotal thyroidectomy for Graves' disease is unstable. When followed over 12 years, 79% of patients changed thyroid status (118). Of patients euthyroid at 1 year after surgery, 50% remained euthyroid, but 35% spontaneously developed subclinical hypothyroidism, 6% clinical hypothyroidism, and 8% hyperthyroidism by the 6th year after surgery. Of patients euthyroid at the 6th year after surgery, 70% remained euthyroid, but 11% spontaneously developed subclinical hypothyroidism, 4% clinical hypothyroidism, and 15% hyperthyroidism by the 12th year after surgery.

As discussed previously, temporary subclinical hypothyroidism occurred often (in 46% of patients) and throughout a long period of follow-up (12 years) (118). After treatment for Graves' disease, patients require long-term monitoring of thyroid function.

Temporary hypothyroidism lasting several months after thyroidectomy for Graves' disease, toxic solitary nodule, and toxic multinodular goiter is caused by suppression of the pituitary–thyroid axis. Long-term instability of thyroid function after bilateral subtotal thyroidectomy for Graves' is a result of changes in iodine intake, thyroid-stimulating antibodies, or autonomy of the thyroid remnant. Long-term changes in thyroid function are not observed after total thyroidectomy for Graves' disease (leaving no remnant), after surgery for toxic solitary nodule and toxic multinodular goiter (which are not under the influence of thyroid-stimulating antibodies), and after hemithyroidectomy for nodules (141).

Prevention

The following principles can be used to decide the extent of thyroidectomy for hyperthyroidism. In the treatment of hyperthyroidism, thyroid cancer, nodules, and other pathologies, as discussed in this chapter and in Chapter 37, hypothyroidism is not a complication but an expected sequela of surgery. However, recurrent hyperthyroidism is a complication; in fact, it represents a colossal failure of surgery, because recurrent hyperthyroidism will require treatment with ^{131}I, which was avoided in the first place in favor of surgery.

The goal in surgery for hyperthyroidism is to ensure permanent euthyroidism by leaving behind a certain thyroid remnant, while at the same time eliminating all chance of hypothyroidism or recurrent hyperthyroidism. Unfortunately, this goal is seldom realized because it is self-contradictory. Manipulating the size of the thyroid remnant does not produce euthyroidism in any predictable way but still leads to significant hypothyroidism. (The data that lead to this conclusion and to those that follow are presented in Chapter 17.) In addition, leaving behind any thyroid remnant leads to some cases of recurrent hyperthyroidism, an unacceptable complication. Therefore, it seems illogical to leave behind a thyroid remnant, because hypothyroidism is not predictably avoided and hyperthyroidism will tend to occur. However, a thyroid remnant is often left behind to avoid hypoparathyroidism. To reduce the chance of recurrent hyperthyroidism, it is necessary to leave a progressively smaller remnant while performing bilateral subtotal thyroidectomy, although even very small remnants will occasionally be associated with recurrence. Total thyroidectomy by completely eliminating the remnant offers the least chance of recurrent hyperthyroidism and is the operation of choice for Graves' disease. As discussed in Chapter 17 (in the sections on thyroid remnant and risks of thyroid surgery, and a logical approach to the extent of surgery), total thyroidectomy should be the goal of thyroid surgery in Graves' disease. If there is a question of parathyroid preservation, then bilateral subtotal thyroidectomy or total lobectomy and contralateral lobectomy can be performed.

Autotransplantation of thyroid tissue was performed in patients with Graves' disease in order to prevent postoperative hypothyroidism because the remnant thyroid tissue was too small. Tissue was autotransplanted into the sternocleidomastoid or strap muscles. After a 2- to 7-year follow-up, transplanted tissue was alive and functioning in 80% of patients as determined by uptake of iodine-123 in the transplant and by normal or slightly elevated serum TSH levels (142).

Treatment

The treatment of hypothyroidism (overt, mild, subclinical) is presented in Chapter 27. Recurrent hyperthyroidism after surgery for Graves' disease is treated with medical therapy (Chapter 15) and/or ^{131}I (Chapter 16) and generally not with surgery because of a threefold greater risk of complications of recurrent laryngeal nerve injury and hypoparathyroidism after reoperation.

ACKNOWLEDGMENTS

The author wishes to thank Lee Reussner, M.D., and Ronald Pulli, M.D., for their excellent suggestions during the preparation of this manuscript.

REFERENCES

1. Halstad WS, Evans HM. The parathyroid glandules: their blood supply and their preservation in operation upon the thyroid gland. *Ann Surg* 1907;47:489.
2. Curtis GM. The blood supply of the human parathyroids. *Surg Gynecol Obstet* 1930;51:805–809.
3. Johansson K, Ander S, Lennquist S, et al. Human parathyroid blood supply determined by laser-Doppler flowmetry. *World J Surg* 1994; 18:417–421.
4. Alveryd A. Parathyroid glands in thyroid surgery: I. Anatomy of parathyroid glands. *Acta Chir Scand Suppl* 1968;389:1–49.
5. Attie JN, Khafif RA. Preservation of parathyroid glands during total thyroidectomy: improved technique utilizing microsurgery. *Am J Surg* 1975;130:399–404.
6. Thompson NW, Olsen WR, Hoffman GL. The continuing development of the technique of thyroidectomy. *Surgery* 1973;73:913–927.
7. Jacobs JK, Aland JW, Ballinger IF. Total thyroidectomy, a review of 213 patients. *Ann Surg* 1983;197:542–549.
8. Falk SA, Birken EA, Baran DT. Temporary postthyroidectomy hypocalcemia. *Arch Otolaryngol Head Neck Surg* 1988;114:168–174.
9. Alveryd A. Parathyroid glands in thyroid surgery: II. Postoperative hypoparathyroidism: identification and autotransplantation of parathyroid glands. *Acta Chir Scand Suppl* 1968;389:53–120.
10. Cakmakli S, Aydintug S, Erdem E. Post-thyroidectomy hypocalcemia: does arterial ligation play a significant role. *Int Surg* 1992;77:284–286.
11. Nies C, Sitter H, Zielke A, et al. Parathyroid function following ligation of the inferior thyroid arteries during bilateral subtotal thyroidectomy. *Br J Surg* 1994;81:1757–1759.
12. Reyes HM, Wright JK, Rosenfield RL. Prevention of hypocalcemia in children due to parathyroid infarction after thyroidectomy. *Surg Gynecol Obstet* 1979;148:76–78.
13. Farnell MB, VanHeerden JA, MCohaney WM, et al. Hypothyroidism after thyroidectomy for Graves' disease. *Am J Surg* 1981;142:535–538.
14. Cusick EL, Krukowski ZH, Matheson NA. Outcome of surgery for Graves' disease re-examined. *Br J Surg* 1987;74:780–783.
15. Hedley AJ, Bewsher PD, Jones SJ, et al. Late onset hypothyroidism after subtotal thyroidectomy for hyperthyroidism: implications for long term follow up. *Br J Surg* 1983;70:740–743.
16. Ramus NI. Hypocalcemia after subtotal thyroidectomy for thyrotoxicosis. *Br J Surg* 1984;71:589–590.
17. Yanagisawa M, Kurihara H, Kimura S, et al. A novel potent vasoconstrictor peptide produced by vascular endothelial cells. *Nature* 1988; 332:411–415.
18. Nomura K, Yamashita J, Ogawa M. Endothelin 1 is involved in the transient hypoparathyroidism seen in patients undergoing thyroid surgery. *J Endocrinol* 1994;143:343–351.
19. Falk SA, Reussner L. Hypothermia causes temporary hypoparathyroidism after thyroid surgery. Proceedings of the 4th International Conference on Head and Neck Cancer, 1996, p. 226.
20. Mosekilde L, Christensen MS. Decreased parathyroid function in hyperthyroidism: interrelationships between serum parathyroid hormone, calcium phosphorus metabolism and thyroid function. *Acta Endocrinol (Copenh)* 1977;84:566–575.
21. Golding Sr, Krane SM. Organ system manifestations of thyrotoxicosis: the skeletal system. In: Ingbar SH, Braverman LE, eds. *Werner's the thyroid.* Philadelphia: JB Lippincott, 1986;chap 40.
22. Skrabanek P. Hypocalcemia after thyroidectomy. *Lancet* 1976;2:1080.
23. Toft AD, Irvine WJ, McIntosh D, et al. Propranolol in the treatment of thyrotoxicosis by subtotal thyroidectomy. *J Clin Endocrinol Metab* 1976;43:1312–1316.
24. Auderberg B, Kagedal B, Hilsson OR, et al. Propranolol and thyroid resection for hyperthyroidism. *Acta Chir Scand* 1979;145:297–303.
25. Wolfe JH, Voelkel EF, Tashjian AH. Distribution of calcitonin-containing cells in the normal adult human thyroid gland: a correlation of morphology with peptide content. *J Clin Endocrinol Metab* 1974;38:688–694.
26. Franz RC, Joubert E, Lodder JV. Transient postthyroidectomy hypocalcemia—the role of parathormone, calcitonin, and plasma albumin. *S Afr J Surg* 1987;25:45–49.
27. Rasmusson B, Borgeskov S, Holm-Hansen B. Changes in serum calcitonin in patients undergoing thyroid surgery. *Acta Chir Scand* 1980; 146:15–17.
28. Watson CG, Steed DL, Robinson AG, Deftos LJ. The role of calcitonin and parathyroid hormone in the pathogenesis of postthyroidectomy hypocalcemia. *Metabolism* 1981;30:588–589.
29. Pottgen P, Davie ER, Post-thyroidectomy hypocalcemia. *Lancet* 1977; 1:1217.
30. Percival RC, Hargreaves AW, Kanis JA. The mechanism of hypocalcemia following thyroidectomy. *Acta Endocrinol (Copenh)* 1985;109:220–226.
31. Sawers J, Kellett H, Brown N, et al. Does calcitonin cause hypocalcemia after thyroidectomy? *Br J Surg* 1982;69:456–458.
32. Hamada N, Mimura T, Suzuki A, et al. Serum parathyroid hormone concentration measured by highly sensitive assay in post-thyroidectomy hypocalcemia of patients with Graves' disease. *Endocrinol Jpn* 1989;36:281–288.
33. Wingert DJ, Friesen SR, Iliopoulos JI, et al. Post-thyroidectomy hypocalcemia: incidence and risk factors. *Am J Surg* 1986;152:606–610.
34. Demeester-Mirkine N, Hooghe L, Van Geertruyden J, et al. Hypocalcemia after thyroidectomy. *Arch Surg* 1992;127:854–848.
35. Bourrel C, Uzzan B, Tison P, et al. Transient hypocalcemia after thyroidectomy. *Ann Otol Rhinol Laryngol* 1993;102:496–501.
36. Hermann M, Richter B, Roka R, et al. Thyroid surgery in untreated severe hyperthyroidism: perioperative kinetics of free thyroid hormones in the glandular venous effluent and peripheral blood. *Surgery* 1994;115:240–245.
37. Mitchie W, Stowers JM, Duncan T, et al. Mechanism of hypocalcemia after thyroidectomy for thyrotoxicosis. *Lancet* 1971;1:508–513.
38. Wartofsky L. Osteoporosis: a growing concern for the thyroidologist. *Thyroid Today* 1988;11(4):1–11.
39. Laitinen O. Hypocalcemia following thyroidectomy. *Lancet* 1976;2:859–860.
40. Wilkin TJ, Isles TE, Paterson CR, Crooks J, Beck JS. Postthyroidectomy hypocalcemia: a feature of the operation or the thyroid disorder? *Lancet* 1977;1:621–623.
41. Brasier AR, Nussbaum SR. Hungry bone syndrome: clinical and biochemical predictors of its occurrence after parathyroid surgery. *Am J Med* 1988;84:654–660.

42. Gann DS. Endocrine and metabolic responses to injury. In: Schwartz SI, ed. *Principles of surgery*. New York: McGraw-Hill, 1979;chap 1.
43. Grant JP. Septic and metabolic complications: recognition and management. In: *Handbook of total parenteral nutrition*, 1st ed. Philadelphia: WB Saunders, 1980;chap 9.
44. Wandall JH. Concentrations of serum proteins during and immediately after surgical trauma. *Acta Chir Scand* 1974;140:171–179.
45. Gilmour IR. The gross anatomy of the parathyroid glands. *J Pathol* 1938;46:133–148.
46. Farrar WB, Cooperman M, James AG. Surgical management of papillary and follicular carcinoma of the thyroid. *Ann Surg* 1980;192:701–704.
47. Thompson NW, Harness JK. Complications of total thyroidectomy for carcinoma. *Surg Gynecol Obstet* 1970;131:861–868.
48. Karlan MS, Catz B, Dunkelman D, et al. A safe technique for thyroidectomy with complete nerve dissection and parathyroid preservation. *Head Neck Surg* 1984;6:1014–1019.
49. Winsa B, Rastad J, Akerstrom G, et al. Retrospective evaluation of subtotal and total thyroidectomy in Graves' disease with and without endocrine ophthalmopathy. *Eur J Endocrinol* 1995;132:406–412.
50. Mazzaferri EL, Young RL, Oertal JE, et al. Papillary thyroid carcinoma: the impact of therapy in 576 patients. *Medicine (Baltimore)* 1977;56:171–196.
51. Flynn MB, Lyons KJ, Tarter JW, et al. Local complications after surgical resection for thyroid carcinoma. *Am J Surg* 1994;168:404–407.
52. De Leo S, Giustozzi GM, Boselli C, et al. Complications after total thyroidectomy in thyroid carcinoma. *Minerva Chir* 1991;46:1251–1254.
53. Wanebo HI, Andrews W, Kaiser DL. Thyroid cancer: some basic considerations. *Am J Surg* 1981;142:474–479.
54. Winsa B, Rastad J, Larrson E, et al. Total thyroidectomy in therapy-resistant Graves' disease. *Surgery* 1994;116:1068–1075.
55. Patwardan NA, Moront M, Rao S, et al. Surgery still has a role in Graves' hyperthyroidism. *Surgery* 1993;114:1108–1113.
56. Sawyers JL, Martin CE, Byrd BF, et al. Thyroidectomy for hyperthyroidism. *Ann Surg* 1972;175:939–947.
57. Andaker L, Johansson K, Smeds S, et al. Surgery for hyperthyroidism: hemithyroidectomy plus contralateral resection or bilateral resection? A prospective randomized study of postoperative complications and long-term results. *World J Surg* 1992;16:765–769.
58. Bergenfelz A, Ahren B. Calcium metabolism after hemithyroidectomy. *Horm Res* 1993;39:56–60.
59. McHenry CR, Pollard A, Walfish PG, et al. Intraoperative parathormone level measurement in the management of hyperparathyroidism. *Surgery* 1990;108:801–807.
60. Lehmann JB, Leidy JW. A post-thyroidectomy convulsion: an unusual presentation of chronic hypoparathyroidism. *West Va Med J* 1994;90:420–421.
61. Tami TA, Parker GS, Griggs JA, et al. Post-thyroidectomy hypocalcemia during lactation. *Ear Nose Throat J* 1990;69:773–774.
62. Murakami T, Tajiri J, Noguchi S. Prediction of the outcome of postoperative hypocalcemia in Graves' disease. *Endocrinol Jpn* 1992;39:103–107.
63. Claussen MS, Pehling GB, Kisken WA. Delayed recovery from post-thyroidectomy hypoparathyroidism: a case report. *Wis Med J* 1993;92:331–334.
64. Fonseca VA, Bloom RD, Dick R, Dandona P. Tetany despite normocalcemia and normomagnesemia following parathyroidectomy. *Postgrad Med J* 1987;63:885–886.
65. Mineoi K, Matsuoka H, Sumimoto T, et al. Torsade de pointes induced by hypocalcemia in a postoperative patient with thyrotoxicosis. *Jpn Heart J* 1992;33:735–738.
66. Halsted WS. Hypoparathyreosis, status parathyroprivous and transplantation of the parathyroid glands. *Am J Med Sci* 1907;134:1–12.
67. Paloyan E, Lawrence Am, Paloyan D. Successful autotransplantation of the parathyroid glands during total thyroidectomy for carcinoma. *Surg Gynecol Obstet* 1977;145:364–368.
68. Paloyan E, Lawrence AM, Brooks MH, et al. Total thyroidectomy and parathyroid autotransplantation for radiation associated thyroid cancer. *Surgery* 1976;80:70–76.
69. Salander H, Tisell LE. Incidence of hypoparathyroidism after radical surgery for thyroid carcinoma and autotransplantation of parathyroid glands. *Am J Surg* 1977;134:358–362.
70. Salander H, Tisell LE. Latent hypoparathyroidism in patients with autotransplanted parathyroid glands. *Am J Surg* 1980;139:385–388.
71. Smith MA, Jarosz H, Hessel P, et al. Parathyroid autotransplantation in total thyroidectomy. *Am Surg* 1990;56:404–406.
72. Katz AD. Parathyroid autotransplantation in patients with parathyroid disease and total thyroidectomy. *Am J Surg* 1981;142:490–493.
73. Ohman U, Granberg PO, Lindell B. Function of the parathyroid glands after total thyroidectomy. *Surg Gynecol Obstet* 1978;146:773–778.
74. Gann DS, Paone JF. Delayed hypocalcemia after thyroidectomy for Graves' disease is prevented by parathyroid autotransplantation. *Ann Surg* 1979;190 508–513.
75. Funahashi H, Satoh Y, Imai T, et al. Our technique of parathyroid autotransplantation in operation for papillary thyroid carcinoma. *Surgery* 1993;114:92–96.
76. Wells SA, Gunnells JC, Shelburne JD, et al. Transplantation of the parathyroid glands in man: clinical indications and results. *Surgery* 1975;78:34–44.
77. Diethelm AG, Adams PL, Murad TM, et al. Treatment of secondary hyperparathyroidism in patients with chronic renal failure by total parathyroidectomy and parathyroid autograft. *Ann Surg* 1981;193:777–793.
78. Edis AJ, Linos DA, Kao PC. Parathyroid autotransplantation at the time of reoperation for persistent hyperparathyroidism. *Surgery* 1980;88:588–593.
79. Saxe AW, Spiegel AM, Marx SJ, Brennan MF. Deferred parathyroid autografts with cryopreserved tissue after reoperative parathyroid surgery. *Arch Surg* 1982;117:538–543.
80. Max MH, Flint LM, Richardson JD, et al. Total parathyroidectomy and parathyroid autotransplantation in patients with chronic renal failure. *Surg Gynecol Obstet* 1981;153:177–180.
81. Wells SA, Farndon JR, Dale JK, et al. Long-term evaluation of patients with primary parathyroid hyperplasia managed by total parathyroidectomy and heterotopic autotransplantation. *Ann Surg* 1980;192:451–458.
82. Cordell LJ, Maxwell JG, Warden GD. Parathyroidectomy in chronic renal failure. *Am J Surg* 1979;138:951–956.
83. Kunori T, Tsuchiya T, Itoh J, et al. Improvement of postoperative hypocalcemia by repeated allotransplantation of parathyroid tissue without anti-rejection therapy. *Tohoku J Exp Med* 1991;165:33–40.
84. Kiprenskii I, Piakhin IS, Podshivalin AV. The transplantation of a segment of pancreas and thyroid-parathyroid complex by using a microsurgical technic. *Vestn Khir I I Grek* 1990;145:108–110.
85. Segerberg EC, Grubb WG, Herndenson AE. The first successful parathyroid transplant from an identical twin for the cure of permanent postoperative hypoparathyroidism. *Surgery* 1992;111:357–358.
86. Cramarossa L, Misasi G, La Motta B, et al. The pathogenesis of hypocalcemia after thyroidectomy. *Ann Ital Chir* 1993;64:271–274.
87. Copp DH, Cameron EC, Cheney BA, et al. Evidence for calcitonin—a new hormone from the parathyroid that lowers blood calcium. *Endocrinology* 1962;70:638–649.
88. Copp DH. Calcitonin: discovery, development and clinical application. *Clin Invest Med* 1994;17:268–277.
89. Lewis P, Rafferty B, Shelley M, et al. A suggested role for calcitonin: the protection of the skeleton during pregnancy and lactation. *J Endocrinol* 1970;49:9–10.
90. Gray TK, Munson PL. Thyrocalcitonin—evidence for a physiological function. *Science* 1969;166:1512–1513.
91. Heersche JNM. Calcitonin effects on osteoclastic resorption: the escape phenomenon revisited. *Bone Miner* 1992;16:174–177.
92. Gennari C, Agnusdei D, Camporeale A. Long term treatment with calcitonin in osteoporosis. *Horm Metab Res* 1993;25:484–485.
93. Wallach S, Farley JR, Baylink DJ, et al. Effects of calcitonin on bone quality and osteoblastic function. *Calcif Tissue Int* 1993;52:335–339.
94. Silva OL, Wisnecki LA, Cyrus J, Snider RH, Moore CF, Becker KL. Calcitonin in thyroidectomized patients. *Am J Med Sci* 1978;275:159–164.
95. Lowery WD, Thomas CG, Aubrey BJ, Rosenstein BD, Talmage RV. The late effect of subtotal thyroidectomy and radioactive iodine therapy on calcitonin secretion and bone mineral density in women treated for Graves' disease. *Surgery* 1986;100:1142–1149.
96. Sianesi M, Cervellin GF, Palummeri E, et al. Calcitonin deficit syndrome in thyroidectomized patients. *Ital J Surg Sci* 1985;15:145–148.
97. Body JJ, Heath H. Estimates of circulating monomeric calcitonin: physiological studies in normal and thyroidectomized man. *J Clin Endocrinol Metab* 1983;57:897–903.
98. Teigs RD, Body JJ, Barta JM, et al. Secretion and metabolism of

monomeric human calcitonin: effects of age, sex and thyroid damage. *J Bone Miner Res* 1986;1:339-49.
99. Sugino K, Kure Y, Iwasaki H, et al. Does total thyroidectomy induce metabolic bone disturbance? *Int Surg* 1992;77:178–180.
100. Body JJ, Demeester-Mirkine N, Corvilain J. Calcitonin deficiency after radioactive iodine treatment. *Ann Int Med* 1988;109:590–591.
101. Tzanela M, Thalassinos NC, Nikou A, et al. Effect of ^{131}I treatment on the calcitonin response to calcium infusion in hyperthyroid patients. *Clin Endocrinol* 1993;38:25–28.
102. Body JJ, Demeester-Mirkine N, Borkowski A, et al. Calcitonin deficiency in primary hypothyroidism. *J Clin Endocrinol Metab* 1986;62:700–703.
103. Demeester-Mirkine N, Bergmann P, Body JJ, et al. Calcitonin and bone mass status in congenital hypothyroidism. *Calcif Tissue Int* 1990;46:222–226.
104. Mundy GR. Osteopenia. *Dis Mon* 1987;23:539–600.
105. Body JJ. Calcitonin: from the determination of circulating levels in various physiological and pathological conditions to the demonstration of lymphocyte receptors. *Horm Res* 1993;39:166–170.
106. Ettinger B, Wingerd J. Thyroid supplements: effect on bone mass. *West J Med* 1986;136:473–476.
107. Fallon MD, Perry HM, Bergfeld M, et al. Exogenous hyperthyroidism with osteoporosis. *Arch Intern Med* 1983;143:442–444.
108. Coindre JM, David JP, Rivere L, et al. Bone loss in hypothyroidism with hormone replacement: a histomorphometric study. *Arch Intern Med* 1986;146:48–53.
109. Ross DS, Neer RM, Ridgway EC, Daniels GH. Subclinical hyperthyroidism and reduced bone density as a possible result of prolonged suppression of the pituitary-thyroid axis with L-thyroxine. *Am J Med* 1987;82:1167–1170.
110. Paul TL, Kerrigan J, Kelly AM, et al. Longterm L-thyroxine therapy is associated with decreased hip bone density in premenopausal women. *JAMA* 1988;259:3137–3141.
111. Ross DS. Hyperthyroidism, thyroid hormone therapy and bone. *Thyroid* 1994;4:319–326.
112. Faber J, Galloe AM. Changes in bone mass during prolonged subclinical hyperthyroidism due to L-thyroxine treatment: a meta-analysis. *Eur J Endocrinol* 1994;130:350–356.
113. Burman KD. How serious are the risks of thyroid hormone over-replacement? *Thyroid Today* 1995;18:1–9.
114. Gonzalez DC, Mautalen CA, Correa A, et al. Bone mass in totally thyroidectomized patients: role of calcitonin deficiency and exogenous thyroid treatment. *Acta Endocrinol* 1991;124:521–525.
115. McDermott MT, Kidd GS, Blue P, Ghaed V, Hofeldt FD. Reduced bone mineral content in totally thyroidectomized patients: possible effect of calcitonin deficiency. *J Clin Endocrinol Metab* 1983;56:936–939.
116. Burmeister LA, Goumaz MO, Mariash CN, et al. Levothyroxine dose requirements for thyrotropin suppression in the treatment of differentiated thyroid cancer. *J Clin Endocrinol Metab* 1992;75:344–350.
117. Berglund J, Bondeson L, Christensen SB, et al. The influence of different degrees of chronic lymphocytic thyroiditis on thyroid function after surgery for benign, non-toxic goitre. *Eur J Surg* 1991;157:257–260.
118. Kuma K, Matsuzuka F, Kobayashi A, et al. Natural course of Graves' disease after subtotal thyroidectomy and management of patients with postoperative thyroid dysfunction. *Am J Med Sci* 1991;302:8–12.
119. Toft AD, Irvine WJ, Sinclair I, et al. Thyroid function after surgical treatment of thyrotoxicosis: a report of 100 cases treated with propanolol before surgery. *N Engl J Med* 1978;298:643–647.
120. Cusick EL, Krukowski ZH, Matheson HA. Outcome of surgery for Graves' disease re-examined. *Br J Surg* 1987;74:780–783.
121. Makiuchi M, Miyakawa M, Sugenoya A, et al. An evaluation of several prognostic factors in the surgical treatment of thyrotoxicosis. *Surg Gynecol Obstet* 1981;152:639–641.
122. Sanchez-Franco F, Garcia MD, Cacicedo L, et al. Transient lack of thyrotropin response to thyrotropin-releasing hormone in treated hyperthyroid patients with low serum thyroxine and triiodothyroxine. *J Clin Endocrinol Metab* 1974;38:1098–1102.
123. Sawers JSA, Toft AD, Irvine WJ, et al. Transient hypothyroidism after iodine-131 treatment of thyrotoxicosis. *J Clin Endocrinol Metab* 1980;50:226–229.
124. Toft AD, Irvine WJ, Hunter M, et al. Anomalous plasma TSH levels in patients developing hypothyroidism in the early months after ^{131}I therapy for thyrotoxicosis. *J Clin Endocrinol Metab* 1974;39:607.
125. Vagenakis AB, Braverman LE, et al. Recovery of pituitary thyrotropic function after withdrawal of prolonged thyroid-suppression therapy. *N Engl J Med* 1975;293:681–684.
126. Duick DS, Stein RB, Warren DW, et al. The significance of partial suppressibility of serum thyroxine by triiodothyronine administration in euthyroid man. *J Clin Endocrinol Metab* 1975;41:229–234.
127. Noh SH, Soh EY, Park CS, et al. Evaluation of thyroid function after bilateral subtotal thyroidectomy for Graves' disease—a long term follow-up of 100 patients. *Yonsei Med J* 1994;35:177–183.
128. Okamoto T, Fujimoto Y, Obara T, et al. Retrospective analysis of prognostic factors affecting the thyroid functional status after subtotal thyroidectomy for Graves' disease. *World J Surg* 1992;16:690–695.
129. Reid DJ. Hyperthyroidism and hypothyroidism complicating the treatment of thyrotoxicosis. *Br J Surg* 1987;74:1060–1062.
130. Cusick EL, Krukowski ZH, Matheson NA. Outcome of surgery for Graves' disease re-examined. *Br J Surg* 1987;74:780–783.
131. Sugrue DD, Drury MI, McEvoy M, Heffernan SJ, O'Malley E. Long term follow up of hyperthyroid patients treated by subtotal thyroidectomy. *Br J Surg* 1983;70:408–411.
132. Takai Y. Clinical evaluations of subtotal thyroidectomy for Graves' disease. *Folia Endocrinol Jpn* 1995;71:27–38.
133. Leese GP, Jung RT, Scott A, et al. Long term follow-up of treated hyperthyroid and hypothyroid patients. *Health Bull* 1993;51:177–183.
134. Simms JM, Talbot CH. Surgery for thyrotoxicosis. *Br J Surg* 1983;70:581–583.
135. Jortso E, Lennquist S, Lundstrom B, Norrby K, Smeds S. The influence of remnant size, antithyroid antibodies, thyroid morphology, and lymphocyte infiltration on thyroid function after subtotal resection for hyperthyroidism. *World J Surg* 1987;11:365–371.
136. Blondeau P. Surgical treatment of hyperthyroidism. *Bull Acad Natl Med* 1991;175:1065–1073.
137. Sugino K, Mimura T, Toshima K, et al. Follow-up evaluation of patients with Graves' disease treated by subtotal thyroidectomy and risk factor analysis for post-operative thyroid dysfunction. *J Endocrinol Invest* 1993;16:195–199.
138. Kasuga Y, Sugenoya A, Kobayashi S, et al. Significance of values of thyrotropin binding inhibitor immunoglobulins and appearance of intrathyroidal lymphocytes at subtotal thyroidectomy for Graves' disease. *J Am Coll Surg* 1994;178:589–594.
139. Csaky G, Balazs G, Bako G, et al. Late results of thyroid surgery for hyperthyroidism performed in childhood. *Prog Ped Surg* 1991;26:31–40.
140. Melliere D, Etienne G, Becquemin JP. Operations for hyperthyroidism. *Am J Surg* 1988;155:395–399.
141. Matte R, Ste-Marie LG, Comtois R, et al. The pituitary thyroid axis after hemithyroidectomy in euthyroid man. *J Clin Endocrinol Metab* 1981;53:377–380.
142. Okamoto T, Fujimoto Y, Obara T, et al. Trial of thyroid autotransplantation in patients with Graves' disease whose remnant thyroid has unintentionally been made too small at subtotal thyroidectomy. *Endocrinol Jpn* 1990;37:95–101.

though CHAPTER 40

Complications of Thyroid Surgery: Thyrotoxic Storm

Leonard Wartofsky and Mark E. Peele

The syndrome of thyrotoxic storm, or crisis, is a life-threatening complication of hyperthyroidism that fortunately occurs only rarely in the perioperative setting. The diagnosis should be considered in the thyrotoxic patient with fever, marked tachycardia, congestive heart failure, diarrhea, and central nervous system signs that may vary from confusion to coma. Thyrotoxic storm is a state of disordered homeostasis resulting from acute decompensation of the cardiovascular, central nervous, gastrointestinal, and hepatorenal systems in the thyrotoxic patient. The superimposition of systemic (nonthyroidal) illness or operative stress may represent the underlying pathophysiology that converts uncomplicated thyrotoxicosis into storm. This is so because these conditions are associated with increases in free, or unbound, thyroid hormones, whereas total hormone levels may not differ significantly from those in uncomplicated thyrotoxicosis.

Although the incidence of storm may approximate only 1% to 2% of all hospitalizations for thyrotoxicosis, the reported mortality rates in large inpatient series have ranged from 28% to 100% (1–8). The clinical presentation is often dramatic, with signs of hypermetabolism and multiple organ system failure, which are associated with high mortality despite vigorous therapy.

Development of an optimal approach to management requires an understanding of the pathophysiology underlying decompensation of thyrotoxicosis into thyrotoxic storm. Because of the occasional presentation of thyroid storm in the peri- or postoperative setting after both thyroid and nonthyroid surgery, surgeons must maintain a heightened awareness of the potential for storm in their patients with thyroid disease.

The natural history of untreated thyrotoxic storm is largely unknown or anecdotal. Historically, thyrotoxic storm after thyroidectomy, thoracoabdominal surgery, or obstetric procedures in thyrotoxic patients was a common complication and major cause of mortality. The development of crisis in this clinical setting was referred to as surgical storm, to emphasize the presumed underlying etiology. Indeed, earlier reports indicated that the most common clinical setting for storm was postsurgical (1–4). Today, in contrast, thyrotoxic storm develops most frequently in the setting of systemic illness such as infection (i.e., medical storm) (5,6). Early diagnosis and improved preoperative medical treatment of the thyrotoxic individual is a likely explanation for the decline in the incidence of surgical storm. However, precipitation of storm in the perioperative period still remains a potential problem today (9).

CLINICAL FEATURES

The *sine qua non* for successful therapy of thyrotoxic storm is early diagnosis. Unfortunately, differentiation of storm from severe, otherwise uncomplicated thyrotoxicosis on the basis of laboratory test results is impossible. Early diagnosis requires both a high index of suspicion and astute recognition of heralding clinical signs common to storm yet unusual in uncomplicated thyrotoxicosis. Clinical judgment will provide the ability to diagnose the thyrotoxic individual in the early stages of incipient storm when therapy is most effective. The diagnosis is most obvious with a classic and dramatic presentation of fully developed storm, which includes fever (>38.5°C), altered mental status, congestive heart failure, and frequent watery stools, but by the time of this presentation,

L. Wartofsky: Department of Medicine, Washington Hospital Center, Washington, D.C. 20010.
M. E. Peele: Division of Cardiology, Brooke Medical Center, Fort Sam Houston, San Antonio, Texas 78234-5012.

the prognosis may be significantly reduced. Burch and Wartofsky (10) proposed a scoring system to assist in the distinction between severe thyrotoxicosis and thyrotoxic storm (Table 1).

Thermogenesis in thyrotoxicosis is enhanced in part because of the elevated basal metabolic rate (BMR). The cellular mechanisms augmenting thermogenesis in states of excess thyroid hormone action may involve increased sodium–potassium (Na-K) adenosine triphosphatase (ATPase) activity, decreased coupling of oxidative phosphorylation to chemical energy formation, or amplification of catecholaminergic responses (6). Indeed, many of the signs and symptoms of thyrotoxicosis are believed to be related to a thyroid hormone–catecholamine interaction, and the sympathetic nervous system can play a role in the pathogenesis of thyroid storm (11). Despite augmented thermogenesis, core body temperature is normal in uncomplicated thyrotoxicosis, largely because of cutaneous vasodilatation with resultant increases in radiant heat losses. The warm, moist extremities and the preference of thyrotoxic patients for cool local environments and light clothing reflect physical and behavioral alterations that serve to improve radiant heat loss.

Defective thermoregulation arises almost universally in thyrotoxic storm (8). The clinical experience reported by Mazzaferri and Skillman (5) and Nelson and Becker (12) indicates that fever greater than 38°C was present in all patients for whom temperature data were available. Whether the febrile response characteristic of storm represents defective central nervous system thermoregulation or elevation of thermogenesis and BMR to levels beyond cutaneous heat radiation capacity is unknown. Measurements of BMR in individuals with storm have averaged twice the level seen in similarly thyrotoxic individuals prior to development of storm (3). These data suggest that the increases in thermogenesis seen in storm are caused in part by elevations of BMR beyond the level encountered in uncomplicated thyrotoxicosis.

Alteration in central nervous system function in thyrotoxic storm is uniformly present, although a spectrum of mental statuses and behavioral abnormalities may exist. Central nervous system symptoms of tremor, restlessness, irritability, and emotional lability are characteristic of thyrotoxicosis. However, confusion, lethargy, and psychosis culminating in stupor and coma are quite typical of storm but unusual in uncomplicated thyrotoxicosis without premorbid psychopathology. Indeed, preservation of normal mentation in a febrile thyrotoxic is strong clinical evidence against impending storm (13) and may suggest merely a superimposed mild infection.

Clinical reports of large series of patients with thyrotoxic storm reveal additional characteristic features. Diarrhea is the most common gastrointestinal complaint in storm, although abdominal pain, nausea, and vomiting are not uncommon. Hepatic function is variably affected; mild degrees of liver dysfunction are the rule, but frank hepatic failure is seen occasionally (14). An often overlooked clinical feature of individuals progressing to storm is severe weight loss and malnutrition. Weight loss, often exceeding 20 kg, is common and reflects presence of the underlying catabolic state (1,3,5). Additionally, hypoglycemia and hypoalbuminemia may be seen in storm and are a further indication of longstanding severe caloric defects (5).

Having made a diagnosis of thyroid storm, the clinician is required to carefully search for a precipitating event or illness, which is fundamental to the evolution of uncomplicated thyrotoxicosis into storm (Table 2). Infection, which often may be occult, is the most important precipitating event in the development of storm today. Vigorous therapeutic intervention aimed at eliminating the precipitating event is required for successful treatment of storm.

TABLE 1. *Diagnostic criteria for thyroid storm (findings, and points assigned to each)*

Thermoregulatory dysfunction		
Temperature:	99–99.9	5
	100–100.9	10
	101–101.9	15
	102–102.9	20
	103–103.9	25
	≥104	30
Central nervous system effects		
Absent		0
Mild agitation		10
Delirium, psychosis, lethargy		20
Seizure or coma		30
Gastrointestinal dysfunction		
Absent		0
Diarrhea, nausea, vomiting, or abdominal pain		10
Unexplained jaundice		20
Cardiovascular dysfunction		
Tachycardia:	90–109	5
	110–119	10
	120–129	15
	130–139	20
	≥140	25
CHF: Absent		0
Mild (edema)		5
Moderate (bibasilar rales)		10
Severe (pulmonary edema)		15
Atrial fibrillation		
Absent		0
Present		10
History of precipitating event (surgery, infection, etc.)		
Absent		0
Present		10

Points are assigned and the scores totalled. When it is not possible to determine whether a finding is caused by an intercurrent illness or by thyrotoxicosis, the higher point score is given so as to favor empirical therapy.
Interpretation: Based on the total score, the likelihood that the diagnosis is thyrotoxic storm is:
Unlikely <25
Impending 25–44
Highly likely >45

TABLE 2. *Clinical disorders underlying thyrotoxic crisis*

Infection (bronchopneumonia, pharyngitis, meningitis, sepsis)
Surgery
Iodine administration (iodinated contrast dye, oral iodine)
Hypoglycemia
Parturition
Trauma (including vigorous and repetitive thyroid palpation)
Emotional stress
Thiourea withdrawal
[131]I therapy
Diabetic ketoacidosis
Pulmonary thromboembolism
Cerebrovascular accidents

PATHOPHYSIOLOGY

Modern mechanisms for the action of thyroid hormone are predicated on hormone entry into the target cell nucleus. Specific thyroid hormone receptors are present in the nucleus closely related to the genetic material. Interaction of thyroid hormone with specific nuclear receptors influences tissue-specific gene expression, with subsequent alteration in cellular metabolism. The clinical expression of excessive thyroid hormone action represents an altered thyroid hormone–nuclear receptor interaction at the molecular level. Enhanced availability of thyroid hormone to enter the cell and interact with nuclear receptors is a potential mechanism for the development of thyrotoxic storm.

A quantitative increase in thyroidal release of thyroxine (T_4) and triiodothyronine (T_3) has not been generally accepted to be central to the development of thyrotoxic storm. Circulating total T_4 and T_3 concentrations usually are no higher in storm than in uncomplicated thyrotoxicosis (15–17). There are instances, however, when storm appears after vigorous gland palpation, iodine-131 (^{131}I) therapy, and iodine administration (4,18,19), which suggests that augmented glandular hormone release was responsible, at least in part. Perhaps more characteristic, in storm, reduced affinity of T_4 and T_3 for their binding proteins results in an increased free fraction of circulating hormone available for cellular entry. The presence of an underlying nonthyroidal illness in storm is common, and altered protein binding of thyroid hormone, with resultant increases in the percent of free dialyzable T_4 and T_3, has been well described for many nonthyroidal illnesses in sick but otherwise euthyroid patients (20–22). Indeed, Brooks and Waldstein (17) demonstrated a twofold increase in the percent of dialyzable T_4 and total free T_4 concentration in storm compared to uncomplicated severe thyrotoxicosis. In another case report (16), total and free T_4 were normal but total and free T_3 were elevated in a patient experiencing surgical storm after a subtotal thyroidectomy. Increased total thyroid hormone concentration and/or lowered protein binding greatly enhances the entry of free hormone (both T_4 and T_3) into target cells.

Other aspects of the pathophysiology of storm may relate to novel changes in thyroid hormone clearance caused by alterations in the kinetics and character of T_4 metabolism. The deiodination of T_4 to lesser iodinated iodothyronines, and the deamination of T_4 or T_3 to tetrac or triac, respectively, are major pathways of clearance. Interestingly, the presence of nonthyroidal illness (including the perioperative state) and the associated caloric deprivation (especially carbohydrate) result in reduced T_4 clearance. For example, infection may be associated with a greater than 50% reduction in T_4 clearance (23). A relatively fasting state as a result of NPO (nothing *per os*) status in the pre- or postoperative patient, or to anorexia and nausea, are common in storm and associated with further reductions in deiodination and clearance of T_4 (20,24,25). This inhibition of deiodination occurs in the liver and kidney, where approximately 60% of T_4 is cleared. The reduction in T_4 deiodinative clearance in fasting, perhaps caused by low hepatic reduced glutathione levels, is coupled loosely to augmented nondeiodinative thyroid hormone metabolism with increased formation of triac, a metabolically active congener of T_3 (24,26).

Although the exact pathophysiology of thyrotoxic storm is not known, substantial inferences can be drawn. The dramatic elevation of free thyroxine concentration, decreased clearance of iodothyronines by the liver, and augmented formation of normally minimally important iodothyronines (triac) in storm are the consequence of complicating medical, surgical, or dietary stresses. These metabolic abnormalities occurring in the thyrotoxic patient appear fundamental to the decompensated clinical presentation of storm.

TREATMENT

Our understanding of the causes and pathophysiology of thyrotoxic storm forms the basis for its treatment. That the cumulative clinical experiences of multiple reported series of patients with thyrotoxic storm over time (1–5) reflect a declining mortality suggests greater success with more recent approaches to therapy (4).

We believe that the therapy of established storm should be directed at four therapeutic goals: (a) to reduce hormone synthesis and release from the thyroid; (b) to antagonize peripheral actions of existing excesses of circulating hormone; (c) to provide supportive care and avoid homeostatic decompensation; and (d) to define and treat any precipitating or complicating underlying conditions (8).

Therapy Directed Against the Thyroid Gland

The inhibition of thyroidal hormone synthesis and release is the classic cornerstone of treatment. The thionamides propylthiouracil (PTU) and methimazole (Tapazole) are potent inhibitors of organification of iodine.

Provided adequate dose and frequency of dosage are used, thionamides will profoundly reduce hormone synthesis in all but the rarest of individuals. Although the onset of action is rapid after oral administration, significant clinical improvement early in the course depends on other therapies. PTU also inhibits peripheral conversion of T_4 to the much more active T_3, thereby facilitating a more rapid fall in serum T_3 concentration, an effect not shared by methimazole. This is important because T_3 is some 10 to 15 times more active than T_4, leading some authors to suggest that T_4 serves primarily as a "prohormone." Initially, we prefer to administer PTU in a dose of 1200 to 1500 mg/day given orally (200–250 mg every 4 hr). Methimazole 120 mg/day given orally (20 mg every 4 hr) is also suitable. Although the use of a thionamide in a patient with previous thionamide-related hepatocellular dysfunction or agranulocytosis cannot be recommended, a history of minor rash or urticaria with these agents should not prevent their use in storm. Unfortunately, no suitable intravenous preparation of either PTU or methimazole is available. Formulation of either drug into a suppository for rectal administration is an effective route to achieve therapeutic blood levels in the patient in whom oral agents are contraindicated or impractical (27,28).

Although further synthesis of iodothyronines in the thyroid may be effectively blocked by thionamides, continued release of preformed hormone from glandular stores will persist unabated during thionamide treatment. Addition of another agent, such as stable iodine or lithium carbonate, is necessary to inhibit thyroidal release of preformed hormone. Because Lugol's iodine therapy alone will augment and enrich hormonal stores in the thyroid, care must be taken to ensure that an adequate thionamide organification block is present prior to initiation of stable iodine therapy. Failure to initiate thionamide therapy prior to iodine treatment can result in worsening of thyrotoxicosis, especially if iodine is inadvertently withdrawn or has to be continued for more than a few weeks (after which escape from the iodine inhibition of hormone release may occur). Lugol's solution 8 minims (approximately 0.5 mL) orally every 6 hr is effective. An intravenous infusion of sodium iodide (1 g every 24 hr) is equally effective and eliminates potential concerns of variable gut absorption. Commercial preparations of the latter are no longer available in the United States and have to be specifically formulated. In contrast to the slow decline in serum levels of T_4 and T_3 seen with sole thionamide therapy, the levels fall rapidly after iodine therapy, with near-normal values often reached in 3 to 5 days (29).

Iodinated radiographic contrast dyes (Oragrafin or ipodate) have been used increasingly in the management of thyrotoxicosis. Ipodate is effective in inhibiting glandular iodine release because of the large amount of stable iodine present in this compound (approximately 65% by weight). Ipodate is also a potent inhibitor of T_4 to T_3 conversion in many tissues. Although the efficacy of ipodate for thyrotoxic storm has not been extensively studied, a rapid decline in circulating T_4 and T_3 levels is typically seen in thyrotoxicosis (30). Ipodate in a daily dose of 1 to 3 g orally in addition to adequate thionamide treatment should be effective.

Occasionally, a patient with thyrotoxic storm is encountered in whom the use of iodine is contraindicated for fear of systemic anaphylaxis, thereby presenting a therapeutic dilemma. In such a patient, lithium carbonate should be considered, as it has been used successfully in the treatment of thyrotoxicosis (31). Lithium carbonate, initially at a dose of 300 mg every 6 hr, should be effective at inhibiting thyroidal hormone release. To avoid lithium toxicity, serum levels must be monitored daily, and dosages titrated to maintain a plasma lithium level of approximately 1.0 mEq/L. Some caution must be exercised, however, because postoperative surgical storm has been reported after subtotal thyroidectomy in a patient prepared with lithium carbonate and beta-blockade (32). This patient had received iodine previously, however, which likely served (in the absence of thioureas) to enrich hormone stores, a complication discussed previously.

Therapy Directed Against Systemic Decompensation

The level of health care and monitoring necessary in thyrotoxic storm mandates admission to a critical care ward, such as a surgical intensive care unit (ICU) for the postoperative patient. The need for aggressive treatment of fever cannot be overemphasized, and acetaminophen is the indicated antipyretic. Salicylates may displace thyroxine from serum binding sites and cannot be recommended because the resultant increase in free hormone could theoretically worsen the clinical picture. Aggressive cooling measures, including alcohol washes, cooling blankets, and ice packs, may be required. Adequate thermoregulation should considerably ameliorate the apparent hypermetabolism present in storm (33). Because of the fever and a possible history of diarrhea and vomiting, fluid losses are large and must be vigorously replaced to prevent potential cardiovascular collapse. Volume status must be monitored carefully (e.g., Swan-Ganz monitoring of central hemodynamics), as overhydration is also a problem in storm. Depleted hepatic glycogen stores and water-soluble vitamin deficiency also require replacement. Typically, 10% dextrose supplied in hypotonic saline at a rate of 3 to 4 liters each day with vitamin supplementation is adequate. The development of congestive heart failure is commonly present because of atrial tachyarrhythmias, impaired myocardial contractility, and volume overload. Therapy with digitalis and diuretics is beneficial, although the required dose of digoxin may be quite high because of altered distribution and metabolism of digitalis.

Glucocorticoids have been used for decades on empirical grounds for thyrotoxic storm (34). The review of

Waldstein et al. (4) suggests a role for exogenous steroids in reducing storm mortality. The use of steroids in storm was prompted by concern over potential impaired adrenocortical reserve. Indeed, plasma clearance rates for cortisol in thyrotoxicosis patients are twice those in euthyroid controls (35). There is also some concern for an inappropriately reduced response of the storm patient to stress, because the response of urinary 17-hydroxycorticosteroids to adrenocorticotropic hormone (ACTH) infusions may be blunted in thyrotoxicosis (36). An additional benefit of steroid treatment is its inhibition of T_4 to T_3 conversion; in this regard, it is similar to PTU and ipodate. An initial dose of 300 mg hydrocortisone followed by 100 mg every 8 to 12 hr should be adequate.

Therapy Directed Against Ongoing Effects of Thyroid Hormone in the Periphery

The activity of the sympathetic nervous system is greatly enhanced in thyrotoxic storm. This hyperadrenergic state may contribute importantly to the apparent elevated metabolic rate present in storm. The use of adrenergic antagonists (beta-blockers) is effective in ameliorating the hypermetabolism of storm. Prior to availability of modern beta-blockers, reserpine (37) and guanethidine (5) were used successfully for the treatment of storm, but efficacy was limited by the side effects of sedation, depression, and hypotension. Specific β-adrenergic receptor antagonists, especially propranolol, have become the drugs of choice (7,38,39). Propranolol, 40 to 80 mg every 6 hr orally, is quite efficacious in reducing sympathetic nervous system activity in storm. Plasma propranolol levels approximating 50 ng/mL may be required to maintain effective blockade. Frequently, larger doses are required to achieve this adequate therapeutic effect in storm, because of variable serum levels after customarily employed doses (38). Propranolol also inhibits T_4 to T_3 conversion modestly, and it may be of some selective advantage over other β-adrenergic receptor antagonists. This advantage may be more theoretical than real: in one study, no reduction in serum T_3 was seen after propranolol therapy (40). In the highly critical initial management, intravenous propranolol in doses of 1 to 2 mg may be used until effective serum levels are achieved after oral administration (39). The ultra-short-acting β-adrenergic blocking agent esmolol may be used for the perioperative management of thyroid storm as well. A loading dose of 250 to 500 µg/kg, followed by a continuous infusion at a rate of 50 to 100 µg/kg per minute, has been shown to be effective (41–43).

The role of propranolol when congestive heart failure is present in storm is arguable. However, careful titration of propranolol dose to allow amelioration of the adrenergic overactivity present in storm, with simultaneous monitoring of hemodynamic cardiovascular function, may be of benefit in selected cases.

Shortly after the initial publication of the successful management of thyrotoxicosis with propranolol, additional reports appeared describing performance of thyroidectomy without complication after no preparation other than propranolol alone (44,45) or propranolol with iodine (40). In the authors' view, such management is usually unnecessary and potentially dangerous, requiring extraordinarily close monitoring of vital signs with repetitive doses indicated to keep pulse rates at 80 to 90 per minute. Given the short half-life (2 to 4 hr) and duration of action (4 to 6 hr) of the drug in the thyrotoxic patient, intravenous dosage is generally required. Occasionally, despite heroic doses of propranolol, adequate control of clinical thyrotoxicosis is not achieved. We have seen one hospitalized patient on a total daily dose of 800 mg of propranolol, who had a persistent tachycardia unresponsive even to additional intravenous doses of the drug. More commonly, the catecholaminergic signs of thyrotoxicosis are blocked by propranolol and the patient appears clinically euthyroid. However, as discussed, propranolol has no effect on thyroid hormone synthesis or release (46), which therefore continue unabated in the absence of thiourea and iodine therapy. Theoretically, it could have been predicted that patients so treated would be vulnerable to storm should a pathophysiologic event increasing free hormone occur (such as perioperative infection). Indeed, this has been confirmed, and enough cases of thyroid storm [sometimes fatal (45)] have occurred in patients on propranolol blockade (47–50) that the surgeon should be wary of preparation with beta-blockade alone. In the patient allergic to thioureas, for whom radioiodine ablation may not be an option (e.g., during pregnancy), surgery may be performed under beta-blockade, albeit more safely with simultaneous iodine or ipodate administration (40).

Attempts may be made to reduce the burden of the excessive circulating concentrations of T_4 and T_3 by either peritoneal dialysis or plasmapheresis (51–54). Hemoperfusion through a resin bed has been shown to be effective experimentally (55), and charcoal columns may be similarly employed (56). Finally, some removal of circulating T_4 and T_3 may be effected safely by the use of cholestyramine resin (57); this agent binds thyroid hormone entering the gastrointestinal tract via enterohepatic recirculation.

Therapy Directed Against the Precipitating Illness

The precipitating cause of thyrotoxic storm is often readily apparent in cases presenting after trauma, thyroidectomy, and parturition. No specific therapy need be reserved for these causes once the initial insult has passed. Hypoglycemia, ketoacidosis, pulmonary emboli, or stroke complicating storm will require the same specific therapy generally reserved for these conditions in the absence of storm. In the stuporous individual, a high index of suspicion for these (often occult) precipitating events must be maintained.

Fever may occur in thyrotoxic storm in the absence of apparent infection, presumably representing the hypermetabolic state (see preceding) or perhaps occult subclinical infection. The serious prognosis of storm emphasizes the need to exclude underlying infection.

Empiric broad-spectrum antibiotic coverage should be discouraged. Collection of blood, urine, and sputum for culture, as well as lumbar puncture in the obtunded patient, is mandatory. A short course of broad-spectrum antibiotics may be initiated, guided by the clinician's best impression of the most likely site of infection, with subsequent tailoring of coverage based on culture results.

Definitive Therapy

Rapid clinical diagnosis of early thyrotoxic storm and aggressive therapeutic intervention provide the best chance for successful resolution of storm. Clinical improvement allows graded withdrawal of treatment modalities. Steroids should be rapidly tapered. Appropriate antibiotic treatment is guided by standard recommendations based on site of infection and etiologic agent. The withdrawal of thioureas, stable iodine, and β-blockers is a difficult clinical decision. In the postthyroidectomy patient, the duration of storm should be self-limited, because most of the source of the new thyroid hormone release was ostensibly excised. In the event that only a lobectomy or a lobectomy and isthmusectomy were performed, medical therapy with thioureas and beta-blockade will have to be continued, gradually tapered, and monitored according to standard recommendations for medical therapy in the preoperative patient (58).

In cases of storm occurring outside the perioperative period, definitive treatment of the underlying thyroid disorder is strongly recommended. A slow taper of thioureas after gradual iodine withdrawal in hopes of a longstanding remission seems unduly optimistic in most cases. The large doses of stable iodine that were already administered will flood the body pool of iodine, diminishing thyroidal radioiodine uptake, thereby making radioiodine ablation a choice of definitive therapy only at some remote future date. In the majority of such cases, surgical treatment 2 to 4 weeks after resolution of storm during continued aggressive therapy with thioureas, iodine, and β-blockers, as well as careful follow-up, seem preferable.

REFERENCES

1. Lahey FH. The crisis of exophthalmic goiter. *N Engl J Med* 1928;199: 255–257.
2. Bayley RH. Thyroid crisis. *Surg Gynecol Obstet* 1934;59:41–47.
3. McArthur JW, Rawson RVV, Means JH, Cope O. Thyrotoxic crisis. *JAMA* 1947;134:868–874.
4. Waldstein SS, Sheldon JS, Kaganiec GI, Bronsky D. A clinical study of thyroid storm. *Ann Intern Med* 1960;52:626–642.
5. Mazzaferri EL, Skillman TG. Thyroid storm. *Arch Intern Med* 1969; 124:584–690.
6. Mackin JF, Canary JJ, Pittman CS. Thyroid storm and its management. *N Engl J Med* 1974;291:1396–1398.
7. Wartofsky L. Thyrotoxic storm. In: Braverman LE, Utiger RE, eds. *The thyroid: a fundamental and clinical text,* 7th ed. Philadelphia: J.B. Lippincott Co., 1996:701–707.
8. Ingbar SH. Thyrotoxic storm. *N Engl J Med* 1966;274:1252–1254.
9. Bennett MH, Wainwright AP. Acute thyroid crisis on induction of anesthesia. *Anaesthesia* 1989;44:28–31.
10. Burch HB, Wartofsky L. Life-threatening thyrotoxicosis: thyroid storm. *Endocrinol Metab Clin North Am* 1993;22:263–277.
11. Wilson BE, Hobbs WN. Psuedoephedrine-associated thyroid storm: thyroid hormone-catecholamine interactions. *Am J Med Sci* 1993;306: 317–319.
12. Nelson NC, Becker WF. Thyroid crisis: diagnosis and treatment. *Ann Surg* 1969;170:263–273.
13. Nicoloff JT. Thyroid storm and myxedema coma. In: Kaplan MM, Larsen PR, eds. *Med Clin North Am* 1985;69:1005–1017.
14. Ficarra BJ, Naclerio EA. Thyroid crisis: pathogenesis of hepatic origin. *Am J Surg* 1945;69:325–337.
15. Brooks MH, Waldstein SS, Bronsky D, Sterling K. Serum triiodothyronine concentrations in thyroid storm. *J Clin Endocrinol Metab* 1975; 40:339–341.
16. Jacobs HS, Eastman CJ, Ekins RP, Mackie DB, Ellis SM, McHardy-Young S. Total and free triiodothyronine and thyroxine levels in thyroid storm and recurrent hyperthyroidism. *Lancet* 1973;2:236–238.
17. Brooks MH, Waldstein SS. Free thyroxine concentrations in thyroid storm. *Ann Intern Med* 1980;90:694–697.
18. McDermott MT, Kidd GS, Dodson LE, Hofeldt FD. Radioiodine-induced thyroid storm. *Am J Med* 1983;75:353–359.
19. Blum M, Kranjac T, Park CM, Engleman RM. Thyroid storm after cardiac angiography with iodinated contrast media. *JAMA* 1976;235: 2324–2325.
20. Wartofsky L, Burman KD. Alterations in thyroid function in patients with systemic illness: the "euthyroid sick syndrome." *Endocr Rev* 1982; 3:164–217.
21. Wartofsky L. Update 1994: the euthyroid sick syndrome. In: Braverman LE, Refetoff S, eds. *Endocrine reviews monographs. 3. Clinical and molecular aspects of diseases of the thyroid.* Bethesda, MD: The Endocrine Society, 1994;248–251.
22. Chopra IJ, Hershman JM, Pardridge WM, Nicoloff JT. Thyroid function in nonthyroidal illnesses. *Ann Intern Med* 1983;98:946–957.
23. Wartofsky L, Martin D, Earll JM. Alterations in thyroid iodine release and the peripheral metabolism of thyroxine during acute falciparum malaria infection in man. *J Clin Invest* 1972;51:2215–2232.
24. Engler D, Burger AG. The deiodination of the iodothyronines and of their derivatives in man. *Endocr Rev* 1984;5:151–184.
25. Kohrle J, Hesch RD, Leonard JL. Intracellular pathways of iodothyronine metabolism. In: Ingbar SH, Braverman LE, eds. *The thyroid,* 6th ed. Philadelphia: JB Lippincott, 1991;144–189.
26. Chopra IJ. Nature, sources, and relative biologic significance of thyroid circulating hormones. In: Ingbar SH, Braverman LE, eds. *The thyroid,* 6th ed. Philadelphia: JB Lippincott, 1986;126–143.
27. Nareem N, Miner DJ, Amatruda JM. Methimazole: an alternative route of administration. *J Clin Endocrinol Metab* 1982;54:180–181.
28. Walter RM, Bartle WR. Rectal administration of propylthiouracil in the treatment of Graves' disease. *Am J Med* 1990;88:69–70.
29. Wartofsky L, Ransil BJ, Ingbar SH. Inhibition by iodine of the release of thyroxine from the thyroid glands of patients with thyrotoxicosis. *J Clin Invest* 1970;49:78–86.
30. Wu S-Y, Chopra IJ, Solomon DH, Johnson DE. The effect of repeated administration of ipodate (Oragrafin) in hyperthyroidism. *J Clin Endocrinol Metab* 1978;47:1358–1361.
31. Lazarus JH, Addison GM, Richards AR, Owen GM. Treatment of thyrotoxicosis with lithium carbonate. *Lancet* 1974;2:1160–1163.
32. Reed J, Bradley EL. Postoperative thyroid storm after lithium preparation. *Surgery* 1985;98:983–986.
33. Hoffenberg R, Louw JH, Voss TJ. Thyroidectomy under hypothermia in a patient with thyroid crisis. *Lancet* 1961;2:687–689.
34. Szilagyi DE, McGraw AB, Smyth NPD. The effects of adrenocortical stimulation on thyroid function: clinical observations in thyrotoxic crisis and hyperthyroidism. *Ann Surg* 1952;136:555–577.
35. Peterson RE. The influence of the thyroid on adrenal cortical function. *J Clin Invest* 1958;37:736–743.

36. Felber JP, Reddy WJ, Selenkow HA, Thorn GW. Adrenocortical response on the 48-hour ACTH infusion test in myxedema and hyperthyroidism. *J Clin Endocrinol Metab* 1959;19:895–906.
37. Dillon PT, Babe J, Meloni CR, Canary JJ. Reserpine in thyrotoxic crisis. *N Engl J Med* 1970;283:1020–1023.
38. Feely J, Forrest A, Gunn A, Hamilton W, Stevenson I, Crooks J. Propranolol dosage in thyrotoxicosis. *J Clin Endocrinol Metab* 1980;51:658–661.
39. Das G, Krieger M. Treatment of thyrotoxic storm with intravenous administration of propranolol. *Ann Intern Med* 1969;70:985–988.
40. Feek CM, Sawers JSA, Irvine WJ, Beckett GJ, Ratcliffe WA, Toft AD. Combination of potassium iodide and propranolol in preparation of patients with Graves' disease for thyroid surgery. *N Engl J Med* 1980;302:883–885.
41. Thorne AC, Bedford RF. Esmolol for perioperative management of thyrotoxic goiter. *Anesthesiology* 1989;71:291–294.
42. Isley WL, Dahl S, Gibbs H. Use of esmolol in managing a thyrotoxic patient needing emergency surgery. *Am J Med* 1990;89:122–123.
43. Brunette DD, Rothong C. Emergency department management of thyrotoxic crisis with esmolol. *Am J Emerg Med* 1991;9:232–234.
44. Zonszein J, Santangelo RP, Mackin JF, Lee TC, Coffey RJ, Canary JJ. Propranolol therapy in thyrotoxicosis. A review of 84 patients undergoing surgery. *Am J Med* 1979;66:411–416.
45. Lee KS, Kim K, Hur KB, Kim CK. The role of propranolol in the preoperative preparation of patients with Graves' disease. *Surg Gynecol Obstet* 1986;162:365–369.
46. Wartofsky L, Dimond RC, Noel GL, Frantz AG, Earll JM. Failure of propranolol to alter thyroid iodine release, thyroxine turnover, or the TSH and PRL responses to TRH in patients with thyrotoxicosis. *J Clin Endocrinol Metab* 1975;41:427–432.
47. Eriksson M, Rubenfeld S, Garber AK, Kohler PO. Propranolol does not prevent thyroid storm. *N Engl J Med* 1977;296:263–264.
48. Jamison MH, Done HJ. Post-operative thyrotoxic crisis in a patient prepared for thyroidectomy with propranolol. *Br J Clin Pract* 1979;33:82–83.
49. Jones DK, Solomon S. Thyrotoxic crisis masked by treatment with beta-blockers. *Br Med J [Clin Res]* 1981;283:659–660.
50. Strube PJ. Thyroid storm during beta blockade. *Anaesthesia* 1984;39:343–346.
51. Ashkar FS, Katims RB, Smoak WM, Gilson AJ. Thyroid storm treatment with blood exchange and plasmapheresis. *JAMA* 1970;214:1275–1279.
52. Herrman J, Hilger P, Rusche HJ, Kruskemper HL. Plasmapheresis in the treatment of thyrotoxic crisis. *Dtsch Med Woschenschr* 1974;99:888–892.
53. Herrman J, Kruskemper HL, Grosser KD. Peritoneal-dialyse in der behandlung der thyreotoxischen krise. *Dtsch Med Woschenschr* 1971;96:742–745.
54. Tajiri J, Katsuya H, Kiyokaya T, et al. Successful treatment of thyrotoxic crisis with plasma exchange. *Crit Care Med* 1984;12:536–537.
55. Burman KD, Yeager HC, Briggs WA, et al. Resin hemoperfusion: a method of removing circulating thyroid hormones. *J Clin Endocrinol Metab* 1976;42:70–78.
56. Candrina R, DiStefano O, Spandrio S, et al. Treatment of thyrotoxic storm by charcoal plasmaperfusion. *J Endocrinol Invest* 1989;12:133–134.
57. Solomon BL, Wartofsky L, Burman KD. Adjunctive cholestyramine therapy for thyrotoxicosis. *Clin Endocrinol (Oxf)* 1993;38:39–43.
58. Burch HB, Wartofsky L. Hyperthyroidism. In: Bardin CW, ed. *Current therapy in endocrinology and metabolism*, 5th ed. Philadelphia: BC Decker, 1994;64–70.

Subject Index

A

ABCC study. *See* Atomic Bomb Casualty Commission study
Abscess, thyroid, 468, 469*f*
Acetylcholinesterase (ACHE), 350
Acropachy, thyroid, 242*f* 243
ACTH (adrenocorticotropic hormone), 245, 481
ADCC assay, of autoantibodies in TAO, 348, 349–350
Addison's disease, antithyroperoxidase in, 47
Adenocarcinoma. *See* Papillary or follicular carcinoma
Adenoma
  C-cell, 84
  cellular, diagnosis by fine-needle biopsy, 109
  diagnosis, by fine-needle biopsy, 109
  follicular. *See* Follicular adenoma
  GsP mutations in, 235, 236*f*
  hyalinizing trabecular, 88
  malignant. *See* Adenocarcinoma
  microfollicular, 109
  nodular, hyperthyroidism of, 76
  papillary, 75
  pituitary, 250
  radioisotope imaging of, 122, 124*f*
  thyroid cancer and, 70–71
  toxic
    clinical features of, 250
    radionuclide scintigraphy of, 413
    with toxic multinodular goiter. *See* Plummer's disease
Adenosine 3',5'-cyclic monophosphate (cAMP), PTH-induced production, 55
Adenyl cyclase, 194, 547
ADHD (attention deficit hyperactivity disorder), 229
Adhesion molecules, 352
Adrenal gland
  hormones, thyroid hormones and, 667
  in hypothyroidism, 386
  insufficiency, hypercalcemia and, 58
Adrenergic antagonists. *See* Alpha-adrenergic blockers; Beta-adrenergic blockers
Adrenocorticotropic hormone (ACTH), 245, 481
Aerodigestive tract invasion, upper
  endoscopy, 659
  imaging, 659, 661
  symptoms, 659, 662*f*
Age
  incidence
    of recurrent hyperthyroidism and, 331
    of solitary nodules and, 412, 565

of substernal goiters and, 449
of thyroid cancer and, 509
prognosis
  of medullary carcinoma and, 84
  of papillary carcinoma and, 571
  of thyroid cancer and, 506, 507
treatment
  of hyperthyroidism and, 276–277
  of thyroid cancer and, 497, 510
  thyroxine replacement and, 480
Airway, involvement in thyroid disorders
  asymptomatic, 457
  compression
    with displacement, 457, 458*f*
    from substernal goiter, 450
    without displacement, 458, 460*f*, 461*f*
  by direct process, 457–458, 458*f*–461*f*
  displacement
    with compression, 457, 458*f*
    with infiltration and/or compression, 458, 459*f*, 460*f*
    without compression, 457–458, 459*f*
  dysfunction, management of, 459, 461
  incidence of, 457
  by indirect process, 459
  invasion, by thyroid cancer, 657
  investigations for, 461–462
  obstruction
    from ectopic thyroid, 473
    postoperative, 713
  reconstruction, 465–466
  surgical management of, 462–463, 465–466, 462*f*–466*f*
  symptomatic, 457
  without displacement, 458
AJCC cancer staging system, 499, 500*f*, 505
Akron experiment, 4
Albright's hereditary osteodystrophy syndrome, 381
Albumin
  binding ability of, 33
  postoperative serum levels, 724
  structure, 33–34
Aldomet (alpha-methyldopa), 670
Alfentanil, 672–673
Alkaline phosphatase, in hungry-bone syndrome, 722, 723
Alpha-adrenergic blockers, for hyperthyroidism
  with beta-adrenergic blockers, 670–671
  in thyroid-associated ophthalmopathy, 369
Alpha-interferon, thyroid function effects, 49–50
Alpha-methyldopa (Aldomet), 670

Aluminum-hydroxide-containing antacids, thyroid function effects, 50
AMA (antimicrosomal antibodies). *See* Antithyroperoxidase
Amenorrhea, in hypothyroidism, 386
American Joint Committee on Cancer staging system, 499, 500*f*, 505
Aminoglutethimide, thyroid function effects, 50
L-Aminotransferase, 35*f*
Amiodarone
  hyperthyroidism-induced by, 9, 69, 249
    medical therapy for, 282–283, 283*f*, 284
    surgical treatment of, 324
  hypothyroidism-induced by, 69, 382
  structure, 282*f*
  thyroid function effects, 43*t*, 49, 50
AMP, 667
Amphetamines, thyroid function effects, 43*t*, 49
Amyloidosis, 69–70, 382
Anaplastic carcinoma
  age of presentation, 503
  biology, cellular, 231, 646–647
  epidemiology, 645
  etiology, 504
  histopathology, 503–504
    giant cell, 542, 647
    small cell, 85, 542
    spindle cell, 542, 647
    squamous, 647
  incidence, 504
  local behavior, 647
  metastases, 174*f*, 515, 647
  precursor lesions, 503
  prognosis, 85–86, 647
  radionuclide imaging, 121, 167*f*
  symptoms, 645–646, 646*t*, 647
  thyroglobulin levels and, 415
  transformation, 503–504
  treatment, 650
    chemotherapy, 647–650
    multimodality, 648–649
ANAs (antinuclear antibodies), 349
Androgen receptors, 550
Androgens
  interaction with thyroxine, 482
  thyroid cancer and, 549
  thyroid function effects, 43*t*, 50
Anemia
  in hyperthyroidism, 243
  in hypothyroidism, 385
Anesthesia
  airway involvement from thyroiditis and, 462–463

hepatotoxicity, hyperthyroidism and, 672
historical aspects, 2
hypothyroidism and, 675–676
induction, 672
minimal alveolar concentration, 668
monitoring, 673
for nodule removal, 420
serum thyroxine levels and, 668
Aneuploidy
  in anaplastic carcinoma, 646
  in medullary carcinoma, 84
ANF (atrial natriuretic factor), 245
Angiography, 143, 148f–149f
Animal models of thyroid cancer
  growth-controlling mechanism in, 552–555
  thymic dysplastic mouse, 554–555
  transplantation studies, 554
  tumor induction methods, 553
Ansa cervicalis anastomosis, for recurrent laryngeal nerve paralysis, 712
Antibody-dependent cell-mediated cytotoxicity assay, of autoantibodies in TAO, 348, 349–350
Antigens, target, in thyroid-associated ophthalmopathy, 351, 352
Antimicrosomal antibodies (AMA). See Antithyroperoxidase
Antinuclear antibodies (ANAs), 349
Antipituicyte antibodies, 383
Antipyrine, 668
Anti-thyroglobulin autoantibodies (ATA), 47, 396, 587
Antithyroid antibodies, with goiter, 435
Antithyroid drugs. See Thionamides
Antithyroperoxidase (anti-TPO; antimicrosomal antibodies)
  in autoimmune thyroid diseases, 380
  elevated titers, 47
  in painless thyroiditis, 396
  in postpartum thyroiditis, 279
Anti-TSH receptor autoantibodies, TSH receptor binding sites for, 214–215
Arytenoid dislocation, postoperative, 713
Askanazy cells, 404, 502
L-Asparaginase, thyroid function effects, 43t
Aspartate transaminase, 385
ATA (antithyroglobulin antibodies), 47, 396, 587
Atenolol, for hyperthyroidism, 670
Atomic Bomb Casualty Commission study (ABCC study)
  death rates, 533
  follow-up data, 524t
  nuclear fallout and, 532
  occult thyroid cancer incidence in, 522–523
  testing methods, 522
ATP, 547
Atrial fibrillation
  in elderly, 282
  medical therapy, 281
Atrial natriuretic factor (ANF), 245
Attention deficit hyperactivity disorder (ADHD), 229
Autoantibodies
  in Hashimoto's thyroiditis, 414–415
  in postpartum hypothyroidism, 380
  replacement therapy and, 482
  in solitary nodules, 414–415
  in subacute thyroiditis, 402
  in thyroid-associated ophthalmopathy, 348–350, 348f
Autoimmune disorders. See also specific autoimmune disorders
  in Hashimoto's thyroiditis, 404
  in painless thyroiditis, 398
  TSH receptor and, 216–217
Autoimmune thyroiditis
  achlorhydria and, 385
  antithyroperoxidase in, 47
  atrophic variant, 380
  etiology, 67
  goitrous variant. See Hashimoto's thyroiditis
  ophthalmopathy and, 341, 350–351
  pathogenesis, 380
  pathology, 67–68, 68f
  pernicious anemia and, 47, 385
  during pregnancy, 279
  prevalence, 379–380
  subclinical hypothyroidism and, 387
Autologous lipoinjection, for unilateral vocal fold paralysis, 711
Autotransplantation
  for ectopic thyroid, 473
  of thyroid tissue, 735–736

B

Bacteria, in acute suppurative thyroiditis, 393
Basal metabolic rate (BMR), in thyroid storm, 740
B-cell lymphoma, Hashimoto's thyroiditis and, 404
BEI test (butanol extractable iodine test), 41
Bequerel, 301
Berry's ligament
  anatomy, 22f
  recurrent laryngeal nerve and, 25, 26f, 707
Beta-adrenergic blockers. See also Propranolol
  actions, 261–262
  classification, 328
  contraindications, 262
  for hyperthyroidism, 670
    with alpha-adrenergic blockers, 670–671
    dosing, 262
    in elderly, 277
    of Graves' disease, 243, 328–329
    with iodine and thionamides, 326–327, 327f
    inhibition of parathyroid hormone secretion, 55
    in preoperative regimens, 326–329, 327f
    side effects, 328–329
    thyroid hormone metabolism and, 261
Beta-agonists, parathyroid hormone secretion and, 55
Beta antagonists. See Beta-adrenergic blockers
Betamethasone, 329
Beta particles, 300, 301
Bile acid sequestrants, 267, 478
Bisphosphonates, for hypercalcemia, 58, 58t
Black thyroid, 70
Blood-group antigens, 543
BMR (basal metabolic rate), in thyroid storm, 740
Bone metabolism, in hyperthyroidism, 242f 243, 242t
Bone metastases, 180f, 521
Bone resorption, calcitonin and, 56
Botulinum-A toxin, in thyroid-associated ophthalmopathy, 369
Bovine thyrotoxicosis (hamburger-induced thyrotoxicosis), 285, 400, 400t
Brachial arch apparatus, embryologic development, 15
Branchial cysts, 468
Breast cancer, thyroid cancer and, 537–538, 567
Breast milk, thyroxine excretion in, 479
Brevibloc (esmolol), for hyperthyroidism, 670
Bromocriptine, for TSH-dependent hyperthyroidism, 276
Bronchocele, 1, 2
Butanol extractable iodine test (BEI test), 41

C

Calcification
  in papillary carcinoma, 105, 105f
  patterns, on radiographs, 137
  psammomatous. See Psammoma bodies
  in substernal goiters, 451
  ultrasonography, 138
Calcitonin
  bone resorption and, 56
  calcium reabsorption and, 723
  characterization, 619
  deficiency, 56
  dietary sources, 731
  discovery, 731
  extrathyroidal expression, 619
  functions, 56, 620
  osteoporosis development and, 56
  pharmacology, 731–732
  physiology, 731
  production, 56, 620, 622f
  resistance, 722
  serum levels
    elevated, 48, 632
    in medullary carcinoma, 84, 504–505, 632
    with nodule, 415
    persistently elevated, management of, 635–636
    postoperative reduction of, 731–733
    in temporary hypocalcemia, 721
  therapy
    for hypercalcemia, 58t
    indications for, 56
Calcitonin gene-related peptide, 619, 620
Calcitriol (1,25-dihydroxyvitamin D3)
  in calcium homeostasis, 53, 54, 55
  in hyperthyroidism, 242
  for hypocalcemia, 60
  serum levels
    elevated, 55, 56
    low, 56
Calcium. See also Hypercalcemia; Hypocalcemia
  absorption, 53, 54f
  dietary intake, 53, 54f
  distribution, 53, 54f
  excretion, 53, 54f
  homeostasis, 53
    calcitriol in, 53, 54, 55
    hormonal regulation of, 54–55, 54f
    magnesium and, 54

parathyroid hormone and, 54–55, 54f, 55
phosphate and, 53
vitamin D and, 54–55, 54f, 55–56
in hyperthyroidism, 242–243, 242t
interaction with magnesium, 726
ionized or free, 724
for postoperative hypocalcemia, 729, 731, 730f
postoperative serum levels, 428
preoperative assessment, 418
reabsorption, 53, 723
supplementation, 60, 61t, 729, 731, 730f
total, 724, 724t
Calcium carbonate, for hypocalcemia, 60, 61t
Calcium channel blockers, for hyperthyroidism, 670
Calcium chloride, for hypocalcemia, 60
Calcium gluconate, for hypocalcemia, 60, 61t
Calcium oxalate, in thyroid gland, 66, 66f
Calcium/pentagastrin test, 632
cAMP response element-binding protein (CREB), 194
cAMP response element (CRE), 213
cAMP response element modulator (CREM), 213
Carbamexine, thyroid function effects, 50
Carbimazole
  hypothyroidism induced by, 381
  structure, 255f
Carcinoembryonic antigen (CEA)
  in medullary carcinoma, 84, 505, 510
  tumor virulence and, 542
Carcinosarcoma, 86
Cardiac failure, symptoms, 674t
Cardiac output
  in hypothyroidism, 384
  in thyrotoxicosis, 281
Cardiomyopathy, with thyrotoxicosis, 244
Cardiovascular system, clinical manifestations
  in hyperthyroidism, 242t, 243–245, 280–282
  in hypothyroidism, 384
Carotid artery, 20, 24
Carotid sheaths, 18
CASTLE tumor, 88
Catecholamines
  in hyperthyroidism, 244
  parathyroid hormone secretion and, 55
C cells. See Parafollicular cells
CEA. See Carcinoembryonic antigen
Cell life cycle, 231, 232f
Cellular biology, central paradigm of, 183–184, 184f
Cellular immunity, TSH receptor and, 217
Central compartment node dissection, for medullary carcinoma, 634, 634f
Central nervous system, dysfunction, in hypothyroidism, 384
Cerebellar ataxia, 384
Cervical ranulas, 468
Cervical spine examination, preoperative, 418
Chemical hyperthyroidism, 9
Chemotherapy
  for distant metastases, 521, 613, 640
  with radiotherapy, for thyroid lymphoma, 652–653
  for thyroid cancer, 647–648
    combination, 649–650

medullary type, 640
single agent, 649
Chernobyl nuclear accident, 532, 533–534
Chest x-ray
  of pulmonary metastases, 520
  of substernal goiter, 451, 451f
Cholecystographic agents, oral
  action, 265–266
  pharmacokinetics, 265–266, 265f
  side effects, 266
  structure, 264, 265f
Cholestipol, thyroid function effects, 43t, 50
Cholestyramine
  for hyperthyroidism
    dosage of, 254t
  thyroid function effects, 43t, 50
  thyroid hormone binding, 478
Chondrosarcoma, 86
Choriocarcinoma
  hyperthyroidism in, 250–251
  secretion of nonthyroid thyrotropin, 320
  treatment, 274–275
Chvostek's sign, 59, 428, 726
Chylothorax, in substernal goiter, 450
Chylous fistula, postoperative, 714
Cirrhosis, TBG elevation and, 33
CLA (common leukocyte antigen), 650
Clear cell tumors, 87
Clinical trials, prospective randomized, 501–502
Clofibrate
  thyroid-binding globulin elevation and, 33
  thyroid function effects, 43t, 50
Cohnheim, benign metastasizing goiter of, 523
Colestipol, for hyperthyroidism, 254t, 284
Collagen injection, for unilateral vocal fold paralysis, 711
Common carotid artery, 20, 24
Common leukocyte antigen (CLA), 650
Computed tomography (CT)
  after goiter removal, 445f
  of congenital lesions, 138, 147f
  indications, 138
  of invasive carcinoma, 661
  of nodule, 125, 413–414, 418, 418f
  orbital, in hyperthyroidism, 245
  in preoperative workup, 139, 148f–149f, 418, 418f
  principles of, 138
  of substernal goiter, 443f, 451–452, 452f
  of thyroglossal duct abnormalities, 469, 470f
  of thyroid masses, 138, 172f, 174f, 176f, 177f
  vs. magnetic resonance imaging, 141
Congenital abnormalities. See also Ectopic thyroid
  anatomic, 467
  biosynthetic defects, 381
  computed tomography of, 138
  endocrine, 467
  hypothyroidism. See Cretinism
  radioisotope imaging of, 130, 130f, 131f, 142
  thyroglossal duct, 467
    imaging of, 468–469
    thyroid function tests in, 469
    treatment of, 469–471, 471f
  thyroid cysts, 473
  in thyroid hormone synthesis, 7

Congestive heart failure, medical therapy, 281
Connective tissue disorder, thyroid-associated ophthalmopathy as, 351–352
Contrast materials
  iodinated dyes, in clinical medicine, 283–284, 283t
  radioactive iodine uptake test and, 117
  for thyroid storm imaging, 742
Cornea involvement, in thyroid-associated ophthalmopathy, 363
Corticosteroids
  action, 264, 264f
  for hyperthyroidism, 264, 264f, 670
  side effects, 264
  suppression of TSH secretion, 667
  for thyroid-associated ophthalmopathy, 369–370, 371–372
  for thyroiditis, 276
Cortisol
  clearance, 481
  secretion, low, 480–481
Cowden's disease, thyroid cancer and, 567
Creatine kinase, in hypothyroidism, 383–384
Creatine phosphokinase, 669
CREB (cAMP response element-binding protein), 194
CRE (cAMP response element), 213
CREM (cAMP response element modulator), 213
Cretinism (congenital hypothyroidism)
  etiology, 381, 382
  goitrous, 432, 484
  historical aspects, 379
  incidence, 388
  iodine deficiency and, 382
  thyroid hormone replacement therapy for, 484
Cricothyroid muscles, 24–25
Cricothyrotomy, 461
CT. See Computed tomography
Curie (Ci), 301
Cyclic AMP (cAMP), 194, 547
Cyclosporine, for thyroid-associated ophthalmopathy, 369–370
Cysteine, 198f
Cystinosis, 382
Cysts
  branchial, 468
  dermoid, 468
  parathyroid, 468
  thyroglossal duct, 467
    carcinoma in, 471
    differential diagnosis of, 467–468, 468f, 469f
    epithelial lining of, 467
    location of, 467
    radioisotope imaging of, 130
    recurrence of, 471
    surgical management of, 469–471, 471f
  thyroid. See Thyroid cysts
  vallecular, 472
Cytochrome P-450, 668
Cytokines, in autoimmune orbital inflammation, 346, 347
Cytology, thyroid, 9, 90–91, 108–109
Cytomel (liothyronine), 388, 476t

D

Danazole, thyroid function effects, 43t
Dantrolene, for hyperthyroidism, 674
Death
    from differentiated thyroid cancer, 512–513
    from radiation-induced thyroid cancer, 533–534
Deep fascia, of neck, 17f, 18
Deiodinases
    expression, 196
    functions, 196–197
    incorporation of selenocysteine, 197, 198f
    regulation, 196–197
    structural features, 197, 197f
    thyroid hormone release and, 31
    type I, 36, 36t
    type II, 36, 36t
    type III, 36, 36t
Delphian lymph nodes, 20
De Quervain's thyroiditis, 320, 382
Dermoid cysts, 468
Dexamethasone
    for Graves' disease, in pregnancy, 279
    for hyperthyroidism, 254t, 670
DHT (dihydrotachysterol), 60
Diabetes insipidus, hypothyroidism and, 383
Diabetes mellitus, type I, 47
Diagnostic imaging. *See also specific imaging modalities*
    conventional, 136
    qualitative, 135
    quantitative, 135
Dibenzyline (phenoxybenzamine), 670
Diet, thyroid cancer and, 530–531
Differentiated thyroid carcinoma (DTC). *See also* Follicular carcinoma; Papillary thyroid carcinoma
    death from, 512–513
    DNA ploidy and, 545–546
    end-stage. *See* Anaplastic carcinoma
    etiology
        immunogenetic studies of, 538–539
        immunologic studies of, 538–539
        oncogenes and, 539
    histopathology, 502–503
    metastases
        cervical, 556
        distant, significance of, 518–519
        positive regional lymph nodes and, 517–518
        pulmonary, 519–521, 520t
    natural history, 512, 604
    prognosis, 513–514, 603–604, 604t, 605f
    treatment
        age and, 510
        controversies in, 496
        external radiotherapy for, 603
        radioiodine for, 601
    TSH receptors in, 602–603
    tumor burden and, 508–509
Diffuse thyroid disorders, radionuclide imaging of, 142
Digital subtraction angiography (DSA), 143, 148f–149f, 172f
Dihydrotachysterol (DHT), 60
1,25-Dihydroxyvitamin D3. *See* Calcitriol
Diiodotyrosines (DITs), 3, 30, 31f
Diltiazem, for hyperthyroidism, 254t
DIMIT, for TSH-dependent hyperthyroidism, 276
Dinitrophenol, 381
Disintegration, radioactive, 314
DITs (diiodotyrosines), 3, 30, 31f
Diuretics, for hypercalcemia, 58, 58t
DNA, nuclear content, papillary carcinoma prognosis and, 575
DNA flow cytometry, for cellular ploidy assessment, 545
DNA index, in anaplastic carcinoma, 646
DNA ploidy
    in anaplastic carcinoma, 646
    as tumor marker, 544–546
DNA repair proteins, 237
L-Dopa, thyroid function effects, 43t
Dopamine, thyroid function effects, 43t, 49
Dopamine receptor agonists, for hyperthyroidism, 267, 276
Doxorubicin, for thyroid carcinoma, 649
Drugs. *See also specific drugs*
    hypothalamic-pituitary-thyroid axis effects, 49
    thyroid function effects, 43, 49f50
DSA (digital subtraction angiography), 143, 148f–149f, 172f
DTC. *See* Differentiated thyroid carcinoma (DTC)
Dysalbuminemia, familial, 9
Dysembryogenesis. *See* Ectopic thyroid
Dyshormogenesis, radioisotope imaging of, 130, 131f
Dysphagia, from substernal goiter, 450
Dyspnea
    of hyperthyroidism, 243
    from substernal goiter, 450

E

Eastern Cooperative Oncology Group (ECOG), chemotherapy trial, 649
EAT (experimental autoimmune thyroiditis), 217
ECOG (Eastern Cooperative Oncology Group), chemotherapy trial, 649
Ectopic thyroid
    dysgenetic, 469
    embryology, 472
    hypothyroidism and, 472
    lingual
        etiology, 65
        histology, 89
        incidence of, 20, 89
        location of, 16, 89
        radionuclide imaging of, 130, 130f, 145f, 146f
    location, 65
    pathophysiology, 472
    radioisotope imaging of, 130, 130f
    sublingual, 473
    symptoms, 472–473
    thyroglossal, 473
    treatment, 473
EGF (epidermal growth factor), 541, 548
ELAM-1 (endothelial leukocyte adhesion molecule-1), 345
Elderly
    hyperthyroidism in
        medical therapy for, 277
        subclinical, 282
        thyrotoxicosis, 669
    hypothyroidism in, 379
Electrolytes, in hypothyroidism, 386–387
ELISA (enzyme-linked immunosorbent assay), of thyroglobulin, 587
Eltroxin. *See* Levothyroxine
Embryology
    of ectopic thyroid, 472
    of neck, 15–16, 16f
Embryonal carcinoma, 250–251
Endemic goiter
    in animal models, 553
    geographic locations of, 432
    goitrogens and, 432
    iodine deficiency and, 432
    iodine excess and, 432
    malnutrition and, 432
    prevention of, 432f433
    thyroglobulin serum levels in, 591
    thyroid cancer and, 529–530, 551–552, 567
Endocrine system
    in hyperthyroidism, 245
    in hypothyroidism, 385–387
Endoscopy
    postoperative, 427
    surgical techniques, 420
        for bilateral vocal cord paralysis, 712
        for unilateral recurrent laryngeal nerve paralysis, 710–711
    of upper aerodigestive tract invasion, 659
Endothelial leukocyte adhesion molecule-1 (ELAM-1),, 345
Endothelin 1, release, temporary hypocalcemia and, 719–720
Endotracheal tube
    endoscopy, postoperative, 427
    extubation, postoperative, 426
Enzyme-linked immunosorbent assay (ELISA), of thyroglobulin, 587
EORTC. *See* European Organization for Research on Thyroid Cancer
Epidermal growth factor (EGF), 541, 548
Epidermal growth factor-receptors, in thyroid cancer, 548
Epinephrine, in pheochromocytoma, 625, 625f
Epstein-Barr virus, lymphoma and, 651
c-*erb* A gene, 541
Ergocalciferol, for hypocalcemia, 60, 61t
Esmolol (Brevibloc), for hyperthyroidism, 670
Esophagram, of substernal goiter, 452
Esophagus
    anatomy, 27
    blood supply, 27
    innervation, 27
    invasion by thyroid cancer, surgical procedures for, 664
    pressure, from substernal goiter, 450
Estrogen receptors, 550
Estrogens
    interaction with thyroxine, 482
    thyroid cancer and, 549–551, 567
    thyroid function effects, 43t, 50
Ethanol intralesional injections, for Plummer's disease, 274

Ether anesthesia, 668
Ethnicity, thyroid cancer incidence and, 526–527
Etidronate, for hypercalcemia, 58, 58t
European Organization for Research on Thyroid Cancer (EORTC)
    prognostic index for thyroid cancer, 500, 508t, 573
    thyroid cancer prognosis study, 507–508, 509
Euthyroid patient
    with asymptomatic nodule, management of, 416–417, 417f
    with autonomous nodule, 416
    elevated serum total T4 in, 41
    goiter in, thyroid hormone replacement therapy for, 436
    thyroglobulin and, 380
    thyroid enlargement in. See Goiter, sporadic
    thyroid peroxidase and, 380
Euthyroid sick syndrome, thyroid replacement therapy, 485
Exophthalmos, 6, 362, 364f. See also Opthalmopathy, thyroid-associated
Experimental autoimmune thyroiditis (EAT), 217
External carotid artery, 20, 24
Extraocular muscles
    anatomy of, 343–344
    in thyroid-associated ophthalmopathy, 352, 363, 365f, 366f
        histologic changes of, 344
    inflammation of, 342–343, 342f, 343f
Eye, in hyperthyroidism, 245
Eyelid
    changes, in thyroid-associated ophthalmopathy, 343
    surgical treatment, for thyroid-associated ophthalmopathy, 372–373
    in thyroid-associated ophthalmopathy, 361–362, 362f
Eye muscle antigens, autoantibodies against, 348–349, 348f

F

Factitious hyperthyroidism, 255t, 320–321
False thyroid capsule, 19
Familial adenomatous polyposis of colon, papillary thyroid carcinoma and, 538
Familial dysalbuminemic hyperthyroxinemia (FDH), 10, 41
Familial hypocalciuric hypercalcemia (FHH), 57
Familial medullary thyroid carcinoma
    clinical course, 638–640, 639f
    diagnosis, 238, 621–623, 621f–623f
    forms of, 82
    genetic abnormalities, 628–629, 629f, 630t
Familial multiple endocrine neoplasia. See Multiple endocrine neoplasia
Fascia, of neck, 17f, 18
Fascial compartments, in neck, 17f18, 17f
FDG ([18F]-2-deoxy-2-fluoro-D-glucose), 143
FDH. See Familial dysalbuminemic hyperthyroxinemia (FDH)
Fenclofenac, thyroid function effects, 43t
Fentanil, 672
Ferrous sulfate, thyroid function effects, 50
Fetus, maternal Graves' disease and, 277–278

FHH (familial hypocalciuric hypercalcemia), 57
Fibroblasts
    orbital
        autoantibodies against, 349
        radiosensitivity, 370
        retroorbital, autoimmune inflammation and, 346
        in thyroid-associated ophthalmopathy, 351, 361
Fibrosarcoma, 86
Fine-needle aspiration (FNA)
    with biopsy. See Fine-needle biopsy (FNB)
    of nodule, 127
    preoperative, 702
    ultrasound-assisted, 413
Fine-needle biopsy (FNB)
    advantages, 106
    complications, 108–109
    cytology, 9, 90–91, 108–109
    diagnosis
        of benign thyroid disease, 110
        of follicular carcinoma, 571
        of medullary carcinoma, 623, 624f
        of multinodular goiter, 437
        of nodule, 414, 417f
        of papillary carcinoma, 571
        of thyroid cancer, 110
    findings
        negative, 571
        in operative planning, 110–111
        in thyroid nodule management, 105–106, 109
    repeat, 110
    sampling adequacy, 108–109
Fluids, in hypothyroidism, 386–387
5-Fluorouracil, TBG elevation and, 33
FNA. See Fine-needle aspiration
FNB. See Fine-needle biopsy
Follicle-stimulating hormone (FSH), 245
Follicular adenoma
    atypical, 78
    with cystic changes and hemorrhage, 161f
    diagnosis
        computed tomography scan for, 158f
        fine-needle biopsy for, 109
        radiography for, 158f
        radionuclide imaging for, 155f–156f, 159f
        ultrasonography for, 159f–161f
        ultrasound-guided fine-needle aspiration for, 156f–157f
    histology, 77–78, 77f
    with parathyroid adenoma, 161f
    vs. follicular carcinoma, 503
Follicular carcinoma. See also Hürthle cell carcinoma
    age at diagnosis, 574
    benign vs. malignant, 503
    cellular biology, 231
    diagnosis, 571
    epidemiology, 565–567
    histopathology, 502–503, 581
    incidence, 78
    medical treatment, 583–584
    metastases, 78, 488, 570, 582
        capsular involvement, 78–80, 79f, 80f, 503
        distant, 518–519
        extracapsular, 503

        extrathyroidal extension of, 578–579
        lymph node, 515, 579–580
        minimally invasive vs. capsular invasive, 78–80, 79f, 80f
    mortality, 572, 581–582, 604
    natural history, 604
    pathology, 78–80, 79f
    prognosis, 78, 603–604, 604t, 605f
        AGES scoring system, 575
        AMES scoring system, 572–575
        DAMES scoring system, 575
        influencing factors for, 571–577
        MACIS scoring system, 575, 604
    radiation-induced, sex hormones and, 551
    recurrence, 572
    risk factors, 572–573, 576
    surgical treatment, 577–581
        extent of surgery and, 577
        postoperative radiotherapy and, 580–581
        results of, 583–584
        thyroidectomy for, 78
    survival, 581, 604
    symptoms, 570–571
    TSH receptors, 602–603
    vs. follicular adenomas, 503
Follicular cell secretion, 3
Follicular goiter, 76–77, 76f
Food
    goitrogenic, 382, 529–530
    thyroid hormone absorption and, 478
Food-induced thyrotoxicosis, 400, 400t
Free thyroxine (FT4)
    estimation methods, 42
    in hyperthyroxinemia without hyperthyroidism, 42
    measurement methods, 42
Free thyroxine index (FT4I)
    calculation, 42
    in hyperthyroxinemia without hyperthyroidism, 42
    in pregnancy, 279
    in thyrotoxicity, 481–482
Free triiodothyronine (FT3), 37
Free triiodothyronine index (FT3I), 42
Frozen section, 91, 110
FSH (follicle-stimulating hormone), 245
FT4. See Free T4
FT3 (free triiodothyronine), 37
FT4I. See Free thyroxine index
FT3I (free T3 index), 42
Fungi, in acute suppurative thyroiditis, 393–394

G

GAG (glycosaminoglycans), 344, 362
Gallamine, 672
Gallium, for hypercalcemia, 58t, 59
Gamma camera imaging, for radioactive iodine uptake test, 118, 118f
Gamma ray emission, from iodine-131, 300f, 301
Gardner's syndrome, thyroid cancer and, 538, 567
Gastrin, 56
Gastrointestinal system, clinical manifestations
    in hyperthyroidism, 242t, 243
    in hypothyroidism, 385
GBq (gigabequerel), 301

GDNF (glial cell line-derived neurotrophic factor), 640
Gender differences
　in papillary carcinoma prognosis, 576
　in substernal goiter incidence, 449
　in thyroid-associated ophthalmopathy, 342, 359
　in thyroid cancer incidence, 540
Gene expression regulation
　central paradigm, 183–184, 184f
　steroid/thyroid hormone nuclear receptor superfamily and, 186–187, 186f
　thyroid hormone receptor binding proteins and, 190
　thyroid hormone receptor response elements and, 188–190, 189f
Generalized resistance to thyroid hormone (GRTH)
　characteristics, clinical, 487
　diagnosis, 223, 224f
　ß receptor mutations in, 223–224
　treatment, 229, 487
　variability, molecular mechanisms of, 227–228
Genes
　basal transcriptional apparatus, 184–185, 185f
　damage from radioiodine therapy, 614–615
　house-keeping, 183
　promoter region, 184–185, 185f
　response elements, 185–186, 186f
　structural organization of, 184, 184f
　transcriptional activity, 183
　transcription factors, 185–186, 186f
Genetic factors
　in radiation-induced thyroid cancer, 534
　screening for, in medullary carcinoma, 636
Genetic studies, thyroid cancer, 538–539
Gestational trophoblastic neoplasms (GTNs), 274–275
Giant cell thyroiditis, 320
Glial cell line-derived neurotrophic factor (GDNF), 640
Glucocorticoids
　for hypercalcemia, 58, 58t
　for subacute thyroiditis, 402
　thyroid function effects, 43t, 49, 50
　for thyroid storm, 742–743
Glucose, metabolism, in hypothyroidism, 387
Glycosaminoglycans (GAG), 344, 362
GNRP (guanyl nucleotide regulatory protein), 547
Goiter
　airway displacement with compression, 457, 458f
　amyloid, 69
　assessment
　　of thyroid function, 435
　　of thyroid size, 435
　benign, 105, 523
　with calcific nodule, 155f
　classification, 431–432
　of Cohnheim, 523
　congenital, 278
　defined, 431
　diagnosis
　　by fine-needle biopsy, 110
　　radionuclide imaging for, 123, 124f, 148f–149f
　dyshormonogenetic, 552
　endemic. See Endemic goiter
　etiology, 274
　　diet and, 529–530
　　iodide deficiency and, 30
　exophthalmic. See Graves' disease
　familial syndromes, 432
　fear of cancer and, 437–438
　follicular, 76–77, 76f
　historical aspects, 1, 431
　hyperthyroidism in, 435
　incidence, geographic, 431
　medical treatment
　　clinical approach to, 434–435
　　in euthyroid patient, 436
　　iodine for, 4, 431
　　radioactive iodine therapy for, 436
　　suppressive therapy for, 44, 486–487
　psammoma bodies in, 438f
　sporadic, 433
　substernal. See Substernal goiter
　surgical treatment
　　changes in thyroid and, 436–437
　　indications for, 436–438, 437f–439f
　　patient selection for, 436
　　postoperative care for, 445–446, 445f
　　preoperative computed tomography for, 139, 148f–149f
　　surgical anatomy and, 438f 440, 440f, 441f
　　technique for, 440–443, 445, 440f–445f
　symptoms, 334
　　cosmetic, 437
　　dysfunctional, 437
　　mechanical, 437, 437f–439f
　thyroid cancer and, 123
　thyroid cancer risk, 7, 528, 529–530, 552
　　case-controlled studies of, 525
　　endemic, 529–530, 551–552, 567
　　in Hashimoto's thyroiditis, 528
　　multinodularity and, 433–435, 434f
　toxic, 68
　　clinical features of, 249–250
　　diffuse. See Graves' disease
　　extent of surgery for, 336–337
　　hyperthyroidism of, 76
　　multinodular with toxic adenoma. See Plummer's disease
　　pathogenesis of, 333–334
　　preoperative preparation, 335
　　radioactive iodine uptake in, 118
　　surgical treatment for, 321
　　treatment of, 255t, 335
Goitrogens
　cocarcinogenesis, 553
　discovery of, 553
　elimination of, 434
　endemic goiter and, 432
　exposure to, 434
　hypothyroidism and, 381
G protein-coupled receptor kinases (GPKs), 210
G-protein-mediated second messenger systems, 194–195
G proteins, TSH receptor signal transduction and, 215
Granulomatous thyroiditis
　subacute, 67, 275, 382
　　etiology of, 67
　　laboratory data for, 400t
　symptoms, 406
Graves' disease
　antinuclear antibodies in, 349
　antithyroperoxidase in, 47
　diagnosis, 414
　　characteristic features in, 247–248
　　of ophthalmopathy in, 360
　　during pregnancy, 48
　　by radioactive iodine uptake, 118, 127, 127f
　　TBII test for, 48
　　by thyroid stimulation test, 120
　differential diagnosis, 397, 398f, 406
　etiology, 7, 67
　genetic predisposition, 75
　hematologic disorders in, 243, 244f
　histology, 75
　hyperthyroidism in, 590
　hypocalcemia and, 59
　medical treatment, 255t
　　for adolescent, 276–277
　　agent selection for, 270–272, 271t
　　in children, 276–277
　　corticosteroids for, 264
　　dosing strategies for, 270–272, 272f
　　histologic changes from, 75
　　hypothyroidism from, 381
　　with lithium, 266
　　lymphoid infiltration in, 68
　　modality selection for, 268–270
　　monitoring of, 272–273
　　for neonate, 280
　　perchlorate for, 267
　　for postpartum patient, 280
　　posttherapeutic hypothyroidism and, 483
　　predisposition to ophthalmopathy and, 342
　　in pregnancy, 277–279, 278f
　　radioiodine for, 7, 297–298, 367–368, 381, 535
　　selection of, 268–270
　　strategy for, 273t
　　for TAO, 367–368
　　thionamides for, 255–256, 257, 269
　　thyroid-associated ophthalmopathy and, 360
　ophthalmopathy. See Ophthalmopathy, thyroid-associated
　pathogenesis, 47–48
　pathophysiology, 668
　postpartum, 279, 280
　during pregnancy, 48
　recurrence
　　after surgery, 322
　　ipodate-thionamide therapy and, 265–266
　　prevention, suppressive therapy for, 488
　remission, spontaneous, 248
　surgical treatment, 321
　　for amiodarone-induced thyrotoxicosis, 324
　　benefits of, 321–324
　　disadvantages of, 326
　　extent of, 329–333
　　modality selection for, 268–270

for noncompliant patient, 324
postoperative follow-up, 333
postoperative hypothyroidism and, 381
preoperative preparation for, 326–329, 327f
progression of TAO and, 324–326
success of, 322–323
thyroidectomy for, 381, 735
thyroid gland enlargement in, 245–246
thyroid stimulating immunoglobulins in, 234, 234f
for thyroid storm, 324
thyroid volume estimation for, 137
symptoms, 359
cardiovascular, 669
muscular weakness, 243
postpartum, 280
pretibial myxedema, 351–352
temporary parathyroid suppression, 721–722
thyroid cancer in
incidence of, 323
papillary, 70
prevalence of, 535
prognosis of, 323–324
risk for, 234, 234f, 528–529
Green retractor, 681, 682f
Growth signal transduction
model of, 232, 232f
in thyroid cells, 232–234, 233f
GRTH. See Generalized resistance to thyroid hormone
GsP (guanine nucleotide stimulatory protein), 232
GTNs (gestational trophoblastic neoplasms), 274–275
GTP (guanosine triphosphate), 232
Guanethidine, 7
Guanine nucleotide stimulatory protein (GsP), 232
Guanosine triphosphate (GTP), 232
Guanyl nucleotide regulatory protein (GNRP), 547
Gull's disease, 380
Gynecomastia, in hyperthyroidism, 245

H

Hair, clinical manifestations
in hyperthyroidism, 242, 242t
in hypothyroidism, 385
Halothane, 668
Hamburger-induced thyrotoxicosis (bovine thyrotoxicosis), 285, 400, 400t
Hashimoto's thyroiditis
amiodarone and, 49
antibodies, 380
antithyroid, 435
antithyroperoxidase, 47
autoantibodies, 414–415
autoimmune disease and, 404
diagnosis
cytologic, 404
elevated T4 levels in, 41
by fine-needle biopsy, 110
laboratory data in, 400t, 404
by radioactive iodine uptake, 118
by radionuclide scanning, 128, 129f, 142
etiology, 30, 67, 403
fibrosing variant, 67–68
histology, 380
Hürthle cells in, 404
hypocalcemia and, 59
incidence, 403
with lymphoma, 105–106, 106f, 404, 645, 651
nodules, 105, 414–415, 418
ophthalmopathy of. See Ophthalmopathy, thyroid-associated
pathogenesis, 7, 403
pathology, 67, 68f, 404, 406
Reidel's struma and, 405, 405t
symptoms, 403–404
thyroid cancer and, 528
thyroid replacement therapy, 483
thyrotoxicosis of, 320
Hashitoxicosis, 320
HBS (hungry bone syndrome), 59, 722–723
HDL, in hypothyroidism, 386
Heat shock proteins, in thyroid-associated ophthalmopathy, 345
Hemangioma, 88
Hematologic disorders, in hyperthyroidism, 242t, 243, 244f
Hematopoietic system
clinical manifestations, in hypothyroidism, 385
thyroid lesions, 87. See also specific hematopoietic lesions
Hemithyroidectomy. See Subtotal thyroidectomy
Hemochromatosis, 382
Hemoptysis, invasive carcinoma and, 659, 662f
Hemorrhage, postoperative, 419, 702, 713
Hemostasis, 2
Heparin, thyroid function effects, 43t
Hepatitis, TBG elevation and, 33
Hepatocellular carcinoma, TBG elevation and, 33
Hereditary hypothyroid myotonia, 383
Heroin
TBG elevation and, 33
thyroid function effects, 43t
High-density lipoprotein, in hypothyroidism 386
HIV, TBG concentration and, 33
HLAs. See Human leukocyte antigens (HLAs)
HL-60 cells, vitamin D stimulation of, 56
Hoffman syndrome, 383
Horner's syndrome
postoperative, 713–714
in substernal goiter, 450
Human chorionic gonadotropin, overproduction, 251
Human immunodeficiency virus, TBG concentration and, 33
Human leukocyte antigens (HLAs)
Hashimoto's thyroiditis and, 403
painless thyroiditis and, 398, 406
thyroid-associated ophthalmopathy and, 341–342, 345
thyroid cancer and, 538
Humoral immunity, TSH receptor and, 216–217
Hungry bone syndrome (HBS), 59, 722–723
Hürthle cell carcinoma
with benign disease, 582
clincial behavior, 80–81, 81f
diagnosis, by fine-needle biopsy, 109
histology, 582
incidence, 582
metastases, 582
surgical treatment, 582–583
Hürthle cells, in Hashimoto's thyroiditis, 404
Hydatidiform mole
hyperthyroidism in, 250–251
secretion of nonthyroid thyrotropin, 320
treatment, 274–275
Hydrocortisone, for hyperthyroidism, 670
Hygromas, cystic, 468
Hypercalcemia
acute, 53
adrenal insufficiency and, 58
chronic, 53
classification, 58t
etiology, 57
hyperthyroidism and, 57–58
lithium carbonate and, 57
malignancy-associated, 57
mediator, 57
pheochromocytoma and, 58
therapy, 58–59, 58t
vitamin D levels in, 56
Hypercarbia, symptoms, 674t
Hypercholesterolemia, hypothyroidism and, 386
Hyperemesis gravidarum, 251, 320
Hyperparathyroidism
medullary thyroid carcinoma and, 626–627
in MEN type I, 636
in MEN type IIA, 636
neonatal severe, 57
primary
etiology of, 57
hypercalcemia and, 57
symptoms of, 57
secondary, 53, 57
Hyperphosphatemia, 53
Hyperplasia
C-cell, 84–85, 622
iodine-131 induced, 534
papillary, differential diagnosis of, 75
parathyroid, papillary thyroid cancer and, 71
TSH-induced, 555
Hyperprolactinemia, 385
Hyperthyroidism. See also Thyrotoxicosis
accelerated, 255t, 281–282
apathetic, 241, 277
autoimmune, 75
chemical, 9
classification, 319–321
clinical, 734
defined, 319
diagnosis
history in, 246
laboratory tests in, 246–247
onset of Graves' ophthalmopathy and, 360, 360f
physical examination in, 246
radioactive iodine uptake in, 127, 127f
differential diagnosis, 246–251, 246t
ectopic, 250
etiology, 246, 246t
drug-induced, 249
iodine excess and, 262, 399

Hyperthyroidism *(contd.)*
  rare, 284–285
  experimental, 669
  factitious, 249, 284
  fetal, 279
  Graves'. *See* Graves' disease
  histology, 75
  historical aspects, 2
  hypercalcemia and, 57–58
  iatrogenic, 249, 267, 268f
  with inappropriate TSH secretion, 45
  incidence
    after thyroidectomy, 735
    autoimmune, 75
  iodine-induced, 262, 399
    clinical features of, 249
    medical therapy for, 255t, 284
  medical treatment, 253, 267–268, 255t, 276
    adjunctive therapy with radioiodine, 285
    adrenergic antagonists for, 261–262
    agents used in, 254t
    age-related variations in, 276–277
    antithyroid drugs for, 298–299
    cardiac disease and, 280–282
    cholestyramine for, 267, 268f
    complementary role of options, 321
    conservative, 284
    corticosteroids for, 264, 264f
    in elderly, 277
    intraoperative, 671–673, 672f
    with iodine-131. *See* Radioiodine, therapy
    for iodine-induced disorders, 255t
    for iodine-induced disroders, 282–284, 283f, 283t
    oral cholecystographic agents for, 264–266, 265f
    perchlorate for, 267
    perioperative, 285–286, 286f
    for postpartum syndromes, 279–280, 280f
    in pregnancy, 277–279, 278f
    preoperative, 669–671
    primary, 254f
    radioiodine for, 113, 553
    thionamides. *See* Thionamides
    in thyroid-associated ophthalmopathy, 368–372, 371f
    thyroid cancer from, 533
    for T3 toxicosis, 274
  in multinodular goiter, 435
  with nodular thyroid disease, 75–76
  osteoporosis and, 733
  with painless thyroiditis, 68
  pathogenesis, 319–321
  pathophysiology, 668
  postoperative, 675
  postpartum, 279
  preoperative assessment, 670
  recurrent, thyroid remnant and, 330–332
  subclinical, 735
    diagnosis of, 44
    in elderly, 282
    osteoporosis and, 732–733
    in toxic multinodular goiter, 333–334
  surgical treatment
    complementary role of options, 321
    extent of, 735
    intraoperative complications of, 675
    intraoperative management, 671–673, 672f
    other treatment options and, 321
    special considerations for, 337
  symptoms, 668–669
    bone/calcium metabolism, 242–243, 242t
    cardiovascular, 242t, 243–245
    endocrine, 242t, 245
    gastrointestinal, 242t, 243
    general systemic, 241, 241t
    glucose intolerance, 241
    hair, 242, 242t
    heat intolerance, 241
    hematologic, 242t, 243, 244f
    immunologic, 242t, 243
    nails, 242, 242t
    neuromuscular, 242t, 243
    ocular, 242t, 245, 669
    renal, 242t, 245
    respiratory, 242t, 243
    skin, 242, 242t
  with thyroid cancer, 250
  with thyrotoxicosis, 319–320
  TSH-dependent, 276
  without thyrotoxicosis, 320–321
Hyperthyroxinemia, without hyperthyroidism, 42t
Hypoadrenalism, with hypothyroidism, 386
Hypocalcemia
  acute, 53
  chronic, 53
  diagnosis, 60
  differential diagnosis, 59t
  etiology, 59
  hypomagnesemia and, 60
  hypoparathyroidism and, 59–60
  postoperative. *See* Postoperative hypocalcemia
  pseudohypoparathyroidism and, 60
  risk factors for, 59
  symptoms, 59
  temporary
    calcitonin release and, 721
    endothelin 1 release and, 719–720
    hypothermia and, 720–721
    parathyroid suppression and, 721–722, 721f
  therapy, 60, 62, 61t
Hypocalcitonemia, postoperative, 731–733
Hypoglycemia, in myxedema coma, 388
Hypomagnesemia, hypocalcemia and, 60
Hyponatremia
  euvolemic, in hypothyroidism, 386–387
  in myxedema coma, 388
Hypoparathyroidism
  hereditary medullary carcinoma and, 636, 637
  postoperative
    pathophysiology of, 724–726
    permanent, 698, 726
    prevention, 728–729
    spurious, 724
    temporary, 698, 725
    thyroid remnant and, 332
    treatment, 729
  primary, 59–60
  in Reidel's struma, 405
  secondary, 721–722, 721f
Hypophosphatemia, 53
Hypophysectomy, 534
Hypotension, induction of general anesthesia in, 673
Hypothalamic disorders, hypothyroidism and, 383
Hypothalamic-pituitary-thyroid axis
  drug effects on, 43, 49
  feedback mechanism failure, 525
  functions, 29
  integration of, 38–39
  negative feedback mechanism, 38f39, 38f, 39f
  suppression, 45, 733–734
Hypothermia, temporary hypocalcemia and, 720–721
Hypothyroidism. *See also* Myxedema
  antithyroperoxidase in, 47
  associated disorders
    benign goiter, 105
    coronary atherosclerosis, 480
    hypercholesterolemia, 386
  central or secondary, 45
    etiology of, 382–383
    vs. primary, 480–481
  congenital. *See* Cretinism
  defined, 379
  diagnosis, 46f, 733
    neonatal screening for, 388
    radioactive iodine uptake in, 126f, 127
    radioiodine renal clearance and, 602
  in elderly, 379
  etiology, 30, 379, 380t
    central, 382–383
    drug-induced, 49–50
    ectopic thyroid and, 472
    Hashimoto's thyroiditis. *See* Hashimoto's thyroiditis
    iodide deficiency and, 30
    iodine-131 treatment, 299
    primary, 379f382
  fetal, 8–9
  historical aspects, 379
  iatrogenic, 270
  incidence, 379, 735
  juvenile, 484
  medical treatment, 483–484, 736. *See also* Thyroxine, replacement therapy
  metabolism in, 387
  myasthenia gravis and, 383
  neonatal, 7, 388
  pathophysiology, 733
  permanent, after 131I and surgery, 322
  postablative, 380–381
  postoperative, 322, 381, 697–698
  postpartum, 380
  posttherapeutic, 483–484
  primary, 379–382
    diagnosis of, 44
    vs. central, 480–481
  silent, 380
  spontaneous recovery from, 381
  subclinical, 379, 675
    etiology of, 387
    thyroid replacement therapy for, 387, 484–485

surgical treatment
  anesthesia for, 675–767
  intraoperative management, 676
  monitoring of anesthesia for, 676
symptoms, 383–387, 481, 675
  cardiovascular, 384
  endocrine, 385–387
  gastrointestinal, 385
  hematopoietic, 385
  integumentary, 385
  metabolic, 387
  neuromuscular, 383–384
  respiratory, 384
  skeletal, 385
temporary, 735
  incidence of, 734
  management of, 734
  pathogenesis of, 733–734
thyroid remnant and, 330
transient, 298, 380
Hypovolemia, symptoms, 674t

I
ICAMs (intracellular adhesion molecules), 345, 346
Idiopathic hypothyroidism, 380
IgGs (immunoglobulin G), 9
Imaging
  diagnostic, in chronic suppression therapy, 489–490
  radiologic, for thyroid volume determination, 303, 304f
Immune system
  in hyperthyroidism, 242t, 243
  in pathophysiology, of thyroid-associated ophthalmopathy, 361
  thionamide effects on, 256–257, 256t
Immunity
  cell-mediated, in TAO, 346
  humoral, in thyroid-associated ophthalmopathy, 347
Immunoassay, for antithyroperoxidase antibodies, 47
Immunoglobulin G (IgG), 9
Immunohistochemical technique, for tumor marker identification, 542
Immunometric method, for TSH assays, 44
Immunoradiometric assay (IRMA)
  parathyroid hormone, 55
  of thyroglobulin, 587
Immunosuppressive agents, for thyroid-associated ophthalmopathy, 369–370
Indomethacin, for hypercalcemia, 59
Infections, of thyroid gland, 382
Inferior thyroid artery, 718, 718f, 719
Inferior thyroid vein, 21
Informed consent, for thyroid surgery, 420
Infrahyoid muscles
  anatomy, 18–19, 19f
  blood supply, 19, 19f
  embryology, 15
  innervation, 18
Insular carcinoma, 88, 542, 647
Integument, clinical manifestations, in hypothyroidism, 385
Interferon-Î, 380
Interleukin-2, 49, 69

Interleukin-6, in amiodarone-induced thyroiditis, 283, 283f
Internal carotid artery, 24
Internal jugular vein, 24
Intracellular adhesion molecules (ICAMs), 345, 346
Intracellular messenger proteins, 235
Intraoperative nerve monitoring, 708
Intubation, fiberoptic nasotracheal, 671–672
Invasive fibrous thyroiditis. See Riedel's struma
Iodides
  actions, 262–263, 263t
  body pool, total, 30
  deficiency, 30
  dietary sources, 29–30
  dosing, 263
  excessive intake, 30, 320. See also Jod-Basedow phenomenon
  metabolism, 29–30
  pharmacokinetics, 263
  side effects, 263
  therapy
    indications for, 263–264
    oral, for hyperthyroidism, 669
    for thyroid storm, 674
  thyroid function effects, 43t, 49
  transport, 30
Iodinated agents, in clinical medicine, 283–284, 283t
Iodination, of thyroglobulin, 30
Iodine. See also Iodides
  allergic reactions, 433
  compound solution. See Lugol's solution
  daily requirements, 263
  deficiency, 381–382
    cancer protective effect of, 434
    cretinism and, 382
    endemic goiter and, 432
    experimental thyroid cancer and, 554
    radioactive iodine uptake in, 118
    thyroid cancer and, 530–531, 567
  excess
    endemic goiter from, 432
    hyperthyroidism and, 399
    extraction by thyrocytes, 297
    postoperative intake, recurrent hyperthyroidism and, 331
  quantitative analysis, 4–5
  radioactive. See Radioiodine
  therapy, 382
    for goiter, 1, 431
    for Graves' disease, 279, 327–328
    historical aspects of, 4–5
    for perioperative hyperthyroidism, 285
    with thionamides
      and beta-blockers, preoperative regimen of, 326–327, 327f
      preoperative regimen of, 326–327, 327f
    toxicity, 1
Iodine-123
  pharmacology, 114, 114t, 141
  for radioactive iodine uptake test, 314
Iodine-131
  contraindications, 299–300
  dosage
    ablative, 605

    calculation for uptake test, 299
    for testing, 609
    for thyroid cancer, 121, 122f, 142–143
    tracer, 142
  half-life, 312, 315, 601
    biologic, 302
    effective, 302
  hyperplasia induction, 534
  imaging with. See Radionuclide imaging
  pharmacology, 113–114, 114t, 141–142
  physical properties, 300–301, 300f
  radiation dose delivered, factors in, 301–302
  radiation dosimetry. See Radioiodine, dosimetry
  radiation safety, 315–316
  renal clearance, 602
  therapy with. See Radioiodine, therapy
  thyroid cancer risk and, 322, 535, 537
  total-body scan, 544, 609–611, 610f
  for toxic nodule, 335, 336
  uptake test. See Radioactive iodine uptake
"Iodine escape" phenomenon, 6
131I-meta-Iodobenzylguanidine scanning, 626
Iodothyronine deiodinases
  expression, 196
  functions, 196–197
  kinetics, 36
  pharmacology, 36t
  regulation, 196–197
Iodothyronine metabolism, regulation of, 36–37
Iopanoic acid
  for preoperative preparation, in Graves' disease, 329
  structure, 265f
  thyroid function effects, 43t, 50
Ipodate
  action, 265
  for hyperthyroidism, dosage of, 254t
  side effects, 266
  structure, 265f
  with thionamides, 265–266
  thyroid function effects, 43t
  for thyroiditis, 276
IRMA (immunoradiometric assay), 55, 587
Isoflurane, 668

J
Jod-Basedow phenomenon
  etiology, 282, 435, 668
  exacerbation by iodides, in toxic multinodular goiter, 334
  in "goiter belts," 399
  ipodate and, 266
  in nodular goiter, 262, 327
  radioiodine uptake in, 142
  thyrotoxicosis without hyperthyroidism in, 320
Juvenile myxedema, thyroid hormone replacement therapy for, 484

K
Keloid formation, 714
Ketamine, 672
Ketoconazole, thyroid function effects, 43t, 49
Kidney, in hyperthyroidism, 242t, 245
Killian's space, 705
Kocker-Debré-Sémélaigne syndrome, 383

L

Labetalol, for hyperthyroidism, 670
Lacrimal gland, in thyroid-associated ophthalmopathy, 351
Lactation suppressants, thyroid cancer and, 550
LAK cell therapy, 69
LAK cell therapy, drug-associated thyroiditis, 69
Laryngeal framework surgery, for unilateral recurrent laryngeal nerve paralysis, 711
Laryngeal mask airway (LMA), 673
Laryngeal nerve
 anatomy, 24–26
 injuries, rehabilitation for, 710
 paralysis, 658
Laryngeal pacing research, 714–715
Laryngeal paralysis, laryngeal pacing research for, 714–715
Laryngeal rehabilitation, 710
Larynx, invasion
 by thyroid cancer, surgical procedures for, 661–662, 664f
 by thyroid tumor, 658, 658f
Lateral aberrant thyroid, 65, 515
LDL, in hypothyroidism, 386
Leiomyoma, 88
Leukemogenesis, of radioiodine therapy, 615
Leukoregulin, in retro-orbital fibroblasts, 346
Levator glandulae thyroideae, 19, 20
Levator palpebrate superioris muscle, in thyroid-associated ophthalmopathy, 344
Levodopa, thyroid function effects, 49
Levothroid. See Levothyroxine
Levothyroxine (Levoxyl)
 absorption, drug effects on, 50
 dosage, 490
 historical aspects, 475
 pharmacology, 477, 476t
 therapeutic assessment, TSH assay for, 44
 therapy
  for myxedema coma, 388
  for nodule, 417
  phenytoin and, 50
  thyrotropin serum levels and, 45
  thyroxine serum levels and, 45
LH, in hyperthyroidism, 245
Libido, in hyperthyroidism, 245
Lingual thyroid. See Ectopic thyroid, lingual
Liothyronine (Cytomel), 388, 476t
Liotrix (Thyrolar), 476, 477
Lipoinjection, for unilateral vocal fold paralysis, 711
Lipoproteins, in hypothyroidism, 386
Lithium
 action, 266
 dosage, 266
 drug-associated thyroiditis, 69
 hypercalcemia and, 57
 hyperthyroidism-induced by, 249
 hypothyroidism-induced by, 381
 pharmacokinetics, 266
 side effects, 266–267, 267t
 therapy
  for hyperthyroidism, 254t, 266, 669
  indications for, 267
  for perioperative hyperthyroidism, 286, 286f
  for preoperative preparation, in Graves' disease, 329
  with radioiodine therapy, 285
  for thyroid storm, 742
 thyroid function effects, 43t, 49
 thyroid replacement therapy and, 483
 toxicity, 266–267
Liver disease, TBG elevation and, 33
LMA (laryngeal mask airway), 673
Lobectomy
 contralateral subtotal, advantages of, 332–333
 for follicular and papillary carcinoma, 577
 near-total, 681
 partial, 681
 postoperative follow-up, 333
 subtotal, 681
 thyroid remnant. See Remnant, thyroid
 total, advantages of, 332–333
 unilateral, 681
Lobectomy-isthmectomy, 110
Long-acting thyroid stimulator (LATS), 7, 47–48, 528
Low-density lipoprotein, in hypothyroidism, 386
Low triiodothyronine state, 37
Lugol's solution
 for hyperthyroidism, 254t, 669
 for neonatal Graves' disease, 280
 for thyroid storm, 742
Lupus erythematosus, antithyroperoxidase in, 47
Luteinizing hormone, in hyperthyroidism, 245
Lymphadenopathy, 141, 468
Lymph nodes
 central compartment dissection, 634, 634f
 Delphian, 20
 metastases
  cervical, 514–517, 715f
  in differentiated carcinoma, 516
  distant, 517–518
  management in medullary thyroid carcinoma, 635
  regional, 514, 514t
 paratracheal, 658
 regional, 514, 514t, 516–518
 thyroid region, 515f
Lymphocytic lesions, of thyroid, 86–87
Lymphokine-activated killer cell therapy, 69
Lymphoma
 classification, 651
 common leukocyte antigen in, 650
 diagnosis, 650
 epidemiology, 645
 etiology, 651
 Hashimoto's thyroiditis and, 404
 histiocytic, 173f
 histopathology, 651
 incidence, 650
 malignant
  histology of, 86–87
  incidence of, 86
  treatment of, 87
 mucosa-associated lymphoid tissue, 651
 radioactive iodine uptake in, 128
 staging, 650–651
 symptoms, 645–646, 646t
 thyroid cancer and, 529
 treatment, 651–653
  by combined modalities, 652–653
  radiotherapy, 652
  radiotherapy with surgery, 652
 tumor markers, 650

M

McCabe facial nerve dissector, 681, 682f
MACIS prognostic scoring system, for follicular carcinoma, 575, 604
MAC (minimal alveolar concentration), 668
Macro-orchidism, 386
Magnesium
 calcium homeostasis and, 54, 726
 deficiency, 54
 distribution, 54
 homeostasis, 54
 parathyroid hormone secretion and, 55
 replacement therapy, 54
  for hypocalcemia, 60, 62, 61t
  for postoperative hypocalcemia, 730f, 731
Magnetic resonance imaging (MRI)
 of diffuse parenchymal disease, 140
 of invasive carcinoma, 661
 of nodule, 140–141, 413–414
 role of, 125, 139–140
 of substernal goiters, 452
 terminology, 140
 vs. computed tomography, 141
Major histocompatibility complex (MHC), 345, 539, 380
Malabsorption syndromes, 478
Malignant hyperthermia, symptoms, 674t
Malnutrition, endemic goiter and, 432
MALT lymphoma, 86–87, 651
MAPK (ras/mitogen-activated protein kinase), 195
MBq (megabequerel), 301, 303
Mediastinal thyroid carcinoma, 90
Medullary thyroid carcinoma (MTC)
 adjunctive treatment, 640
 amyloid deposition in, 69
 associated disorders, 623–624
  adrenal medullary disease, 625–626, 625f
  hyperparathyroidism, 626–627
  multiple endocrine neoplasia, 504, 624, 627, 628f
 calcitonin in, 48, 56, 510
  persistent elevation, management of, 635–636
  prognosis and, 504–505
 carcinoembryonic antigen in, 505, 510
 C-cell lesions and, 81–82
 clinical course, 637–640, 638f, 639f
 diagnosis
  earliest age for, 631
  by fine-needle biopsy, 623, 624f
  by radionuclide imaging, 121, 167f, 143
  screening tests for, 630–633
 epidemiology, 567
 etiology
  cellular, 231
  genetic inheritance, 538
  oncogenes in, 539, 541
 familial. See Familial medullary thyroid carcinoma

future research, 640
hereditary. *See* Familial medullary thyroid carcinoma
histopathology, 83–84, 504–505
incidence, 82, 234, 502
metastases
   lymphatic, 633
   prognosis and, 515
mixed follicular-medullary type, 84
nerve growth factor and, 548–549
pathogenesis, 512
pathology, 82–84, 83f, 620–623
prognosis, 84, 510, 542
Ret receptor in, 235, 235f
signal receptor proteins in, 234–235
sporadic
   clinical course of, 638, 639f
   diagnosis of, 621–623, 621f–623f, 624
   familial screening for, 632–633
   genetic abnormalities in, 629
   management of, 636, 637
   screening tests for, 633
   surgical treatment, 633–637, 634f
     adrenal gland considerations in, 637
     central compartment node dissection for, 634, 634f
     of lateral cervical lymphatics, 635
     parathyroid gland considerations in, 636–637
     total thyroidectomy for, 633–634
symptoms of, 82
tumor markers, 542–543, 621
undifferentiated, thyroglobulin levels and, 415
Megabequerel (MBq), 301, 303
MEN. *See* Multiple endocrine neoplasia
Men, nodules in, 411
Merseburg triad, 2
Mesenchymal lesions, 88
Messenger RNA synthesis, 184, 184f
Metabolic insufficiency, 7
Metaplastic squamous lesions, of thyroid, 89
Metastases
adjuvant therapy, 664–665
airway involvement, 459
anaplastic carcinoma, 647
biology, hypotheses of, 514, 514t
bone, 180f, 521
cervical, 471
differentiated carcinoma, 514–517, 514t, 515f
distant, 515
   in differentiated thyroid cancer, 518–519
   incidence of, 612
   pre-treatment evaluation of, 612
   prognostic factors for, 613–614, 615t
   treatment results for, 613–614, 614t
   treatment strategies for, 612–613
ectopic thyroid hormone secretion, 320
extracapsular spread, 515–516
follicular carcinoma, 570, 582
Hürthle cell carcinoma, 582
incidence, 523
long-term follow-up, 607
medullary carcinoma
   adjunctive therapy for, 640
   persistent, management of, 635–636
mixed papillary-follicular carcinoma, 175f
mortality, 664

papillary carcinoma, 176f, 177f, 519, 570–571
pulmonary, 519–521, 520t
   in papillary carcinoma, 519
   thyroglobulin levels in, 607, 608f
of pyriform sinus, 659f
radionuclide imaging of, 121–122, 175f–180f
to recurrent laryngeal nerve, 658, 659f
resectability and, 661
shave technique for, 661
sites of, 657, 658t
surgical techniques for, 661–664, 663f, 664f
surgical treatment, mortality of, 664
survival and, 658–659
thyroglobulin levels in, 543, 607f 609, 608f
to thyroid, 87–88
treatment planning for, 661
of TSH-dependent thyroid cancer, 551
tumor heterogeneity and, 511
Methadone, 33, 43t
Methimazole (MMI)
actions, 254, 256, 257
for amiodarone-induced thyroiditis, 283, 283f
for Graves' disease, 298–299
   dosing strategies, 270–272, 271t
   postpartum, 280
   in pregnancy, 278–279, 278f
for hyperthyroidism, 260, 669
   dosage of, 254t
   iodine-induced, 284
hypothyroidism induced by, 381
immune system effects, 256–257, 256t
pharmacokinetics, 258, 258f
with radioiodine therapy, 285
side effects, 259–260, 259t
structure, 253–254, 255f
thyroid function effects, 43t
for thyroid storm, 741–742
vs. propylthiouracil, 261t
Methoxyflurane (Penthrane), 668, 672
Methylthiouracil, 255f
Metoclopramide, thyroid function effects, 43t, 49
Metoprolol, for hyperthyroidism, 670
MHC (major histocompatibility complex), 380, 345, 539
Microcarcinoma, papillary, 71, 521, 566
Microfollicular adenoma, 109
Micropapillary carcinoma, 565
Middle thyroid vein, 21
Migration inhibition factor (MIF), 346
Minimal alveolar concentration (MAC), 668
Minocycline, black thyroid and, 70
Mithramycin, for hypercalcemia, 58, 58t
MITs (monoiodotyrosines), 30, 31f
Mixed follicular-medullary carcinoma, 84
Mixed papillary-follicular carcinoma
   classification, 502
   with metastases, 175f
   mortality rates, 572
   radioisotope imaging of, 121f
MMI. *See* Methimazole
Molecular biology, central paradigm, 183–184, 184f
Monoclonal antibodies, 542
Monoclonal gammopathy, benign, 41

Monoiodotyrosines (MITs), 30, 31f
Mortality rate, accelerated hyperthyroidism, 281
Mounding phenomenon, 383
MRI. *See* Magnetic resonance imaging
Mucoepidermoid carcinoma, 89
Mucosa-associated lymphoid tissue lymphoma, 86–87, 651
Mucosal neuroma syndrome. *See* Multiple endocrine neoplasia (MEN), type IIB
Müller muscle, in thyroid-associated ophthalmopathy, 344
Multifactorial analyses, *vs.* univariate analysis, 501
Multinodular goiter. *See* Goiter
Multiple endocrine neoplasia (MEN)
type II, 58
type IIA, 234–235, 504
   genetic abnormalities in, 628, 629f
   hyperparathyroidism and, 626–627
   medullary thyroid carcinoma and, 624
   pheochromocytoma and, 625
   prognosis, 84
   screening tests, 630–631, 631f
   thyroidectomy for, 630, 631
   variant forms of, 627
type IIB, 82, 627, 628f
   clinical course of, 640
   genetic abnormalities in, 629, 630t
   medullary thyroid carcinoma and, 235, 504
   prognosis, 84
   screening tests for, 631
Multiple myeloma, 57, 87
Muscle relaxants, 672
Mutations
from environmental exposure, 231
gain-of-function or activating, 232, 235–236
germline, 231
somatic, 231–232
spontaneous, 231
Myasthenia gravis, hypothyroidism and, 383
c-myc oncogene, 540–541
N-myc proto-oncogene, 541
Myocardial infarction, symptoms, 674t
Myoedema, 383
Myopathy
ocular, 343
thyroid, 383, 669
Myxedema
coma
   precipitants of, 388, 388t
   symptoms of, 388
   thyroid hormone replacement therapy for, 481
   treatment, 388
corticosteroids for, 6
defined, 379
historical aspects, 9
idiopathic, 68
madness, 384
pretibial, 242, 351
primary, 380

N

Nadolol, for hyperthyroidism, 670
Nails, in hyperthyroidism, 242, 242t
Narcotics, 672

National Cancer Institute Surveillance, Epidemiology, and End Results Program, 498
Natural killer cells, 538
NCI Surveillance, Epidemiology, and End Results Program, 498
Neck
　anatomy, 19f
　dissections, for papillary carcinoma, 515
　embryology of, 15–16, 16f
　fascial compartments, 17–18, 17f
　irradiation, solitary nodules and, 412
　metastases, 514–517, 515f
　muscles, anterior, 18–21
Neck phantom, 312
Neonates
　Graves' disease in, medical therapy for, 280
　thyroglobulin serum levels, 587–589, 589f
Nerve growth factor, thyroid cancer and, 548–549
Nerve monitoring, intraoperative, 708
Neurilemmoma, 88
Neuromuscular system, clinical manifestations
　in hyperthyroidism, 242t, 243
　in hypothyroidism, 383–384
Nicotinic acid, 33, 50
Nodules, multiple. See Goiter
Nodules, solitary
　aspiration, fine-needle, 127
　asymptomatic in euthyroid patient, 416–417, 417f
　autonomous, 333, 415–416
　　determination of, 486
　　treatment of, 334–335
　benign, suppressive therapy for, 487–488
　calcified, 152ff155f
　categories, functional, 142
　clinical considerations, 411–413, 412t
　cold/nonfunctioning, 162f, 416
　cystic. See Thyroid cysts
　diagnosis
　　cytologic, 414
　　by frozen section vs. FNA, 91
　　imaging methods for, 413–414
　　physical examination for, 412–413
　　radioactive iodine uptake test of, 113
　　radionuclide scanning for, 142–143
　　by thyroid stimulation test, 120
　　by ultrasonography, 137–138
　false-functioning, 165f
　fine-needle biopsy, 105, 414
　　circumferential sampling of, 107
　　needles for, 107
　　repeat procedure, inadequate sample and, 109
　　technique for, 106–108, 106f, 107f
　follicular
　　adenomatous, 77–78, 77f, 79f
　　carcinoma, 78–80, 79f
　　nodular goiter and, 76–77, 76f
　　papillary hyperplasia with, 75
　follow-up, 109–110
　formation, 432, 433f
　functional assessment, 122
　hot/functioning, 333
　　radionuclide imaging of, 163f–165f
　　treatment of, 334–335

　of Hürthle cell lesions, 80–81, 81f
　hyperfunctioning
　　nonsuppressible, 123, 125, 126f
　　radioisotope imaging of, 123, 125, 125f, 126f
　hyperthyroidism and, 105, 319–320
　hypofunctioning, 122, 123f
　incidence, 411, 412, 565
　laboratory evaluation, 414–415
　malignant, 122. See also Thyroid cancer
　　clinical suspicion of, 416–417
　　incidence of, 411, 416
　　symptoms associated with, 105
　　ultrasonography of, 138
　medical treatment
　　ethanol intralesional injections for, 274
　　fine-needle biopsy findings in, 105–106, 109
　　thyroxine suppression therapy for, 416
　mixed cystic/solid, 416
　papillary thyroid cancer and, 70–71
　in pregnancy, 550
　in radiated children, 531
　regression, 336
　risk, after radiation exposure, 533
　solid, 416
　surgical treatment, 321, 416
　　anesthesia for, 420
　　clinical examination for, 417–418
　　endoscopy, intraoperative, 420
　　imaging for, 418, 418f, 419f
　　indications for, 417
　　informed consent for, 420
　　patient preparation for, 418–419
　　positioning for, 420
　　postoperative considerations, 426–428
　　risks of, 419
　　technique for, 420–421, 423–425, 421f–425f
　thyroglobulin levels and, 543
　thyroid cancer risk and, 525, 565
　toxic, 333
　　clinical features of, 334
　　hyperthyroidism of, 76
　　pathogenesis of, 334
　　treatment of, 335–336
　warm, 249
Non-G-protein-mediated second messenger systems, 195
Non-Hodgkin's lymphomas, epidemiology, 567
Nonsteroidal anti-inflammatory drugs, for hyperthyroidism, 267
Nonthyroid illnesses (NTIs)
　serum thyrotropin and, 44–45
　serum total thyroxine levels in, 41–42
　thyroid replacement therapy for, 485
Norepinephrine
　in hypothyroidism, 386
　in pheochromocytoma, 625, 625f
NOSPECS, 367, 367f
NTIs. See Nonthyroid illnesses

O

Obstructive sleep apnea, in hypothyroidism, 384
Occult papillary carcinoma (papillary microcarcinoma), 71, 521, 566
Octreotide

　for hyperthyroidism, 254t
　thyroid function effects, 49
Ocular myopathy, in thyroid-associated ophthalmopathy, 343
Omohyoid muscles, anatomy, 18
Oncogenes
　activation, 646
　dominant expression, 232
　growth signal transduction and, 232, 232f
　in thyroid cancer, 232f, 233f, 234
　　diagnosis, 238
　　multiple hits in, 237–238, 237t, 237f
　　prognosis, 238
　　research studies, 539–541
　　treatment, 238
Oncogenesis, 195f196, 196f
Ophthalmopathy, thyroid-associated
　autoimmune thyroid disease and, 9, 341
　classification, 367, 367f
　clinical features, 342–343, 342f, 343f
　　cornea, 363
　　extraocular muscles, 363, 365f, 366f
　　eyelids, 361–362, 362f
　　globe, 362–363, 363f, 364f
　　optic neuropathy, 363–364, 366–367, 367f
　defined, 341
　diagnosis, 360
　distribution, bimodal, 359
　etiology, 360
　genetic predisposition, 360
　Graves' disease treatment and, 360
　histology, 344–345
　immunohistochemistry, 345–346
　　antibodies against eye muscle antigens and, 348–349, 348f
　　autoantibodies against orbital fibroblasts, 349
　　biological activity of autoantibodies, 349–350
　　cell-mediated immunity and, 346
　　circulating T-cells and, 346–347
　　humoral immunity and, 347–348
　　organ nonspecific antibodies in Graves' disease, 349
　　retrobulbar T-cells and, 347
　　in vitro studies, 346
　incidence, 359
　macroscopic changes in, 344
　medical treatment, 368
　　alpha-adrenergic blocking agents for, 369
　　botulinum-A for, 369
　　corticosteroids for, 369–370, 371–372
　　hyperthyroidism control in, 368–369
　　immunosuppressive agents for, 370
　　iodine-131 for, 299
　　orbital radiation for, 370–371, 371f, 372f
　onset, hyperthyroidism diagnosis and, 360, 360f, 361t
　orbital involvement, 343, 359, 360
　pathogenic mechanisms, 350–353
　pathophysiology, 361
　predisposing factors, 341–342
　pretibial myxedema and, 242
　prognosis, pretreatment T3 and, 368
　progression, after thyroidectomy, 324–326
　recurrent hyperthyroidism and, 331

risk, 245
  cigarette smoking, 245
  gender differences in, 359
 stages, clinical, 368, 376–377
 surgical treatment, 372
  of eyelid, 372–373
   orbital decompression, 373–374
   for strabismus, 374–376, 375f, 376f
 symptoms, 359
 terminology, 341
 thyroid status and, 367–368
Optic neuritis, in thyroid-associated ophthalmopathy, 343
Optic neuropathy, in thyroid-associated ophthalmopathy, 363–364, 366–367, 367f
Oral contraceptives
 thyroid cancer and, 550
 thyroid function effects, 50
Orbit
 anatomy of, 343–344
 fibroblasts, autoantibodies against, 349
 histology of, 343–344
 inflammation in TAO
  mechanism of localization for, 352
  in vitro studies of, 346
Orbital connective tissue, in thyroid-associated ophthalmopathy, 343
Orbital decompression, for thyroid-associated ophthalmopathy, 373–374
Osteodystrophy, thyrotoxic, 722–723
Osteoporosis
 calcitonin and, 56
 hyperthyroidism and, 242
 hyperthyroidism with hypocalcitonemia and, 733
 hypocalcitonemia in, 732
 risk, 9, 482
Osteosarcoma, 86
Oxprenolol, for hyperthyroidism, 670
Oxyphil carcinoma, 502

P

Painless thyroiditis (silent)
 classification, 394t, 394
 course, 394, 395f
 diagnosis
  laboratory data in, 396, 400t
  radioiodine uptake test for, 113
 differential diagnosis, 399–401
 etiology, 397–399, 399f
 with hyperthyroidism, 68
 incidence, 395
 medical treatment, 395
 pathology, 405–406
 postpartum, 396t, 397
 prognosis, 396–397
 symptoms, 248, 395, 406
Palpation thyroiditis, 67
Pamidronate, for hypercalcemia, 58, 58t
Pancuronium, 672
Papillary hyperplasia
 differential diagnosis of, 75
 in follicular nodule, 75
Papillary microcarcinoma, 71, 521, 566. *See also* Papillary thyroid carcinoma
Papillary thyroid carcinoma (PTC)
 age and, 70

calcification, 105, 105f
 with cystic neck mass, 176f
death rates, 581
diagnosis, 571
 age at, 574
 radionuclide imaging for, 168f–171f
epidemiology, 565–567
etiology
 cellular, 231
 diet and, 530–531
 factors in, 70–71
 radiation exposure and, 504
giant cell metaplasia in, 567, 572
histopathology, 502
 columnar cell variant, 74, 567
 diffuse sclerosis variant, 74, 567
 encapsulated variant, 74–75
 follicular variant, 72–73, 72f, 74
 tall cell variant, 74, 74f
incidence, 70
intrathyroidal, 573
medical treatment, results of, 583–584
metastases, 570–571, 574
 extracapsular extension, 170f
 extrathyroidal extension, 578–579
 isthmus involvement, 168f
 lung, 519
 lymph node, 177f, 572, 579–580
 neck, dissections for, 515
 recurrent laryngeal nerve involvement, 171f
 tracheal, 462–463, 465–466, 462f–466f, 658, 660f
 of upper aerodigestive tract, 657, 658t
minimal or occult, 521
multifocality, 73
natural history, 604
oncogenes, 540
pathogenesis, 567–569
pathology, 71–74, 71f, 72f, 567
prognosis, 70, 73–74, 603–604, 604t
 extent of disease and, 573
 influencing factors for, 571–577
 treatment and, 573–574
recurrence, 568, 572
Ret receptor in, 235, 235f
risk factors, 572–573
sclerosing, 171f
small, 71
spindle cell metaplasia in, 567, 572
surgical treatment, 577–581
 extent of surgery and, 577
 lymph node dissection in, 578
 postoperative radiotherapy and, 580–581
 results of, 583–584
 of tracheal infiltration, 462–463, 465–466, 462f–466f
survival, 572
symptoms, 569–571
tall cell variant, 567
thyroglossal duct-associated, 90
 with thyroid cyst, 168f
tumor size, 570
Parafollicular cells (C cells)
 adenomas, 84
 anatomy, 619
 calcitonin production, 48, 56

discovery of, 3
 distribution, 619, 621f
 embryology, 65
 extrathyroidal, 56
 function, 619–620
 histology, 619, 620f
 hyperplasia, 84–85, 622
 lesions, 81–82
 normal, 66, 66f
 secretory products, 619–620. *See also* Calcitonin
 ultimobranchial cells and, 16
Paraganglioma, 88
Parasitic infections, in acute suppurative thyroiditis, 394
Parathyroid adenomas, radiation exposure and, 534
Parathyroid gland
 abscess, 473
 adenoma
  papillary thyroid cancer and, 71
  simulation of intrinsic cold nodule, 162f
 anatomy, 21, 23–24, 22f–24f
 blood supply, 24, 718–719, 718f
 cysts, 414, 468
 damage, from thyroid surgery, 419
 disease with nodules, 418, 425
 dissection, in cervical approach thyroidectomy, 686–687, 687f
 embryology, 16
 in goiter surgery, 441–442
 histopathological confirmation, during thyroidectomy, 423
 hyperplasia, papillary thyroid cancer and, 71
 identification, in thyroidectomy, 719
 inferior, 23, 24
 ischemia, temporary hypocalcemia and, 717–719, 718f
 location/positions of, 21, 23–24, 23f, 24f
 in medullary thyroid carcinoma management, 636–637
 postoperative hypocalcemia and, 59
 preservation
  surgical, with small thyroid remnant, 332
  in thyroidectomy, 719
 removal, during thyroidectomy, 675
 superior, 23, 24
 suppression, temporary hypocalcemia and, 721–722, 721f
 tissue, intrathyroidal, 87
Parathyroid hormone (PTH). *See also* Hyperparathyroidism; Hypoparathyroidism
 anabolic effects, 55
 calcium homeostasis and, 53–55, 54f
 catabolic effects, 55
 in hyperthyroidism, 242
 in hypothyroidism, 385
 postoperative levels, 726
 production, 55
 radioimmunoassays, 55
 renal reabsorption of calcium, 723
Parathyroid hormone related peptide (PTHrp), 57
Paroxysmal atrial tachycardia, symptoms, 674t
Partial molar pregnancy, 275
PBI test (protein-bound iodine test), 41, 396
PCT (polymerase chain reaction), 209

PDGF (platelet-derived growth factor receptors), 549
Pendred's syndrome, 381
Pentagastrin, calcitonin stimulation, 56
Pentagastrin test
　in multiple endocrine neoplasia IIA, 630, 632
　persistent calcitonin elevation from, 635–636
Penthrane (methoxyflurane), 668, 672
Perchlorate, for hyperthyroidism, 254t, 267
Perchlorate discharge test, 120, 381
Pergolide, for TSH-dependent hyperthyroidism, 276
Pericardial effusion, in hypothyroidism, 384
Perithyroid sheath, 19
Pernicious anemia, 47, 385
Perphenazine, thyroid function effects, 43t, 50
Pertechnetate. See Technetium-99m pertechnetate
PET (positron emission tomography), 143
Pharmacologic agents. See Drugs
Pharyngeal pouch, 15, 16f
Pharynx, thyroid cancer in, surgical procedures for, 663–664
Phenobarbital, thyroid function effects, 43t, 50
Phenolsulfotransferase (PST), 35f
Phenoxybenzamine (Dibenzyline), 670
Phenylbutazine, 43t
Phenylbutazone, 43t
Phenylthiourea, 6
Phenytoin
　interaction with thyroxine, 482
　thyroid function effects, 43t, 50
Pheochromocytoma
　familial, thyroid cancer and, 7
　hypercalcemia and, 58
　hypertensive crisis and, 329
　medullary thyroid carcinoma and, 625–626, 625f, 637
　screening tests, 632
Phosphate
　absorption, 53
　excretion, 53
　metabolism, 53
　oral, for hypercalcemia, 58, 58t
Phospholipase C (PL-C), 194
Phosphorus, serum levels, 53
Pigments, in thyroid, 70
Pituitary gland
　hormones, thyroid hormones and, 667
　in hypothyroidism, 385
　tumors
　　hyperthyroidism and, 320
　　TSH-secreting, 45
Pituitary resistance to thyroid hormone (PRTH)
　diagnosis, 223, 224f
　medical treatment, 228–229, 276
　suppression therapy, 487
　variability, molecular mechanisms of, 227–228
PK-A (protein kinase A), 194
PK-C (protein kinase C), 194
Plasma cell tumors, extramedullary, 87
Plasmapheresis, for Graves' disease, 329
Platelet-derived growth factor receptors (PDGF receptors), 549
PLAT (paraganglionic-like adenoma of thyroid), 88

PL-C (phospholipase C), 194
Pleural effusion, in hypothyroidism, 384
Plummer's disease
　clinical manifestations, 435
　development, 273–274
　pathophysiology, 668
　treatment, 274
Pneumocystis carinii infection, acute suppurative thyroiditis and, 394
Polymerase chain reaction (PCR), 209
Positron-emission tomography (PET), 143, 303
Postirradiation polyglandular neoplasia syndrome, 534
Postoperative hypocalcemia
　diagnosis, 726–728, 727t
　incidence, 59, 724
　laboratory evaluation, 727, 727t, 727–728
　pathophysiology, 717–724, 718t, 718f, 721f
　permanent, 725
　risk factors, 59
　symptoms, 59, 726
　temporary, 698, 725
　　pathophysiology of, 717–724, 718t, 718f, 721f
　　vs. permanent, 726
　treatment
　　medical, 729, 731, 730t
　　surgical, 729
Postpartum thyrocarditis, 255t
Postpartum thyroiditis
　differential diagnosis, 397, 398f
　etiology, 397–398, 398
　medical treatment, 279–280
　patterns, 280f
　prevalence, 396t, 397
　transient thyrotoxicosis and, 483
Postpartum thyrotoxicosis, etiology, 406–407
Potassium iodide, with propranolol, for hyperthyroidism, 670
Potassium perchlorate discharge test, 120
Prednisolone
　for hyperthyroidism, 670
　for iodine-induced hyperthyroidism, 284
Prednisone
　for hyperthyroidism, 254t
　for iodine-induced hyperthyroidism, 284
　for thyroid-associated ophthalmopathy, 371–372
　for thyroiditis, 276
Pregnancy
　Graves' disease in, 277–279, 278f
　hyperthyroidism and, 251
　hyperthyroxinemia, normal, 277
　nodular disease in, 550
　thyroxine replacement therapy in, 484
Pretracheal fascia, of neck, 17f, 18, 19
Prevertebral fascia, of neck, 17f, 18
Primary myxedema, 380
Pro-oncogenes, mutations
　of DNA repair proteins, 237
　of regulatory proteins, 237
Propranolol
　for Graves' disease
　　in pregnancy, 279
　　preoperative preparation and, 328–329
　for hyperthyroidism, 261–262, 670
　　dosage of, 254t

iodine-induced, 284
perioperative management of, 286
for painless or silent thyroiditis, 395
thyroid function effects, 43t, 50
for thyroid storm, 674
Proptosis, in thyroid-associated ophthalmopathy, 343
Propylthiouracil (PTU)
　actions, 254, 257
　for Graves' disease, 298–299
　　dosing strategies in, 270–272, 271t
　　postpartum, 280
　　in pregnancy, 278–279, 278f
　for hyperthyroidism, 257t, 260, 669
　　dosage of, 254t
　　iodine-induced, 284
　hypothyroidism induced by, 381
　immune system effects, 256–257, 256t
　pharmacokinetics, 257–258, 257t
　with radioiodine therapy, 285
　side effects, 259–260, 259t
　structure, 253–254, 255f
　thyroid function effects, 43t
　for thyroid storm, 674, 741–742
　vs. methimazole, 261t
Prostacyclin I2, 547
Prostaglandin E2, 361
Protein-bound iodine test (PBI test), 41, 396
Protein kinase A (PK-A), 194
Protein kinase C (PK-C), 194
Proteins, thyroid-orbital shared, 350
Protirelin, for thyrotropin-releasing hormone test, 48
Proton magnetic spectroscopy, of nodule, 414
Proto-oncogenes
　function of, 231
　mutated. See Oncogenes
　in thyroid cancer, 539
PRTH. See Pituitary resistance to thyroid hormone
Psammoma bodies
　in goiter, 438f
　in Hashimoto's thyroiditis, 404
　in papillary thyroid carcinoma, 71–73, 74, 137
Pseudoanemia, of hyperthyroidism, 243
Pseudohypoparathyroidism, types, 60
Psoriasis, vitamin D for, 56
PST (phenolsulfotransferase), 35f
PTH. See Parathyroid hormone
PTHrp (parathyroid hormone related peptide), 57
PTU. See Propylthiouracil
p53 tumor suppressor gene, mutations of, 236, 236f
Pulmonary embolus, symptoms, 674t
Pulmonary metastases
　in differentiated thyroid carcinoma, 519–521, 520t
　survival rates, 520, 520t
　treatment, age and, 520
Pyriform sinus, invasion by thyroid cancer, 659f

R

Race, thyroid-associated ophthalmopathy and, 341
Radiation-associated thyroid cancers (RATC), 531

Radiation exposure. *See also* Thyroid cancer, radiation-induced
  of adults, carcinogenicity of, 531–532
  in childhood, thyroid cancer and, 525, 531
  conditions associated with, 534–535
  fibrosis from, 69
  mechanism of action, in thyroid cancer, 534
  nodule development and, 412, 533, 565
  from nuclear fallout, 532
    thyroid cancer and, 535, 537
  papillary thyroid carcinoma and, 70, 504
  safety considerations, 315–316
  thyroid abnormalities and, 566
  thyroid cancer risk, 6
    in animals, 554
Radiation therapy, external, thyroid cancer risk, 322
Radioactive iodine. *See* Radioiodine
Radioactive iodine uptake (RAIU)
  applications, 113
  benign adenomas and, 122, 124*f*
  in congenital lesions, 130
  correction factors, 314
  description, 48
  elevated, without hypothyroidism symptoms, 486
  exogenous thyroid preparations and, 116
  in goiter, 435
  in hyperthyroidism, 127, 127*f*, 247
  in hypothyroidism, 126*f*, 127
  imaging
    rectilinear scanner for, 115, 115*f*
    scintillation camera for, 115–116, 116*f*
  indications, 118
  instrumentation, 115
  interference
    from contrast materials, 117
    from exogenous thyroid preparations, 116
  interpretation, 117–118
  for iodine-131 dosage calculation, 299
  iodine-123 for, 314
  in metastatic thyroid tumors, 581
  patient preparation, 116
  probe, 312, 313*f*
  in pulmonary metastases, 519, 520
  stimulation by TSH, 603
  technique, 117, 117*f*, 118, 118*f*, 312–315
  thyroglobulin synthesis and, 543
  in thyroid cysts, 130
  in thyrotoxicosis, 380, 399
Radiography
  chest
    of pulmonary metastases, 520
    of substernal goiter, 451, 451*f*
  contrast dyes, for thyroid storm, 742
  role of, 137
  of solitary nodule, 413
Radioimmunoassay (RIA)
  historical aspects, 5
  of parathyroid hormone, 55
  of thyroglobulin, 587
Radioiodine. *See also* Iodine-131
  carcinogenicity, 615
  complications, 299, 614–615
    acute side effects, 614
    carcinogenesis, 615
    genetic defects, 614–615

  hypocalcitonemia, 731
  infertility, 614–615
  leukemogenesis, 615
  ophthalmopathy, 342
  pulmonary fibrosis, 615
  thyroid cancer, 535, 537
  contraindications, 284, 299–300
  dosimetry, 301, 601–603, 602*t*
    biologic half-life and, 302, 303–304, 305*f*–306*f*
    dosage schemes, 302
    effective half-life and, 303–304, 305*f*–306*f*, 307
    examples of, 307, 309, 312, 308*f*, 310*f*–311*f*
    half-life of radionuclide and, 302
    maximum uptake and, 303, 307
    methods, 301–304, 307, 305*f*–306*f*
    thyroid volume and, 303, 304*f*
    treatment goals and, 302–303
  failure, 298
  historical aspects, 5
  iodine-123, 114, 114*t*, 141, 314
  postoperative, 604–606
    recurrence rates and, 605
    routine administrations, 605
    survival rates and, 605, 606*t*
  radiation dosimetry. *See* Radioiodine, dosimetry
  radiation safety and, 315–316
  teratogenicity, 277–278
  therapy
    adjunctive, 285
    calculated dose method for, 297, 298
    for childhood Graves' disease, 277
    for distant metastases, 612–613
    for follicular carcinoma, 574
    for goiter, 297, 335, 436
    for Graves' disease, 367–368, 381
    for hyperthyroidism, 268–269, 297, 302*f* 303
    for local recurrence, 611–612
    low-dose method, 297
    methods for, 312–315, 313*f*
    for nodules, 297
    for papillary carcinoma, 568, 574
    for Plummer's disease, 274
    for pulmonary metastases, 519
    single high-dose method, 297, 298
    for thyroid cancer, 121, 122*f*, 142–143
Radionuclide imaging
  clinical uses of
    congenital disorders, 142
    diffuse disorders, 142
    nodules, 142–143
  radiopharmaceuticals for, 141–142
  role of, 141
  scintigraphy
    indications for, 414
    for I131 total-body scanning, 609–611, 610*f*
    of solitary nodule, 413
    of substernal goiters, 452
  of thyroglossal duct abnormalities, 469
Radiopharmaceuticals. *See also specific radiopharmaceuticals*

  for anatomical evaluations, 113
  for functional evaluations, 113
  for imaging, 141–142. *See also* Radionuclide imaging
  investigational, 143
  types of, 113–115, 114*t*
Radiotherapy
  with chemotherapy, for thyroid lymphoma, 652–653
  external
    for differentiated thyroid carcinoma, 603
    for distant metastases, 613
    for invasive thyroid cancer, 664–665
    for local recurrence, 612
    to neck, relapse-free survival rate for, 606–607, 606*t*
    postablative hypothyroidism and, 381
    for thyroid-associated ophthalmopathy, 370–371, 371*f*, 372*f*
    for thyroid lymphoma, 652
  preoperative, 648
  with surgery
    for anaplastic carcinoma, 648–649
    for thyroid lymphoma, 652
RAIU. *See* Radioactive iodine uptake
Ras/mitogen-activativated protein kinase (MAPK), 195
ras oncogene family, in thyroid cancer, 540
Ras protein, mutations, 235, 236*f*
Ras signaling system, 233–234, 233*f*
RATC (radiation-associated thyroid cancers), 531
REAL classification (Revised European-American Lymphoma classification), 651
Rectilinear scanner, for radioactive iodine uptake test, 115, 115*f*
Recurrent laryngeal nerve
  anatomy, 25–26, 26*f*, 705–706, 706*f*
  dissection, in cervical approach thyroidectomy, 684–686, 686*f*
  identification
    methods for, 707
    in substernal goiter removal, 454, 454*f*
    during thyroidectomy, 425, 426*f*, 427*f*
  injury, 708
    bilateral, 709, 712
    rehabilitation for, 710
    with superior laryngeal nerve injury, 710, 712
    from thyroid surgery, 419
    unilateral, 708–709
  intraoperative monitoring, 708
  invasion by thyroid cancer, 658, 659*f*, 662, 664*f*
  in multinodular goiter, 439
  risks, in goiter surgery, 442
  traction neuropraxia, 459
  unilateral paralysis, treatment of, 710–712
Referral centers, thyroid cancer studies from, 498
Regulatory proteins, 237
Reidel's struma
  association with Hashimoto's thyroiditis, 405, 405*t*
  pathology, 405
  symptoms, 405
  treatment, 405

Reinnervation technique, for recurrent laryngeal nerve paralysis, 711–712
Relaxed skin tension line (RSTL), 682
Remnant, thyroid
　after bilateral subtotal thyroidectomy, 699
　after total thyroidectomy, 699
　autonomy, 331
　calcitonin leak from, 722
　computed tomography of, 138
　etiology, 457
　hypothyroidism and, 330
　posttherapeutic hypothyroidism and, 483–484
　recurrent hyperthyroidism and, 330–332
　size
　　ideal, 329–330
　　recurrent hyperthyroidism and, 331–332
　　small as possible, 332
　　surgical risks and, 332
　vascularity, 329
　weight, 329
Renal cancer metastases, to thyroid gland, 87
Replacement therapy, 490. *See also under specific thyroid hormones*
　assessment, TSH assay for, 44
　bone loss and, 9
　effect on radioactive iodine uptake test, 116
　for euthyroid goiter, 436
　for Graves' disease, in pregnancy, 279
　indications
　　cretinism, 484
　　juvenile myxedema, 484
　　nonthyroid illness, 485
　maintenance dosage, 481–482
　overreplacement, osteoporosis and, 732–733
　for subclinical hypothyroidism, 387
　for substernal goiter, 453
　toxicity, symptoms of, 481
　withdrawal of, prior to radioisotope imaging, 121
Reproductive system, in hypothyroidism, 386
Reserpine, 7
Resorcinol, 381
Respiratory system
　clinical manifestations
　　in hyperthyroidism, 242t, 243
　　in hypothyroidism, 384
　　in substernal goiter, 450
　compromise, with goiter, 434
　thyroid remnants in, 457
Ret proto-oncogene, 624
　blood screening, 632
　mutations, in hereditary medullary thyroid carcinoma, 629, 630t
　point mutations, 628–629, 629f
　transformation mechanism, 629
Ret receptor, 233, 233f, 235, 235f
Reverse transcription-PCR, 211–212
Reverse triiodothyronine (rT3)
　in nonthyroid illness, 37
　structure, 31f
　synthesis, 35, 35f, 36
Revised European-American Lymphoma classification (REAL classification), 651
Rheumatoid arthritis, antithyroperoxidase in, 47
RIA. *See* Radioimmunoassay
Rickets, 56

Riedel's struma
　conditions associated with, 382
　incidence, 69, 404–405
　symptoms, 382
Rifampin
　interaction with thyroxine, 482
　thyroid function effects, 43t, 50
RNA processing, alternative, 619, 622f
Rocuronium, 672
RSTL (relaxed skin tension line), 682
rT3. *See* Reverse triiodothyronine

S
Salicylate, thyroid function effects, 50
Salicylates
　for hyperthyroidism, 267
　thyroid function effects, 43t, 50
Saline hydration, for hypercalcemia, 58, 58t
Salivary gland tumors, radiation exposure and, 534
Salsalate, thyroid function effects, 50
Salt, iodinized, 432–433, 530
Sarcoidosis, 382
Sarcoma, thyroid, 86, 653
Saturated solution of potassium iodide (SSKI), 254t, 263, 327
Scarring, hypertrophic, 714
Schmidt syndrome, 481
Schwannoma, 86, 88
Scintigraphy. *See* Radionuclide imaging, scintigraphy
Scintillation camera, for radioactive iodine uptake test, 115–116, 116f
Scleroderma, thyroid dysfunction in, 70
Sclerosing mucoepidermoid carcinoma with eosinophilia, 89
Sclerosis, progressive systemic, 382
Second messenger systems
　G-protein-mediated, 194–195
　non-G-protein-mediated, 195
Selenocysteine, 197, 198f
Sepsis
　postoperative, 702
　symptoms, 674t
Serum binding proteins, 33–34
Serum total thyroxine, 41–42
SETTLE lesion, 88
Sevoflurane, 672
Sex hormone-binding globulin, 245, 386
Sex hormones, thyroid cancer development and, 549–551
Sex predilection, of substernal goiters, 449
Sex variation
　in follicular carcinoma risk, 576
　in nodule incidence, 565
　in papillary carcinoma risk, 576
Shave technique, for invasive thyroid cancer, 661
Sick euthyroid syndrome, serum thyrotropin and, 44–45
Signal proteins, 234
Signal receptor proteins, 234–235
Silent thyroiditis. *See* Painless thyroiditis
Single photon emission computed tomography (SPECT), 113
Sipple's syndrome. *See* Multiple endocrine neoplasia (MEN), type IIA

Sistrunk procedure, 90, 471
Sjögren's syndrome, antithyroperoxidase in, 47
Skeletal muscle
　disorder, thyroid-associated ophthalmopathy as, 351–352
　in hyperthyroidism, 243
Skeletal system, in hypothyroidism, 385
Skin
　in hyperthyroidism, 242, 242t
　in hypothyroidism, 385
Skin flap necrosis, postoperative, 714
Small cell carcinoma, 85
Smoking
　subclinical hypothyroidism and, 485
　thyroglobulin serum levels and, 589
　thyroid-associated ophthalmopathy and, 342, 360
　thyroid function and, 50
Sodium thiocyanate, 6
Sotalol, for hyperthyroidism, 670
Soybean flour, thyroid function effects, 43t
SPECT (single photon emission computed tomography), 113
Spontaneous resolving hyperthyroidism (SRH), 275
Squamous cell thyroid carcinoma, 88–89, 89, 653
SRH (spontaneous resolving hyperthyroidism), 275
SSKI (saturated solution of potassium iodide), 254t, 263, 327
Staphylococcus, acute suppurative thyroiditis and, 393
Statistical issues
　in thyroid cancer literature, problems with, 499–500
　univariate *vs.* multivariate analysis, 501
Sternohyoid muscles, anatomy, 18
Sternothyroid muscles, anatomy, 18
Sternotomy
　complete median, 691–692, 693f
　upper partial median, 691, 692f, 693f
Steroid hormone receptors, 188
Steroids
　for amiodarone-induced thyroiditis, 283, 283f
　for perioperative management of hyperthyroidism, 286
Steroid/thyroid hormone nuclear receptor superfamily, 186–187, 186f
Strabismus surgery, for thyroid-associated ophthalmopathy, 374–376, 375f, 376f
Strap muscles. *See* Infrahyoid muscles
Stress, thyroid storm and, 743
Struma ovarii, 284–285, 320
Subclavian artery, right aberrant, 706
Substernal goiter
　age and, 449
　classification, 447–448
　diagnosis
　　computed tomography for, 443f
　　methods for, 451–452, 452f
　etiology, 447
　functional activity and, 450–451
　gender differences and, 449
　incidence, 447, 448t
　intrathoracic, 448
　location, 449

mediastinal, 448
pathology, 448–449, 449f
surgical treatment
    cervical approach for, 453, 453f
    complications of, 455
    median sternotomy for, 453
    operative approach selection for, 453–454
    reasons for, 452–453
    technique for, 454–455, 454f
    thoracotomy for, 453
symptoms, 449–450
thyroid hormone replacement, 453
Subtotal thyroidectomy (hemithyroidectomy), 442–443
bilateral, 329
    complications from, 699
    postoperative permanent hypocalcemia and, 725
    postoperative temporary hypocalcemia and, 725
    selection of, 699–700
    thyroid function after, 735
for childhood Graves' disease, 277
for follicular and papillary carcinoma, 577
indications, 442–443
temporary hypoparathyroidism after, 725
Succinylcholine, 672
Sufentanil, 672
Sulfonamides, thyroid function effects, 43t
Sulfonylureas, thyroid function effects, 43t
Superficial fascia, of neck, 17, 17f
Superior laryngeal nerve
anatomy, 706–707, 707f
identification methods, 707–708
injury, 18–19
    with recurrent laryngeal nerve injury, 710
    rehabilitation for, 710
    treatment of, 712
intraoperative monitoring, 708
    with recurrent laryngeal nerve injury, treatment of, 712
Superior thyroid artery, parathyroid gland blood supply and, 718, 718f
Superior thyroid vein, 21
Superior vena cava syndrome, 245
Superior vena obstruction, from substernal goiter, 450
Suppression therapy, 490. See also under specific thyroid hormones
assessment, TSH assay for, 44
chronic, diagnostic imaging in, 489–490
diagnostic, 486–487, 486t
indications, 486t
    benign nodules, 487–488
    Graves's disease recurrence prevention, 488
    nontoxic goiter, 486–487
    thyroid cancer, 488–489
interruption of, 489
physiologic basis, 485
Suppurative thyroiditis, acute
differential diagnosis, 468
etiology, 393–394
laboratory data, 393, 394t
prevalence, 393
symptoms, 393
Suprasternal space of Burns, 17

Surgery, thyroid. See also Lobectomy; Subtotal thyroidectomy; Thyroidectomy
changing trends in, 701–702
for childhood Graves' disease, 277
complications
    airway obstruction, 713
    arytenoid dislocation, 713
    chylous fistula, 714
    from completion or reoperation, 700–701, 701t
    current statistics, 703
    hemorrhage, 702, 713
    historical aspects of, 702–703
    hypocalcemia. See Postoperative hypocalcemia
    hypoparathyroidism. See Hypoparathyroidism, postoperative
    incidence of, 697
    minor nonneural, 714
    mortality rate, 702
    neural injury, 708–710
    preoperative preparation and, 697
    sepsis, 702
    skin flap necrosis, 714
    sympathetic nerve injury, 713–714
    tetany, 702–703
    thyroid storm. See Thyroid storm
    total vs. bilateral subtotal thyroidectomy, 699
    tracheoesophageal blood supply, 714
    vs. natural sequelae, 697–699
for distant metastases, 612
extent, for toxic multinodular goiter, 336–337
general anesthesia, 329
for hyperthyroidism
    extent of, 329–333
    selection of, 268–269
    special considerations in, 337
Hypocalcitonemia from, 731–733
informed consent, 420
for invasive carcinoma
in nineteenth century, 2
with radiotherapy, for anaplastic carcinoma, 648–649
risks, thyroid remnant and, 332
for thyrotoxicosis, 276
for toxic multinodular goiter, 335
for toxic solitary nodule, 335, 336
Surveillance, Epidemiology, and End Results Program (SEER), 498
Suspensory ligament (Berry's ligament), 25
Sympathetic nerve injury, postoperative, 713–714
Synthroid, 479. See also Levothyroxine

T

T3. See Triiodothyronine
T4. See Thyroxine
3,3'-T2, structure, 31f
Tamoxifen, 550
TAO. See Ophthalmopathy, thyroid-associated
TBG (thyroid-binding globulin), 10, 34t
T4-binding protein. See Thyroxine-binding globulin
T-cells
circulating, in thyroid-associated ophthalmopathy, 346–347

retrobulbar, in thyroid-associated ophthalmopathy, 347
Technetium-99m pertechnetate
imaging
    of nodules, 142
    simulation of abnormality on, 145f
    of substernal goiters, 452
    technique for, 118–119, 119f, 120f
    of thyroglossal duct abnormalities, 469
pharmacology, 114, 114t, 141
Teflon injection, for unilateral vocal fold paralysis, 710–711
Teratomas, 88
Testes, embryonal carcinoma of, 320
Testicular feminization syndrome, 191–192
Testosterone, 386
T2 formation, 36–37
Tg. See Thyroglobulin
Tg antibodies, 350
Tg receptor promoters, 213, 213f
Thallium-201 (Tl-201), 115, 143
Thermogenesis, in thyrotoxicosis, 740
Thiocyanate, 381
Thionamides. See also specific thionamides
action
    extrathyroidal, 257
    intrathyroidal, 254–257, 256f, 256t
development of, 5–6
for Graves' disease, 298–299
    in childhood, 277
    dosing strategies in, 270–272, 271t
    neonatal, 280
    postpartum, 280
    in pregnancy, 278–279, 278f
for hyperthyroidism, 260, 669
    advantages of, 268–269
    iodine-induced, 284
    perioperative, 285–286
    relapse rate and, 269
with iodine
    and beta-blockers, preoperative regimen of, 326–327, 327f
    preoperative regimen of, 326–327
with ipodate, 265–266
pharmacokinetics, 257–259, 257t, 258t
for Plummer's disease, 274
prolonged therapy, risk of, 322
radioactive iodine uptake test and, 118
with radioiodine therapy, 285
side effects, 259–260, 259t
sites of action, 268, 269f
structures, 253–254, 255f
for toxic solitary nodule, 335, 336
withdrawal, relapse from, 322
Thiopental sodium, 672
Thiouracil, 255f
Thiourea, 255f
Thiourylene, 668
Thoracotomy
anterior, 694–695, 694f
posterolateral, 695, 695f
for substernal goiter, 453
Thymic remnants, 88
Thymoma, 88
Thymus gland, anatomy, 26
Thyrocardiac disease, treatment of, 255t
Thyrocytes, iodine extraction by, 297

Thyroglobulin (Tg)
  in autoimmune thyroiditis, 380
  congenital biosynthetic defects, 381
  interaction with thionamides, 255
  iodination, 30, 32f
  serum levels
    in adults, 589–590
    assay methods for, 587
    assay of, 48
    elevated or rising, 48
    in endemic goiter, 591
    in Graves' disease, 590
    indications for measurement, 596
    in lymphocytic thyroiditis, 591
    in neonates, 587–589, 589f
    with nodule, 415
    normal values for, 587, 588t
    in subacute thyroiditis, 591
    during suppression therapy, 489–490
  synthesis, 29, 30
  in thyroid cancer
    assay methods for, 591–592, 592f
    diagnostic significance of, 592–593, 593f
    for follow-up, 594–595
    need for total-body scans and, 593–594, 594f
    production of, 543, 602
    release mechanism for, 595–596
  as tumor marker, 543–544
Thyroglobulin antibodies, in Hashimoto's thyroiditis, 403
Thyroglossal duct
  carcinoma associated with, 89–90
  congenital abnormalities, 467
    imaging of, 468–469
    thyroid function tests in, 469
    treatment of, 469–471, 471f
  course of, 16, 16f
  cysts, 65, 90
    carcinoma in, 471
    computed tomography of, 138, 147f
    radionuclide imaging of, 130, 147f
    thyroid carcinoma associated with, 90
  remnants, 88, 458f
Thyrohyoid muscles, 18
Thyroid antibodies, serologic tests for, 47
Thyroid artery
  inferior, 21, 22f, 23, 24, 25
  superior, 20–21, 23
Thyroid-associated ophthalmopathy. See Ophthalmopathy, thyroid-associated
Thyroid-binding globulin (TBG)
  deficits, 10
  serum levels
    elevation of, 34t
    reduction of, 34t
Thyroid binding proteins, drug effects on, 50
Thyroid cancer, 7. See also specific carcinomas
  age and, 412
  associated disorders, 527, 567
    breast cancer, 537–538
    endemic goiter, 529–530, 551–552, 567
    goiter, 433–435, 434f, 527, 528, 529–530
    Graves' disease, 234, 234f, 528–529
    nodules, 527
    thyroiditis, 527–528
    thyroid lymphoma, 529

death rate, 500
diagnosis
  by fine-needle biopsy, 110
  oncogenes and, 238
  tumor suppressor genes and, 238
epidemiology, 565–567
etiology, 506t, 525–526, 556, 566–567
  antithyroid drugs and, 537
  diet and, 530–531
  immunological factors in, 528
experimental, growth-controlling mechanism in, 552–555
fear, goiter and, 437–438
follow-up, thyroglobulin levels for, 594–595, 607–609, 608t, 608f
genetic aberrations in, 237–238, 237t, 237f
histopathology, 502
  interpretation problems, 499, 500f
human leukocyte antigens and, 538
with hyperthyroidism, 250, 284
hypocalcemia and, 59
incidence, 526, 565
  age and, 509
  ethnicity and, 526–527
  gender differences in, 411–412
  geographic patterns of, 566
  in Graves' disease, 323
  racial patterns of, 566
intralaryngeal, 90
intratracheal, 90
literature, problems with, 497
  end results reporting, 499
  histopathologic interpretation, 499, 500f
  lengthy accrual periods, 498–499
  prospective randomized clinical trials and, 501–502
  referral bias, 498
  statistical issues, 499–500
  study population heterogeneity, 497–498
  tumor registries, 498
  univariate vs. multivariate analysis, 501
medical treatment, 556, 557
  age and, 510
  assessment for suppression therapy, 44
  controversies, 496–497
  diagnostic imaging for, 489–490
  outcome of, 499
  suppressive therapy for, 488–489
  tumor heterogeneity and, 511
metastatic invasion. See Metastases
mortality, 526, 657
natural history, 511, 512, 556
nodular, hyperthyroidism of, 76
occult
  diagnosis of, 521
  geographic incidence of, 522–523
  histology of, 523
  incidence of, 565
  metastatic disease of, 523
  prevalence of, 521–524, 522t, 523t
  prognosis of, 524, 524t
  treatment for, 524–525
oncogenes, 237–238, 237t, 237f
outcome, tumor heterogeneity and, 511–512
pathogenesis, 495–496, 512
  molecular, 195–196, 196f
prevalence, sex variations in, 555–556

prognosis, 505–508, 506t, 513–514, 556
  age and, 509
  biochemical phenotyping of, 510–511
  DNA ploidy and, 545
  in Graves' disease, 323–324
  oncogenes and, 238
  prostacyclin I2 and, 547
  sex variations in, 555–556
  tumor burden and, 508–509
  tumor suppressor genes and, 238
radiation-induced, 6, 412, 531–532
  death rates from, 533–534
  dosage effects, 532
  histologic changes in, 532
  incidence of, 533
  latency period for, 532–533
  management of, 535, 536f
  mechanism of action, 534
radioisotope imaging of
  interpretation of, 122–123, 125, 127, 123f–126f
  method for, 120–122, 121f, 122f
recurrence
  detection of, 544
  local, treatment of, 611–612
research, 556
  genetic studies, 538–539
  growth-controlling mechanisms, 551–555
  methods, 555
  oncogene studies, 539–541
  receptor studies, 546–551
  tumor markers, 542–546
risk, 507–508, 507t, 508t, 509f, 525
staging, 499, 500f, 505
surgical treatment
  age and, 604, 604t
  with external radiotherapy, 603
  prognosis after, 513–514
  radical neck dissection for, 7
survival, 526, 658–659
thyroglobulin in
  assay methods for, 591–592, 592f
  diagnostic significance of, 592–593, 593f
  for follow-up, 594–595
  need for total-body scans and, 593–594, 594f
  production of, 543
  release mechanism for, 595–596
  thyroid hormone therapy and, 593–594, 594f
thyroglossal duct-associated, 89–90, 471
with tracheal invasion, 166f, 175f
transcription factors, 235–237, 236f
TSH-dependent, metastases of, 551
tumor diameter, 565
tumor heterogeneity, 511–512
types, 231
undifferentiated. See Anaplastic carcinoma
vasoactive intestinal polypeptide and, 549
Thyroid cysts
  aspiration of, 415
  benign, 150f–154f
  congenital, 473
  fine-needle biopsy and, 111
  fluid of, 414
  hemorrhagic, 151f
  incidence, 415

with papillary carcinoma, 168f
postaspiration imaging of, 150f
preaspiration imaging of, 150f
radioactive iodine uptake in, 130
radionuclide imaging of, 147f
recurrent, 415
solid benign, 155f–162f
symptoms, 415
ultrasonography of, 138
Thyroid disease. *See also specific thyroid disorders*
autoimmune. *See* Autoimmune thyroiditis
with diffuse lesions, 65
autoimmune disease, 67–69, 68f
fibrous variants, 69–70
pigmentation, 70
thyroiditides, 66–67
molecular basis, 198
regulation of gene expression, 183–187, 184f–186f
signaling cascades from cell surface and, 193–195
nodular, 65, 70
C-cell lesions, 81–82
with follicular architecture, 75–86, 76f, 77f, 79f–81f, 83f
Hürthle cell lesions, 80–81, 81f
with hyperthyroidism, 75–76
lymphocytic, 86–87
medullary carcinomas, 82–84, 83f
with papillary pattern, 70–75, 71f, 72f, 74f
substernal. *See* Substernal goiter
Thyroidea ima artery, anatomy, 705
Thyroidectomy. *See also* Subtotal thyroidectomy
cervical technique
division of isthmus and lobe removal, 689, 690f
flap elevation, 682–683, 684f
incision marking for, 682, 683f
instrumentation for, 681–682, 682f, 682t
parathyroid gland dissection, 686–687, 687f
patient positioning for, 682, 683f
postoperative care, 690
recurrent laryngeal nerve dissection, 684–686, 686f
superior pole dissection, 687–688, 689f
thyroid gland exposure, 683, 684f, 685f
thyroid gland mobilization, 683–684, 685f
wound closure, 689–690, 691f
closure, 425, 427f
completion, 700–701, 701t
complications, vs. natural sequelae, 697–699
en bloc total, 463f, 465
end-stage angina pectoris and, 4
for follicular carcinoma, 78
of goiter, thyroid cancer frequency and, 530
for Graves' disease, 321–324
historical aspects, 2
incisions, 420, 421f, 422f
for goiter removal, 444f
McPhee, 424–425, 425f
mobilization process for, 421, 423, 423f, 424f
for multiple endocrine neoplasia type IIA, 630, 631

near-total, 443
advantages of, 700
for follicular and papillary carcinoma, 577
for nodule
clinical examination of, 417–418
endoscopy, intraoperative, 420
imaging of, 418, 418f, 419f
indications for, 417
informed consent for, 420
patient preparation for, 418–419
positioning for, 420
risks of, 419
technique for, 420–421, 423–425, 421f–425f
parathyroid histopathological confirmation, 423
partial, 552
postoperative
care, 426–428, 445–446, 445f
follow-up, 333
hypocalcaemia. *See* Postoperative hypocalcemia
hypoparathyroidism. *See* Hypoparathyroidism, postoperative
hypothyroidism, 322, 381, 697–698
recurrent laryngeal nerve identification for, 425, 426f, 427f
skin flaps for, 420–421
sternotomy, 425
technique for goiter removal, 440–443, 445, 440f–445f
thoracic technique, 690–691
anterior thoracotomy for, 694–695, 694f
complete median sternotomy, 691–692, 693f
posterolateral thoracotomy for, 695, 695f
upper partial median sternotomy, 691, 692f, 693f
thyroid-associated ophthalmopathy progression and, 324–326
thyroid function after, 735
total, 329, 552
advantages of, 700
completeness of, 569
complications from, 568, 699
contraindications for, 578
for medullary thyroid carcinoma, 633
morbidity of, 497
for papillary carcinoma, 568–569
with parathyroid preservation and small remnant, 332
postoperative permanent hypocalcemia and, 725
postoperative radioiodine and, 568, 569
postoperative temporary hypocalcemia and, 725
risks from, 332
selection of, 699–700
technique for, 633–634
vs. conservative procedures, 496–497
Thyroid function tests. *See also specific tests*
in goiter assessment, 435
preoperative, for nodule removal, 418
screening, 45, 46f
serological, 47–48
for solitary nodule, 414
in thyroglossal duct abnormalities, 469

in vitro, 41–47, 42t
in vivo, 48–49, 42t
Thyroid gland. *See also specific thyroid gland disorders*
accessory, 19, 20
anatomy, 16f, 19–20, 65–66, 66f, 705
upper aerodigestive structures and, 657–658, 658f
variations in, 20, 21f
anomalous development, 65
blood supply, 20–21, 20f, 22f
cells, signal transduction in, 232–234, 233f
connective tissue capsule, 19–20
development, 457
diffusely enlarged, fine-needle biopsy for, 111
drug effects on, 49–50
ectopic, 65
edema, from iodine-131 treatment, 299
embryologic development of, 15–16, 65
enlargement, 431. *See also* Goiter; Nodules
in hyperthyroidism, 245–246
fascia, 19, 20
gender differences, 555–556
growth, 432, 433f
hormones. *See* Thyroid hormones
infections, 382
innervation, 20f
mal-descent, 65
mobilization, in thyroidectomy, 683–684, 685f
morphology, in dyshormonogenesis, 75
normal
imaging of, 143f–145f
magnetic resonance imaging of, 140
preoperative examination, 418
pyramidal lobe, radionuclide imaging of, 144f
size, 19, 431, 435
status
changing, serum thyrotropin and, 45
thyroid-associated ophthalmopathy and, 367–368
surgical exposure, in thyroidectomy, 683, 684f, 685f
ultimobranchial body residuum, 65
unilateral, 415
volume, 431
determination, for radiation dosimetry, 303, 304f
ultrasonic scanning assessment of, 137
weight, 65
Thyroid hormone receptor binding proteins, 190, 247
Thyroid hormone receptor gene, ß mutations, 226f–27f
Bercu patients and, 225, 228f
as dominant negative proteins, 225, 227
in generalized resistance to thyroid hormone, 223–224
Refetoff patients and, 225, 228f
Thyroid hormone receptor response elements (TREs), 188–190, 189f
Thyroid hormone receptors (TRs), 194
function, T3 in, 190–191, 191f
ligand binding, 190–191, 191f
mutant, 191–192, 192f
subtypes, 187–188, 187f

Thyroid hormone resistance, 10
  attention deficit hyperactivity disorder and, 229
  central, 45
  clinical definitions of, 223
  clinical forms of, 223, 224f
  generalized. *See* Generalized resistance to thyroid hormone
  β mutations, 226f–27f
    Bercu patients and, 225, 228f
    as dominant negative proteins, 225, 227
    Refetoff patients and, 225, 228f
  phenotypes, 223
  pituitary. *See* Pituitary resistance to thyroid hormone
  variable, molecular mechanisms of, 227–228
Thyroid hormones. *See also specific hormones*
  action
    complexity of, 193t
    mechanism of, 192–193, 192f
  adrenal hormones and, 667
  biosynthesis, 29–32, 32f
    acquired defects, 381–382
    congenital defects, 381
    defective, 10
    iodides and, 263
  cell uptake, drug effects on, 50
  exogenous, thyrotoxicosis from, 320–321
  gastrointestinal absorption, drug effects on, 50
  kinetics, 34t
  mechanisms of action, 37
  metabolism, 4, 34, 37
    drug effects on, 50
    molecular aspects of, 196–198, 197f, 198f
    in nonthyroid illness, 37
    peripheral, 32–37
    selenium deficiency and, 198
  neoplastic growth and, 551
  peripheral resistance to, 41
  pharmacologic interactions, 668
  physiologic effects, 667
  pituitary hormones and, 667
  preparations, commercially available, 475, 477, 476t
    animal-derived, 477
    for clinical use, 477–478
    synthetic, 477
  release, 31–32, 263
  steroid/thyroid hormone nuclear receptor superfamily, 186–187, 186f
  in subacute thyroiditis, 401
  suppression. *See* Suppression therapy
  synthesis, inhibition of, 741–742
  therapy. *See also* Replacement therapy; Suppression therapy
    historical aspects, 475
    pharmacokinetics, 478–479, 479t
    in thyroid cancer, thyroglobulin serum levels and, 593–594, 594f
  transport, 33, 33f
  withdrawal, thyroglobulin levels after, 609, 609t
Thyroid ima artery
  anatomy, 21
  goiter surgery and, 443, 445, 444f

Thyroiditis
  acute
    etiology of, 67
    radioisotope imaging of, 127
    suppurative, 393–394, 394t, 468
  autoimmune. *See* Autoimmune thyroiditis
  classification, 393, 394t
  de Quervain's, 382
  diffuse thyroid enlargement and, 66–67
  drug-associated, 68–69
  etiology, iodine-131 treatment, 299
  experimental autoimmune, 217
  focal nonspecific, 68
  Hashimoto's. *See* Hashimoto's thyroiditis
  hypothyroidism-associated lymphocytic. *See* Hashimoto's thyroiditis
  invasive fibrous. *See* Riedel's struma
  ligneous, 69. *See also* Riedel's struma
  lymphocytic, 275, 406, 406f. *See also* Painless thyroiditis
    differential diagnosis of, 406
    thyroglobulin in, 591
    medical management, 275–276
    murine model of, 256
  nonsuppurative, 382
  palpation, 67
  pathology, interrelationships of, 405–407, 406f
  Pneumocystis carinii, fine-needle biopsy of, 111
  postpartum, differential diagnosis of, 399–401
  radiation-induced
    clinical features of, 248
    symptoms of, 614
  silent. *See* Painless thyroiditis
  subacute, 275, 320. *See also* Granulomatous thyroiditis, subacute; Painless thyroiditis
    clinical features of, 248
    differential diagnosis of, 402, 402t
    etiology of, 67
    incidence of, 401
    laboratory data for, 400t
    pathogenesis of, 402–403
    pathology of, 401–402
    phases of, 401
    radioisotope imaging of, 127–128, 128f
    symptoms of, 382, 401
    thyroglobulin in, 591
    treatment of, 402
  subclinical, ophthalmopathy associated with, 349
  thyroid cancer and, 527–528
  treatment of, 255t
Thyroidology
  historical aspects, 1–3
  in twentieth century, 3–10
Thyroid peroxidase (TPO), 30
  in autoimmune thyroiditis, 380
  interaction with thionamides, 254–255
  receptor promoters, 213, 213f
Thyroid receptor auxiliary proteins (TRAPs), 190
Thyroid receptor immunoglobulins (TRAbs), 75
Thyroid receptor intermediary proteins (TRIPs), 190

Thyroid receptor uncoupling proteins (TRUPs), 190
Thyroid remnant. *See* Remnant, thyroid
Thyroid-stimulating antibodies (TSAbs)
  assays
    cAMP-generating, 48. *See also* Thyroid-stimulating immunoglobulin (TSI)
    TSH-binding inhibition. *See* TSH-binding inhibition (TBII)
  historical aspects, 8, 9
  long-acting thyroid stimulator, 47–48, 528
  in thyroid cancer, 528–529
Thyroid-stimulating antibody inhibitors (TSHI-Abs), 9
Thyroid-stimulating hormone. *See* Thyrotropin
Thyroid-stimulating hormone receptor. *See* TSH receptor
Thyroid-stimulating hormone receptor antibodies (TSHR-Abs)
  in Graves' disease, 247–248, 279
  serum levels, 270
  thionamides and, 257
  transplacental transfer, 280
  in treatment monitoring, 273, 273f
Thyroid-stimulating hormone receptor gene mutations, 111
Thyroid-stimulating hormone-receptor (TSH-R), 547
Thyroid stimulating hormone (TSH). *See* Thyrotropin
Thyroid-stimulating immunoglobulin (TSI)
  in Graves' disease, 234, 234f, 590
  in hyperthyroidism, 48
  in neonatal hyperthyroidism, 319
  recurrent hyperthyroidism and, 331
  in thyroid cancer, 529
Thyroid stimulation test, 120
Thyroid storm
  associated disorders, 741t
  defined, 673, 739
  diagnosis, 740t
  differential diagnosis, 674, 674t
  duration, 675
  etiology, 299
  historical aspects, 739
  incidence, 328
  pathophysiology, 741, 741t
  postoperative, 703
  symptoms, 673, 739–740, 740t
  treatment, 674–675, 741–744
  unresponsive to medical therapy, surgery for, 324
Thyroid suppression test
  method for, 119–120
  purpose of, 119
Thyroid uptake test, 42. *See also* Radioactive iodine uptake
  indications for, 118
  interpretation of, 117f, 118
  pharmacologic intervention, 119–120, 381
  technique for, 117, 117f
  using iodine. *See* Radioactive iodine uptake
  using Tc-99m pertechnetate, 118–119, 119f, 120f
Thyroid veins, 21
Thyrolar (liotrix), 476, 477

Thyroperoxidase gene mutations, 10
Thyroplasty, medialization, 711
Thyrotoxicity, symptoms, 481
Thyrotoxicosis
 bovine, 285
 with cardiomyopathy, 244
 cardiovascular problems and, 482
 correction, thyroid-associated ophthalmopathy and, 367–368
 defined, 319
 destruction-induced. See Thyroiditis, postpartum
 in elderly, 669
 with hyperthyroidism, 319–321
 hypothyroidism and, 380
 iodide-induced, 6
 iodine-induced, 282, 435
  laboratory data for, 400t
  medical treatment for, 282–284, 283f, 283t
 medical treatment, 275–276
  for iodine-induced disease, 282–284, 283f, 283t
 lithium for, 267
 persistent. See Graves' disease
 surgical treatment, 276, 321
 symptoms, 241, 249, 674t
 transient, 381
 without hyperthyroidism, 320–321
Thyrotropin (TSH), 121
 assay
  clinical applications of, 44
  development of, 43–44
  pitfalls of, 44–45
  as screening test, 45, 46f
 beta, 10
 circulating level, 38
 deficiency, 382–383
 excessive secretion
  nonpituitary, 320
  pituitary, 320
  in pituitary adenomas, 250
  in thyroid cancer, 551–552
 functions, 29, 485
 goiter and, 433
 growth signal transduction and, 232–233, 233f
 in hyperthyroxinemia without hyperthyroidism, 42
 in hypothyroidism, subclinical, 387
 identification, 4
 inappropriate secretion of, 8
 nonneoplastic pituitary secretion of, 250
 in painless thyroiditis, 396
 release, regulation of, 38, 38f
 secretion, 38
  inhibition of, 485. See also Suppression therapy
  suppression of, 667
 serum levels
  with goiter, 435
  in hyperthyroidism, 246
  with solitary nodule, 414
  during thyroxine replacement therapy, 480
  in subclinical hypothyroidism, 379
 subunits, 38
 suppression. See also Suppression therapy
  by iodine-131, 297

 synthesis, 38
 in thyroid hormone replacement therapy, 482
 TSH receptor binding sites for, 214–215
 unresponsiveness, 381
 vs. LATS, 7
Thyrotropin receptor. See TSH receptor
Thyrotropin receptor autoantibodies, 483
Thyrotropin receptor (TSH-R), 10
Thyrotropin-releasing hormone (TRH)
 functions, 38
 test, indications for, 48
 TSH response to, 333
 TSH synthesis and, 38
Thyroxin-binding globulin (TBG), 32, 33, 33f
Thyroxine (T4)
 absorption, 478
 actions, 5, 29
 assay, indications for, 45, 47, 47f
 biosynthesis, 30
 in central hypothyroidism, 45
 commercially available preparations, 475, 476t
 conjugation with sulfate, 35
 conversion to T3, 34
 drug interactions, 482–483
 free. See Free thyroxine
 function, 3
 in hyperthyroxinemia without hyperthyroidism, 42
 for hypothyroidism, 109
 interactions, pharmacologic, 668
 metabolism, 37, 261
 oral preparations, 7, 478
 oxidative phosphorylation process and, 669
 pharmacokinetics, 478–479, 479t
 physiologic effects, 667
 reduction
  with ipodate, 265
  in nonthyroid illness, 37
 release, 31–32
 replacement therapy
  age and, 480
  average daily requirements for, 479–480
  for benign nodules, 487–488
  changes in requirements, 483
  concomitant adrenal insufficiency and, 480–481
  indications for, 479, 480t
  initiation of, 480
  for myxedema coma, 481
  in posttherapeutic hypothyroidism, 483–484
  in pregnancy, 484
  radioactive iodine uptake test and, 116
 serum free, elevated, 41
 serum levels
  anesthetics and, 668
  in hyperthyroidism, 246–247
  levothyroxine replacement therapy and, 45
  during thyroxine replacement therapy, 480
  total, 41–42
 structure, 31f, 265f
 synthesis, 34
 therapy, thyroglobulin levels and, 544
 with thionamides, for Graves' disease, 271t
 in thyroid storm, 741
 in TSH-suppressive therapy, 552

 unbound, 33
Thyroxine-binding globulin (TBG)
 elevation, 33, 34, 41
 interactions, 33
 reduction, 33, 34, 41
 serum, estimation methods, 42
 structure, 33
Thyroxine-binding pre-albumin (TBPA), 32
Thyroxine suppression therapy, for nodules, 416
Total-body scans
 with iodine-131, 609–611, 610f
 in thyroid cancer, thyroglobulin serum levels and, 593–594, 594f
TPO. See Thyroid peroxidase
TRAbs (thyroid receptor immunoglobulins), 75
Trachea
 anatomic relationship, to recurrent laryngeal nerves, 25
 anatomy, 27
 blood supply, 27
 compression, 459
 infiltration, with papillary carcinoma, surgical management of, 462–463, 465–466, 462f–466f
 innervation, 27
 invasion
  by papillary carcinoma, 658, 660f
  by thyroid cancer, surgical procedures for, 663, 665f
Tracheoesophageal blood supply, postoperative, 714
Tracheoesophageal groove, 25
Tracheomalacia, 714
Transcription, 183
Transcription factors, 235–237, 236f
Transforming growth factor-alpha, 541
Transforming growth factor-beta (TGF-ß), in retro-orbital fibroblasts, 346
Transfusion reactions, symptoms, 674t
Transmembrane receptors, 193–194, 193f
Transthyretin (TTR), 32, 33
TRAPs (thyroid receptor auxiliary proteins), 190
T3 receptors, 37
TREs (thyroid hormone receptor response elements), 188–190, 189f
TRH testing, of thyroid suppressive therapy, 488
TRIAC (3,5,3'-triiodothyroacetic acid), 37
 for hyperthyroidism, 267
 structure, 31f
 for TSH-dependent hyperthyroidism, 276
3,5,3'-Triiodothyroacetic acid. See TRIAC
Triiodothyronine (T3)
 absorption, 478
 actions, 5, 6, 29
 assay, indications for, 45, 47, 47f
 biosynthesis, 30, 34
 commercially available preparations, 475, 476t
 conjugation with sulfate, 35
 free or unbound, 37
 in hyperthyroidism, 247
 in hyperthyroxinemia without hyperthyroidism, 42
 metabolism, 37, 261
 oral, 7

Triiodothyronine (T3) *(contd.)*
 physiologic effects, 667
 production, extrathyroidal, 32
 reduction
  with ipodate, 265
  in nonthyroid illness, 37
 release, 31–32
 replacement therapy, 477
  for depression, 485
  for myxedema coma, 481
  radioactive iodine uptake test and, 116
 serum levels
  pretreatment, TAO prognosis and, 368
  total, 42–43
  with toxic solitary nodule, 334
 structure, 31*f*
 synthesis, 34–35
 thyroid hormone receptor function and, 190–191, 191*f*
 in thyroid storm, 741
 for thyroid suppression test, 119–120
 toxicosis, 43
  medical management, 274
  nodules, 415
  treatment of, 255*t*
 unbound, 33
Triiodothyronine suppression test
 contraindications, 48–49
 indications for, 48
 method for, 48
Triiodothyronine uptake test (T3U), 5, 42
TRIPs (thyroid receptor intermediary proteins), 190
Trophoblastic disease
 hyperthyroidism and, 250–251
 medical management, 274
 treatment of, 255*t*
Trousseau's test, 428
TRUPs (thyroid receptor uncoupling proteins), 190
TSAbs. *See* Thyroid-stimulating antibodies
TSH. *See* Thyrotropin
TSH-binding inhibition (TBII), 48
TSHIAbs (thyroid-stimulating antibody inhibitors), 9
TSHR-Abs. *See* Thyroid-stimulating hormone receptor antibodies
TSH receptor, 234
 autoimmity and, 209
 autoimmunity and, 216–217
 binding sites, 209
  for anti-TSH receptor autoantibodies, 214–215
  for thyrotropin, 214–215
 endocytosis and internalization, 215–216
 gene expression, 211–214, 212*f*, 213*f*

 regulation of, 212–214, 213*f*
 growth signal transduction and, 232–233, 233*f*
 molecular cloning of, 209
 mRNA, tissue distribution of, 211–212
 mutations
  gain-of-function, 217, 218*f*
  loss-of-function, 217–218
 ophthalmopathy and, 350
 protein expression, 214
 signal transduction, 215
 structure, 210*f*
  alternative splicing and, 212, 212*f*
  extracellular domain, 210, 211*f*
  genomic, 211, 212*f*
  of subunits, 216, 216*f*
  transmembrane/cytoplasmic regions, 210, 210*f*
 structure-function relationship, 214–216, 216*f*
TSH-R (thyroid-stimulating hormone-receptor), 547
TSH-secreting pituitary tumors, 45
TSH stimulation, of autonomous nodule, 415
TSI. *See* Thyroid-stimulating immunoglobulin
T3 sulfate, 31*f*
TTR. *See* Transthyretin (TTR)
Tumor markers. *See also specific tumor markers*
 immunocytohistochemical methods for, 542
 ploidy, 544–546
 thyroglobulin, 543–544
Tumor necrosis factor ‡, 380
Tumor registries, 498
Tumors, thyroid
 central hypothyroidism and, 383
 in unusual locations, 89–90
Tumor suppressor genes, 231
 in anaplastic carcinoma, 646
 inactivation, 232
 oncogenesis and, 195–196, 196*f*
 predisposition to tumor formation, growth signal transduction and, 232, 232*f*
 in thyroid cancer
  diagnosis, 238
  prognosis, 238
  treatment, 238
T3 uptake test (T3U), 5, 42
Turner's syndrome, 386

U

UBB (ultimobranchial body), 16, 89, 473
Ulex europaeus I lecithin, 503
Ultimobranchial body (UBB), 16, 89, 473
Ultrasonography
 B-mode, 469
 indications, 125, 137–138

 of nodule, 415, 418, 419*f*
 of normal thyroid, 143*f*
 of solitary nodule, 413
 of substernal goiter, 452
 of thyroglossal duct abnormalities, 469

V

Vagus nerve, 24
Vallecular cysts, 472
Vascular cell adhesion molecule-1 (VCAM-1), 345
Vasoactive intestinal polypeptide (VIP), 549
VCAM-1 (vascular cell adhesion molecule-1), 345
Vencuronium, 672
Verapamil, for hyperthyroidism, 670
VIP (vasoactive intestinal polypeptide), 549
Viral Harvey *ras* oncogene, 541
Viral infections, in subacute thyroiditis, 402–403
Vision loss, from thyroid-associated ophthalmopathy, 366
Vitamin D
 calcium homeostasis and, 54–55, 54*f*
 physiological effects, 55–56
 replacement therapy
  for hypocalcemia, 60
  for postoperative hypocalcemia, 730*f*, 731
Vitamin D receptor, 56
Vocal cord
 anatomy, 672*f*
 paralysis
  bilateral, 709, 712
  postoperative risk of, 321–322
  preoperative, 709
  from substernal goiter, 450
  thyroid remnant and, 332
  treatment of, 712
Voice, after thyroid surgery, 428
Von Graefe's sign, 362

W

Waldenstrom's macroglobulinemia, 41
WHO cancer staging system, 499, 505
Wolff-Chaikoff effect, 258, 262, 282, 669
Women, nodules in, 411
World Health Organization cancer staging system, 499, 505

X

X-ray fluorescent imaging, 125

Z

Zinn's annulus, in thyroid-associated ophthalmopathy, 344, 345
Zuckerkandl, tubercles of, 19